Head, Neck, and Neuroanatomy

THIEME Atlas of Anatomy

Fourth Edition

Thieme

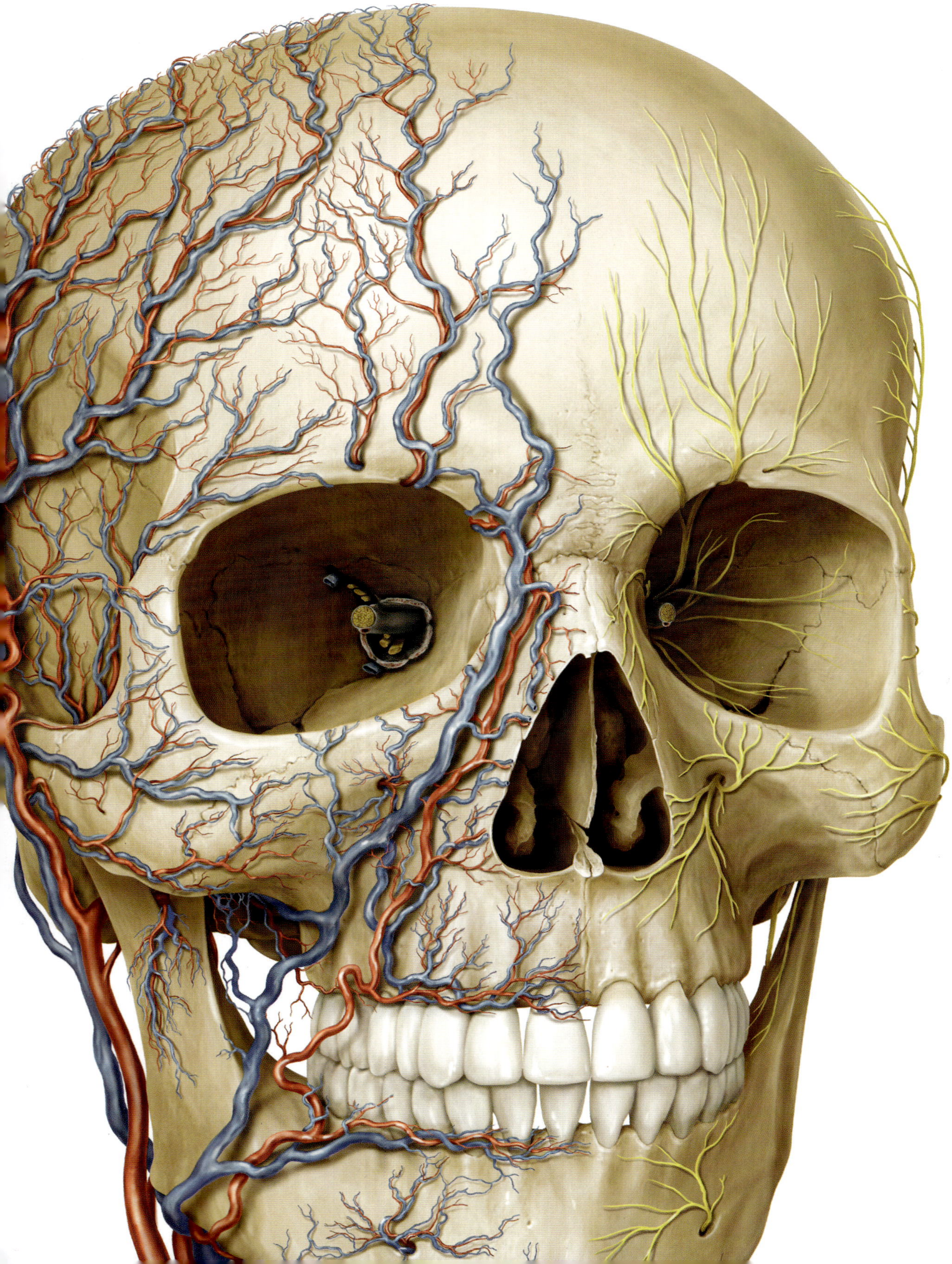

Head, Neck, and Neuroanatomy

THIEME Atlas of Anatomy

Fourth Edition

Authors

Michael Schuenke, MD, PhD
Institute of Anatomy
Christian Albrechts University, Kiel

Erik Schulte, MD
Institute of Functional and
Clinical Anatomy
Johannes Gutenberg University,
Mainz

Udo Schumacher, MD
FRCPath, CBiol, FIBiol, DSc
MSB Medical School, Berlin

Consulting Editor

Cristian Stefan, MD
Department of Molecular
Pathobiology
New York University College of
Dentistry

Illustrations by
Markus Voll
Karl Wesker

1801 Illustrations

Thieme
New York • Stuttgart • Delhi • Rio de Janeiro

Translators: Terry Telger, John Grossman, and Judith Tomat
Illustrators: Markus Voll and Karl Wesker
Compositor: DiTech Process Solutions

Library of Congress Cataloging-in-Publication Data is available from the publisher.

Important note: Medicine is an ever-changing science undergoing continual development. Research and clinical experience are continually expanding our knowledge, in particular our knowledge of proper treatment and drug therapy. Insofar as this book mentions any dosage or application, readers may rest assured that the authors, editors, and publishers have made every effort to ensure that such references are in accordance with the **state of knowledge at the time of production of the book**.

Nevertheless, this does not involve, imply, or express any guarantee or responsibility on the part of the publishers in respect to any dosage instructions and forms of applications stated in the book. **Every user is requested to examine carefully** the manufacturers' leaflets accompanying each drug and to check, if necessary in consultation with a physician or specialist, whether the dosage schedules mentioned therein or the contraindications stated by the manufacturers differ from the statements made in the present book. Such examination is particularly important with drugs that are either rarely used or have been newly released on the market. Every dosage schedule or every form of application used is entirely at the user's own risk and responsibility. The authors and publishers request every user to report to the publishers any discrepancies or inaccuracies noticed. If errors in this work are found after publication, errata will be posted at www.thieme.com on the product description page.

Some of the product names, patents, and registered designs referred to in this book are in fact registered trademarks or proprietary names even though specific reference to this fact is not always made in the text. Therefore, the appearance of a name without designation as proprietary is not to be construed as a representation by the publisher that it is in the public domain.

Thieme addresses people of all gender identities equally. We encourage our authors to use gender neutral or gender-equal expressions wherever the context allows.

Thieme Medical Publishers, Inc.
Thieme Publishers New York
333 Seventh Avenue, New York, NY 10001 USA
+1 800 782 3488, customerservice@thieme.com

Cover design: © Thieme
Cover art: © Karl Wesker, Berlin

Typesetting: DiTech Process Solutions

Printed in India by Replika Press Pvt. Ltd. 5 4 3 2 1

DOI: 10.1055/b000000914
ISBN: 978-1-68420-594-3
Also available as eBook:
eISBN (PDF) 978-1-68420-595-0
eISBN (epub) 978-1-68420-596-7

MIX
Paper | Supporting responsible forestry
FSC™ C016779

Foreword

Each of the authors of the single volume *Thieme Atlas of Anatomy* was impressed with the extraordinary detail, accuracy, and beauty of the illustrations that were created for the *Thieme* three-volume series of anatomy atlases. We felt these images were one of the most significant additions to anatomic education in the past 50 years. The effective pedagogical approach of this series, with two-page learning units that combined the outstanding illustrations and captions that emphasized the functional and clinical significance of structures, coupled with the numerous tables summarizing key information, was unique. We also felt that the overall organization of each region, with structures presented first systemically — musculoskeletal, vascular, and nervous — and then topographically, supported classroom learning and active dissection in the laboratory.

This series combines the best of a clinically oriented text and an atlas. Its detail and pedagogical presentation make it a complete support for classroom and laboratory instruction and a reference for life in all the medical, dental, and allied health fields. Each of the volumes — *General Anatomy and Musculoskeletal System*, *Internal Organs*, and *Head, Neck, and Neuroanatomy* — can also be used as a stand-alone text/atlas for an in-depth study of systems often involved in the allied health/medical specialty fields.

We were delighted when *Thieme* asked us to work with them to create a single-volume atlas from this groundbreaking series, and we owe a great debt to the authors and illustrators of this series inasmuch as their materials and vision formed the general framework for the single volume *Thieme Atlas of Anatomy*.

We thank the authors and illustrators for this very special contribution to the teaching of anatomy and recommend it for thorough mastery of anatomy and its clinically functional importance in all fields of health care-related specialties.

Lawrence M. Ross, Brian R. MacPherson, and Anne M. Gilroy

Preface of the Authors and Illustrators

When Thieme started planning the first edition of this atlas, they sought the opinions of students and instructors alike in both the United States and Europe on what constituted an "ideal" atlas of anatomy—ideal to learn from, to master extensive amounts of information while on a busy class schedule, and, in the process, to acquire sound, up-to date knowledge. The result of our work in response to what Thieme had learned is this atlas. The *Thieme Atlas of Anatomy*, unlike most other atlases, is a comprehensive educational tool that combines illustrations with explanatory text and summary tables, introducing clinical applications throughout, and presenting anatomic concepts in a step-by-step sequence that includes system-by-system and topographical views.

For the first edition we had hoped that our *Atlas of Anatomy* would help the medical student to understand the anatomical basis of clinical medicine. This indeed was accepted by the students all over the world and soon a second edition had to come on the market in Germany, which was extensively extended and revised, followed by further third, fourth, fifth, and sixth editions. More and more information has been added over these editions, including spreads on important foundational information on the common imaging planes for plain film, MRI, and CT scans, the structure of and function of muscle fasciae, the structure and chemical composition of hyaline cartilage, and the regeneration of peripheral nerves, bone marrow, and paraganglia, as well as new graphical summaries in neuroanatomy and new sections describing internal female genitalia and surgical interventions with respect to female genitalia. This atlas takes special care to cover variants in human anatomy such as blood vessels whose courses deviate from the "norm," or anomalous positions of organs. Hence the sixth German edition looks ever more distinctly different from the first one. Of course, we have also checked, corrected, and updated all of the information in this atlas.

We are grateful to the American branch of Thieme that they have made this fourth English edition possible. We hope that this updated version will serve the medical students and practitioners of medicine alike in helping them to understand human morphology which is indispensable for diagnosis and therapy.

Michael Schünke, Erik Schulte, Udo Schumacher,
Markus Voll, and Karl Wesker

Acknowledgments

First we wish to thank our families. This atlas is dedicated to them.

Since the publication of the first volume of the *Thieme Atlas of Anatomy* in 2006, we have received numerous suggestions for refinements and additions. We would like to take this opportunity to express our sincere thanks to all those who through the years have helped us to improve the Thieme Atlas of Anatomy in one way or another. Specifically, this includes Kirsten Hattermann, Ph.D.; Runhild Lucius, D.D.S.; Prof. Renate Lüllmann-Rauch, M.D.; Prof. Jobst Sievers, M.D.; Ali Therany, D.D.S.; Prof. Thilo Wedel, M.D. (all at the Anatomic Institute of Christian Albrecht University of Kiel); as well as Prof. Christoph Düber, M.D. (University of Mainz Medical School); Christian Friedrichs, D.D.S. (Practice for Tooth Preservation and Endodontics, Kiel); Prof. Reinhart Gossrau, M.D. (Charité Berlin, Institute of Anatomy); Prof. Daniel Haag-Wackernagel, Ph.D. (Basel); Johannes-Martin Hahn, M.D., (Tübingen); Prof. Stefan Müller-Hülsbeck, M.D. (DIAKO Krankenhaus gGmbH Flensburg); Róbert Késmárszky, M.D.; Prof. Susanne Klutmann (UKE Hamburg); Michael Kriwat (Kiel); Prof. Paul Peter Lunkenheimer, M.D. (Westphalian Wilhelm University Münster); Dr. Janos Mester, professor (UKE Hamburg); Dr. Jörg Detlev Moritz, associate professor (Klinik für Radiologie und Neuroradiologie Kiel); Dr. Thomas Müller, associate professor (University of Mainz Medical School); Dan mon O'Dey, M.D., associate professor (Luisenhospital Aachen); Dr. Kai-Hinrich Olms, Fußchirurgie Bad Schwartau, Daniel Paech, M.D., M.S. (physics) (Deutsches Krebsforschungszentrum Heidelberg); Dr. Thilo Schwalenberg, senior physician (Urologische Klinik des Universitätsklinikums Leipzig); Hans-Peter Sobotta, M.D. (Stiftung Herzogin Elisabeth Hospital Braunschweig); Dr. Katharina Spanel-Borowski, professor emeritus (University of Leipzig); Dr. Jürgen Specht (Orthopaedicum Frankfurt); Prof. Christoph Viebahn, Ph.D. (Georg-August-Universität Göttingen); Imke Weyers, M.D. (Univ. Lübeck).

For extensive corrections, especially in the first edition, we thank Gabriele Schünke, M.S. biology; Jakob Fay, M.D.; as well as medical students Claudia Dücker, Simin Rassouli, Heike Teichmann, Susanne Tippmann, and dental student Sylvia Zilles; also, Julia Jörns-Kuhnke, M.D., especially for her assistance with the figure labels.

We extend special thanks to Stephanie Gay and Bert Sender, who prepared the layouts. Their ability to arrange the text and illustrations on facing pages for maximum clarity has contributed greatly to the quality of the atlas.

We particularly acknowledge the efforts of those who handled this project on the publishing side:

Jürgen Lüthje, M.D., Ph.D., executive editor at Thieme Medical Publishers, has "made the impossible possible." He not only reconciled the wishes of the authors and artists with the demands of reality but also managed to keep a team of five people working together for years on a project whose goal was known to us from the beginning but whose full dimensions we only came to appreciate over time. For this he has earned our deepest heartfelt gratitude. Since Dr. Jürgen Lüthje retired in 2018, Dr. Jochen Neuberger has taken over and has shown great initiative in continuing and further developing the Thieme Atlas of Anatomy.

Sabine Bartl, developmental editor, became a touchstone for the authors in the best sense of the word. She has, as a humanities scholar, not a doctor, reviewed the text and, in connection with the illustrations, was able to determine whether a beginning student, and thus one who is not (yet) a physician, could clearly appreciate the logic of the presentation. Based on her suggestions topics were also reformulated and redesigned. It is not only the authors who are indebted to her, but also the reader benefits from her didactic talent.

We owe a great debt of thanks to Martin Spencker, who was at the time of publication of the first edition managing director of Educational Publications at Thieme, especially to his ability to make quick and unconventional decisions when dealing with problems and uncertainties. His openness to all the concerns of the authors and artists and the transparency and fairness in all discussions gave the project momentum and established conditions for a cooperative partnership. We also owe him a huge debt of gratitude.

We are grateful to Antje Bühl, who was there from the beginning as project assistant, working "behind the scenes" on numerous tasks such as repeated proofreading and helping to arrange the figure labels.

We are also indebted to Yvonne Strassburg, Michael Zepf, and Laura Diemand who saw to it that the *Thieme Atlas of Anatomy* was printed and bound on schedule, and that the project benefited from the best practical expertise throughout the entire process of publication. We also thank Susanne Tochtermann-Wenzel and Anja Jahn for their assistance with technical issues involving every aspect of the illustrations; Julia Fersch who ensured that the *Thieme Atlas of Anatomy* is also accessible via eRef; Almut Leopold and Dr. Wilhelm Kuhn for the exceptional index; Marie-Luise Kürschner and Nina Jentschke for the appealing cover design; as well as Dr. Thomas Krimmer, Liesa Arendt, Birgit Carlsen, Stephanie Eilmann, Marion Hamm, and Anne Döbler, representing all those now and previously involved in the marketing, sale, and promotion of the *Thieme Atlas of Anatomy*.

The authors, August 2022

As consulting editor I was asked to review, for accuracy and appropria teness, the English translation of the *Thieme Atlas of Anatomy: Head, Neck, and Neuroanatomy*, Fourth Edition. My work involved a review and edit of the translation, conversion of nomenclature to terms in common usage in English, and some small changes in presentation to reflect accepted approaches to certain anatomic structures in North American anatomy programs. This task was eased greatly by the clear organization of the original text. In all of this, I have tried diligently to remain faithful to the intentions and insights of the authors and illustrators, whom I wish to thank for this outstanding revision.

In remembrance of Ancuta (Anca) M. Stefan, M.D.

Cristian Stefan

The people behind the Thieme Atlas of Anatomy

A work such as the *Thieme Atlas of Anatomy* can only arise when the people involved in the project work hand in hand. The integrated educational and artistic work you now hold in your hands is the product of an intensive discourse between anatomy professors Michael Schünke, Erik Schulte, and Udo Schumacher and anatomic illustrators Markus Voll and Karl Wesker.

Creating learning units that comprehensively treat a topic on a two-page spread is a challenge in itself. The authors must carefully select the content, assemble it, and add explanatory legends. Yet how this content is presented in the atlas, how appealing and memorable it is, depends largely on the illustrations. And the *Thieme Atlas of Anatomy* now includes a good 5,000 of them. In creating them, Markus Voll and Karl Wesker drew on many years of experience in anatomic illustration, visited anatomic collections, studied specimens, and immersed themselves in old and new works of anatomy. This was the foundation on which the *Thieme Atlas of Anatomy* arose.

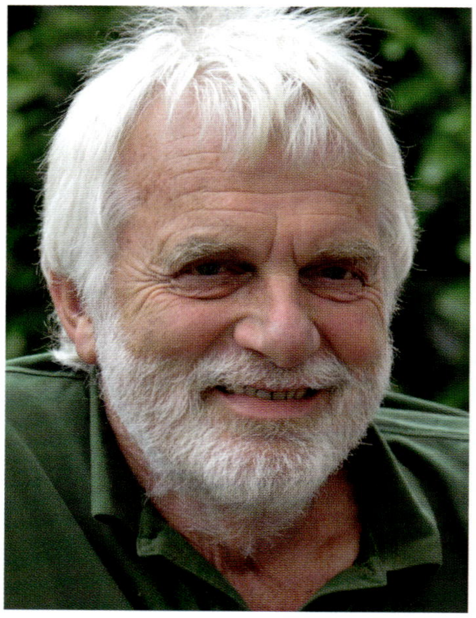

Photo: private

Michael Schuenke, MD, PhD, professor

Institute of Anatomy of the University of Kiel; studied biology and medicine in Tübingen and Kiel; extensive teaching of medical students and physical therapists; author and translator of other textbooks.

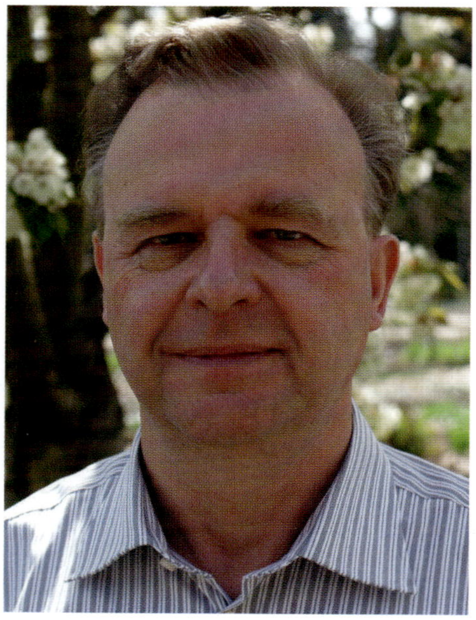

Photo: Kristina Schäfer

Erik Schulte, MD, professor

Institute of Functional and Clinical Anatomy of the Johannes Gutenberg University of Mainz; studied medicine in Freiburg; extensive teaching of medical students; award for excellence in teaching in Mainz.

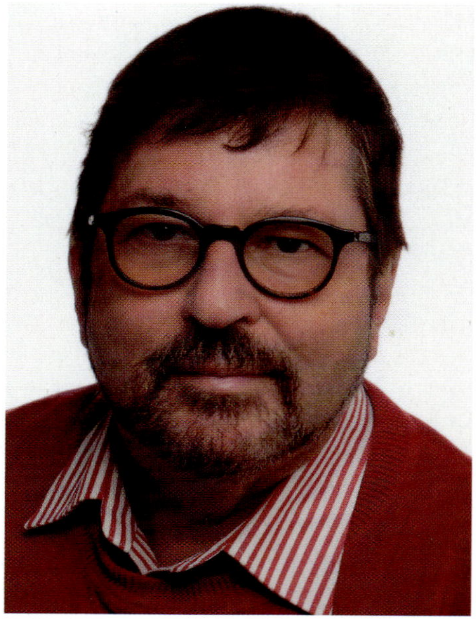

Photo: private

Udo Schumacher, MD, professor

MSB Medical School Berlin; studied medicine in Kiel, and a one-year sojourn at the Wistar Institute of Anatomy and Biology, Philadelphia; intensive experience in teaching medical students, physical therapists, and specialty candidates (FRCS). Spent several years in Southampton and gained experience in integrated interdisciplinary instruction.

It guides the reader through anatomy step by step, revealing what a crucial role anatomy will later play in medical practice. This was a particularly important consideration for the authors. Whether performing bowel surgery for a tumor, puncturing the tympanic membrane in a middle ear infection, or examining a pregnant patient, no physician lacking knowledge of anatomy is a good physician.

Even the *Thieme Atlas of Anatomy* cannot spare you the effort of learning, yet the authors and illustrators can assure you that it will make it a lot more pleasant.

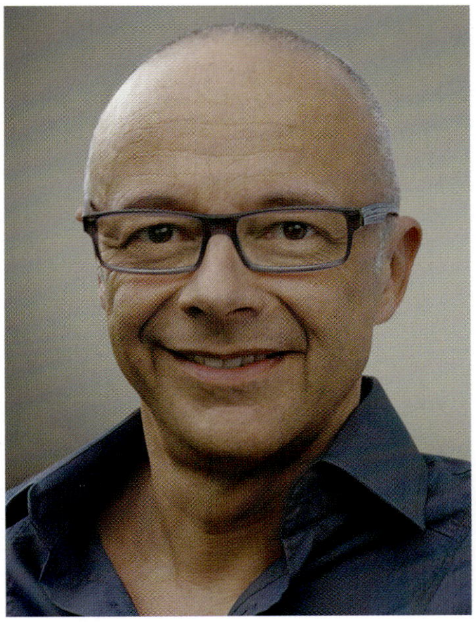

Photo: private

Markus Voll

Freelance illustrator and graphic artist in Munich, trained as an artist at the Blocherer School of Design in Munich, studied medicine at the University of Munich. He has decades of experience as a scientific illustrator for numerous book projects.

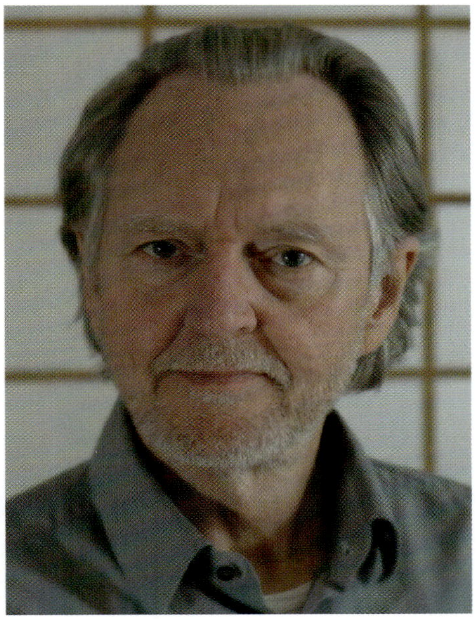

Photo: private

Karl Wesker

Freelance painter and graphic artist in Berlin. Apprenticeship as a plate etcher and lithographer, studied visual communication at the University of Applied Sciences in Münster and at the Berlin University of the Arts and art science at the Technical University of Berlin. He has worked for decades as a freelance painter and graphic scientific artist, including book projects in anatomy.

Contents

A Head and Neck

B Neuroanatomy

C Glossary and Synopsis

1 Glossary

2 Synopsis

Appendix

A Head and Neck

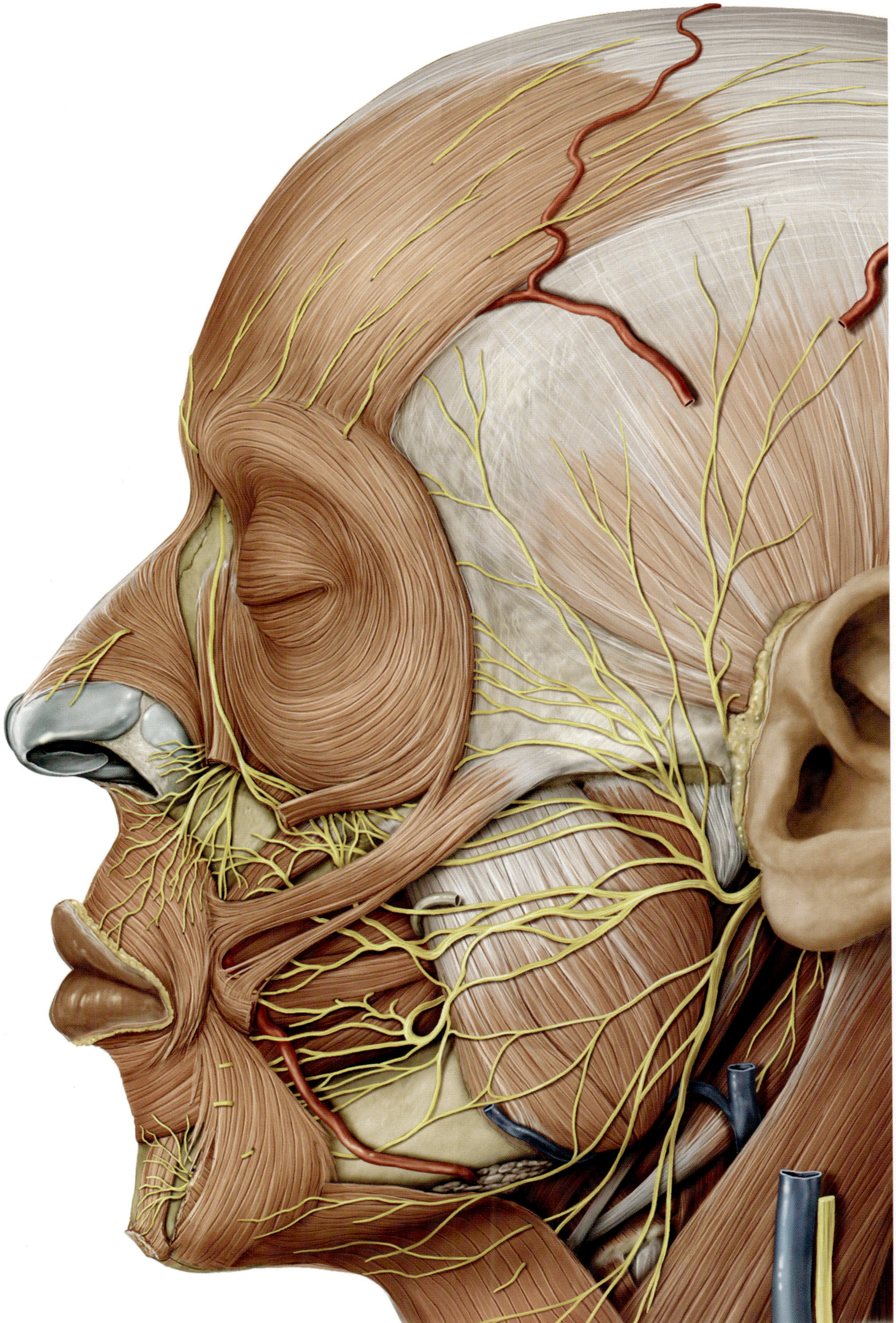

1.1 Regions and Palpable Bony Landmarks

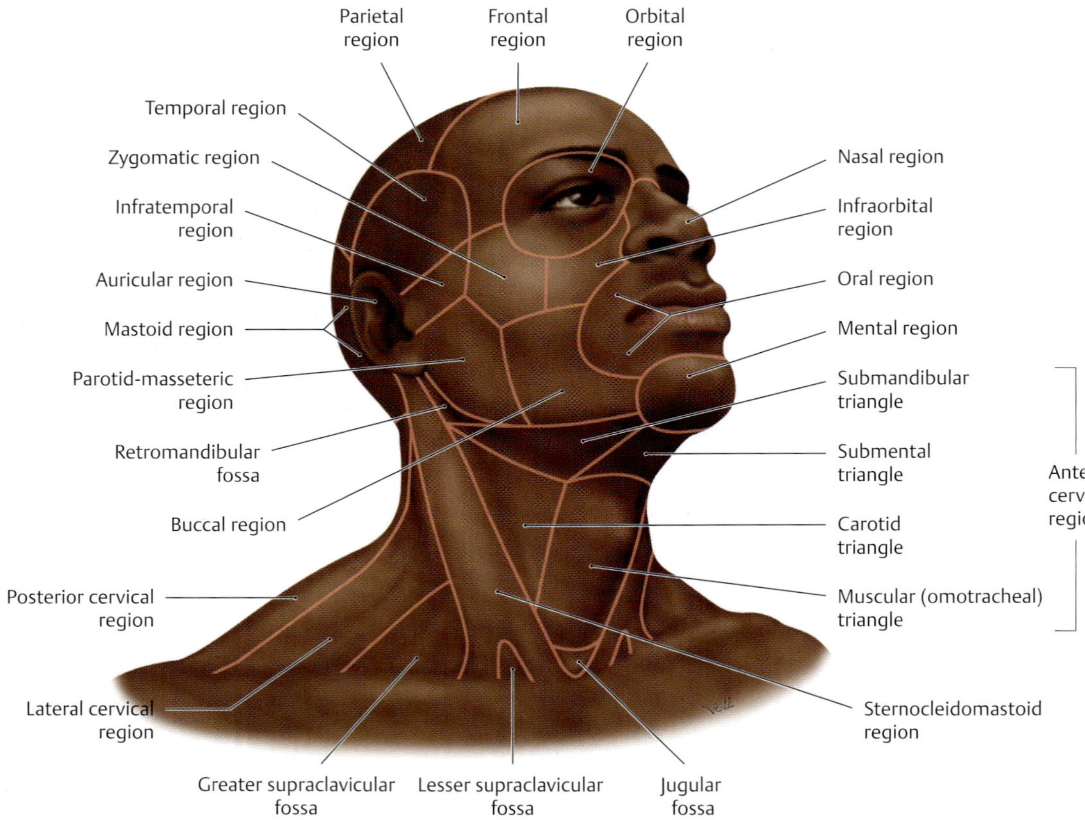

A Head and neck regions
Right anterior view.

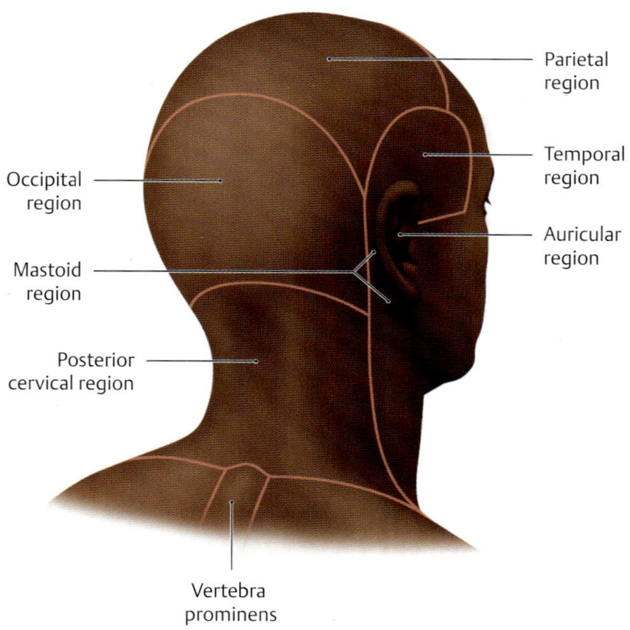

B Head and neck regions
Right posterior view.

C Head and neck regions

Head regions	Neck regions
• Frontal region • Parietal region • Occipital region • Temporal region • Auricular region • Mastoid region • Facial region – Orbital region – Infraorbital region – Buccal region – Parotid-masseteric region – Zygomatic region – Nasal region – Oral region – Mental region	• Anterior cervical regions – Submandibular triangle – Carotid triangle – Muscular (omotracheal) triangle – Submental triangle • Sternocleidomastoid region – Lesser supraclavicular fossa • Lateral cervical region – Omoclavicular triangle (major supraclavicular fossa) • Posterior cervical region

The regions of the head and neck are clinically important since they can exhibit many skin lesions, the location of which must be precisely described. This is particularly important for skin cancer given that the tissue fluid, through which the tumor cells spread, drains into different groups of lymph nodes named for their location.

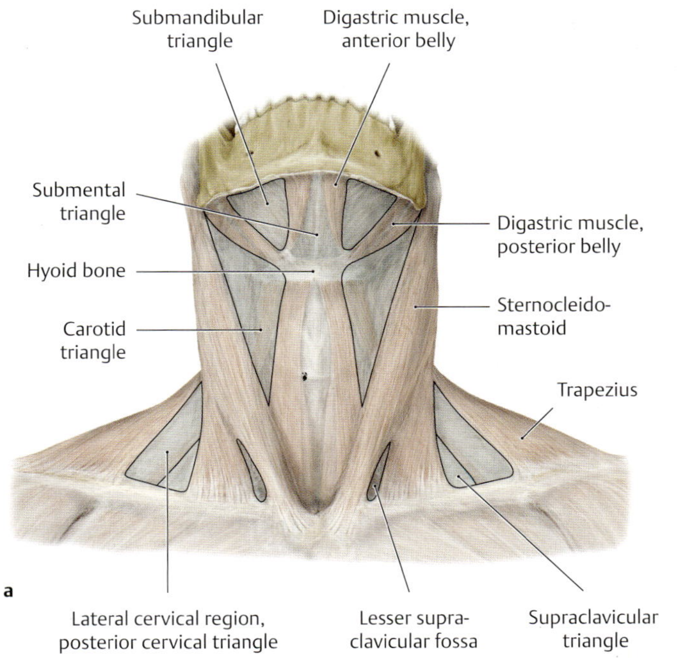

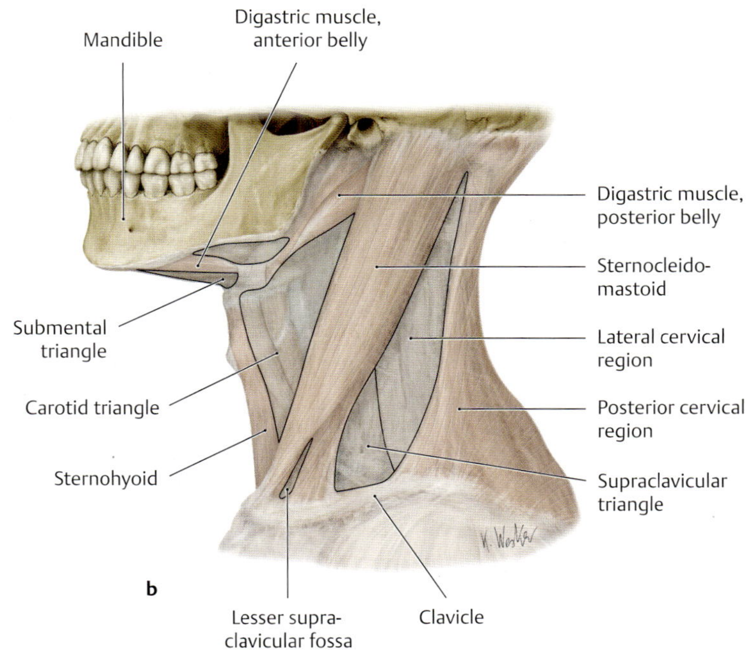

D Regions of the neck (cervical regions)
a Right lateral view, **b** left posterior oblique view.

These neck muscles are easily visible and palpable making them suitable as landmarks for a topographical classification of the neck.

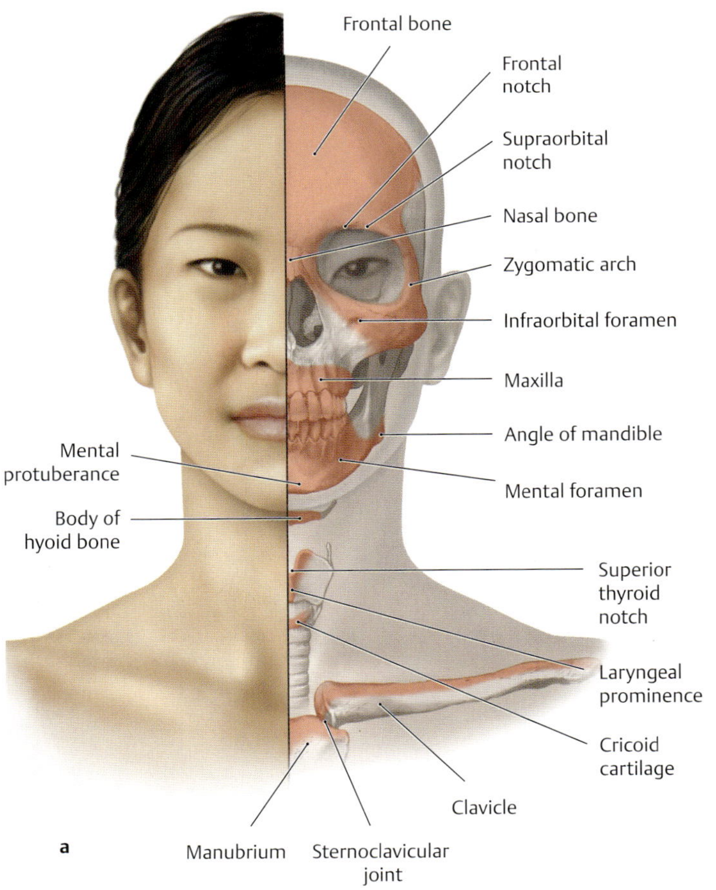

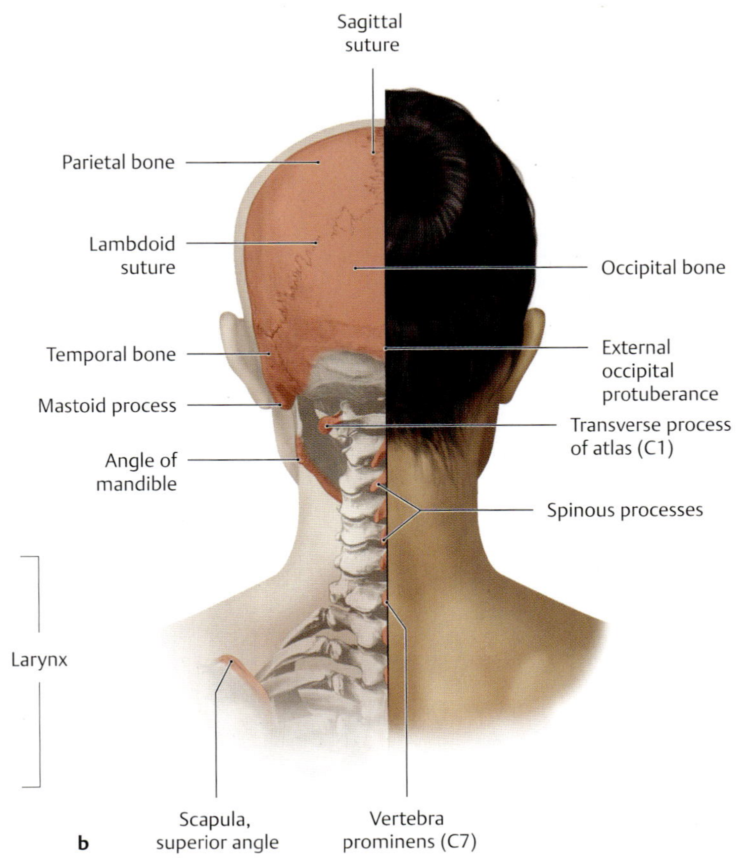

E Palpable bony landmarks at the head and neck
a Frontal view; **b** Dorsal view.

1.2 Head and Neck and Cervical Fasciae

The head and neck form an anatomical and functional unit with the neck connecting the head and the trunk. The neck contains many pathways to which the cervical viscera are indirectly attached. In the head however, there is only visceral fascia around the parotid gland but no general fasciae. Multiple fascial layers subdivide the neck into compartments which will be referred to when describing the location of structures within the neck.

A Sequence of topics in this chaper about the head and neck

Overview	• Regions and palpable bony landmarks • Head and neck with cervical fasciae • Clinical anatomy of the head and neck • Embryology of the face • Embryology of the neck
Bones	• Cranial bones • Teeth • Cervical spine • Ligaments • Joints
Muscles	• Muscles of facial expression • Masticatory muscles • Neck muscles
Classification of pathways	• Arteries • Veins • Lymphatics • Nerves
Organs and their pathways	• Ear • Eye • Nose • Oral cavity • Pharynx • Parotid gland • Larynx • Thyroid and parathyroid glands
Topographical anatomy	• Anterior facial region • Neck, anterior view, superficial layers • Neck, anterior view, deep layers • Lateral head: superficial layer • Lateral head: middle and deeper layer • Infratemporal fossa • Pterygopalatine fossa • Posterior cervical triangle • Superior thoracic aperture, carotid triangle and deep lateral cervical region • Posterior neck and occiput regions • Cross section of the head and neck

B Cervical fascia

Deep to the skin is the superficial cervical fascia (subcutaneous tissue) which contains the platysma muscle anterolaterally. Deep to the superficial are the following layers of deep cervical fascia:

1. Investing layer: envelops the entire neck, and splits to enclose the sternocleidomastoid and trapezius muscles.
2. Pretracheal layer: the muscular portion encloses the infrahyoid muscles, while the visceral portion surrounds the thyroid gland, larynx, trachea, pharynx, and esophagus.
3. Prevertebral layer: surrounds the cervical vertebral column, and the muscles associated with it.
4. Carotid sheath: encloses the common carotid artery, internal jugular vein, and vagus nerve.
5. Visceral fascia: encloses the larynx, trachea, pharynx, esophagus and thyroid.

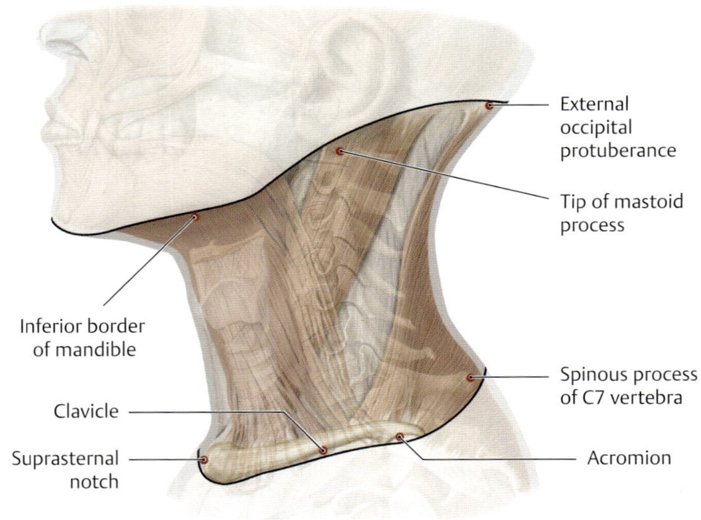

C Superficial and inferior boundaries of the neck

Left lateral view. The following palpable structures define the superior and inferior boundaries of the neck:

- Superior boundaries: inferior border of the mandible, tip of the mastoid process, and external occipital protuberance
- Inferior boundaries: suprasternal notch, clavicle, acromion, and spinous process of the C7 vertebra.

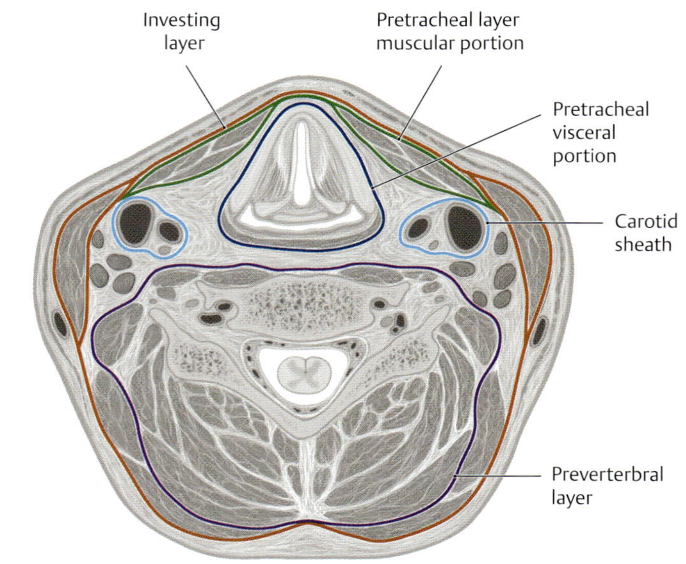

D Relationships of the deep fascia in the neck. Transverse section at the level of the C5 vertebra

The full extent of the cervical fascia is best appreciated in a transverse section of the neck:

- The *muscle fascia* splits into three layers:
  - Superficial lamina (orange),
  - Pretracheal lamina (green), and
  - Prevertebral lamina (violet).
- There is also a neurovascular fascia, called the *carotid sheath* (light blue), and
- a *visceral fascia* (dark blue).

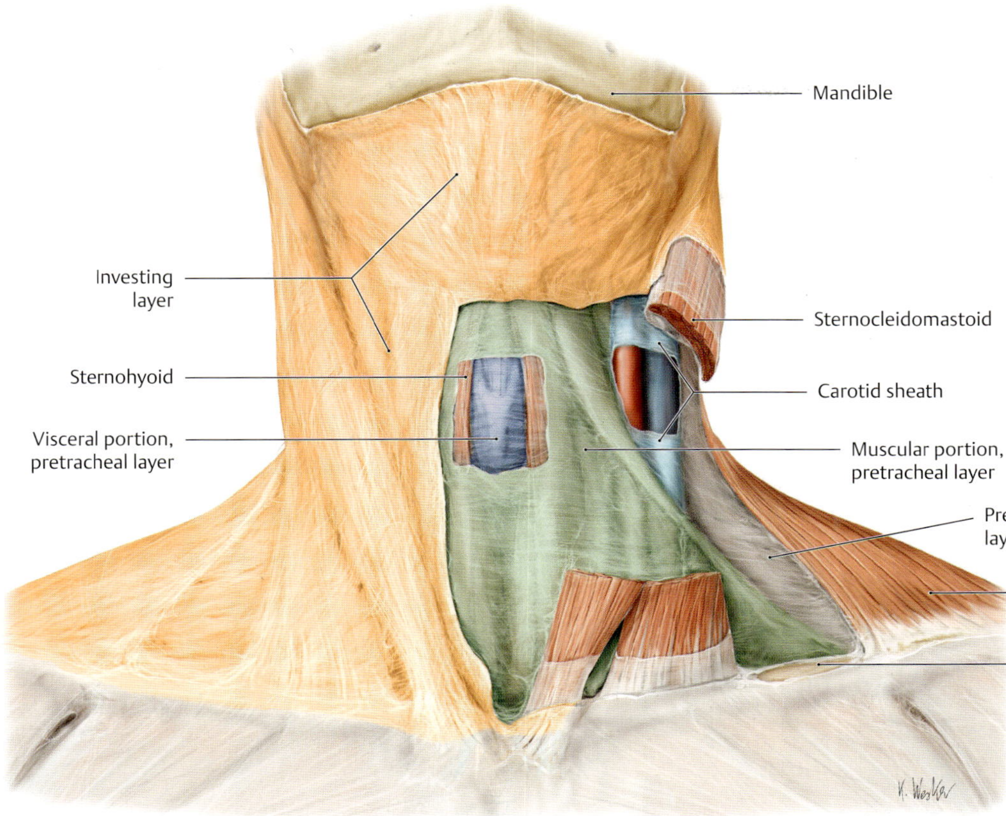

a

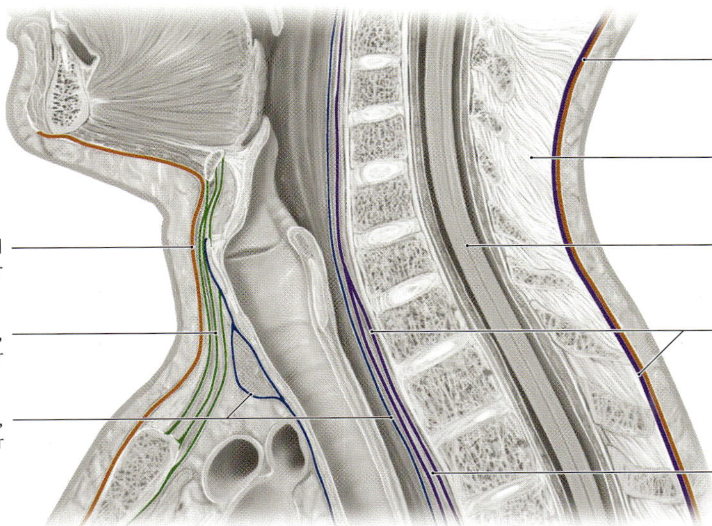

b

E Fascial relationships in the neck

a Anterior view. The cutaneous muscle of the neck, the platysma, is highly variable in its development and is subcutaneous in location, overlying the superficial cervical fascia. In the dissection shown, the platysma has been removed at the level of the inferior mandibular border on each side. The cervical fasciae form a fibrous sheet that encloses the muscles, neurovascular structures, and cervical viscera (see **B** for further details). These fasciae subdivide the neck into spaces, some of which are open superiorly and inferiorly for the passage of neurovascular structures. The *investing layer* of the deep cervical fascia has been removed at left center in this dissection. Just deep to the investing layer is the *muscular portion of the pretreacheal layer*, part of which has been removed to display the *visceral portion of the pretracheal layer*. The neurovascular structures are surrounded by a condensation of the cervical fascia called the *carotid sheath*. The deepest layer of the deep cervical fascia, called the *prevertebral layer*, is visible posteriorly on the left side. These fascia-bounded connective-tissue spaces in the neck are important clinically because they provide routes for the spread of inflammatory processes, although the inflammation may (at least initially) remain confined to the affected compartment

b Left lateral view. This midsagittal section shows that the deepest layer of the deep cervical fascia, the prevertebral layer, directly overlies the vertebral column in the median plane and is split into two parts. With tuberculous osteomyelitis of the cervical spine, for example, a gravitation abscess may develop in the "danger space" along the prevertebral fascia (retropharyngeal abscess). This fascia encloses muscles laterally and posteriorly (see **D**). The carotid sheath is located farther laterally and does not appear in the midsagittal section.

1.3 Clinical Anatomy

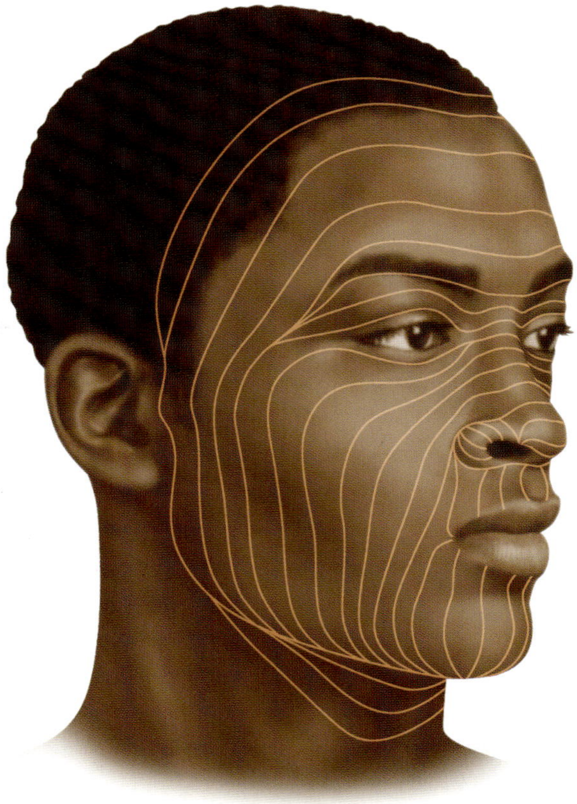

A Cleavage or tension lines
Anterior oblique view.
Skin and its subcutaneous tissue are under tension explaining why a small, round needle hole can result in a small longish slit in the skin aligned along the tension lines in the area around the incision. To promote swift healing and reduce visible scarring, incisions in the head region are aligned along these tension lines. Knowledge of the tension line patterns in the face and neck are critically important in plastic surgery to minimize scarring in these highly visible areas.

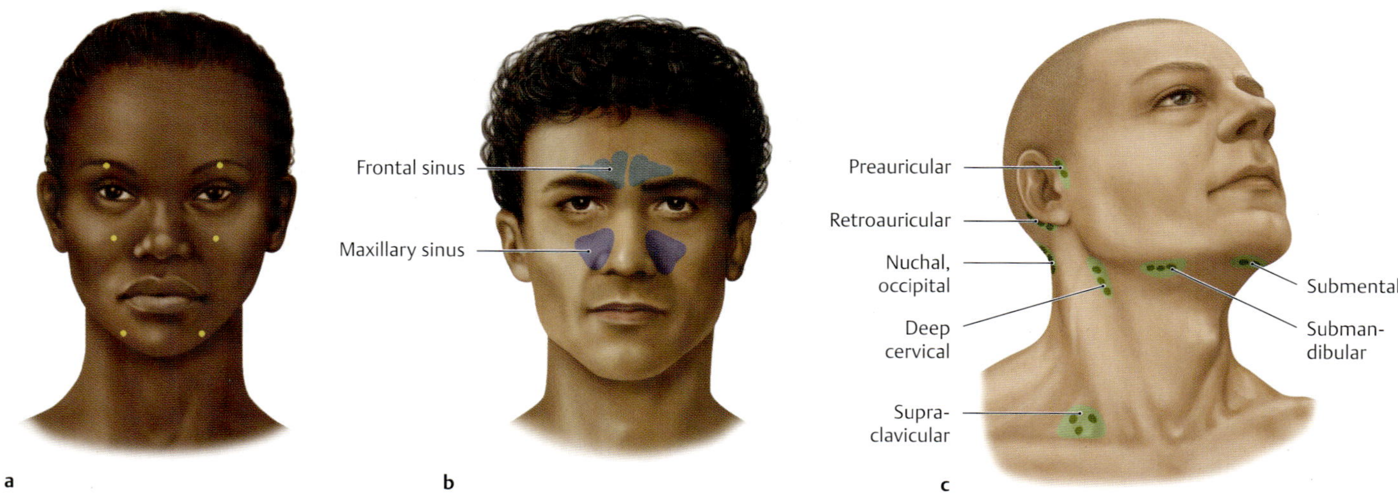

B Projection of clinically important structures onto the head and neck
Frontal view (**a** and **b**) and right lateral view (**c**).

a Exit points of the trigeminal nerve (CN V - sensory): These points are important for sensory testing of the head. If the pressure of a fingertip placed at these exit points causes pain, the respective branch of the trigeminal nerve is stimulated.

b Skin areas above the paranasal sinuses: When paranasal sinuses are inflamed, the skin areas above them are sensitive to pressure causing pain.

c Superficial lymph nodes at the junction between head and neck: The most important of lymph node groups are shown here. If the lymph nodes are enlarged, the cause can be related to inflammation or a tumor in the tributary area of the nodes. During a clinical examination of the head, these lymph node groups are always palpated.

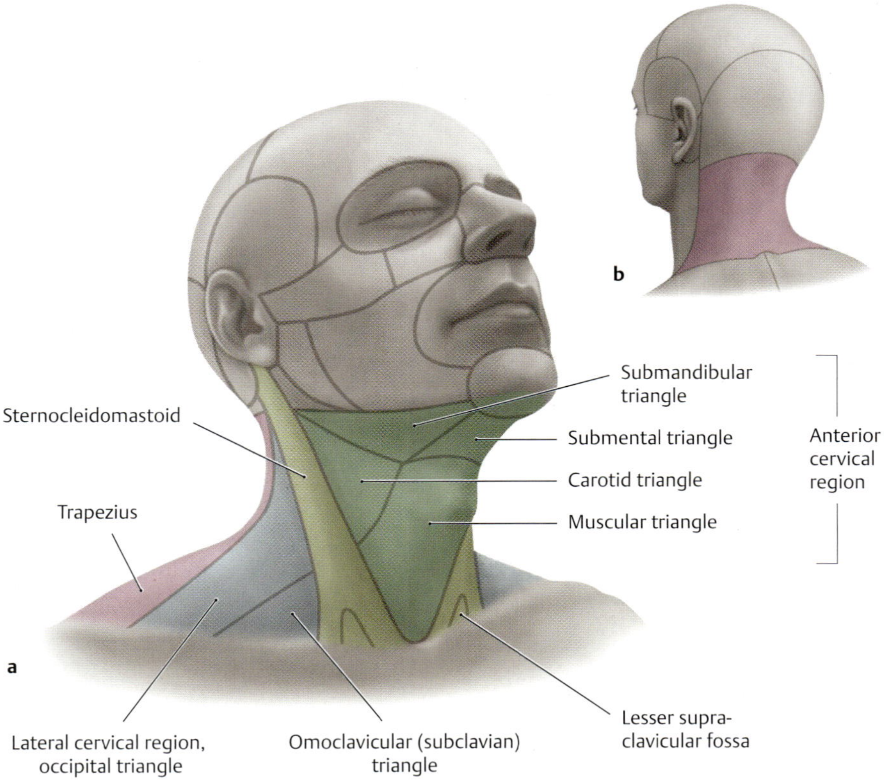

C Localization of important anatomic structures with respect to the topographical areas and regions of the neck

a Right anterior view; **b** Left posterior view.
Certain deeper structures of the neck project onto other regions. Conversely, pathological changes in one region can be referred to the underlying anatomical structure. Carotid body (glomus) tumors occur in the carotid triangle.

Anterior cervical region

- Submandibular triangle
  - Submandibular lymph nodes
  - Submandibular gland
  - Hypoglossal nerve
  - Parotid gland (posterior)
- Carotid triangle
  - Carotid bifurcation
  - Carotid body
  - Hypoglossal nerve
- Muscular triangle
  - Thyroid gland
  - Larynx
  - Trachea
  - Esophagus
- Submental triangle
  - Submental lymph nodes

Sternocleidomastoid region

- Sternocleidomastoid muscle
- Carotid artery
- Internal jugular vein
- Vagus nerve
- Jugular lymph nodes

Lateral cervical region

- Lateral lymph nodes
- Accessory nerve
- Cervical plexus
- Brachial plexus

Regio cervicalis posterior

- Neck muscles
- Trigonum arteriae vertebralis

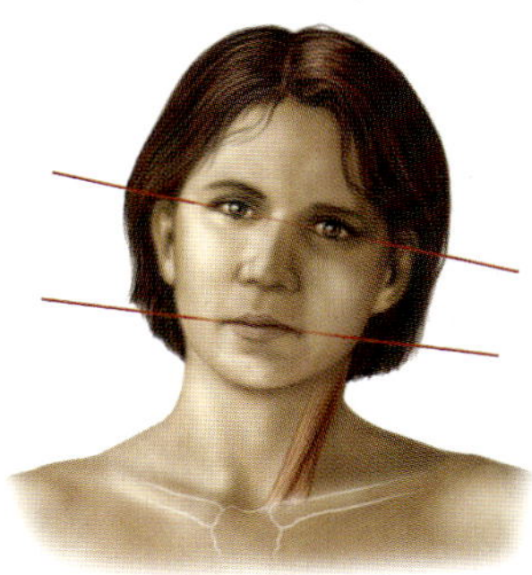

D Left-sided muscular torticollis

Torticollis and struma (swellings of the neck, see **E**) can be readily diagnosed by visual examination. In the case of torticollis, the sternocleidomastoid muscle is shortened—most commonly as a result of intrauterine malposition in infants. The head is tilted toward the affected side and is slightly rotated toward the opposite side. Without therapy (physical therapy/surgery) torticollis secondarily leads to asymmetrical growth of spinal column and facial skeleton. The effects of the cranial asymmetry may include a convergence of the facial planes toward the affected side (see lines).

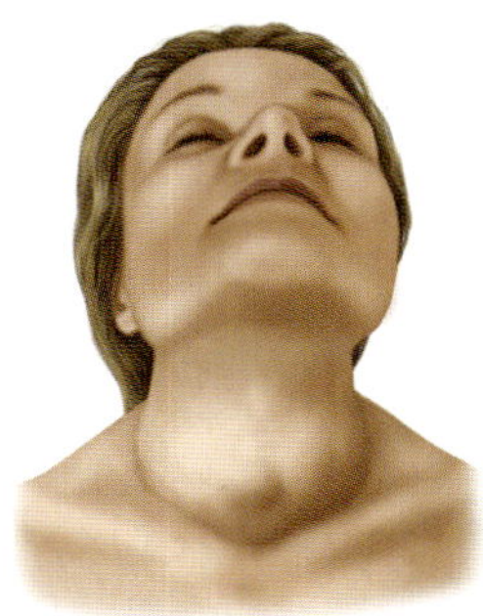

E Retrosternal goiter

A goiter that arises from the inferior poles (see p. 224) of the thyroid gland may extend to the thoracic inlet and compress the cervical veins at that level. The result of this is venous congestion and dilation in the head and neck region.

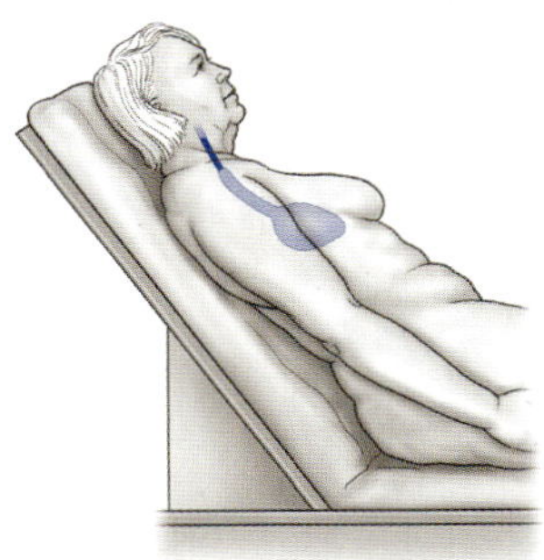

F Assessing the central venous pressure in the neck in a semi-upright position

Normally the cervical veins are collapsed in the sitting position. But in a patient with rightsided heart failure, there is diminished venous return to the right heart, causing distention of the jugular veins. The extent of the venous congestion is indicated by the level of pulsations in the external jugular vein (the "venous pulse," upper end of the blue line). The higher the level of jugular pulsation, the greater the backup of blood into the vein. This provides a means of assessing the severity of right-sided heart failure.

1.4 Embryology of the Face

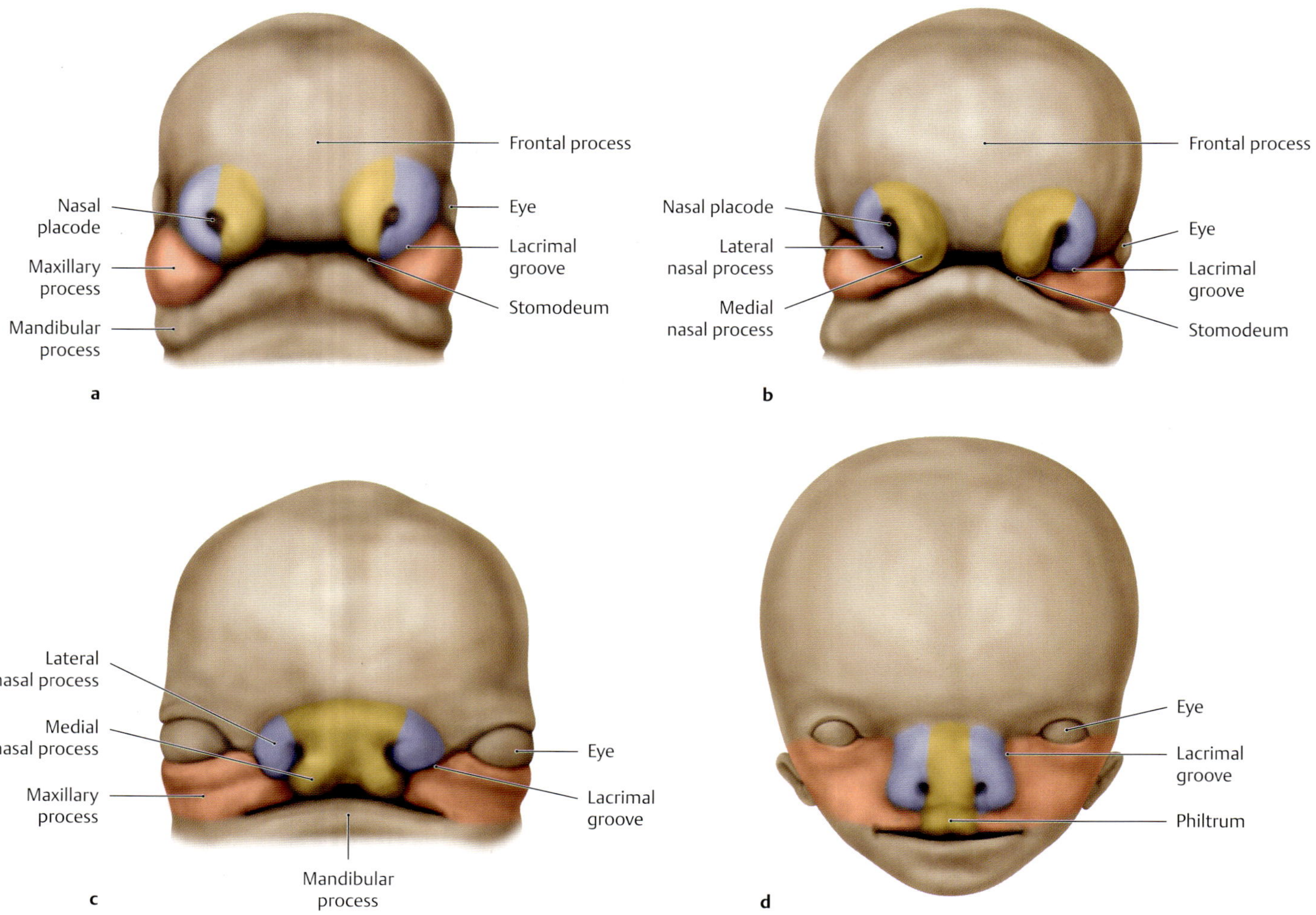

A Fusion of facial prominences
Frontal view. Understanding the clinically important development of the cleft lip, jaw, and palate (**c**) requires knowledge of facial evelopment.

a Embryo at five weeks. The surface ectoderm of the 1st branchial arch invaginates to form the stomodeum which later connects to the endodermal epithelium of the oral cavity. The facial outline develops from facial prominences, the tissue of which arises from the 1st branchial arch or neural crest mesenchyme. The mandibular processes are located caudal to the stomodeum with the maxillary processes located lateral to it. Superomedial to the maxillary processes are the medial and lateral nasal process. Both medial nasal processes border the frontal process.

b Embryo at six weeks. A furrow separates the nasal processes from the maxillary process.

c Embryo at seven weeks. The medial nasal processes have fused along the midline and their inferolateral margins contact the maxillary processes on either side.

d Embryo at ten weeks. Cell migration is completed.

B Facial prominences and their derivatives

Facial prominence	Derivative
Frontal process	Forehead, bridge of nose, medial and lateral nasal process
Maxillary process	Cheeks, lateral parts of upper lip
Medial nasal process	Philtrum, tip of the nose and ridge of the nose
Lateral nasal process	Nasal wing
Mandibular process	Lower lip

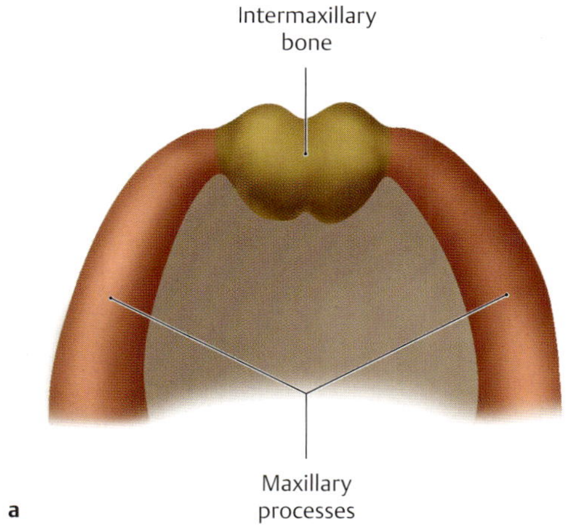

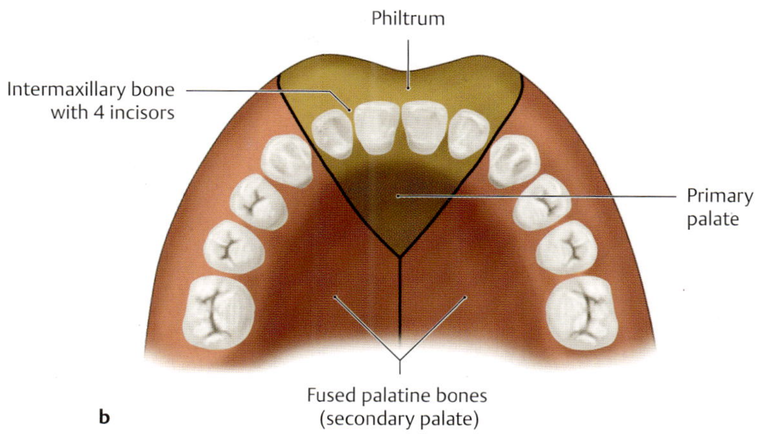

C Intermaxillary segment
a and **b** Caudal view of palate.

a The medial nasal processes develop bone tissue that fuses along the midline and gives rise to a separate bone, the intermaxillary bone.

b The philtrum also arises from tissue of the medial nasal process along with intermaxillary bone and its four incisors. The bone of the primary palate fuses with the maxillary processes (secondary palate) and is no longer a separate bone in adults.

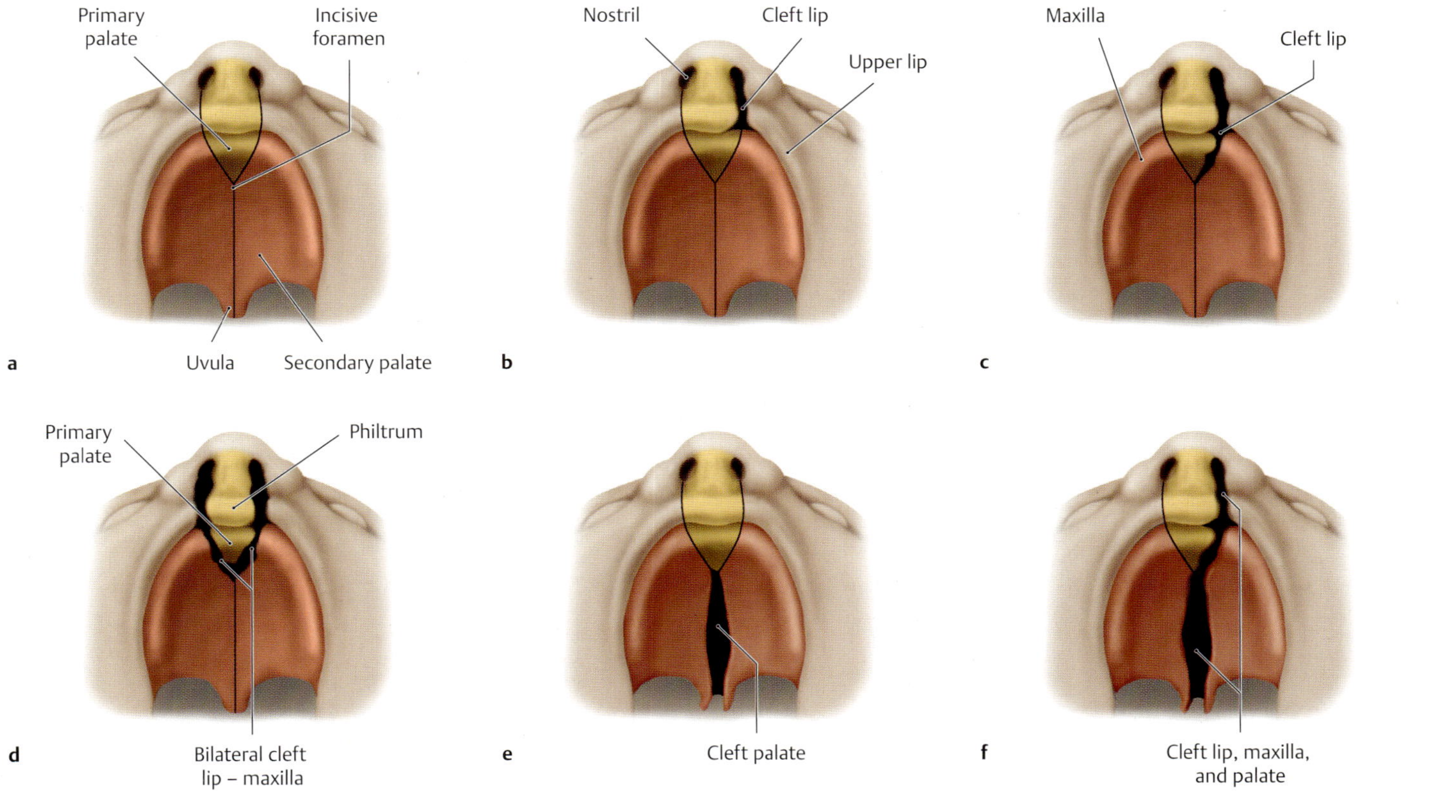

D Formation of facial clefts
a–f Caudal and ventral view.

a Normal condition. The palatine bones and the maxillary processes have fused with the primary palate. The surface epithelium forms oral mucosa that lines the roof of the oral cavity. The bony palate beneath the oral mucosa separates the oral and nasal cavities.

b Cheiloschisis. A cleft lip that extends up to the nose (harelip) occurs on the left side if the tissue of the upper lip does not fuse on the left side.

c Cheilognathoschisis. A cleft lip and maxilla occurs if the fusion of primary and secondary palates on the left side does not occur.

d Cleft formation can also occur bilaterally: bilateral cleft lip and maxilla.

e Palatoschisis. Incomplete fusion of the primary and secondary palates on both sides results in an isolated cleft palate.

f Cheilognathopalatoschisis. Combination of all three: unilateral cleft lip, maxilla, and palate. If it occurs bilaterally it is known as cleft palate.

1.5 Embryology of the Neck

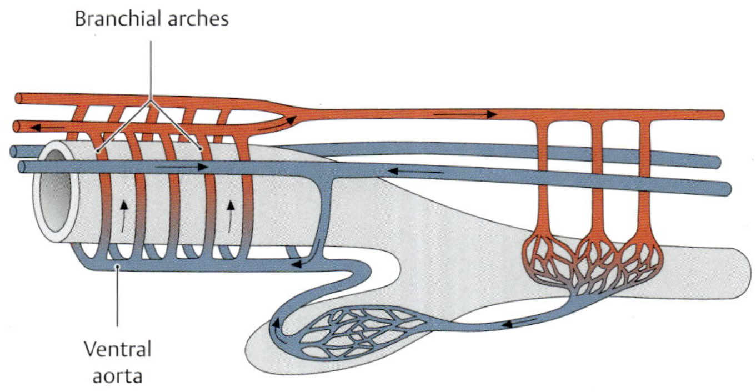

A The branchial arches of the lancelet
Left lateral view. This simplified schematic of the circulatory system of a lancelet fish illustrates the basic relation between the vascular tree and the branchial arches in chordates, including the vertebrates. Oxygen-depleted blood (in blue) is pumped rostrally (toward the head) through a ventral aorta to a series of branchial arches, where it passes through gills, picks up oxygen (red), and then is distributed to the body (compare this paired, segmental arterial arch with the thoracic segment in humans). A similar anatomical organization and circulatory pattern is seen in the human embryo, where the gills and branchial arches are transformed into pharyngeal arches which develop into various structures in the head and neck. Errors during this developmental process give rise to a series of relatively common anatomical anomalies in the neck (see **G**).

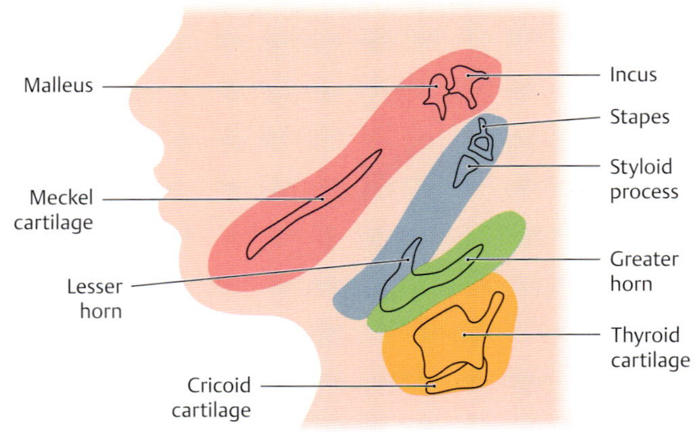

C Derivation of musculoskeletal structures from the pharyngeal arches in the adult
Left lateral view. Besides the cartilaginous rudiments of the skeleton (see labels), the muscles and their associated nerves can be traced embryologically to specific pharyngeal arches. The first pharyngeal arch gives rise to the masticatory muscles, the mylohyoid muscle, the anterior belly of the digastric muscle, the tensor veli palatini, and the tensor tympani. The second pharyngeal arch gives origin to the muscles of facial expression, the posterior belly of the digastric, the stylohyoid muscle, and the stapedius. The stylopharyngeus muscle is derived from the third pharyngeal arch. The fourth and sixth pharyngeal arches give rise to the cricothyroid muscle, levator levi palatini, constrictor pharyngis, and the intrinsic muscles of the larynx. The nerve supply to the muscles can also be explained in terms of their embryologic origins (see **D**).

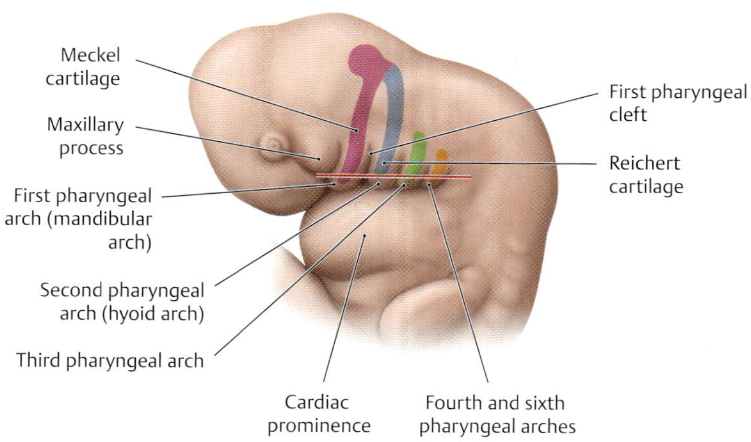

B Pharyngeal arches and pharyngeal clefts of a 4-week-old embryo
Left lateral view. The human embryo has four pharyngeal arches separated by intervening pharyngeal clefts. The cartilages of the four pharyngeal arches are shown in different colors. Like other tissues of the pharyngeal arches, they migrate with further development to form various skeletal and ligamentous elements in the adult (see **C**).

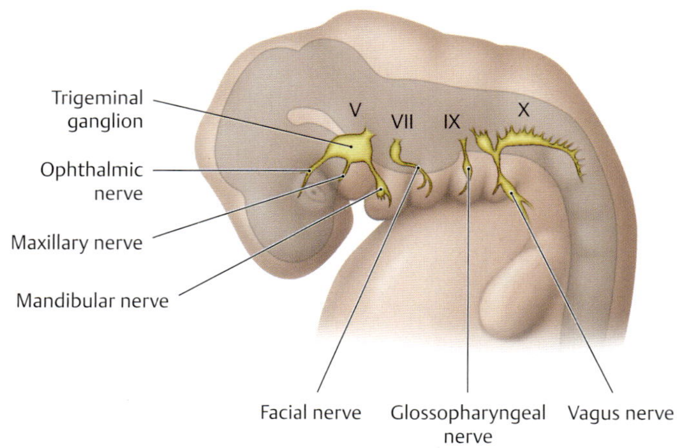

D Innervation of the pharyngeal arches
Left lateral view. Each of the pharyngeal arches is associated with a cranial nerve:

First pharyngeal arch	Trigeminal nerve (CN V) (mandibular nerve)
Second pharyngeal arch	Facial nerve (CN VII)
Third pharyngeal arch	Glossopharyngeal nerve (CN IX)
Fourth and sixth pharyngeal Vagus nerve	Vagus nerve (CN X) (superior and recurrent laryngeal nerves) (CN X) arches

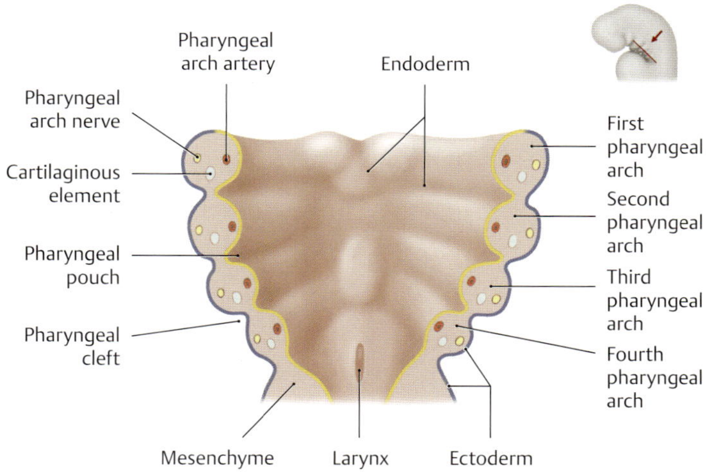

E Internal structure of the pharyngeal arches

Posterior view. The pharyngeal arches are covered externally by ectoderm and internally by endoderm. Each pharyngeal arch contains an arch artery, an arch nerve, and a cartilaginous element, all of which are surrounded by mesodermal and muscular tissue. The external furrows are called the pharyngeal clefts, and the internal furrows are called the pharyngeal pouches. The endodermal lining of the pharingeal pouches develops into endocrine glands of the neck, a process which may involve significant migration of cells from their site of origin.

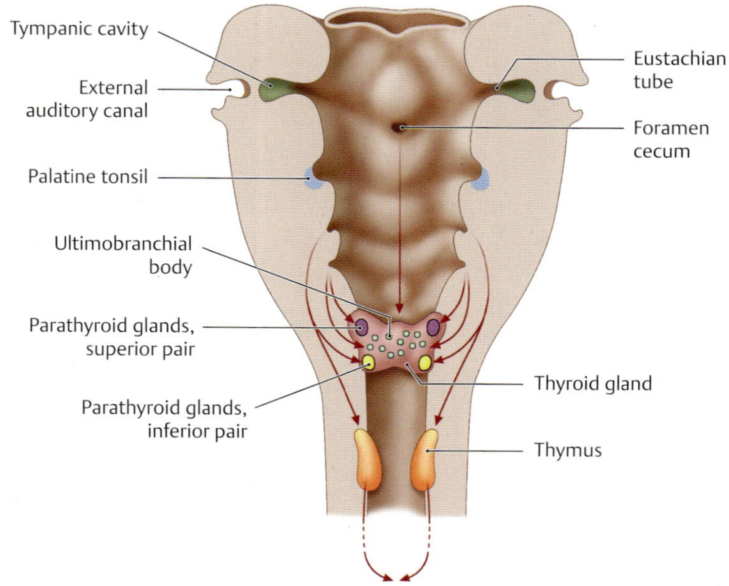

F Migratory movements of the pharyngeal arch tissues (after Sadler)

Anterior view. During embryonic development, the epithelium from which the thyroid gland is formed migrates from its site of origin on the basal midline of the tongue to the level of the first tracheal cartilage, where the thyroid gland is located in postnatal life. As the thyroid tissue buds off from the tongue base, it leaves a vestigial depression on the dorsum of the tongue, the foramen cecum. The parathyroid glands are derived from the fourth pharyngeal arch (superior pair) or third pharyngeal arch (inferior pair), which also gives origin to the thymus. The ultimobranchial body, whose cells migrate into the thyroid gland to form the calcitonin-producing C cells or parafollicular cells, is derived from the fifth, vestigial, pharyngeal arch. The latter arch is the last to develop and is usually considered part of the fourth pharyngeal arch. The external auditory canal is derived from the first pharyngeal cleft, the tym-panic cavity and eustachian tube from the first pharyngeal pouch, and the palatine tonsil from the second pharyngeal pouch.

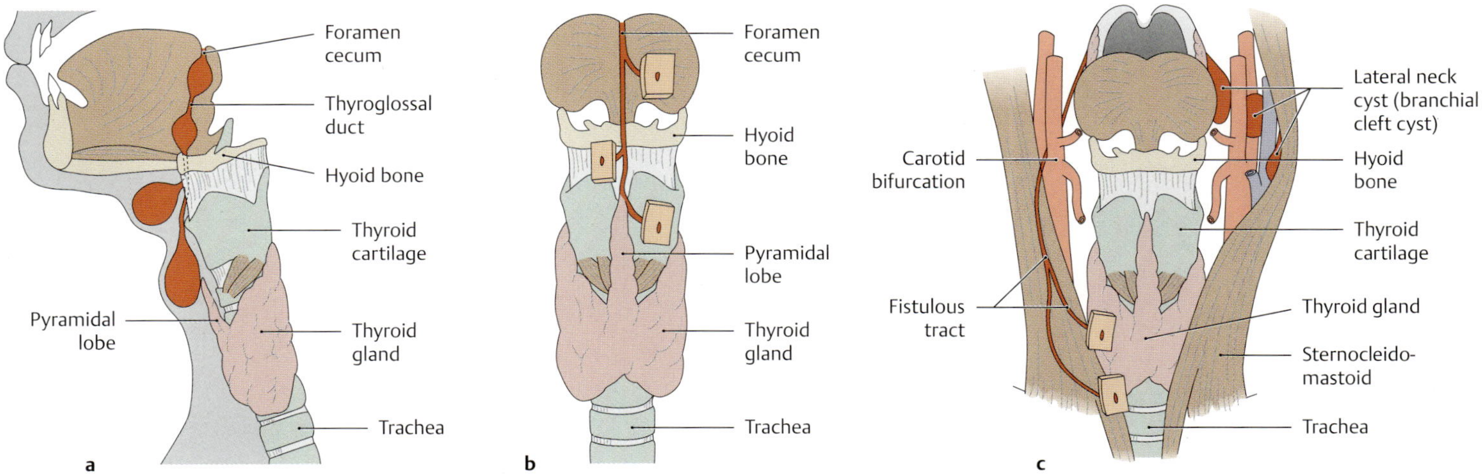

G Location of cysts and fistulas in the neck

a Median cysts, **b** median fistulas, **c** lateral fistulas and cysts.

Median cysts and fistulas in the neck (**a**, **b**) are remnants of the thyroglossal duct. Failure of this duct to regress completely may lead to the formation of a mucus-filled cavity (cyst), which presents clinically as a firm neck mass.

Lateral cysts and fistulas in the neck are anomalous remnants of the ductal portions of the cervical sinus, which forms as a result of tissue migration during embryonic development. If epithelium-lined remnants persist, neck cysts (right) or fistulas (left) may appear in postnatal life (**c**). A complete fistula opens into the pharynx and onto the surface of the skin, whereas an incomplete (blind) fistula is open at one end only. The external orifice of a lateral cervical fistula is typically located at the anterior border of the sternocleidomastoid muscle.

2.1 Skull, Lateral View

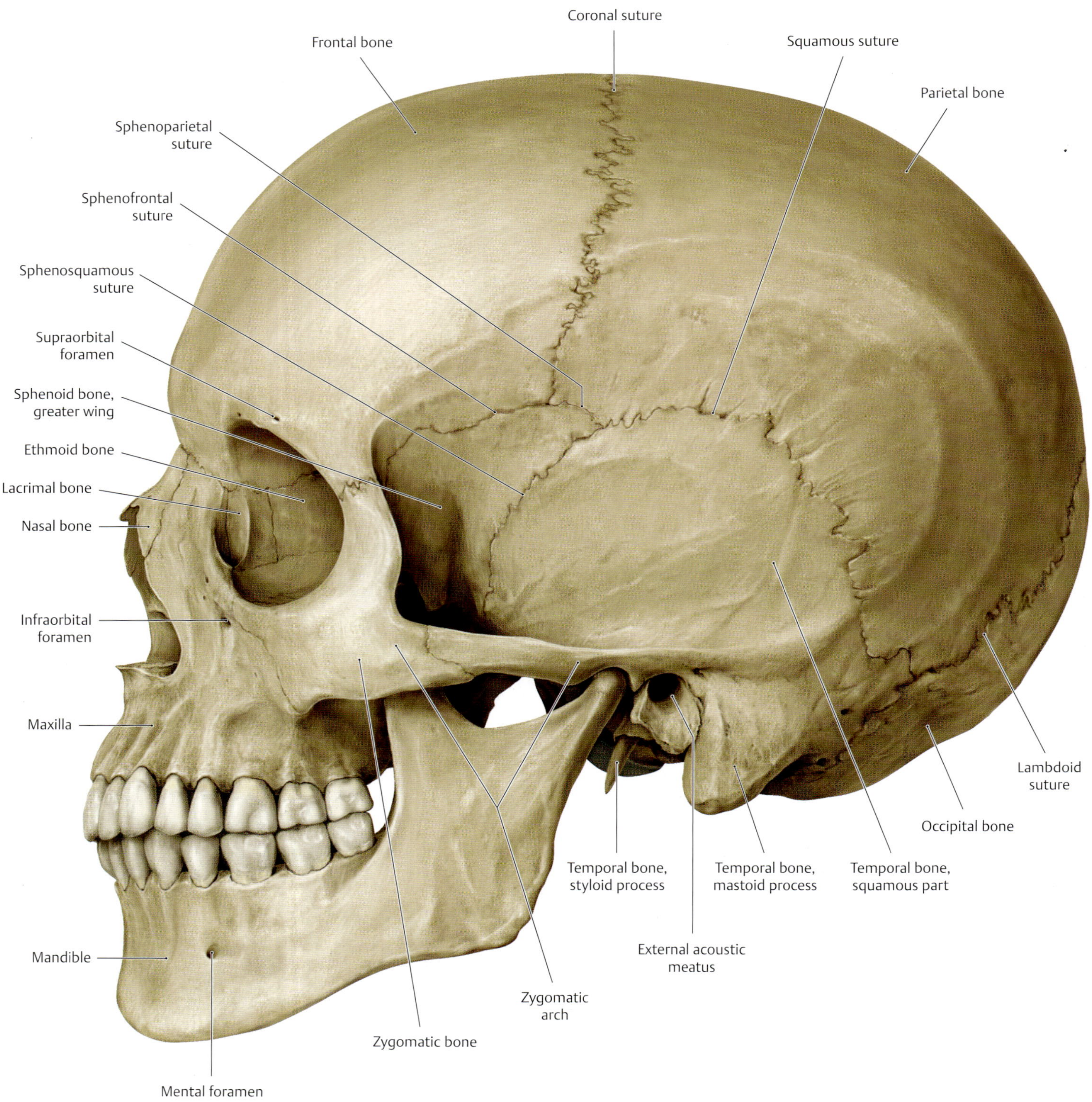

A Lateral view of the skull (cranium)
Left lateral view. This view was selected as an introduction to the skull because it displays the greatest number of cranial bones (indicated by different colors in **B**). The individual bones and their salient features as well as the cranial sutures and apertures are described in the units that follow. This unit reviews the principal structures of the lateral aspect of the skull. The chapter as a whole is intended to familiarize the reader with the names of the cranial bones before proceeding to finer anatomical details and the relationships of the bones to one another. The teeth are described in a separate unit (see p. 48 ff).

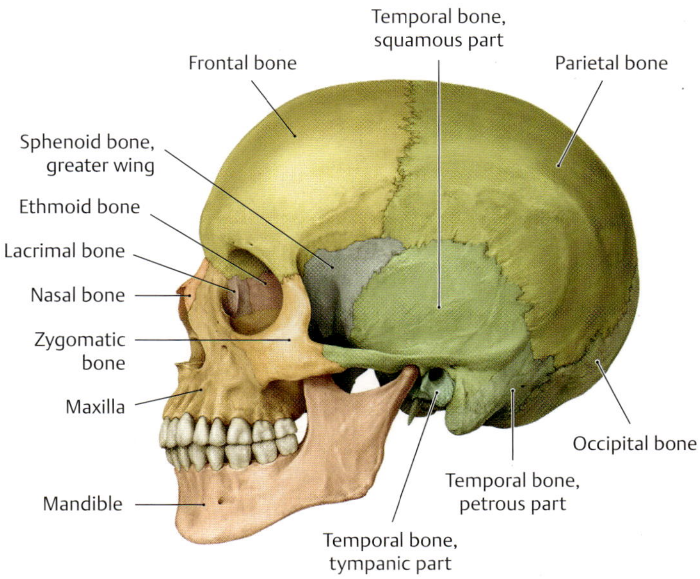

B Lateral view of the cranial bones
Left lateral view. The bones are shown in different colors to demonstrate more clearly their extents and boundaries.

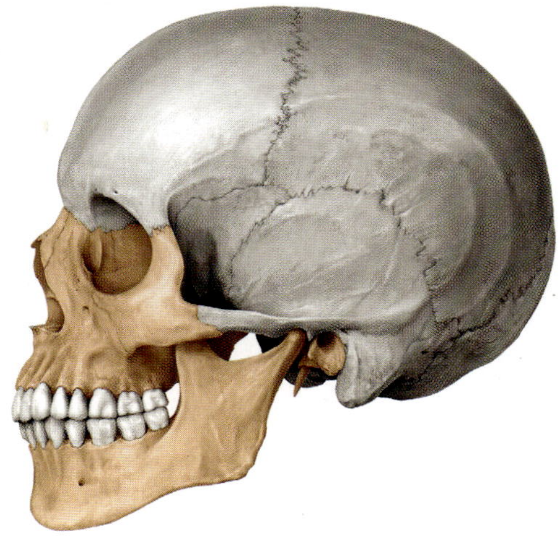

C Bones of the neurocranium (gray) and viscerocranium (orange)
Left lateral view. The skull forms a bony capsule that encloses the brain, sensory organs, and viscera of the head. The greater size of the neurocranium (cranial vault) relative to the viscerocranium (facial skeleton) is a typical primate feature directly correlated with the larger primate brain.

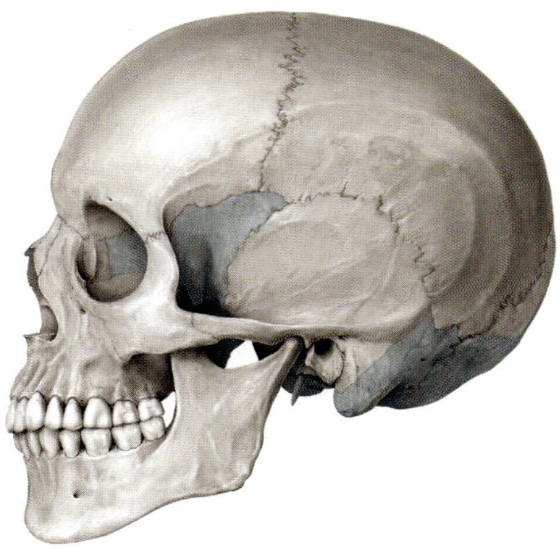

D Ossification of the cranial bones
Left lateral view. The bones of the skull either develop directly from mesenchymal connective tissue (intramembranous ossification, gray) or form indirectly by the ossification of a cartilaginous model (enchondral ossification, blue). Elements derived from intramembranous and endochondral ossification (desmocranium and chondrocranium respectively) may fuse together to form a single bone (e.g., the occipital bone, temporal bone, and sphenoid bone).
The clavicle is the only tubular bone that undergoes membranous ossification. This explains why congenital defects of intramembranous ossification affect both the skull and clavicle (*cleidocranial dysostosis*).

E Bones of the neurocranium and viscerocranium

Neurocranium (gray)	**Viscerocranium** (orange)
• Frontal bone • Sphenoid bone (excluding the pterygoid process) • Temporal bone (squamous part, petrous part) • Parietal bone • Occipital bone • Ethmoid bone (cribriform plate) • Auditory ossicles	• Nasal bone • Lacrimal bone • Ethmoid bone (excluding the cribriform plate) • Sphenoid bone (pterygoid process) • Maxilla • Zygomatic bone • Temporal bone (tympanic part, styloid process) • Mandible • Vomer • Inferior nasal turbinate • Palatine bone • Hyoid bone (see p. 47)

F Bones of the desmocranium and chondrocranium

Desmocranium (gray)	**Chondrocranium** (blue)
• Nasal bone • Lacrimal bone • Maxilla • Mandible • Zygomatic bone • Frontal bone • Parietal bone • Occipital bone (upper part of the squama) • Temporal bone (squamous part, tympanic part) • Palatine bone • Vomer	• Ethmoid bone • Sphenoid bone (excluding the medial plate of the pterygoid process) • Temporal bone (petrous and mastoid parts, styloid process) • Occipital bone (excluding the upper part of the squama) • Inferior nasal turbinate • Hyoid bone (see p. 47) • Auditory ossicles

2.2 Skull, Anterior View

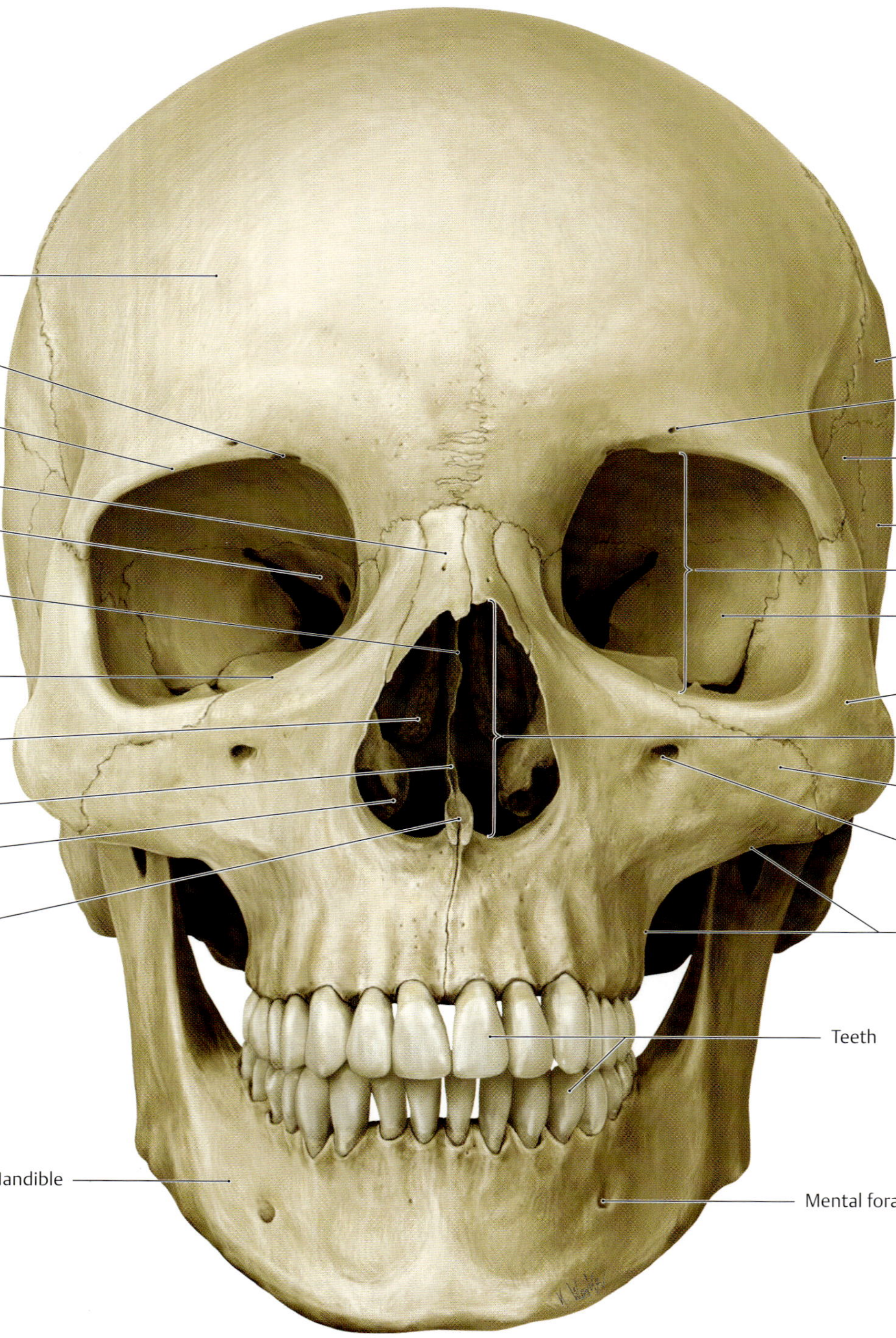

A Anterior view of the skull
The boundaries of the facial skeleton (viscerocranium) can be clearly appreciated in this view (the individual bones are shown in **B**). The bony margins of the anterior nasal aperture mark the start of the respiratory tract in the skull. The nasal cavity, like the orbits, contains a sensory organ (the olfactory mucosa). The *paranasal sinuses* are shown schematically in **C**. The anterior view of the skull also displays the three clinically important openings through which sensory nerves pass to supply the face: the supraorbital foramen, infraorbital foramen, and mental foramen (see p. 123 and 227).
Note: In cases of suspected midfacial fracture (mainly Le Fort I and II) intraoral palpation of the zygomatic-alveolar line is recommended for a possible step off and change in maxilla mobility against the skull in the case of dislodged zygomatic bone fractures.

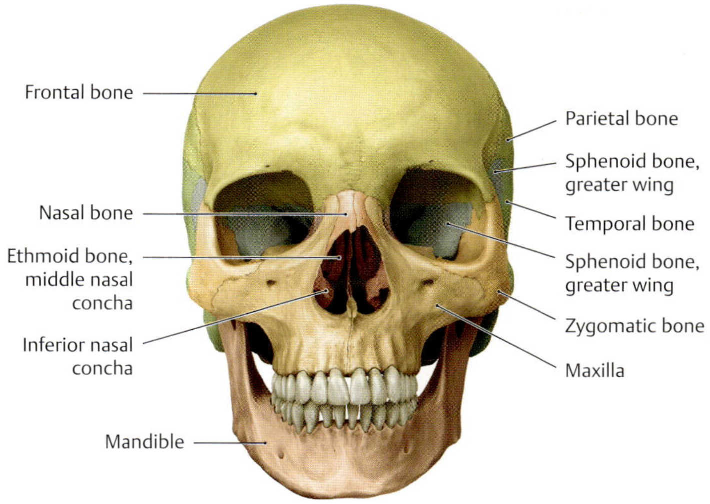

B Cranial bones, anterior view

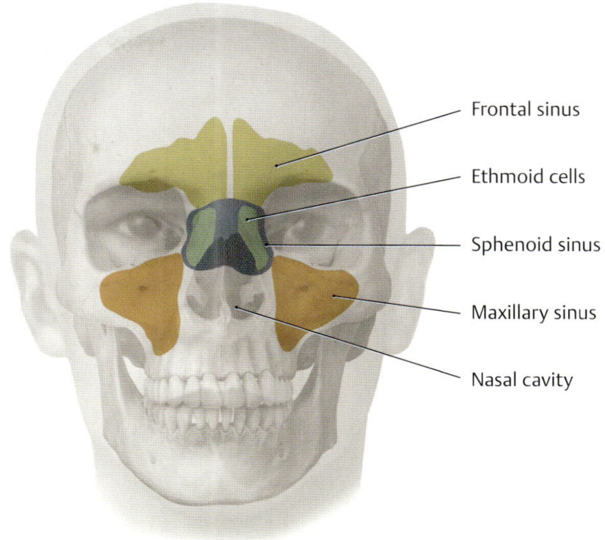

C Paranasal sinuses: pneumatization lightens the bone

Anterior view. Some of the bones of the facial skeleton are pneumatized (i.e., they contain air-filled cavities that reduce the total weight of the bone). These cavities, called the paranasal sinuses, communicate with the nasal cavity and, like it, are lined by ciliated respiratory epithelium. Inflammations of the paranasal sinuses (sinusitis) and associated complaints are very common. Because some of the pain of sinusitis is projected to the skin overlying the sinuses, it is helpful to know the projections of the sinuses onto the surface of the skull.

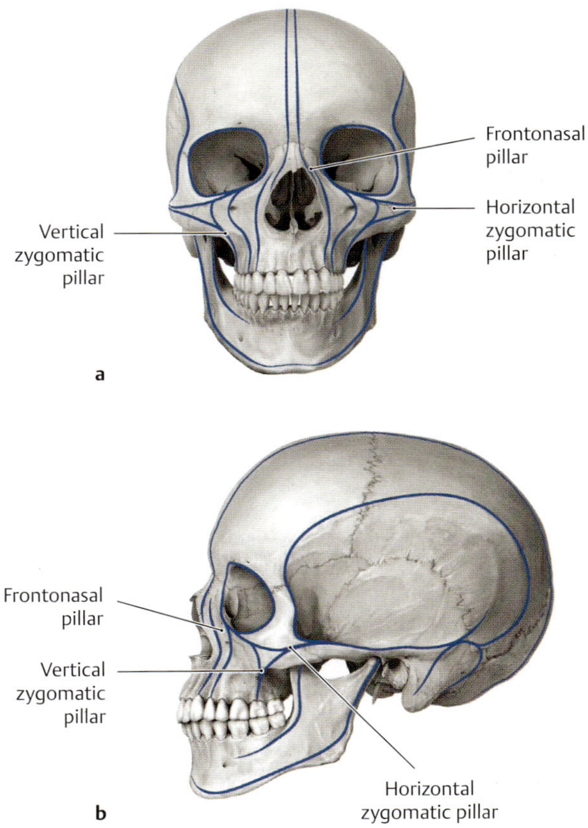

D Principal lines of force (blue) in the facial skeleton

a Anterior view, **b** lateral view. The pneumatized paranasal sinuses (**C**) have a mechanical counterpart in the thickened bony "pillars" of the facial skeleton, which partially bound the sinuses. These pillars develop along the principal lines of force in response to local mechanical stresses (e.g., masticatory pressures). In visual terms, the frame-like construction of the facial skeleton may be likened to that of a frame house: The paranasal sinuses represent the rooms while the pillars (placed along major lines of force) represent the supporting columns.

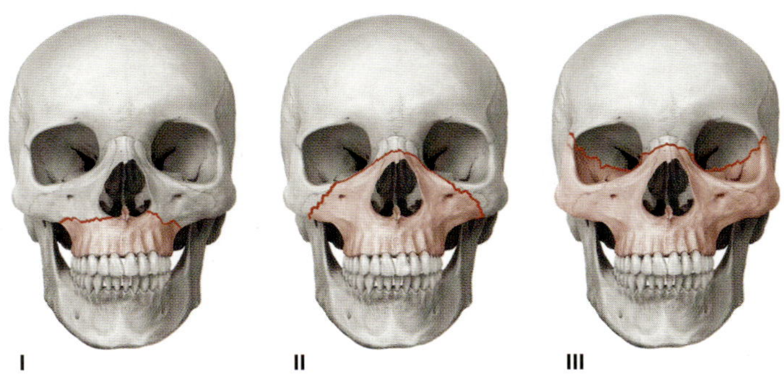

E LeFort classification of midfacial fractures

The frame-like construction of the facial skeleton leads to characteristic patterns of fracture lines in the midfacial region (LeFort I, II, and III).

LeFort I: This fracture line runs across the maxilla and above the hard palate. The maxilla is separated from the upper facial skeleton, disrupting the integrity of the maxillary sinus (*low transverse fracture*).

LeFort II: The fracture line passes across the nasal root, ethmoid bone, maxilla, and zygomatic bone, creating a *pyramid fracture* that disrupts the integrity of the orbit.

LeFort III: The facial skeleton is separated from the base of the skull. The main fracture line passes through the orbits, and the fracture may additionally involve the ethmoid bones, frontal sinuses, sphenoid sinuses, and zygomatic bones.

2.3 Skull, Posterior View, and Cranial Sutures

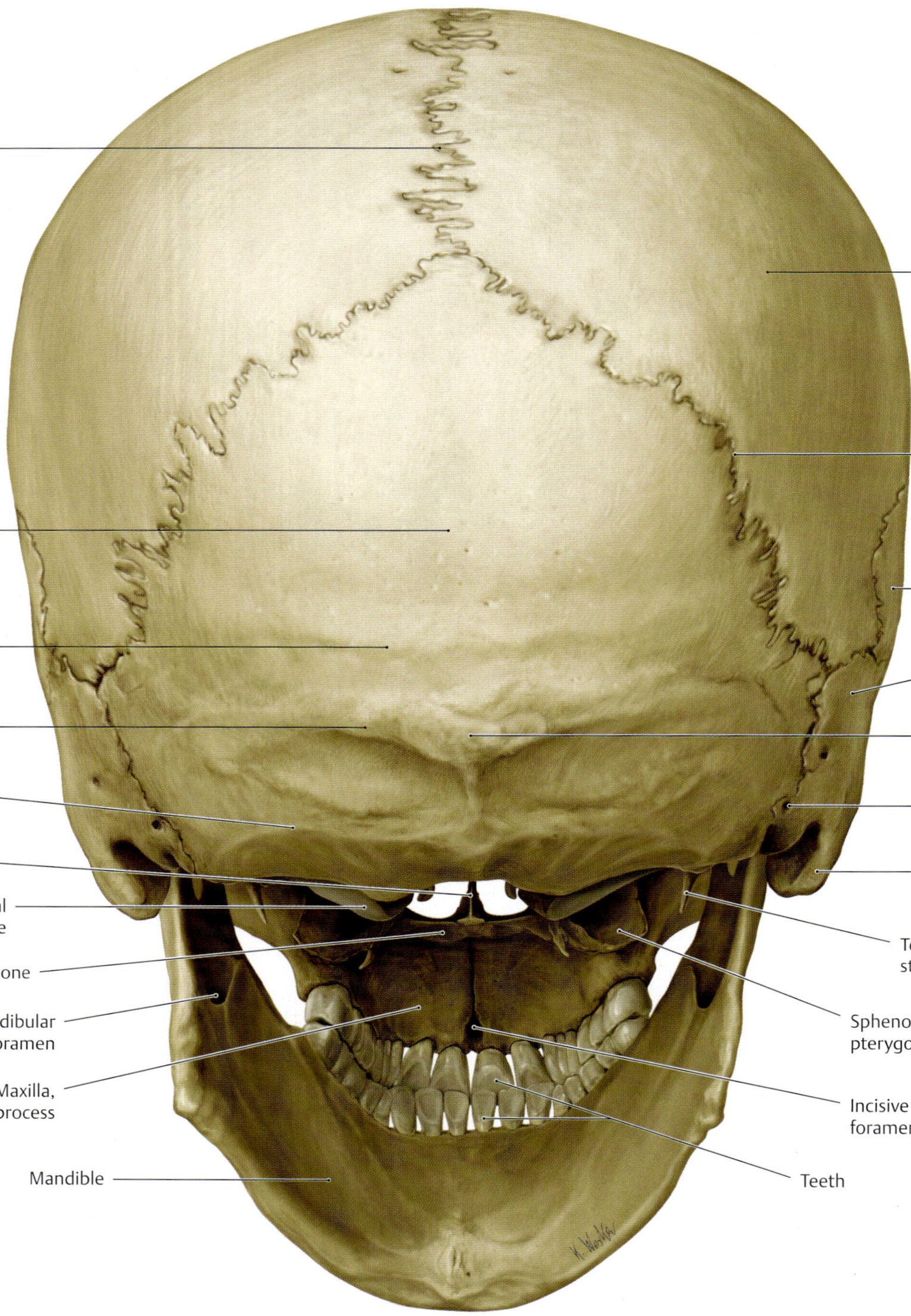

A Posterior view of the skull

The occipital bone, which is dominant in this view, articulates with the parietal bones, to which it is connected by the lambdoid suture. The cranial sutures are a special type of syndesmosis (= ligamentous attachments that ossify with age, see **F**). The outer surface of the occipital bone is contoured by muscular origins and insertions: the inferior, superior, and supreme nuchal lines. The *external occipital protuberance* serves as an anatomical reference point: It is palpable at the back of the head. The mastoid foramen provides a point of an emergence of a vein (see p. 19).

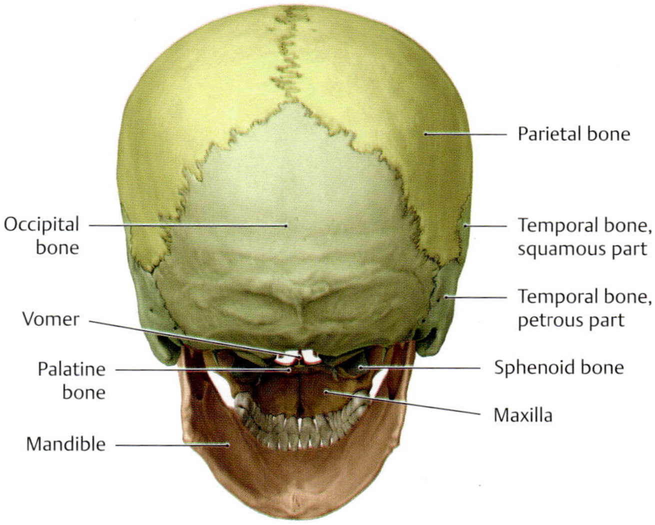

B Posterior view of the cranial bones

Note: The temporal bone consists of two main parts based on its embryonic development: a squamous part and a petrous part (cf. p. 28).

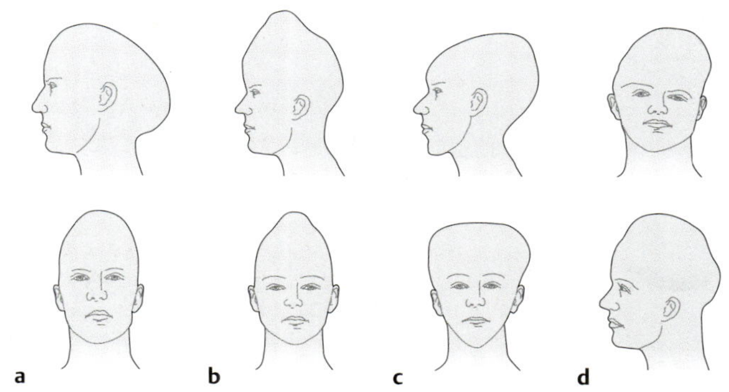

D Cranial deformities due to the premature closure of cranial sutures

The premature closure of a cranial suture (craniosynostosis) may lead to characteristic cranial deformities, which are normal variants of no clinical significance. The following sutures may close prematurely, resulting in various cranial shapes:

a Sagittal suture: scaphocephaly (long, narrow skull)
b Coronal suture: oxycephaly (pointed skull)
c Frontal suture: trigonocephaly (triangular skull)
d Asymmetrical suture closure, usually involving the coronal suture: plagiocephaly (asymmetrical skull).

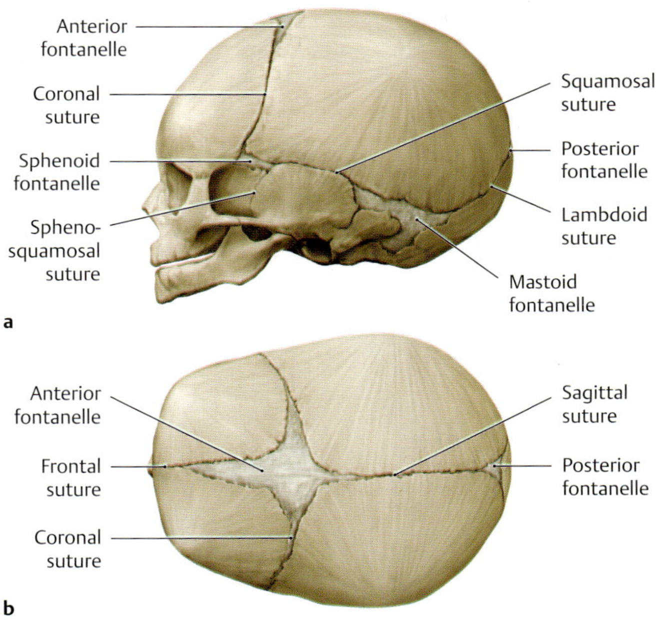

C The neonatal skull

a Left lateral view, **b** superior view.

The flat cranial bones must grow as the brain expands, and so the sutures between them must remain open for some time (see **F**). In the neonate, there are areas between the still-growing cranial bones that are not occupied by bone: the fontanelles. They close at different times (the sphenoid fontanelle in about the 6th month of life, the mastoid fontanelle in the 18th month, the anterior fontanelle in the 36th month). The *posterior fontanelle* provides a reference point for describing the position of the fetal head during childbirth, and the *anterior fontanelle* provides a possible access site for drawing a cerebrospinal fluid sample in infants (e.g., in suspected meningitis).

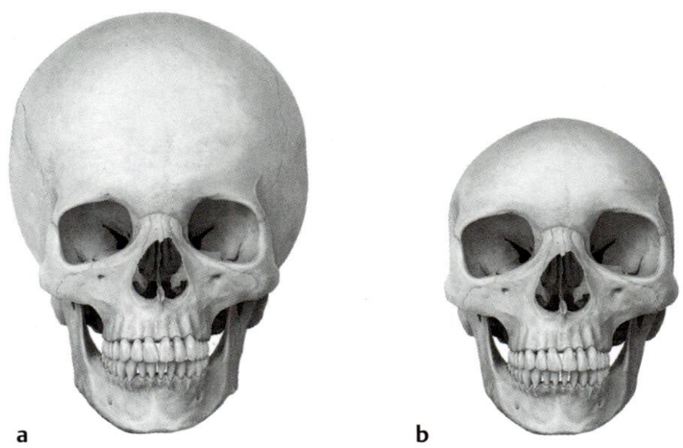

E Hydrocephalus and microcephaly

a Characteristic cranial morphology in *hydrocephalus*. When the brain becomes dilated due to cerebrospinal fluid accumulation *before* the cranial sutures ossify (hydrocephalus, "water on the brain"), the neurocranium will expand while the facial skeleton remains unchanged.
b *Microcephaly* results from premature closure of the cranial sutures. It is characterized by a small neurocranium with relatively large orbits.

F Age at which the principal sutures ossify

Suture	Age at ossification
Frontal suture	Childhood
Sagittal suture	20–30 years of age
Coronal suture	30–40 years of age
Lambdoid suture	40–50 years of age

2.4 Exterior and Interior of the Calvarium

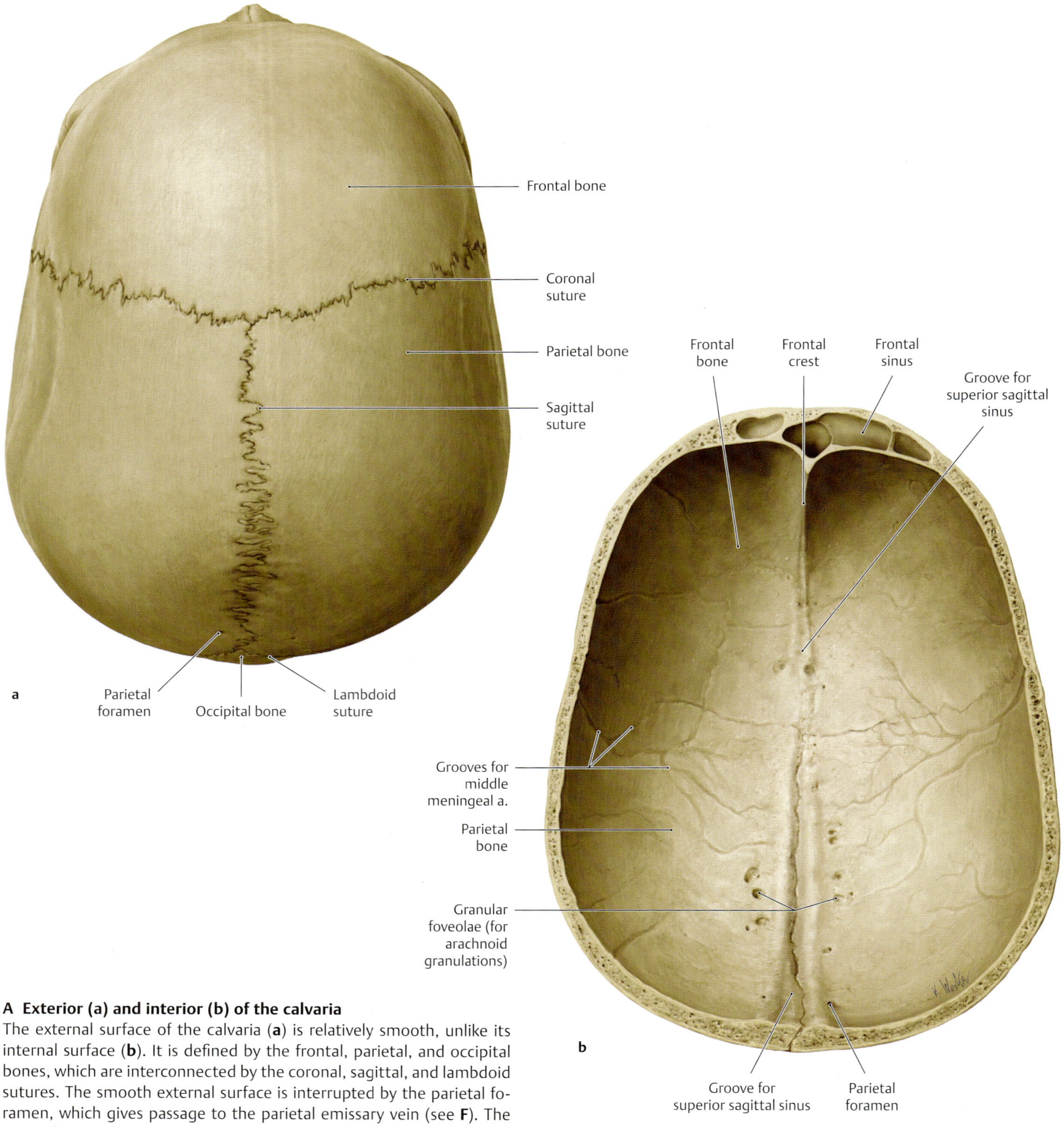

A Exterior (a) and interior (b) of the calvaria
The external surface of the calvaria (**a**) is relatively smooth, unlike its internal surface (**b**). It is defined by the frontal, parietal, and occipital bones, which are interconnected by the coronal, sagittal, and lambdoid sutures. The smooth external surface is interrupted by the parietal foramen, which gives passage to the parietal emissary vein (see **F**). The internal surface of the calvaria also bears a number of pits and grooves:

- The granular foveolae (small pits in the inner surface of the skull caused by saccular protrusions of the arachnoid membrane covering the brain)
- The groove for the superior sagittal sinus (a dural venous sinus of the brain)
- The arterial grooves (which mark the positions of the arterial vessels of the dura mater, such as the middle meningeal artery which supplies most of the dura mater and overlying bone)
- The frontal crest (which gives attachment to the falx cerebri, a sickle-shaped fold of dura mater between the cerebral hemispheres, see p. 308).

The frontal sinus in the frontal bone is also visible in the interior view.

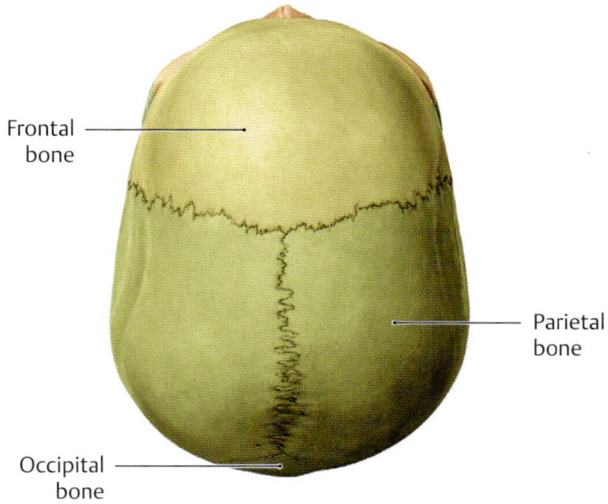

B Exterior of the calvaria viewed from above

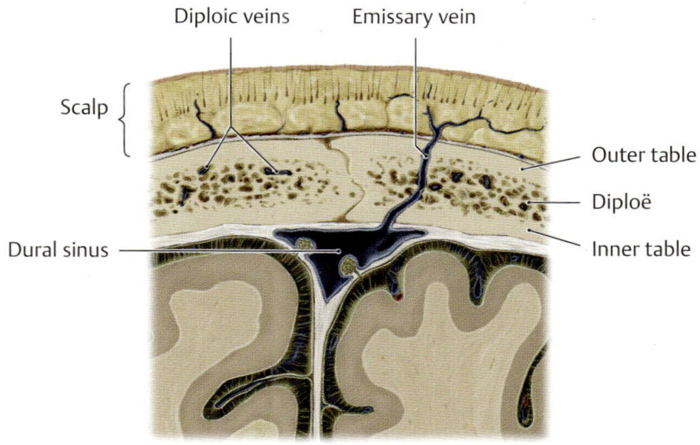

C The scalp and calvaria

Note the three-layered structure of the calvaria, consisting of the outer table, the diploë, and the inner table.

The diploë has a spongy structure and contains red (blood-forming) bone marrow. With a plasmacytoma (malignant transformation of certain white blood cells), many small nests of tumor cells may destroy the surrounding bony trabeculae, and radiographs will demonstrate multiple lucent areas ("punched-out lesions") in the skull. Vessels called *emissary veins* may pass through the calvaria to connect the venous sinuses of the brain with the veins of the scalp (see panels **E** and **F**).

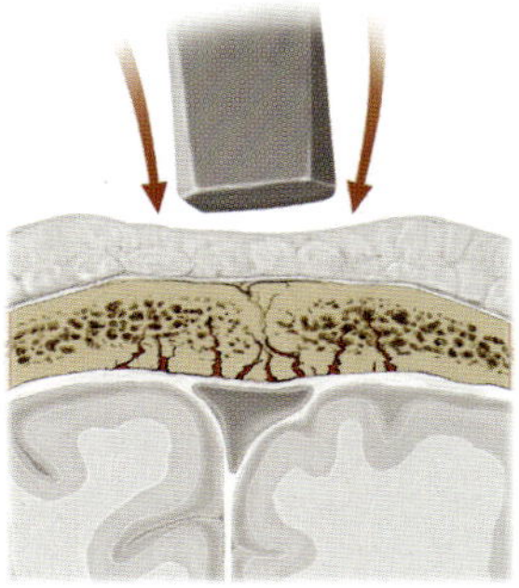

D Sensitivity of the inner table to trauma

The inner table of the calvaria is very sensitive to external trauma and may fracture even when the outer table remains intact (look for corresponding evidence on CT images).

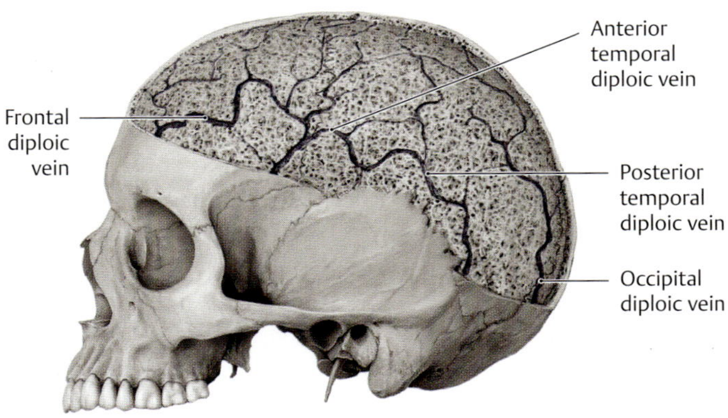

E Diploic veins in the calvaria

The diploic veins are located in the cancellous or spongy tissue of the cranial bones (the diploë) and are visible when the outer table is removed. The diploic veins communicate with the dural venous sinuses and scalp veins by way of the emissary veins, which create a potential route for the spread of infection.

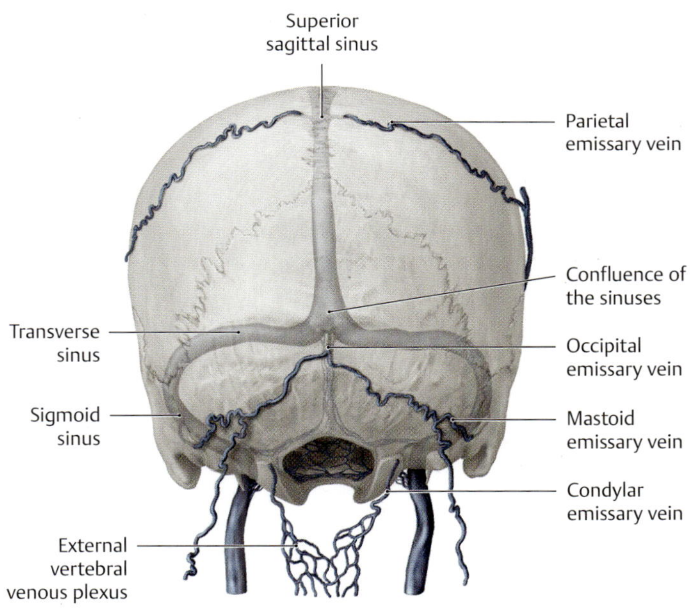

F Emissary veins of the occiput

Emissary veins establish a direct connection between the dural venous sinuses and the extracranial veins. They pass through preformed cranial openings such as the parietal foramen and mastoid foramen. The emissary veins are of clinical interest because they may allow bacteria from the scalp to enter the skull along these veins and infect the dura mater, causing meningitis.

2.5 Base of the Skull, External View

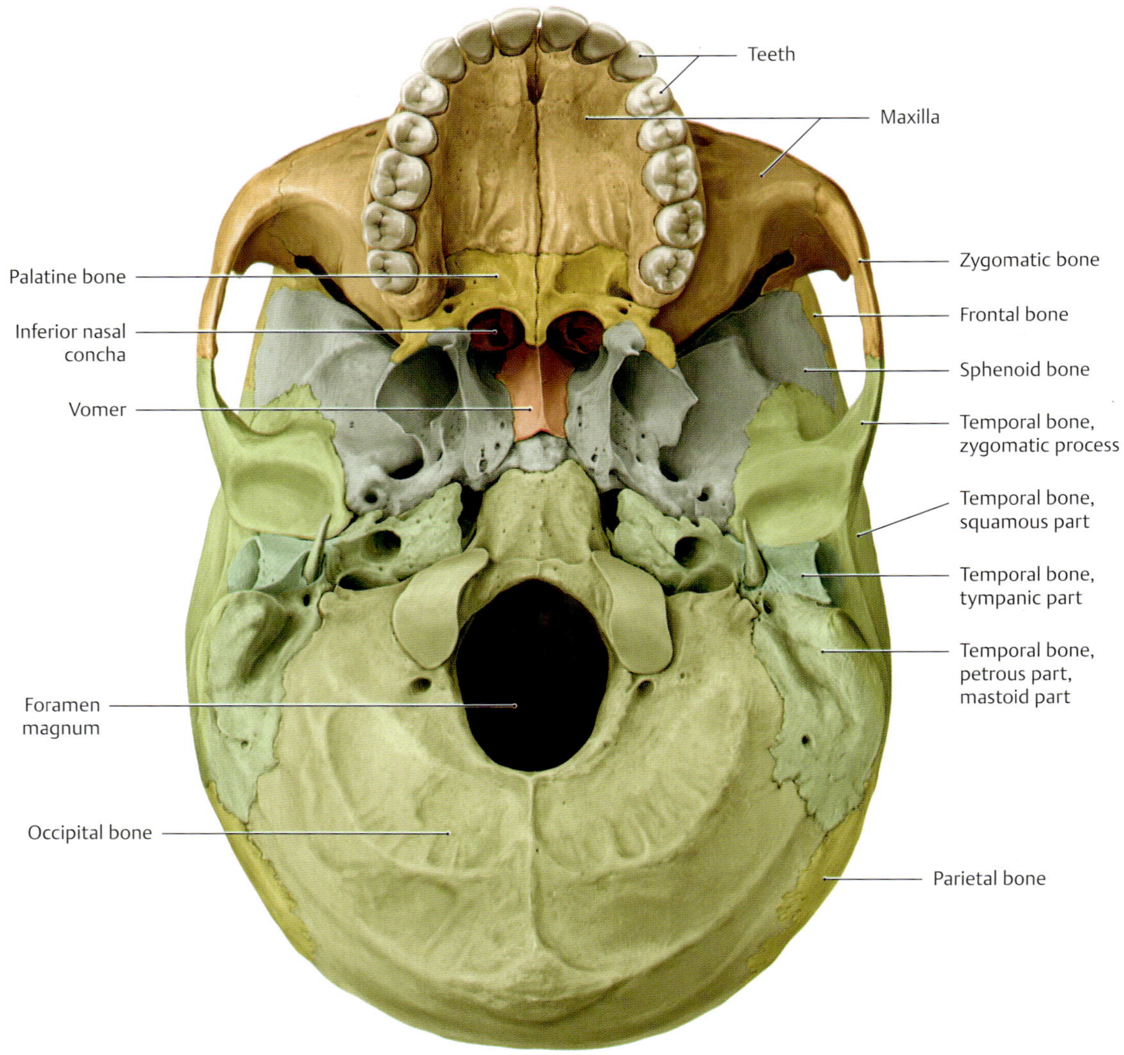

A Bones of the base of the skull
Inferior view. The base of the skull is composed of a mosaic-like assembly of various bones. It is helpful to review the shape and location of these bones before studying further details.

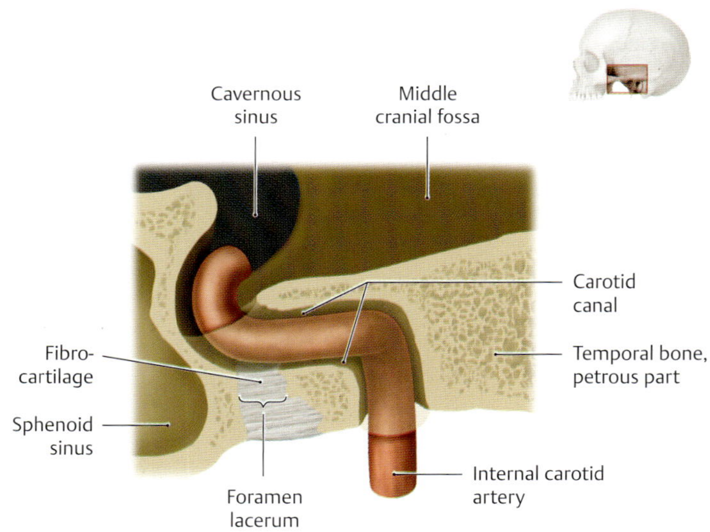

B Relationship of the foramen lacerum to the carotid canal and internal carotid artery
Left lateral view. The foramen lacerum is not a true aperture, being occluded in life by a layer of fibrocartilage; it appears as an opening only in the dried skull. The foramen lacerum is closely related to the carotid canal and to the internal carotid artery that traverses the canal. The greater petrosal nerve and deep petrosal nerve pass through the foramen lacerum (see pp. 127, 131, and 136).

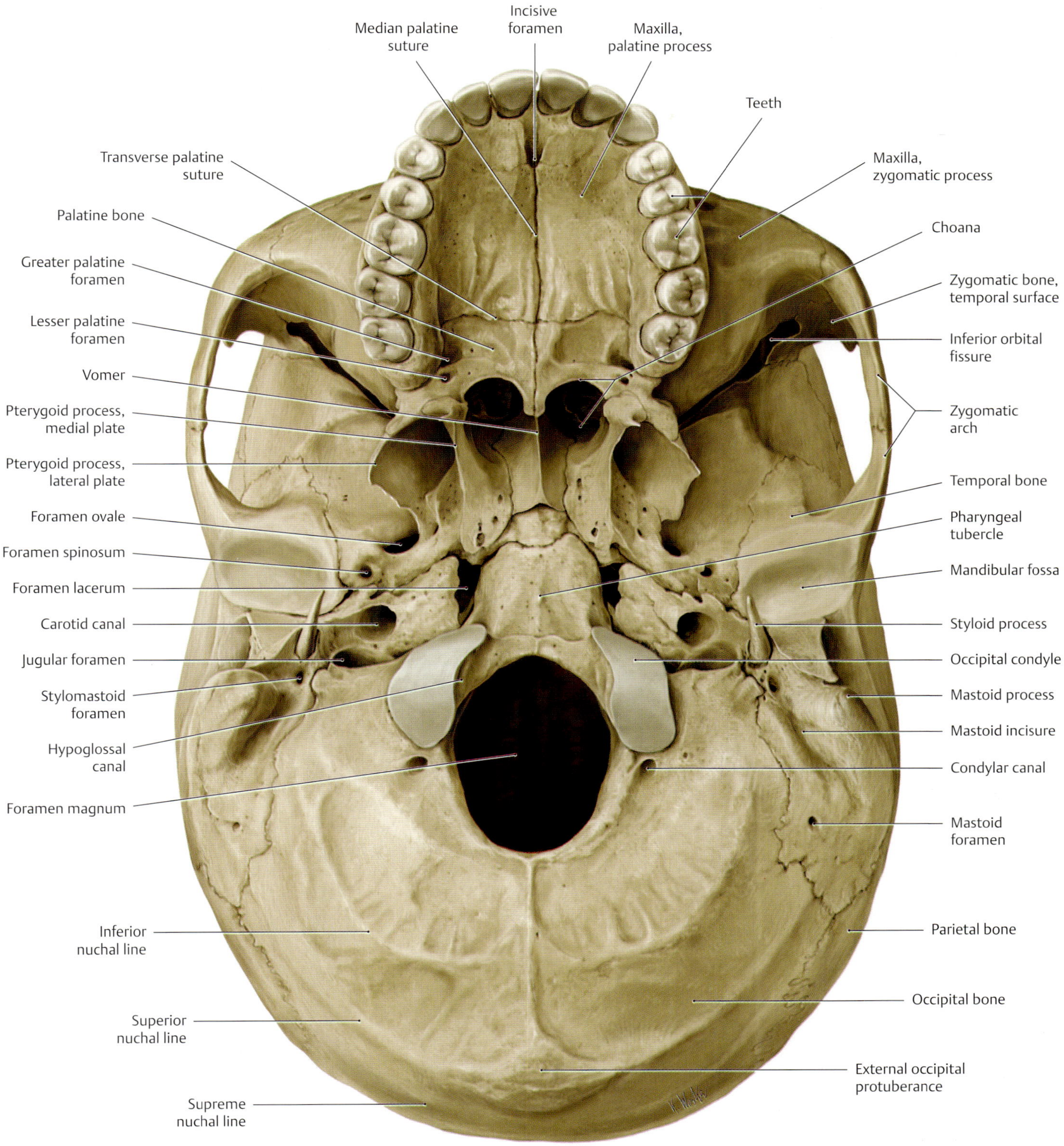

C The basal aspect of the skull

Inferior view. The principal external features of the base of the skull are labeled. Note particularly the openings that transmit nerves and vessels. With abnormalities of bone growth, these openings may remain too small or may become narrowed, compressing the neurovascular structures that pass through them. If the optic canal fails to grow normally, it may compress and damage the optic nerve, resulting in visual field defects. The symptoms associated with these lesions depend on the affected opening. All of the structures depicted here will be considered in more detail in subsequent pages.

2.6 Base of the Skull, Internal View

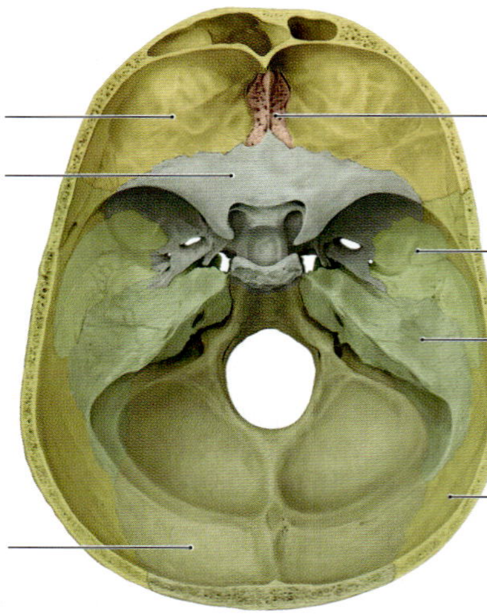

A Bones of the base of the skull, internal view
Different colors are used here to highlight the arrangement of bones in the base of the skull as seen from within the cranium.

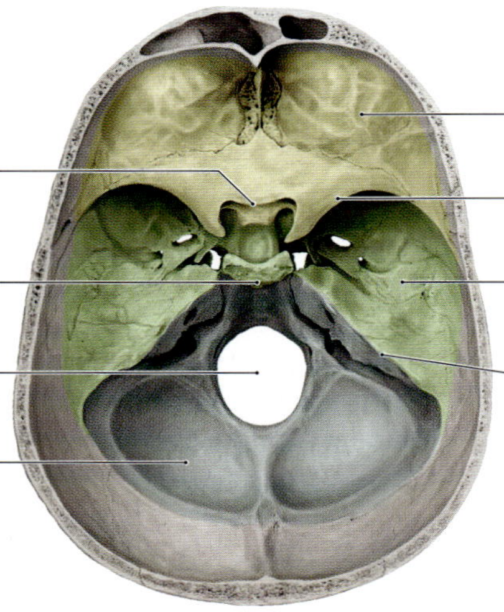

a

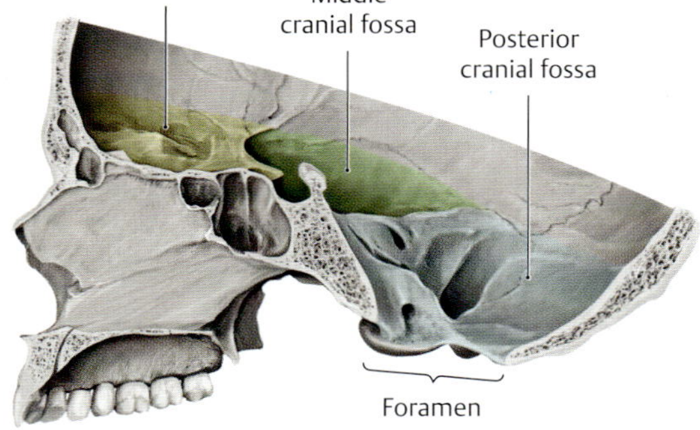

b

B The cranial fossae
a Interior view, **b** midsagittal section. The interior of the skull base is not flat but is deepened to form three successive fossae: the anterior, middle, and posterior cranial fossae. These depressions become progressively deeper in the frontal-to-occipital direction, forming a terraced arrangement that is displayed most clearly in **b**.
The cranial fossae are bounded by the following structures:

- Anterior to middle: the lesser wings of the sphenoid bone and the jugum sphenoidale.
- Middle to posterior: the superior border (ridge) of the petrous part of the temporal bone and the dorsum sellae.

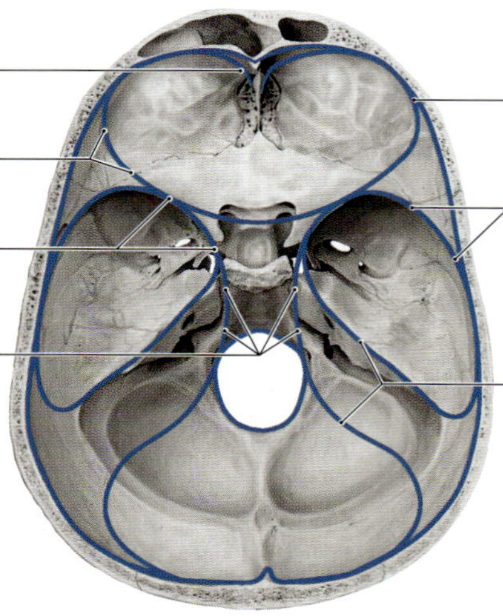

a

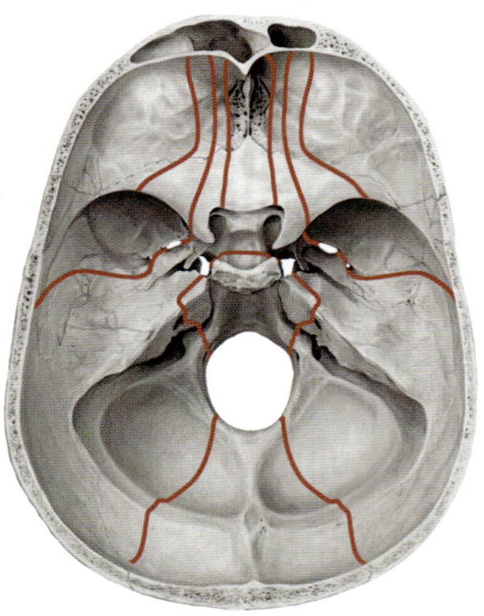

b

C Base of the skull: principal lines of force and common fracture lines
a Principal lines of force, **b** common fracture lines (interior views). In response to masticatory pressures and other mechanical stresses, the bones of the skull base are thickened to form "pillars" along the principal lines of force (compare with the force distribution in the anterior view on p. 15). The intervening areas that are not thickened are sites of predilection for bone fractures, resulting in the typical patterns of basal skull fracture lines shown here. An analogous phenomenon of typical fracture lines is found in the midfacial region (see the anterior views of LeFort fractures on p. 15).

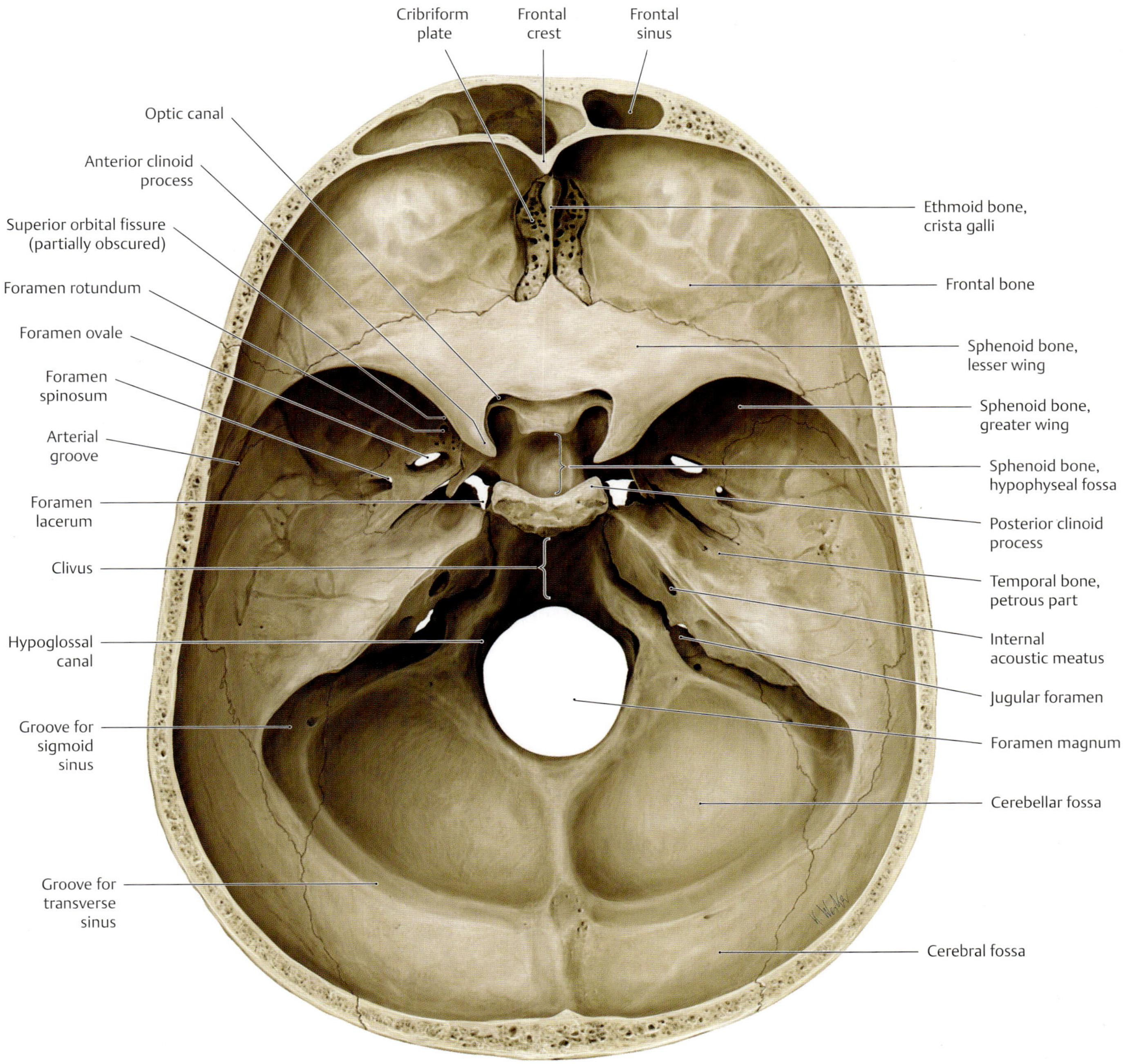

D Interior of the base of the skull

It is interesting to compare the openings in the interior of the base of the skull with the openings visible in the external view (see p. 21). These openings do not always coincide because some neurovascular structures change direction when passing through the bone or pursue a relatively long intraosseous course. An example of this is the internal acoustic meatus, through which the facial nerve, among other structures, passes from the interior of the skull into the petrous part of the temporal bone. Most of its fibers then leave the petrous bone through the stylomastoid foramen, which is visible from the external aspect (see pp. 126, 137, and 151).

In learning the sites where neurovascular structures pass through the base of the skull, it is helpful initially to note whether these sites are located in the anterior, middle, or posterior cranial fossa. The arrangement of the cranial fossae is shown in **B**. The cribriform plate of the ethmoid bone connects the nasal cavity with the anterior cranial fossa and is perforated by numerous foramina for the passage of the olfactory fibers (see p. 182).

Note: Because the bone is so thin in this area, a frontal head injury may easily fracture the cribriform plate and lacerate the dura mater, allowing cerebrospinal fluid to enter the nose. This poses a risk of meningitis, as bacteria from the nonsterile nasal cavity may enter the sterile cerebrospinal fluid.

2.7 Occipital Bone and Ethmoid Bones

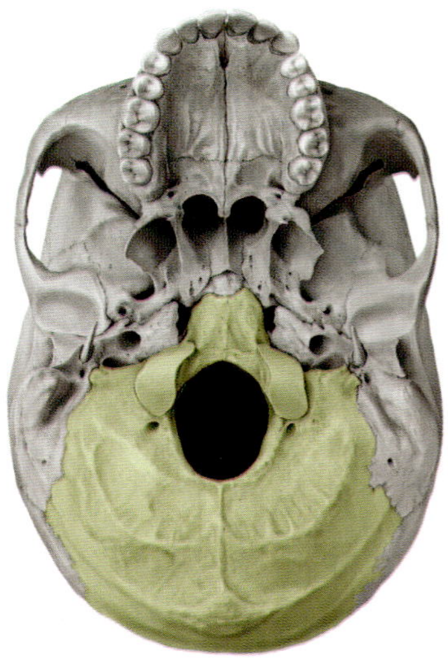

A Integration of the occipital bone into the external base of the skull

Inferior view. Note the relationship of the occipital bone to the adjacent bones.

The occipital bone fuses with the sphenoid bone during puberty to form the "tribasilar bone."

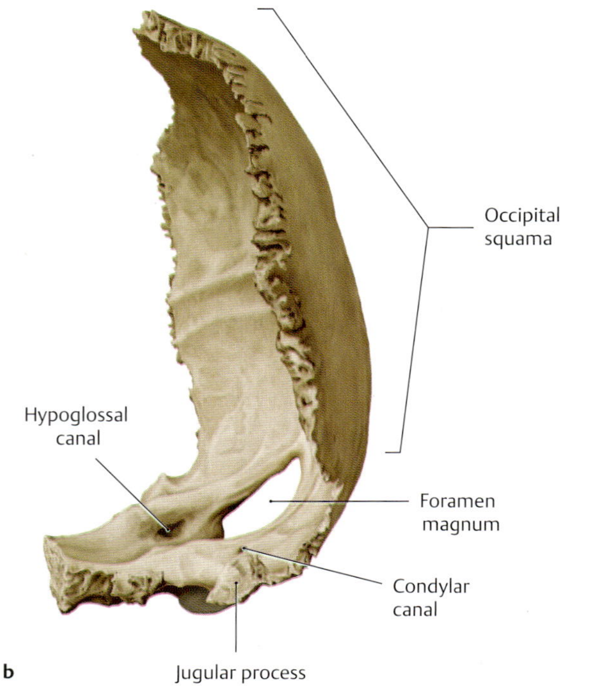

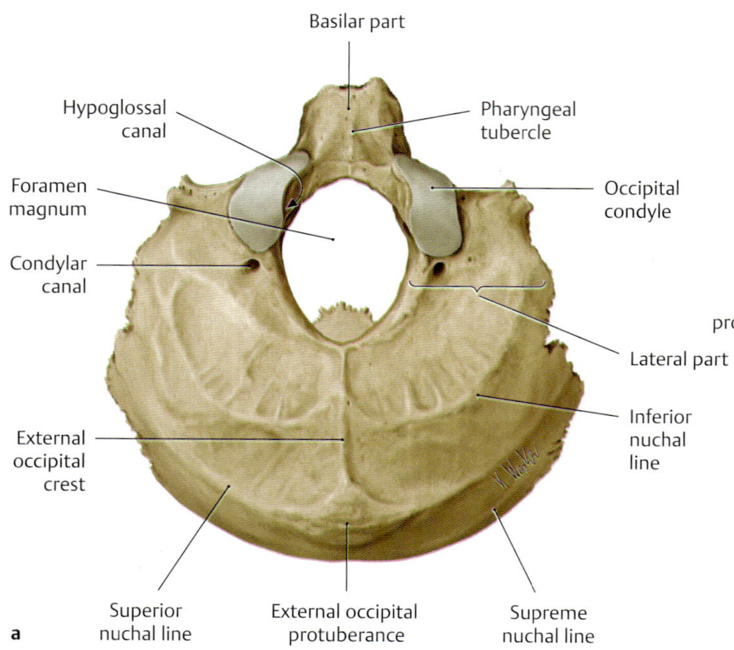

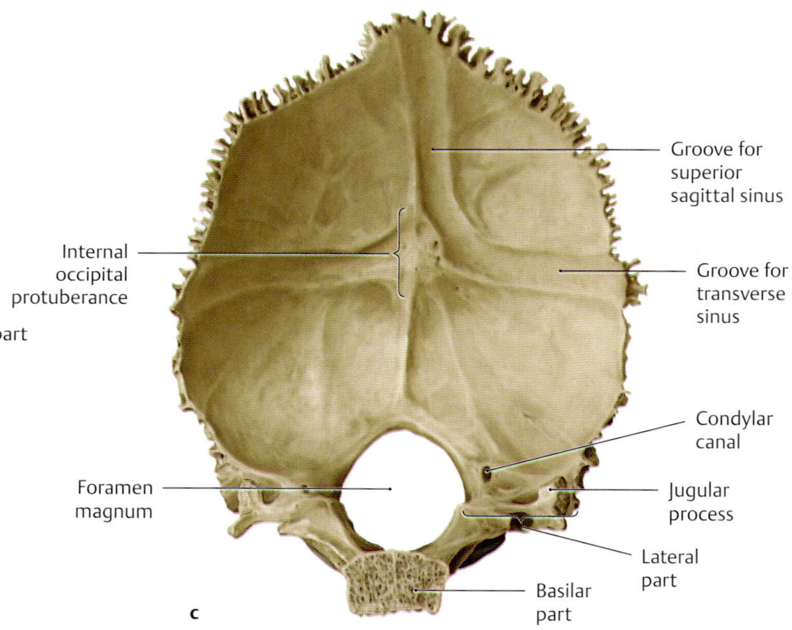

B Isolated occipital bone

a Inferior view. This view shows the basilar part of the occipital bone, whose anterior portion is fused to the sphenoid bone. The condylar canal terminates posterior to the occipital condyles, while the hypoglossal canal passes superior to the occipital condyles. The former contains the emmissary condylar v., which begins in the sigmoid sinus and ends in the external vertebral venous plexus (emissary veins, see p. 19). The latter, in addition to the venous plexus, contains the hypoglossal n. (CN XII). The pharyngeal tubercle gives attachment to the superior pharyngeal constrictor while the external occipital protuberance provides a palpable bony landmark on the occiput.

b Left lateral view. The extent of the occipital squama, which lies above the foramen magnum, is clearly appreciated in this view. The internal openings of the condylar canal and hypoglossal canal are visible along with the jugular process, which forms part of the wall of the jugular foramen (see p. 21). This process is analogous to the transverse process of a vertebra.

c Internal surface. The grooves for the dural venous sinuses of the brain can be identified in this view. The internal occipital protuberance (cruciform eminence) overlies the confluence of the superior sagittal sinus and transverse sinuses. The configuration of the eminence shows that in some cases the sagittal sinus drains predominantly into the left transverse sinus (see p. 384).

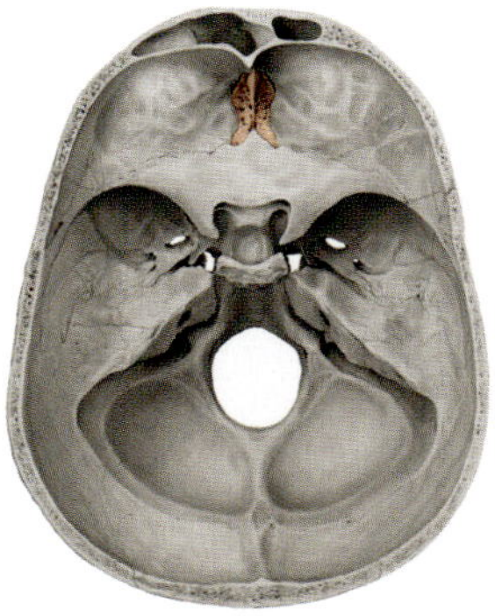

C Integration of the ethmoid bone into the internal base of the skull
Superior view. The upper portion of the ethmoid bone forms part of the anterior cranial fossa, while its lower portions contribute structurally to the nasal cavities. The ethmoid bone is bordered by the frontal and sphenoid bones.

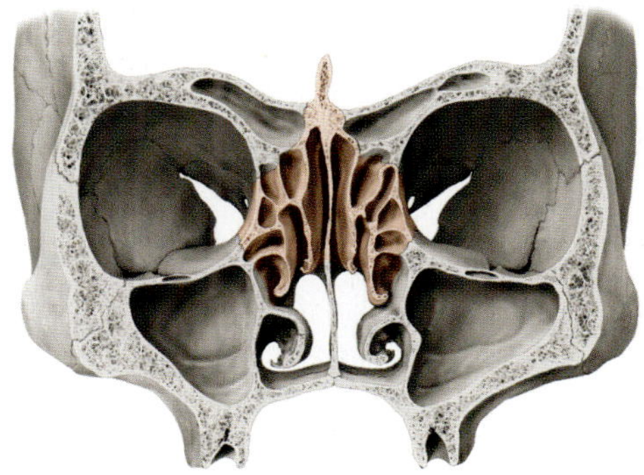

D Integration of the ethmoid bone into the facial skeleton
Anterior view. The ethmoid bone is the central bone of the nose and paranasal sinuses.

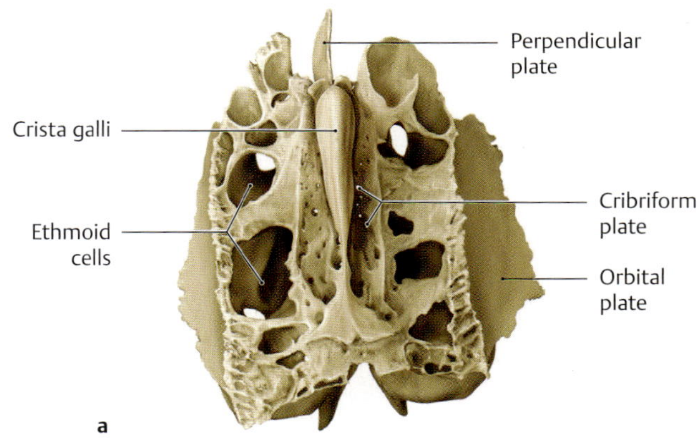

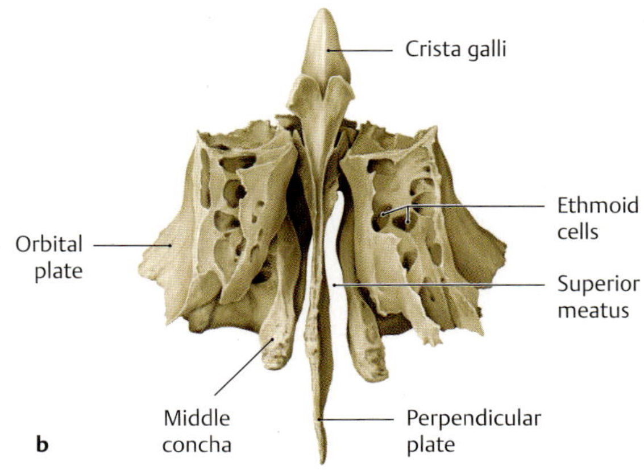

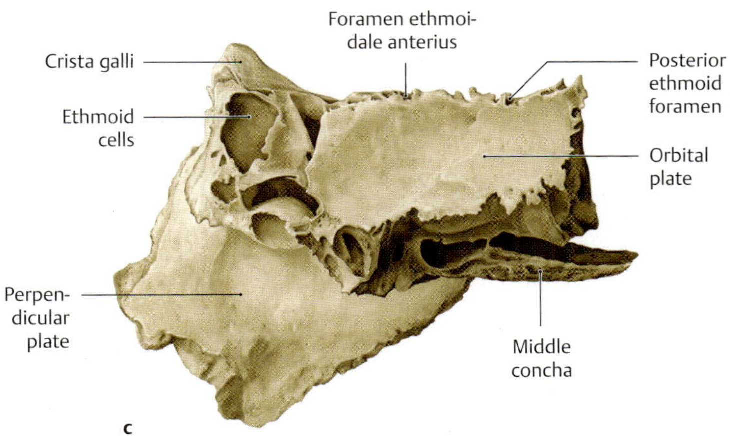

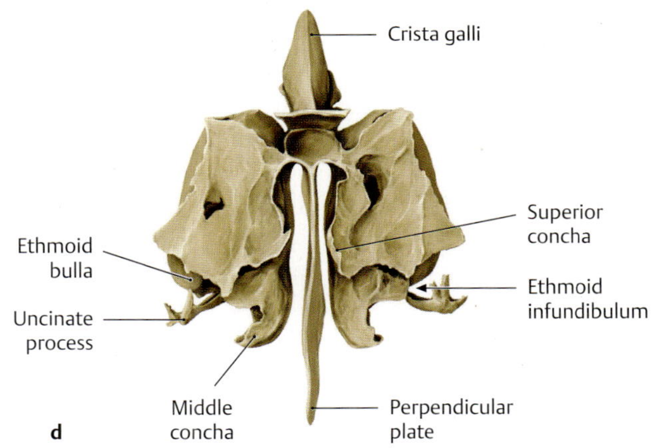

E Isolated ethmoid bone

a Superior view. This view demonstrates the crista galli, which gives attachment to the falx cerebri (see p. 308) and the horizontally directed cribriform plate. The latter is perforated by foramina through which the olfactory fibers pass from the nasal cavity into the anterior cranial fossa. With its numerous foramina, the cribriform plate is a mechanically weak structure that fractures easily in response to trauma. This type of fracture is manifested clinically by cerebrospinal fluid leakage from the nose ("runny nose" in a patient with head injury).

b Anterior view. The anterior view displays the midline structure that separates the two nasal cavities: the perpendicular plate (which resembles the pendulum of a grandfather clock). Note also the middle concha, which is part of the ethmoid bone (of the conchae, only the inferior concha is a separate bone), and the ethmoid cells, which are clustered on both sides of the middle conchae.

c Left lateral view. Viewing the bone from the left side, we observe the perpendicular plate and the opened anterior ethmoid cells. The orbit is separated from the ethmoid cells by a thin sheet of bone called the orbital plate.

d Posterior view. This is the only view that displays the uncinate process, which is almost completely covered by the middle concha when in situ. It partially occludes the entrance to the maxillary sinus, the semilunar hiatus, and it is an important landmark during endoscopic surgery of the maxillary sinus. The narrow depression between the middle concha and uncinate process is called the ethmoid infundibulum. The frontal sinus, maxillary sinus, and anterior ethmoid cells open into this "funnel." The superior concha is located at the posterior end of the ethmoid bone.

2.8 Frontal and Parietal Bones

A Frontal bone
a Anterior view (external surface), **b** inferior view (orbital surface), and **c** posterior view (internal surface).
The **frontal bone** forms the bony base of the anterior calvaria (see p. 14 and 34 for its position in the skull). It develops from two bones that fuse in the midline. The dividing line between the two bones is still detectable in adolescents as the frontal suture; in adults it is usually completely ossified, obliterating the suture. The frontal bone comprises the following parts:

- squama frontalis (the bony base of the forehead),
- two horizontal orbital parts (the greater portion of the bony base of the roof of each orbit), and
- the pars nasalis that lies between them and forms the superior bony part of the nose.

The squama frontalis has external and internal surfaces; the latter forms part of the anterior cranial fossa. It curves to become the temporal surface on both sides.
Clinically important features of the frontal bone include the paired frontal sinuses which are separated by a bony septum and form part of the roof of each orbit. Infections can spread from this site (see **C**). Fractures play a role as well. They usually occur as a result of occupational and traffic accidents involving frontal trauma (for example when the skull hits the windshield in a rear-end collision). The result is a frontobasal or anterior skull base fracture. These fractures are classified after Escher according to the anatomic region involved (see **B**).

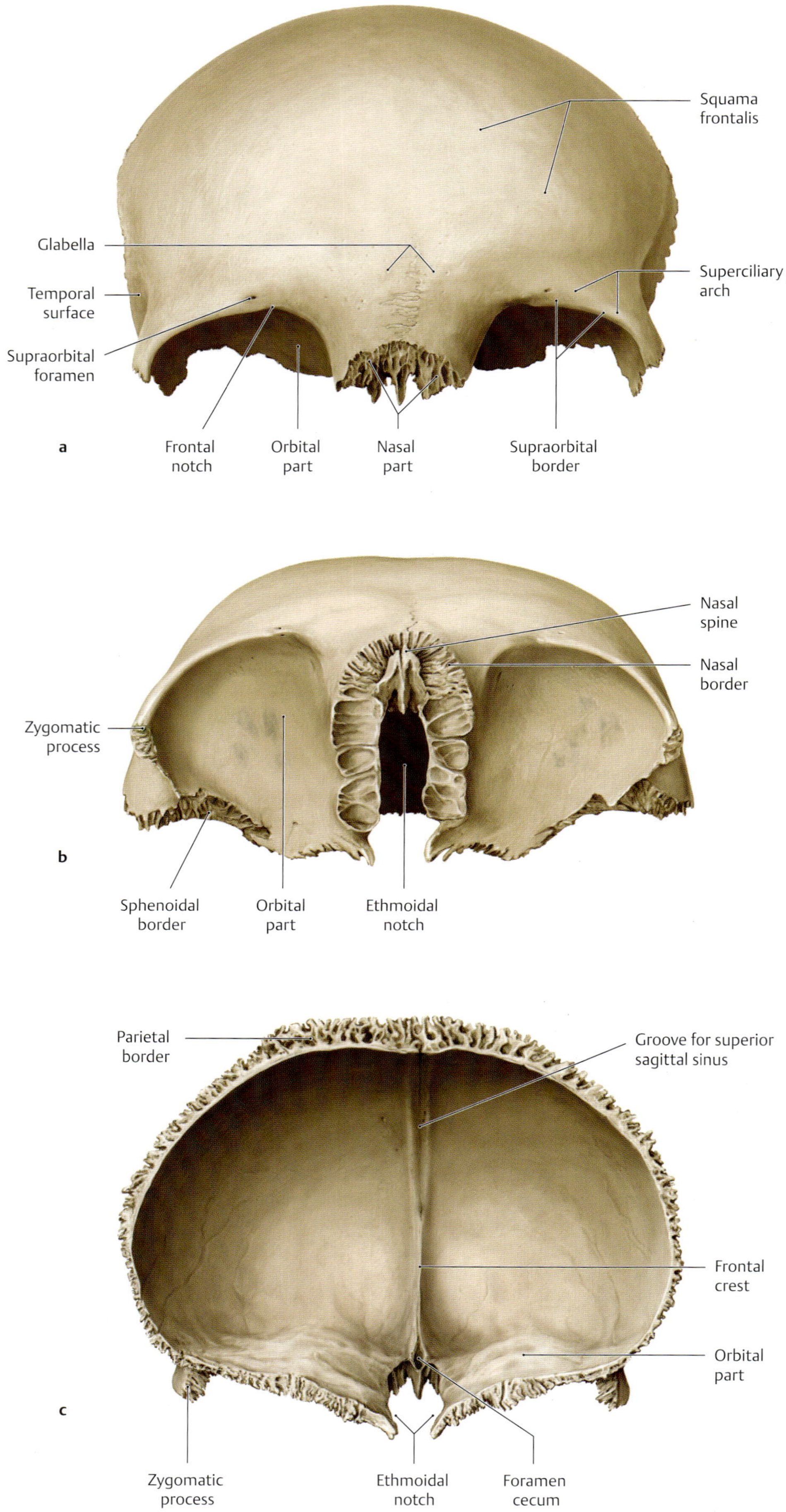

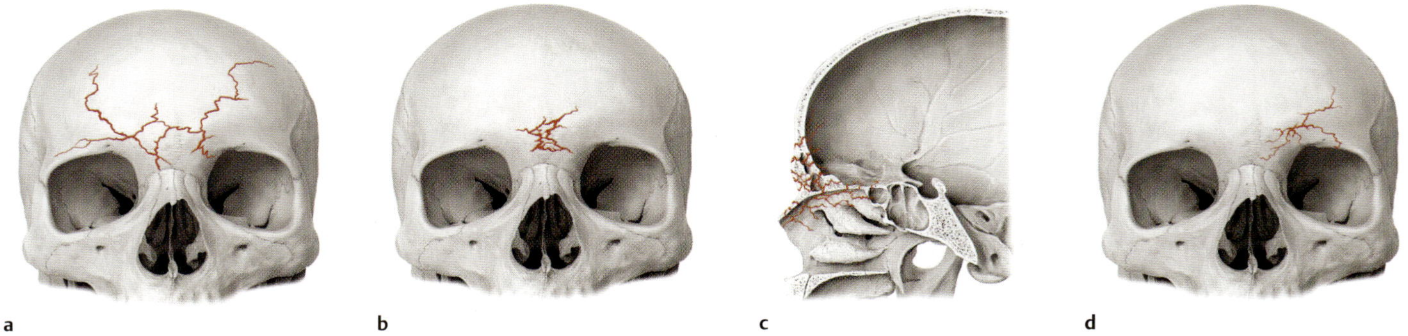

B Classification of frontobasal fractures after Escher

a Type I: High frontobasal fracture: force is directed against the superior portions of the squama frontalis. The fracture lines extend into the frontal sinuses from above.

b Type II: Middle frontobasal fracture: Force directed against the forehead and base of the nose leads to an impression fracture of the frontal sinus, the ethmoid bone, and in applicable cases the sphenoid sinus as well. When the dura mater is torn, cerebrospinal fluid flows out through the nose (nasal liquorrhea; risk of retrograde bacterial infection with meningitis).

c Type III: Deep frontobasal fracture: central anterior trauma. The midface is avulsed off the skull base, merging into vertical or transverse midface fractures (Le Fort III, see p. 15).

d Type IV: Lateral orbital fractures: These result from anterolateral incident force. The frontal sinus and orbital roof are involved.

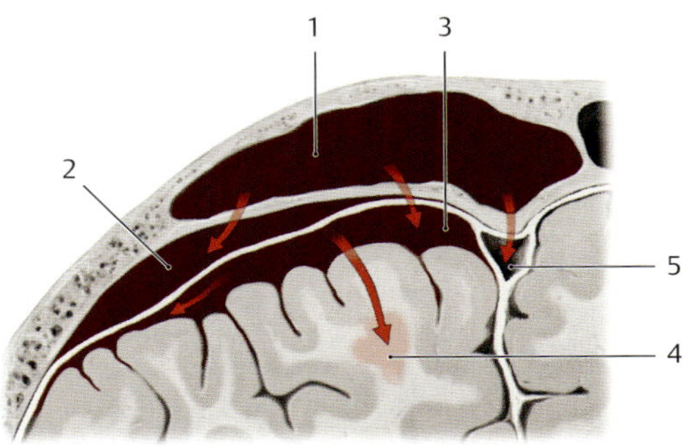

C Anatomic basis of complications involving bacterial frontal sinus infection.

Superior view of the frontal bone (cut away). The close proximity of the frontal sinus (as a part of the frontal bone) to the brain means that infections of the frontal sinus can easily spread to vital structures. The frontal sinus itself can fill with pus (empyema; 1). The pus can break through the bone to the dura mater (epidural abscess; 2). Penetration of the dura mater results in meningitis (3). If this infection enters the brain, it will lead to formation of an abscess (4). Spread of the infection to the superior sagittal sinus leads to sagittal sinus thrombosis (5).

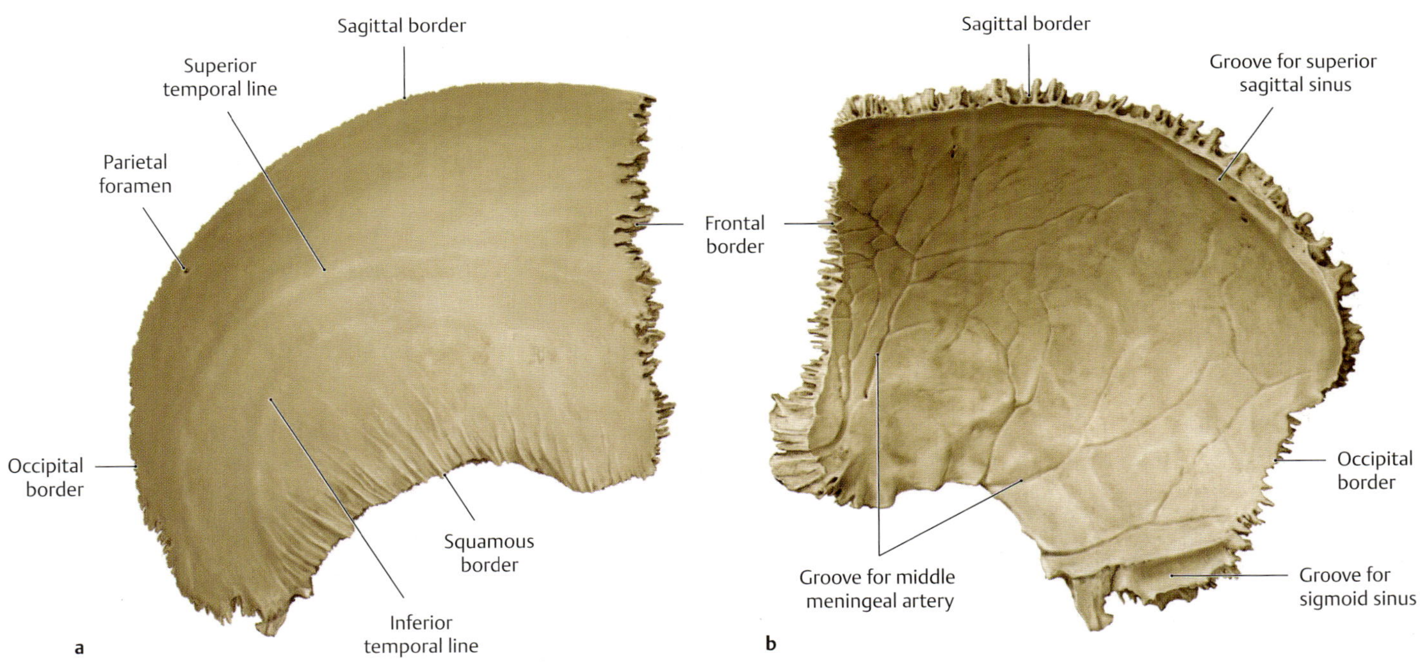

D Parietal bone

a Right parietal bone, lateral view (external surface); **b** right parietal bone, medial view (internal surface).

The two parietal bones form the middle portion of the calvaria with its highest portion, the apex. The parietal bone is divided into an external surface and an internal surface. The groove for the middle meningeal artery is visible on the internal surface. The medial meningeal artery plays an important role in epidural hematomas (see p. 390).

2.9 Temporal Bone

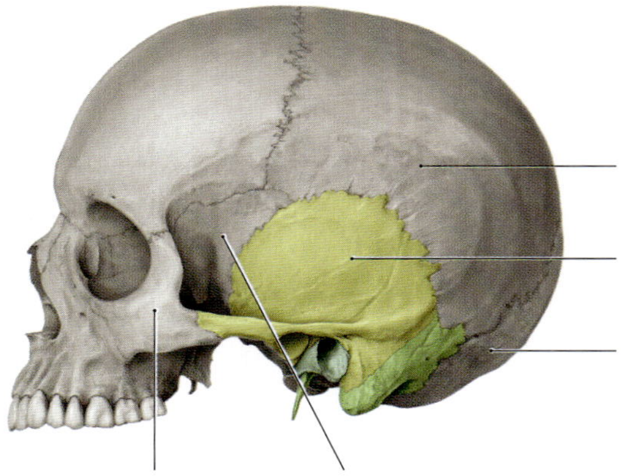

A Position of the temporal bone in the skull
Left lateral view. The temporal bone is a major component of the base of the skull. It forms the bony housing for the auditory and vestibular apparatus and bears the articular fossa of the temporomandibular joint.

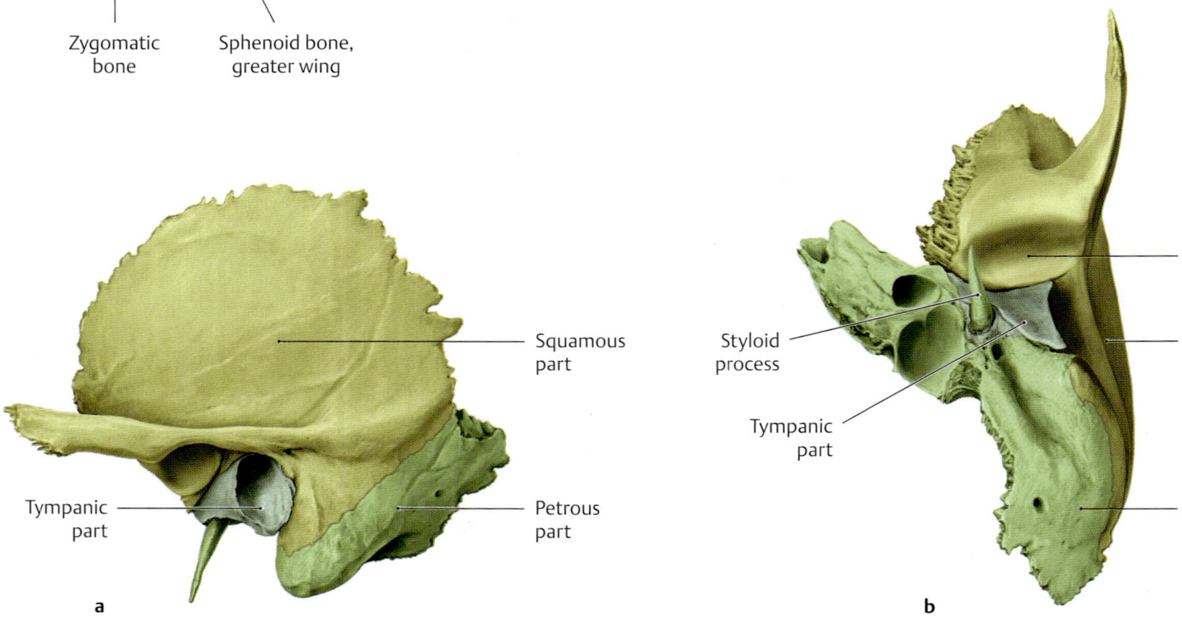

B Ossification centers of the left temporal bone
a Left lateral view; **b** inferior view.
The temporal bone develops from three centers that fuse to form a single bone:

- The squamous part, or temporal squama (light green), bears the articular fossa of the temporomandibular joint (mandibular fossa).
- The petrous part, or petrous bone (pale green), contains the auditory and vestibular apparatus.
- The tympanic part (darker green) forms large portions of the external auditory canal.

Note: The styloid process appears to belong to the tympanic part of the temporal bone because of its location. Developmentally, however, it is part of the petrous bone.

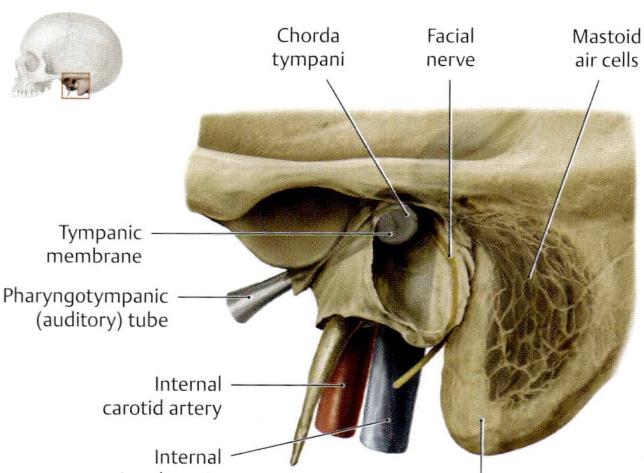

C Projection of clinically important structures onto the left temporal bone
The tympanic membrane is shown translucent in this lateral view. Because the petrous bone contains the middle and inner ear and the tympanic membrane, a knowledge of its anatomy is of key importance in otological surgery. The internal surface of the petrous bone has openings (see **D**) for the passage of the facial nerve, internal carotid artery, and internal jugular vein. A small nerve, the chorda tympani, passes through the tympanic cavity, and lies medial to the tympanic membrane. The chorda tympani arises from the facial nerve, which is susceptible to injury during surgical procedures (cf. **A**, p. 126). The mastoid process of the petrous bone forms air-filled chambers, the mastoid cells, that vary greatly in size. Because these chambers communicate with the middle ear, which in turn communicates with the nasopharynx via the pharyngotympanic (auditory) tube (also called eustachian tube) bacteria in the nasopharynx may pass up the pharyngotympanic tube and gain access to the middle ear. From there they may pass to the mastoid air cells and finally enter the cranial cavity, causing meningitis.

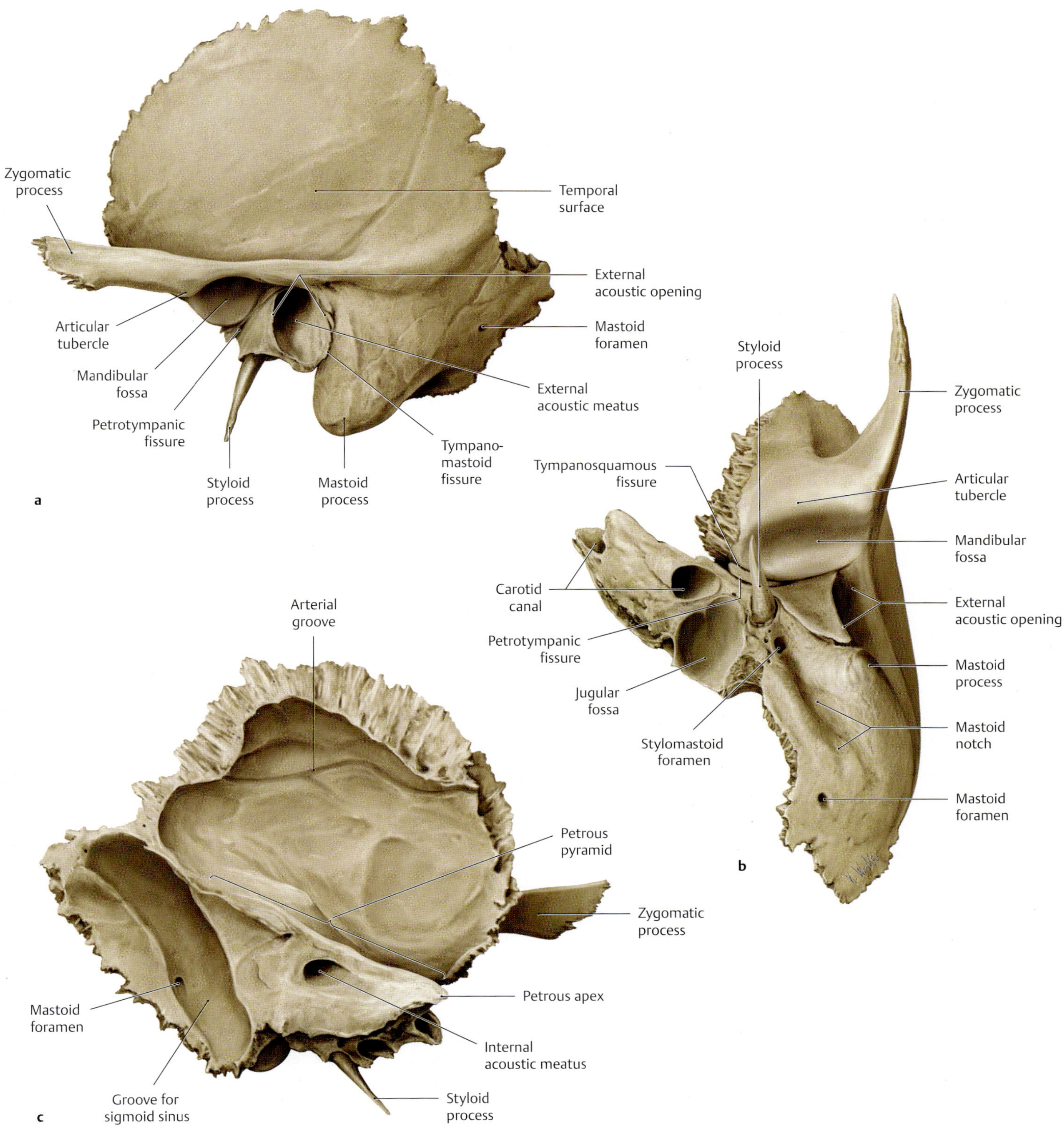

D Left temporal bone

a Lateral view. The principal structures of the temporal bone are labeled in the diagram. An emissary vein (see p. 19 for the emissary veins) passes through the mastoid foramen (external orifice shown in **a**, internal orifice in **c**). The mastoid process develops gradually in life due to traction from the sternocleidomastoid muscle and is pneumatized from the inside (see **C**).

b Inferior view. The shallow articular fossa of the temporomandibular joint (the mandibular fossa) is clearly seen from the inferior view. The facial nerve emerges from the base of the skull through the stylomastoid foramen. The initial part of the internal jugular vein is adherent to the jugular fossa, and the internal carotid artery passes through the carotid canal to enter the skull.

c Medial view. This view displays the internal orifice of the mastoid foramen and the internal acoustic meatus. The facial nerve and vestibulocochlear nerve are among the structures that pass through the internal meatus to enter the petrous bone. The part of the petrous bone shown here is also called the *petrous pyramid*, whose apex (often called the "petrous apex") lies on the interior of the base of the skull.

2.10 Maxilla

A Position of the two maxillae in the skull
Frontal view. The structure of the two maxillae largely determines the shape of the face. They support the superior row of teeth and transfer the pressure of chewing via the frontal process and zygomatic arches to the cranium. In their central position they form part of the orbits (see p. 36) and the wall of the nasal cavity (see p. 40) as well as part of the palate (see p. 44 f). The maxillary sinus in the maxilla is an important paranasal sinus (see p. 41 and 184).

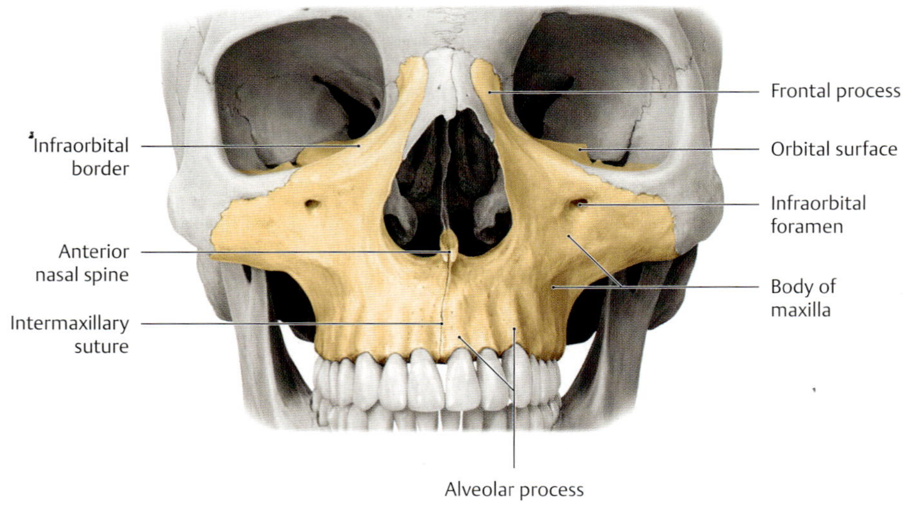

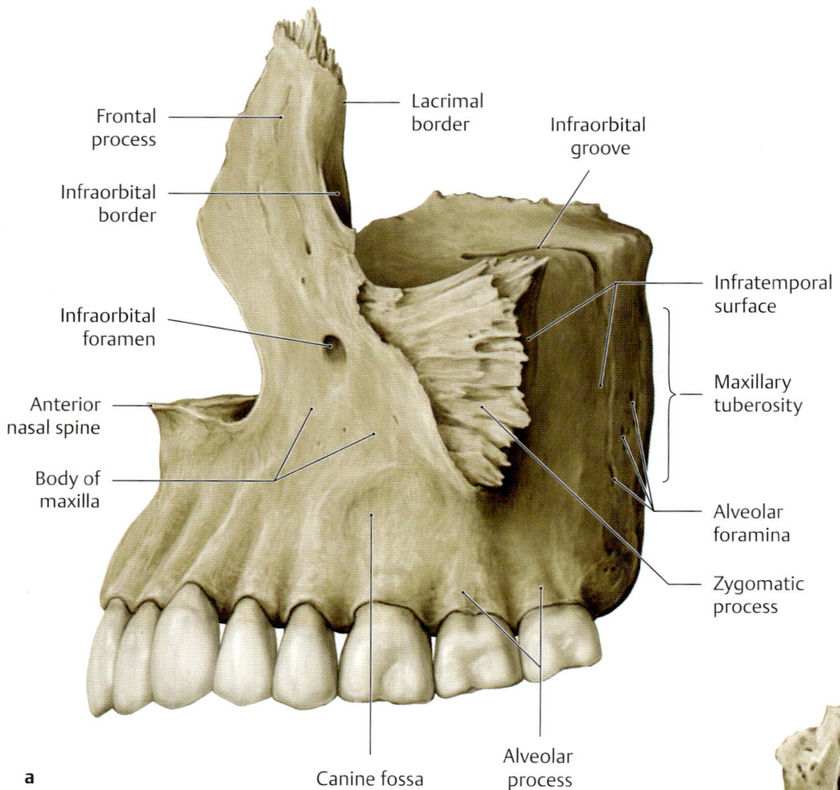

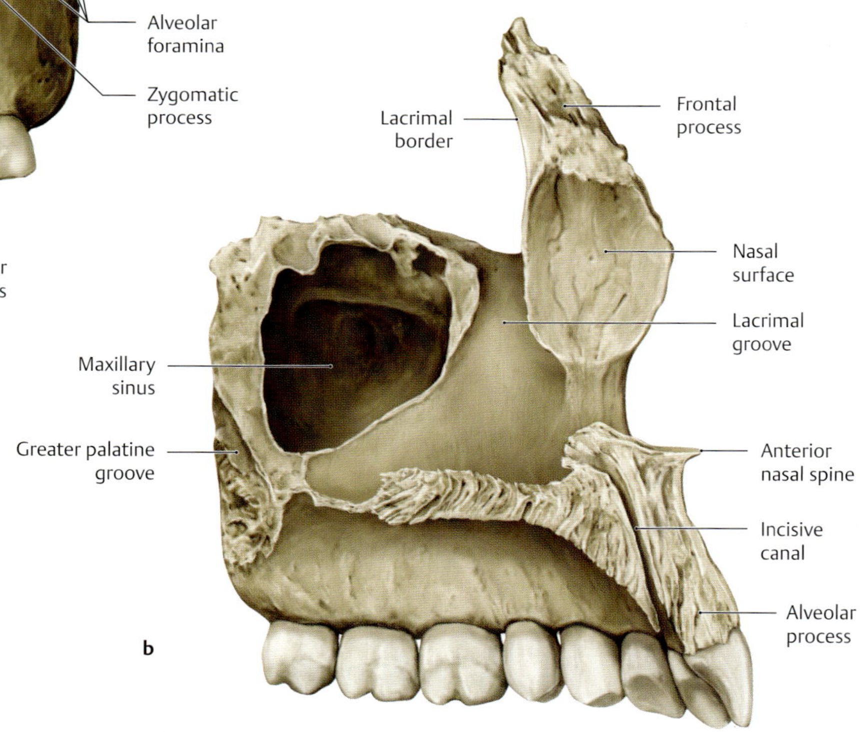

B Isolated maxilla
Lateral view (**a**) and medial view (**b**) with the maxillary sinus opened.

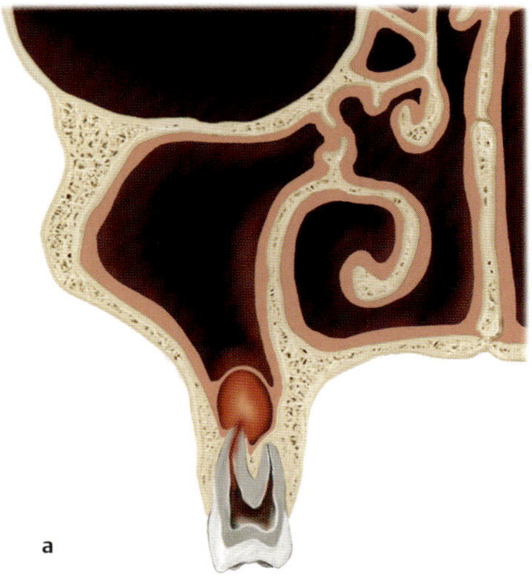

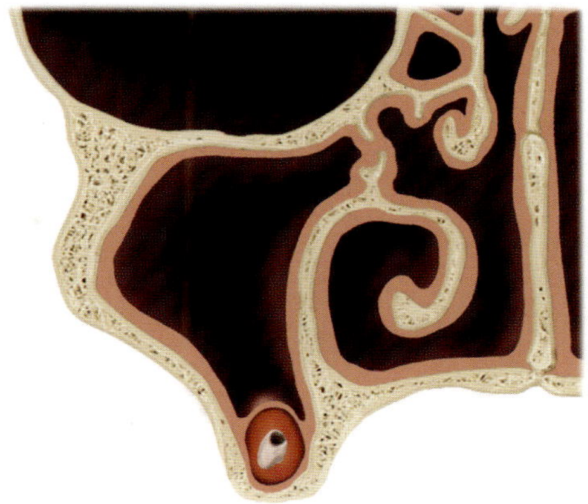

C Odontogenic cysts in the maxilla
Anterior view of a right maxillary sinus. The roots of the superior teeth extend into the maxillary sinus. This anatomic relationship is clinically important as pain referred to the maxillary sinus can be caused by teeth. Conversely, inflammation in the maxillary sinus can spread to the teeth of the upper jaw.

a Radicular cysts develop from the tip of the root of a tooth. Chronic inflammation in the root of the tooth then leads to development of a cyst in the maxillary sinus.

b Follicular cysts occur as a result of expansion of the dental follicle in the coronal region of a tooth that is prevented from erupting (such as a wisdom tooth).

Thus, clinical evaluation of an inflammation of the maxillary sinus must always consider possible causes in the teeth. Because of this, disorders of the maxillary sinus require close cooperation between ear, nose, and throat specialists and dentists.

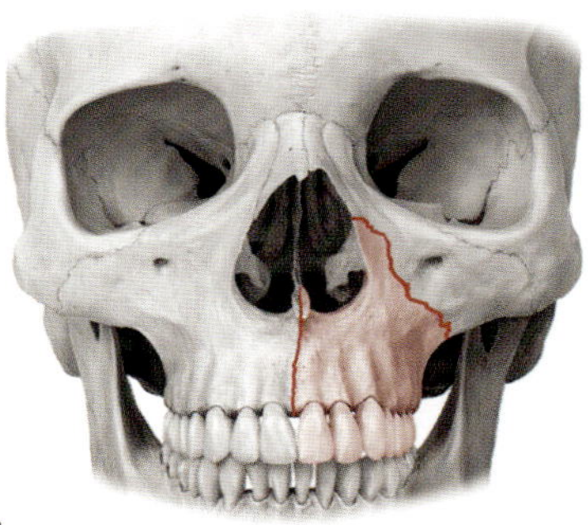

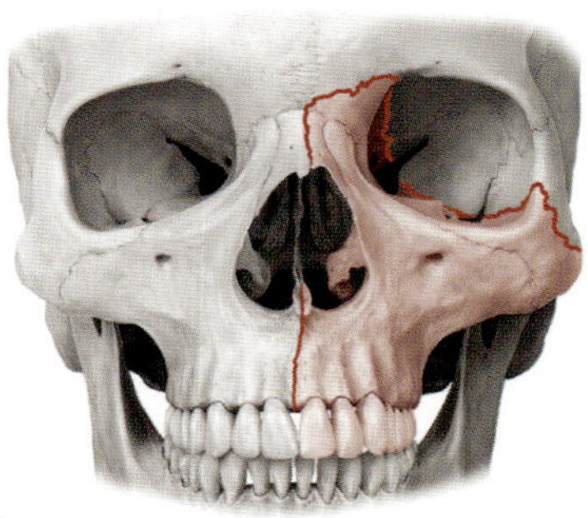

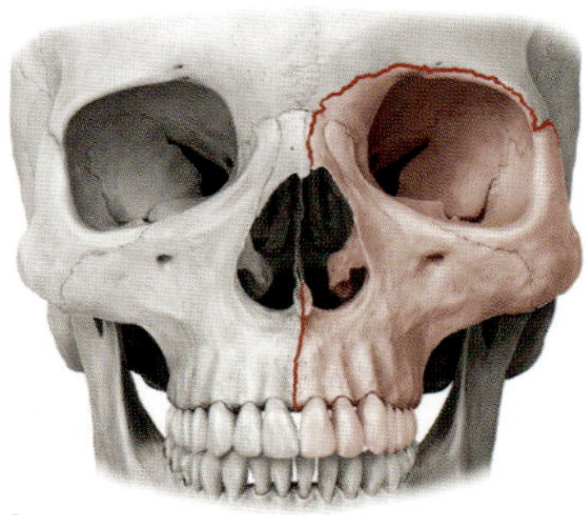

D Maxillary resections
Tumors in the maxillary sinus can be removed surgically. The position and extent of the tumor determine how radical the operation will be. The following procedures are differentiated: a partial resection of the maxilla (**a**), a total resection (**b**), and a total resection combined with removal of the orbit and its contents (orbital exenteration) (**c**).

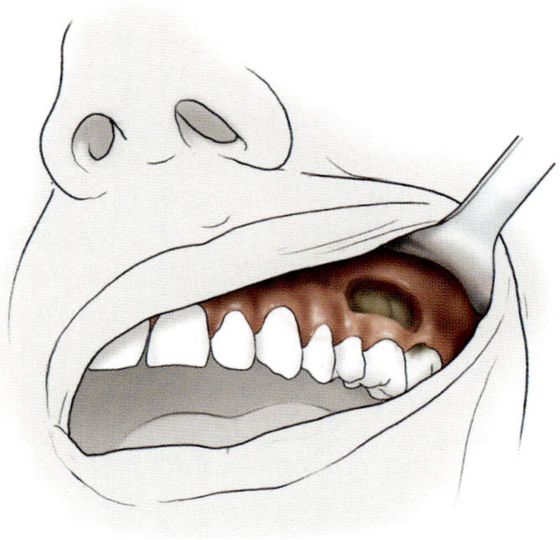

E Surgical approach to the maxillary sinus
An approach through the oral vestibule is often chosen for surgical removal of a tumor. The upper lip is reflected with a retractor and the anterior wall of the maxillary sinus is removed. This exposes the maxillary sinus. Where indicated, this procedure can be expanded into adjacent regions including the ethmoid bone, orbit, and sphenoid sinus. In chronic sinusitis, an endonasal approach is chosen (see **Ed**, p. 25 and **F**, p. 43).

2.11 Zygomatic, Nasal, Vomer, and Palatine Bones

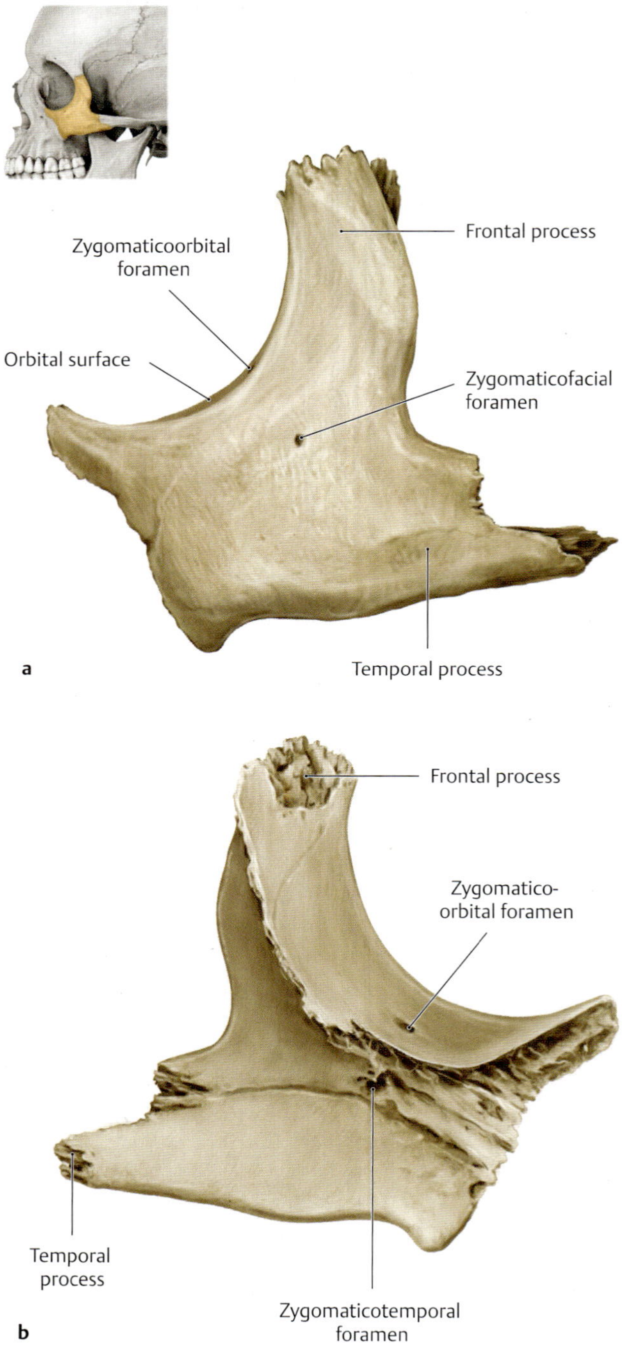

A Zygomatic bone

a Left lateral view (lateral surface) and **b** medial view (temporal surface).

The zygomatic bone forms a bridge between the lateral wall of the skull and the facial bones. It is the bony base of the cheek and as a result it often determines the shape of the face in slender persons. The zygomatic bone has a cheek surface, lateral surface, and orbital and temporal surfaces.

The zygomatico-orbital foramen on the orbital surface represents the inlet of the zygomatic canal. It splits into two canals within the zygomatic bone which terminate at the zygomaticofacial and zygomaticotemporal foramen. The zygomatic branch of the maxillary nerve enters the zygomatic canal, where it splits and courses through the two canals.

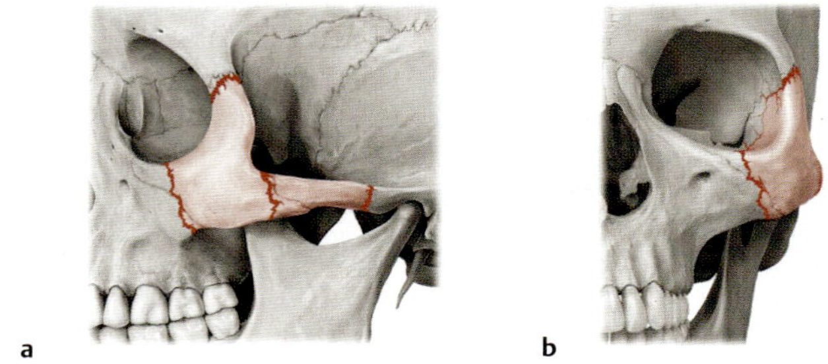

B Fractures of the zygomatic bone

Lateral view (**a**) and frontal view (**b**).

Fractures of the zygomatic bone are relatively common in blunt trauma of the lateral midface. Often the bone breaks at all three junctions with its two adjacent bones. Zygomatic fractures are occasionally obscured by soft-tissue swelling. Therefore, one should always determine whether a zygomatic fracture is present after blunt trauma. This is done by comparing both sides (shape of cheek, motility of the eyeball) and testing for sensory deficits (the zygomatic nerve, which courses through a bony canal, may be injured as well).

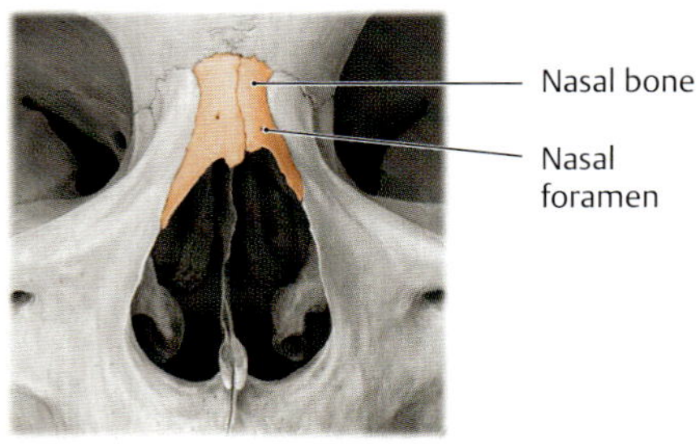

C Nasal bone

The two nasal bones form the bony base of the bridge of the nose. Their superior borders articulate with the frontal bone, their lateral borders with the maxilla. The inferior border is part of the anterior nasal aperture (see p. 14). Fractures of the nasal bone are common and often require reduction.

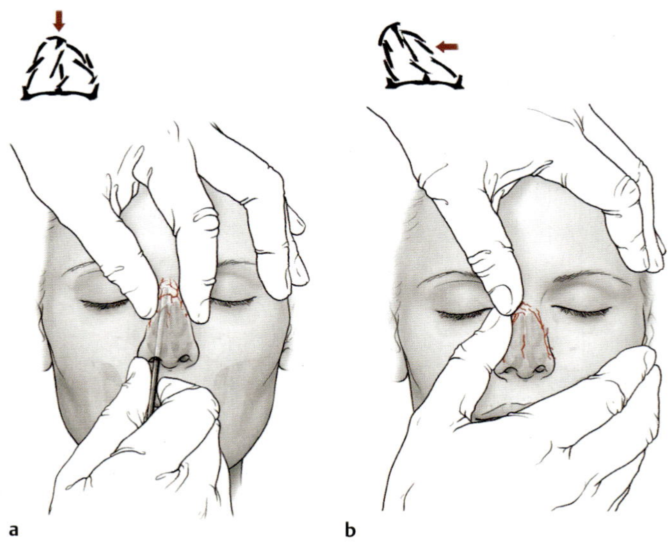

D Principle of the reduction of nasal fractures

In frontal trauma the reduction is performed internally with a retractor (**a**); in lateral trauma external manual reduction is performed (**b**).

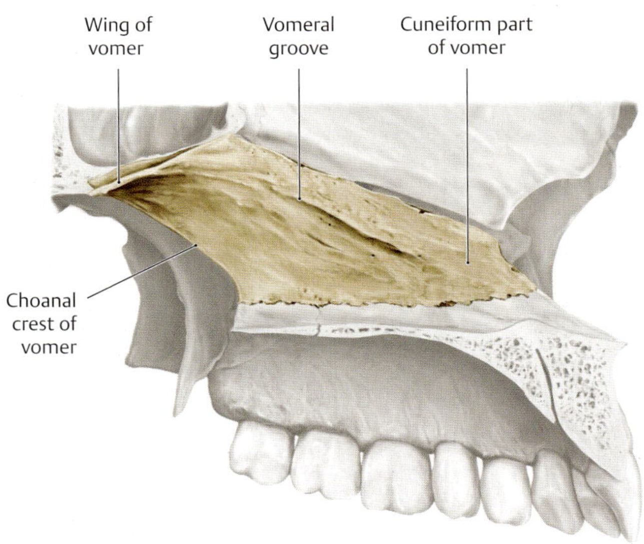

E Vomer bone
Lateral view. The vomer bone and the perpendicular plate of the ethmoid bone together form the bony base of the nasal septum (see p. 14). Along its superior border are two wings (alae vomeris) that form the junction with the body of the sphenoid bone. As a midline structure, it helps to separate the two posterior nasal cavities (choanae; see p. 44 and 185).

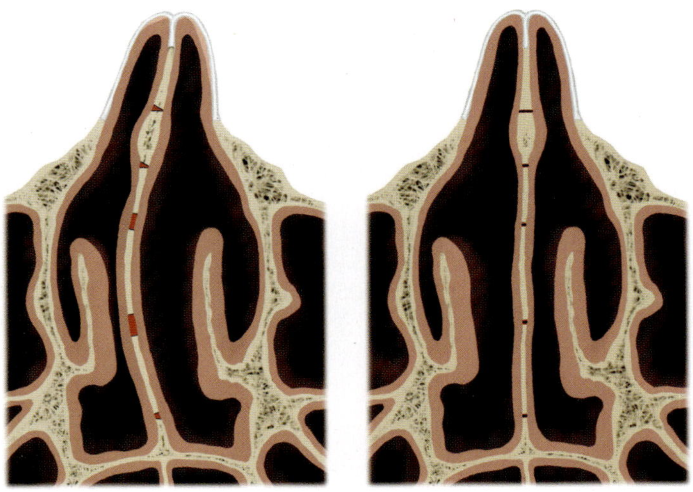

F Correction of the nasal septum
Superior view. Curved nasal septa are a common cause of impaired nasal breathing. Surgical correction can involve removing the nasal septum, straightening it, and reimplanting it.

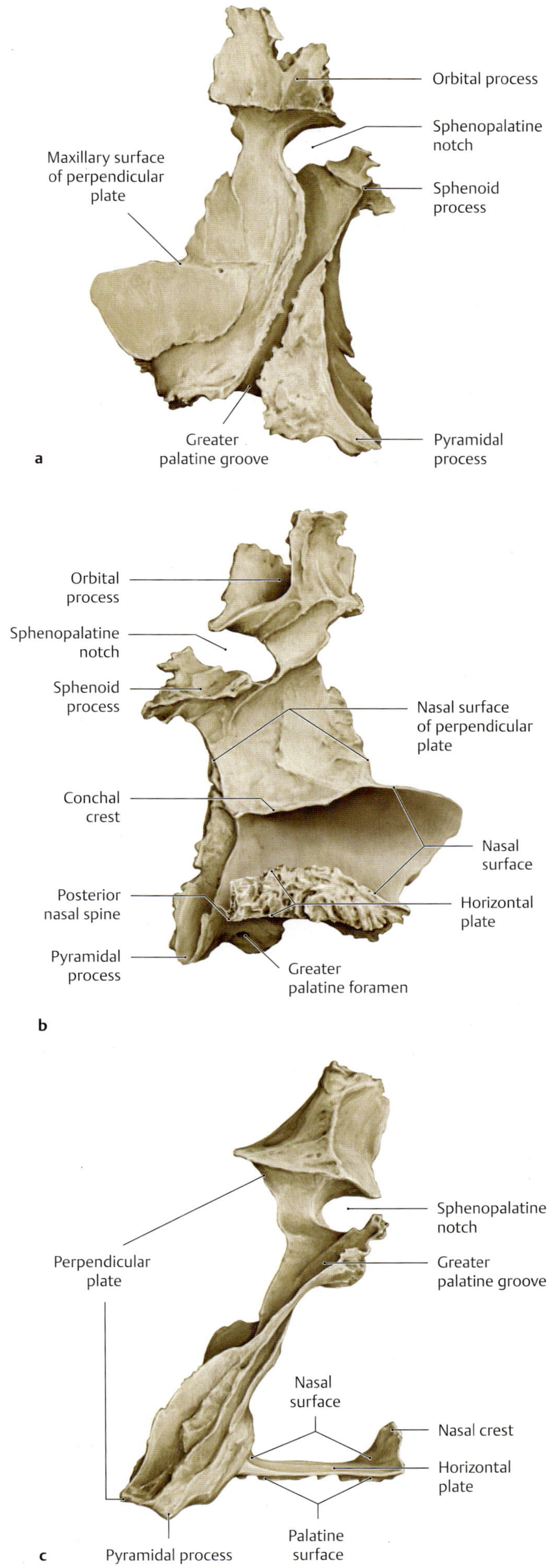

G Palatine bone
a Lateral view of palatine bone, **b** medial view, and **c** posterior view.
The palatine bone consists of a horizontal and a perpendicular plate. The **horizontal plate** is the posterior border of the hard palate (see p. 41); the **perpendicular plate** is the portion of the lateral nasal cavity that lies in front of the pterygoid process. The palatine bone supplements the occipital aspect of the maxilla and with this bone separates the oral cavity from the nasal cavity.

2.12 Sphenoid Bone

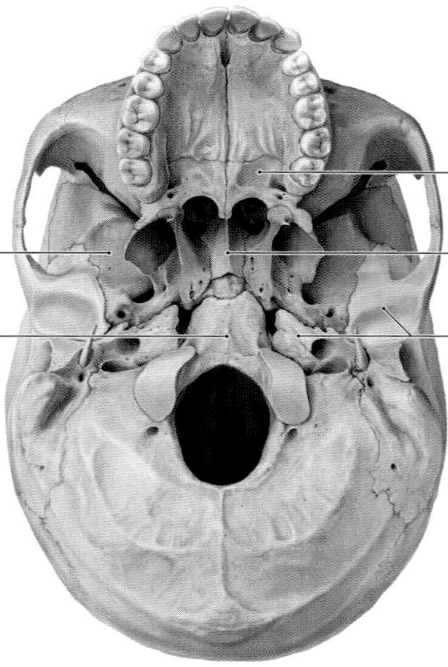

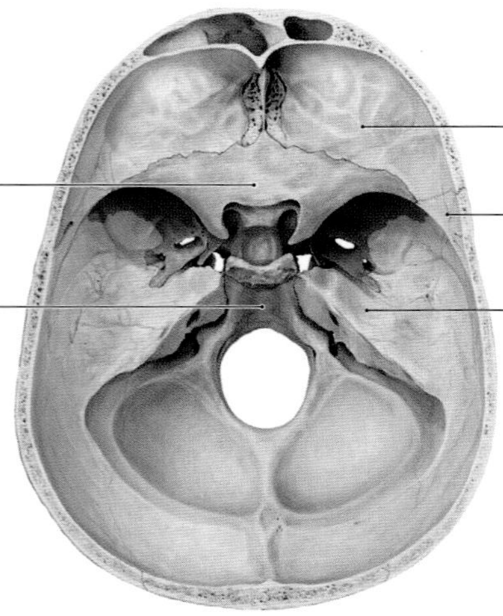

A Position of the sphenoid bone in the skull
The sphenoid bone is the most structurally complex bone in the human body. It must be viewed from various aspects in order to appreciate all its features (see also **B**):

- **a Base of the skull, external aspect.** The sphenoid bone combines with the occipital bone to form the load-bearing midline structure of the skull base.
- **b Base of the skull, internal aspect.** The sphenoid bone forms the boundary between the anterior and middle cranial fossae. The openings for the passage of nerves and vessels are clearly displayed (see details in **B**).
- **c Lateral view.** Portions of the greater wing of the sphenoid bone can be seen above the zygomatic arch, and portions of the pterygoid process can be seen below the zygomatic arch.

Note the bones that border on the sphenoid bone in each view.

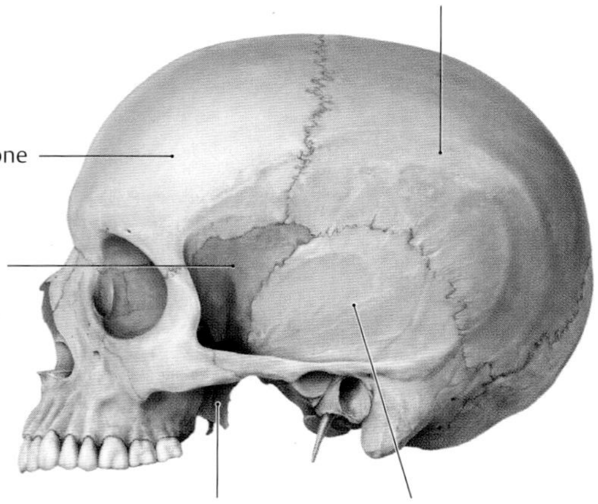

B Isolated sphenoid bone

- **a Inferior view** (its position in situ is shown in **A**). This view demonstrates the medial and lateral plates of the pterygoid process. Between them is the pterygoid fossa, which is occupied by the medial pterygoid muscle. The foramen spinosum and foramen rotundum provide pathways through the base of the skull.
- **b Anterior view.** This view illustrates why the sphenoid bone was originally called the sphecoid bone ("wasp bone") before a transcription error turned it into the sphenoid ("wedge-shaped") bone. The apertures of the sphenoid sinus on each side resemble the eyes of the wasp, and the pterygoid processes of the sphenoid bone form its dangling legs, between which are the pterygoid fossae. This view also displays the superior orbital fissure, which connects the middle cranial fossa with the orbit on each side. The two sphenoid sinuses are separated by an internal septum (see p. 43).
- **c Superior view.** The superior view displays the sella turcica, whose central depression, the hypophyseal fossa, contains the pituitary gland. The foramen spinosum, foramen ovale, and foramen rotundum can be identified posteriorly.
- **d Posterior view.** The superior orbital fissure is seen particularly clearly in this view, while the optic canal is almost completely obscured by the anterior clinoid process. The foramen rotundum is open from the middle cranial fossa to the external base of the skull (the foramen spinosum is not visible in this view; compare with **a**). Because the sphenoid and occipital bones fuse together during puberty ("tribasilar bone"), a suture is no longer present between the two bones. The cancellous trabeculae are exposed and have a porous appearance.

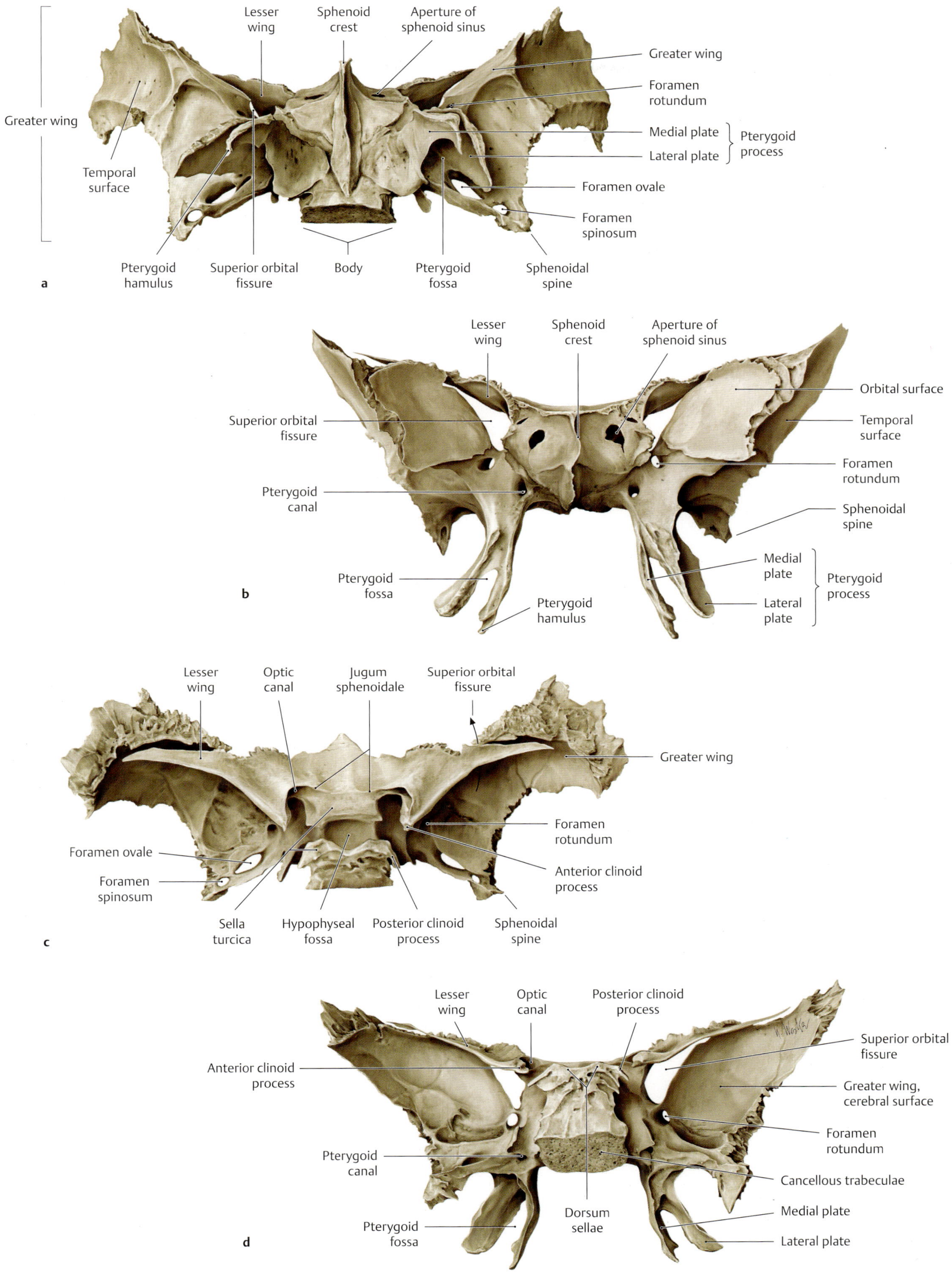
Lesser wing
Sphenoid crest
Aperture of sphenoid sinus
Greater wing
Foramen rotundum
Medial plate
Lateral plate
Pterygoid process
Foramen ovale
Foramen spinosum
Greater wing
Temporal surface
Pterygoid hamulus
Superior orbital fissure
Body
Pterygoid fossa
Sphenoidal spine
a
Lesser wing
Sphenoid crest
Aperture of sphenoid sinus
Orbital surface
Temporal surface
Superior orbital fissure
Foramen rotundum
Pterygoid canal
Sphenoidal spine
Medial plate
Lateral plate
Pterygoid process
Pterygoid fossa
Pterygoid hamulus
b
Lesser wing
Optic canal
Jugum sphenoidale
Superior orbital fissure
Greater wing
Foramen rotundum
Anterior clinoid process
Foramen ovale
Foramen spinosum
Sella turcica
Hypophyseal fossa
Posterior clinoid process
Sphenoidal spine
c
Lesser wing
Optic canal
Posterior clinoid process
Anterior clinoid process
Superior orbital fissure
Greater wing, cerebral surface
Foramen rotundum
Pterygoid canal
Cancellous trabeculae
Dorsum sellae
Medial plate
Lateral plate
Pterygoid fossa
d

2.13 Orbit: Bones and Openings for Neurovascular Structures

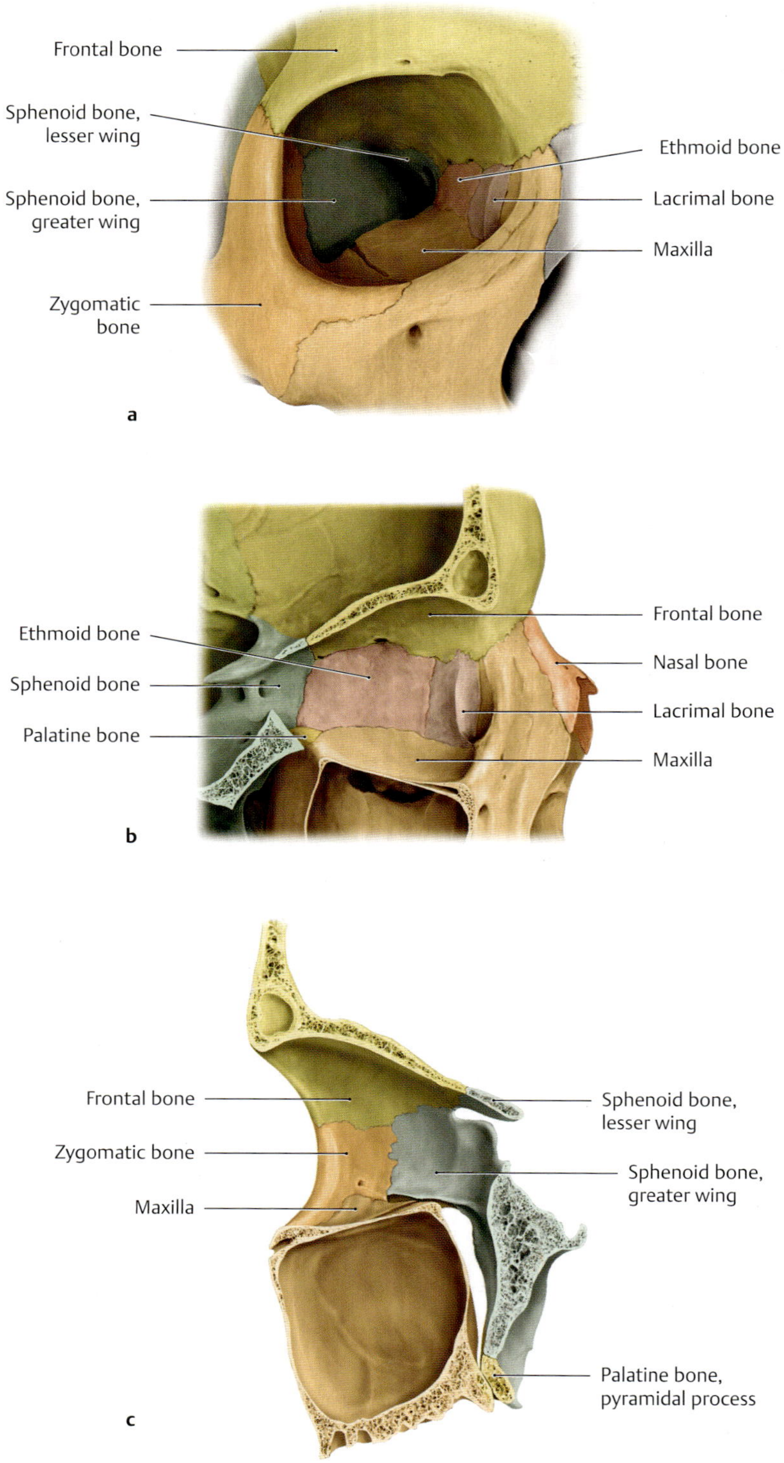

A Bones of the right orbit
Anterior view (**a**), lateral view (**b**), and medial view (**c**). The lateral orbital wall has been removed in **b**, and the medial orbital wall has been removed in **c**.
The orbit is formed by seven different bones (indicated here by color shading): the frontal bone, zygomatic bone, maxilla, ethmoid bone, sphenoid bone (see **a** and **c**), and also the lacrimal bone and palatine bone, which are visible only in the medial view (see **b**).
The present unit deals with the bony anatomy of the orbits themselves. The relationships of the orbits to each other are described in the next unit.

B Openings in the orbita for neurovascular structures
Note: The supraorbital foramen is an important site in routine clinical examinations because the examiner presses on the supraorbital rim with the thumb to test the sensory function of the supraorbital nerve. The supraorbital nerve is a terminal branch of the first division of the trigeminal nerve (CN V_1, see p. 116). When pain is present in the distribution of the trigeminal nerve, tenderness to pressure may be noted at the supraorbital site.

Opening or passage	Neurovascular structures
Optic canal	• Optic nerve (CN II) • Ophthalmic artery
Superior orbital fissure	• Oculomotor nerve (CN III) • Trochlear nerve (CN IV) • Ophthalmic nerve (CN V_1) – Lacrimal nerve – Frontal nerve – Nasociliary nerve • Abducent nerve (CN V_I) • Superior ophthalmic vein
Inferior orbital fissure	• Infraorbital nerve (of CN V_2) • Infraorbital artery, vein, and nerve (of CN V_2) • Orbital branches (of CN V_2) • Inferior ophthalmic vein
Anterior ethmoidal foramen	• Anterior ethmoidal artery, vein, and nerve
Posterior ethmoidal foramen	• Posterior ethmoidal artery, vein, and nerve
Infraorbital canal	• Infraorbital artery, vein, and nerve
Supraorbital foramen	• Supraorbital artery • Supraorbital nerve (lateral branch)
Frontal incisure	• Supratrochlear artery • Supraorbital nerve (medial branch)
Zygomatico-orbital foramen	• Zygomatic nerve (of CN V_2)
Nasolacrimal canal	• Nasolacrimal duct

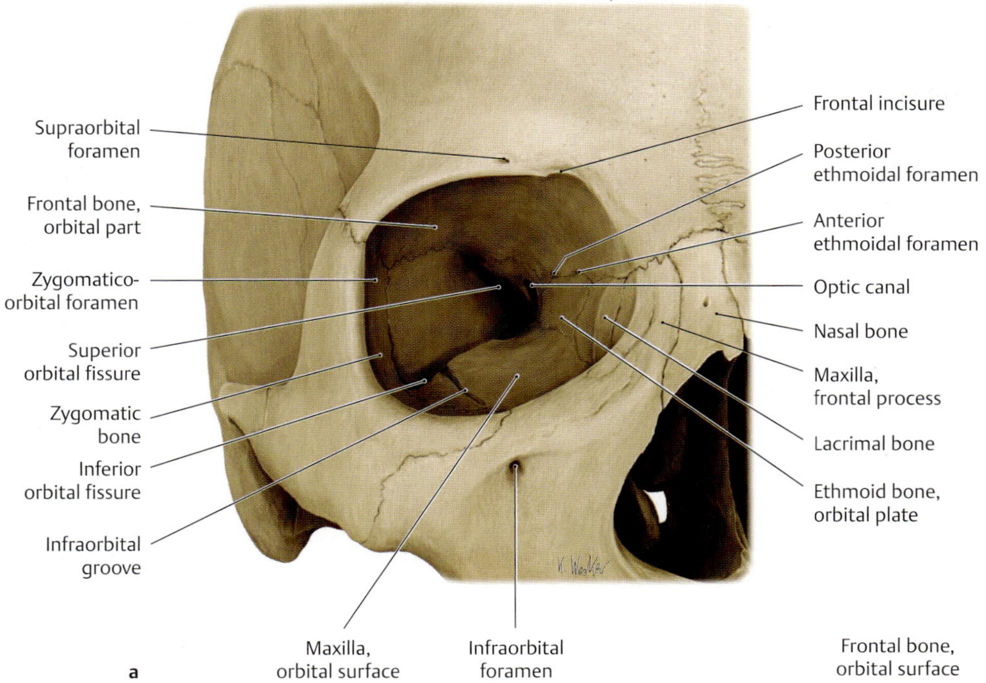

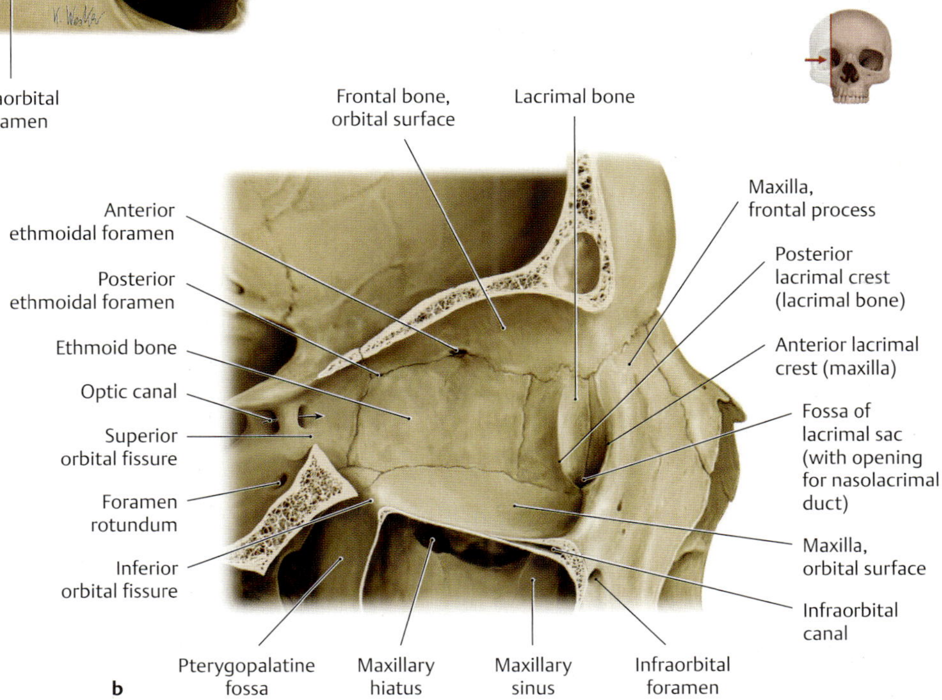

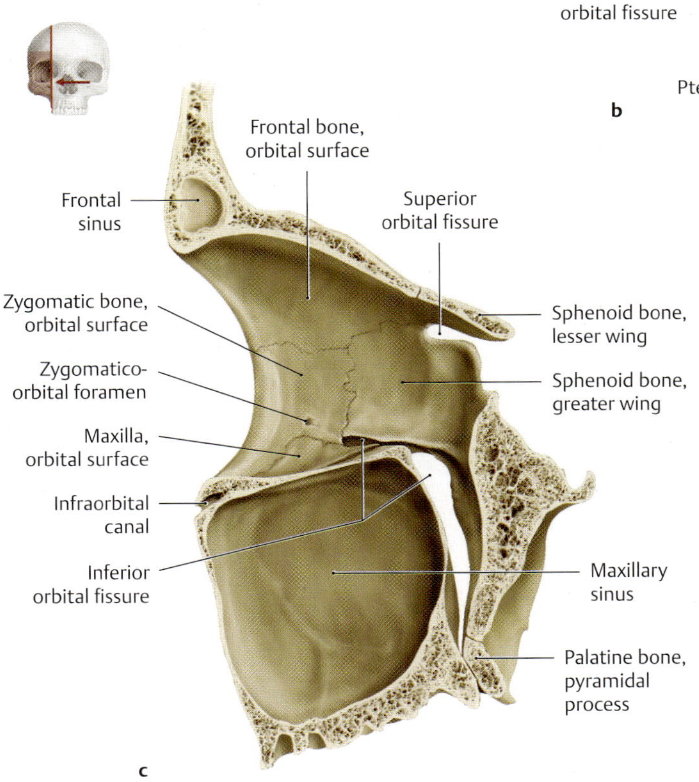

C Openings and pathways for neurovascular structures

Right orbit, anterior view (**a**), lateral view (**b**), and medial view (**c**). The lateral orbital wall has been removed in **b**, the medial orbital wall in **c**. The following openings for the passage of neurovascular structures (see listing in **B**) can be identified: the superior and inferior orbital fissures (**a**–**c**), the optic canal (**a**, **b**), the anterior and posterior ethmoidal foramina (**b**, **c**), the infraorbital groove (**a**), which merges into the infraorbital canal (**b**, **c**) and ends in the infraorbital foramen (**a**, **b**); Supraorbital foramen and frontal incisure (**a**); Zygomatico-orbital foramen (**c**). Diagram **b** shows the orifice of the nasolacrimal duct, by which lacrimal fluid is conveyed to the inferior meatus of the nose (see p. 42).

The lateral view (**b**) demonstrates the funnel-like structure of the orbit, which functions like a socket to contain the eyeball and constrain its movements. The inferior orbital fissure opens into the pterygopalatine fossa, which borders on the posterior wall of the maxillary sinus. It contains the pterygopalatine ganglion, an important component of the parasympathetic nervous system (see pp. 239 and 127). In the maxillary sinus, which has been exposed, the elevated opening of the maxillary sinus (maxillary hiatus) is identifiable. It connects the maxillary sinus located below the middle nasal concha with the nasal cavity.

2.14 Orbit and Neighboring Structures

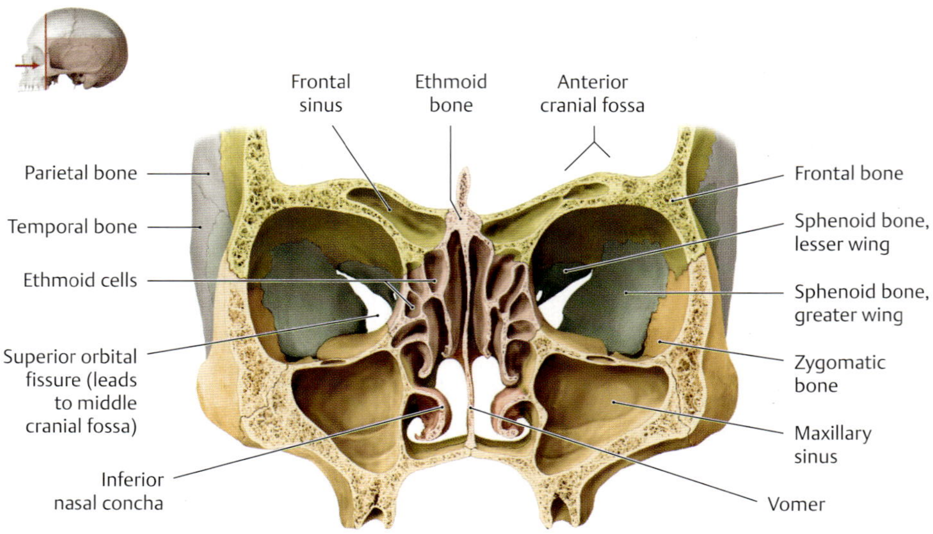

A Bones of the orbit and adjacent cavities
The color-coding here is the same as for the bones of the orbit on pp.14–15. These bones also form portions of the walls of neighboring cavities. The following adjacent structures are visible in the diagram:

- Anterior cranial fossa
- Frontal sinus
- Middle cranial fossa
- Ethmoid cells*
- Maxillary sinus

Disease processes may originate in the orbit and spread to these cavities, or originate in these cavities and spread to the orbit.

* The *Terminologia Anatomica* has dropped the term "ethmoid sinus" in favor of "ethmoid cells."

B Clinically important relationships between the orbits and surrounding structures

Relationship to the orbit	Neighboring structure
Inferior	• Maxillary sinus
Superior	• Frontal sinus • Anterior cranial fossa (contains the frontal lobes of the brain)
Medial	• Ethmoid cells
Deeper structures that have a clinically important relationship to the orbit: • Sphenoid sinus • Middle cranial fossa • Optic chiasm • Pituitary • Cavernous sinus • Pterygopalatine fossa	

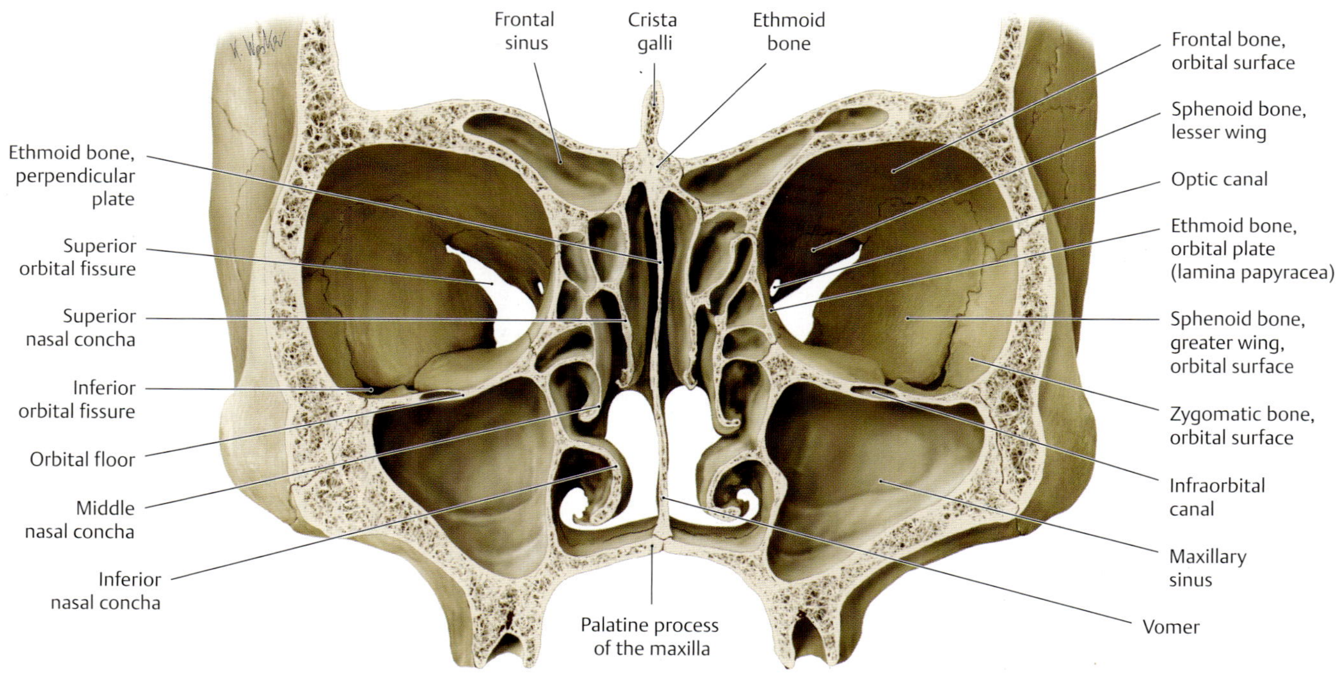

C Orbits and neighboring structures
Coronal section through both orbits, viewed from the front. The walls separating the orbit from the ethmoid cells (0.3 mm, lamina papyracea) and from the maxillary sinus (0.5 mm, orbital floor) are very thin. Thus, both of these walls are susceptible to fractures and provide routes for the spread of tumors and inflammatory processes into or out of the orbit. The superior orbital fissure communicates with the middle cranial fossa, and so several structures that are not pictured here—the sphenoid sinus, pituitary gland, and optic chiasm—are also closely related to the orbit.

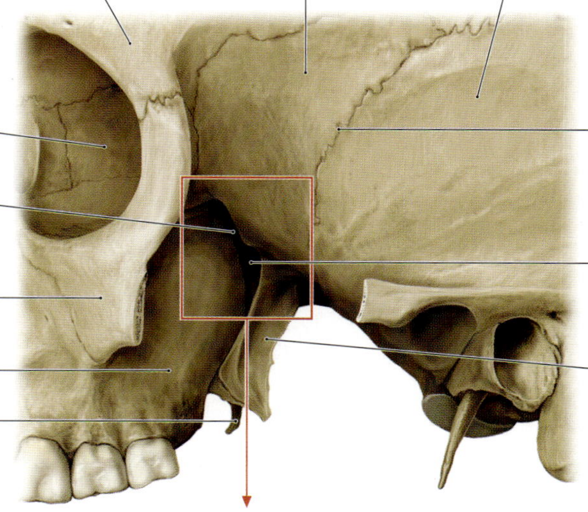

D Close-up view of the left pterygopalatine fossa

Lateral view. The pterygopalatine fossa is a crossroads between the middle cranial fossa, orbit, and nasal cavity, being traversed by many nerves and vessels that supply these regions. The pterygopalatine fossa is continuous laterally with the infratemporal fossa. This diagram shows the lateral approach to the pterygopalatine fossa through the infratemporal fossa, which is utilized in surgical approaches to tumors in this region (e.g., nasopharyngeal fibroma).

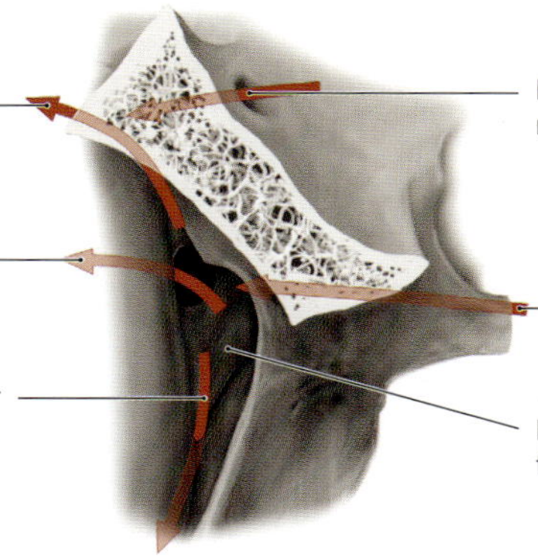

E Connections of the left pterygopalatine fossa with adjacent regions

Detail from **D**. The contents of the pterygopalatine fossa include the pterygopalatine ganglion (see pp. 239 and 127), which is an important parasympathetic ganglion in the autonomic nervous system.

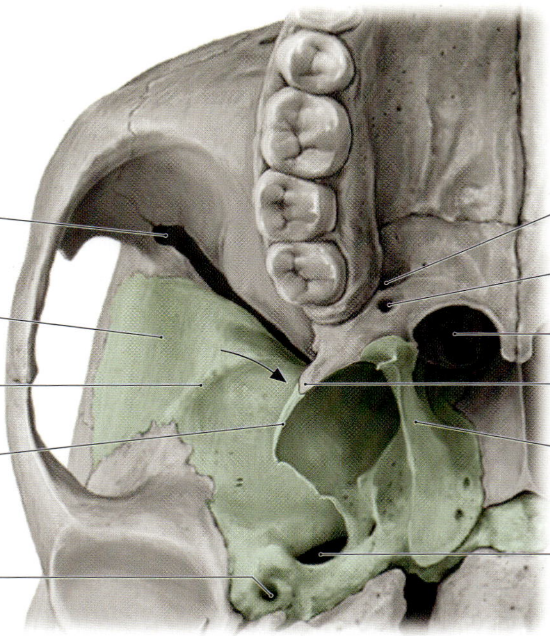

F Structures adjacent to the right pterygopalatine fossa

Inferior view. The arrow indicates the approach to the pterygopalatine fossa via the infratemporal fossa as viewed from the skull base. The fossa itself (not visible in this view) is lateral to the lateral plate of the pterygoid process of the sphenoid bone. In this image the sphenoid bone is shaded green.

For borders of the pterygopalatine fossa as well as access routes and neurovascular structures, see p. 238 f.

2.15 Nose: Nasal Skeleton

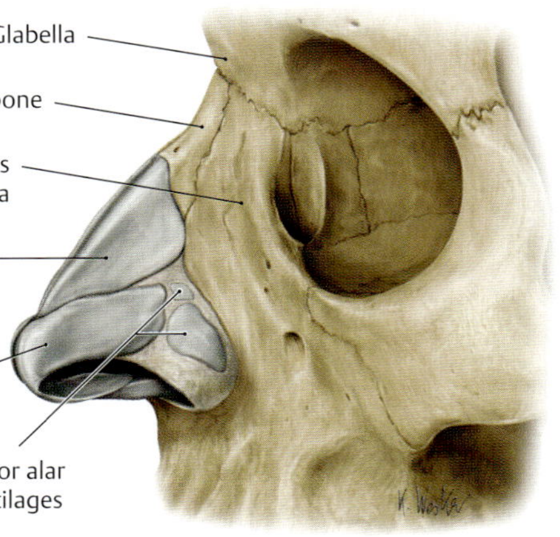

A Skeleton of the external nose

Left lateral view. The skeleton of the nose is composed of bone, cartilage, and connective tissue. Its upper portion is bony and frequently involved in midfacial fractures, while its lower, distal portion is cartilaginous and therefore more elastic and less susceptible to injury. The proximal lower portion of the nostrils (alae) is composed of connective tissue with small embedded pieces of cartilage. The lateral nasal cartilage is a winglike lateral expansion of the cartilaginous nasal septum rather than a separate piece of cartilage.

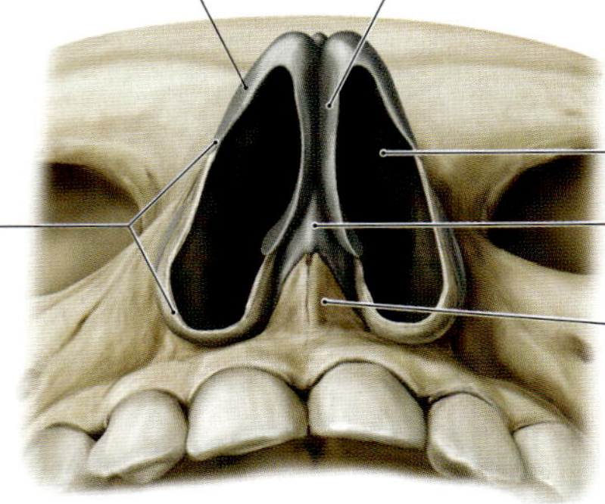

B Nasal cartilage

Inferior view. Viewed from below, each of the major alar cartilages is seen to consist of a medial and lateral crus. This view also displays the two nares, which open into the nasal cavities. The right and left nasal cavities are separated by the nasal septum, whose inferior cartilaginous portion is just visible in the diagram. The wall structure of a single nasal cavity will be described in this unit, and the relationship of the nasal cavity to the paranasal sinuses will be explored in the next unit.

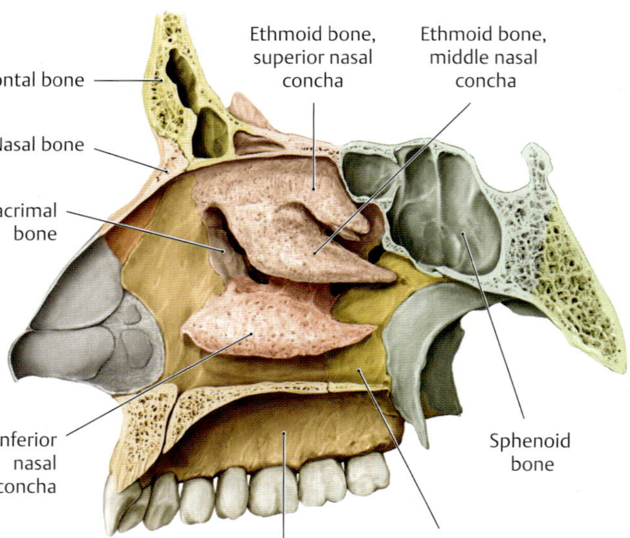

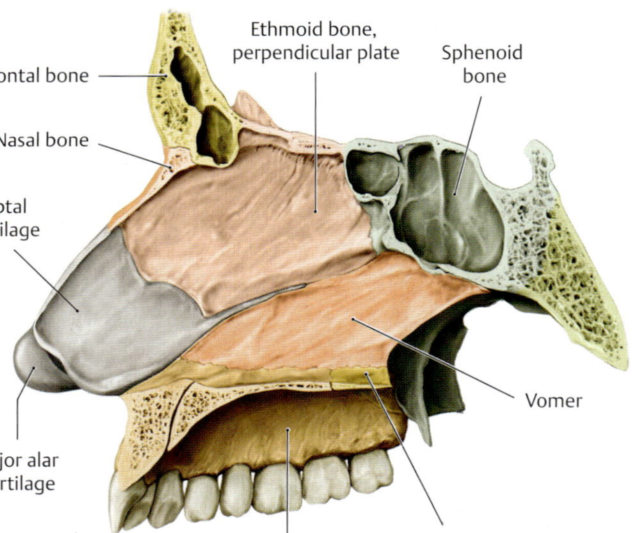

C Bony walls of the nasal cavity

a Right nasal cavity, left lateral view; nasal septum has been removed.
b Paramedian section, left lateral view.
The nasal cavity has four walls:

- the roof (nasal, frontal and ethmoid bones);
- the floor (maxilla and palatine bones);
- the lateral wall including maxilla, nasal, lacrimal, ethmoid, and palatine bones and the inferior nasal concha;
- the medial wall (nasal septum, see **b** and **E**), which is composed of cartilage and the following bones: nasal, ethmoid, vomer, and sphenoid;
- palatine and maxilla, these latter three contributing only small bony projections to the nasal septum.

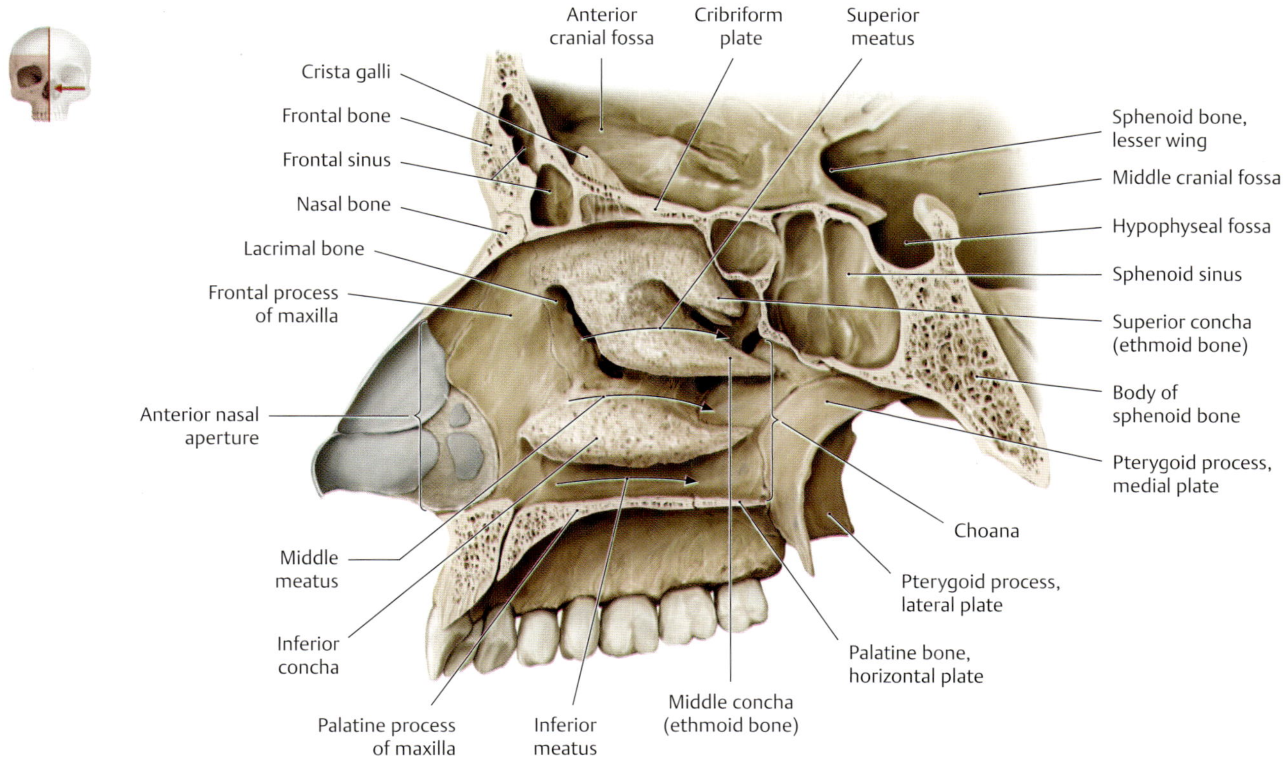

D Nasal cavity with illustration of airflow around the three nasal conchae

Left lateral view. Air enters the bony nasal cavity through the anterior nasal aperture and passes over the three nasal conchae as well as through the spaces under each conchae—the inferior, middle, and superior meatus. Air leaves the nose through the choanae, entering the nasopharynx.

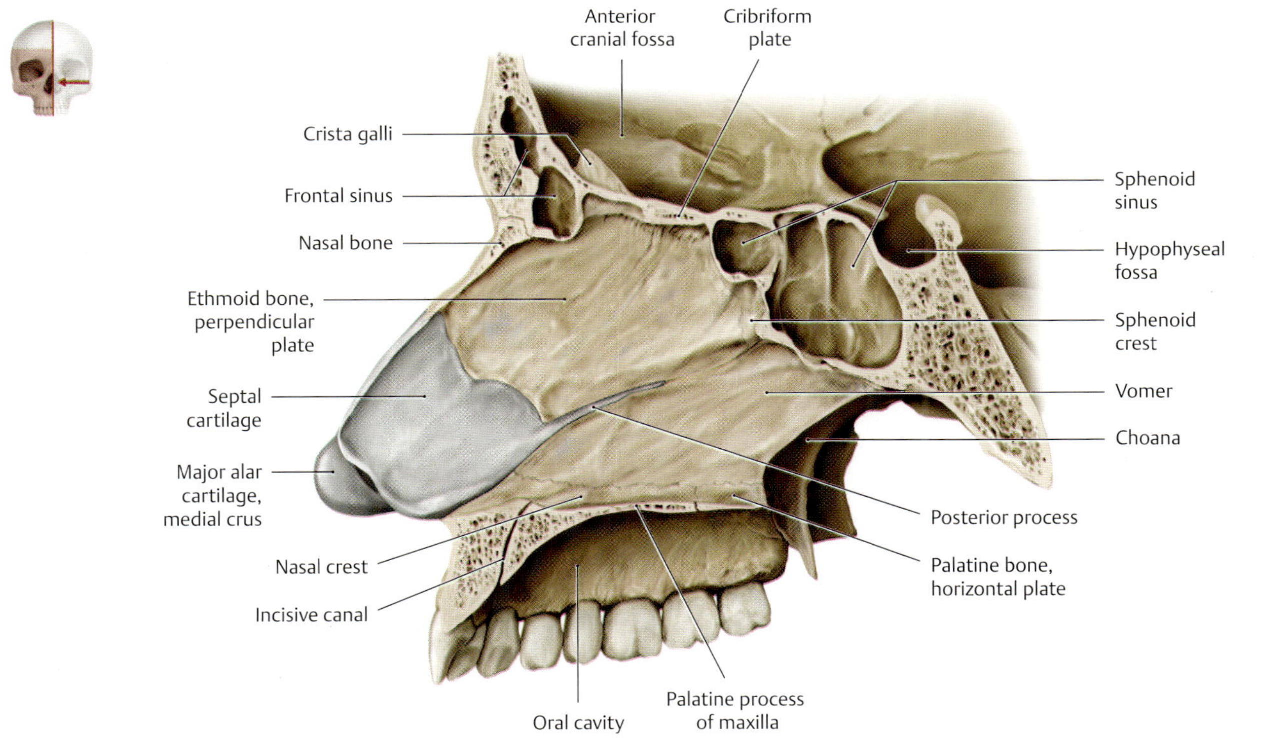

E Nasal septum

Parasagittal section viewed from the left side. The left lateral wall of the nasal cavity has been removed with the adjacent bones. The nasal septum consists of an anterior cartilaginous part, the septal cartilage, and a posterior bony part (see **Cb**). The posterior process of the cartilaginous septum extends deep into the bony septum. Deviations of the nasal septum are common and may involve the cartilaginous part of the septum, the bony part, or both. Cases in which the septal deviation is sufficient to cause obstruction of nasal breathing can be surgically corrected.

2.16 Nose: Paranasal Sinuses

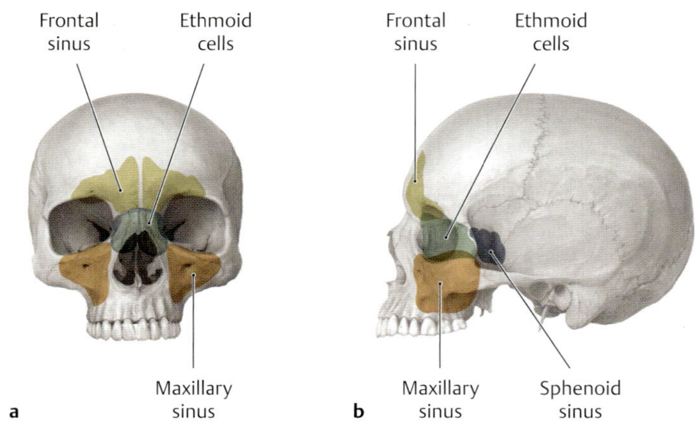

A Projection of the paranasal sinuses onto the skull
a Anterior view, **b** lateral view.
The paranasal sinuses are air-filled cavities that reduce the weight of the skull. Because they are subject to inflammation that may cause pain over the affected sinus (e.g., frontal headache due to frontal sinusitis), knowing the location of the sinuses is helpful in making the correct diagnosis.
Note: The term "ethmoidal (air) cells" has replaced the formerly used term "ethmoidal sinus."

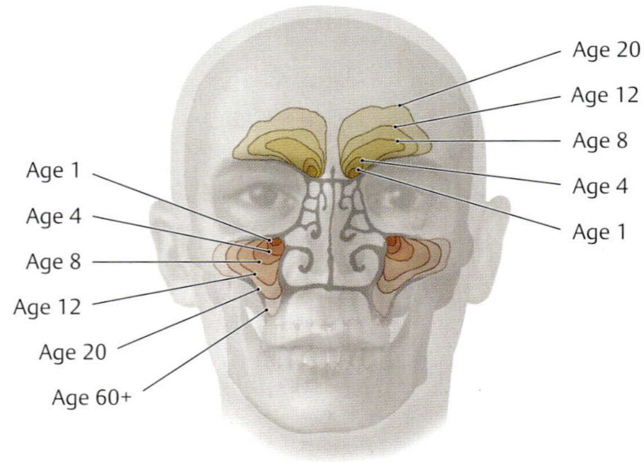

B Pneumatization of the maxillary and frontal sinuses
Anterior view. The frontal and maxillary sinuses develop gradually during the course of cranial growth (pneumatization)—unlike the ethmoid sinuses which are already pneumatized at birth. As a result, sinusitis in children is most likely to involve the ethmoid cells (with risk of orbital penetration: red, swollen eye; see **D**).

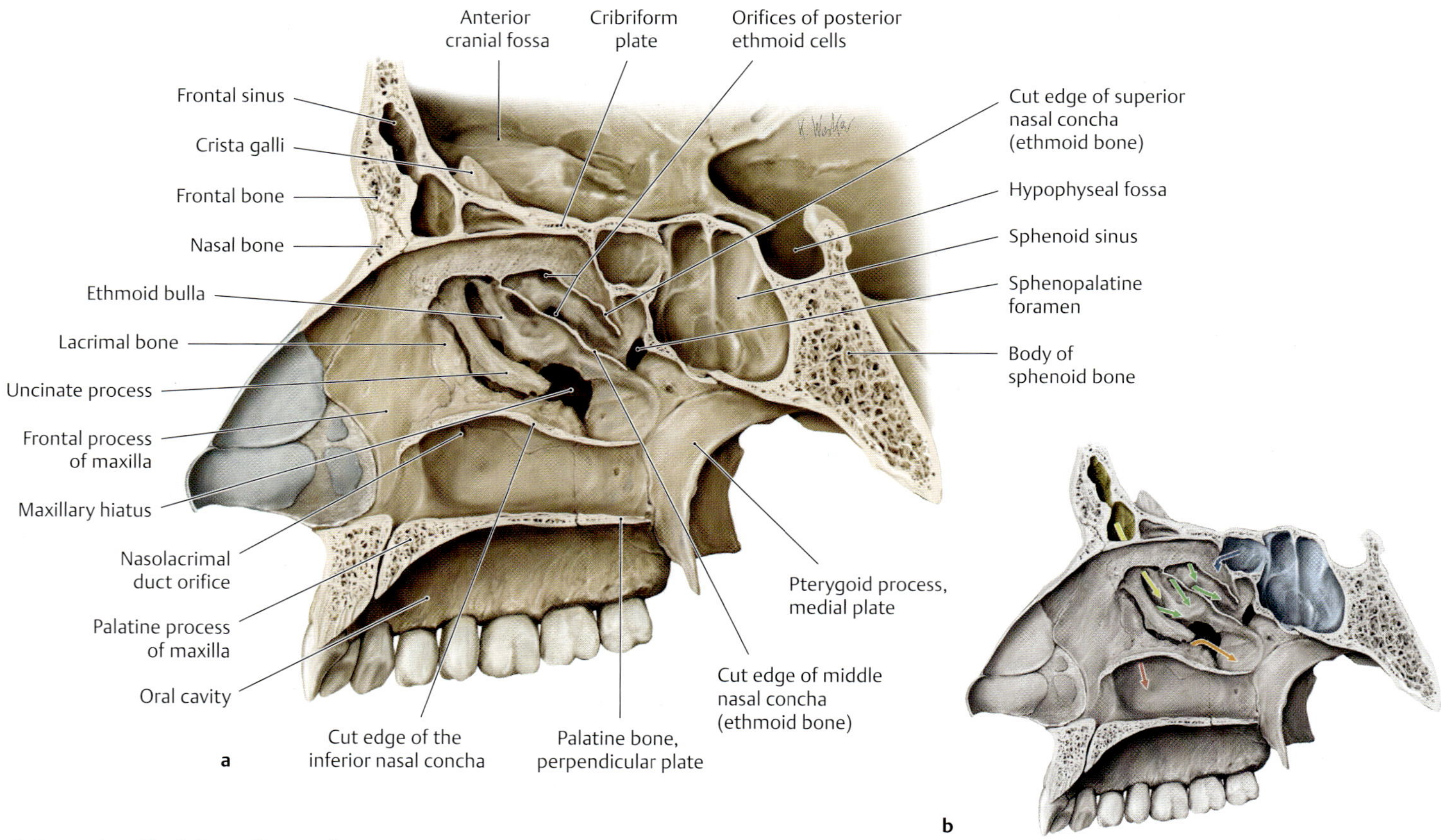

C Lateral wall of the right nasal cavity
a, **b** Midline section viewed from the left with the nasal conchae removed to display the openings in the underlying meatal regions, that is, the nasolacrimal duct and paranasal sinuses emptying into the nasal cavity (see colored arrows in **b**: red = nasolacrimal duct, yellow = frontal sinus, orange = maxillary sinus, green = anterior and posterior ethmoid cells, blue = sphenoid sinus; drainage routes are described in **E**).

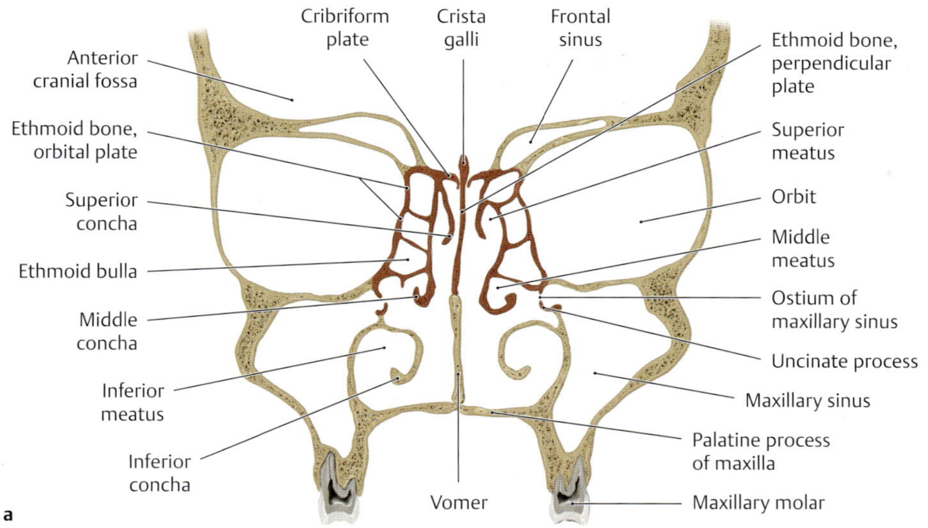

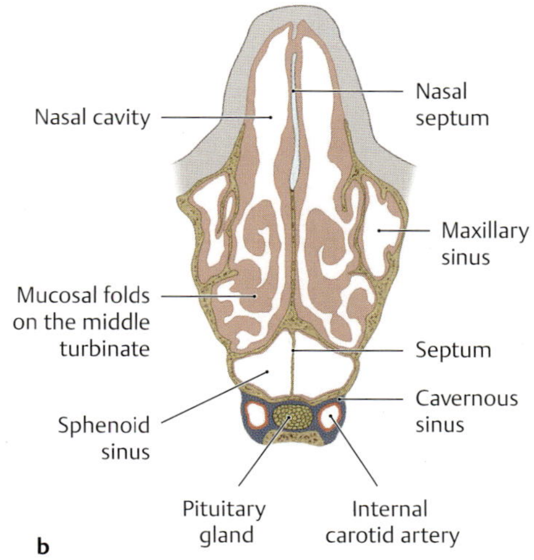

D Bony structure of the paranasal sinuses

a Frontal section; **b** transverse section, mucosa has been left intact, superior view.

The central structure of the *paranasal sinuses* is the ethmoid bone (red). Its cribriform plate forms a portion of the anterior skull base. The frontal and maxillary sinuses are grouped around the ethmoid bone. In the *nasal cavity*, the inferior, middle and superior nasal meatuses are visible. They are each bounded by their analogously named concha. The *middle* concha is a useful landmark in surgical procedures on the anterior ethmoid bone and the maxillary sinus, the bony ostium of which is located *lateral* to the middle concha, and opens into the middle meatus. *Below* this concha, located cranially is the largest chamber in the ethmoid bone, the ethmoidal bullae. At its anterior margin a bony hook is visible. It bounds the maxillary sinus opening anteriorly as the uncinate process. The lateral wall separating the ethmoid bone from the orbit is paper-thin (lamina papyracea) so inflammatory processes and tumors may penetrate this thin plate in either direction.

Note: The deepest point of the maxillary sinus is located in the root area of the maxillary molars (in 30% of people, the distance between maxillary sinus and buccal root is less than 1 mm). Thus, periapical inflammation in this area can extend to the sinus floor. When extracting an upper molar, opening the maxillary sinus is the most likely procedure.

The transverse section (**b**), shows the hypophysis, located behind the sphenoid sinus in the hypophyseal fossa (see **C**), is accessible to transnasal surgical procedures. The surface of the mucosa has been left intact to show how narrow the entire nasal cavity is and how swelling can quickly obstruct it (see **E**).

E Sites where the nasolacrimal duct and paranasal sinuses open into the nasal cavity

Nasal passage	Structures that open into the passage
Inferior meatus	• Nasolacrimal duct
Middle meatus	• Frontal sinus • Maxillary sinus • Anterior ethmoid cells • Middle ethmoid cells
Superior meatus	• Posterior ethmoid cells
Spheno-ethmoid recess	• Sphenoid sinus

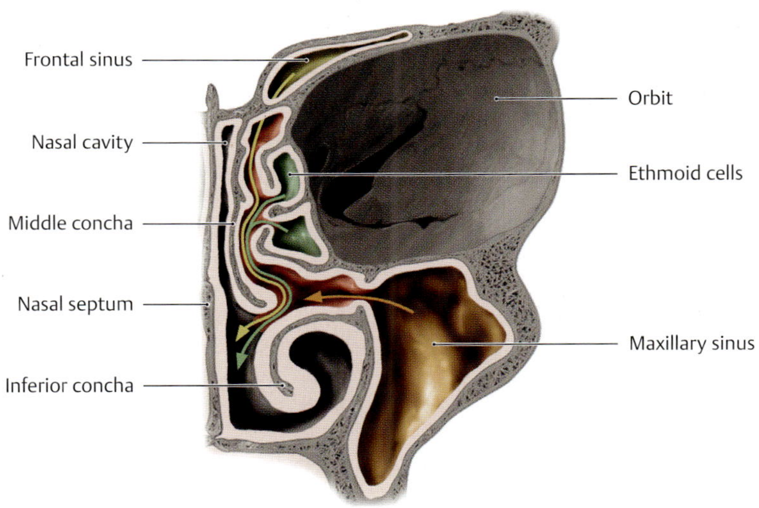

F Ostiomeatal unit on the left side of the nasal cavity

Coronal section. When the mucosa (ciliated respiratory epithelium) in the ethmoid cells (green) becomes swollen due to inflammation (sinusitis), it blocks the flow of secretions (see arrows) from the frontal sinus (yellow) and maxillary sinus (orange) in the ostiomeatal unit (red). Because of this blockage, microorganisms also become trapped in the other sinuses, where they may incite inflammation. Thus, while the anatomical focus of the disease lies in the ethmoid cells, inflammatory symptoms are also manifested in the frontal and maxillary sinuses. In patients with *chronic sinusitis*, the narrow sites can be surgically widened to establish an effective drainage route, alleviating the condition.

2.17 Hard Palate

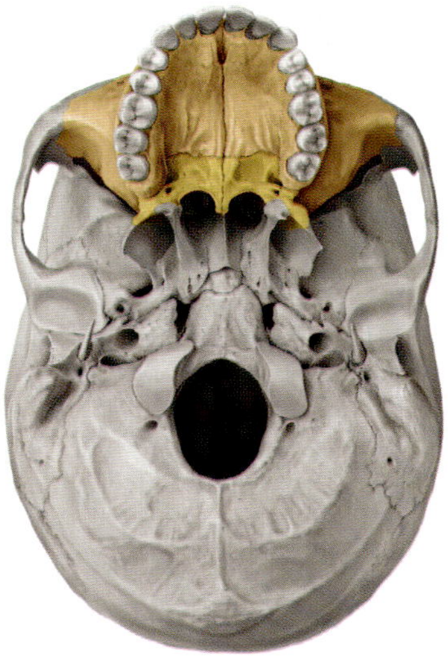

A Integration of the hard palate into the base of the skull
Inferior view.

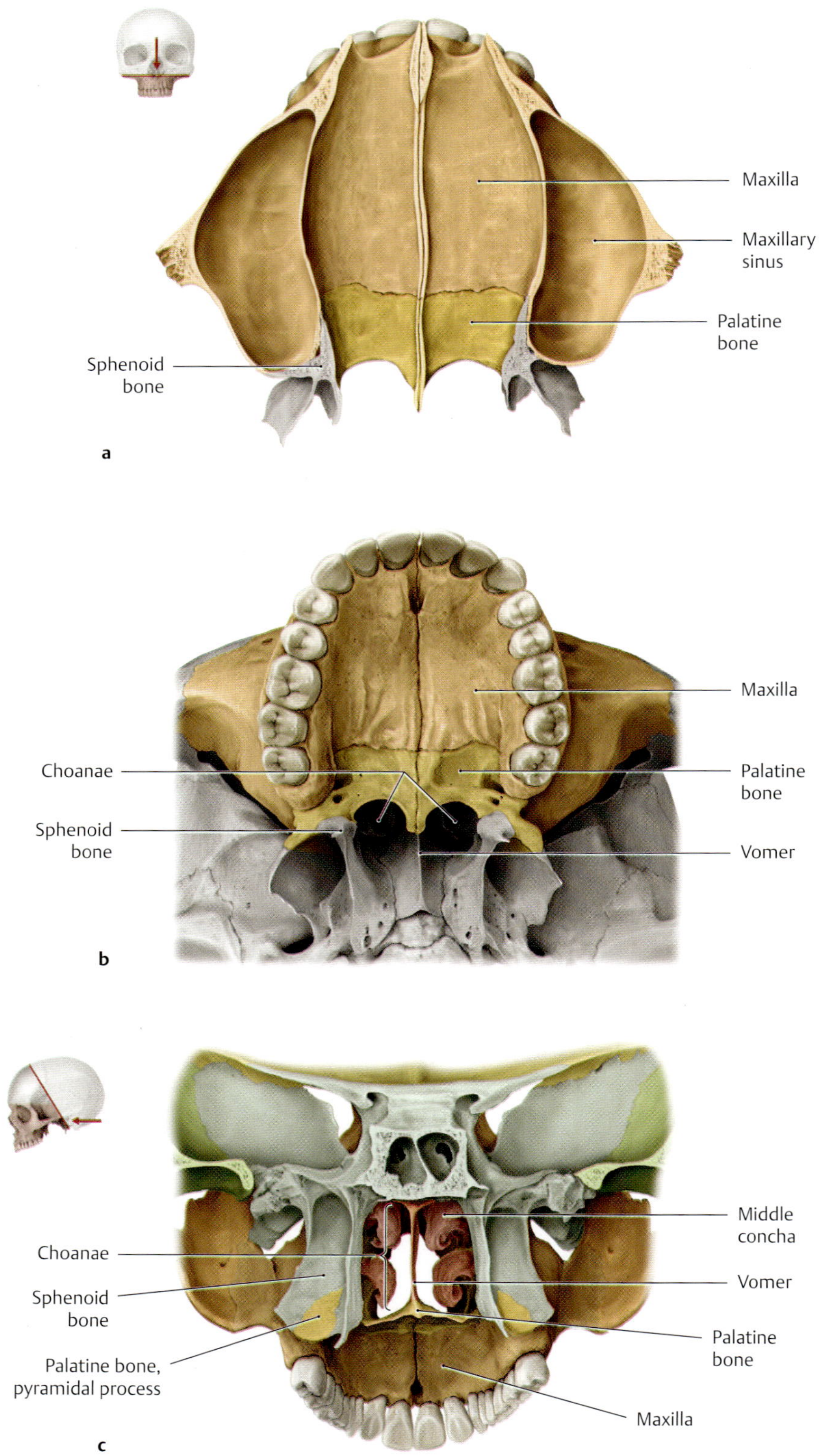

B Bones of the hard palate

a Superior view. The hard palate is a horizontal bony plate formed by parts of the maxilla and palatine bone. It serves as a partition between the oral and nasal cavities. In this view we are looking down at the floor of the nasal cavity, whose inferior surface forms the roof of the oral cavity. The upper portion of the maxilla has been removed. The palatine bone is bordered posteriorly by the sphenoid bone.

b Inferior view. The choanae, the posterior openings of the nasal cavity, begin at the posterior border of the hard palate.

c Oblique posterior view. This view demonstrates the close relationship between the oral and nasal cavities.
Note how the pyramidal process of the palatine bone is integrated into the lateral plate of the pterygoid process of the sphenoid bone.

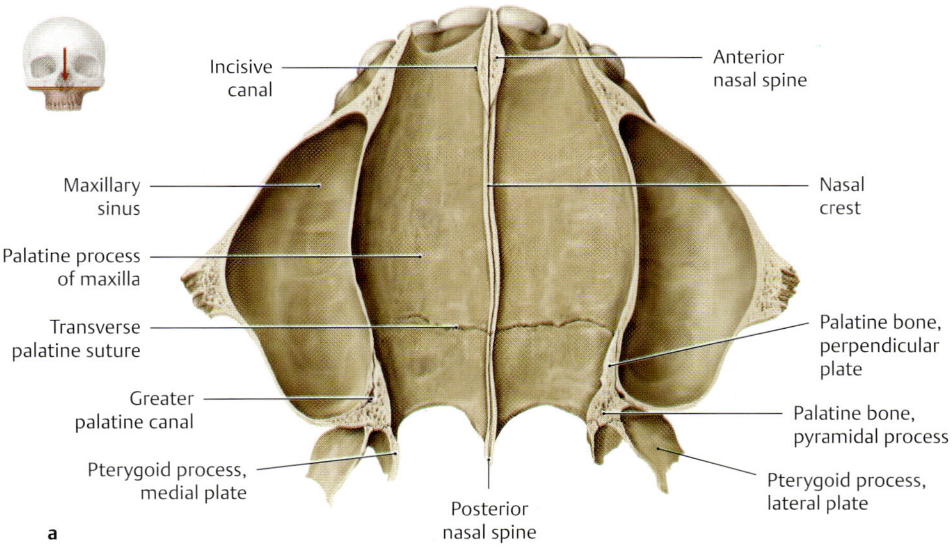

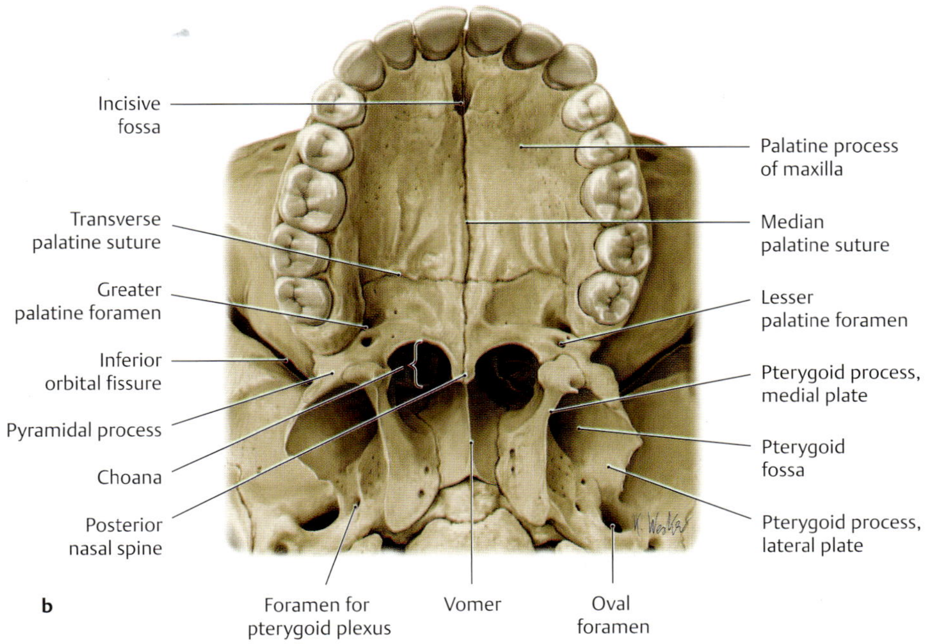

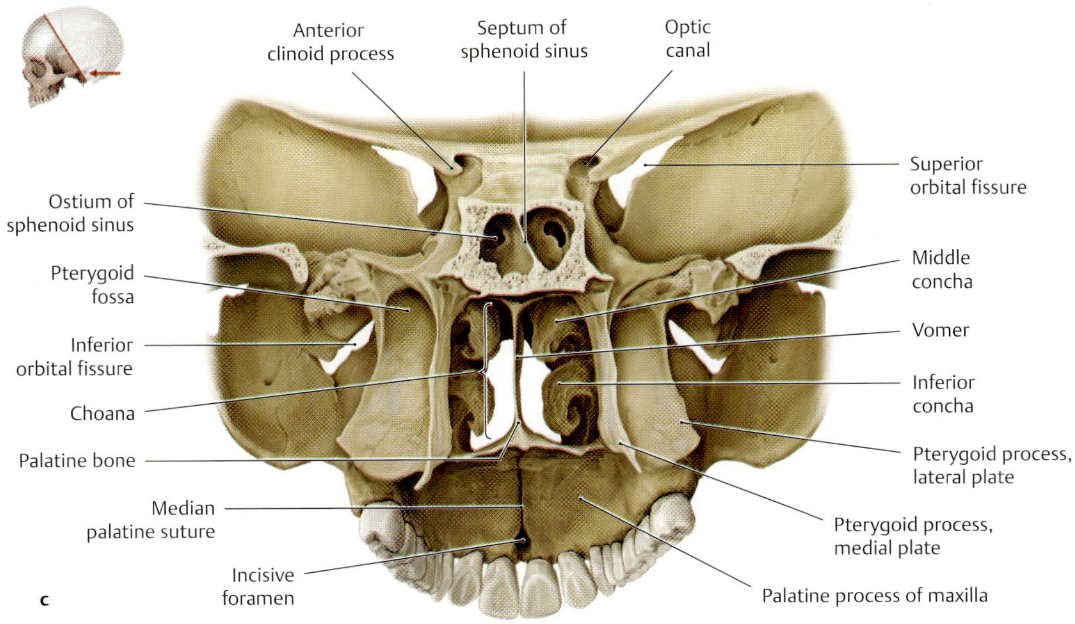

C Hard palate

a Superior view of the floor of the nasal cavity (= upper portion of hard palate) with the upper part of the maxilla removed. The hard palate separates the oral cavity from the nasal cavities. The small canal that links the oral and nasal cavities, the incisive canal (present here on both sides), merges within the bone to form one canal, which opens on the inferior surface by a single orifice, the incisive foramen (see **b**).

b Inferior view. The two horizontal processes of the maxilla, the palatine processes, grow together during development and become fused at the median palatine suture. Failure of this fusion results in a *cleft palate*. The boundary line between anterior clefts (cleft lip, alone or combined with a cleft alveolus) and posterior clefts (cleft palate) is the incisive foramen. These anomalies may also take the form of cleft lip and palate (with a defect involving the lip, alveolus, and palate).
Note: The nasal cavity (whose floor is formed by the hard palate) communicates with the nasopharynx by way of the choanae.

c Oblique posterior view of the posterior part of the sphenoid bone at the level of the sphenoid body, displaying both sphenoid sinuses separated by a septum. The close topographical relationship between the nasal cavity and hard palate can be appreciated in this view. If the hard palate is unfused in a nursing infant due to a cleft anomaly (cf. **b**), some of the ingested milk will be diverted from the oral cavity and will enter the nose. This defect should be closed with a plate immediately after birth to permit satisfactory oral nutrition.

2.18 Mandible and Hyoid Bone

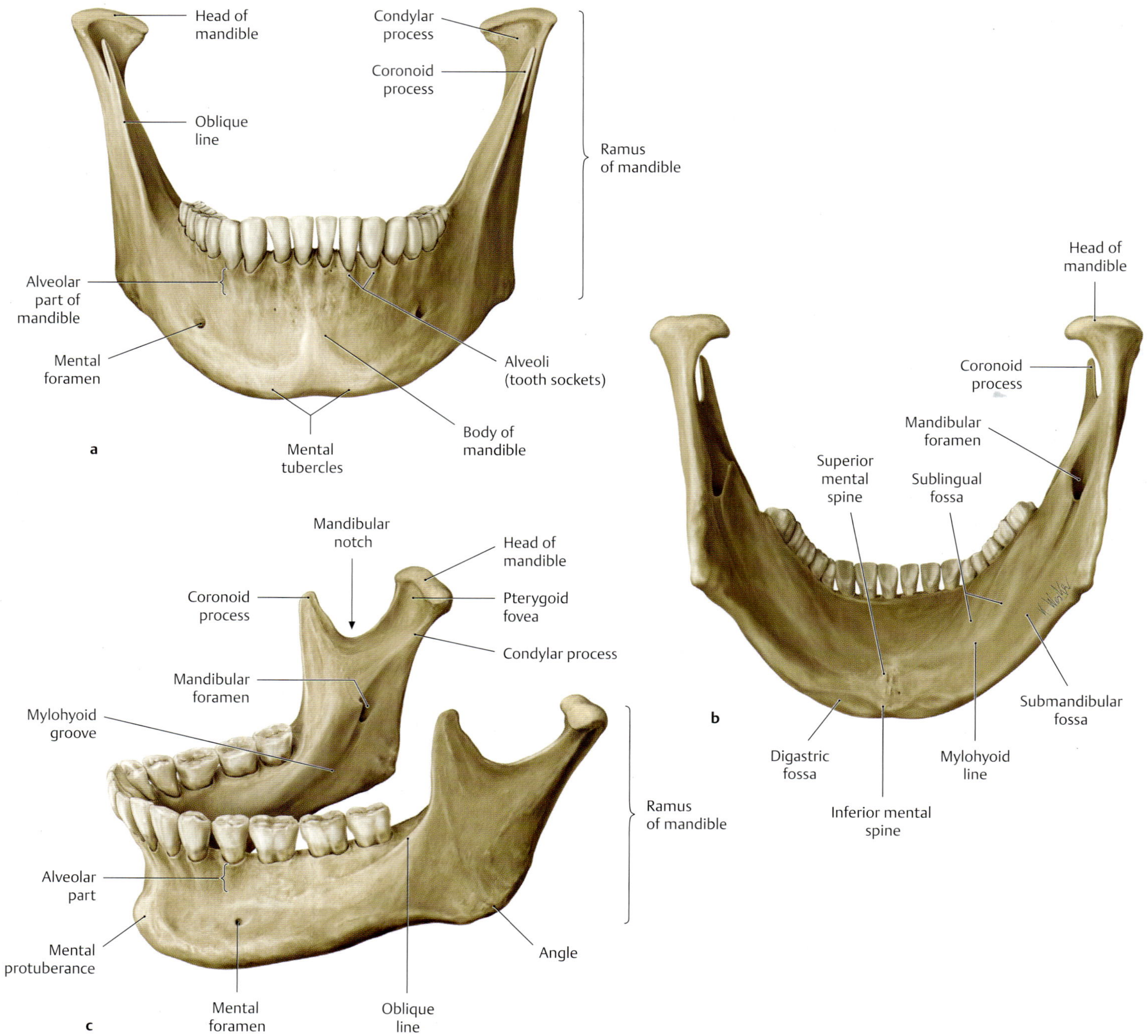

A Mandible

a Anterior view. The mandible, itself a part of the viscerocranium, is connected to the neurocranium by the temporomandibular joint. This "head of the mandible" is situated atop the vertical (ascending) ramus of the mandible, which joins with the body of the mandible at the mandibular angle. The teeth are set in the alveolar processes (alveolar part) along the upper border of the mandibular body. This part of the mandible is subject to typical age-related changes as a result of dental development (see **B**). The mental branch of the trigeminal nerve exits through the mental foramen to enter its bony canal. The location of this foramen is important in clinical examinations, as the tenderness of the nerve to pressure can be tested at that location (e.g., in trigeminal neuralgia, p. 123).

b Posterior view. The mandibular foramen is particularly well displayed in this view. It transmits the inferior alveolar nerve, which supplies sensory innervation to the mandibular teeth. Its terminal branch emerges from the mental foramen. The two mandibular foramina are interconnected by the mandibular canal.

c Oblique left lateral view. This view displays the coronoid process, the condylar process, and the mandibular notch between them. The coronoid process is a site for muscular attachments, while the condylar process bears the head of the mandible, which articulates with the mandibular fossa of the temporal bone. A depression on the medial side of the condylar process, the pterygoid fovea, gives attachment to portions of the lateral pterygoid muscle.

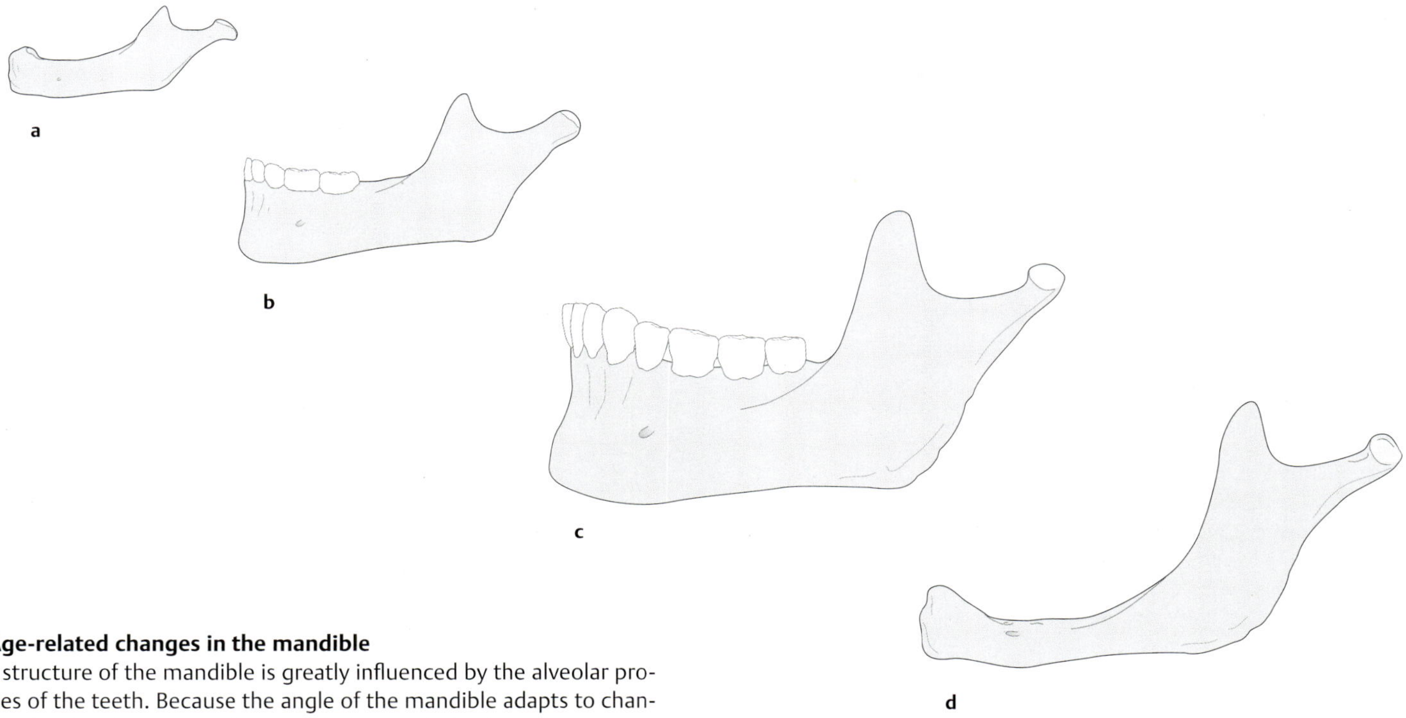

B Age-related changes in the mandible

The structure of the mandible is greatly influenced by the alveolar processes of the teeth. Because the angle of the mandible adapts to changes in the alveolar process, the angle between the body and ramus also varies with age-related changes in the dentition. The angle measures approximately 150° at birth, and approximately 120–130° in adults, decreasing to 140° in the edentulous mandible of old age.

- **a At birth**, the mandible is without teeth and the alveolar part has not yet formed.
- **b In children**, the mandible bears the deciduous teeth. The alveolar part is still relatively poorly developed because the deciduous teeth are considerably smaller than the permanent teeth.
- **c In adults**, the mandible bears the permanent teeth, and the alveolar part of the bone is fully developed.
- **d Old age** is characterized by an edentulous mandible with resorption of the alveolar process.

Note: The resorption of the alveolar process with advanced age leads to a change in the position of the mental foramen (which is normally located below the second premolar tooth, as in **c**). This change must be taken into account in surgery or dissections involving the mental nerve.

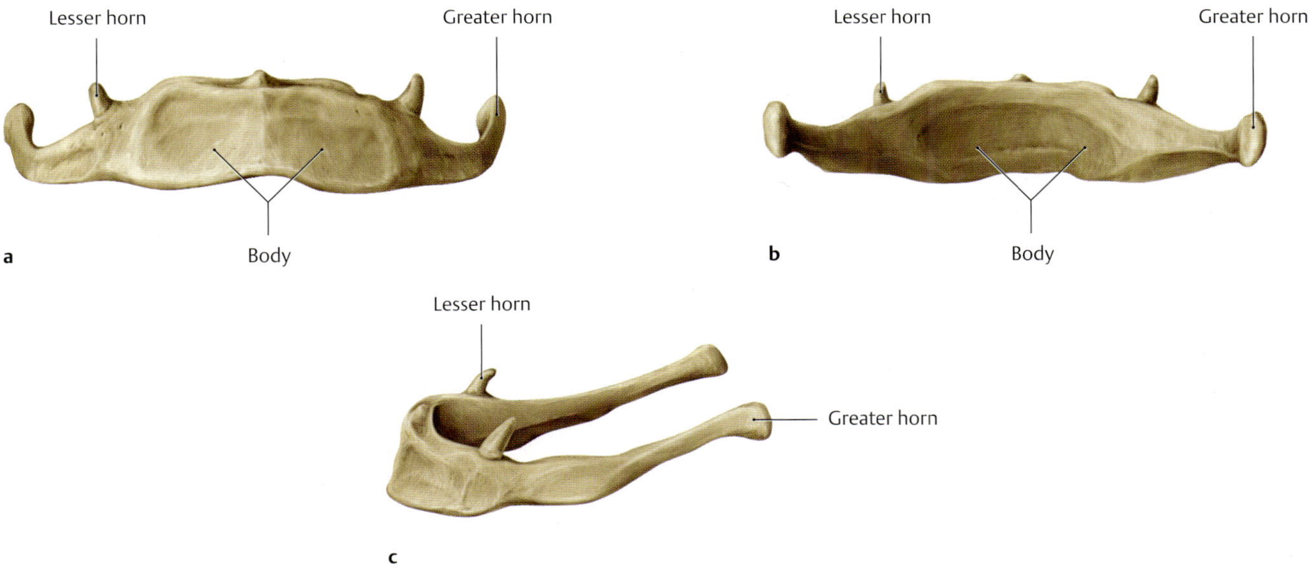

C Hyoid bone

a Anterior view; **b** posterior view; **c** oblique left lateral view. The hyoid bone is suspended by muscles between the oral floor and larynx in the neck (see p. 189), although it is listed among the cranial bones in the *Terminologia Anatomica*. The greater horn and body of the hyoid bone are palpable in the neck. The physiological movement of the hyoid bone during swallowing is also palpable.

2.19 Teeth in situ

A Characteristics of teeth

Human teeth are the result of a long phylogenetic evolution in vertebrates. The typical dentition of a mammal is as follows:

- **heterodont** = four different forms of teeth (incisors, canine, premolars, molars)
- **thecodont** = teeth held in place by a resilient attachment apparatus in the dental alveoli of the jaws
- **diphyodont** = two successive sets of teeth (deciduous teeth and permanent teeth).

Note: In humans diphyodonty pertains only to deciduous teeth (1. tooth generation) and their replacement teeth (2. tooth generation). The accessional teeth (1., 2., and 3. molar), which come through at the back of the gum are *monophyodont* since they do not have primary predecessors.

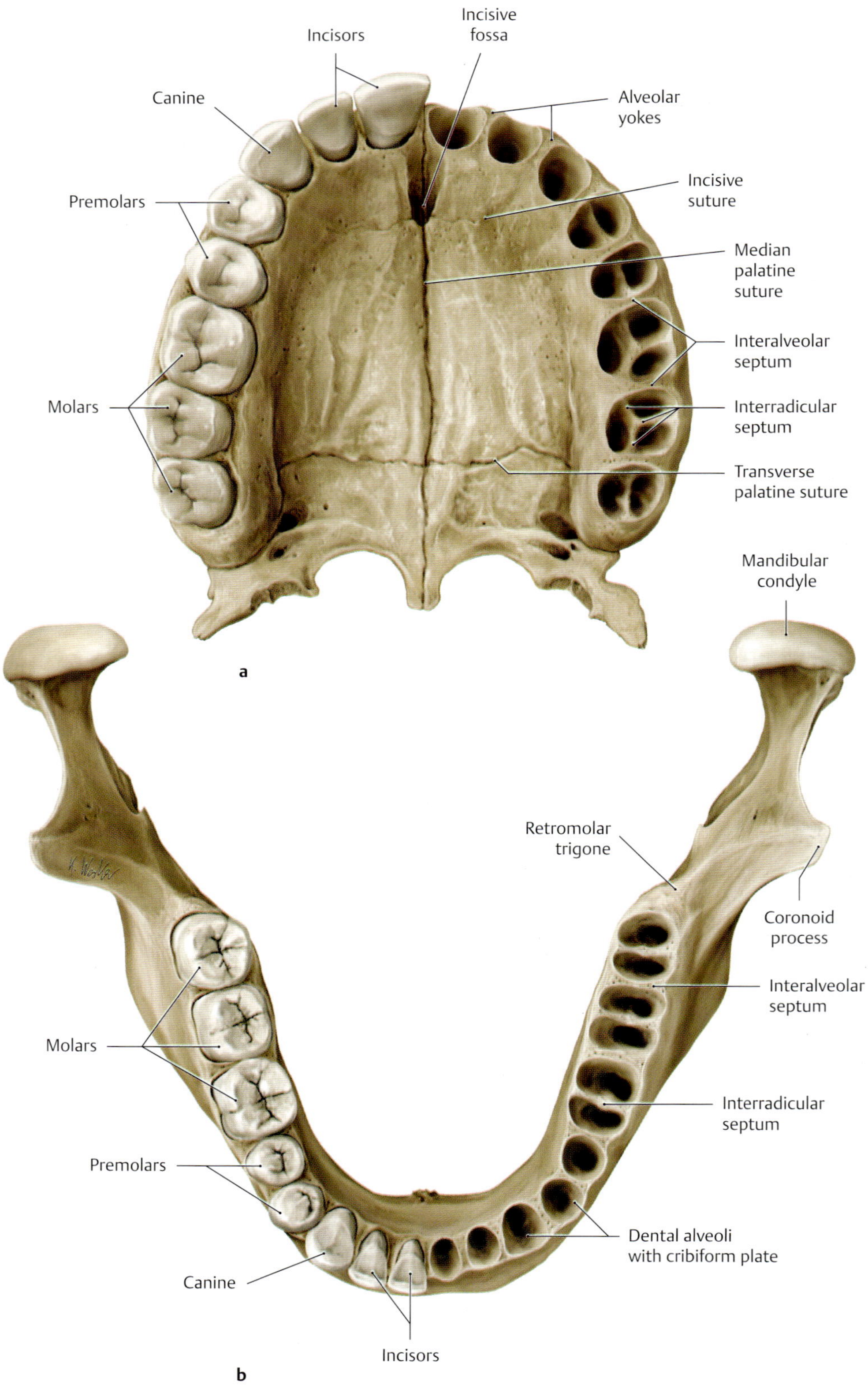

B Permanent teeth in adults

a Maxilla caudal view showing the chewing surfaces. **b Mandibular** cranial view; *right side of both images* shows the alveolar process of maxilla and mandible after removal of teeth.
In human dentition, both the maxilla and mandible each contain 16 teeth, which are aligned in a bilateral-symmetrical fashion and are adjusted to different chewing functions. Each half of both maxilla and mandible consist of

- **Front Teeth:** two incisors and one canine,
- **Side Teeth:** two premolars and three molars.

Note: While the front teeth grab the food and bite off pieces for mastication, it is the side teeth that actually perform mastication. They function in mincing and grinding the food.
After removal of teeth (see left side in each image) the alveolar process, which holds the teeth, becomes visible. Particularly in the front teeth area, the dental roots in the alveoles curve the jawbone in parts heavily to the vestibular to the extent that they become palpable as so-called *juga alveolaria*. At these points, the adjacent compact bone is extremely thin (approximately 0.1 mm). The *septa interalveolaria* separates the alveoles of two adjacent teeth. The *septa interradicularia* separates the tooth chambers of multi-rooted teeth (for structure of the alveolar bone see p. 57).

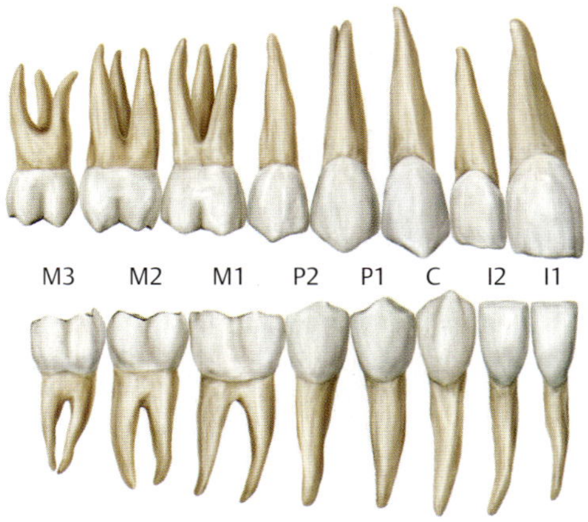

C Tooth shapes of the permanent dentition
The dentition of an adult consists of 8 different shapes of teeth in both the maxilla and mandible. Starting from the front of the jaw, the teeth are arraigned successively to lateral-posterior and without any gaps:

- I1 - middle incisor
- I2 - lateral incisor
- C - canine
- P1 - first premolar
- P2 - second premolar
- M1 - first molar
- M2 - second molar
- M3 - third molar

Note: Molars are the human's largest teeth. They have distinct cusps (tubercles) and fossae. The first molar often possesses an additional cusp, the tuberculum (cusp of) carabelli (see **E** for comparison). For build-up of occlusal surfaces cf. p. 45.

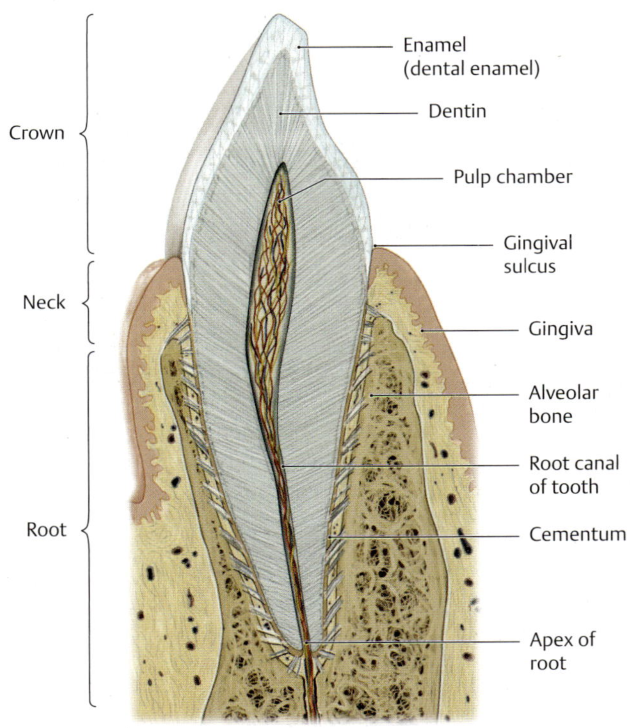

D Histology of a Tooth
A mandibular incisor serves as an example in this image, which depicts both hard substance (dentin, enamel, cementum) and soft tissue (pulp).

E Number of cusps, roots, and root canals of the permanent teeth of the maxilla and mandible
Data about the frequency was taken from Lehmann et al. (2009) and Strub et al. (2003). The area where a root is divided into two branches is called bifurcation and trifurcation for three root branches.

Maxillary Tooth	Number of Cusps	Number of Roots	Number of Root Canals
I1 (11/21)*	incisal edge	1	1
I2 (12/22)	incisal edge	1	1
C (13/23)	1 (cutting edge)	1	1
P1 (14/24)	2	2 (ca. 60%) 1 (ca. 40%) 3 (rare)	2 (ca. 80%) 1 (ca. 20%) 3 (rare)
P2 (15/25)	2	1 (ca. 90%) 2 (ca. 10%)	1 (ca. 60%) 2 (ca. 40%)
M1 (16/26)	4 without tubercle carabelli = additional cusp located on mesiopalatine cusp	3	4 (ca. 55%) 3 (ca. 45%)
M2 (17/27)	4	3	3 (ca. 55%) 4 (ca. 45%)
M3 (18/28)	mostly 3 (extremely inconsistent in shape)	Roots often intermingled (so-called taproots)	irregular
Mandibular Tooth	**Number of Cusps**	**Number of Roots**	**Number of Root Canals**
I1 (31/41)	incisal edge	1	1 (ca. 70%) 2 (ca. 30%) 3 (rare)
I2 (32/42)	incisal edge	1	1 (ca. 70%) 2 (ca. 30%)
C (33/43)	cutting edge	1	1 (ca. 80%) 2 (ca. 20%)
P1 (34/44)	2 (75%) 3 (25%)	1	1 (ca. 75%) 2 (ca. 25%) 3 (rare)
P2 (35/45)	3 (lingual cusp often divided into 2t)	1	1 (ca. 95%) 2 (ca. 5%) 3 (rare)
M1 (36/46)	5	2	3 (ca. 75%) 2 (ca. 25%) 4 (rare)
M2 (37/47)	4	2	3 (ca. 70%) 2 (ca. 30%) 4 (rare)
M3 (38/48)	usually 4 (very variable)	usually 2 (very variable)	irregular

* For identification of teeth with 2-digit numbers see **D**. p. 50

2.20 Terminology, Dental Schema, and Dental Characteristics

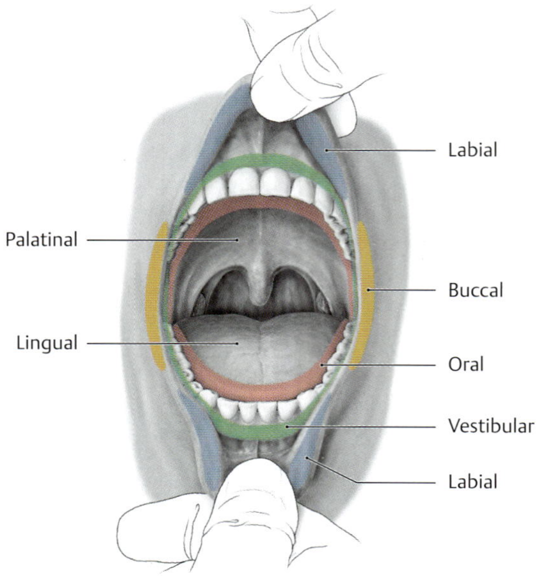

A Directions of the oral cavity

B Anatomical terms of the tooth

Term	Description
mesial	in the dental arch toward the midline
distal	toward the end of dental arch
oral	toward oral cavity
facial	toward the cheek or lips
lingual	toward the tongue
labial	toward the inside of the lip
buccal	toward the inside of the cheek
palatal	toward the palate (only with maxillary teeth)
vestibular	toward vestibule of the mouth
approximal	between two teeth crowns
incisal	toward biting edge
occlusal	on the chewing surface
cervical	toward neck of a tooth
coronal	toward the crown of a tooth
apical	toward the root tip of a tooth
pulpal	toward dental pulp

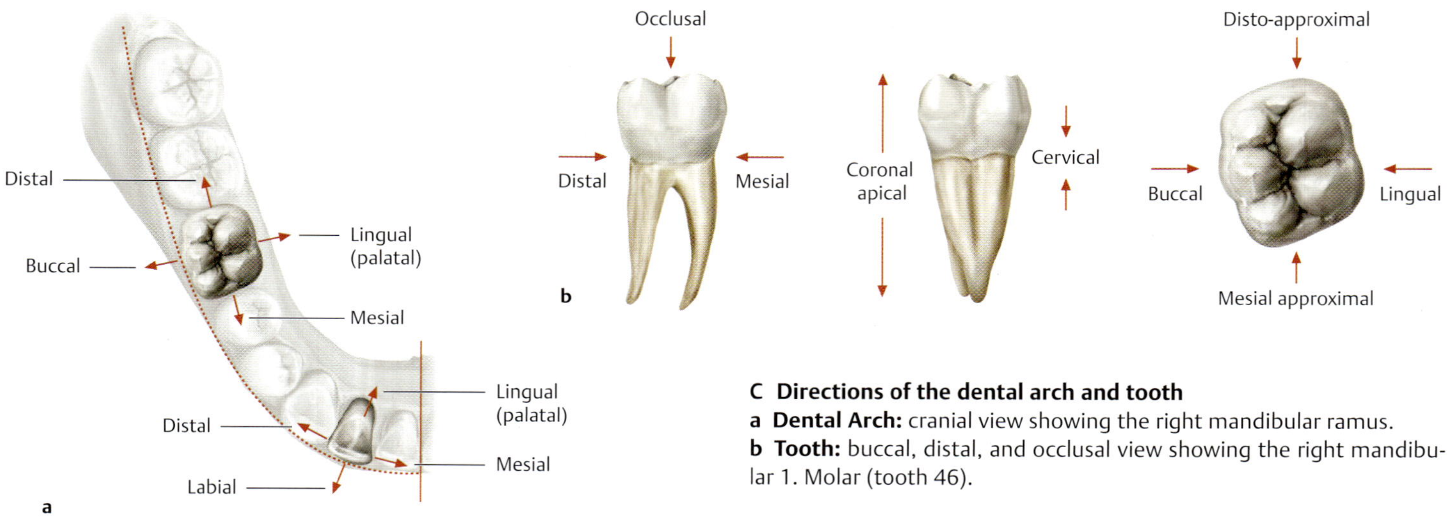

C Directions of the dental arch and tooth
a Dental Arch: cranial view showing the right mandibular ramus.
b Tooth: buccal, distal, and occlusal view showing the right mandibular 1. Molar (tooth 46).

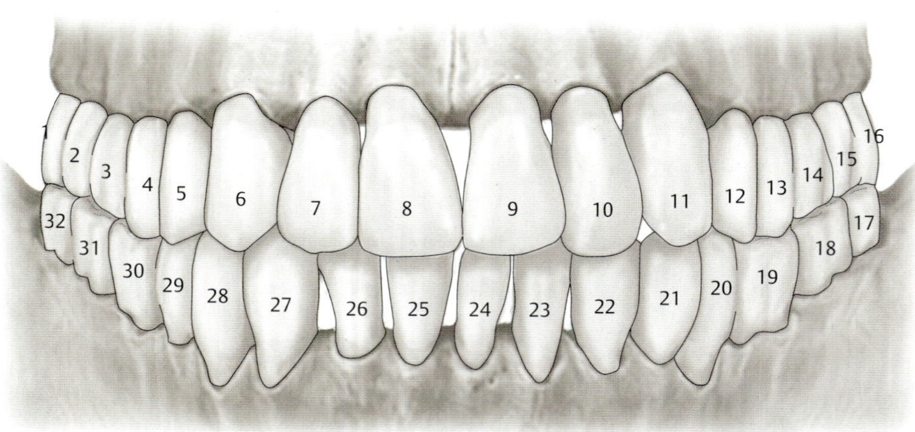

D Coding the permanent teeth
In the United States, the permanent teeth are numbered sequentially, not assigned to quadrants. Progressing in a clockwise fashion (from the perspective of the dentist), the teeth of the upper arc are numbered 1 to 16, and those of the lower are considered 17 to 32.
Note: The third upper molar (wisdom tooth) on the patient's right is considered 1.

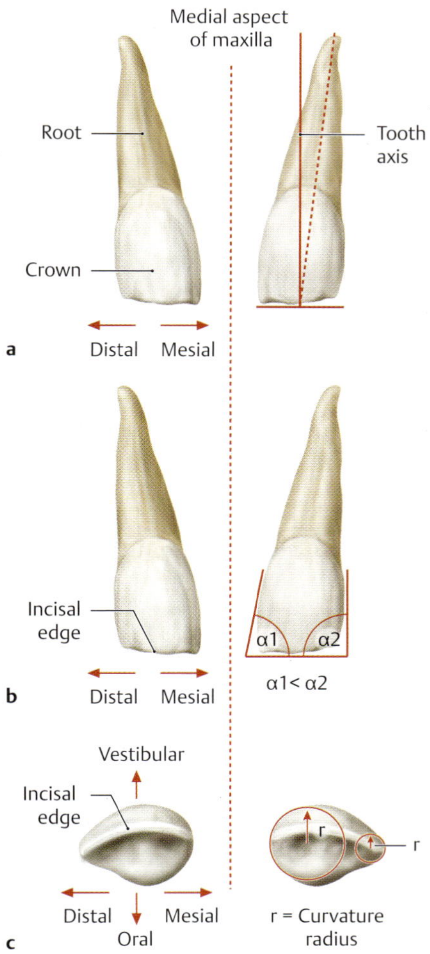

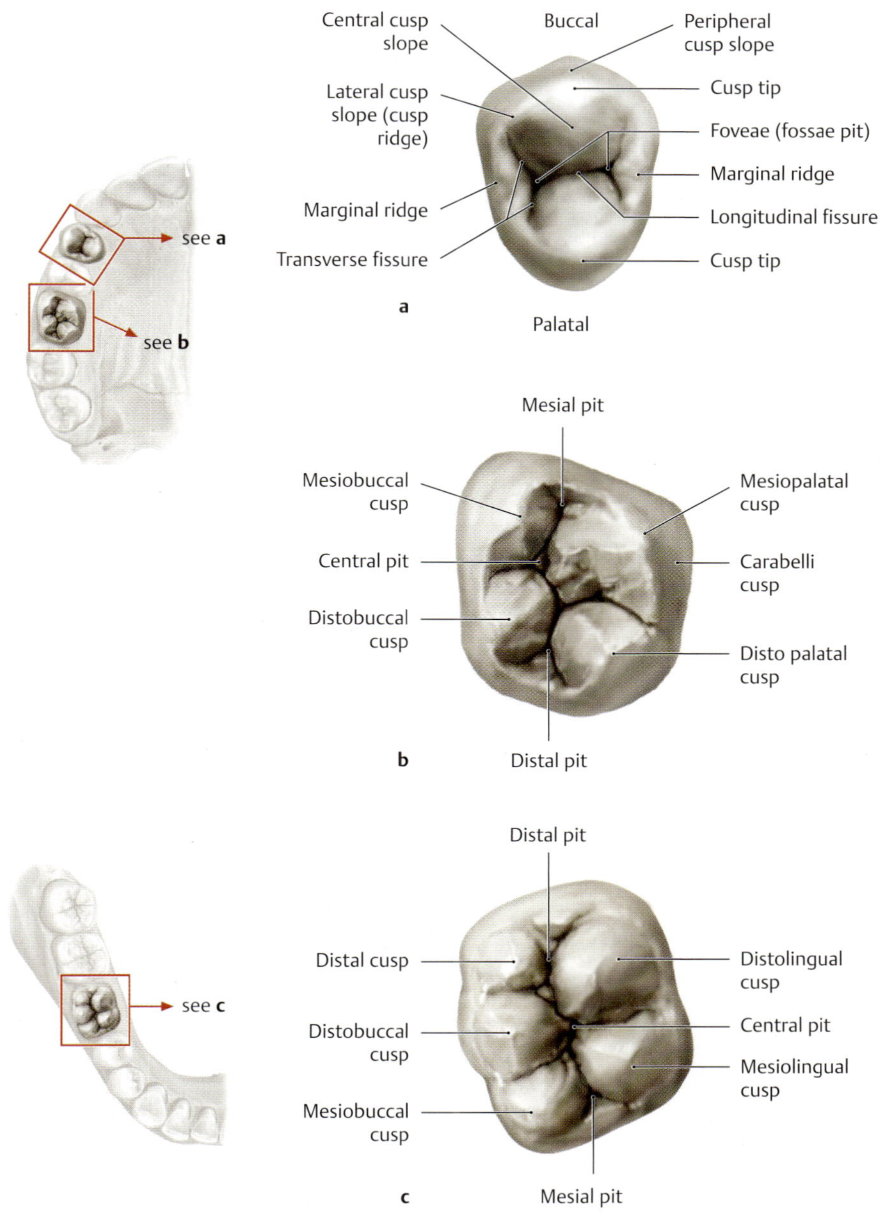

E Common dental characteristics

As early as 1870, Felix Muehlreiter described certain dental characteristics, which all teeth have in common and with the help of which the same teeth can be safely assigned to either the left or the right side respectively:

- **a Root surface characteristic:** Evaluation of tooth from vestibular. It refers to the course of the root of the tooth, which bends distally and thus slightly deviates from the axis of the tooth.
- **b Tooth angle characteristic:** Evaluation of tooth from vestibular. It is particularly pronounced in canines. The angle formed by the incisal edge and the sides of the crown is shorter on the mesial surface compared to the distal surface.
- **c Curvature characteristic:** Evaluation from incisal or occlusal. It shows that the proximal surface radius of curvature is longer on the mesial than on the distal surface, meaning teeth are significantly more dense mesially.

Further distinguishing features include the **cervical line of a tooth** (course of the cementoenamel junction), the **tooth equator** (anatomical equator), the **crown escape** (particularly pronounced in mandibular teeth) as well as the **root cross section**.

F Structure of the chewing surface

- **a** components of the chewing surface illustrated with the help of an upper right premolar (P1 or Tooth 14 respectively), occlusal view
- **b** nomenclature of the cusp of the 1. upper molar (M1) and the right maxilla (tooth 16), cranial view
- **c** nomenclature of the cusp of the 1. lower molar (M1) of the right mandible (tooth 46), cranial view

With the exception of both the upper and lower incisors (dentes incisivi), the chewing surfaces of the human permanent dentition have up to 5 cusps (cuspis dentis). While the canines (dentes canini) have a split incisal edge in the shape of a biting edge composed of a single large cusp, the molars (dentes premolars and molars) all have at least two biting edges (see p. 53). On an individual basis, one distinguishes between cusp tip, cusp ridge, fossae, fissures, and marginal ridge (**a**). Horizontal and vertical fissures separate the individual tooth cusps. Dents at cross points and junctions of the tooth have a predilection to become decayed. Inside the cusps of a chewing surface one distinguishes between supporting and non-supporting cusps (see p. 47). Accessory cusps, so-called tubercula anomalia, are not rare (for example tuberculum carabelli at the mesio-palatal cusp of the 1. upper molar).

Note: While the anatomical chewing surface is defined by both the marginal ridges as well as the ridge of the cusp edge, the functional chewing surface overlaps with the outside surface of the supporting cusps.

2.21 Position of Teeth in Permanent Dentition: Orientation of the Skull and Dental Occlusion

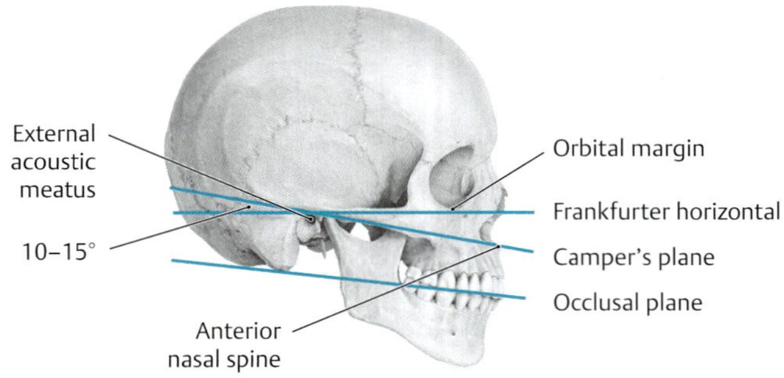

A Occlusal planes of the skull
The following planes help to evaluate the position of teeth in the jaw and orientation of the skull:

- **Frankfurt Horizontal Plane** = passing from the upper edge of the porus acusticus to the lowest point of the orbital rim.
- **Camper Plane** = according to Camper (1792), running from the superior rim of the porus acusticus externus to spina nasalis anterior. Nowadays, its clinical definition describes the plane extending between both the dorsal soft tissue points (left and right tragus) and the anterior subnasale.
- **Occlusal Plane** = running through incisal edge (see **B**) and the highest point of the disto-buccal cusp tips (see **B**) of the 2. left and right mandibular molars.

Note: While the Camper and Frankfurt plane form an angle of 10–15°, the Camper and Occlusal plane run nearly parallel to each other at a posterior angle of approximately 8°.

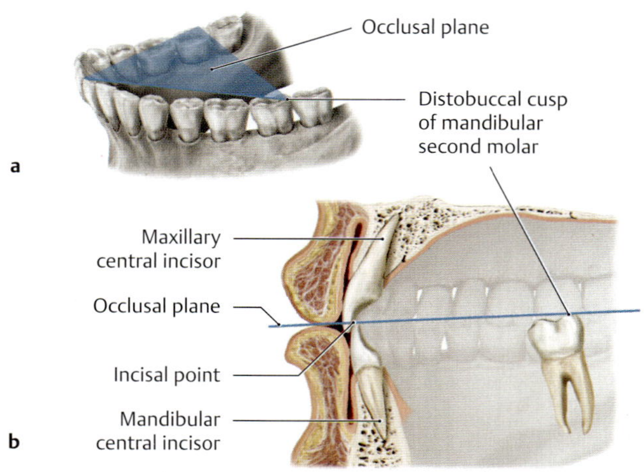

B Occlusal plane
a Left-front and above view of occlusal plane; **b** vestibular view of occlusal plane. The occlusal plane is marked by three reference points in the tooth-bearing region of the mandible:

- Incisal point (where the incisal edges of the two lower middle incisors touch)
- Tip of the disto-buccal cusp of the 2. mandibular right molar (tooth 47)
- Tip of the disto-buccal cusp of the 2. mandibular left molar (tooth 37)

Thus, the occlusal plane is situated at the height of lip closure line and runs parallel to the Camper plane (see **A**).

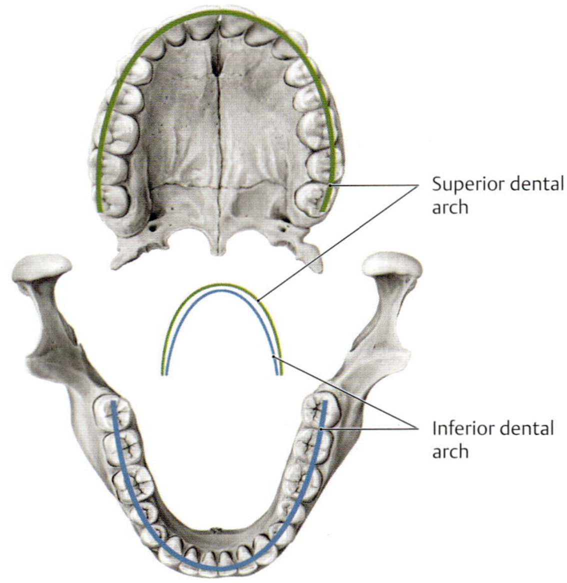

C Upper and lower dental arch
In the maxilla and mandible, the teeth are positioned in the shape of an arch (so-called dental arches: Arcus dentalis superior and inferior respectively). The dental arches relate to the curve formed by the cutting edges of the incisors, crown tips of the molars and buccal cusp tips of the premolars and molars. The Arcus dentalis superior forms a semi-ellipse and the Arcus dentalis inferior a parable. Due to the different shapes of the two dental arches, both the maxillary incisors and molars overhang their mandibular counterparts, thereby covering the incisor edges and the buccal cusps.
Note: Due to the convex proximate surfaces, the teeth forming the dental arch touch only at certain points (so-called proximal contact points). The contact points are usually situated in the upper third of the crown and help to give interdental support and stabilization of two adjacent teeth (see **B**).

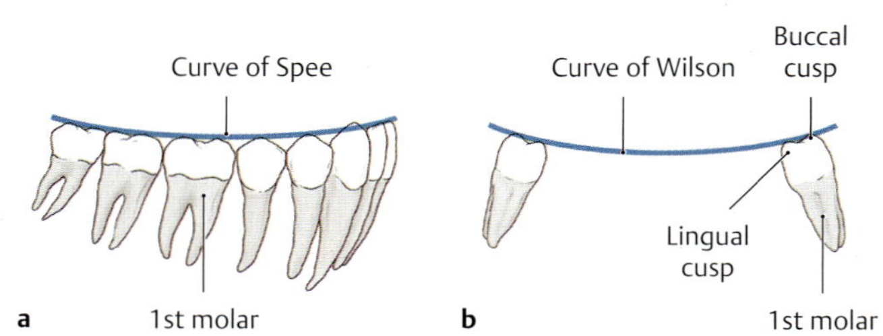

D Sagittal and transversal occlusal curve
a Sagittal occlusal curve (so-called curve of Spee), vestibular view; **b** transversal occlusal curve (so-called curve of Wilson), distal view.
If looking at the cusp tips of the mandibular toothrow from vestibular, the line connecting the buccal cusp tips forms a convex curve the lowest point of which is situated in the area around the 1. molar. According to Spee (1870), that curve touches the anterior area of the temporomandibular joint capsule; its center is supposed to be situated in the middle of the orbita. The course of the transversal occlusal curve is the result of the lingual cusps of the mandibular teeth lying lower than the buccal cusps.
Note: Both the sagittal and transversal occlusal curves are important when installing artificial teeth.

E Different types of occlusal forms

Occlusion means the contact of teeth of the maxilla and mandible. In more detail, one distinguishes between

- **static occlusion** = contacts of teeth when the jaw is not moving,
- **dynamic occlusion** = contacts made when the jaw is moving,
- **habitual occlusion** = alignment of the teeth of the upper and lower jaw when brought together.

Maximal intercuspation refers to the position of the maxilla and mandible when brought into maximum contact, meaning the cusps of the teeth of both arches fully interpose themselves with one another.

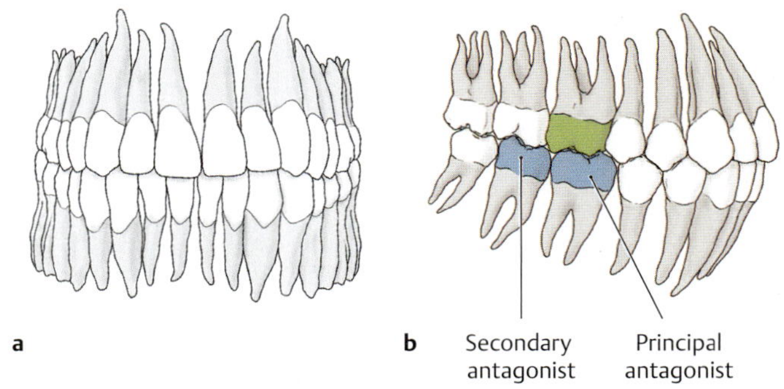

F Occlusion of tooth rows at normal occlusion

a Frontal view; **b** vestibular view.
At normal occlusion, two phenomena become visible:

- Due to the differing sizes of both dental arches, the incisal edges of the upper incisors overlap the lower incisors by approximately 3–4 mm on the vestibular (see **b** and **Ga**). The overlapping of the buccal cusps of the maxillary teeth with the mandibular teeth is attributable to the same cause. It is however not visible (see **Gc** and **d**).
- The upper middle incisor is wider than the lower middle incisor, which results in a mesiodistal shift, which extends to the posterior region (see **b** and **Gb**).

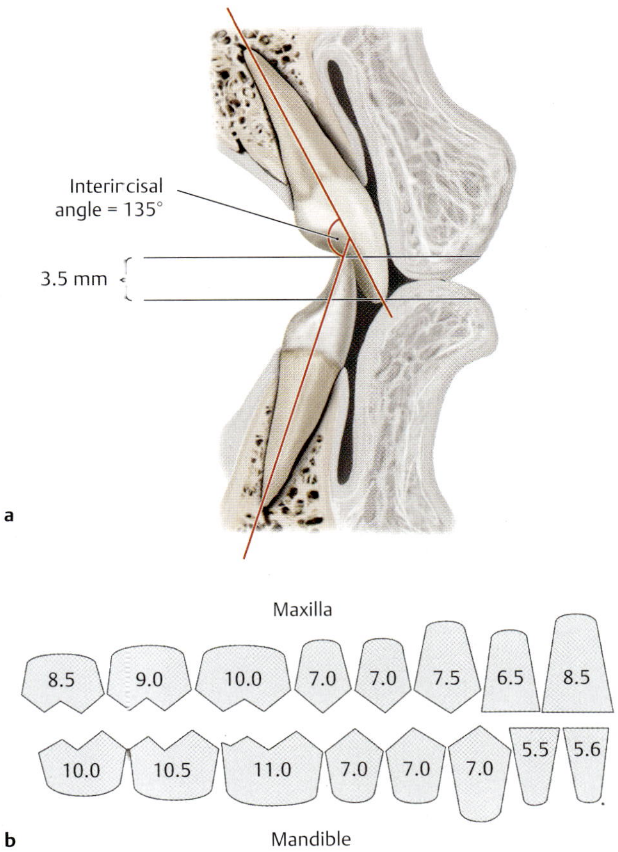

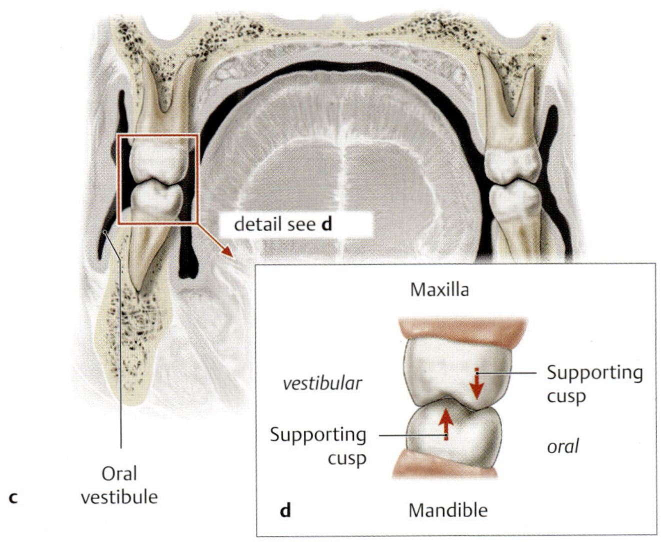

G Position of teeth at normal occlusion

a Occlusion of the upper and lower incisors; **b** schema of the teeth's position in the maxilla and mandible. Stated is the medium mesio-distal width of the teeth in millimeters; **c** normal occlusion, distal view; **d** enlarged section from image **c**.

a In the lateral view, the so-called incisor overbite (see **F**), also known as scissors bite, is clearly visible. The occlusal contacts between the lower incisors and the palatal surfaces of the upper incisors and the axes of the upper and lower incisors are at a 135° angle (*interincisal angle*) to each other.

b In the sagittal direction—with the exception of two teeth (1. lower incisor, and 3. upper molar)—every tooth is in contact with two teeth of the opposing jaw, the primary and secondary antagonist (= **one-tooth to two-teeth relationship in the posterior region**, cf. **F**). The tip of the upper canine is situated between the lower canine and the following lower premolar, the mesiobuccal cusp of the 1. upper molar points toward the mesiobuccal fissure of the 1. lower molar. This tooth position is called neutral occlusion.

c and d In transversal direction, the maxillary and mandibular buccal cusps overlap on the vestibular. The cusps, which reach into the fissure and fossa of their antagonists respectively, are called supporting and working cusp respectively and have a rather round shape unlike the non-supporting cusps. The maxillary supporting cusps are palatal cusps and buccal cusps in the mandible.

Note: The primary function of the chewing surfaces in the posterior tooth region is chopping and grinding food between the cusps. The fissures serve as drain channels for the crushed food and at the same time offer space for the cusps to grind.

2.22 Permanent Teeth Morphology

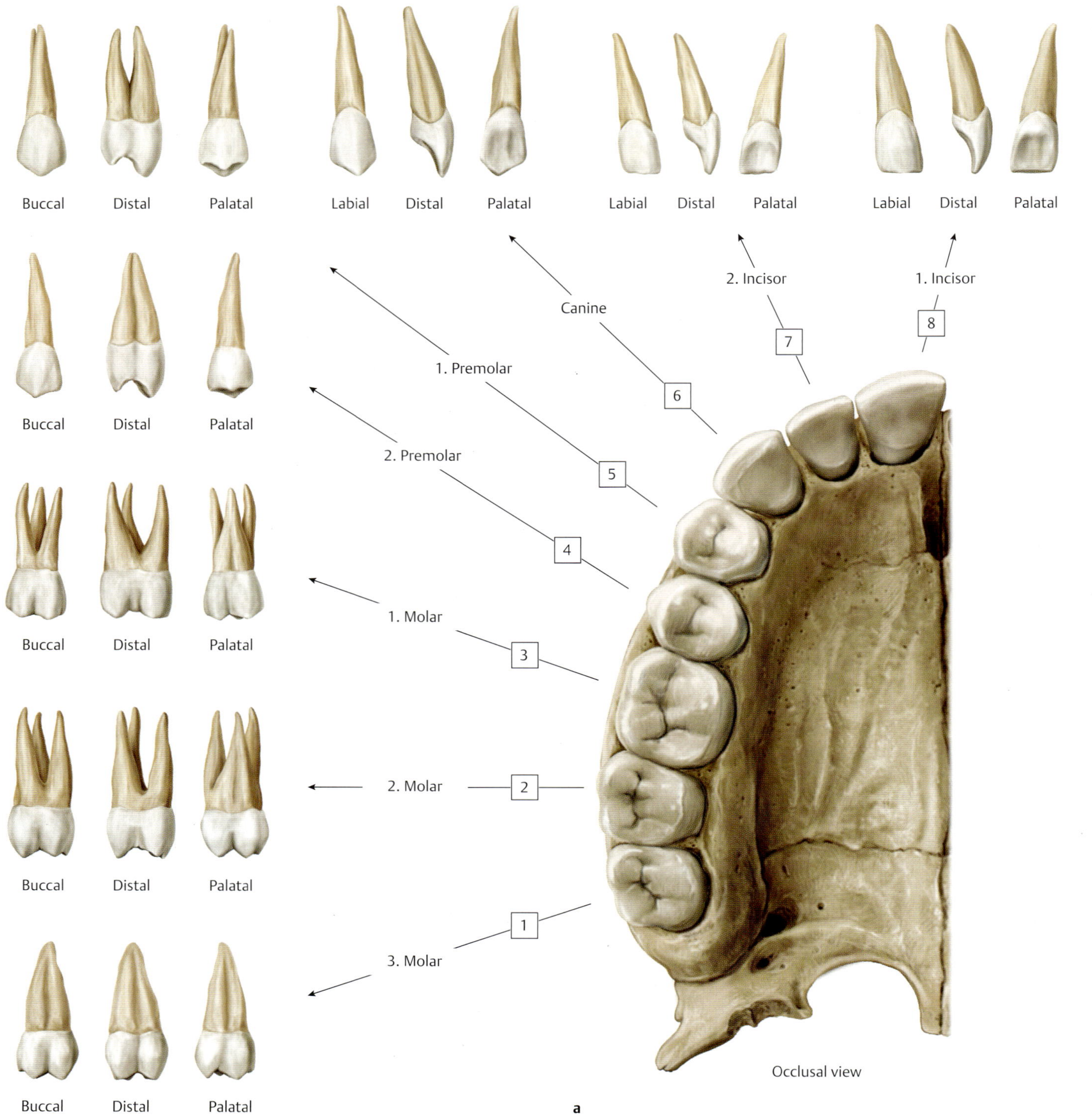

A Morphology of the permanent teeth of the maxilla and mandible

a Right maxilla, occlusal view; **b** right mandible, occlusal view (Isolated teeth shown in various views; for numeration of individual teeth cf. Dental formula, p. 50.)

Incisors (dentes incisivi): Incisors are used for cutting off chunks of food. Accordingly, they are sharp-edged (scoop-shaped). In addition, they largely determine the aesthetic appearance of the oral region. In general, all incisors are single-rooted. The upper medial incisor is the largest, the lower medial the smallest. The palatal surfaces of the two upper incisors have two marginal ridges each, in between which a tuberculum dentis is located in the medial incisor and a foramen cecum in the lateral incisor. Similar characteristics are considerably less distinct in both the lower incisors.

Canines (dentes canini): Canines are the most shape-consistent teeth. Their common characteristic is a single cusp formed by a divided incisal surface. Usually, canines are single-rooted, have a relatively long root and support the incisors (longer and more pointed canines in mammals are considered fangs). While the labial surface has two facets, the oral

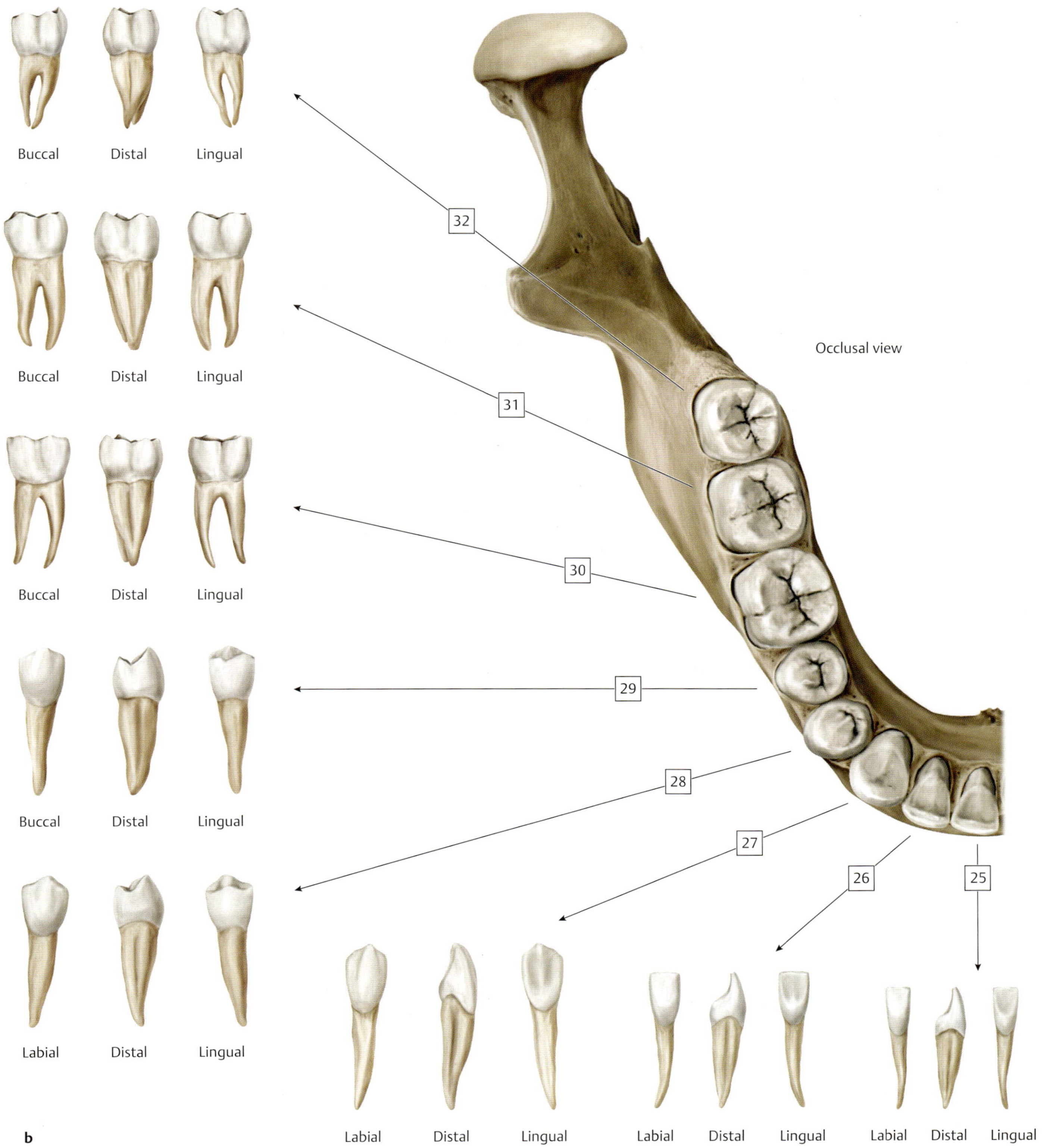

surface has two well pronounced marginal ridges, a median line and a tuberculum dentis. Root surface and curvature characteristic are well defined.

Premolars (dentes premolars): Their common characteristic is a two-cusp morsal surface with a vestibular cusp alignment. Except for the upper premolar, they have a single root. The premolars represent a transitional form from incisors to molars and have cusps and fissures. That is a sign that now it is all about grinding rather than biting off food.

Molars (dentes molars): They are the largest teeth of the permanent dentition and have a morsal suface with multiple cusps. In order to absorb the powerful chewing pressure, the maxillary molars have three roots, compared with usually two in the mandible. Only the roots of the third molars (wisdom teeth, which usually erupt not before age 16—if at all) are often fused together (see **E**, p. 49).

2.23 Periodontium

A Elements and functions of the periodontium

What holds teeth to the jaw bone is a particular form of syndesmosis, the gomphosis (dentoalveolar syndesmosis). The periodontium's functional unit includes all structures, which bind the tooth to its bony socket:

- alveolar bone
- cementum
- periodontal ligament (desmodontium)
- gum (gingiva)

Essential functions of the periodontium:

- anchoring of the tooth in the bone and transforming chewing pressure into tensile stress
- mediating sensation of pain and regulating chewing pressure through nerve fibers and sensitive nerve endings
- defending against infection through efficient separation of oral cavity and dental root region and large number of defense cells
- rapid metabolism and high regenerative capacity (adapting to functional and topographic changes for example in position of teeth as a result of orthodontic treatment) through a generous blood supply.

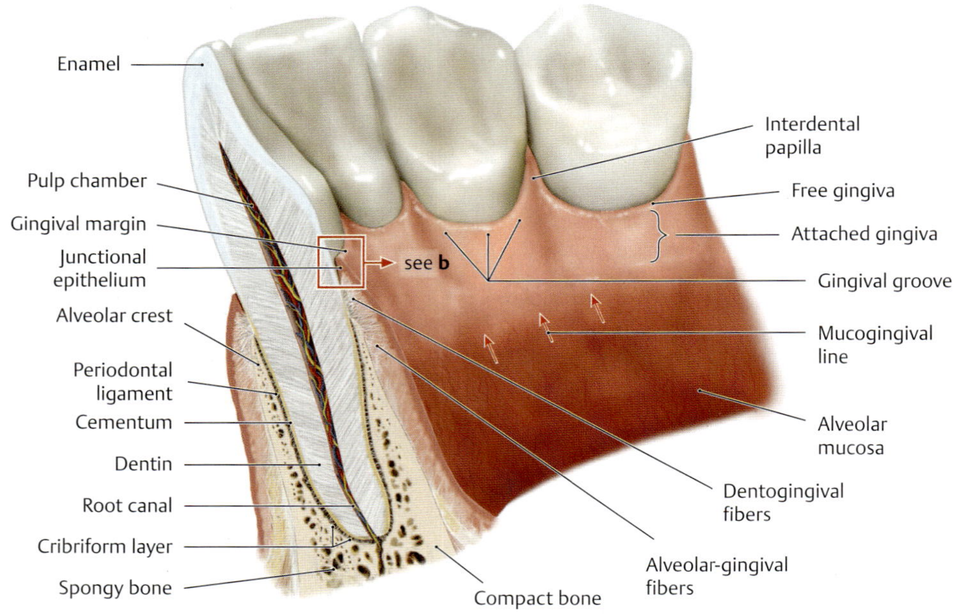

a

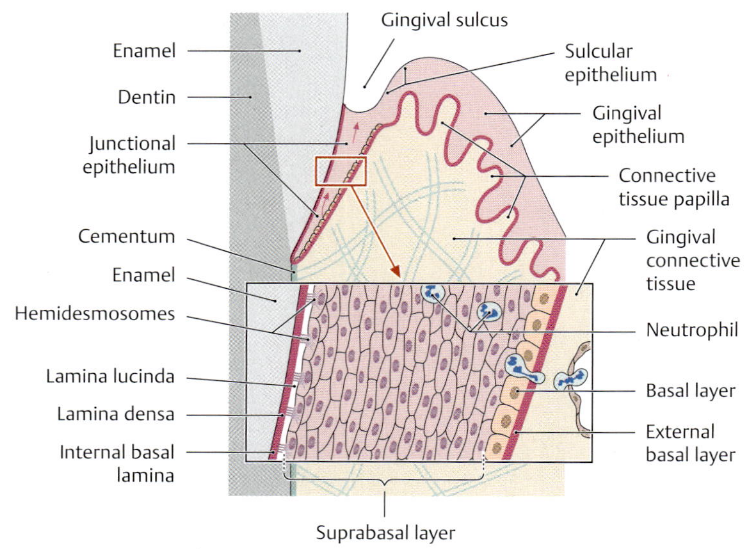

b

B Gingiva

a Gingiva at a glance; **b** junctional epithelium.

a Gingiva is part of the oral mucosa and extends from the gingival margin to the mucogingival border. There, the gingival epithelium (multi-layered, usually parakeratinized stratified squamous epithelium), which has a light pink shade, blends into the considerably more reddish alveolar epithelium (multi-layered, not parakeratinized stratified squamous epithelium). There is a clinical distinction between two sections:

- free gingiva (1–2 mm wide) = gingival margin, surrounds the neck of the tooth like a cuff and is attached to the cervical enamel. The gingival sulcus is a 0.5–1 mm deep channel that extends around the tooth. At the bottom edge of the sulcus is the junctional epithelium (see **b**);
- attached gingiva (3–7 mm wide): begins at the height of the gingival sulcus and extends to the mucogingival border. Since it is attached to both the neck of the tooth and the alveolar crest through dentogingival fibers, which run horizontally, it often has a speckled texture.

b The junctional epithelium attaches to the cementum surface by hemidesmosomes and basal lamina thereby ensuring a complete attachment of the oral mucosa to the tooth surface. It becomes broader in the apical-coronal direction. The deep outer layer of basal lamina represents the border to the gingival connective tissue and further extends to the basal lamina of the oral sulcus epithelium. The junctional epithelium differs from the other epitheliums in the oral cavity in several aspects:

- it consists of only two layers: stratum basale and stratum suprabasale;
- at its base, it lacks connective tissue papillae;
- it has a high cell turnover (formation of new cells every 4–6 days): While the cuboid basal cells are responsible for cell replenishment, the daughter cells differentiate into flattened cells, which are aligned parallel to the tooth surface. Further toward the gingival sulcus where they are rejected, these cell layers constantly form new hemidesmosomes while dissolving old ones;
- it has a particular immune defense (neutrophil granulocytes constantly move around the junctional epithelium).

Note: The integrity of the junctional epithelium is a precondition for the health of the entire periodontium. If bacterial colonization leads to inflammation of the neck of the tooth (typical plaque formation as a result of poor oral hygiene), the junctional epithelium loses its attachment to the tooth and gingival pockets form in the area around the gingival sulcus (periodontosis).

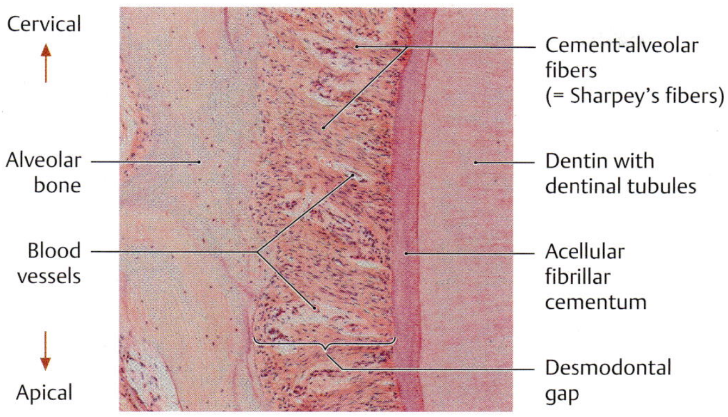

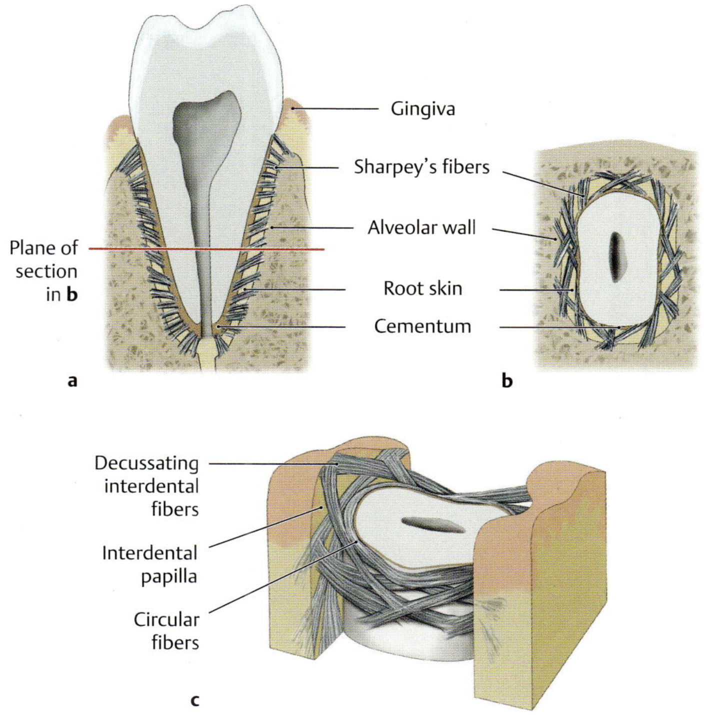

C Periodontal ligament (desmodontium)

The periodontal ligament is a highly vascularized, cell- and fiber-rich connective tissue, which fills the 200µm wide gap between cementum-covered root element and alveolar bone. It consists of a complex system of collagen fibers (cementum or dental alveolar collagen fiber bundles), which holds the tooth in place in the bony socket in a spring-like manner. The collagen fibers, also known as *Sharpey's fibers*, are attached to both the cementum and alveolar bone. The fibers run in different directions (see **D**), which enables them to counteract all movements of the tooth (axial pressure, lateral tilt, and torsional motion) and develop tension. The tensile stress, which is constantly present during the chewing process, helps stimulate permanent regeneration in bones and collagen fibers. In addition, highly active fibroblasts are responsible for a high turnover of collagen fibers in the periodontal ligament. Their collagen synthesis, which is dependent on vitamin C, occurs four times faster compared to skin synthesis (which explains rapid fiber loss as a result of vitamin C deficiency). In a toothless jaw, the alveolar process gradually atrophies, a fact that further underscores the significance of masticatory forces for the bone.

D Course of collagen fibers in the periodontal ligament and gingiva

a and **b** Longitudinal and cross section of the tooth; **c** schematic course of gingival fibers

While the cementoalveolar fiber bundles in the periodontal ligament are usually oriented obliquely (slanted downward) (**a**), the supra-alveolar fiber apparatus consists of mainly bundles, which run in a circular direction around the circumference of the tooth (**c**).

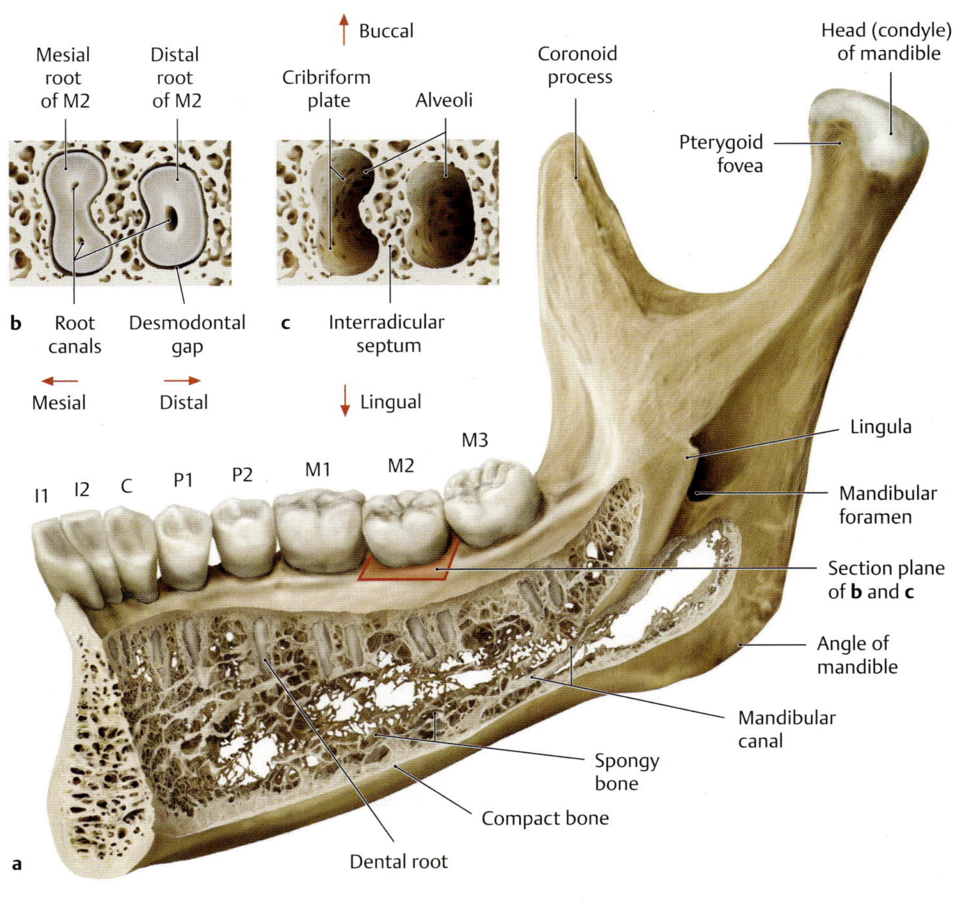

E Structure of the alveolar bone

a Right side of a human mandible, oral view (the compact layer of bone on the mandible is removed); **b** and **c** horizontal section of tooth sockets with (**b**) and without dental roots (**c**). Cranial view (based on prepared specimen slides, part of the anatomical collection of the University of Kiel).

With regard to their structure, the alveolar processes of maxilla and mandible are lamellar bones with an inner (lingual/palatal) and outer (vestibular/buccal) compact layer as well as a central spongy layer, which lies in between. An additional component is the alveolar bone, which forms part of the alveolar pocket (socket). The alveolar sockets resemble cups with numerous holes in their bony walls, the cribriform layer of bone. Blood and lymphatic vessels enter the periodontal ligament through these holes into the desmodontal gap where they form a dense latticework surrounding the dental roots.

2.24 Deciduous Teeth

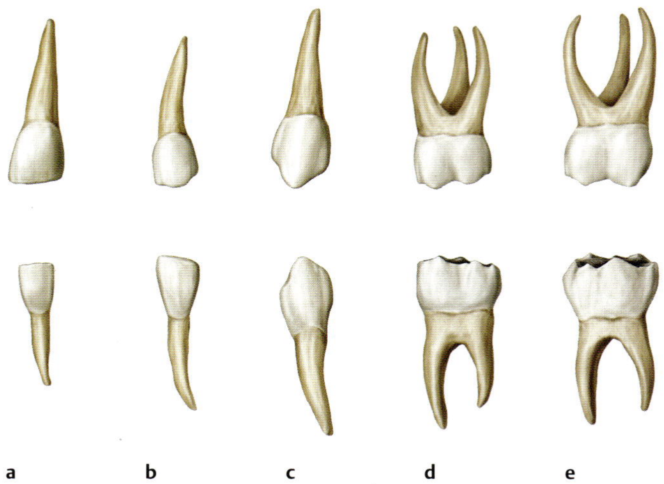

A Deciduous teeth of the left maxilla and mandible
The deciduous dentition consists of 20 teeth. We distinguish between

a medial incisor
b lateral incisor
c canine
d 1st molar
e 2nd molar

B Average age of eruption of teeth (according to Rauber/Kopsch)
Eruption of the deciduous teeth is called primary (1.) dentition and the eruption of the permanent teeth secondary dentition. The last column lists the chronological order in which the teeth erupt. For instance: For the 2. dentition, the anterior molar (tooth 6) is the first to erupt (six-year molar).
Note: Deciduous teeth are given Roman numerals and the permanent teeth Arabic numbers.

1. Dentition	Tooth	Eruption	Order
	I	6–8 months	1
	II	8–12 months	2
	III	15–20 months	4
	IV	12–16 months	3 "1st milk molar"
	V	20–40 months	5 "2nd milk molar"
2. Dentition	Tooth	Eruption	Order
	1	6–9 years	2
	2	7–10 years	3
	3	9–14 years	5
	4	9–13 years	4
	5	11–14 years	6
	6	6–8 years	1 "six-year molar"
	7	10–14 years	7 "twelve-year molar"
	8	16–30 years	8 "wisdom tooth"

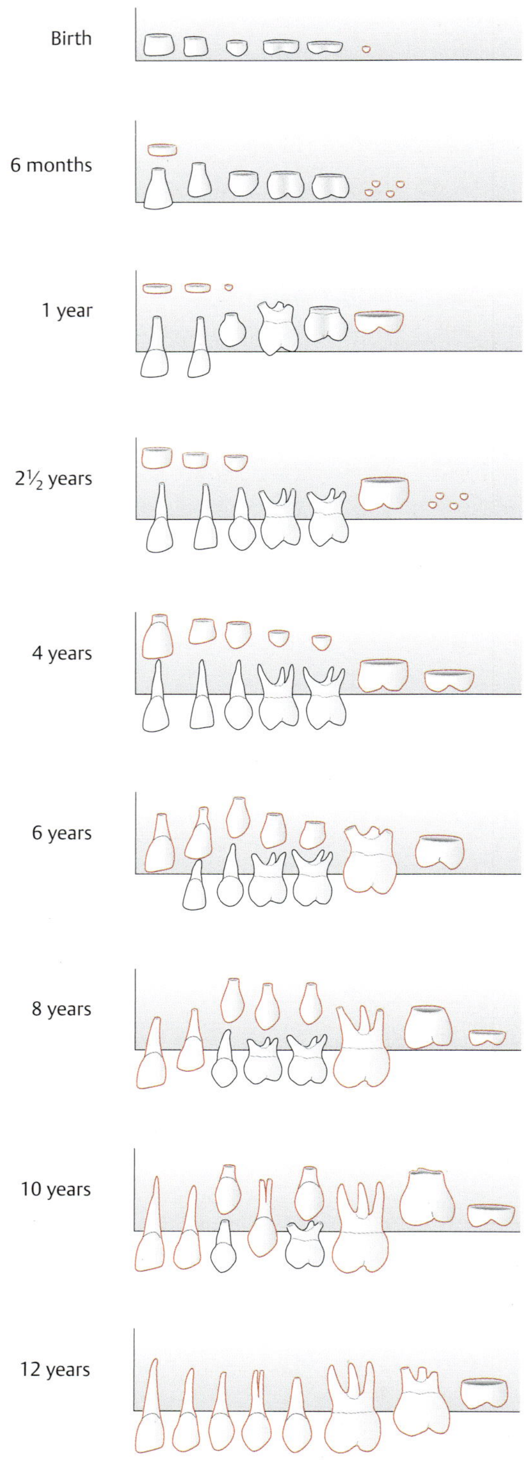

C Eruption of deciduous and permanent teeth
The left maxilla serves as an example to show the tooth eruption pattern (deciduous teeth in black, permanent teeth in red). Knowledge of the eruption pattern is clinically important since corresponding data helps to diagnose growth delay in children.

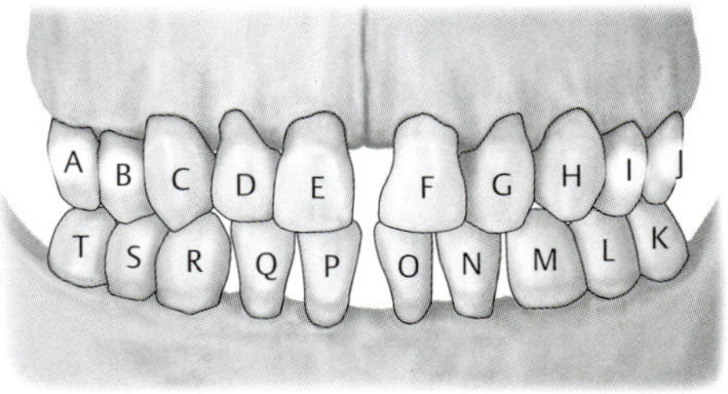

D Dental chart of the deciduous dentition

E Deciduous teeth and underlying permanent teeth in the maxilla and mandible of a 6 year old

a and **b** Frontal view; **c** and **d** left view. The anterior bone lamella above the roots of the deciduous teeth has been removed, the underlying permanent teeth are visible.

A six year old was chosen because at that age all deciduous teeth have erupted and are all still present. Yet, at the same time, the anterior molar has started to erupt as the first permanent tooth (see **C**).

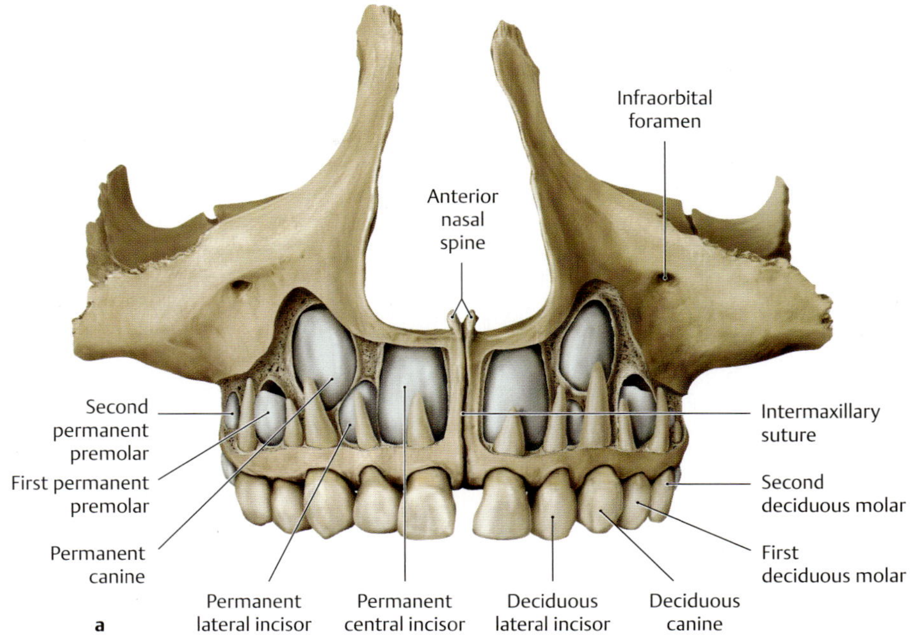

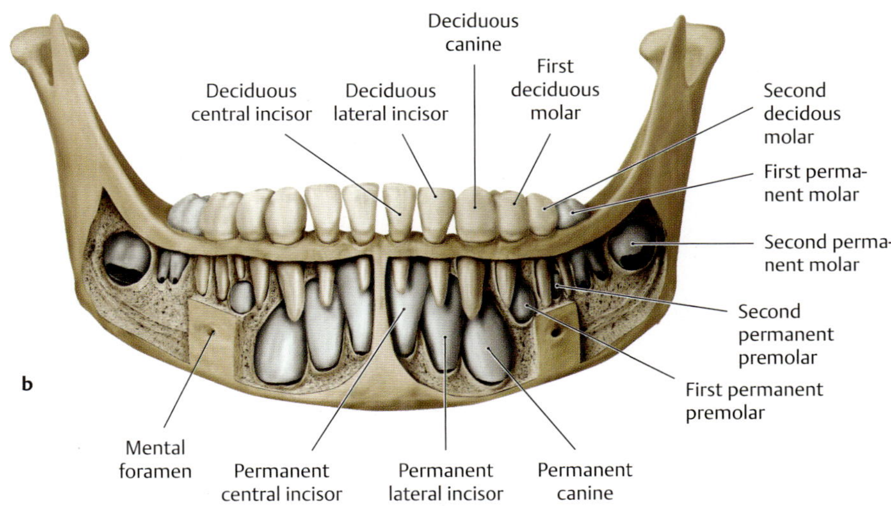

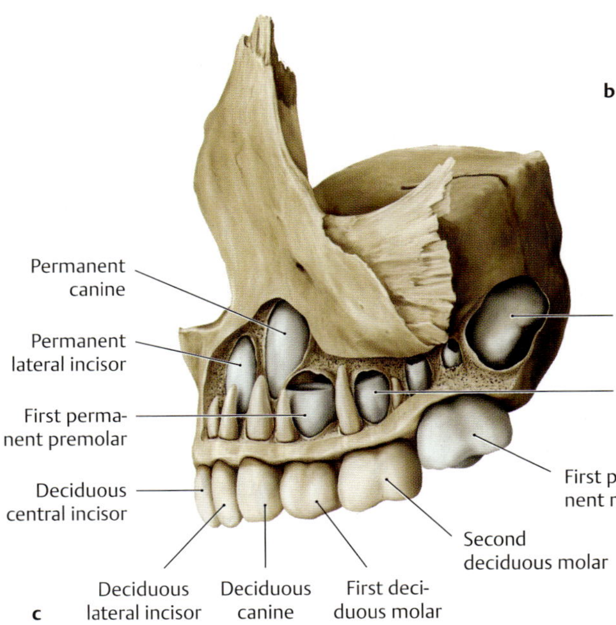

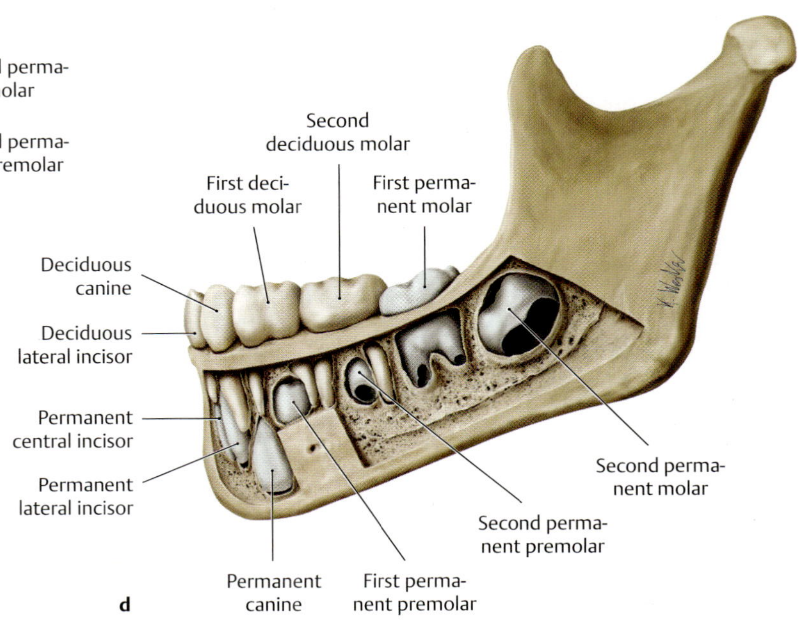

2.25 Tooth Development (Odontogenesis)

A Early stage of tooth development in the mandible of a human embryo
View of a mandible at the beginning of the 7th week of embryonic development (with the coronal cut at the height of the enamel caps of the second primary molar). Localized epithelial thickening presents the first morphologically verifiable sign of the start of tooth development. They run in a horseshoe shape parallel to the lip line and grow into the mesenchyme of the maxilla and mandible of a five-week-old human embryo (cf. **Ba**). In mesial-distal direction, the free margins on both sides of the general dental lamina thickens to form 5 tooth buds each, equal to the 10 primary teeth in both lower and upper jaw. Subsequently, each of these tooth epithelial buds transforms first into cap-shaped and later bell-shaped enamel organs (cf. **Bb** and **c**).

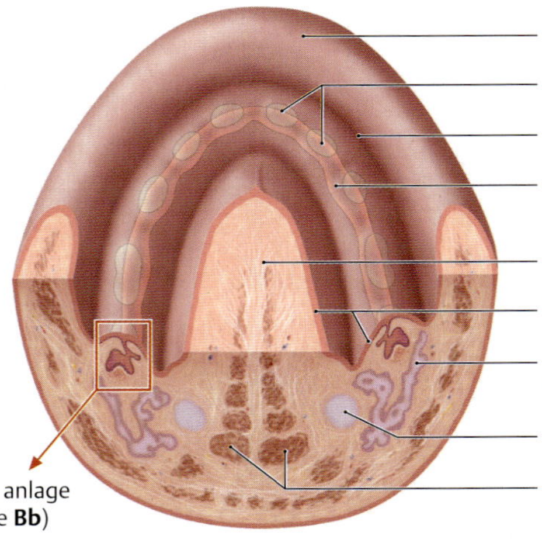

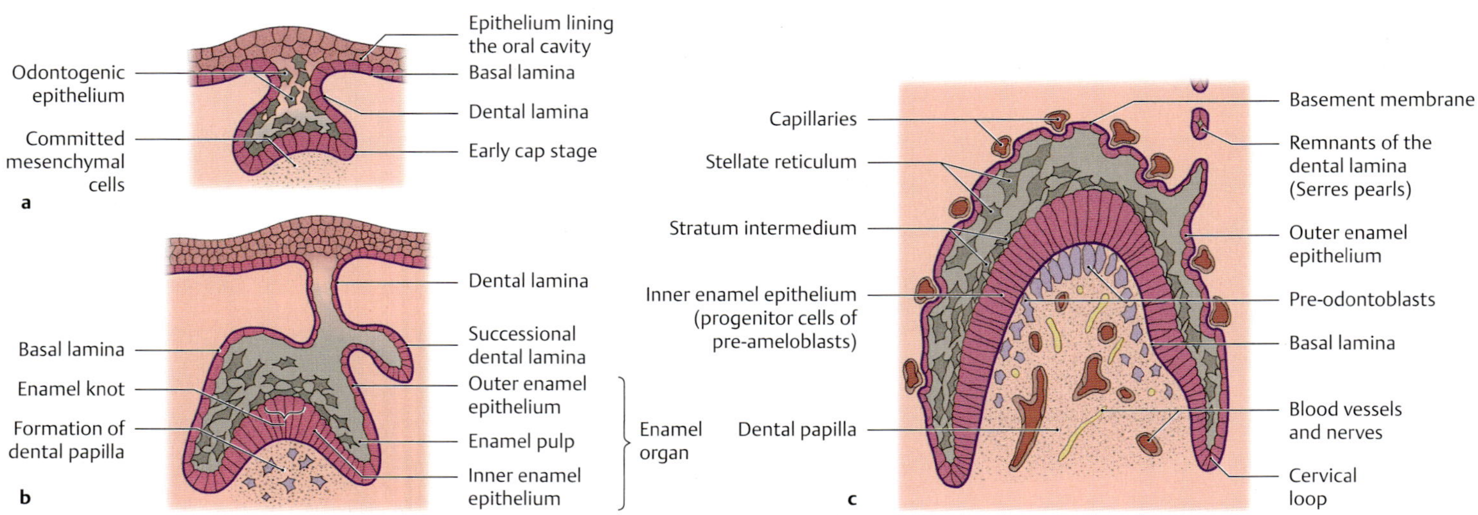

B Early stage of tooth development and formation of tooth germs
a Early cap stage; **b** late cap stage; **c** bell stage (according to Weiss). In the human embryo, primary teeth begin to develop in the 5th week. At around 3 months of gestation (15–19 embryonic week), the hard tissue that surrounds the teeth starts to form.

Early Cap stage: Bud- and cap-shaped collections of cells develop as a result of intensive cell proliferation in the odontogenic epithelium. Their concavity deepens at the far side of the epithelium and starting from the margin they grow around the mesenchyme (see **C**).

Late Cap stage:

- The enamel organ is composed of an inner and outer enamel epithelium and the stellate reticulum, which lies in between. The cells of the inner enamel epithelium grow increasingly columnar-shaped on the basal lamina particularly around the enamel knot. Increasing extracellular matrix production (stellate reticulum) leads to further separation of the outer and inner enamel epithelium layers. Cells of the outer enamel epithelium spread further apart in the enamel pulp.
- Starting from the palatal (maxilla) and lingual (mandible) margin of the dental lamina, the permanent (successional) dental lamina starts to develop and forms the basis for the formation of the permanent teeth of the secondary dentition.

Note: The permanent teeth (molars of the permanent dentition), which are located distally from the primary dentition result from the dental lamina, which elongates distally.

Bell stage:

- The stellate reticulum becomes increasingly more voluminous and divides into a loose mid-zone (stratum reticulum proper) and a cellular layer (stratum intermedium) immediately next to the inner enamel epithelium.
- The cells of the inner enamel epithelium develop into precursor cells for the pre-ameloblasts. Their secretions are responsible for the formation of the adjacent mesenchymal cells into the future pre-odontoblasts.
- The thickening of the basement membrane located between pre-ameloblasts and pre-odontoblasts leads to the transformation of the membrana perforata. In the area around the cervical loop, the basement membrane of the inner enamel epithelium continues into the basement membrane of the outer enamel epithelium thereby covering the entire surface of the enamel organ. Capillaries on the outer layer of the basement membrane provide its nourishment.
- The connection of the developing enamel organ to the dental lamina becomes increasingly weaker until the lamina almost completely dissolves.
- With increasing expansion of the growing tooth bud the loose mesenchymal tissue, which surrounds the enamel organ and dental papilla, thickens into the dental sac from which the periodontium later develops (see **E**).

Shortly before the hard tissue starts to develop (cf. **D**), the tooth bud consists of a bell-shaped enamel organ, dental papilla, and the dental sac.

C Epithelial-mesenchymal interaction (according to Schroeder)
The development of primary teeth results from the interaction of surface ectoderm (epithelium of the primitive oral cavity) and mesenchyme (of the cranial neural crest), which lies underneath. This interaction leads to clusters of highly specialized cells, the odontoblasts and ameloblasts. They in turn, induce secretion of dental hard tissue predentin and enamel matrix through growth and differentiation factors (e.g. BMPs = bone morphogenetic proteins, FGFs = fibroblast growth factors, SHh = sonic hedgehog) (see **D**).
Note: The growth and differentiation factors are concentrated in the enamel knot (see **Bb**), which are the localized thickenings of the dental lamina where the primary teeth will later develop. Thus, enamel knots have a signaling function for tooth development (e.g., for shape of crowns and number of cusps) and resemble the ectodermal ridges, which regulate limb bud development.

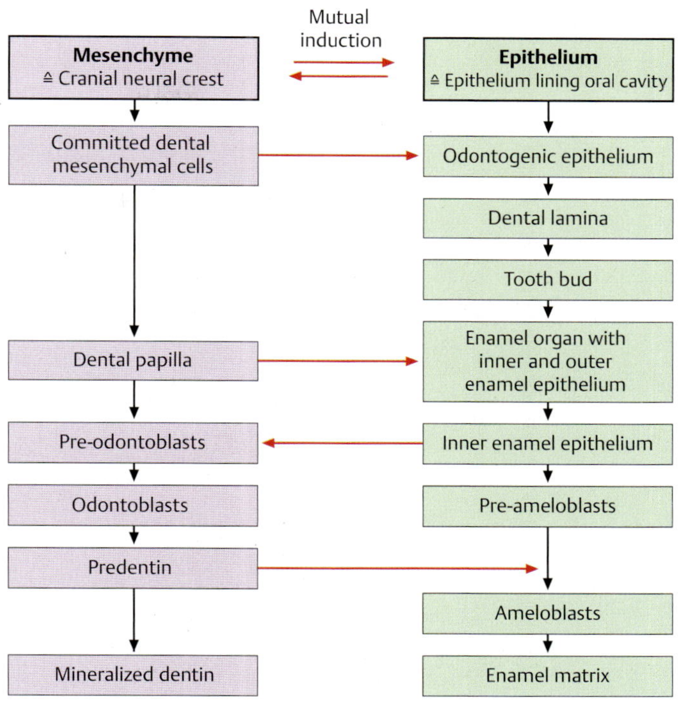

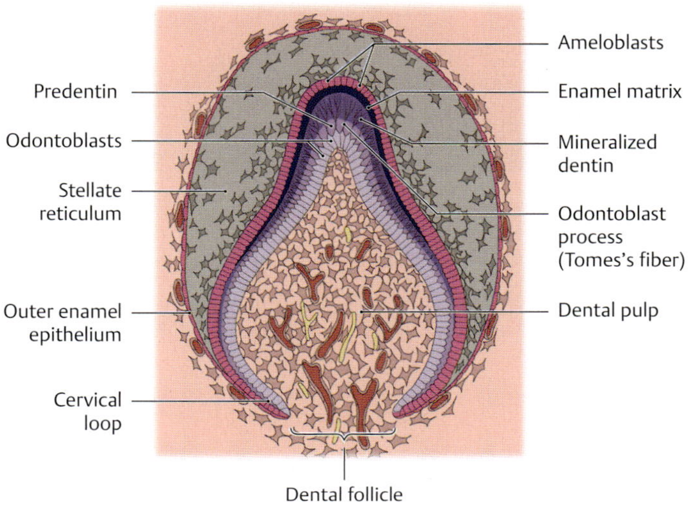

D Formation of dental hard tissues forming the crown
The formation of dental hard tissue around the forming crown is—similar to the early development stages—the result of a series of processes of mutual induction (see **Ba–c**). The thickening of the basement membrane (membrana perforata, see **Bc**) leads to the transformation of pre-odontoblasts into odontoblasts and the start of the synthesis of predentin, which is deposited in the area of the basement membrane. This process, in turn, induces differentiation of pre-ameloblasts into secretory ameloblasts. With the layer of predentin deposited, the ameloblasts start releasing organic enamel matrix. With the dissolution of the basement membrane (membrana perforata), the enamel is now directly adjacent to the dentin and the deposition gradually spreads toward the cervix (neck) of the crown. With the two dental hard tissues continuing to form, the odontoblasts and ameloblasts move further apart in opposite directions. The ameloblasts secrete column-shaped enamel rods, which will later mineralize and extend from the enamel-dentin junction to the enamel surface. The ameloblasts will become inactive when the enamel layer is completed and are eventually sloughed when the tooth erupts. As a result, enamel is cell-free and cannot repair itself. The odontoblasts also recede with increasing formation of dentin, yet leave behind a thin process (odontoblastic process or "Tomes fiber") in a small channel within the dentin (dentinal tubule), which permeates the entire dentin layer. The odontoblast cell bodies are positioned at the pulp-dentin junction and are able to continually form dentin throughout the life of the tooth.
Note: While the crown formation of the primary teeth is complete by the time a baby is between 2 and 6 months old, the formation of the root in the primary dentition takes approximately 2–3 years from the time the tooth erupts.

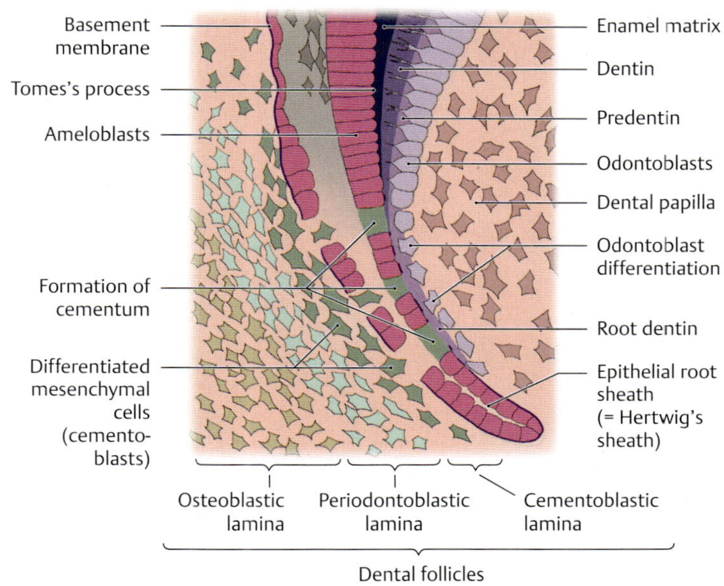

E Root formation and differentiation of the dental sac
The formation of the root begins once enamel and dentin have developed in the area of the crown. It organizes along the epithelial root sheath (Hertwig epithelial root sheath)—a two-layered epithelium (inner and outer enamel epithelium lie directly on top of each other, the stellate reticulum is absent). The epithelial root sheath grows from the cervical loop in an apical direction. In teeth with multiple roots, the epithelial root sheath induces differentiation of odontoblasts, which in turn start to synthesize dentin. The resulting pulp cavity increasingly narrows in an apical direction creating one or more root canals so nerves and vessels can enter and exit the dental pulp. With progressing dissolution of the epithelial root sheath (from cervical to apical), the mesenchyme cells of the dental sac contact the root dentin and start forming cementum (lamina cementoblastica). Further peripheral in the adjacent mesenchyme of the dental sac, the root dentin induces formation of the future periodontal ligament and alveolar bone.

2.26 Dental Radiology

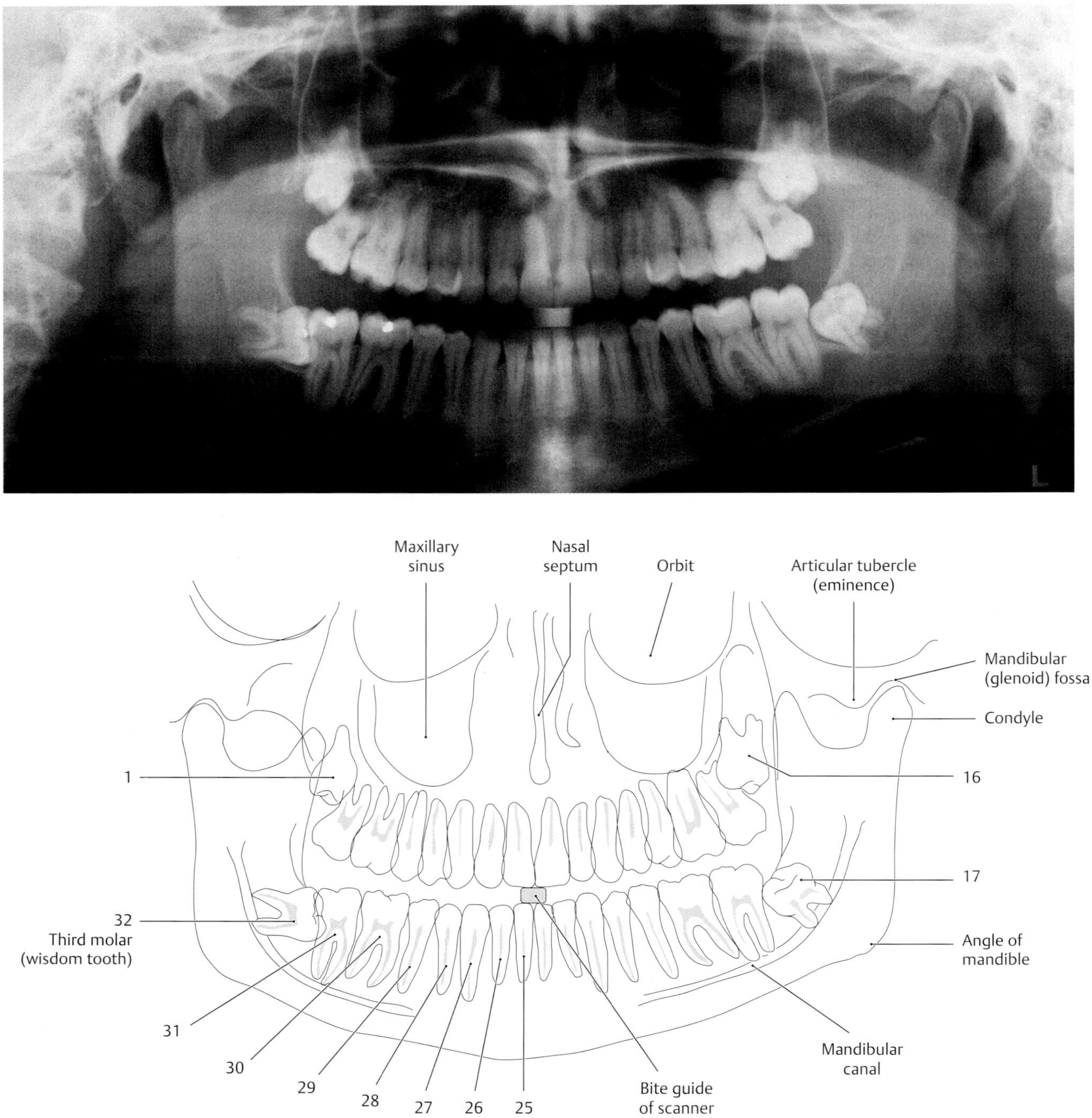

A Panoramic tomogram and orthopanotomogram
The panoramic tomogram is a topogram, which provides a first overview of the temporomandibular joints, cavities and bones as well as the condition of the teeth (carious lesions, position of wisdom teeth). In this imaging technique, X-ray tube and film move around the planes to be shown while blurring the images of the structures lying outside of the focal zone. Corresponding to the shape of the jaw, the plane in the panoramic tomogram is parabolic. The image of the dentition shown here indicates that removal of the wisdom teeth is advisable since they either have not yet fully erupted (1, 16, and 17) or are in transverse position and thus cannot erupt (32). If based on the panoramic tomogram, caries can be suspected, single tooth radiographs of the affected region are taken. Their higher resolution allows for a more refined diagnosis (see **C–H**). In addition to the conventional (analogue) technique, which uses an X-ray film as image receptor, digital X-ray technology is increasingly used, in which a sensor transforms the absorbed X-rays into digital signals and displays them on a computer screen. A substantial advantage of this technology is the lower level of radiation exposure through shorter exposure time and the easy transfer of data.
Note: The upper incisors are wider than the lower incisors leading to the interlocking of cusps and fissures (see p. 53).
(We thank FB Zahnärztliches Röntgen, UKE Hamburg-Eppendorf, Prof. U. J. Rother, D.D.S., and Dr. Christian Scheifele for kindly providing the radiograph on this page.)

B Single tooth radiographs

Single tooth radiographs are detailed X-rays of an individual tooth and its neighboring teeth. Generally, orthoradial images are taken in which the X-ray beam is directed vertically to the tangent to the dental arch or, to put in simpler terms, linearly from outside toward the tooth. Thus, the X-ray shows all structures that follow each other in the beam path consecutively so that they overlap. Thus, in teeth with multiple roots, the individual root canals cannot be clearly evaluated (see **C**). This is only possible with the help of so-called eccentric images, in which the X-ray beam is directed to the tangent in a particular angle, so that consecutive structures are clearly distinguishable. One particular type of single tooth radiograph is the so-called bitewing X-ray (see **H**), in which only an image of the crown is taken instead of the entire tooth. The patient bites the teeth together on a small piece of film, allowing for the display of maxillary and mandibular teeth at the same time, which helps detection of tooth decay underneath fillings or on the contact surfaces.

(Our thanks to Dr. med. Dent. Christian Friedrichs for his permission to use the X-rays on this page.)

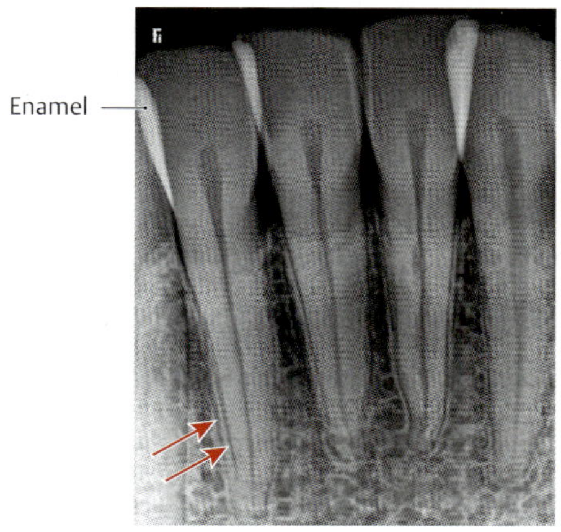

C Mandible front, teeth 23–26

Single-rooted teeth, like the incisors shown here, have two root canals in a third of all cases. The orthoradial image shows a cross section of the dental root and a double periodontal space (see arrows). If the tooth has in fact two root canals, it cannot be determined with the help of the orthoradial image (see **B**).

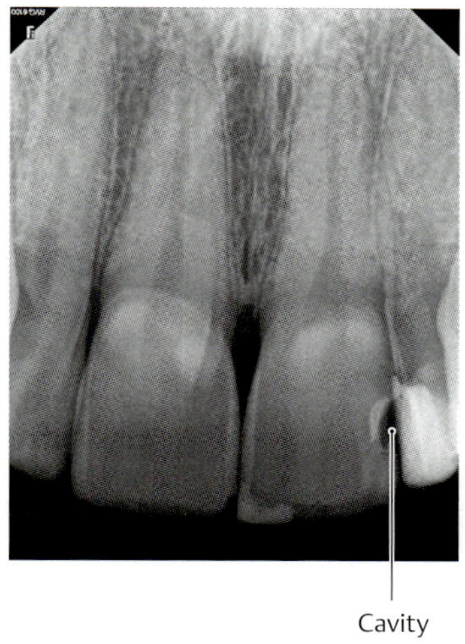

D Maxilla front, teeth 7–10

The bright spots shown here in tooth 9 distal can indicate tooth decay, open cavities or such as in this case, old, non X-ray opaque filling material. Underfilling material is slightly X-ray opaque.

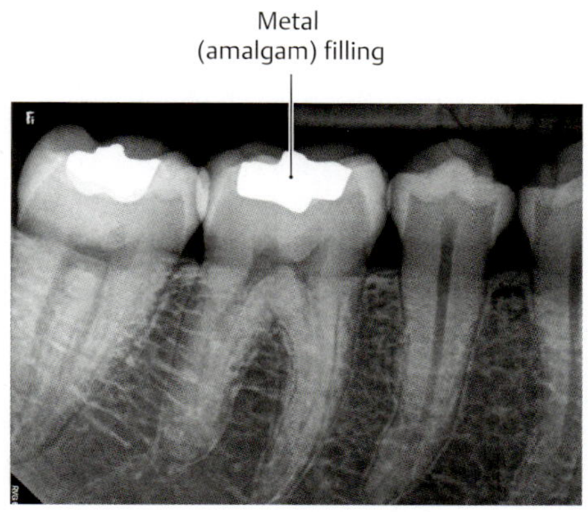

E Mandible side teeth, 28–31

Metal-dense X-ray shadows as those shown here near the crowns of teeth 30 and 31 can be the result of metal inlays, crowns, amalgam fillings, or modern zinc oxide ceramics.

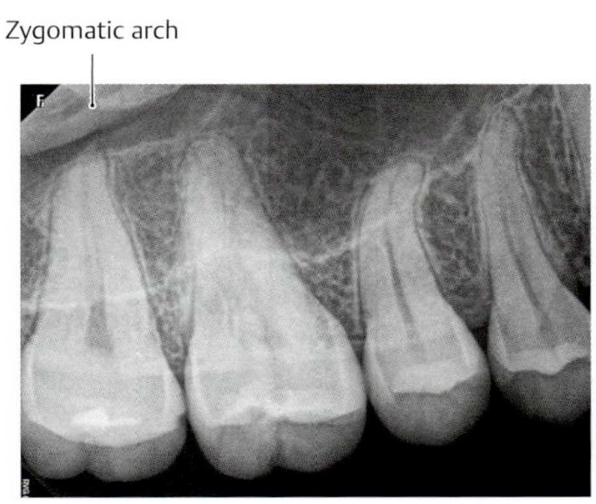

F Maxilla side teeth, 2–5

In the lateral tooth area of the maxilla, superimposition of teeth and zygomatic arch frequently occurs, shown here in the upper left margin. The roots of the molars are less clearly visible.

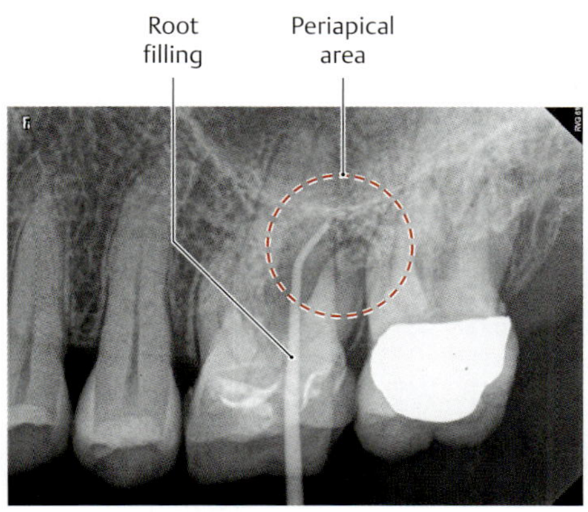

G Maxilla side teeth with pathological finding, teeth 12–15

An infection of the root canal system, which has spread to the periapical bone can lead to the formation of a fistula. In order to be able to exactly locate the infection, a gutta-percha root-filling peg is inserted into the fistula from outside. Around the distobuccal dental root of tooth 14, a bright spot indicating the infection is visible. Tooth 15 has been capped with a crown.

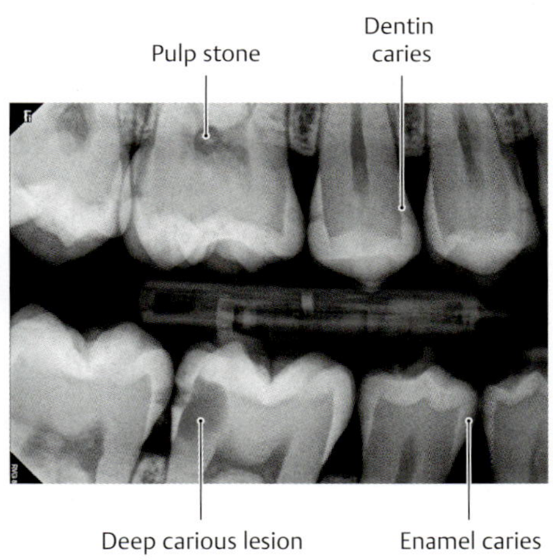

H Bitewing image for caries diagnosis

Massive carious damage at tooth 30 distal. Enamel caries and partial beginning of dentinal caries at the contact points of almost all teeth. In addition to the occlusal planes, the contact points represent typical caries predilection sites. Partly visible in the lumen of the pulp chambers are pulp stones.

2.27 Dental Local Anesthesia

A Anatomical facts and local anesthesia technique

Knowledge of the topographic anatomy of the head and neck is crucial when administering local anesthesia for dental procedures. Of particular significance here is the course of the trigeminal nerve. As the largest cranial nerve, it provides sensory innervation to the tooth-supporting parts of the maxilla and mandible (alveolar bone, teeth, and gingiva). In addition, a thorough understanding of the topography of the osseous structures is indispensable because they are of greater importance for needle direction than the soft tissue. Two of the most popular injection techniques are infiltration- and block anesthesia (see below). Vasoconstrictor is an additional component of local anesthetic solutions (for example adrenaline), which prolongs the local anesthetic duration, prevents increased plasma levels and greater risk of toxicity reactions, and decreases the risk of bleeding. In order to eliminate the risk of an accidental intravascular injection it is important to always aspirate when performing infiltration and block anesthesia. Among the most serious side effects in case of an accidental vascular puncture are cardiovascular and anaphylactic reactions.

a

b

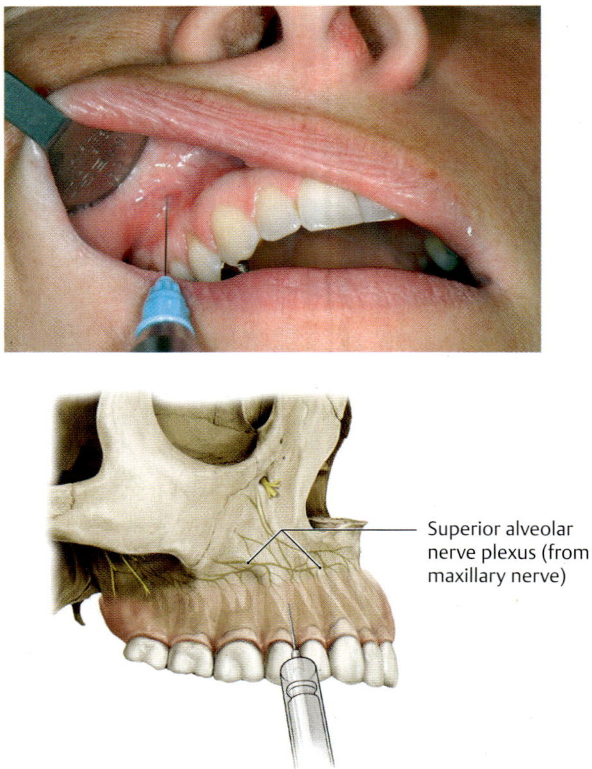

B Principle of infiltration anesthesia

a Injection technique performed on patient; **b** schematic diagram illustrating loss of sensation.

Infiltration anesthesia is the technique most commonly used in odontology (see **C** for injection technique). It is particularly suitable for a range of maxilla procedures. The maxilla is predominantly spongy bone with an extremely thin layer of compact bone facilitating diffusion of the anesthetic through the bone to the apex of the tooth. When administering infiltration anesthesia, local anesthetic solution floods the terminal nerve endings thus blocking them. The anesthetic is usually deposited supraperiosteally in the apical area of the affected tooth.

Note: Due to the significantly thicker cortical bone of the mandible, the diffusion rate surrounding the mandibular molar areas is considerably lower. This is the main reason why block anesthesia is used for mandibular procedures (see **D** and **E**).

C Infiltration anesthesia technique

- penetrate oral mucosa in the area near the apex
- place needle toward bone
- advance the needle until you can feel it meet bony resistance, parallel to the tooth axis in a 30 degree angle to the bone surface
- aspirate area
- slowly inject local anesthetic solution (1ml/30s) while maintaining bone contact
- remove needle from oral cavity
- wait for anesthetic to diffuse while monitoring the patient

D Frequently used methods of block anesthesia in oral and maxillofacial surgery

(From Daublaender M. Lokalanesthesie in der Zahn, Mund – und Kieferheilkunde. In van Aken H, Wulf H. Lokalanaesthesie, Regionalanaesthesie, Regionale Schmerztherapie. 3. Aufl. Stuttgart: Thieme: 2010)

The goal of block anesthesia is the complete and reversible blockage of an entire sensitive peripheral nerve. What is crucial is the exact deposition of a sufficient volume of anesthetic (solution) in an area with close topographical connection to the relevant nerve—for example, where the nerve enters or exits the bone channel.

Nerve	Innervation Area	Injection Site	Volume
Maxilla			
Infraorbital n.	Alveolar extension/ appendage, vestibular mucosa and maxillary front teeth, upper lip, lateral aspect of the nose and anterior cheek	Infraorbital foramen	1–1.5 ml
Nasopalatine n.	Palatal mucosa in area surrounding front teeth	Incisive foramen	0.1–0.2 ml
Greater palatine n.	Palatal mucosa running up to the canine teeth of relevant side	Greater palatine foramen	0.3–0.5 ml
Posterior superior alveolar nn.	Alveolar extension, vestibular mucosa and molar teeth	Maxillary tuberosity	1–1.8 ml
Mandible			
Inferior alveolar n.	Alveolar extension. Lingual mucosa and mandible teeth of respective side, vestibular mucosa in area around front teeth	Mandibular foramen	1.5–2 ml
Buccal n.	Vestibular mucosa in molar area		0.5 ml
Mental n.	Vestibular mucosa in front teeth area	Mental foramen	0.5–1 ml

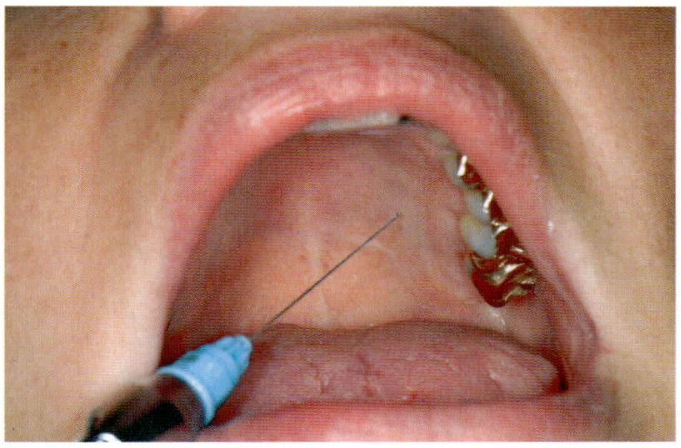

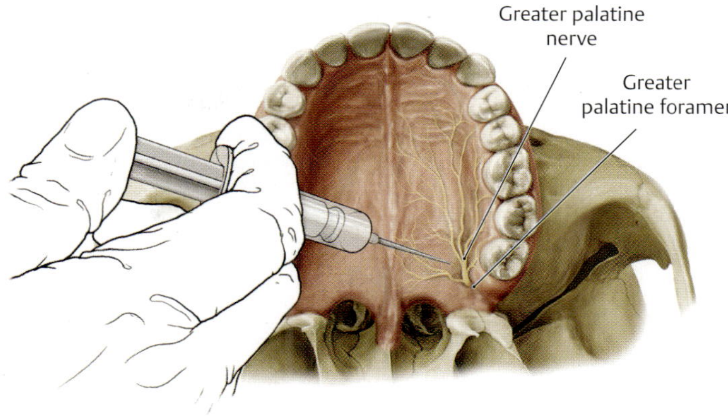

a

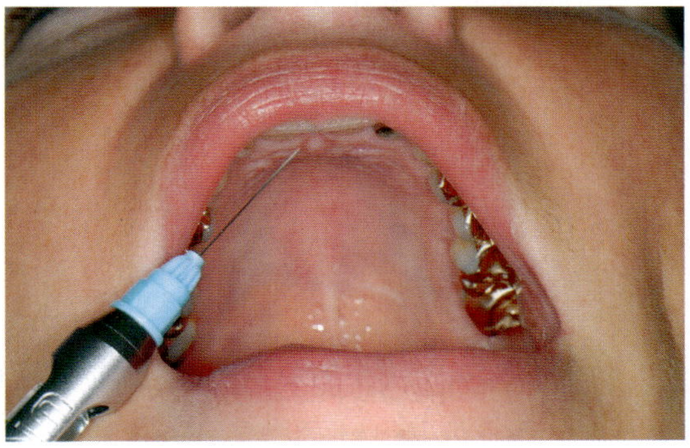

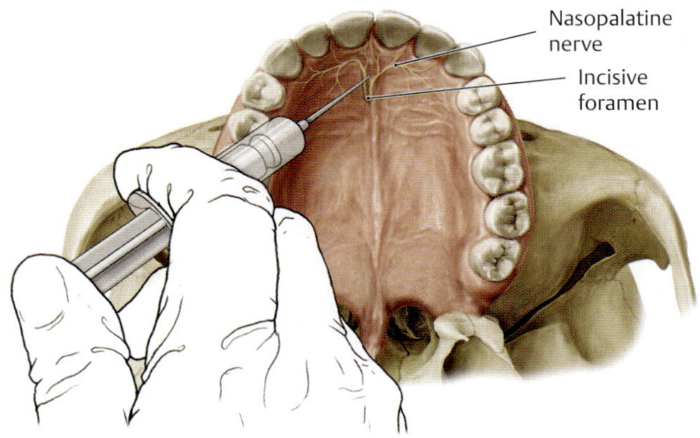

b

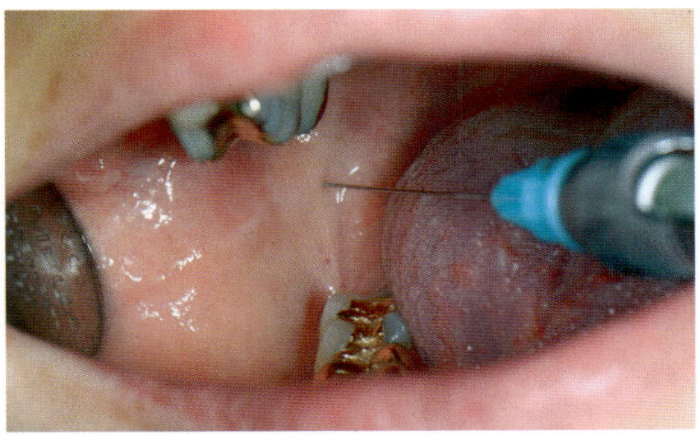

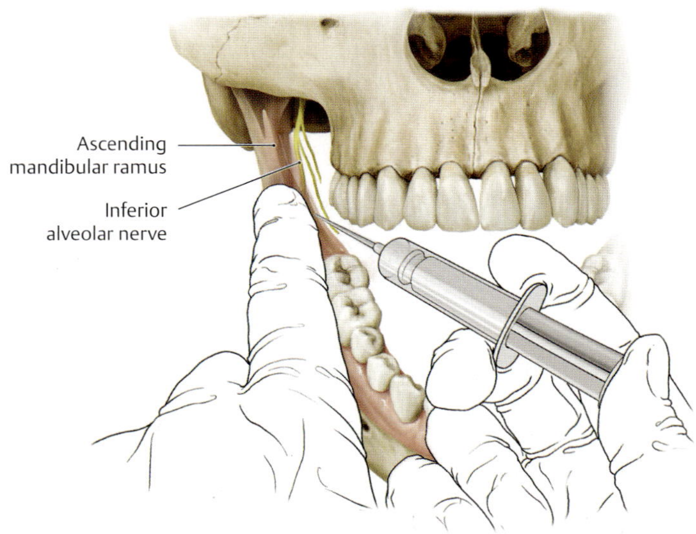

c

E Site of a typical injection for the anesthetic block of maxilla and mandible (Photos by Daubländer M. Lokalanästhesie in der Zahn-, Mund- und Kieferheilkunde. In van Aken H, Wulf H. Lokalanästhesie, Regionalanästhesie, Regionale Schmerztherapie. 3rd ed. Stuttgart: Thieme; 2010)

a Greater palatine foramen (greater palatine n.)
Indication: Painful treatment in the area surrounding the palatal mucosa and the bones in the molar and premolar area of one side of the maxilla.
Technique: Local anesthetic needs to be deposited as close as possible to the greater palatine foramen (area of insertion in children is near the first molar; in adults: more distal near the second and third molar). With the mouth opened wide and the head reclined, the needle—approaching from the premolar area of the contralateral side—is advanced in a 45 degree angle to the palatal surface until it touches the bone.
Clinical considerations: As a result of the injection placed/positioned too far distal the ipsilateral soft palate gets blocked which causes the patient discomfort (difficulty swallowing).

b Incisive foramen (nasopalatine n.)
Indication: Painful treatment in the area of the anterior third of the palate (stretching from the left to the right canine).
Technique: With the mouth wide open and the head reclined, the needle—advancing from a lateral direction—is inserted directly next to the papilla, approximately 1 cm palatal off the gingival edge and further advanced in a medial-distal direction.
Clinical considerations: Compact mucosa requires high injection pressure.

c Mandibular foramen (inferior alveolar n.)
Indication: Painful treatment in the area around mandibular teeth as well as the buccal mucosa mesial of the mental foramen.
Technique: In the wide-open mouth, the therapist palpates with his index finger the leading edge of the ascending mandibular ramus. Approaching from the premolar area of the opposite side, the needle is inserted approximately 1 cm above occlusal plane, lateral to the pterygomandibular fold and reaches the mandibular foramen after advancing another 2.5 cm cranial to the mandibular lingula.
Clinical considerations: In children, the mandibular foramen is on level with the occlusal plane.

2.28 Temporomandibular Joint

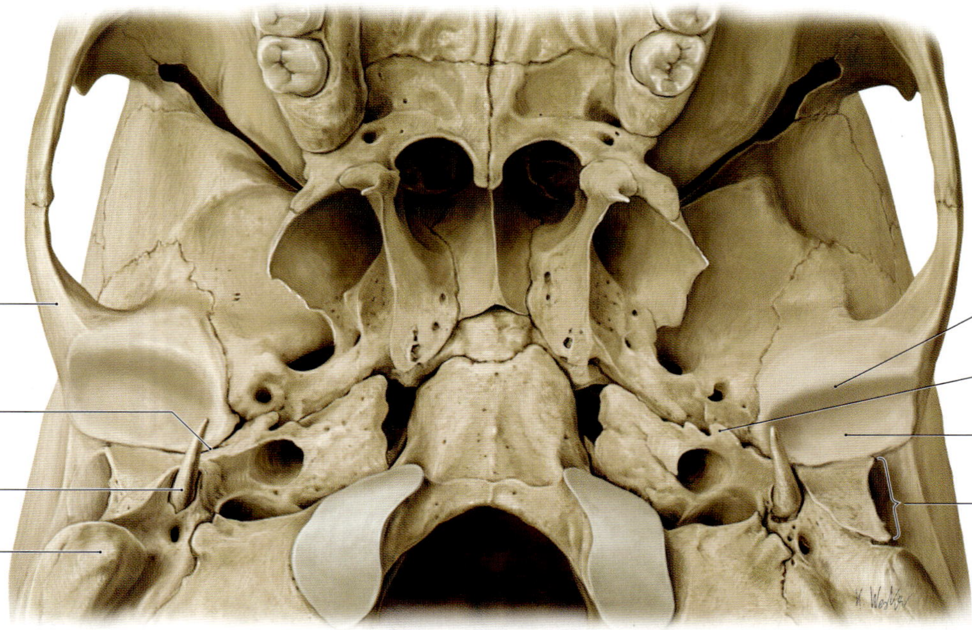

A Mandibular fossa of the temporomandibular joint on the outer skull base
View from below. In the temporomandibular joint, the head of the mandible of the lower jaw articulates with the socket, the mandibular fossa as shown here. It is part of the squamous part of the temporal bone. The articular tubercle, or eminence, is located at the anterior part of the mandibular fossa. Since the joint capsule (see **B**) is considerably smaller than the fossa sufficient motility of the temporomandibular joint is ensured. Unlike other joint surfaces, the mandibular fossa is covered with fibrous cartilage and not hyaline cartilage. The external acoustic meatus is located behind the fossa of the temporomandibular joint. This proximity explains blunt force jaw trauma causing damage to the auditory canal.

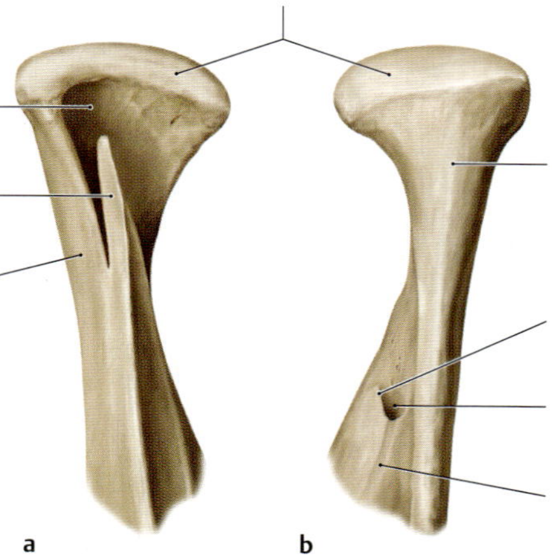

B Head of the mandible of the right temporomandibular joint
Frontal view (**a**) and dorsal view (**b**). The joint capsule of the mandibular head is not only considerably smaller than the socket but it is also cylindrical. This cylinder shape increases head mobility given that it allows rotation around a vertical axis.

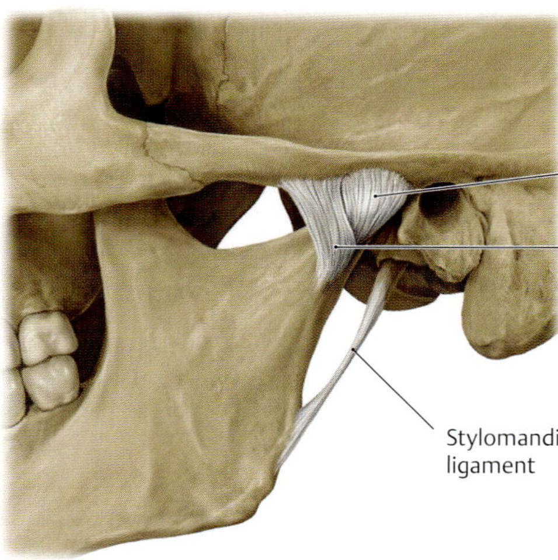

C Left temporomandibular joint with ligamentous apparatus
Lateral view. The temporomandibular joint is surrounded by a relatively atonic capsule (danger of luxation), which extends dorsally up to the petrotympanic fissure (see **A**). It is secured by three ligaments. This lateral view shows the strongest ligament, the lateral ligament, which lies on the capsule and with which it is connected as well as the weaker stylomandibular ligament.

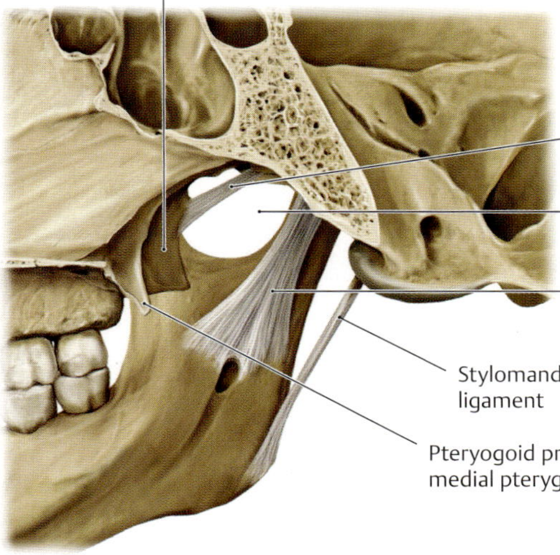

D Right temporomandibular joint with ligamentous apparatus
Medial view. From a medial view, the sphenomandibular ligament is visible, which extends from the sphenoidal spine (see **A**) medial to the mandibular branch.

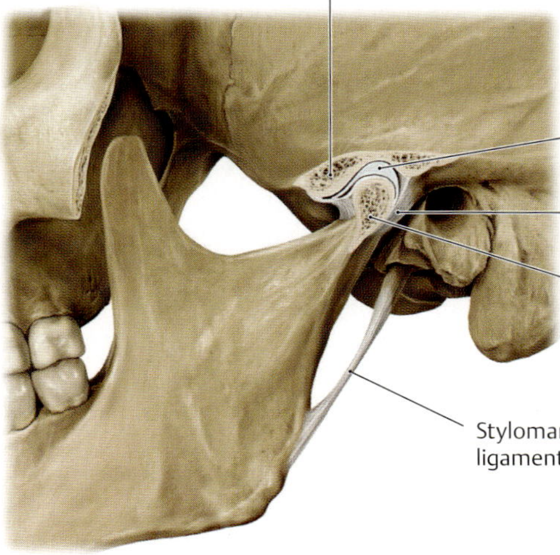

E Opened, left temporomandibular joint
Lateral view. Sagittal section through joint. The capsule extends dorsally to the petrotympanic fissure (not shown here). The articular disk, which is located between head and fossa is visible creating separate superior and inferior synovial cavities. It is attached to the capsule on all sides.

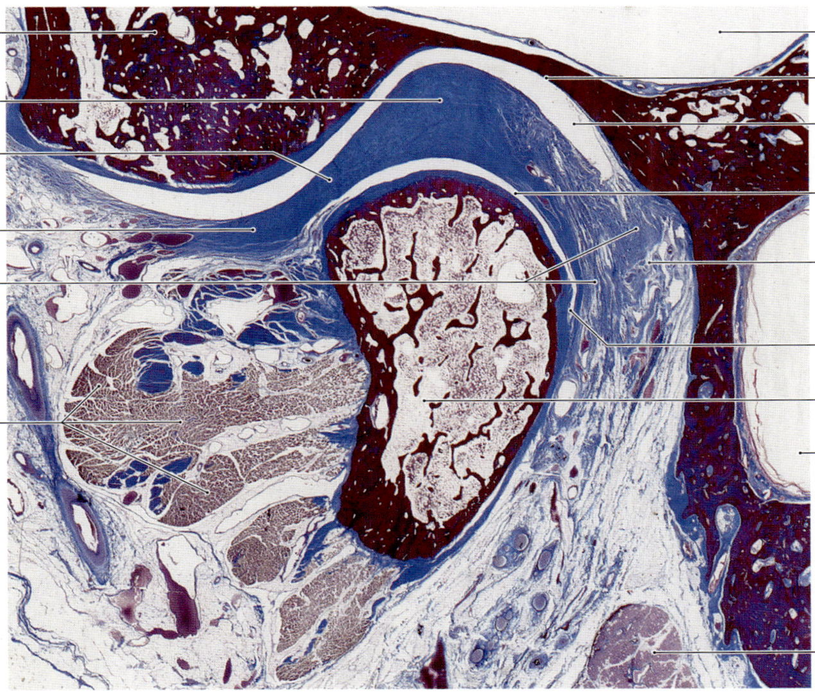

F Histology of the temporomandibular Joint
Sagittal cut showing the lateral area of a human temporomandibular joint, lateral view (original specimen provided by Prof. M. Schünke, M.D., Ph.D., sections stained with azan, 10 µm).
The articular disk divides the temporomandibular joint in two completely separate synovial joint cavities. We distinguish between an anterior, avascular, and collagen rich fiber section and one posterior and vascularized section. While the front section in its entirety shows a biconcave shape, a posterior and anterior ligament and an intermediary zone, the back section is divided into two leaves (called the bilaminar zone). The superior leaf contains elastic fibers and inserts in the area around the petrosquamous fissure, the inferior leaf extends to the neck of the mandible. Located between the two leaves lies the retroarticular cushion. The capsule is rather weak, laterally and is secured medially by collateral ligaments (see **C**).
Note: While the inferior head of the lateral pterygoid m. inserts at the condylar process (mandibular neck), the superior head of the muscle inserts into the articular disk and pulls on it (not shown here).

2.29 Biomechanics of the Temporomandibular Joint

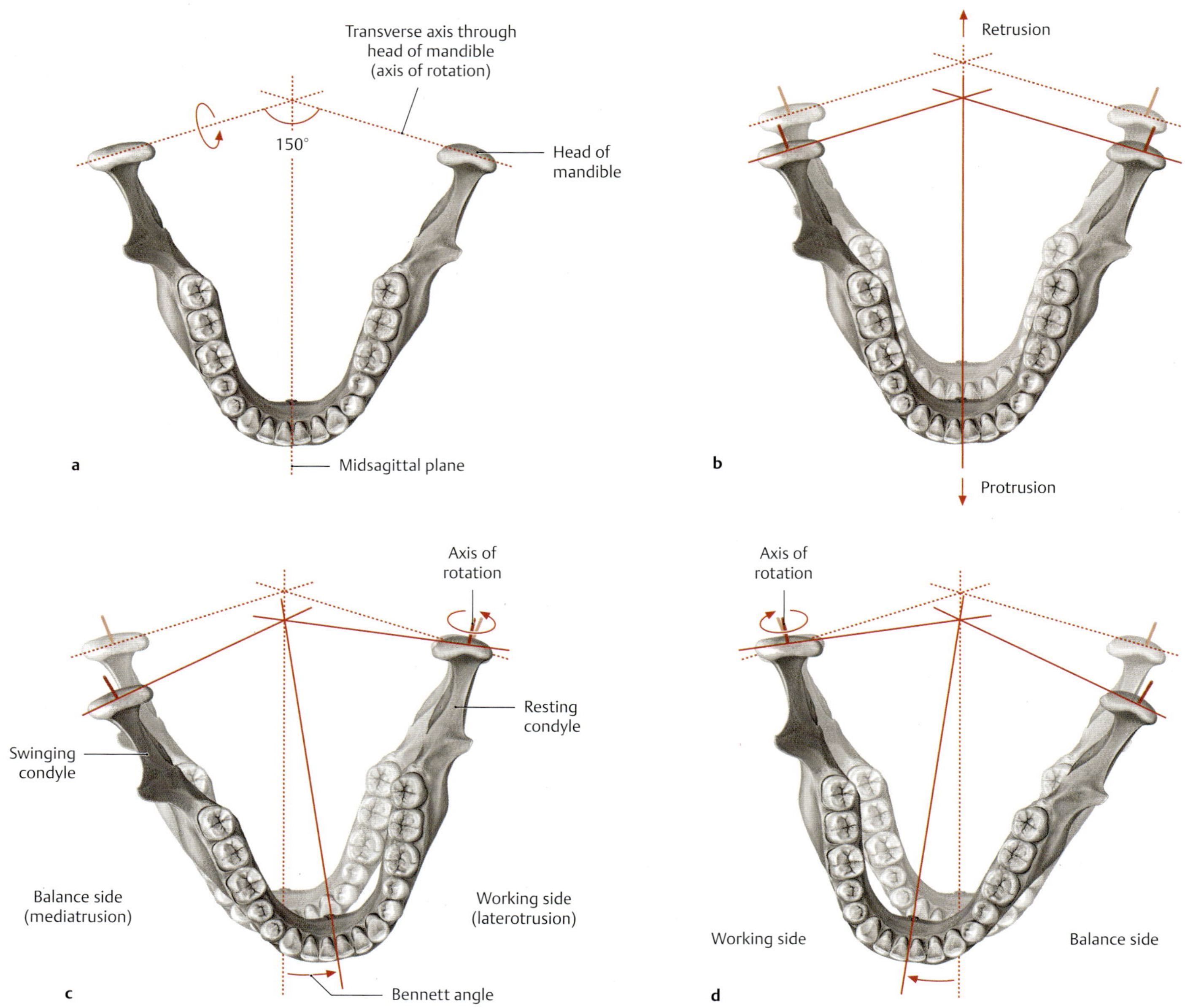

A Movement options of the temporomandibular joint, mandible
View from above. Most of the motions of the temporomandibular joint are combined motions. They can be attributed to three basic motions:

- rotary motion (opening and closing of the mouth)
- translatory motion (feeding motion)
- grinding motion

a Rotary motion. During the rotary motion the joint axis crosses diagonally through both mandibular heads. Both joint axes intersect in an individually variable angle of about 150° (margin of deviation 110–180°). During this motion the temporomandibular joint is a hinge joint (abduction, lowering, and abduction lifting, of the mandible). Such a clean rotary motion usually happens when asleep, when the mouth is slightly open (angle of up to approximately 15°, see **Bb**). During every additional opening of the mouth of more than 15° it is combined with a translatory motion (rotary gliding).

b Translatory motion. During this motion the mandible is pushed forward and pulled back (protrusion and retrusion respectively). The axes during this motion run parallel to the median axis through the center of the mandibular joint capsules.

c Grinding motion in the left temporomandibular joint. During the grinding motion one differentiates the resting and the swinging condyle. The resting condyle on the left working side rotates around a nearly vertical axis (also a rotary axis) through the mandibular head, while the swinging condyle of the right balancing side pans to the front, inner side in the sense of a translatory motion. The extent of the mandible panning is measured in degrees and is called a Bennett angle. During the panning of the mandible a laterotrusion is carried out on the working side and a mediotrusion on the balancing side.

d Grinding motion of the right temporomandibular joint. Now the right temporomandibular joint is the working side, the right resting condyle turns around the nearly vertical rotation axis, while the left condyle pans to the front, inner side: balancing side.

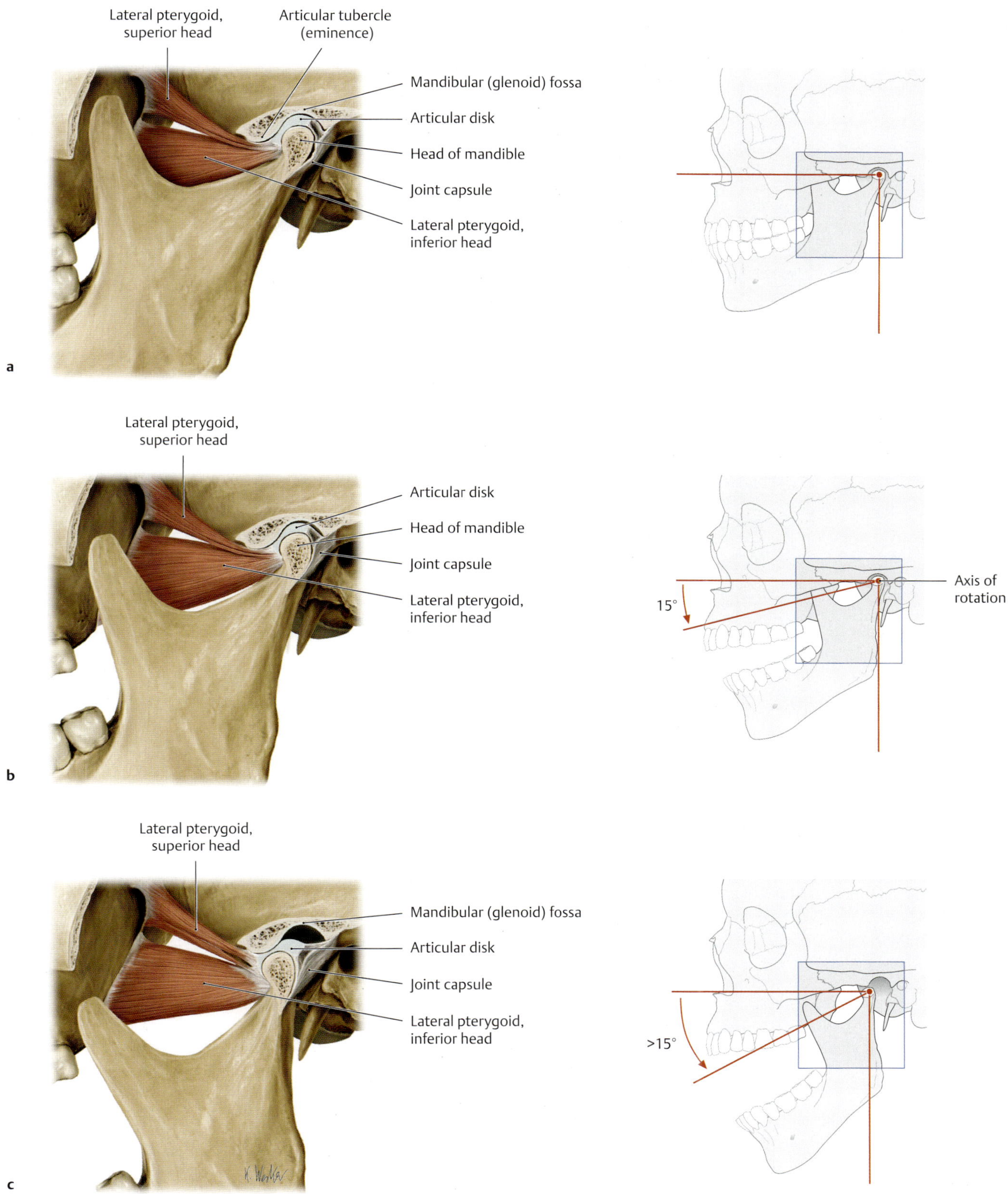

B Temporomandibular joint motions

View from the left lateral side. Depicted on the left side is the joint with the disk and the capsule as well as the lateral pterygoid m. respectively, and on the right side schematic the course of the axis. Muscle, capsule, and disk build a functionally combined musculo-disco-capsulo system that works closely together during the opening and closing of the mouth.

a Closed mouth. In idle position with the mouth closed the mandibular head rests in the mandibular fossa of the temporal bone.

b Mouth opening up to 15°. The mandibular heads stay in the mandibular fossa up to this degree of abduction.

c Mouth opening more than 15°. The mandibular heads shift to the front of the articular eminence; as a result the joint axis that runs diagonally through the mandibular heads shifts ventrally. The articular disk is pulled forward by the superior head of the lateral pterygoid m. The inferior head of the lateral pterygoid m. inserts onto the neck of the condylar process of the mandible.

2.30 The Cervical Spine

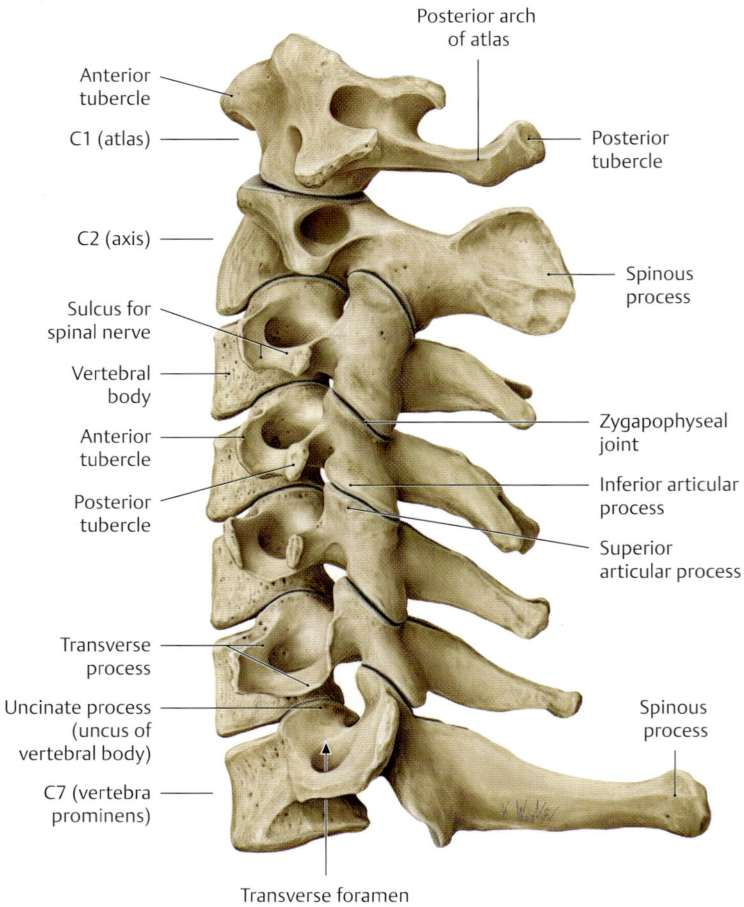

A Cervical spine, left lateral view

The cervical spine consists of seven vertebrae, the upper two of which, the atlas (C1) and axis (C2), differ markedly from the other five vertebrae. They form the atlanto-occipital and atlanto axial joints which will be discussed in the next unit. The remaining five vertebrae are made up of the following components:

- One vertebral body,
- One vertebral arch,
- One spinous process,
- Two transverse processes,
- Four articular processes.

Cervical vertebrae have the following characteristics:

- Bifid spinous processes,
- Transverse foramen on transverse processes,
- Large, triangular vertebral foramen as well as
- Uncovertebral joints (see p. 76 f).

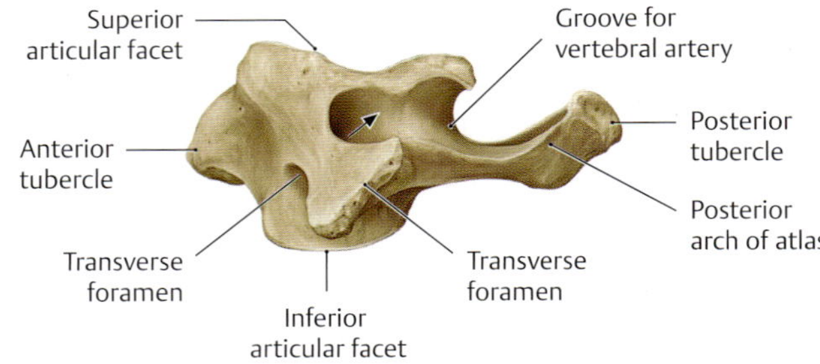

a First cervical vertebra (C1, atlas)

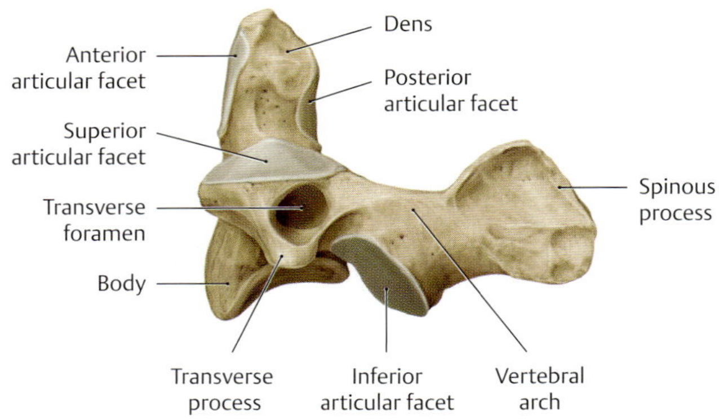

b Second cervical vertebra (C2, axis)

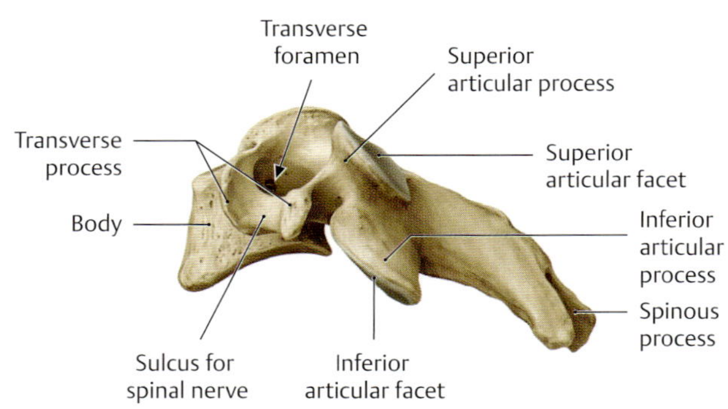

c Fourth cervical vertebra (C4)

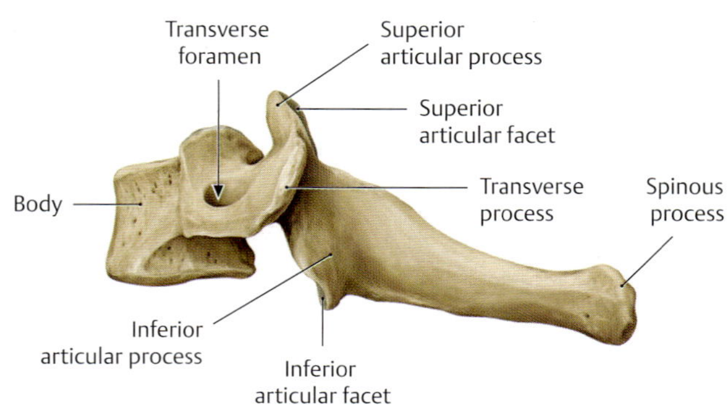

d Seventh cervical vertebra (C7, vertebra prominens)

B Cervical vertebrae, left lateral view

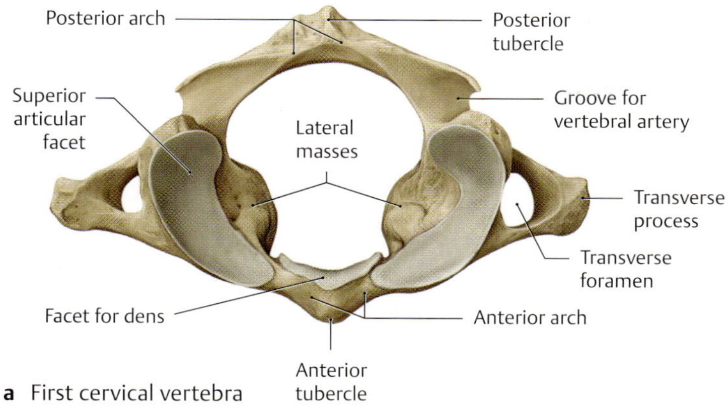

a First cervical vertebra (atlas)

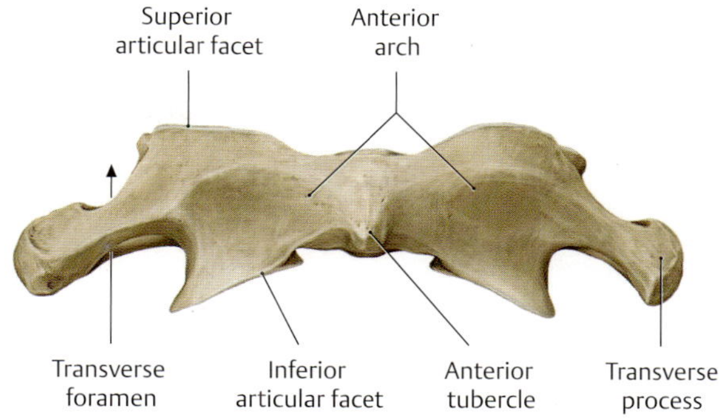

a First cervical vertebra (atlas)

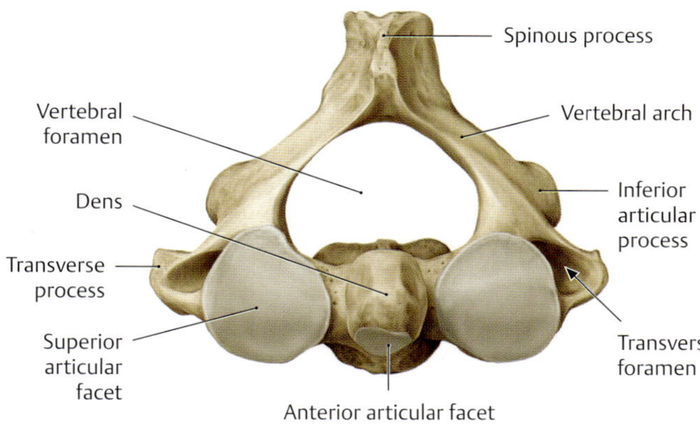

b Second cervical vertebra (axis)

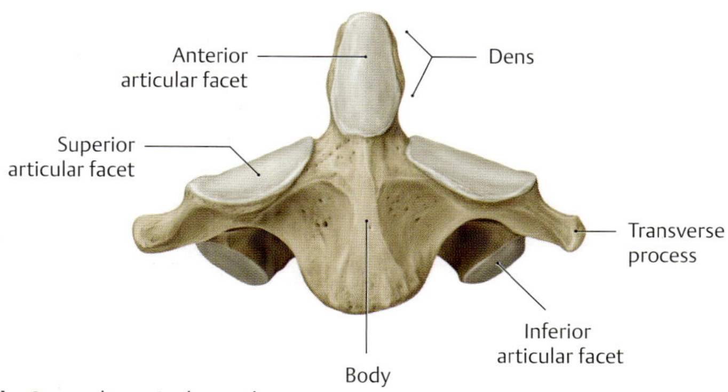

b Second cervical vertebra (axis)

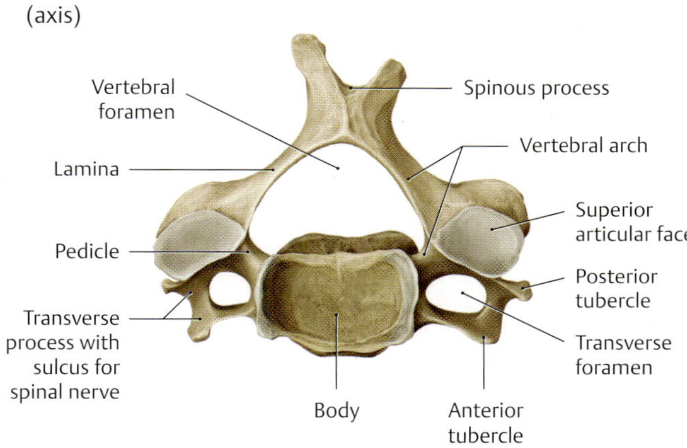

c Fourth cervical vertebra

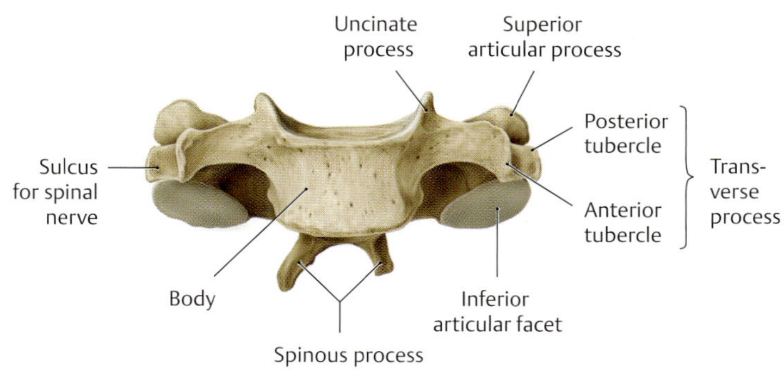

c Fourth cervical vertebra

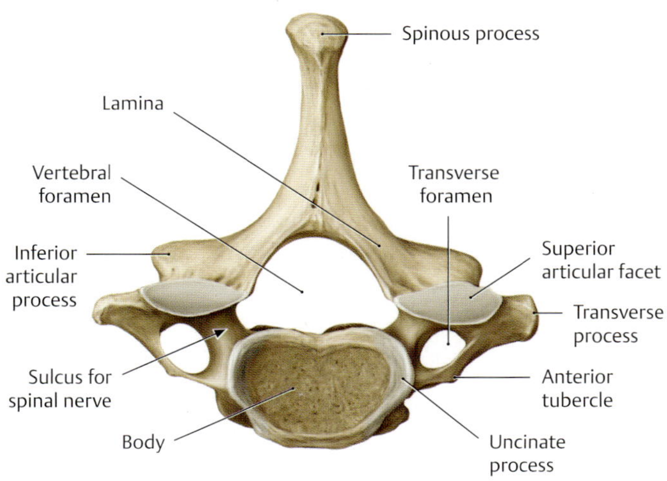

d Seventh cervical vertebra (vertebra prominens)

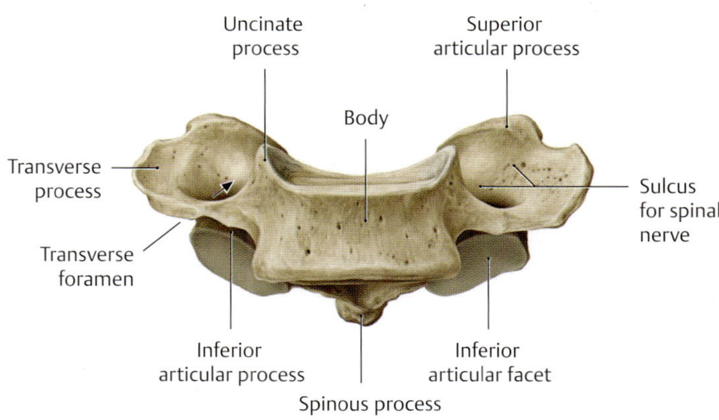

d Seventh cervical vertebra (vertebra prominens)

C Cervical vertebrae, superior view

D Cervical vertebrae, anterior view

2.31 Overview of the Ligaments of the Cervical Spine

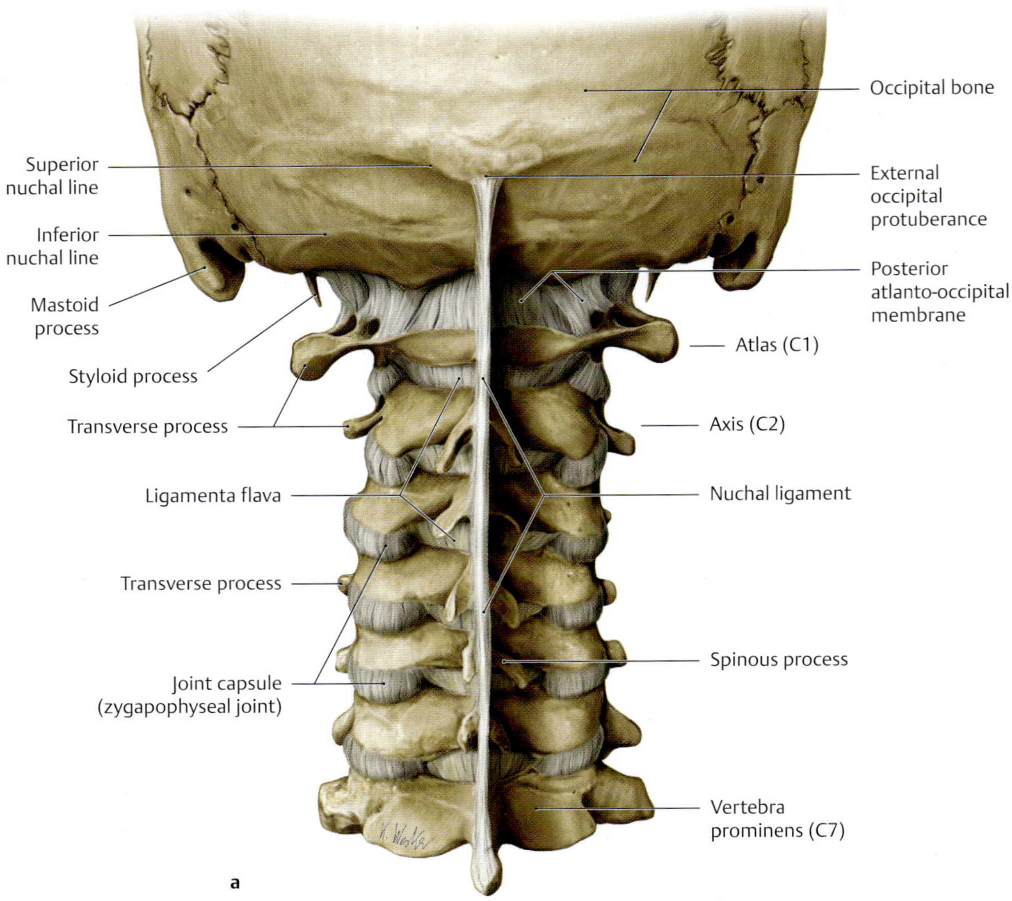

A The ligaments of the cervical spine
a Posterior view
b Anterior view after removal of the anterior skull base (see p. 74 for the ligaments of the upper cervical spine, especially the craniovertebral joints).

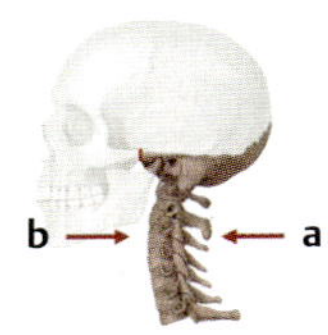

B The craniovertebral joints
The craniovertebral joints are the articulations between the atlas (C1) and occipital bone (atlanto-occipital joints) and between the atlas and axis (C2, atlantoaxial joints). While these joints, which number six in all, are anatomically distinct, they are mechanically interlinked and comprise a functional unit (cf. p. 74).

Atlanto-occipital joints
Paired condyloid joints where the oval, slightly concave superior articular facets of the atlas articulate with the convex occipital condyles
Atlantoaxial joints
• *Lateral atlantoaxial joint* = paired articulation between the inferior articular facets of the atlas and the superior articular facets of the axis • *Median atlantoaxial joint* = unpaired articulation (comprising an anterior and posterior compartment) between the dens of the axis, the fovea of the atlas, and the cartilage-covered anterior surface of the transverse ligament of the atlas (see p. 74)

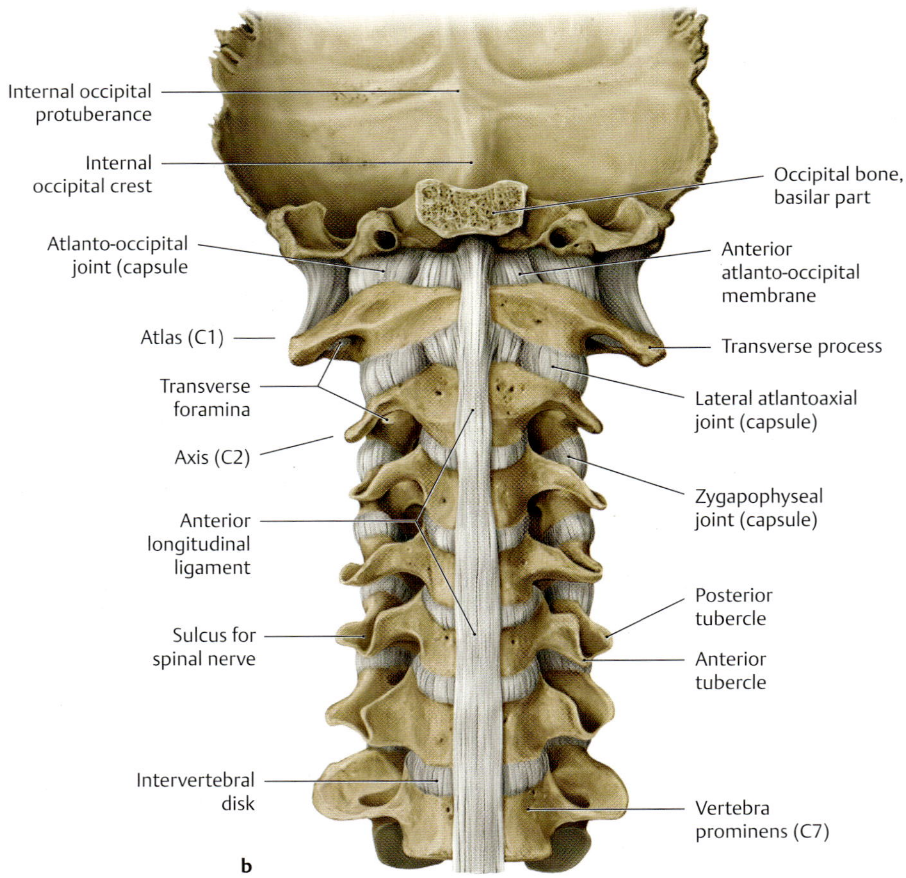

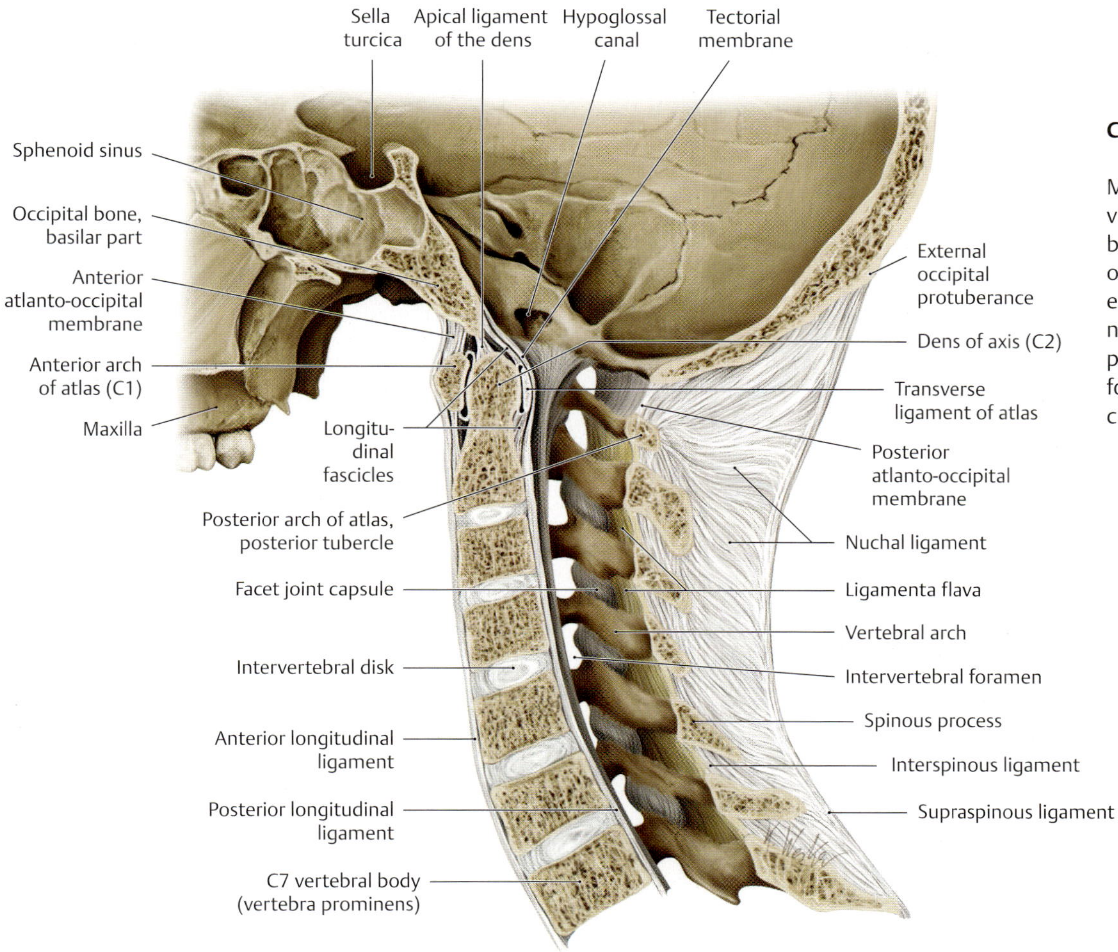

C The ligaments of the cervical spine: nuchal ligament
Midsagittal section, left lateral view. The nuchal ligament is the broadened, sagittally oriented part of the supraspinous ligament that extends from the vertebra prominens (C1) to the external occipital protuberance (see **A**; see also p. 74 for the ligaments of the atlanto-occipital and atlantoaxial joints).

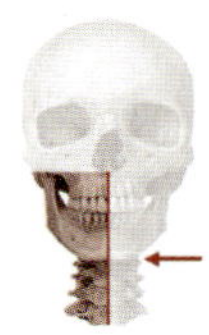

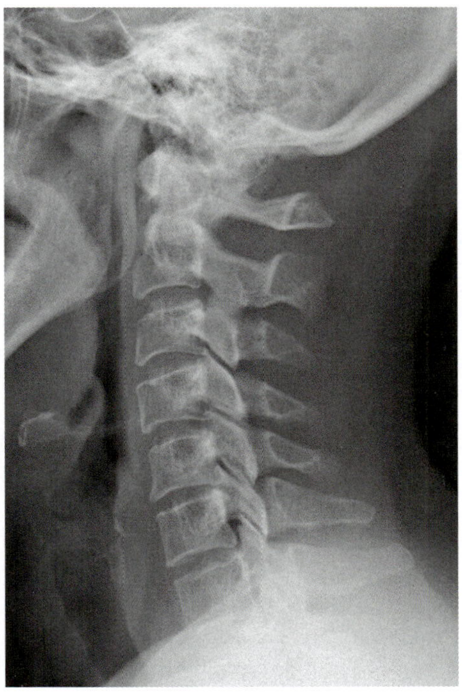

D Plain lateral radiograph of the cervical spine

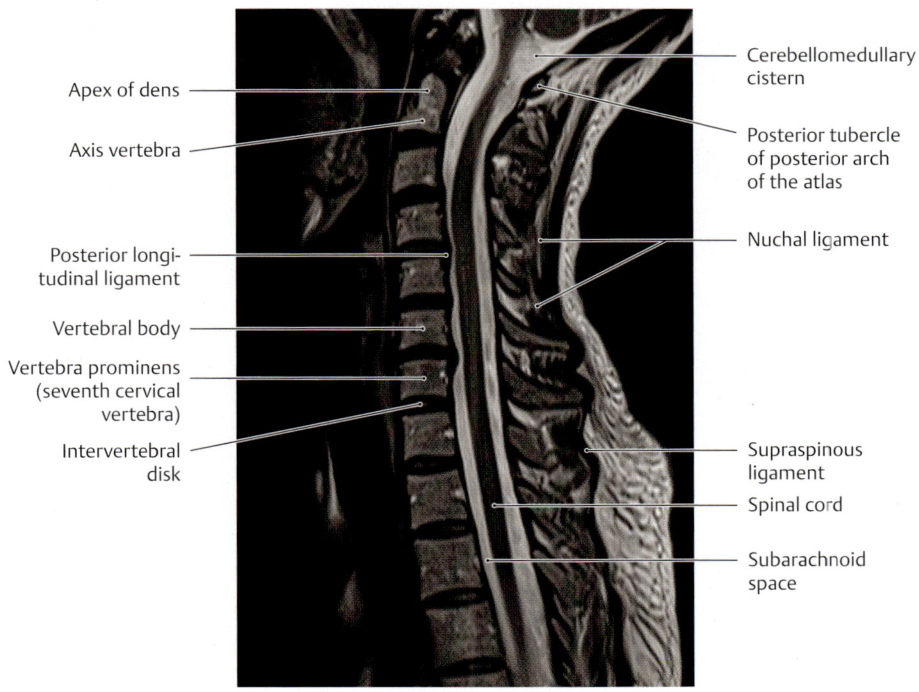

E Magnetic resonance image of the cervical spine
Midsagittal section, left lateral view T2-weighted TSE sequence (original image: Prof. S. Müller-Hülsbeck, M.D., Inst. für Diagnostische und Interventionelle Radiologie/Neuroradiologie, DIAKO Krankenhaus gGmbH Flensburg).

2.32 The Ligaments of the Upper Cervical Spine (Atlanto-occipital and Atlantoaxial Joints)

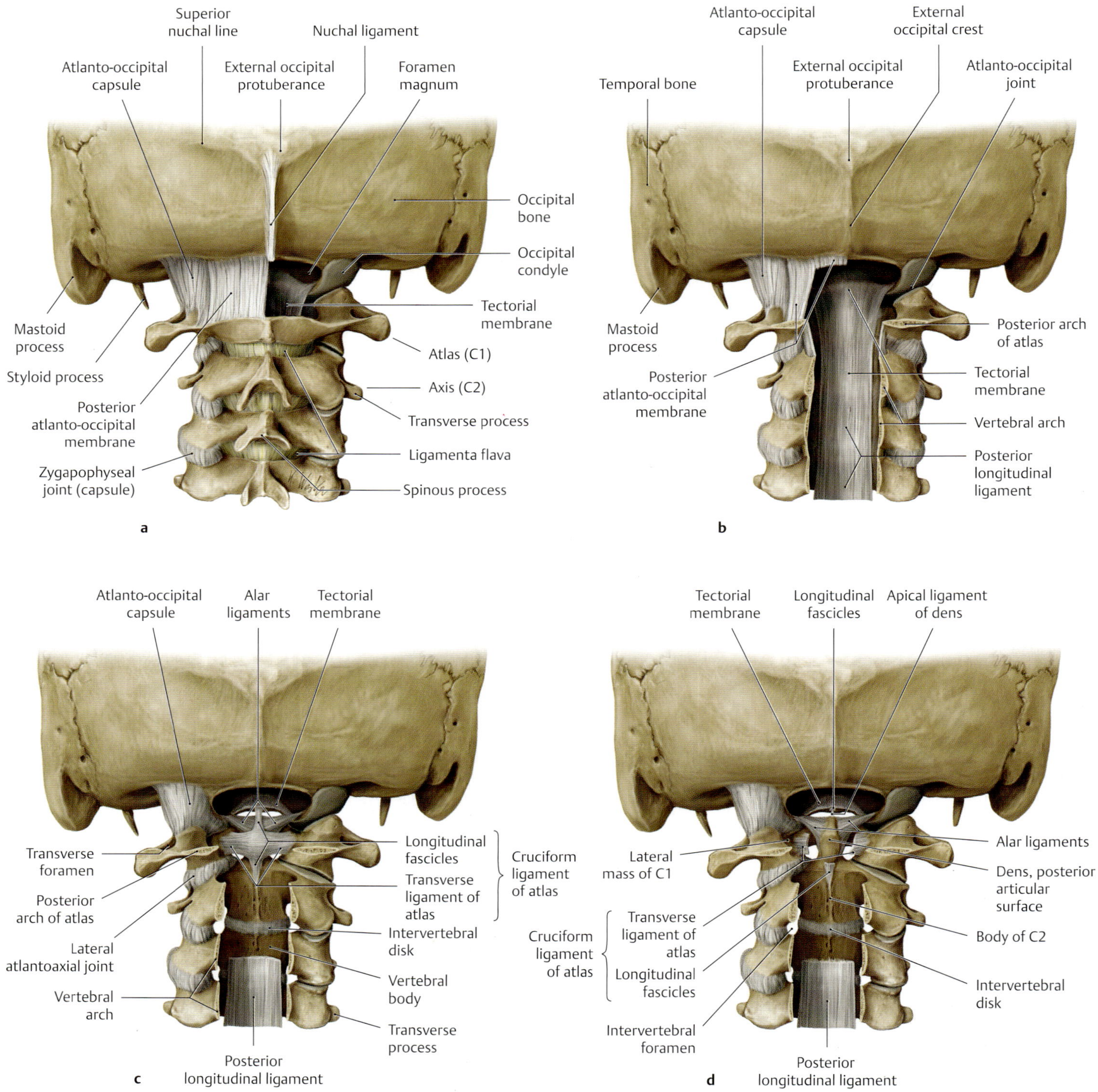

A The ligaments of the craniovertebral joints
Skull and upper cervical spine, posterior view.

a The posterior atlanto-occipital membrane—the "ligamentum flavum" between the atlas and occipital bone (see p. 66)—stretches from the posterior arch of the atlas to the posterior rim of the foramen magnum. This membrane has been removed on the right side.
b With the vertebral canal opened and the spinal cord removed, the tectorial membrane, a broadened expansion of the posterior longitudinal ligament, is seen to form the anterior boundary of the vertebral canal at the level of the craniovertebral joints.
c With the tectorial membrane removed, the cruciform ligament of the atlas can be seen. The transverse ligament of the atlas forms the thick horizontal bar of the cross, and the longitudinal fascicles form the thinner vertical bar.
d The transverse ligament of the atlas and longitudinal fascicles have been partially removed to demonstrate the paired alar ligaments, which extend from the lateral surfaces of the dens to the corresponding inner surfaces of the occipital condyles, and the unpaired apical ligament of the dens, which passes from the tip of the dens to the anterior rim of the foramen magnum.

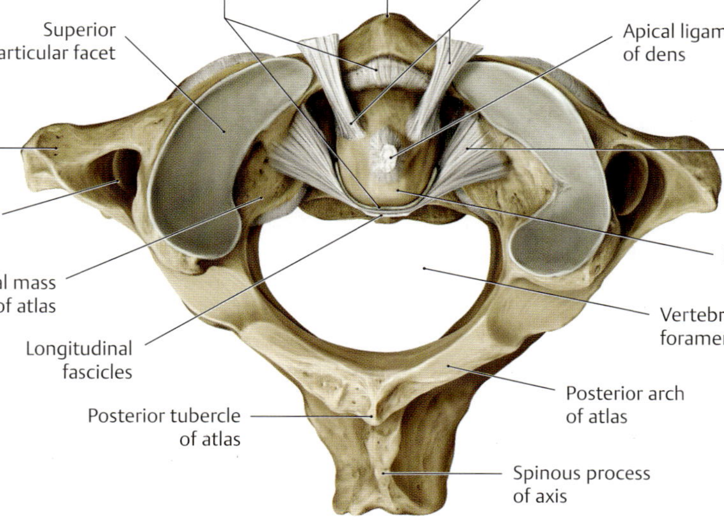

B The ligaments of the median atlantoaxial joint
Atlas and axis, superior view. (The fovea, while part of the median atlantoaxial joint, is hidden by the joint capsule.)

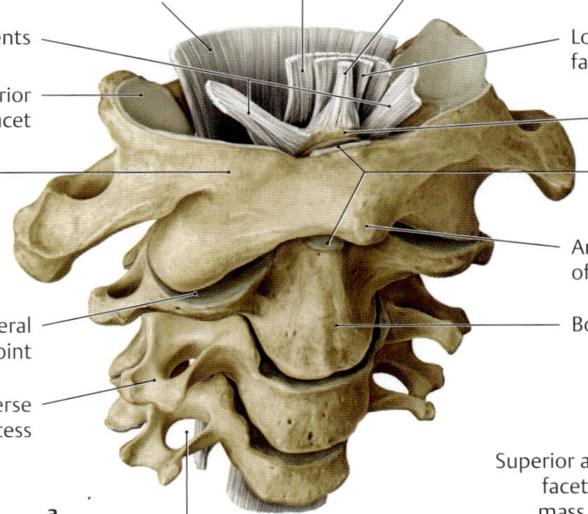

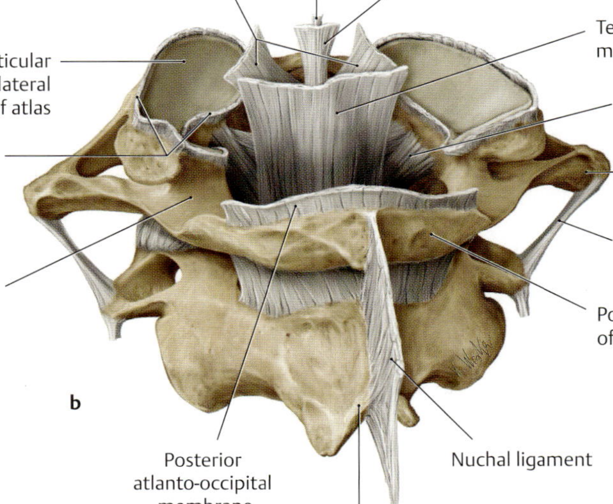

C The ligaments of the craniovertebral joints (joint capsule removed)

a Proximal cervical spine, anterosuperior view with the joint capsule removed;

b Atlas and axis, posterosuperior view.

2.33 The Uncovertebral Joints of the Cervical Spine

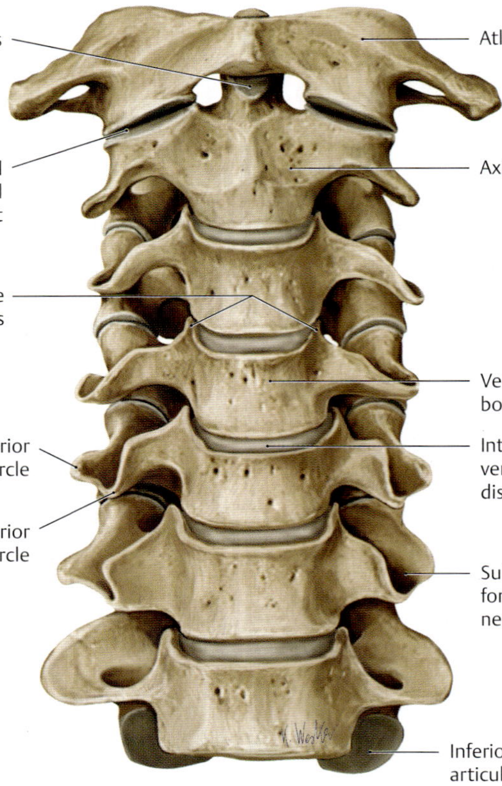

a

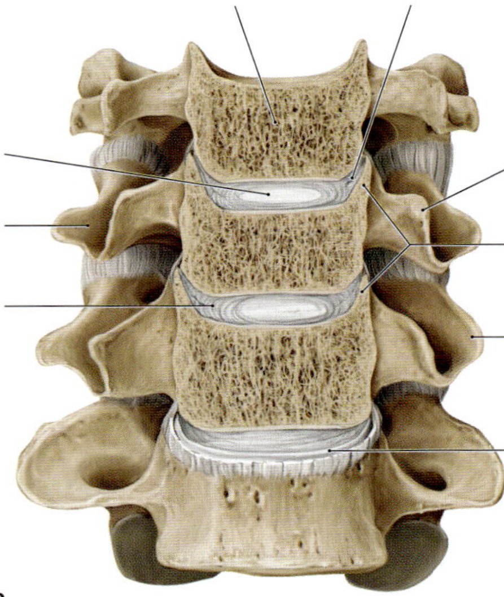

b

A The uncovertebral joints in a young adult
Cervical spine of an 18-year-old man, anterior view

a The upper end plates of the C3 through C7 vertebral bodies have lateral projections (uncinate processes) that develop during childhood. Starting at about 10 years of age, the uncinate processes gradually come into contact with the oblique, crescent-shaped margin on the undersurface of the next higher vertebral body. This results in the formation of lateral clefts (uncovertebral clefts or joints, see **b**) in the outer portions of the intervertebral disks.

b C4 through C7 vertebrae. The bodies of the C4–C6 vertebrae have been sectioned in the coronal plane to demonstrate more clearly the uncovertebral joints or clefts. These clefts are bounded laterally by a connective tissue structure, a kind of joint capsule, which causes them to resemble true joint spaces. These clefts or fissures in the intervertebral disk were first described by the anatomist Hubert von Luschka in 1858, who called them *lateral hemiarthroses*. He interpreted them as primary mechanisms designed to enhance the flexibility of the cervical spine and confer a functional advantage (drawings based on specimens from the Anatomical Collection at Kiel University).

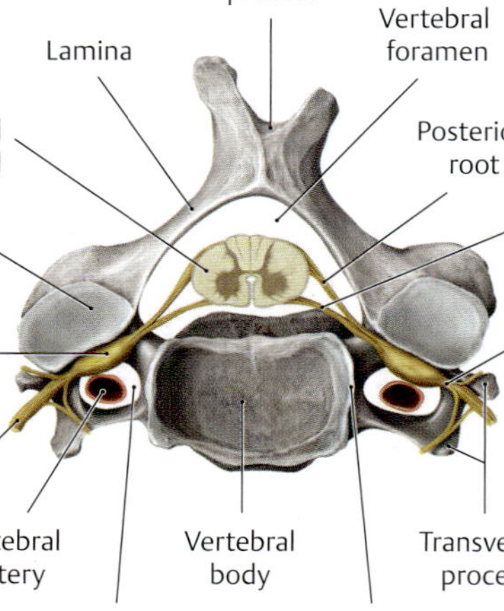

a

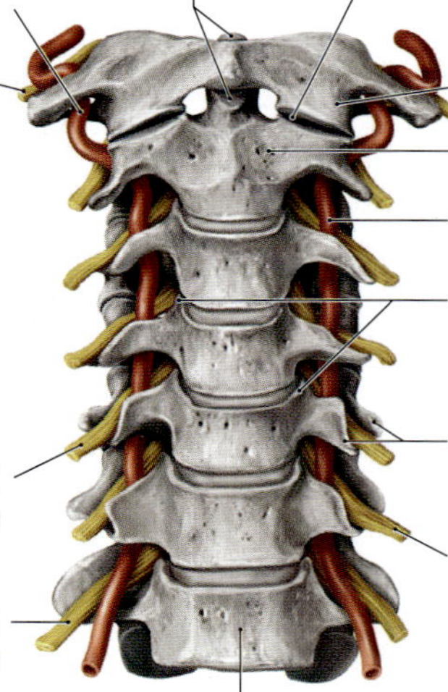

b

B Topographical relationship of the spinal nerve and vertebral artery to the uncinate process

a Fourth cervical vertebra with spinal cord, spinal roots, spinal nerves, and vertebral arteries, superior view;

b Cervical spine with both vertebral arteries and the emerging spinal nerves, anterior view.

Note the course of the vertebral artery through the transverse foramina and the course of the spinal nerve at the level of the intervertebral foramina. Given their close proximity, both the artery and nerve may be compressed by osteophytes (bony outgrowths) caused by uncovertebral arthrosis (cf. **D**).

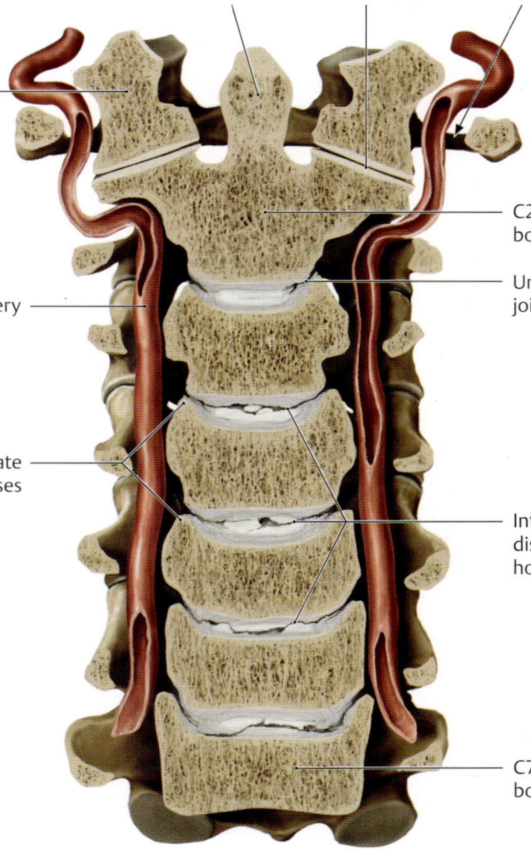

C Degenerative changes in the cervical spine (uncovertebral arthrosis)

Coronal section through the cervical spine of a 35-year-old man, anterior view. Note the course of the vertebral arteries on both sides of the vertebral bodies.

The development of the uncovertebral joints at approximately 10 years of age initiates a process of cleft formation in the intervertebral disks. This process spreads toward the center of the disk with aging, eventually resulting in the formation of complete transverse clefts that subdivide the intervertebral disks into two slabs of roughly equal thickness. The result is a progressive degenerative process marked by flattening of the disks and consequent instability of the motion segments (drawing based on specimens from the Anatomical Collection at Kiel University).

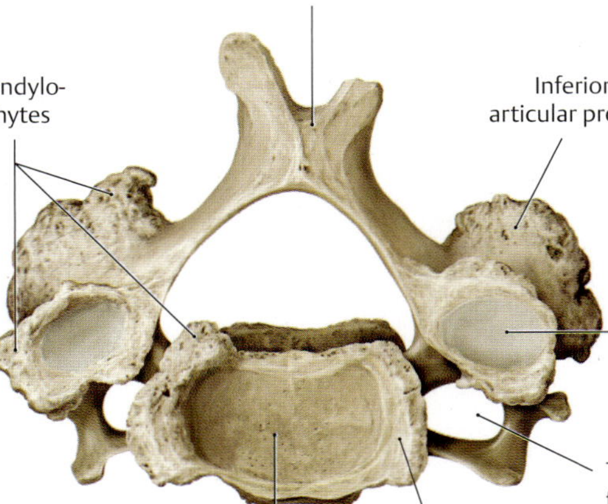

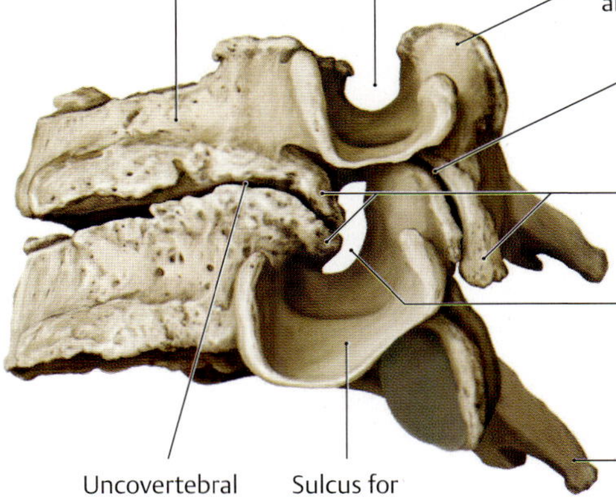

D Advanced uncovertebral arthrosis of the cervical spine

a Fourth cervical vertebra, superior view; **b** Fourth and fifth cervical vertebrae, lateral view (drawings based on specimens from the Anatomical Collection at Kiel University).

The uncovertebral joints undergo degenerative changes comparable to those seen in other joints, including the formation of osteophytes (called spondylophytes when they occur on vertebral bodies). These sites of new bone formation serve to distribute the imposed forces over a larger area, thereby reducing the pressure on the joint. With progressive destabilization of the corresponding motion segment, the facet joints undergo osteoarthritic changes leading to osteophyte formation. Osteophytes of the uncovertebral joints have major clinical importance because of their relation to the intervertebral foramen and vertebral artery (uncovertebral arthrosis). They cause a progressive narrowing of the intervertebral foramen, with increasing compression of the spinal nerve and often of the vertebral artery as well (cf. **C**). Meanwhile, the spinal canal itself may become significantly narrowed (spinal stenosis) by the same process.

3.1 Muscles of Facial Expression: Overview

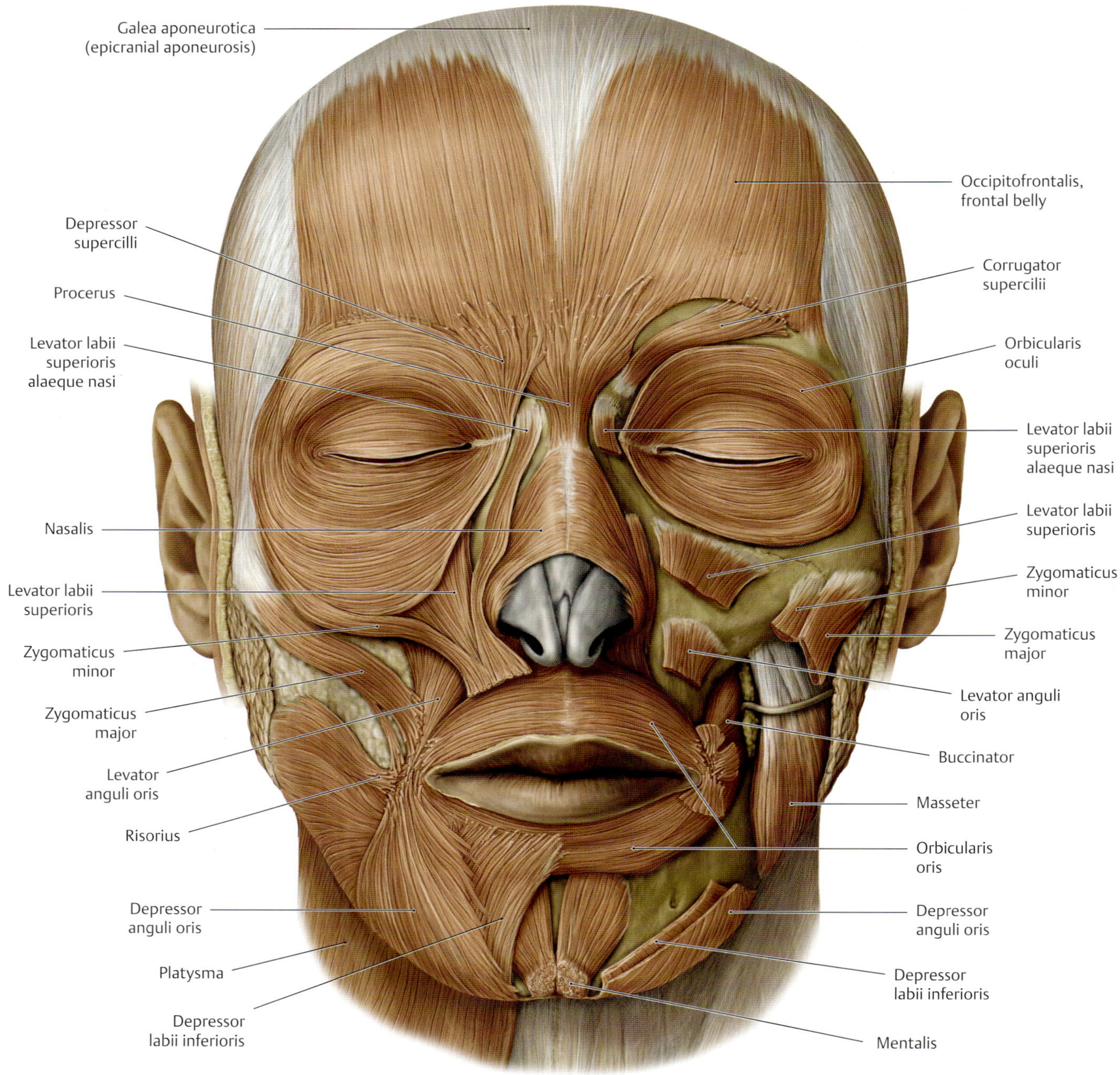

A Muscles of facial expression
Anterior view. The superficial layer of muscles is shown on the right half of the face, the deep layer on the left half. The muscles of facial expression represent the superficial muscle layer in the face and vary greatly in their development among different individuals. They arise either directly from the periosteum or from adjacent muscles to which they are connected, and they insert either onto other facial muscles or directly into the connective tissue of the skin. The classic scheme of classifying the other somatic muscles by their origins and insertions is not so easily adapted to the facial muscles. Because the muscles of facial expression terminate directly in the subcutaneous fat and the superficial body fascia is absent in the face, the surgeon must be particularly careful when dissecting in this region. Due to their cutaneous attachments, the facial muscles are able to move the facial skin (e.g., they can wrinkle the skin, an action temporarily abolished by botulinum toxin injection) and produce a variety of facial expressions. They also serve a protective function (especially for the eyes) through their sphincter-like action and are active during food ingestion (closing the mouth for swallowing). All of the facial muscles are innervated by branches of the facial nerve, while the muscles of mastication (see p. 82) are supplied by motor fibers from the trigeminal nerve (the masseter muscle has been left in place to represent these muscles). A thorough understanding of muscular anatomy in this region is facilitated by dividing the muscles into different groups (see p. 80).

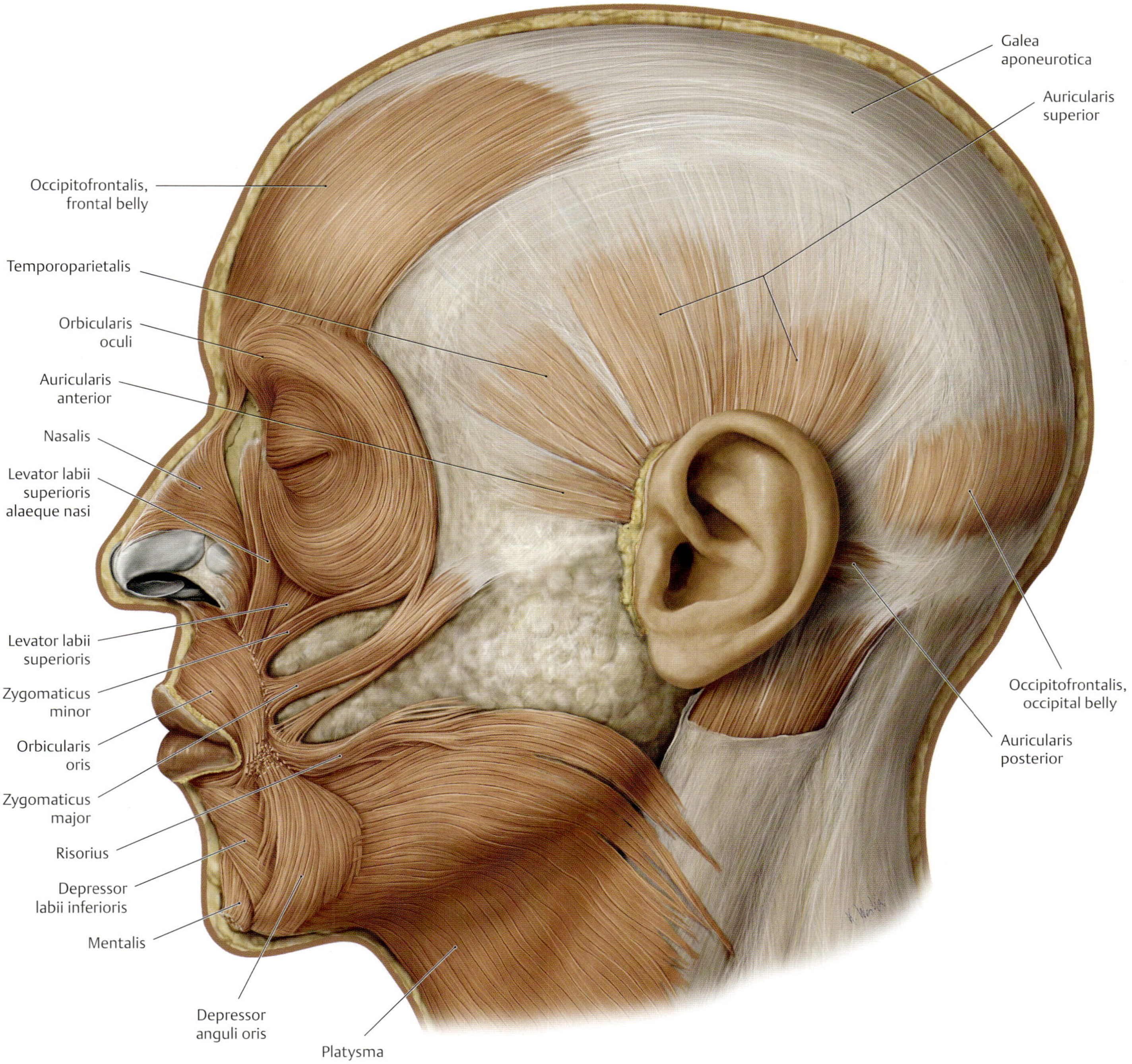

B Muscles of facial expression
Left lateral view. The superficial muscles of the ear and neck are particularly well displayed from this perspective. A tough tendinous sheet, the galea aponeurotica, stretches over the calvaria and is loosely attached to the periosteum. The muscles of the calvaria that arise from the galea aponeurotica are known collectively as the "epicranial muscle." The two bellies of the occipitofrontalis (frontal and occipital) can be clearly identified. The temporoparietalis, whose posterior part is called the auricularis superior arises from the lateral part of the galea aponeurotica. The levator anguli oris is not visible here because it is covered by the levator labii superioris located above it.

3.2 Muscles of Facial Expression: Actions

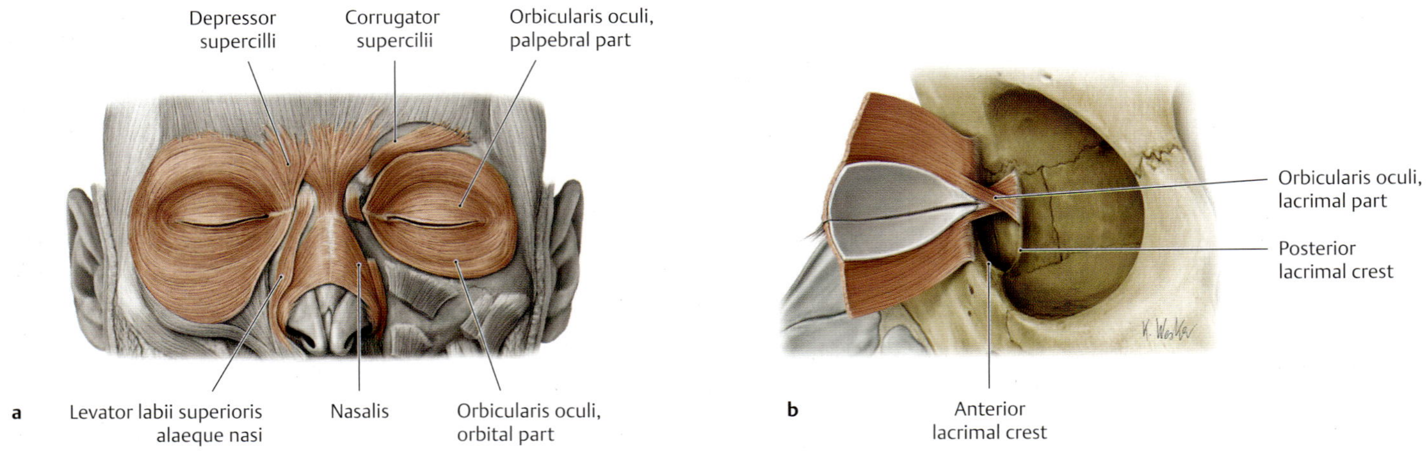

A Muscles of facial expression: palpebral fissure and nose

a Anterior view. The most functionally important muscle is the *orbicularis oculi*, which closes the palpebral fissure as a protective reflex against foreign matter. If the action of the orbicularis oculi is lost because of facial nerve paralysis (see also **D**), the loss of this protective reflex will be accompanied by drying of the eye from prolonged exposure to air without the lubricating nature of being able to blink. The function of the orbicularis oculi is tested by asking the patient to squeeze the eyelids tightly shut.

b The orbicularis oculi has been dissected from the left orbit to the medial canthus of the eye and reflected anteriorly to demonstrate its lacrimal part (Horner's muscle). This part of the orbicularis oculi arises mainly from the posterior lacrimal crest, and its action is a subject of debate (expand or empty the lacrimal sac).

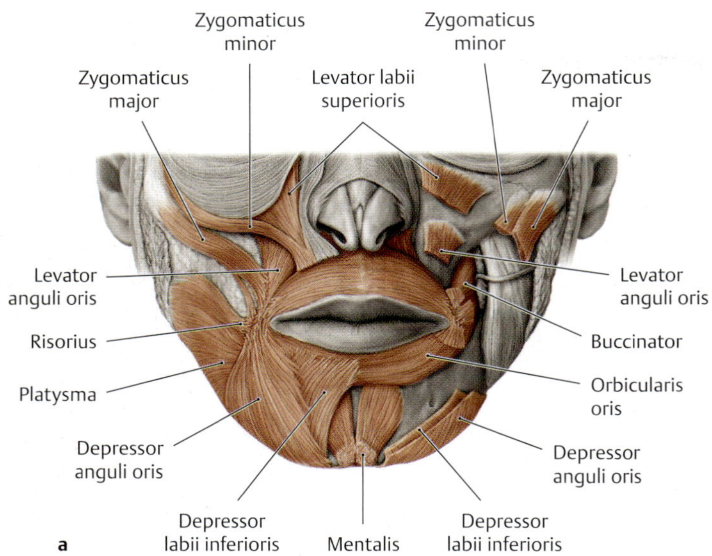

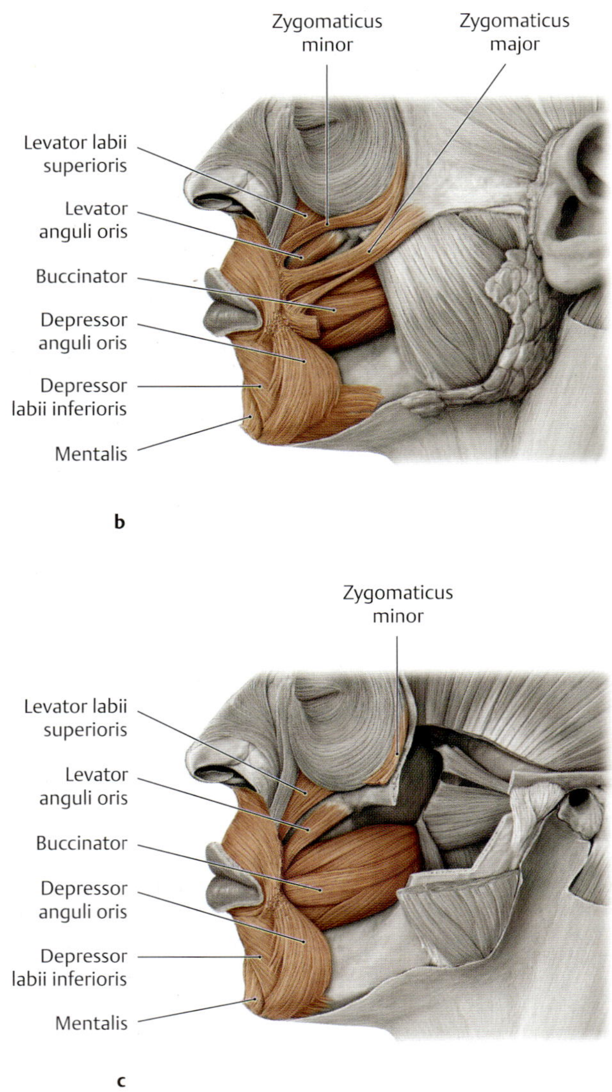

B Muscles of facial expression: mouth

a Anterior view, **b** left lateral view, **c** left lateral view of the deeper lateral layer.

The *orbicularis oris* forms the muscular foundation of the lips, and its contraction closes the oral aperture. Its function can be tested by asking the patient to whistle. Facial nerve paralysis may lead to drinking difficulties because the liquid will trickle back out of the unclosed mouth during swallowing. The *buccinator* lies at a deeper level and forms the foundation of the cheek. During mastication, this muscle moves food between the dental arches from the oral vestibule.

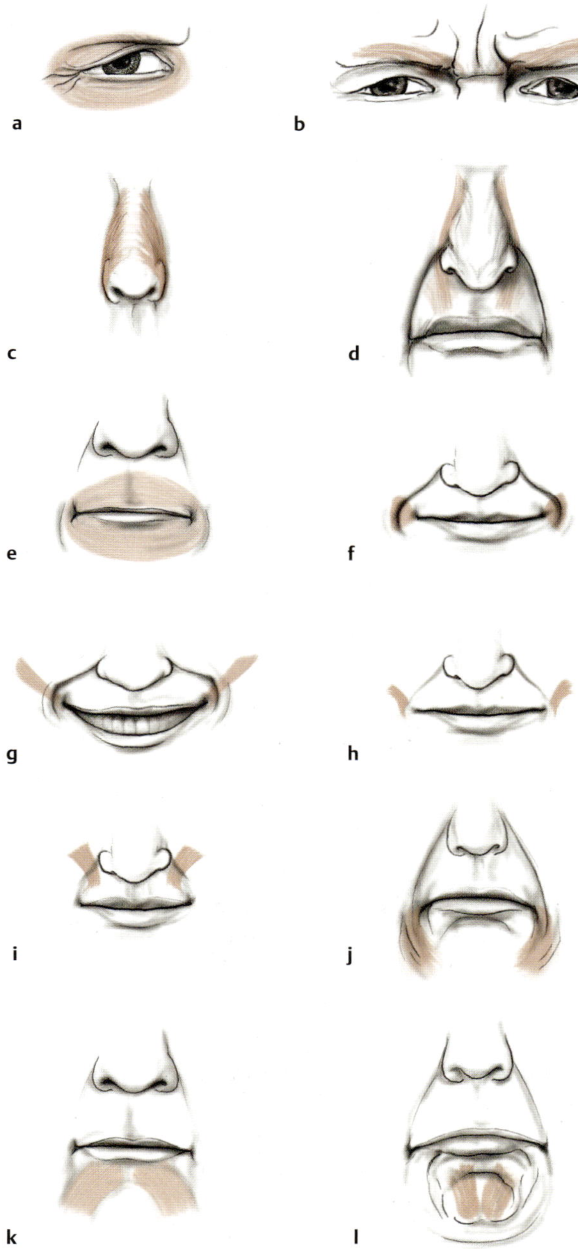

C Changes of facial expression

- **a** Contraction of the orbicularis oculi at the lateral canthus of the eye expresses concern.
- **b** Contraction of the corrugator supercilii occurs in response to bright sunlight: "thoughtful brow."
- **c** Contraction of the nasalis constricts the naris and produces a cheery or lustful facial expression.
- **d** Forceful contraction of the levator labii superioris alaeque nasi on both sides is a sign of disapproval.
- **e** Contraction of the orbicularis oris expresses determination.
- **f** Contraction of the buccinator signals satisfaction.
- **g** The zygomaticus major contracts during smiling.
- **h** Contraction of the risorius reflects purposeful action.
- **i** Contraction of the levator anguli oris signals self-satisfaction.
- **j** Contraction of the depressor anguli oris signals sadness.
- **k** Contraction of the depressor labii inferioris depresses the lower lip and expresses perseverance.
- **l** Contraction of the mentalis expresses indecision.

D Muscles of facial expression: functional groups

The various mimetic muscles are easier to learn when they are studied by regions. It is useful clinically to distinguish between the muscles of the forehead and palpebral fissure and the rest of the mimetic muscles. The muscles of the forehead and palpebral fissure are innervated by the superior branch of the facial nerve, while all the other mimetic muscles are supplied by other facial nerve branches. As a result, patients with central facial nerve paralysis can still close their eyes while patients with peripheral facial nerve paralysis cannot (see p.125 for further details).

Region	Muscle	Remarks
Calvarium	Epicranial muscle, consisting of	Muscle of the calvarium
	– Occipitofrontalis (frontal and occipital bellies)	Wrinkles the forehead
	– Temporoparietalis	Has no mimetic function
Palpebral fissure	Orbicularis oculi, consisting of	Closes the eyelid (**a**)
	– Orbital part	Tightly contracts the skin around the eye
	– Palpebral part	Palpebral reflex
	– Lacrimal part	Acts on the lacrimal sac
	Corrugator supercilii	Wrinkles the eyebrow (**b**)
	Depressor supercilii	Lowers the eyebrow
Nose	Procerus	Wrinkles the root of the nose
	Nasalis	Narrows the naris (**c**)
	Levator labii superioris alaeque nasi	Elevates the upper lip and nasal alae (**d**)
Mouth	Orbicularis oris	Closes the mouth (**e**)
	Buccinator	Muscle of the cheek (important during eating and drinking) (**f**)
	Zygomaticus major	Large muscle of the zygomatic arch (**g**)
	Zygomaticus minor	Small muscle of the zygomatic arch
	Risorius	Muscle of smiling/grinning (**h**)
	Levator labii superioris	Elevates the upper lip
	Levator anguli oris	Pulls the corner of the mouth upward (**i**)
	Depressor anguli oris	Pulls the corner of the mouth downward (**j**)
	Depressor labii inferioris	Pulls the lower lip downward (**k**)
	Mentalis	Pulls the skin of the chin upward (**l**)
Ear	Auricularis anterior	Anterior muscle of the auricle
	Auricularis superior	Superior muscle of the auricle
	Auricularis posterior	Posterior muscle of the auricle
Neck	Platysma	Cutaneous muscle of the neck

3.3 Muscles of Mastication: Overview and Superficial Muscles

Overview of the muscles of mastication
The muscles of mastication in the strict sense consist of four muscles: the masseter, temporalis, medial pterygoid, and lateral pterygoid.
The primary function of all these muscles is to close the mouth and move the upper teeth against the lower teeth in a grinding action during mastication. The lateral pterygoid muscle assists in opening the mouth. The two pterygoid muscles are also active during mastication (for the individual muscle actions, see **A–C**).

The mouth is opened primarily by the suprahyoid muscles and the force of gravity. The masseter and medial pterygoid form a muscular sling in which the mandible is suspended (see p. 84).
Note: All muscles of mastication are innervated by the mandibular nerve (third division of the trigeminal nerve), while the muscles of facial expression are innervated by the facial nerve.

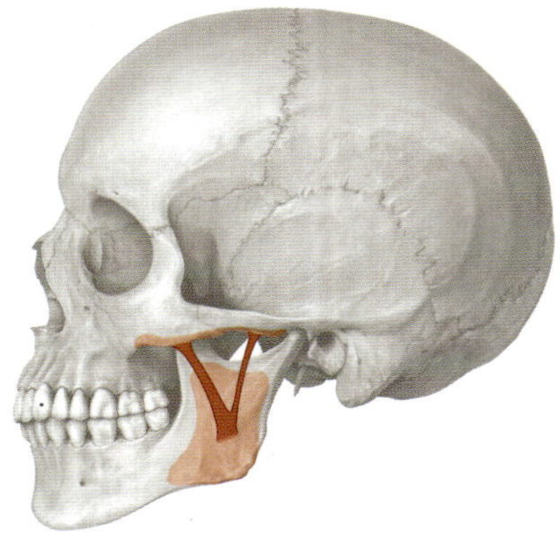

A Schematic of the masseter muscle

Masseter

Origin:	• Superficial part: zygomatic arch (anterior two-thirds) • Deep part: zygomatic arch (posterior third)
Insertion:	• Masseteric tuberosity on the mandibular angle
Actions:	• Elevates the mandible • Protrudes the mandible
Innervation:	Masseteric nerve, a branch of the mandibular division of the trigeminal nerve (CN V_3)

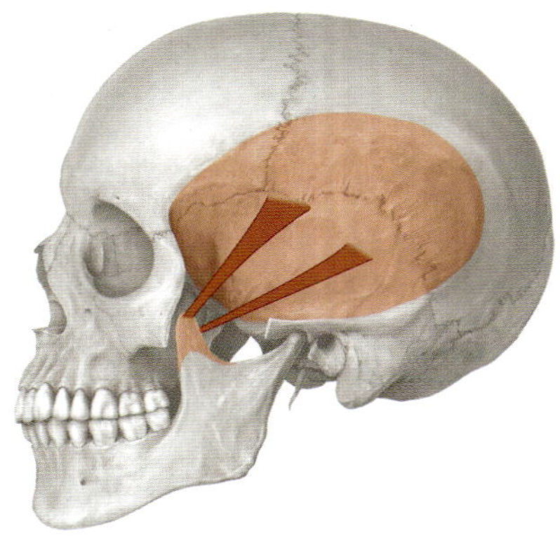

B Schematic of the temporalis muscle

Temporalis

Origin:	Inferior temporal line of the temporal fossa
Insertion:	Apex and medial surface of the coronoid process of the mandible
Actions:	• Elevates the mandible, chiefly with its vertical fibers • Retracts the protruded mandible with its horizontal posterior fibers • Unilateral contraction: mastication (moves the mandibular head on the balance side forward)
Innervation:	Deep temporal nerves, branches of the mandibular division of the trigeminal nerve (CN V_3)

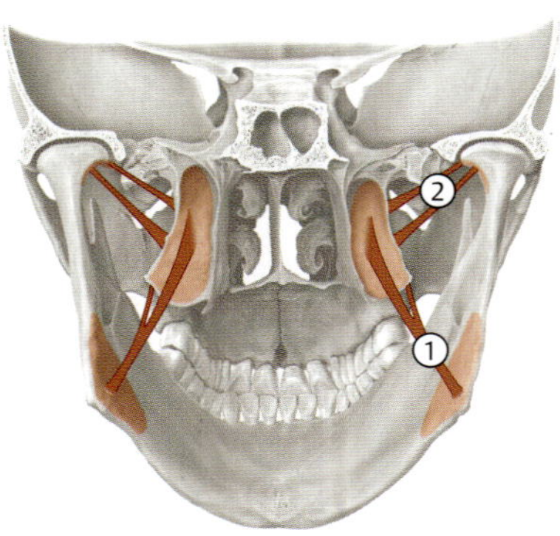

C Schematic of the medial and lateral pterygoid muscles

① Medial pterygoid

Origin:	Pterygoid fossa and medial surface of the lateral plate of the pterygoid process
Insertion:	Medial surface of the mandibular angle (pterygoid tuberosity)
Actions:	Elevates the mandible
Innervation:	Medial pterygoid nerve, a branch of the mandibular division of the trigeminal nerve (CN V_3)

② Lateral pterygoid

Origin:	• Superior head: Infratemporal crest of greater wing of the sphenoid • Inferior head: lateral surface of the lateral pterygoid plate
Insertion:	• Superior head: articular disk of the temporomandibular joint • Inferior head: neck of the condylar process of the mandible
Actions:	• Bilateral contraction: initiates mouth opening by protruding the mandible and moving the articular disk forward • Unilateral contraction: elevates the mandible to the opposite side during mastication
Innervation:	Lateral pterygoid nerve, a branch of the mandibular division of the trigeminal nerve (CN V_3)

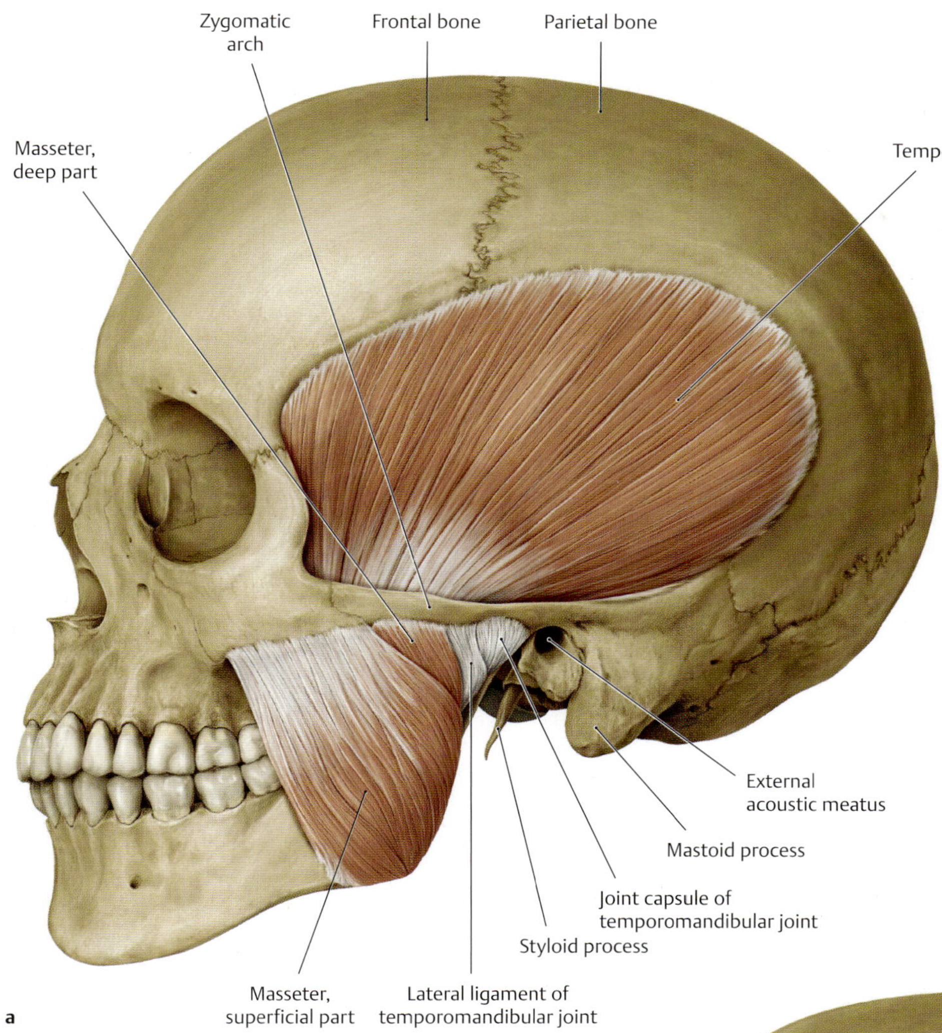

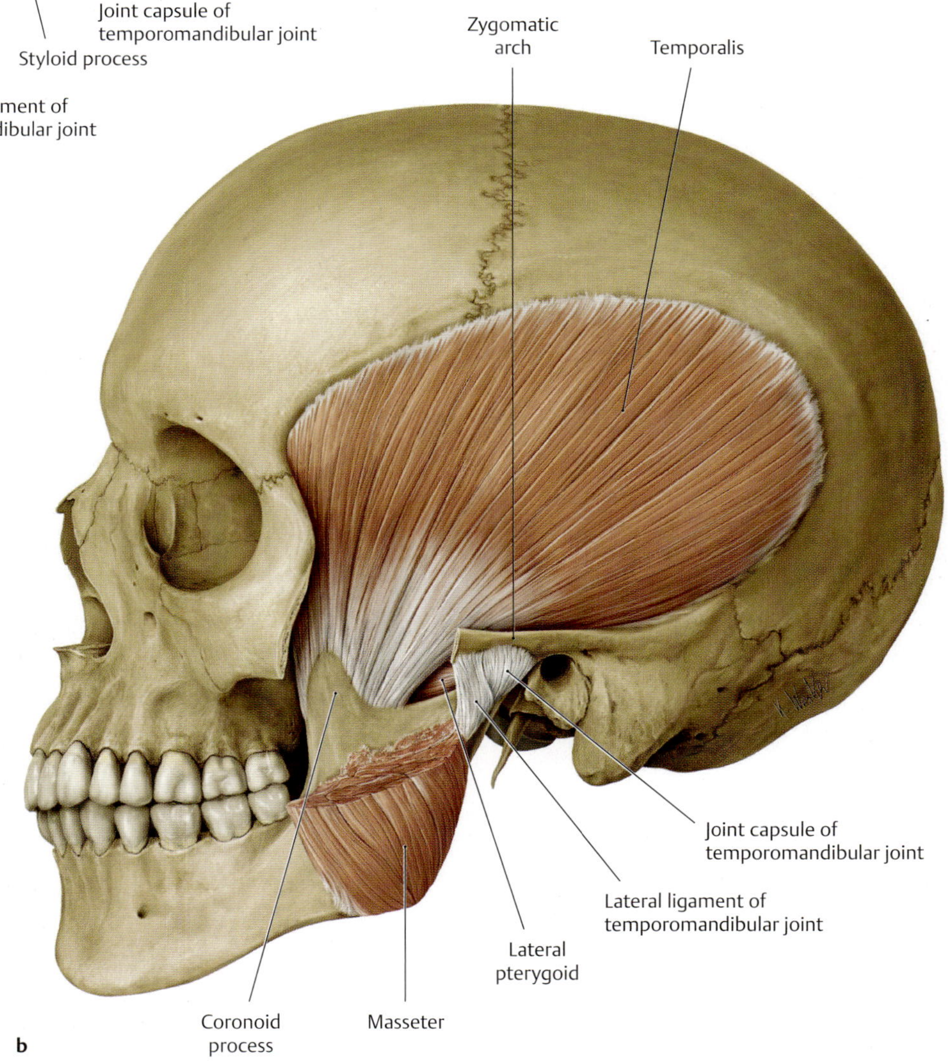

D Temporalis and masseter

Left lateral view. **a** Superficial layer, **b** deep layer. The masseter and zygomatic arch have been partially removed.

The full extent of the *temporalis* is shown in **b**. It is the most powerful muscle of mastication and does approximately half the work of mastication. The *masseter* consists of a superficial part and a deep part. The temporalis and masseter act powerfully in raising the mandible and closing the mouth. A small portion of the lateral pterygoid is visible in **b**.

3.4 Muscles of Mastication: Deep Muscles

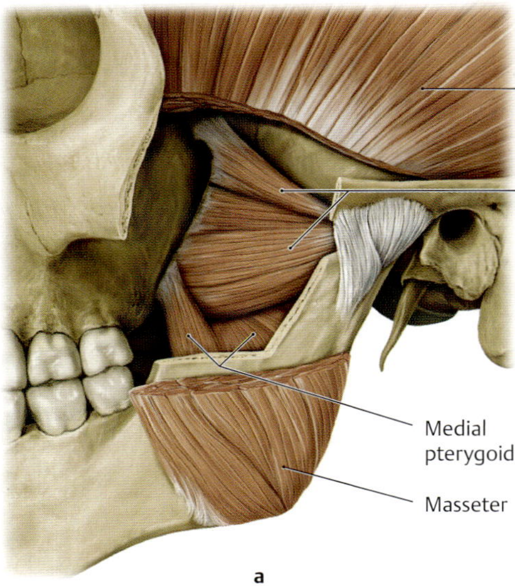

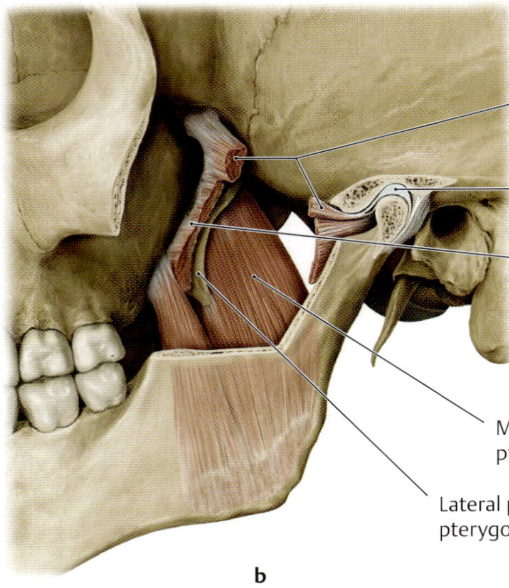

A Lateral and medial pterygoid muscles
Left lateral views.

a The coronoid process of the mandible has been removed here along with the lower part of the temporalis so that both pterygoid muscles can be seen.

b The temporalis has been completely removed, and the inferior part of the lateral pterygoid has been windowed. The lateral pterygoid initiates mouth opening, which is then continued by the suprahyoid muscles. With the temporomandibular joint opened, we can see that fibers from the lateral pterygoid blend with the articular disk of the temporomandibular joint. The lateral pterygoid functions as the guide muscle of the joint. Because its various parts (superior and inferior) are active during all movements, its actions are more complex than those of the other muscles of mastication. The medial pterygoid runs almost perpendicular to the lateral pterygoid and contributes to the formation of a muscular sling that partially encompasses the mandible (see **B**).

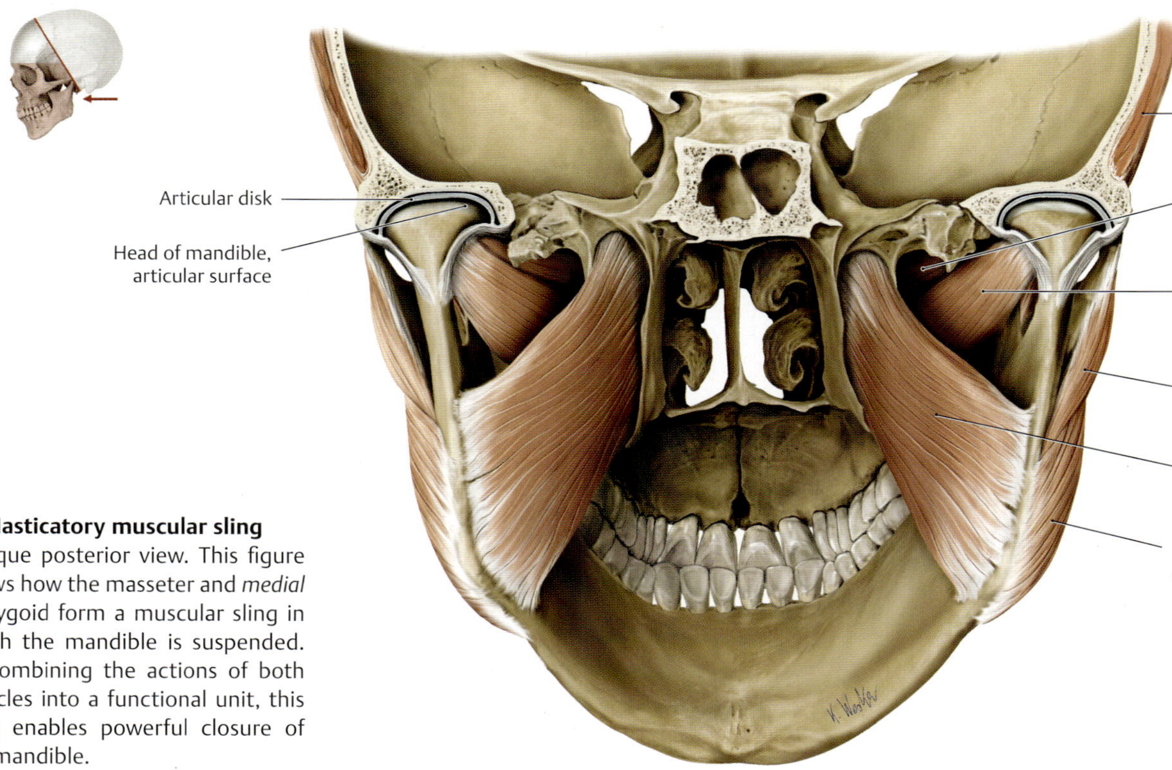

B Masticatory muscular sling
Oblique posterior view. This figure shows how the masseter and *medial* pterygoid form a muscular sling in which the mandible is suspended. By combining the actions of both muscles into a functional unit, this sling enables powerful closure of the mandible.

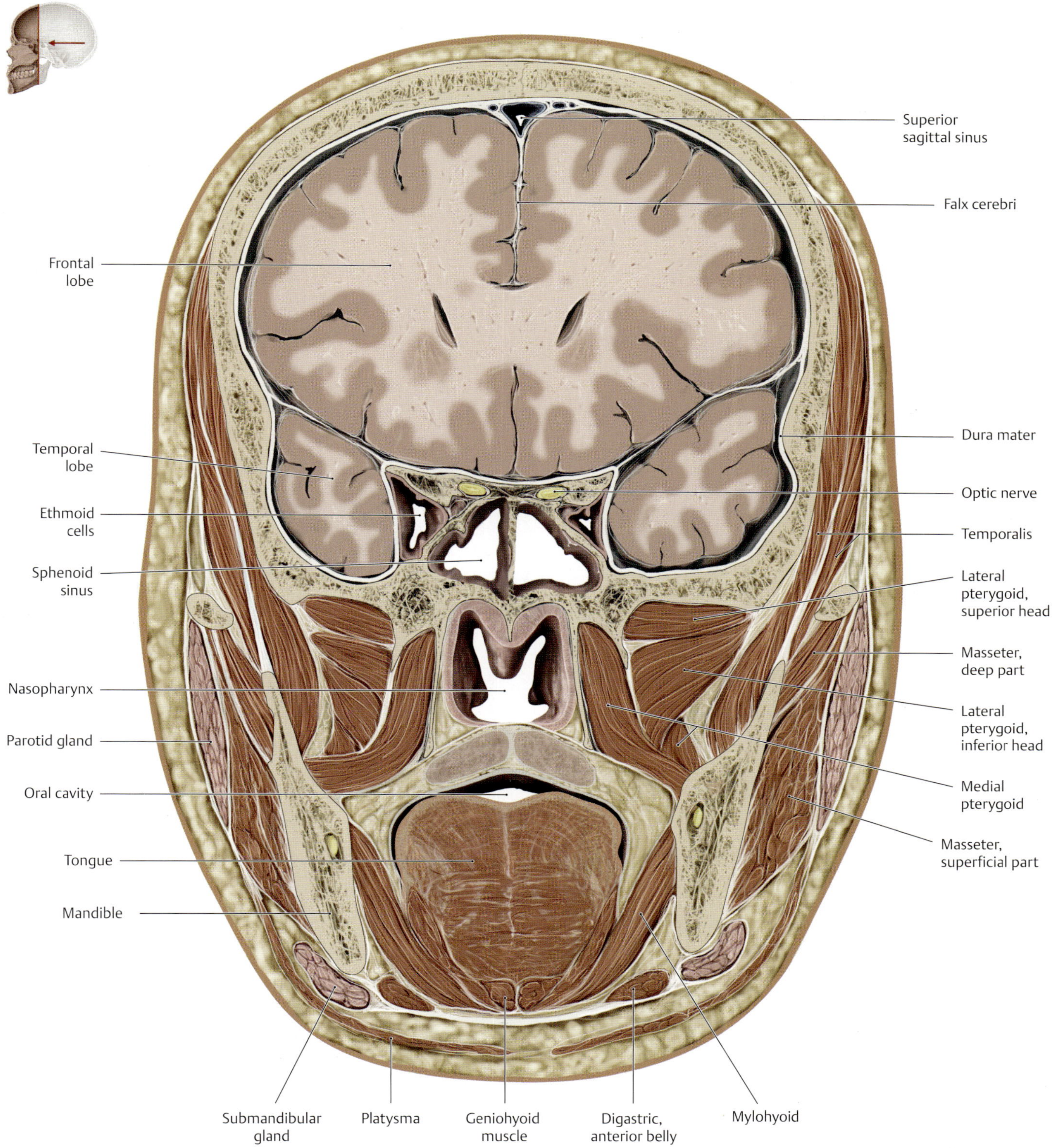

C Muscles of mastication, coronal section at the level of the sphenoid sinus

Posterior view. The topography of the muscles of mastication and neighboring structures is particularly well displayed in this section.

3.5 Muscles of the Head: Origins and Insertions

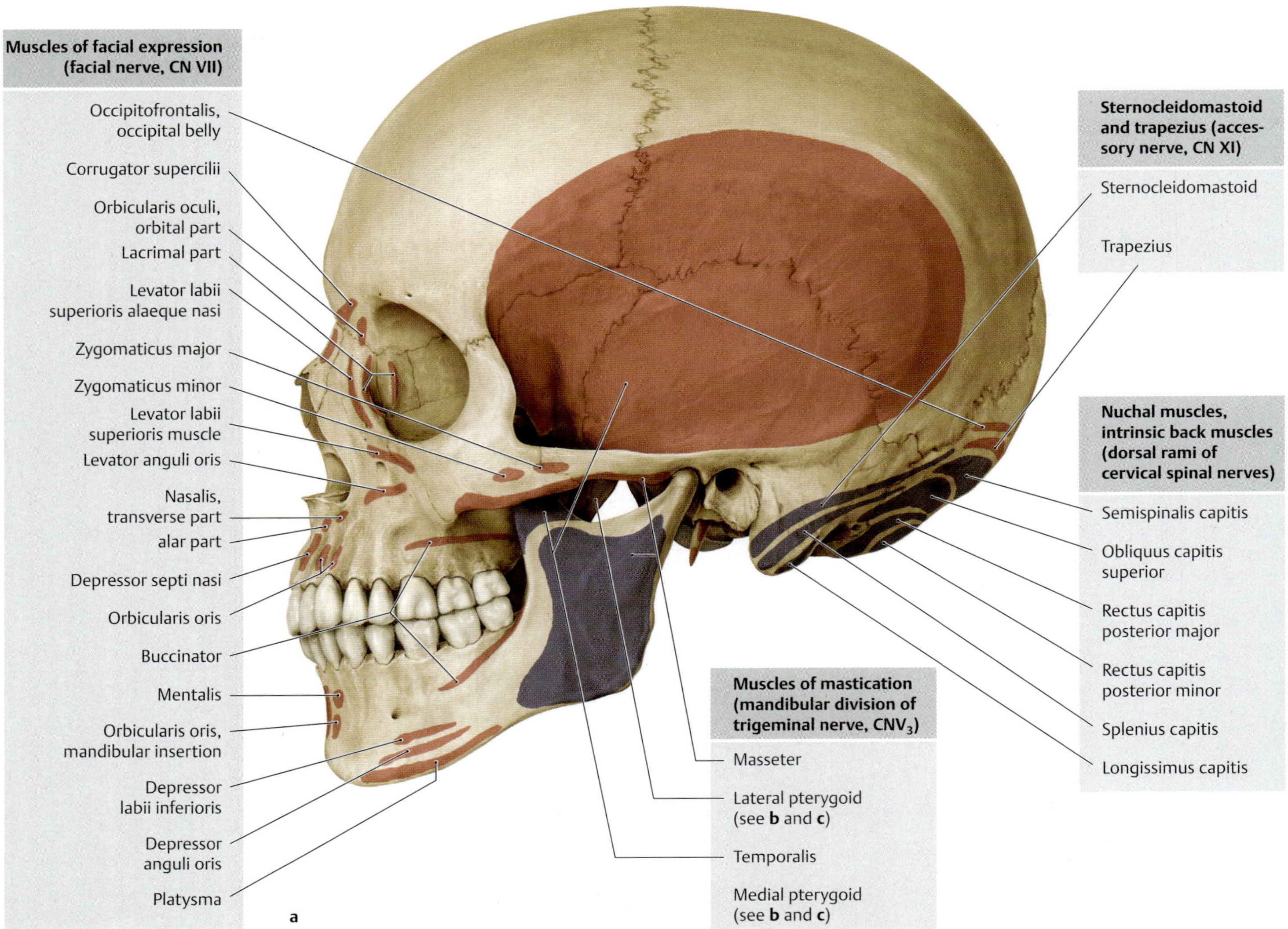

A Muscle origins and insertions on the skull

a Left lateral view, **b** view of the inner surface of the right hemimandible, **c** inferior view of the base of the skull.
The origins and insertions of the muscles are indicated by color shading (origin: red, insertion: blue).

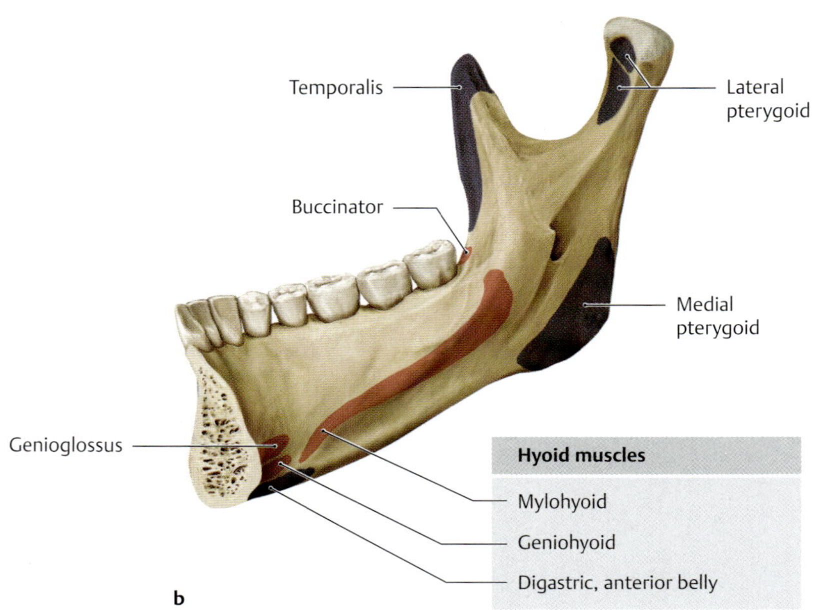

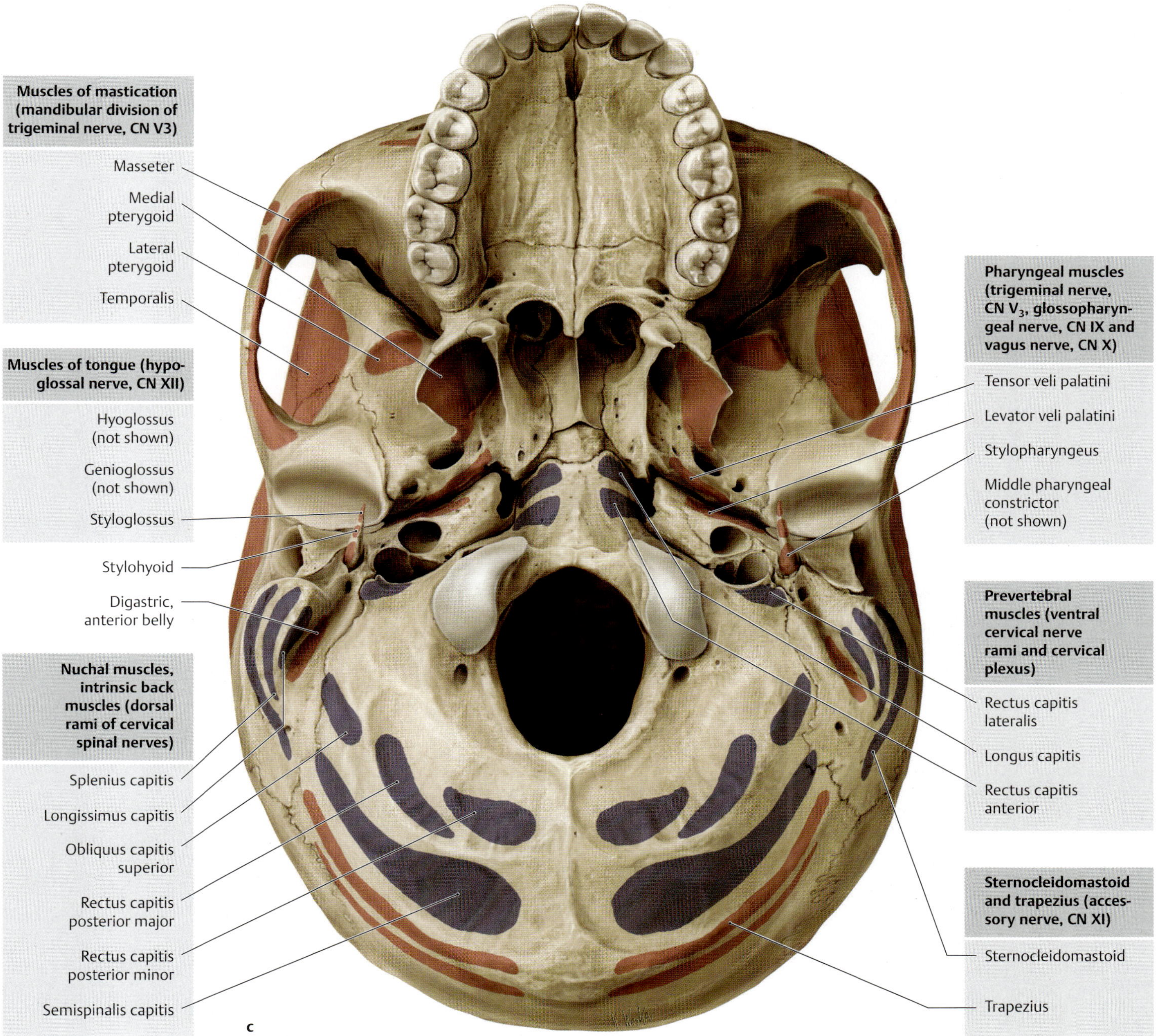
Muscles of mastication (mandibular division of trigeminal nerve, CN V3)
Masseter
Medial pterygoid
Lateral pterygoid
Temporalis
Muscles of tongue (hypoglossal nerve, CN XII)
Hyoglossus (not shown)
Genioglossus (not shown)
Styloglossus
Stylohyoid
Digastric, anterior belly
Nuchal muscles, intrinsic back muscles (dorsal rami of cervical spinal nerves)
Splenius capitis
Longissimus capitis
Obliquus capitis superior
Rectus capitis posterior major
Rectus capitis posterior minor
Semispinalis capitis
c
Pharyngeal muscles (trigeminal nerve, CN V_3, glossopharyngeal nerve, CN IX and vagus nerve, CN X)
Tensor veli palatini
Levator veli palatini
Stylopharyngeus
Middle pharyngeal constrictor (not shown)
Prevertebral muscles (ventral cervical nerve rami and cervical plexus)
Rectus capitis lateralis
Longus capitis
Rectus capitis anterior
Sternocleidomastoid and trapezius (accessory nerve, CN XI)
Sternocleidomastoid
Trapezius

3.6 Neck Muscles: Overview and Superficial Muscles

A Scheme used for classifying the neck muscles into groups

The next few sections follow the outline below, which is based on the topographical anatomy of the neck. Various schemes may be used, however. While the nuchal muscles are classified as neck muscles from a topographical standpoint, they belong functionally to the category of intrinsic back muscles (which are not described here).

Superficial neck muscles
- Platysma
- Sternocleidomastoid
- Trapezius*

Suprahyoid muscles
- Digastric
- Geniohyoid
- Mylohyoid
- Stylohyoid

Infrahyoid muscles
- Sternohyoid
- Sternothyroid
- Thyrohyoid
- Omohyoid

* Not a neck muscle in the strict sense, but included here owing to its topographical importance

Prevertebral muscles (deep strap muscles)
- Longus capitis
- Longus colli
- Rectus capitis anterior
- Rectus capitis lateralis

Lateral (deep) neck muscles
- Scalenus anterior
- Scalenus medius
- Scalenus posterior

Nuchal muscles (intrinsic back muscles)
- Semispinalis capitis
- Semispinalis cervicis
- Splenius capitis
- Splenius cervicis
- Longissimus capitis
- Iliocostalis cervicis
- Suboccipital muscles

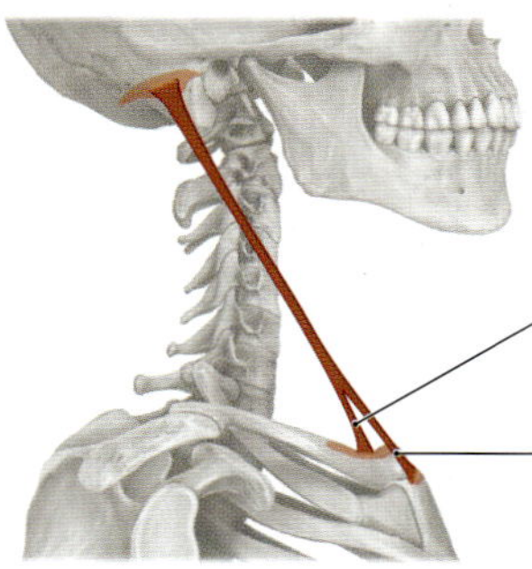

B Schematic of the sternocleidomastoid

Origin:
- Sternal head: manubrium sterni
- Clavicular head: medial third of the clavicle

Insertion: Mastoid process and superior nuchal line

Actions:
- Unilateral:
  - Tilts the head to the same side
  - Rotates the head to the opposite side
- Bilateral:
  - Extends the head
  - Assists in respiration when the head is fixed

Innervation: Accessory nerve (cranial nerve XI [CN XI] and direct branches from the cervical plexus (C1–C2)

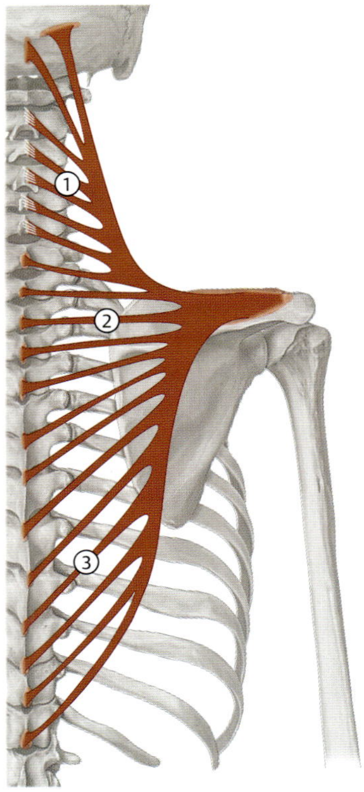

C Schematic of the trapezius

Origin:
① Descending part:
- Occipital bone (superior nuchal line and external occipital protuberance)
- The spinous processes of all cervical vertebrae via the nuchal ligament

② Transverse part:
Broad aponeurosis at the level of the T1–T4 spinous processes

③ Ascending part:
Spinous processes T5–T12

Insertion:
- Lateral third of the clavicle (descending part)
- Acromion (transverse part)
- Scapular spine (ascending part)

Actions:
- Descending part:
  - Draws the scapula obliquely upward and rotates it externally (acting with the inferior part of the serratus anterior)
  - Tilts the head to the same side and rotates it to the opposite side (with the shoulder girdle fixed)
- Transverse part: draws the scapula medially
- Ascending part: draws the scapula medially downward (supports the rotating action of the descending part)
- Entire muscle: stabilizes the scapula on the thorax

Innervation: Accessory nerve (CN XI) and cervical plexus (C2–C4)

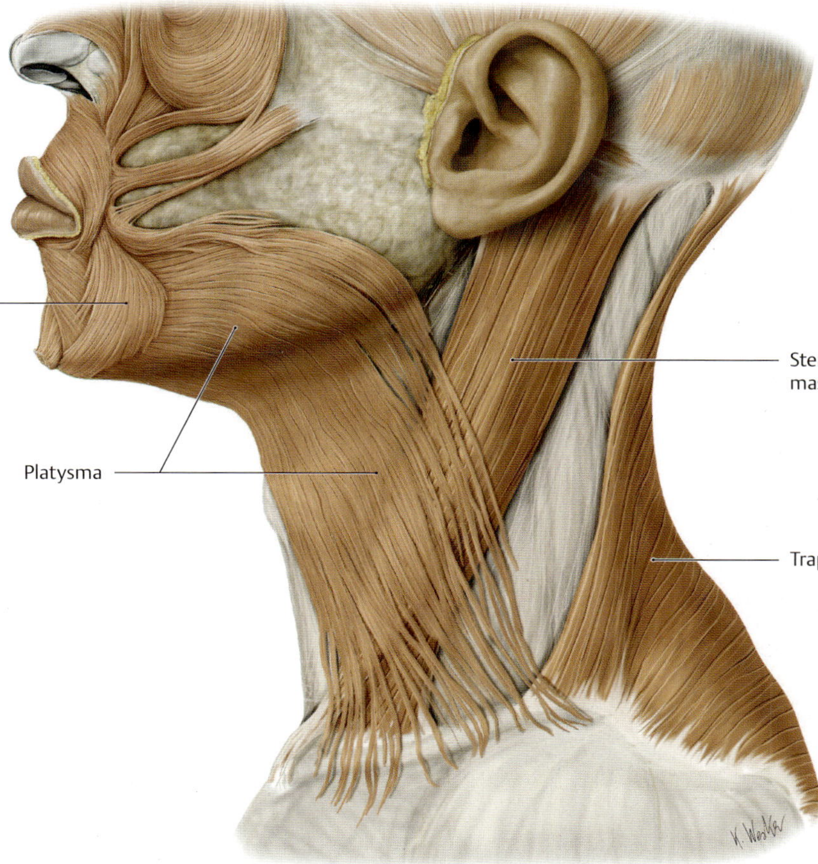

D Cutaneous muscle of the neck (platysma)

Left lateral view. The platysma is a broad, flat, subcutaneous muscular sheet located superficial to the investing layer of the deep cervical fascia. Unlike most muscles, it is not enveloped in its own fascial sheath (see classification scheme in **A**), but is instead directly associated with (and in part inserts into) the skin. This characteristic, which it shares with the muscles of facial expression, makes the platysma difficult to dissect. It also shares with those craniofacial muscles its source of innervation: the facial nerve. The platysma is highly variable in size—its fibers may reach from the lower part of the face to the upper thorax.

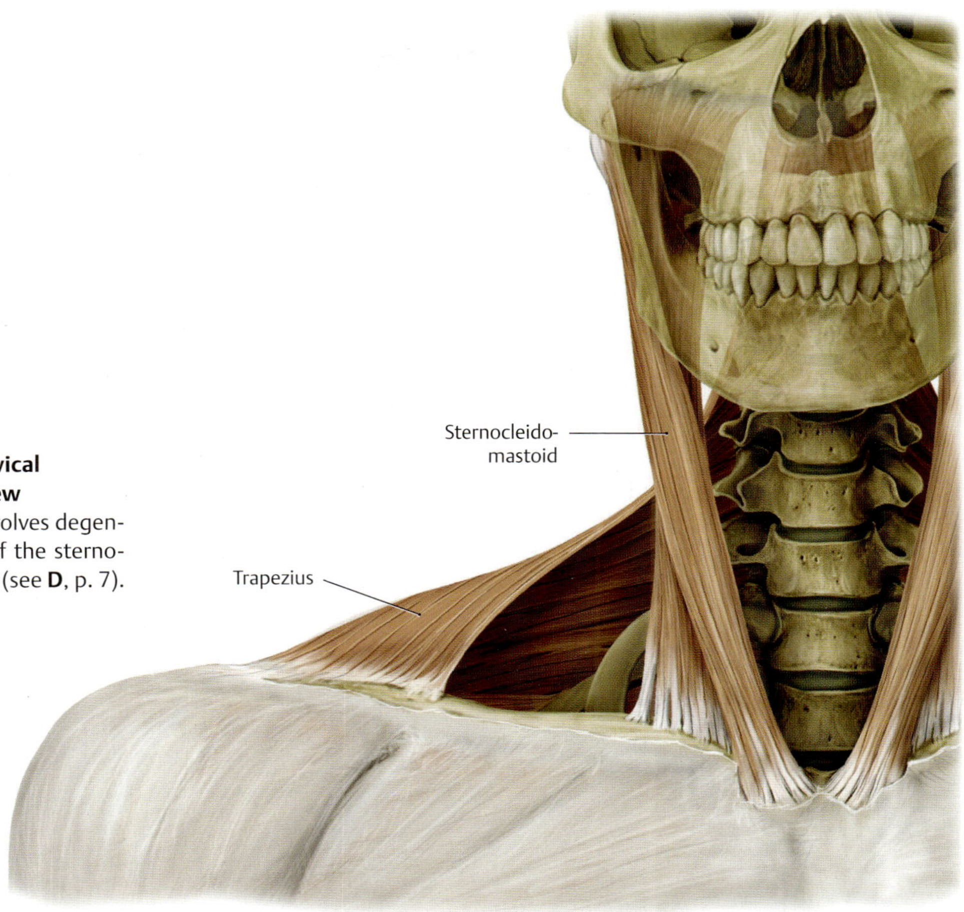

E Superficial neck muscles: sternocleidomastoid and cervical part of trapezius, anterior view

Congenital muscular torticollis involves degenerative scarring and shortening of the sternocleidomastoid muscle on one side (see **D**, p. 7).

3.7 Neck Muscles: Suprahyoid and Infrahyoid Muscles

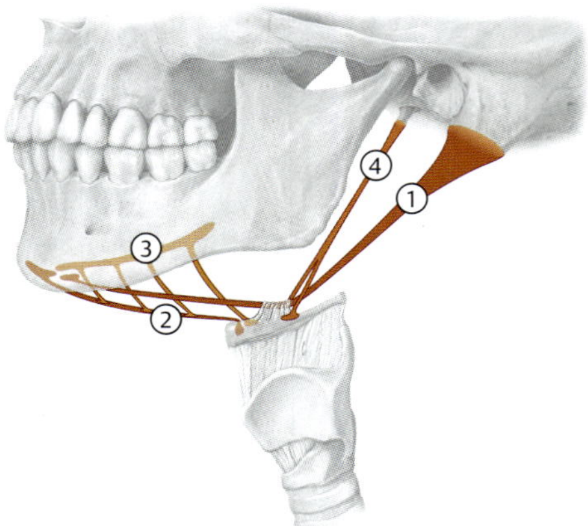

A Overview of the suprahyoid muscles

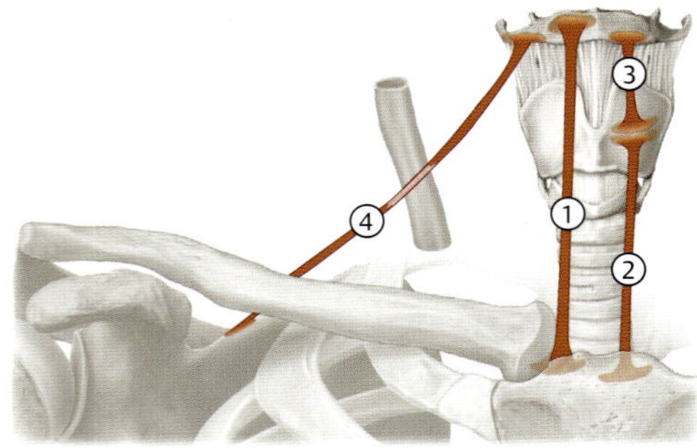

B Schematic of the infrahyoid muscles

① Digastric muscle

Origin:
- Anterior belly: digastric fossa of the mandible
- Posterior belly: medial to the mastoid process (mastoid notch)

Insertion: Body of the hyoid bone via an intermediate tendon with a fibrous loop

Actions:
- Elevates the hyoid bone (during swallowing)
- Assists in opening the mandible

Innervation:
- Anterior belly: nerve to the mylohyoid (from the mandibular nerve of CN V – trigeminal)
- Posterior belly: facial n. (CN VII)

② Geniohyoid muscle

Origin: Inferior mental spine of the mandible

Insertion: Body of the hyoid bone

Actions:
- Draws the hyoid bone forward (during swallowing)
- Assists in opening the mandible

Innervation: Ventral ramus of C1

③ Mylohyoid muscle

Origin: Mylohyoid line of the mandible

Insertion: Body of the hyoid bone by a median tendon of insertion (mylohyoid raphe)

Actions:
- Tightens and elevates the oral floor
- Draws the hyoid bone forward (during swallowing)
- Assists in opening the mandible and moving it from side to side (mastication)

Innervation: Mylohyoid nerve (from the mandibular nerve, a division of CN V)

④ Stylohyoid muscle

Origin: Styloid process of the temporal bone

Insertion: Body of the hyoid bone by a split tendon

Actions:
- Elevates the hyoid bone (during swallowing)
- Assists in opening the mandible

Innervation: Facial nerve (CN VII)

① Sternohyoid muscle

Origin: Posterior surface of the manubrium of the sternum and sternoclavicular joint

Insertion: Body of the hyoid bone

Actions:
- Depresses (fixes) the hyoid bone
- Depresses the larynx and hyoid bone (for phonation and the terminal phase of swallowing)

Innervation: Ansa cervicalis of the cervical plexus (C1–C3) as well as C4

② Sternothyroid muscle

Origin: Posterior surface of the manubrium of the sternum

Insertion: Oblique line of the thyroid

Actions:
- Draws the larynx and hyoid bone downward (fixes the hyoid bone)
- Depresses the larynx and hyoid bone (for phonation and the terminal phase of swallowing)

Innervation: Ansa cervicalis of the cervical plexus (C1–C3) as well as C4

③ Thyrohyoid muscle

Origin: Oblique line of the thyroid

Insertion: Body of the hyoid bone

Actions:
- Depresses and fixes the hyoid bone
- Raises the larynx during swallowing

Innervation: Ventral ramus of C1 as well as C4

④ Omohyoid muscle

Origin: Superior border of the scapula

Insertion: Body of the hyoid bone

Actions:
- Depresses (fixes) the hyoid bone
- Draws the larynx and hyoid bone downward (for phonation and the terminal phase of swallowing)
- Tenses the cervical fascia with its intermediate tendon and maintains patency of the internal jugular vein

Innervation: Ansa cervicalis of the cervical plexus (C1–C3) as well as C4

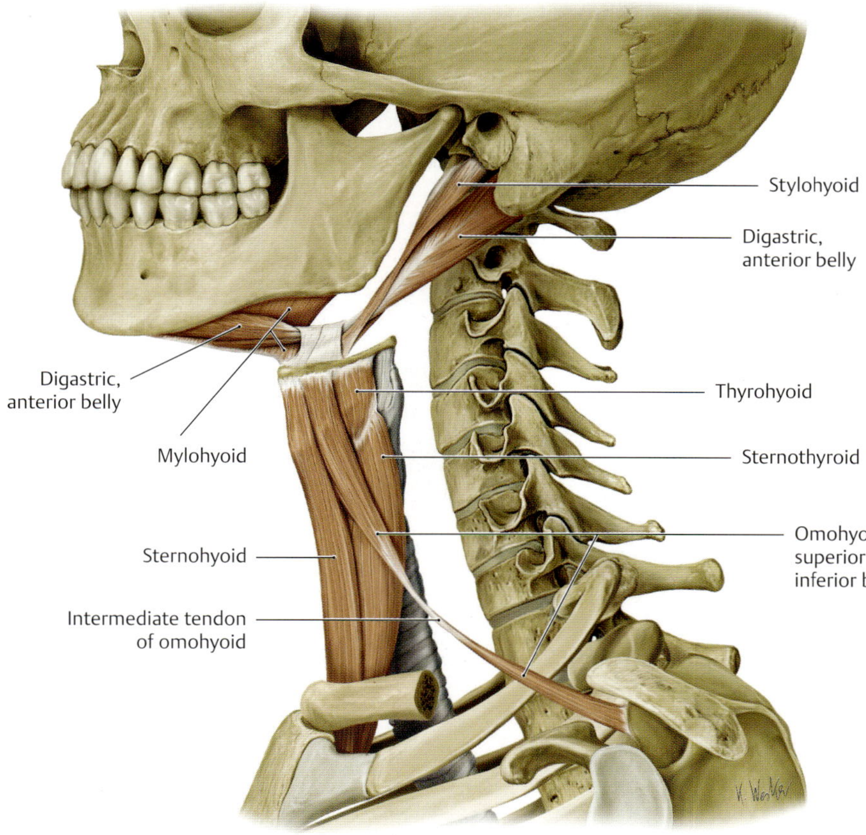

C Supra- and infrahyoid muscles, left lateral view

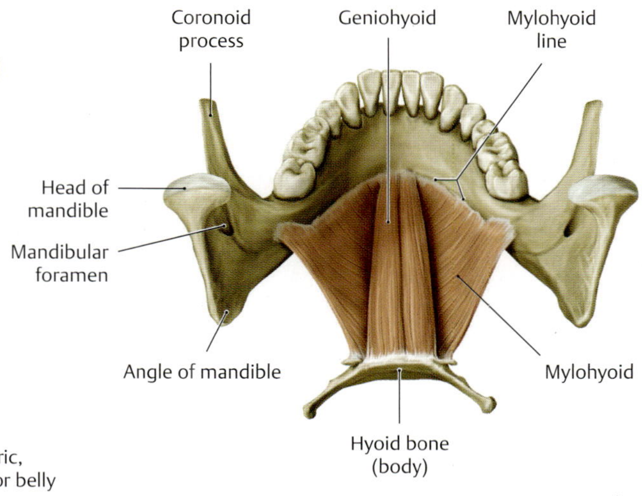

E Suprahyoid muscles: the mylohyoid and geniohyoid, posterosuperior view

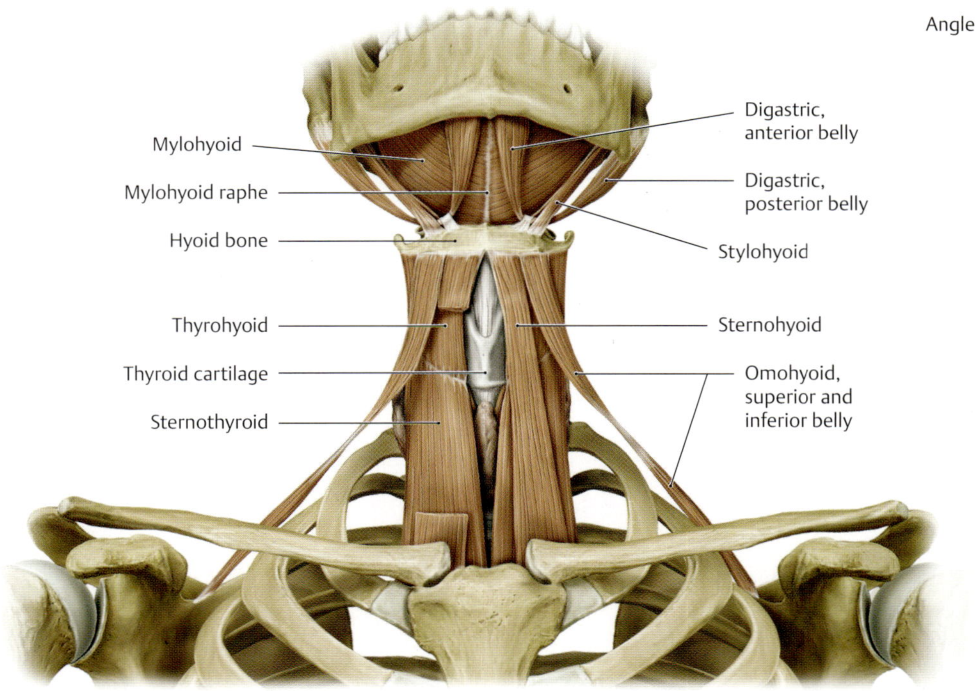

D Supra- and infrahyoid muscles, anterior view
Part of the sternohyoid muscle has been removed on the right side.

3.8 Neck Muscles: Prevertebral and Lateral (Deep) Muscles

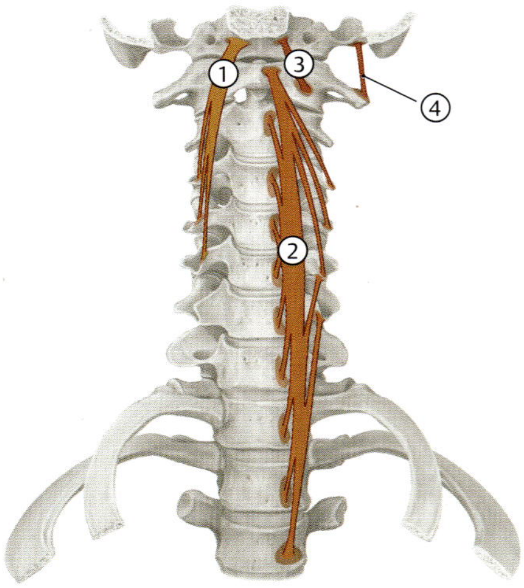

A Schematic of the prevertebral muscles

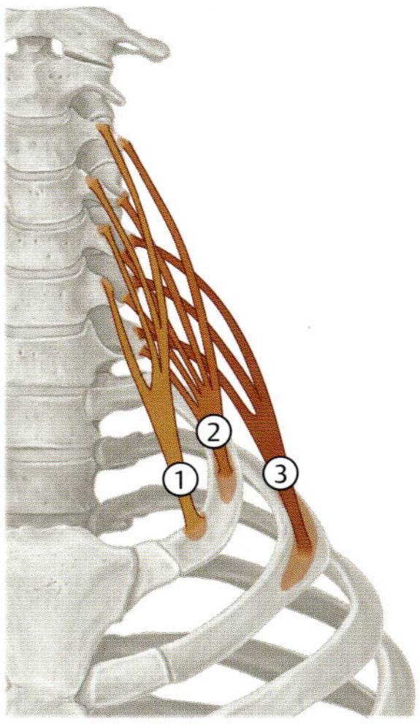

B Schematic of the lateral (deep) neck muscles

① Longus capitis

Origin: Anterior tubercles of the transverse processes of the C3–C6 vertebrae
Insertion: Basilar part of the occipital bone
Actions:
- Unilateral: tilts and slightly rotates the head to the same side
- Bilateral: flexes the head

Innervation: Direct branches from the cervical plexus (C1–C4)

② Longus colli

Origin:
- Vertical (intermediate) part: anterior surfaces of the C5–C7 and T1–T3 vertebral bodies
- Superior oblique part: anterior tubercle of the transverse processes of the C3–C5 vertebrae
- Inferior oblique part: anterior surfaces of the T1–T3 vertebral bodies

Insertion:
- Vertical part: anterior surfaces of the C2–C4 vertebrae
- Superior oblique part: anterior tubercle of the atlas
- Inferior oblique part: anterior tubercles of the transverse processes of the C5 and C6 vertebrae

Actions:
- Unilateral: tilts and rotates and cervical spine to the same side
- Bilateral: flexes the cervical spine

Innervation: Direct branches from the cervical plexus (C2–C4) as well as direct branches from C5, C6

③ Rectus capitis anterior

Origin: Lateral mass of the atlas
Insertion: Basilar part of the occipital bone
Actions:
- Unilateral: lateral flexion at the atlanto-occipital joint
- Bilateral: flexion at the atlanto-occipital joint

Innervation: Ventral rami of C1

④ Rectus capitis lateralis

Origin: Transverse process of the atlas
Insertion: Basilar part of the occipital bone (lateral to the occipital condyles)
Actions:
- Unilateral: lateral flexion at the atlanto-occipital joint
- Bilateral: flexion at the atlanto-occipital joint

Innervation: Ventral rami of C1

Mm. scaleni

Origin:
① Scalenus anterior: anterior tubercle of the transverse processes of the C3–C6 vertebrae
② Scalenus medius: transverse processes of atlas and axis; posterior tubercles of the transverse processes of the C3–C7 vertebrae
③ Scalenus posterior: posterior tubercle of the transverse processes of the C5–C7 vertebrae

Insertion:
- Scalenus anterior: scalene tubercle on the first rib
- Scalenus medius: first rib (posterior to the groove for the subclavian artery)
- Scalenus posterior: outer surface of the second rib

Actions:
- With the ribs mobile: inspiration (elevates the upper ribs)
- With the ribs fixed: bends the cervical spine to the same side (with unilateral contraction)
- Flexes the neck (with bilateral contraction)

Innervation: Direct branches from the cervical plexus and brachial plexus (C3–C6)

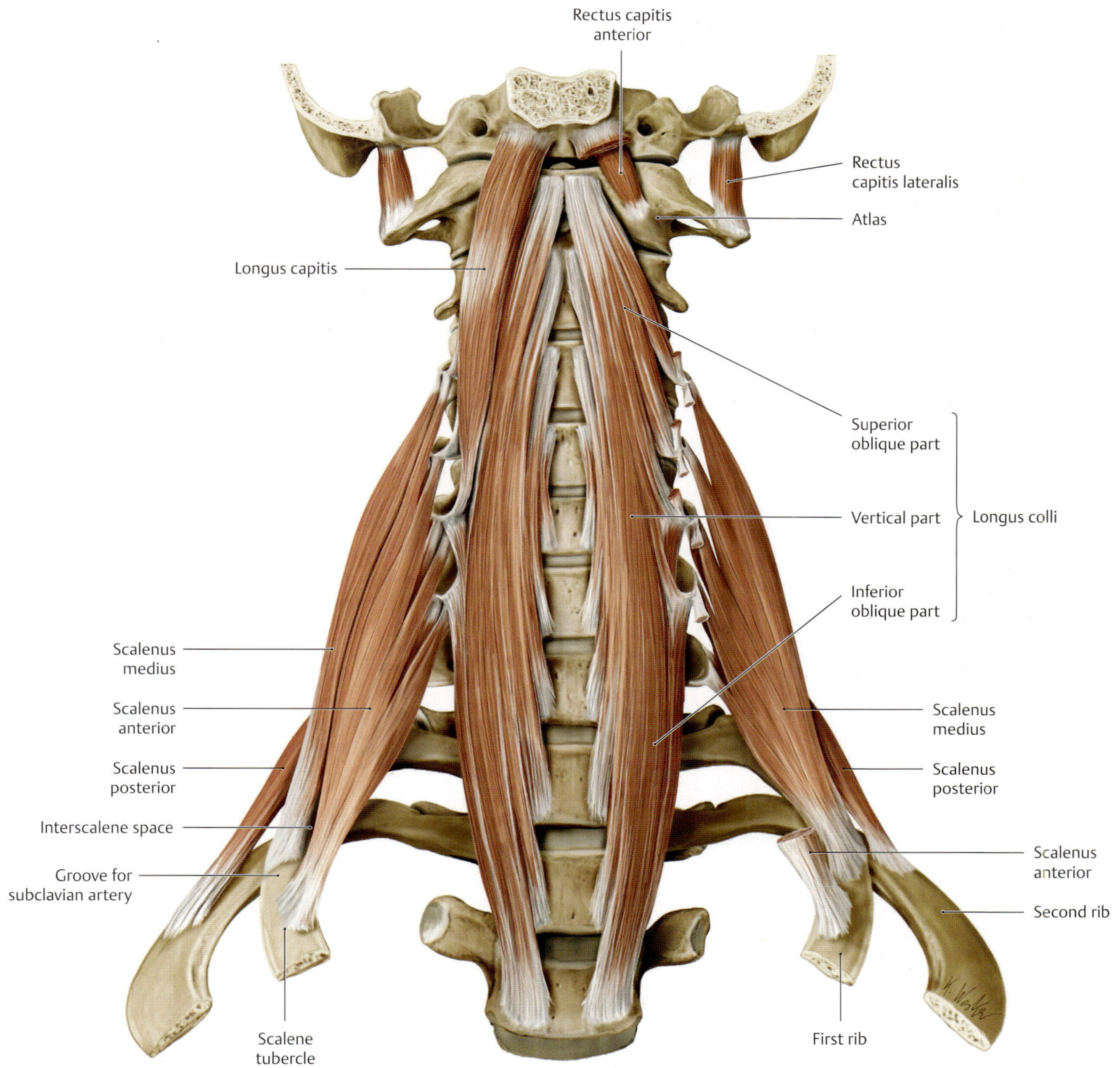

C Prevertebral and lateral (deep) neck muscles, anterior view
The longus capitis and scalenus anterior muscles have been partially removed on the left side. The prevertebral muscles stretch between the cervical spine and skull, acting upon both. The three overlapping scalene muscles are classified as lateral (deep) neck muscles. As they pass between the cervical spine and the upper two ribs, they also assist in respiration. The scalenus anterior and scalenus medius are separated by the *interscalene space*—a topographically important interval that is traversed by the brachial plexus and subclavian artery.

4.1 Classification of the Arteries Supplying the Head and Neck

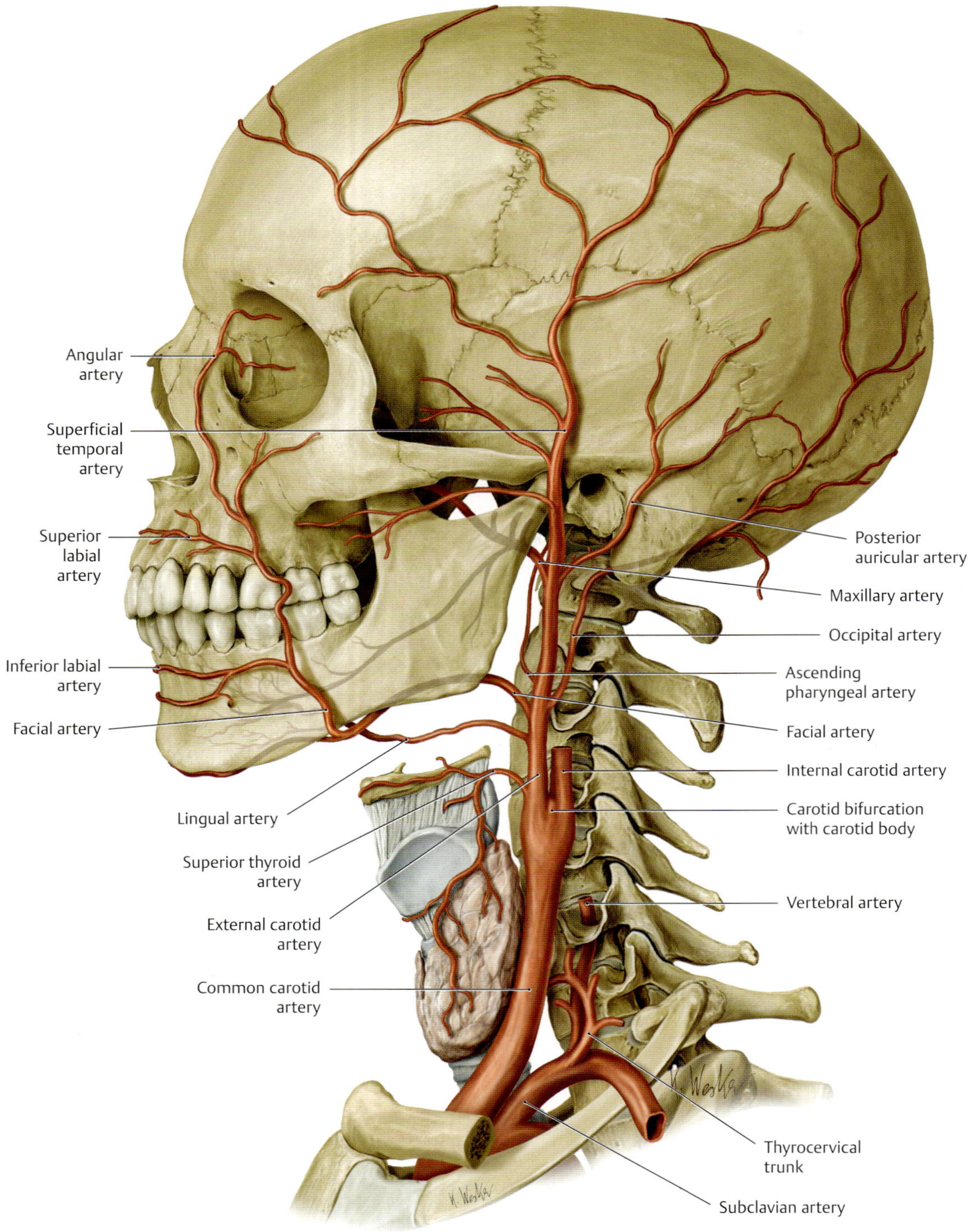

Classification of the arteries supplying the head and neck

Branches of the external carotid artery

Anterior branches
- Superior thyroid artery
  - infrahyoid branch
  - superior laryngeal artery
  - cricothyroid branch
  - sternocleidomastoid branch
  - glandular branch
- lingual artery
- facial artery

Medial branch
- ascending pharyngeal artery

Posterior branches
- occipital artery
- posterior auricular artery

Terminal branches
- maxillary artery
- superficial temporal artery

Branches of the subclavian artery

Internal thoracic artery
- mediastinal branches
- thymic branches
- pericardiacophrenic artery
- mammary branches
- anterior intercostal branches
- musculophrenic artery
- superior epigastric artery

Vertebral artery
- spinal branches
- meningeal branch
- posterior spinal arteries
- anterior spinal artery
- posterior inferior cerebellar artery
- basilar artery

Thyrocervical trunk
- inferior thyroid artery (ascending cervical artery)
- transverse cervical artery
  - superficial branch (superficial cervical artery)
  - deep branch (dorsal scapular artery)
- suprascapular artery

Costocervical trunk
- deep cervical artery
- supreme intercostal artery

A Overview of the arteries of the head and neck
Left lateral view. The head and neck are mainly supplied by the internal and external carotid arteries. They arise from the common carotid artery, which bifurcates in the neck after originating from the aortic arch. The internal and external arteries are connected with each other through anastomoses (see **D**). The internal carotid artery mainly—but not exclusively—supplies the intracranial structures (brain). The external carotid artery supplies the neck and head. In the neck region, the common carotid artery and the external carotid artery give off smaller branches. Additionally, areas near the thorax are also supplied by branches of the subclavian artery.
The carotid body is situated in the carotid bifurcation. It detects hypoxia and pH changes, which is important for the regulation of respiration.

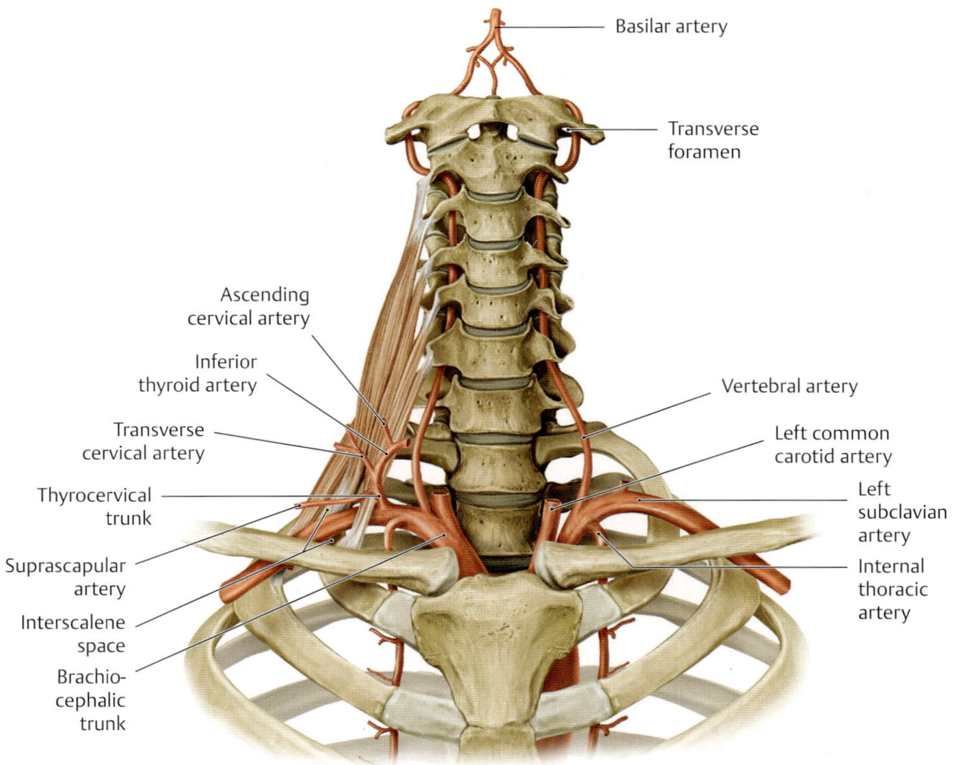

B Subclavian artery and its branches
Anterior view. The subclavian artery distributes a number of branches to structures located at the base of the neck and about the thoracic inlet. Two branches of special importance are the thyrocervical trunk, which gives origin to the transverse cervical artery, and the costocervical trunk (s. **C**).
Note: The branches of the subclavian artery may arise in a variable sequence. After emerging from the thoracic inlet, the subclavian artery passes through the interscalene space (between the scalenus anterior and medius muscles, see p. 93), to the upper limb.
The *vertebral artery* arises from the posterior aspect of the subclavian artery on each side and ascends through the foramina in the transverse processes of the cervical vertebrae. After entering the skull, both vertebral arteries fuse into a single basilar artery which will anastomose with the two internal carotid arteries, forming the arterial circle (of Willis) that has a major clinical importance in supplying blood to the brain.

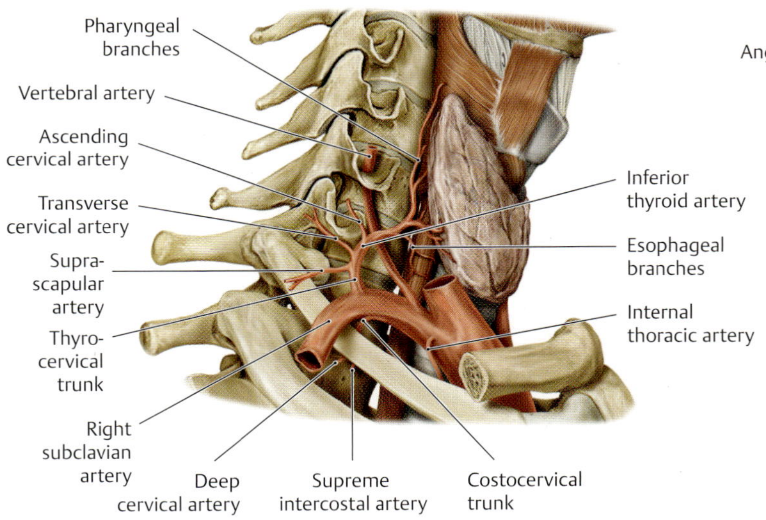

C Thyrocervical trunk, costocervical trunk and their branches
Right lateral view. The thyrocervical trunk arises from the subclavian artery and divides into the inferior thyroid artery, transverse cervical artery, and suprascapular artery. It mainly supplies structures located at the lateral base of the neck and is variable in its development.
The costocervical trunk arises posteriorly from the subclavian artery at the level of the scalenus anterior muscle. It divides into the deep cervical artery and supreme intercostal artery, supplying blood to the posterior neck muscles and the first intercostal space.

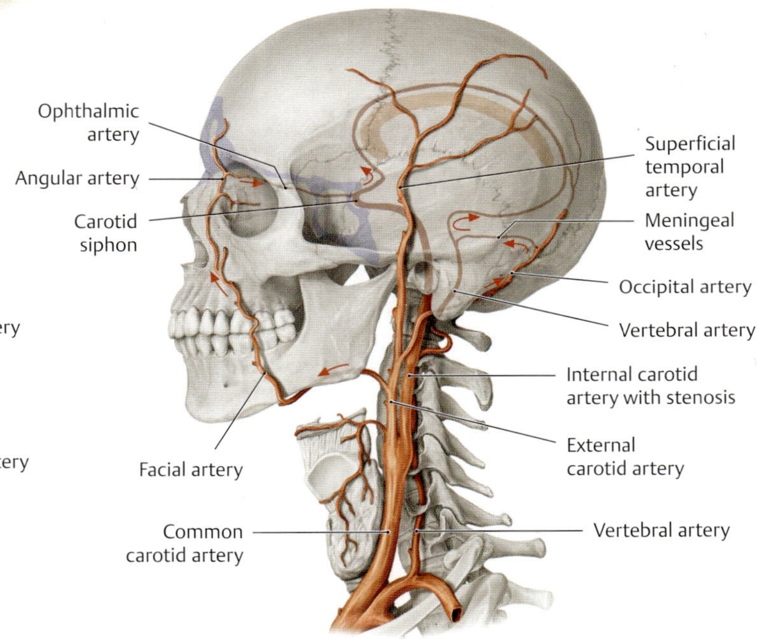

D Collateral pathways that develop in response to internal carotid artery stenosis
Atherosclerosis of the internal carotid artery is a frequent clinical problem. Narrowing of the carotid lumen (stenosis) eventually results in decreased blood flow to the brain. If the lumen is occluded suddenly, the result is a stroke. But if the stenosis develops over time, blood can still reach the brain through the gradual recruitment of collateral channels. As this occurs, the direction of blood flow may become reversed in anastomotic areas close to the brain (see arrows). As long as an adequate collateral circulation is maintained, the stenosis does not produce clinical manifestations.
The principal collateral pathways are as follows:

- Ophthalmic collaterals: external carotid artery → facial artery → angular artery → ophthalmic artery → carotid siphon
- Occipital anastomosis: external carotid artery → occipital artery → small meningeal arteries → vertebral artery

4.2 Internal Carotid Artery and Classification of the Branches of the External Carotid Artery

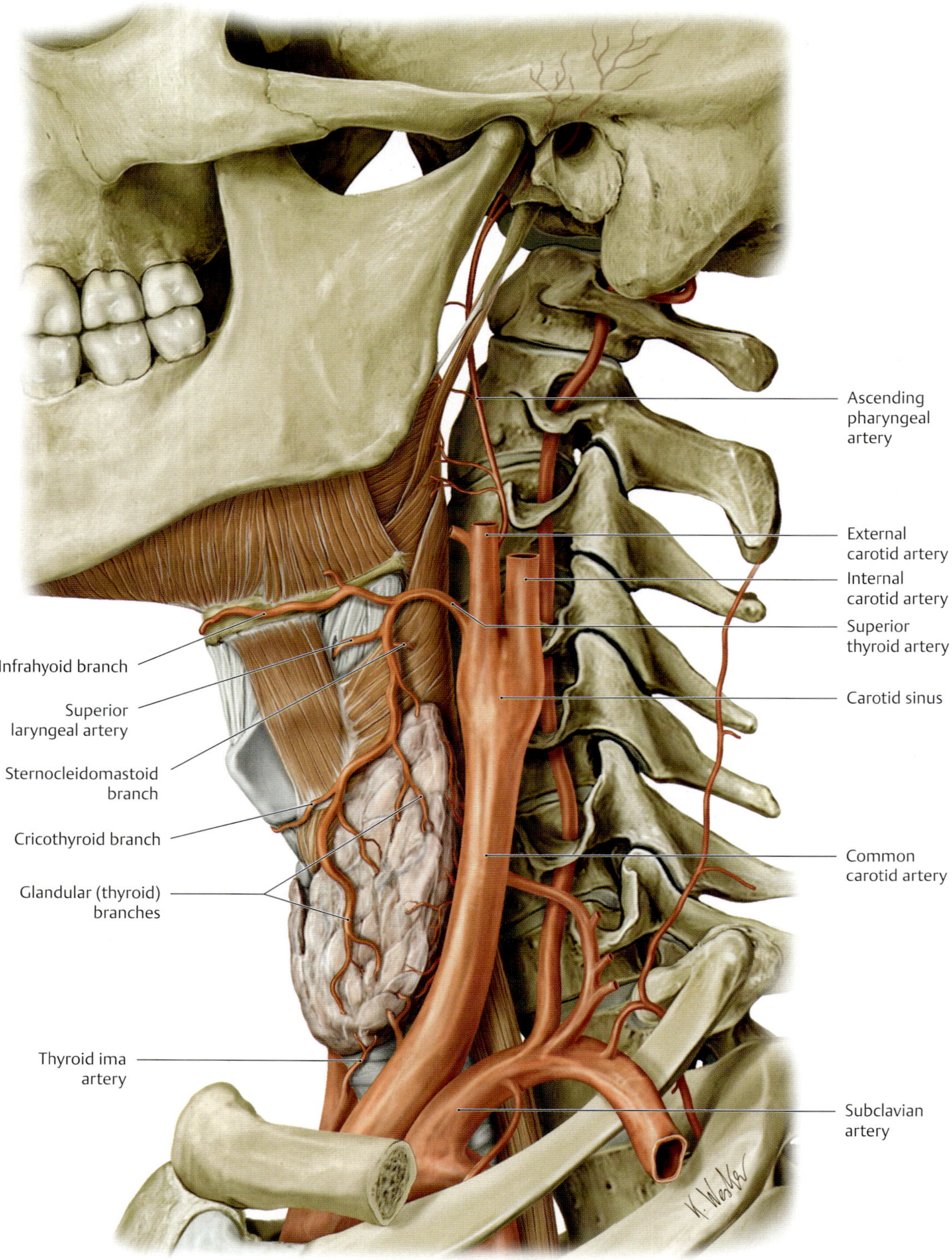

A Common carotid and external carotid arteries and their branches in the neck

Left view. The head and neck are supplied by the common carotid artery. It arises from the brachiocephalic trunk, directly to the left of the aortic arch. The right and left common carotid arteries bifurcate at approximately the level of the C4 vertebral body into the left and right internal and external carotid arteries. The internal carotid artery supplies the brain and orbit (see p. 102 f), giving off no branches in the neck.

The external carotid artery gives off numerous branches in the head and neck (see **B**). In the neck, it primarily supplies the anterior structures including the cervical viscera. The two carotid arteries are invested in a connective-tissue layer of the cervical fascia, the carotid sheath (**B**, p. 4).

Note: The brain is supplied exclusively by the internal carotid arteries and the vertebral arteries.

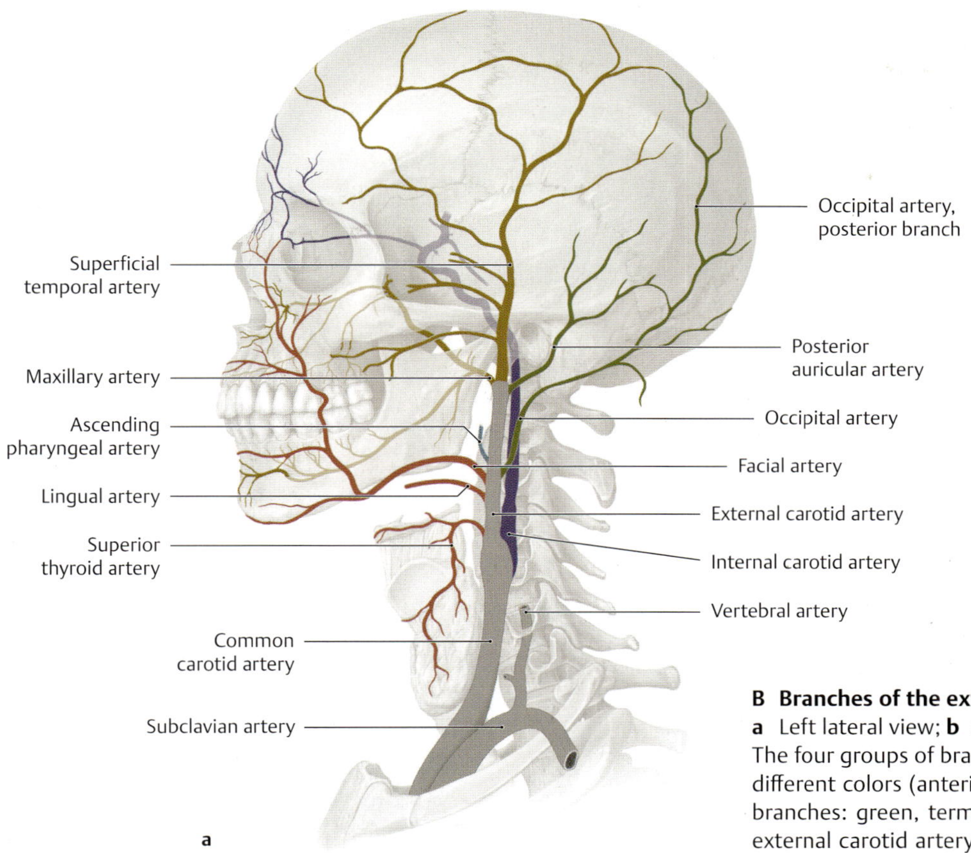

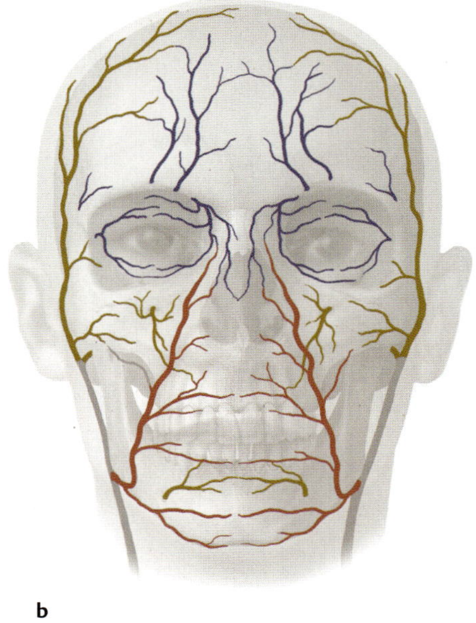

B Branches of the external carotid artery
a Left lateral view; **b** anterior view.
The four groups of branches of the external carotid artery are shown in different colors (anterior branches: red, medial branch: blue, posterior branches: green, terminal branches: brown). Certain branches of the external carotid artery (facial artery, red) communicate with branches of the internal carotid artery (terminal branches of the ophthalmic artery, purple) through anastomoses in the facial region **b**. Extracerebral branches of the internal carotid artery are described on p. 102 f.

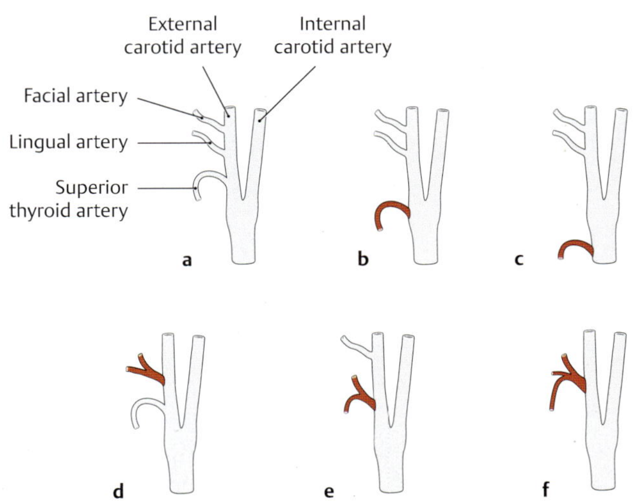

C Branches of the external carotid artery: typical anatomy and variants (after Lippert and Pabst)

a In **typical cases** (50%) the facial artery, lingual artery, and superior thyroid artery arise from the external carotid artery above the carotid bifurcation.

b–f **Variants:**

b, c The superior thyroid artery arises at the level of the carotid bifurcation (20%) or from the common carotid artery (10%).

d–f Two or three branches combine to form a common trunk: linguofacial trunk (18%), thyrolingual trunk (2%), or thyrolinguofacial trunk (1%).

D Overview of the branches of the external carotid artery
(more distal branches are described in the units below)
Subsequent units deal with the arteries of the head as they are grouped in the table below, followed by the branches of the internal carotid artery and the veins.

External carotid branches	Distribution
Anterior:	
• Superior thyroid artery	• Larynx, thyroid gland
• Lingual artery	• Oral floor, tongue
• Facial artery	• Superficial facial region
Medial:	
• Ascending pharyngeal artery	• Plexus to the skull base
Posterior:	
• Occipital artery	• Occiput
• Posterior auricular artery	• Ear
Terminal:	
• Maxillary artery	• Masticatory muscles, posteromedial part of the facial skeleton, meninges
• Superficial temporal artery	• Temporal region, part of the ear

4.3 External Carotid Artery: Anterior, Medial, and Posterior Branches

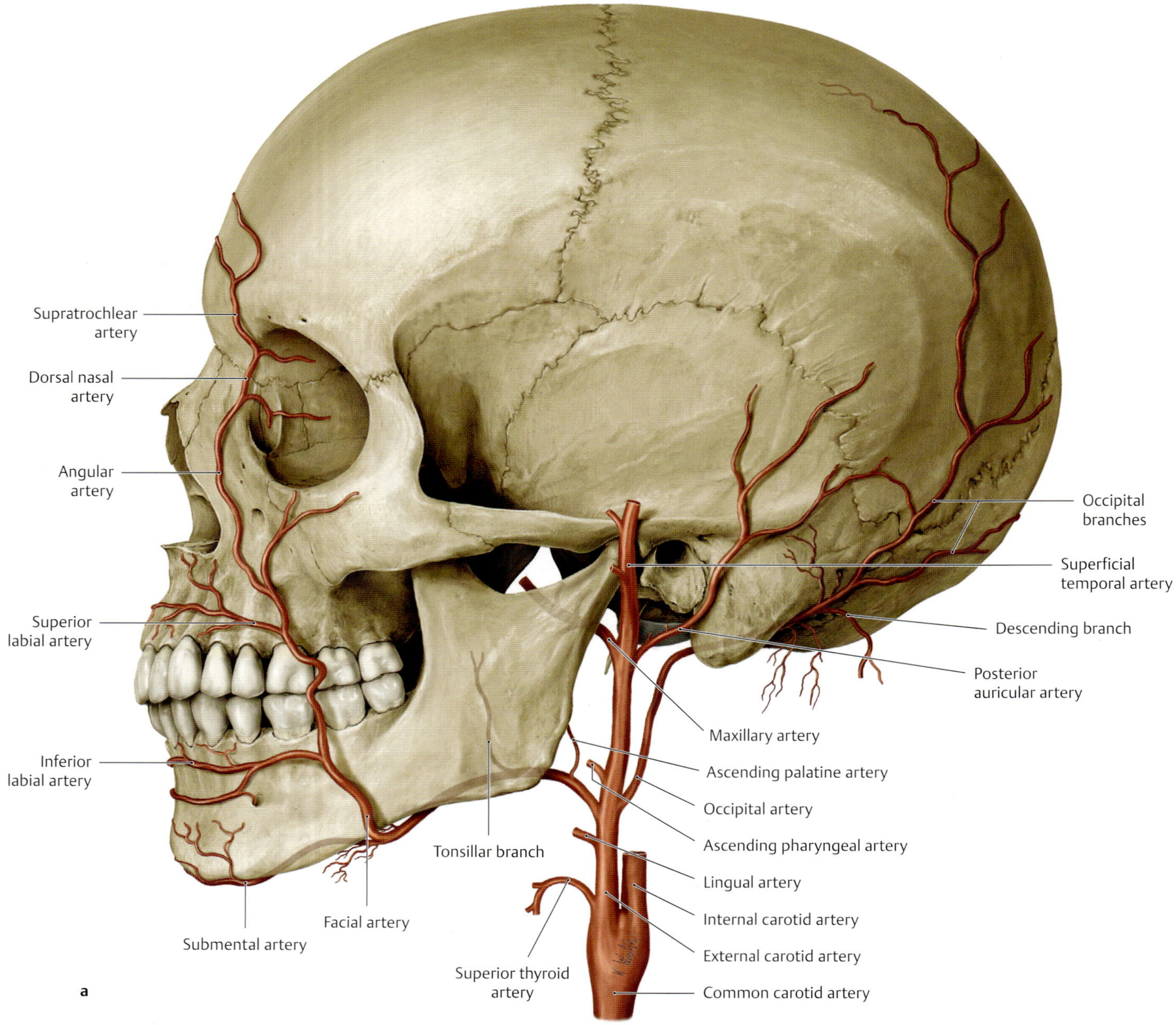

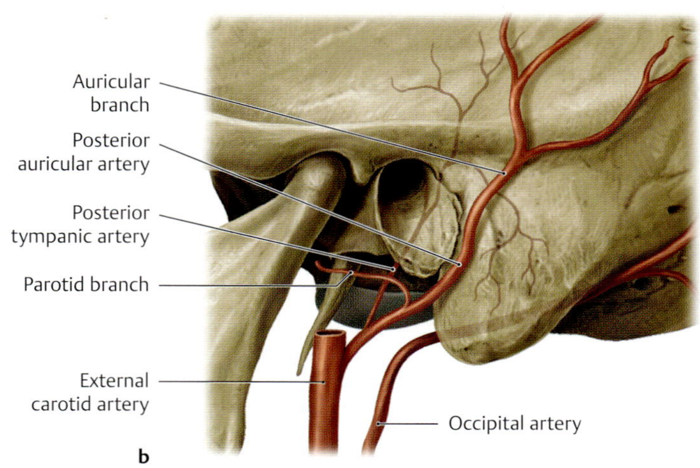

A Facial artery, occipital artery, and posterior auricular artery and their branches

Left lateral view. An important anterior branch of the external carotid is the **facial artery**, which gives off branches in the neck and face. One clinically important *cervical branch* is the ascending palatine artery; the *tonsillar branch* is ligated during tonsillectomy. Of the *facial branches*, the superior and inferior labial arteries combine to form an arterial circle around the mouth. The *terminal branch* of the facial artery, the angular artery, anastomoses with the dorsal nasal artery. The latter vessel is the terminal branch of the ophthalmic artery, which arises from the internal carotid artery. Because of the extensive anastomoses mentioned above, facial injuries have a tendency to bleed profusely but also tend to heal quickly and well owing to the copious blood supply. The pulse of the facial artery is palpable at the anterior border of the masseter muscle insertion on the mandibular ramus. The principal branches of the **posterior auricular artery** include the posterior tympanic artery and the parotid artery. Alternatively, the posterior tympanic artery can arise as a branch of the stylomastoid artery, see **A**, p. 156, and **B**, p. 137.

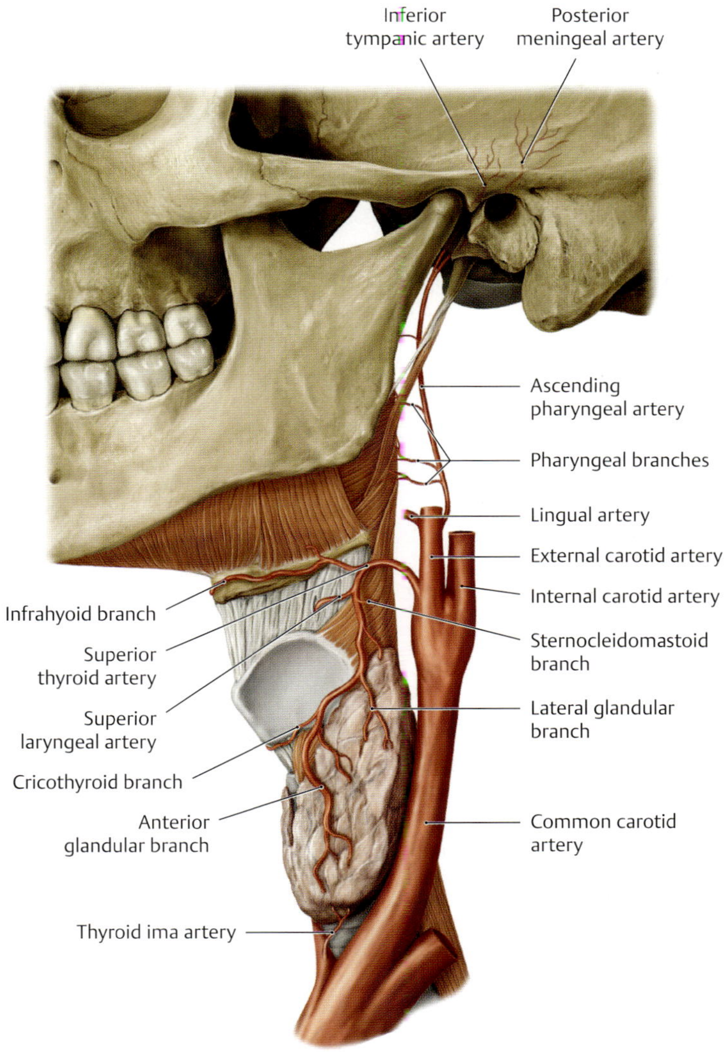

B Superior thyroid artery, ascending pharyngeal artery and their branches

Left lateral view. The superior thyroid artery is typically the first branch to arise from the external carotid artery. One of the anterior branches, it supplies the larynx and thyroid gland. The ascending pharyngeal artery arises from the medial side of the external carotid artery, usually above the level of the superior thyroid artery.

Note: The level at which a vessel branches from the external carotid artery does not necessarily correlate with the course of the vessel.

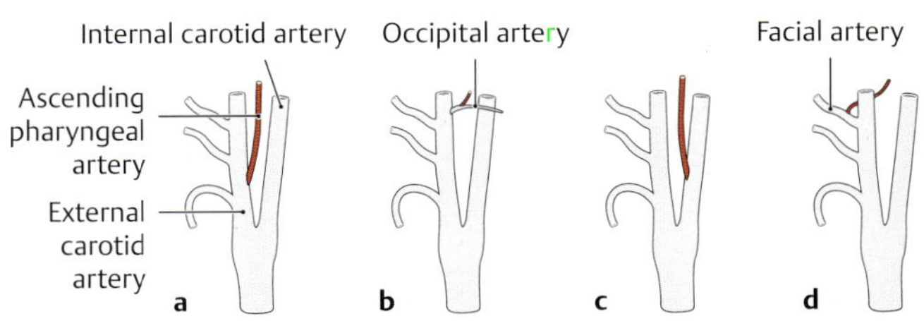

C Origin of the ascending pharyngeal artery: typical case and variants (after Lippert and Pabst)

a In **typical cases** (70%) the ascending pharyngeal artery arises from the external carotid artery.

b–d Variants:

b The ascending pharyngeal artery arises from **b** the occipital artery (20%), **c** the internal carotid artery (8%), or **d** the facial artery (2%).

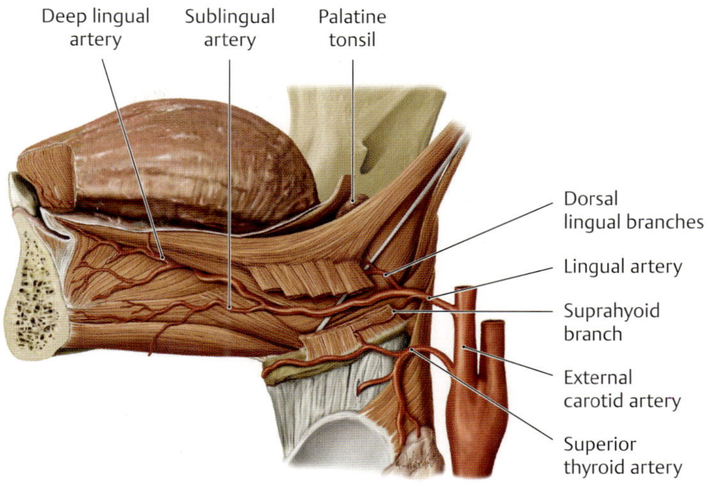

D Lingual artery and its branches

Left lateral view. The lingual artery is the second anterior branch of the external carotid artery. It has a relatively large caliber, providing the tongue with its rich blood supply. It also gives off branches to the pharynx and tonsils.

E Branches of the external carotid artery and their distribution: anterior, medial, and posterior branches with their principal distal branches

Branches of external carotid	Distribution
Anterior:	
• Superior thyroid artery (see **B**)	
– Glandular branches	• Thyroid gland
– Superior laryngeal artery	• Larynx
– Sternocleidomastoid branch	• Sternocleidomastoid muscle
• Lingual artery (see **D**)	
– Dorsal lingual branches	• Base of tongue, epiglottis
– Sublingual artery	• Sublingual gland, tongue, oral floor, oral cavity
– Deep lingual artery	• Tongue
• Facial artery (see **A**)	
– Ascending palatine artery	• Pharyngeal wall, soft palate, pharyngotympanic tube
– Tonsillar branch	• Palatine tonsil (main branch)
– Submental artery	• Oral floor, submandibular gland
– Labial arteries	• Lips
– Angular artery	• Nasal root
Medial:	
• Ascending pharyngeal artery (see **B**)	
– Pharyngeal branches	• Pharyngeal wall
– Inferior tympanic artery	• Mucosa of middle ear
– Posterior meningeal artery	• Dura, posterior cranial fossa
Posterior:	
• Occipital artery (see **A**)	
– Occipital branches	• Scalp, occipital region
– Descending branch	• Posterior neck muscles
• Posterior auricular branch (see **A**)	
– Stylomastoid artery	• Facial nerve in the facial canal
– Posterior tympanic artery	• Tympanic cavity
– Auricular branch	• Posterior side of auricle
– Occipital branch	• Occiput
– Parotid branch	• Parotid gland

4.4 External Carotid Artery: Terminal Branches

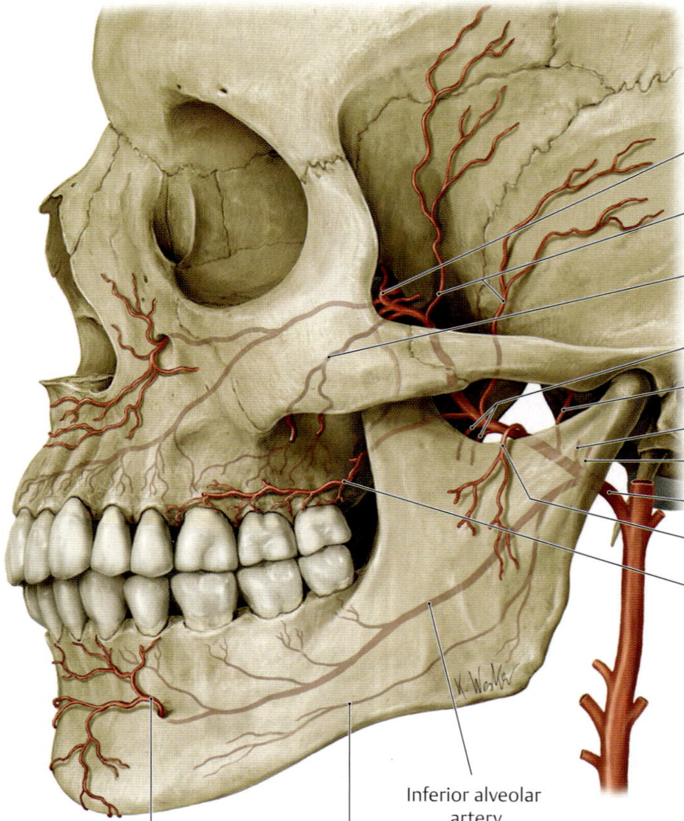

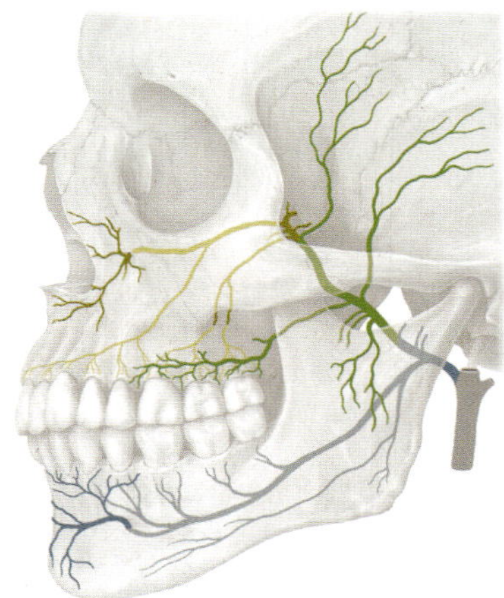

A Maxillary artery and its branches
Left lateral view. The maxillary artery is the larger of the two terminal branches of the external carotid artery. Its origin lies deep to the mandibular ramus (important landmark for locating the vessel). The maxillary artery consists of three parts:

- Mandibular part (blue)
- Pterygoid part (green)
- Pterygopalatine part (yellow)

B The two terminal branches of the external carotid artery with their principal branches

Branch		Distribution
Maxillary artery		
Mandibular part:	• Inferior alveolar artery	• Mandible, teeth, gingiva (the mental branch is its terminal branch)
	• Middle meningeal artery (see **C**)	• Calvaria, dura, anterior and middle cranial fossae
	• Deep auricular artery	• Temporomandibular joint, external auditory canal
	• Anterior tympanic artery	• Tympanic cavity
Pterygoid part:	• Masseteric artery	• Masseter muscle
	• Deep temporal branches	• Temporalis muscle
	• Pterygoid branches	• Pterygoid muscles
	• Buccal artery	• Buccal mucosa
Pterygopalatine part:	• Posterior superior alveolar artery	• Maxillary molars, maxillary sinus, gingiva
	• Infraorbital artery	• Maxillary alveoli
	• Descending palatine artery	
	– Greater palatine artery	• Hard palate
	– Lesser palatine artery	• Soft palate, palatine tonsil, pharyngeal wall
	• Sphenopalatine artery	
	– Lateral posterior nasal arteries	• Lateral wall of the nasal cavity, conchae
	– Posterior septal branches	• Nasal septum
Superficial temporal artery	• Transverse facial artery	• Soft tissues below the zygomatic arch
	• Frontal and parietal branches	• Scalp of the forehead and vertex
	• Zygomatico-orbital artery	• Lateral orbital wall

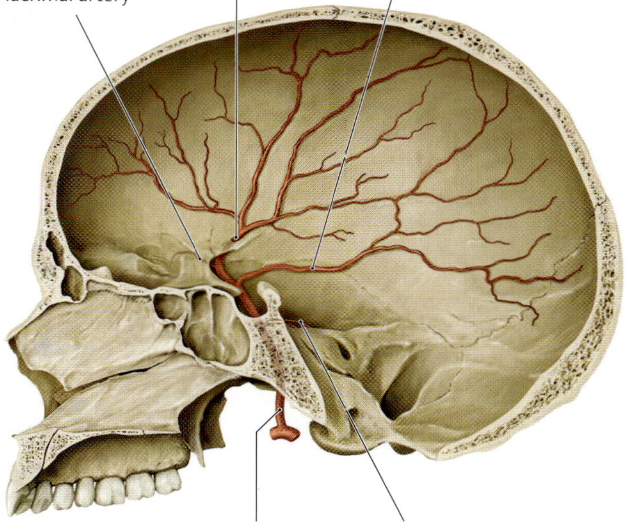

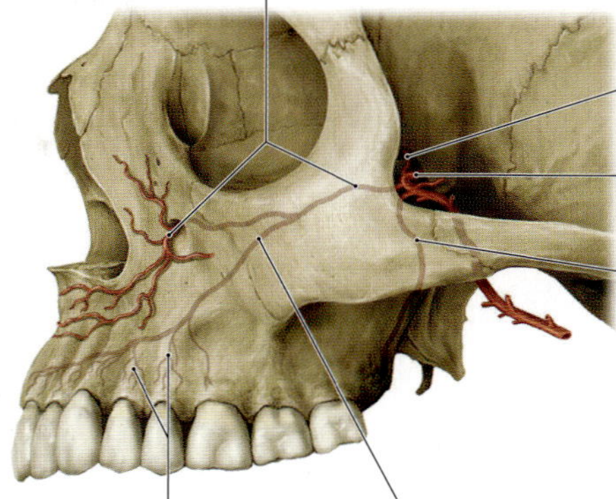

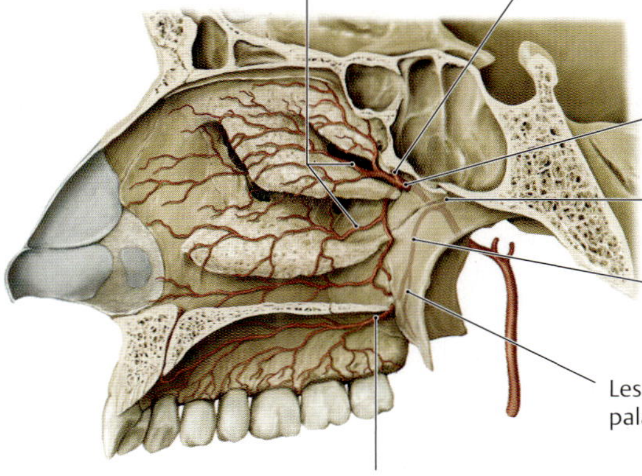

C Selected clinically important branches of the maxillary artery

a Right middle meningeal artery, **b** left infraorbital artery, **c** right sphenopalatine artery with its branches that supply the nasal cavity.

The **middle meningeal artery** passes through the foramen spinosum into the middle cranial fossa. Despite its name, it supplies blood not just to the meninges but also to the overlying calvarium. Rupture of the middle meningeal artery by head trauma results in an epidural hematoma (see p. 390). The **infraorbital artery** is a branch of the maxillary artery and thus of the *external* carotid artery, while the supraorbital artery (a branch of the ophthalmic artery) is a terminal branch of the *internal* carotid artery. These vessels provide a path for a potential anastomosis between the external and internal carotid arteries. When severe nasopharyngeal bleeding occurs from branches of the **sphenopalatine artery** (a branch of the maxillary artery), it may be necessary to ligate the maxillary artery in the pterygopalatine fossa (see **A**, p. 238, as well as **C**, p. 103, and **Gb**, p. 185).

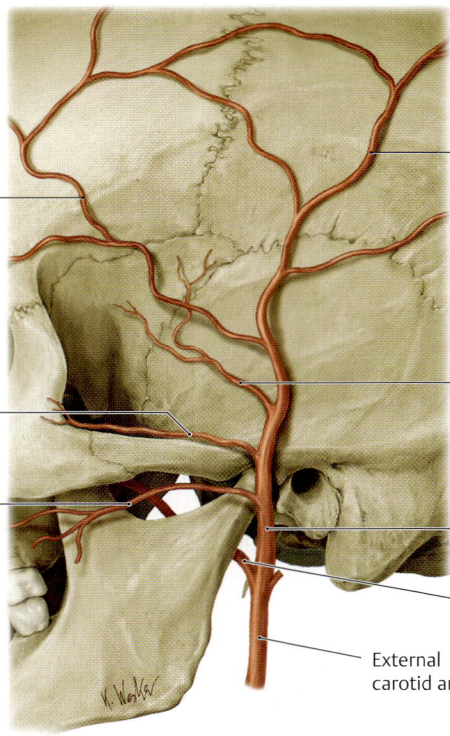

D Superficial temporal artery

Left lateral view. Particularly in elderly or cachectic patients, the often tortuous course of the frontal branch of this vessel can easily be traced across the temple. The superficial temporal artery may be involved in an inflammatory autoimmune disease (temporal arteritis), which can be confirmed by biopsy of the vessel. The patients, usually elderly males, complain of severe headaches.

4.5 Internal Carotid Artery: Branches to Extracerebral Structures

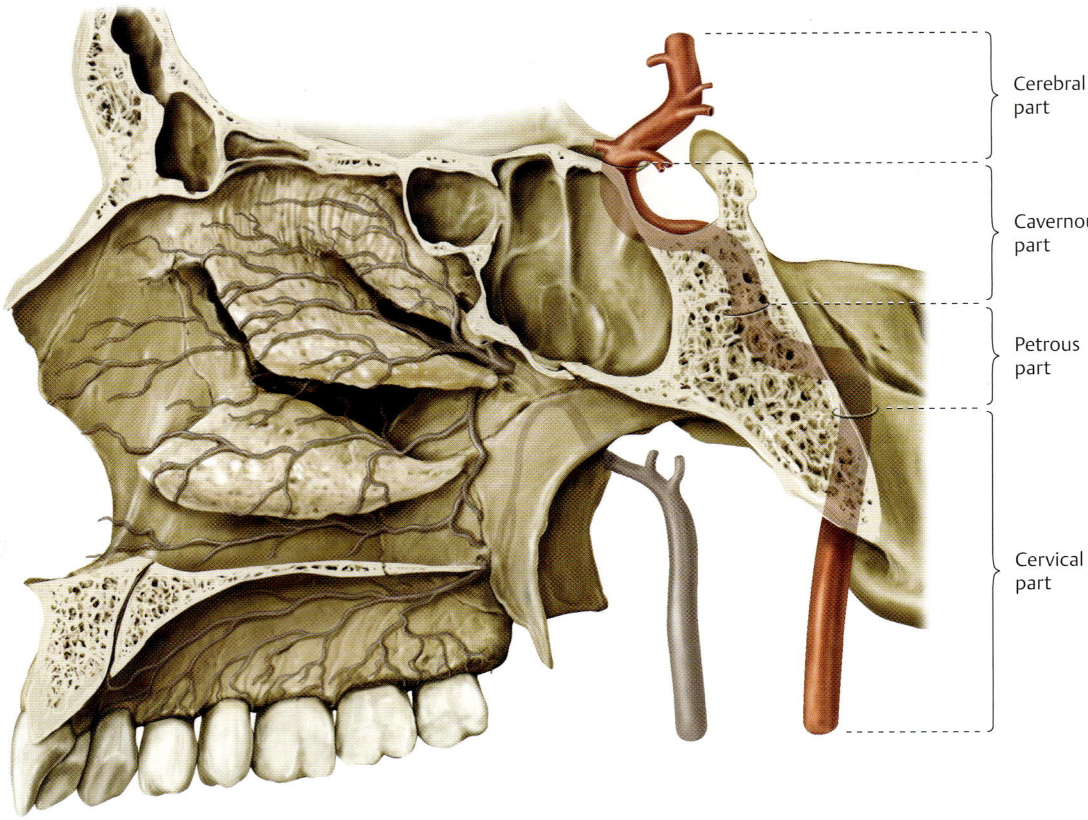

a

A Subdivisions of the internal carotid artery and branches that supply extracerebral structures of the head

a Medial view of the right internal carotid artery in its passage through the bones of the skull. **b** Anatomical segments of the internal carotid artery and their branches.

The internal carotid artery is distributed chiefly to the brain but also supplies extracerebral regions of the head. It consists of four parts (listed from bottom to top):

- Cervical part
- Petrous part
- Cavernous part
- Cerebral part

The petrous part of the internal carotid artery (traversing the carotid canal) and the cavernous part (traversing the cavernous sinus) have a role in supplying extracerebral structures of the head. They give off additional small branches that supply local structures and are usually named for the areas they supply. Only specialists may be expected to have a detailed knowledge of these branches. Of special importance is the *ophthalmic artery*, which arises from the cerebral part of the internal carotid artery (see **B**).

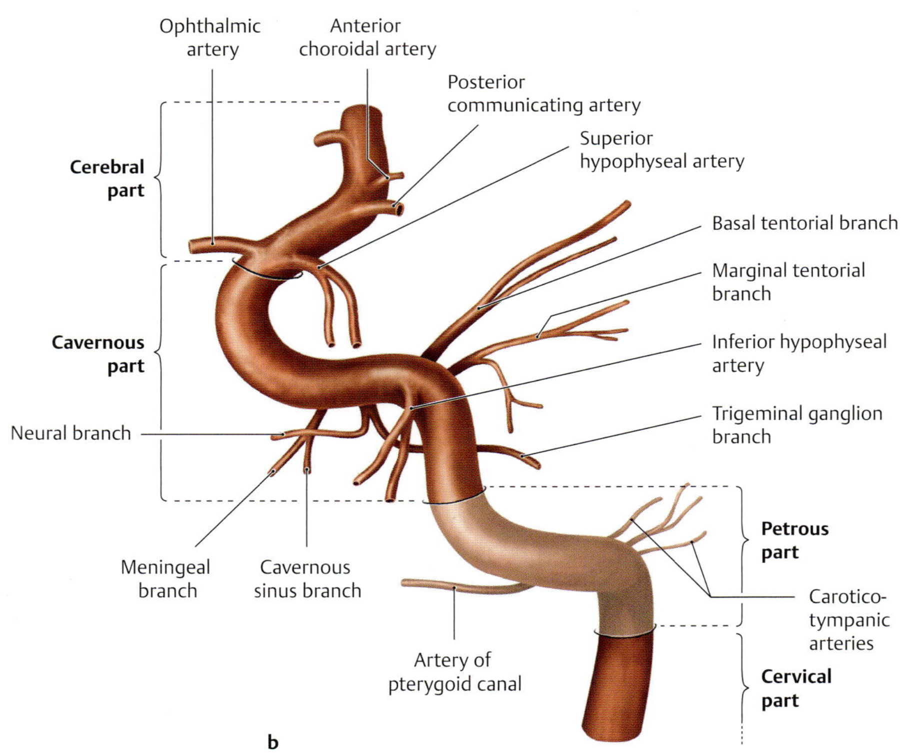

b

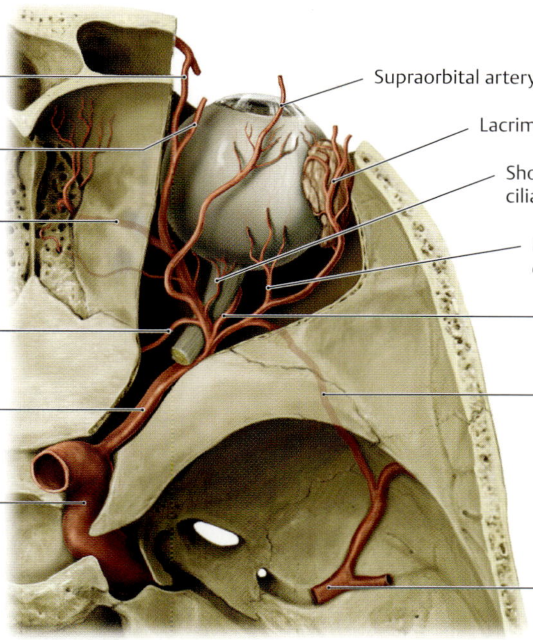

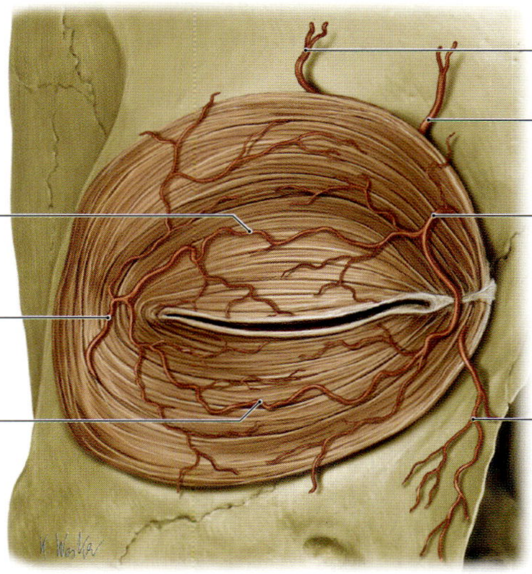

B Ophthalmic artery

a Superior view of the right orbit. **b** Anterior view of the facial branches of the right ophthalmic artery.

Figure **a** shows the origin of the ophthalmic artery from the internal carotid artery. The ophthalmic artery supplies blood to the eyeball itself and to orbital structures. Some of its terminal branches are distributed to the eyelid and portions of the forehead (**b**). Other terminal branches (anterior and posterior ethmoidal arteries) contribute to the supply of the nasal septum (see **C**).

Note: Branches of the lateral palpebral artery and supraorbital artery (**b**) may form an anastomosis with the frontal branch of the superficial temporal artery (territory of the external carotid artery) (see p. 91). With atherosclerosis of the internal carotid artery, this anastomosis may become an important alternative route for blood to the brain.

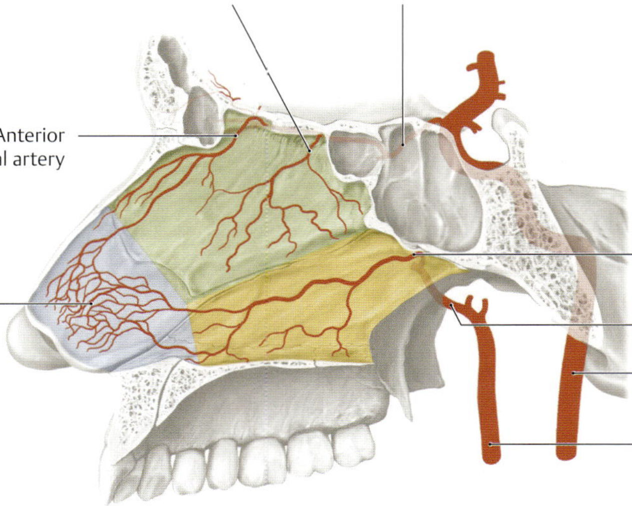

C Vascular supply of the nasal septum

Left lateral view. The nasal septum is another region in which the internal carotid artery (anterior and posterior ethmoidal arteries, green) anastomoses with the external carotid artery (sphenopalatine artery, yellow). A richly vascularized area on the anterior part of the nasal septum, called Kiesselbach's area (blue), is the most common site of nosebleed. Since Kiesselbach's area is an area of anastamosis, it may be necessary to ligate the sphenopalatine/maxillary artery and/or the ethmoidal arteries through an orbital approach, depending on the source of the bleeding.

4.6 Veins of the Head and Neck: Superficial Veins

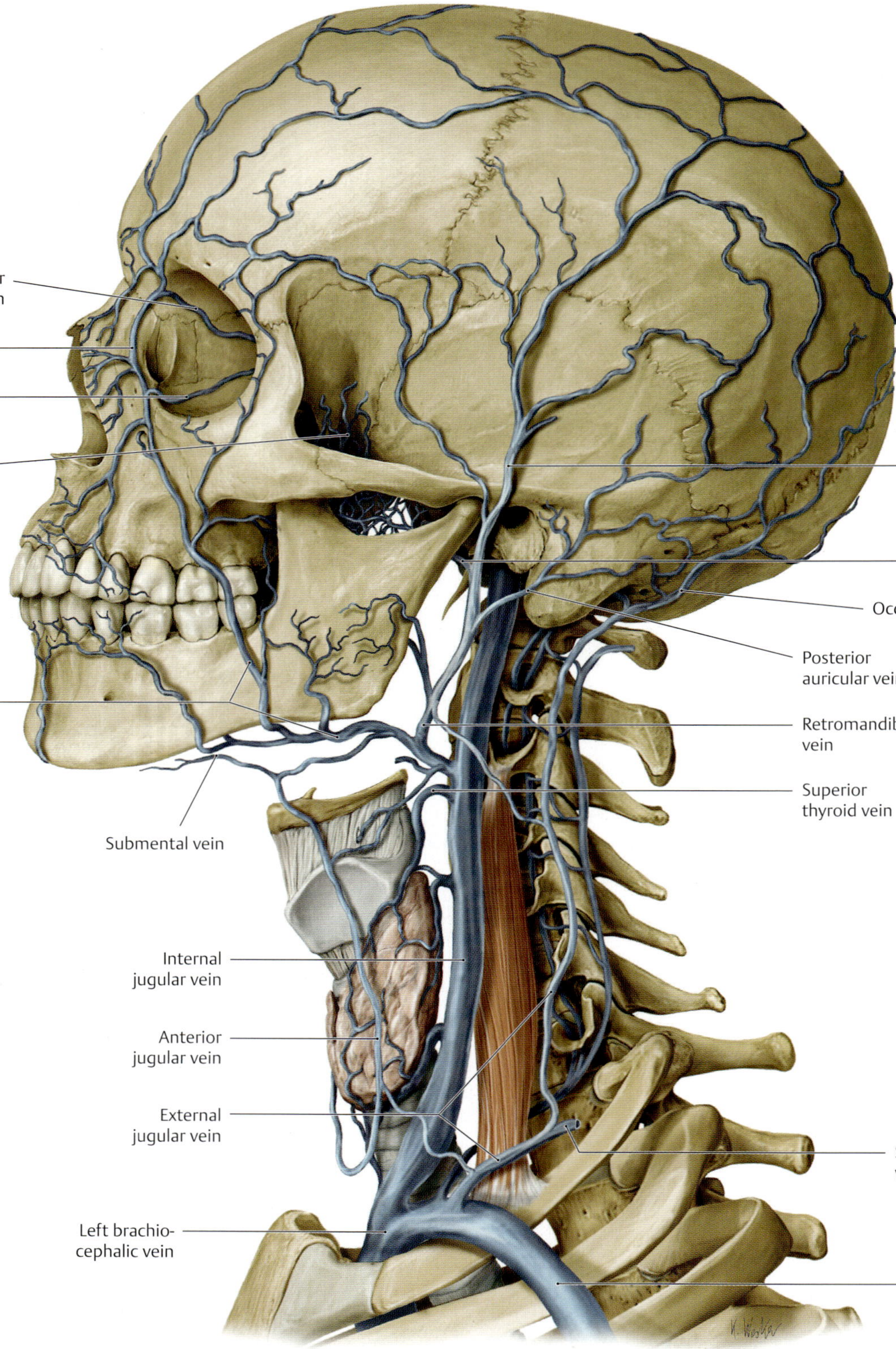

A Superficial head and neck veins and their drainage to the brachiocephalic vein

Left lateral view. The principal vein of the neck is the *internal jugular vein*, which drains blood from the interior of the skull (including the brain). Enclosed in the carotid sheath, the left internal jugular vein descends from the jugular foramen to its union with the subclavian vein to form the brachiocephalic vein. The main tributaries of the internal jugular vein in the head region are the facial and thyroid veins. The *external jugular vein* drains blood from the occiput (occipital vein) and nuchal regions to the subclavian vein, while the *anterior jugular vein* drains the superficial anterior neck region. Besides these superficial veins, there are more deeply situated venous plexuses (orbit, pterygoid plexus, middle cranial fossa) that are described in the next unit.

Note: The superficial veins are most closely related to the deep veins in the area of the angular vein, with an associated risk of spreading infectious organisms intracranially (see p. 107).

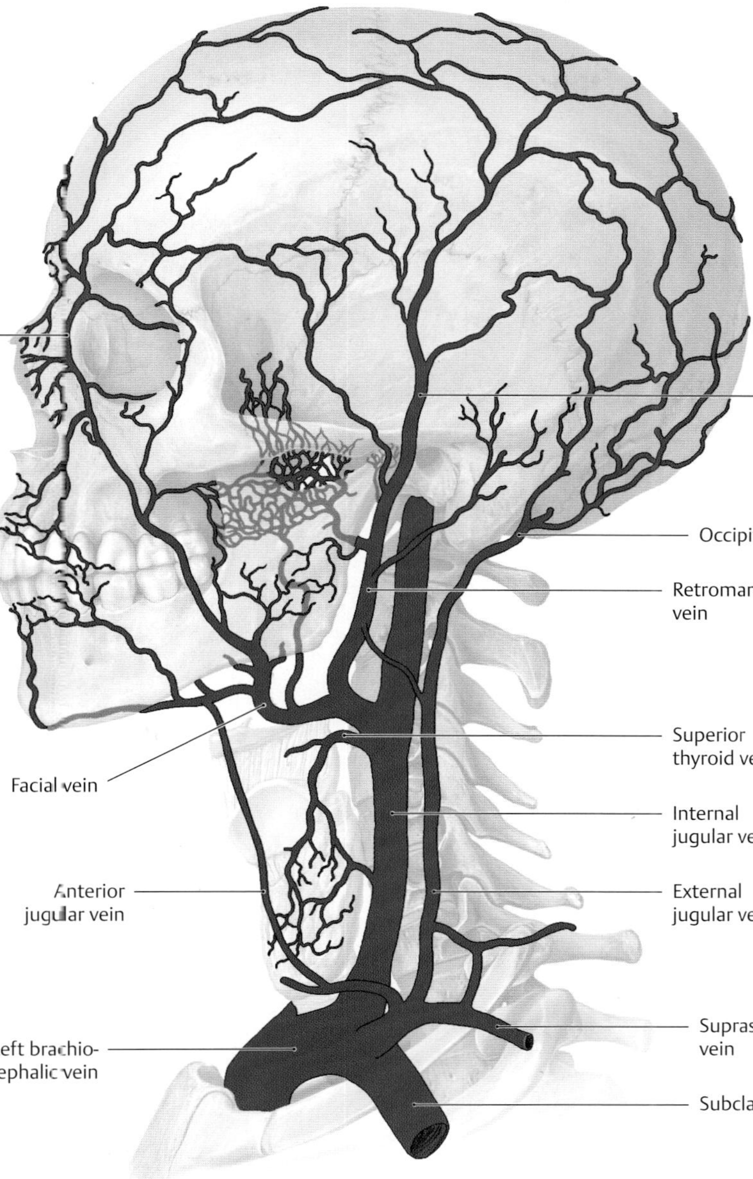

B Overview of the principal veins in the head and neck
Left lateral view. Only the more important veins are labeled in the diagram. As at many other sites in the body the course and caliber of the veins in the head and neck are variable to a certain degree, except for the largest venous trunk. The veins interconnect to form extensive anastomoses, some of which extend to the deep veins (see **A**, pterygoid plexus).

C Drainage of blood from the head and neck
Blood from the head and neck is drained chiefly by three jugular veins: the internal, external, and anterior. These veins have a variable size and course, but the anterior jugular vein is usually the smallest and most variable of the three. The external and internal jugular veins communicate by valveless anastomoses that allow blood to drain from the external jugular vein back into the internal jugular vein. This reflux is clinically significant because it provides a route by which bacteria from the skin of the head may gain access to the meninges (see p. 107 for details). The neck is subdivided into spaces by multiple layers of cervical fascia. One fascia-enclosed space is the carotid sheath, whose contents include the internal jugular vein. The other two jugular veins lie within the superficial cervical fascia.

Vein	Region drained	Relationship to deep cervical fasciae (see p. 4)
• Internal jugular vein	• Interior of the skull (including the brain)	• Within the carotid sheath
• External jugular vein	• Head (superficial)	• Initially, it runs above the superficial layer of the cervical fascia then between superficial and middle layers of the cervical fascia
• Anterior jugular vein	• Neck, portions of the head	• Penetrates the superficial layer of cervical fascia at the posterior edge of the sternocleidomastoid m., and then runs above the middle layer of cervical fascia

4.7 Veins of the Head and Neck: Deep Veins

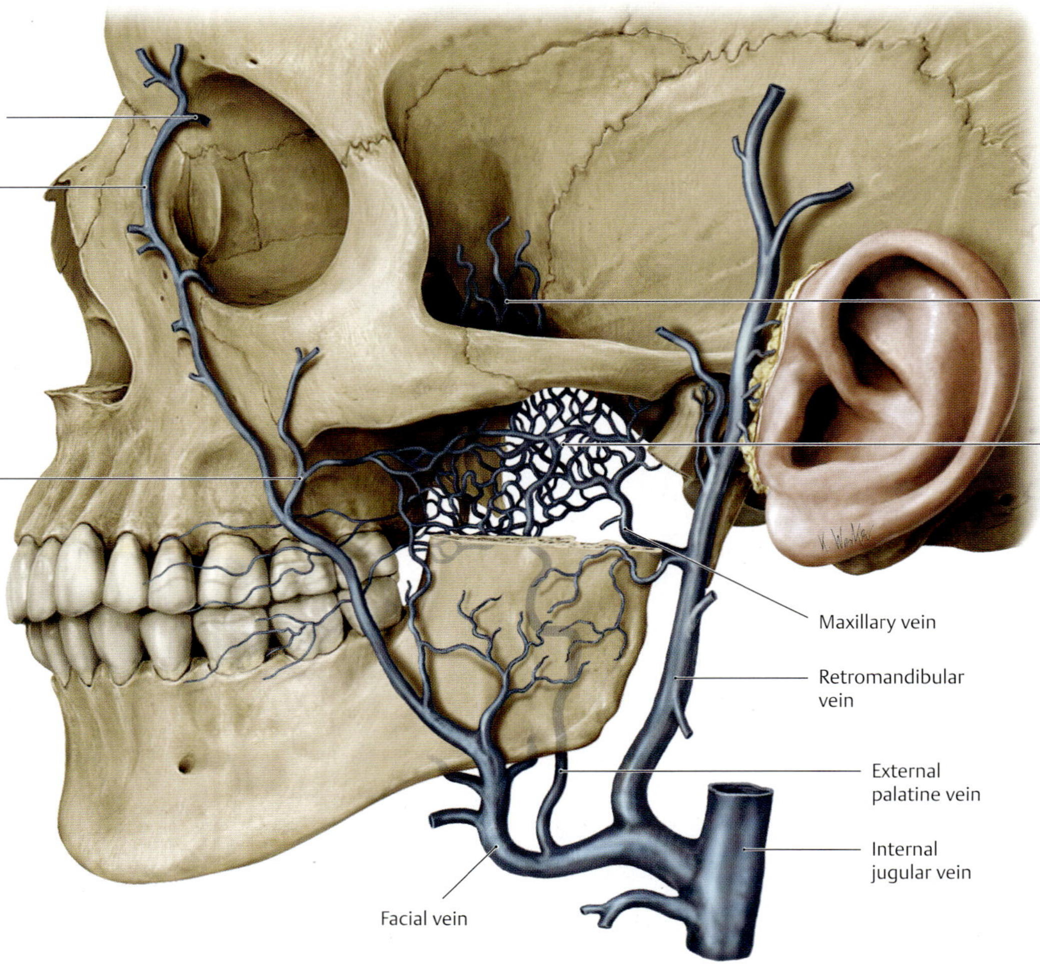

A Deep veins of the head: pterygoid plexus
Left lateral view. The pterygoid plexus is a venous network situated within the infratemporal fossa, behind the mandibular ramus between the muscles of mastication. It has extensive connections with the adjacent veins.

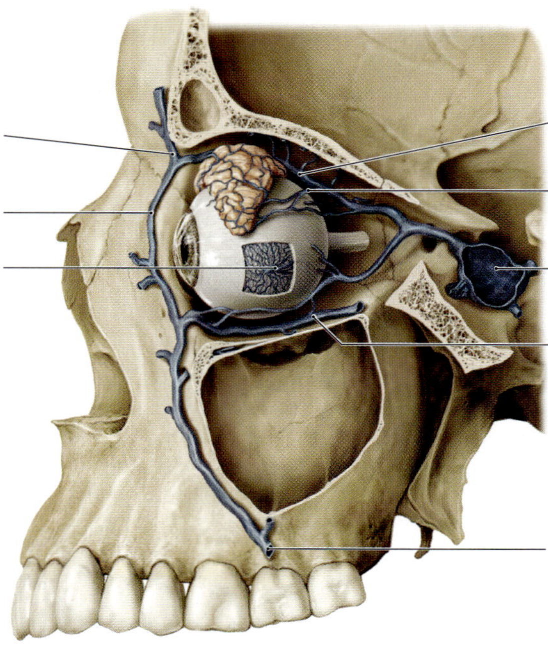

B Deep veins of the head: orbit and middle cranial fossa
Left lateral view. There are two relatively large venous trunks in the orbit, the superior and inferior ophthalmic veins, the latter of which is occasionally absent. They do not run parallel to the arteries. The veins of the orbit drain predominantly into the cavernous sinus. Orbital blood can also drain externally via the angular vein and facial vein. Because the veins are valveless, extracranial bacteria may migrate to the cavernous sinus and cause thrombosis in that venous channel (see **E** and p. 227).

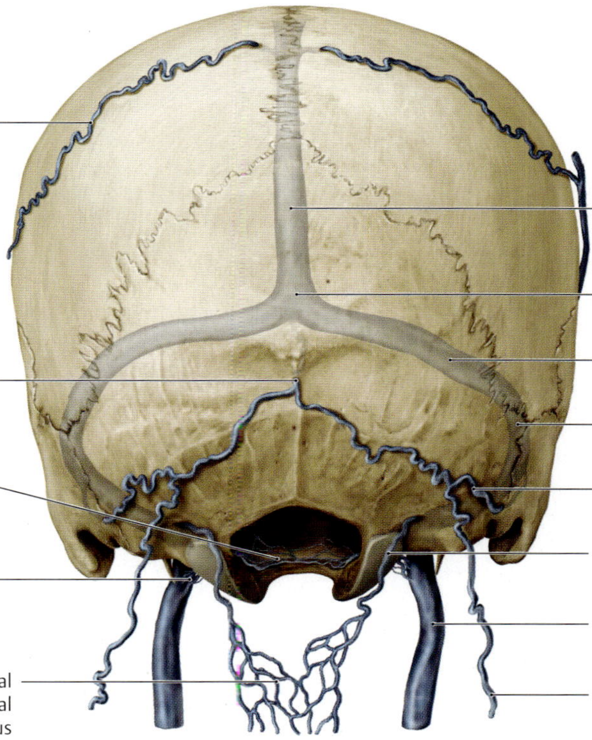

C Veins of the occiput

Posterior view. The superficial veins of the occiput communicate with the dural sinuses by way of the diploic veins. These vessels, called emissary veins, provide a potential route for the spread of infectious organisms into the dural venous sinuses.

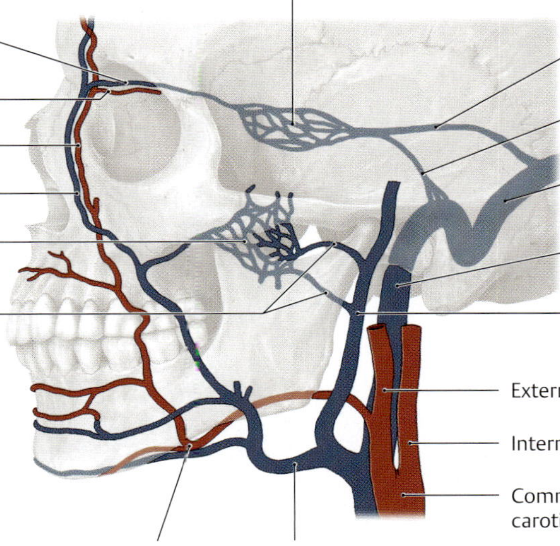

D Clinically important vascular relationships in the facial region

The facial artery and its branches and the terminal branch of the ophthalmic artery, the dorsal nasal artery, are clinically important vessels in the facial region because they may bleed profusely in patients who sustain midfacial fractures. The veins in this region are clinically important because they may allow infectious organisms to enter the cranial cavity. Bacteria from furuncles (boils) on the upper lip or nose may gain access to the cavernous sinus by way of the angular vein (see **E**).

E Venous anastomoses as portals of infection

* Very important clinically because the deep spread of bacterial infection from the facial region may result in cavernous sinus thrombosis (infection leading to clot formation that may occlude the sinus). Bacterial thrombosis is less common at other sites.

Extracranial vein	Connecting vein	Venous sinus
• Angular vein	• Superior ophthalmic vein	• Cavernous sinus*
• Veins of palatine tonsil	• Pterygoid plexus, inferior ophthalmic vein	• Cavernous sinus*
• Superficial temporal vein	• Parietal emissary vein	• Superior sagittal sinus
• Occipital vein	• Occipital emissary vein	• Transverse sinus, confluence of the sinuses
• Occipital vein, posterior auricular vein	• Mastoid emissary vein	• Sigmoid sinus
• External vertebral venous plexus	• Condylar emissary vein	• Sigmoid sinus

4.8 Veins of the Neck

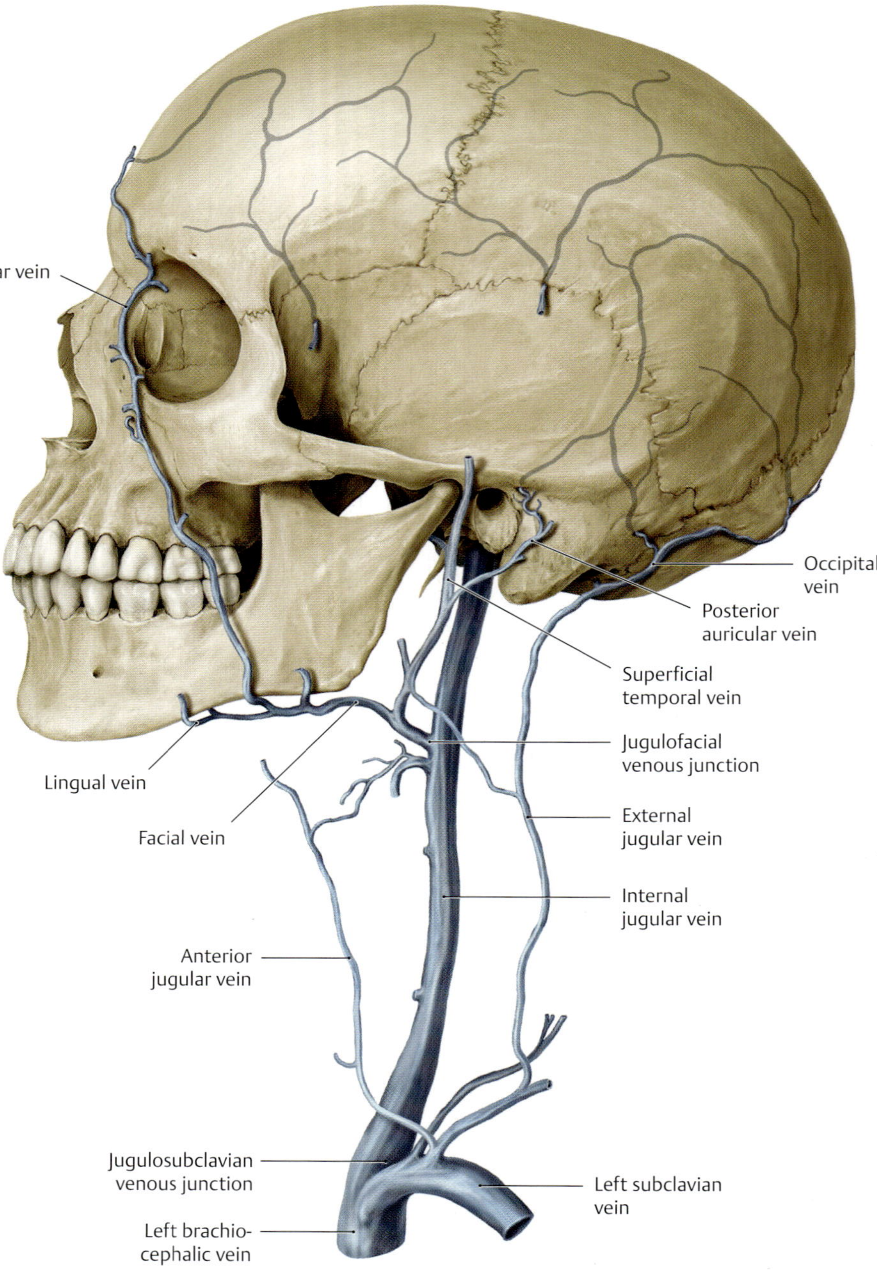

A Principal venous trunks in the neck
Left lateral view. Three jugular veins return blood to the superior vena cava from the head and neck region:

- The large internal jugular vein (located in the carotid sheath) drains blood from the cranial cavity and brain, face, and thyroid gland to the subclavian vein.
- The external jugular v. (smaller than internal jugular v. and may be absent in around 25% of the population) at first lies over the superficial layer of cervical fascia but beneath the platysma. It perforates the fascia to join the subclavian v. draining the superficial area located behind the ear.
- The anterior jugular vein (smallest of the three jugular veins, not always present) begins below the hyoid bone and usually terminates at the external jugular vein. It drains the superficial anterior wall of the neck.

The internal jugular vein and subclavian vein on each side unite to form the brachiocephalic vein (see **D**). The veins on the right and left sides may communicate via the jugular venous arch (see **D**).

B Principal veins in the neck, their tributaries and anastomoses
In addition to the veins listed below, there are a number of smaller veins that drain blood from adjacent structures. Since they are highly variable in their development, they are not listed here.

The cervical veins are interconnected by extensive anastomoses (not all of which are shown here, in some cases because they are too small). As a result, the ligation of one vein will not cause a serious impairment of venous return. A *venous junction* is a site where two larger veins join at an approximately 90° angle. The two principal venous junctions in the neck are the jugulofacial and the jugulosubclavian. The jugulofacial venous junction is smaller than the jugulosubclavian venous junction, which also marks the termination of the thoracic duct (see **A**, p. 242).

Tributaries of the superior vena cava
- Right brachiocephalic vein
- Left brachiocephalic vein

Tributaries of the brachiocephalic vein
- Internal jugular vein
- Subclavian vein
  - External jugular vein
- Thyroid venous plexus (usually drains to left brachiocephalic vein)
- Vertebral vein
- Internal thoracic veins

Tributaries of the internal jugular vein
- Dural sinuses
- Superior thyroid vein
- Facial vein
  - Lingual vein
  - Angular vein (anastomosis with ophthalmic vein)
  - Retromandibular vein
  - Posterior auricular vein (over the retromandibular v.)
  - Superficial temporal veins (anastomoses with pterygoid plexus)
- Posterior auricular vein

Tributaries of the external jugular vein
- Occipital vein

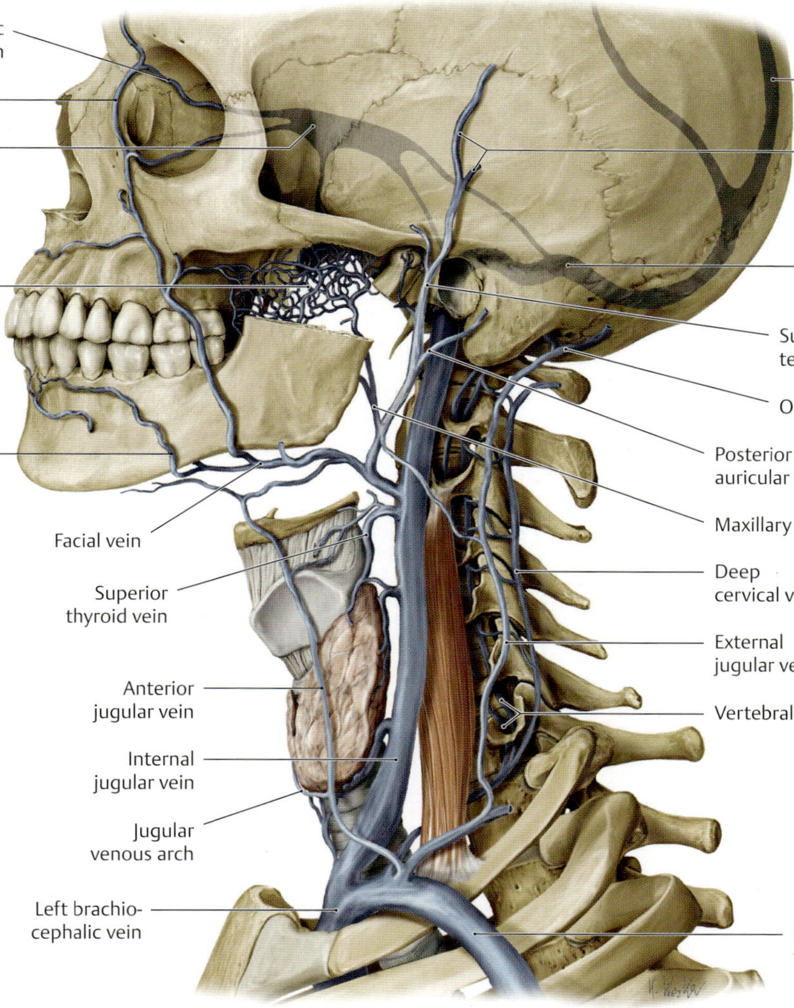

C Cervical veins and their relationship to the veins of the skull and dural sinuses

Left lateral view. The dural venous sinuses collect venous blood from the brain and channel it to the internal jugular vein. When the lymph nodes are removed in a neck dissection for a head and neck malignancy, the internal jugular vein should be ligated on one side only to avoid causing a potentially lethal venous stasis in the brain.

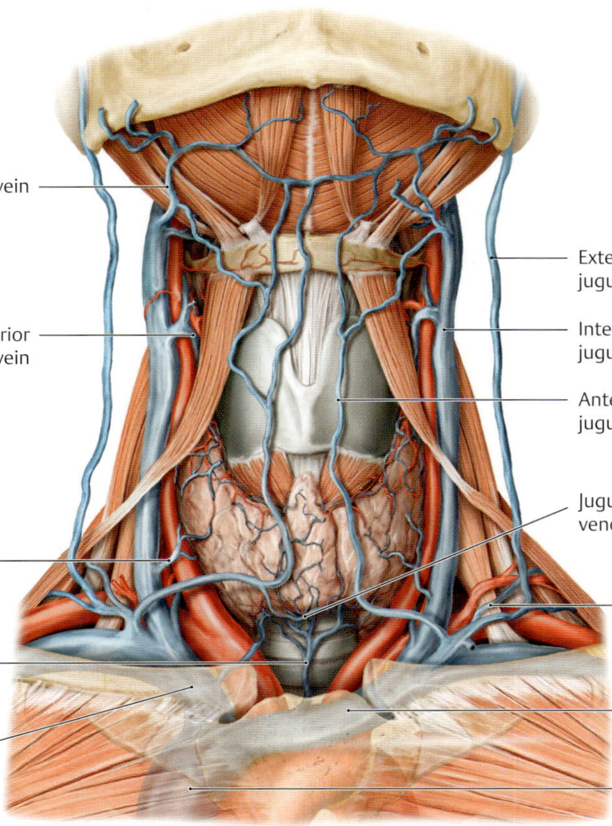

D Cervical veins

Anterior view. Most veins in the neck are valveless "thoroughfares" that drain blood from the head. They are minimally distended and not readily visible above the plane of the heart in both the standing and sitting positions. In the supine position, however, the veins become engorged and are visible even in a healthy individual. Visible distention of cervical veins, specifically the jugular veins, in the standing position is a sign of right-sided heart failure, in which blood collects proximal to the right heart, generally due to improper functioning of the right ventricle. The internal jugular vein is large and is frequently used as an access site for the placement of a central venous catheter in intensive care medicine, making it possible to infuse greater fluid volumes than with a peripheral venous line. The jugular venous arch forms a connecting trunk between the anterior jugular veins on each side, which creates a potential hazard for hemorrhage in tracheostomies.

4.9 Lymph Nodes and Lymphatic Drainage of the Head and Neck

Lymphatic system of the head and neck
A distinction is made between regional lymph nodes, which are associated with a particular organ or region and constitute primary filtering stations, and collecting lymph nodes, which usually receive lymph from multiple regional lymph node groups. Lymph from the head and neck region, gathered in scattered regional nodes, flows through its system of deep cervical collecting lymph nodes, into the right and left jugular trunks, each closely associated with its corresponding internal jugular vein. The jugular trunk on the right side drains into the right lymphatic duct, which terminates at the right jugulosubclavian junction. The jugular trunk on the left side terminates at the thoracic duct, which empties into the left jugulosubclavian junction (cf. **D**).

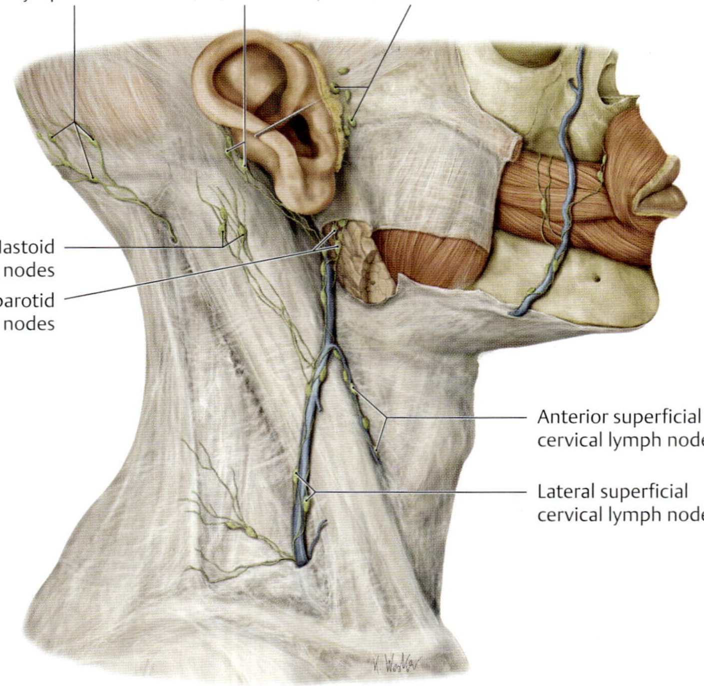

A Superficial lymph nodes in the neck
Right lateral view. It is extremely important to know the distribution of the lymph nodes in the neck because enlarged cervical lymph nodes are a common finding at physical examination. The enlargement of cervical lymph nodes may be caused by inflammation (usually a *painful* enlargement) or neoplasia (usually a *painless* enlargement) in the area drained by the nodes. The superficial cervical lymph nodes are primary drainage locations for lymph from adjacent areas or organs.
Note: Lymph from superficial lymph vessels in the head region drain into lymph nodes in the neck located close to the head.

B Deep cervical lymph nodes
Right lateral view. The deep lymph nodes in the neck consist mainly of collecting nodes. They have major clinical importance as potential sites of metastasis from head and neck tumors (see **D** and **E**). One or more delphian lymph nodes that lie deep to the fascia of the cricothyroid muscle are of particular clinical significance. As metastases can develop in them early, this group of nodes can be regarded as early warning lymph nodes for laryngeal and thyroid carcinoma. Palpation of the thyroid also includes the delphian node. Normally it is too small to be palpated. It is only detectable when it becomes pathologically enlarged.
Affected deep cervical lymph nodes may be surgically removed (neck dissection) or may be treated by regional irradiation. For this purpose the American Academy of Otolaryngology, Head and Neck Surgery has grouped the deep cervical lymph nodes into six levels (Robbins 1991):

I Submental and submandibular lymph nodes
II–IV Deep cervical lymph nodes distributed along the internal jugular vein (lateral jugular lymph nodes):
- **II** Deep cervical lymph nodes (upper lateral group)
- **III** Deep cervical lymph nodes (middle lateral group)
- **IV** Deep cervical lymph nodes (lower lateral group)

V Lymph nodes in the posterior cervical triangle
VI Anterior cervical lymph nodes

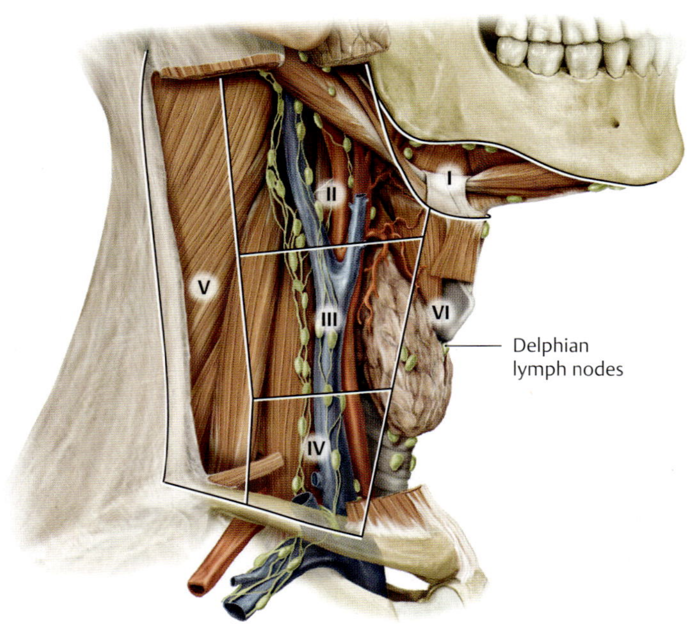

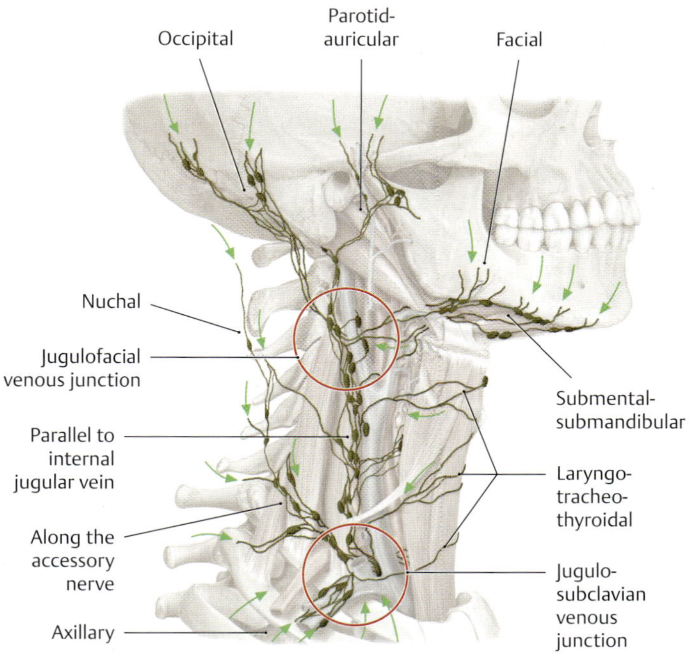

C Directions of lymphatic drainage in the neck

Right lateral view. The principal pattern of lymphatic flow in the neck is depicted. Understanding this pattern is critical to identifying the location of a potential cause of enlarged cervical lymph nodes. There are two main sites in the neck where the lymphatic pathways intersect:

- The jugulofacial venous junction: Lymphatics from the head pass obliquely downward to this site, where the lymph is redirected vertically downward in the neck.
- The jugulosubclavian venous junction: The main lymphatic trunk, the thoracic duct, terminates at this central location, where lymph collected from the left side of the head and neck region is combined with lymph draining from the rest of the body.

If only peripheral nodal groups are affected, this suggests a localized disease process. If the central groups (e.g., those at the venous junctions) are affected, this usually signifies an extensive disease process. Central lymph nodes can be obtained for diagnostic evaluation by prescalene biopsy.

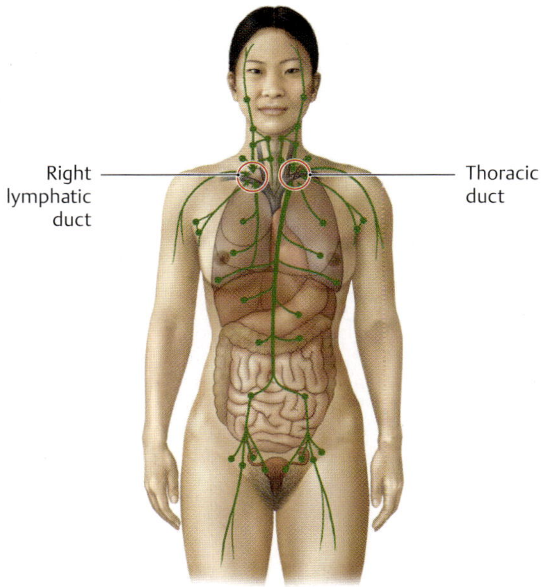

D Relationship of the cervical nodes to the systemic lymphatic circulation

Anterior view. The cervical lymph nodes may be involved by diseases that are not primary to the head and neck region, because lymph from the entire body is channeled to the left and right jugulosubclavian junctions (red circles). This can lead to retrograde involvement of the cervical nodes. The *right lymphatic duct* terminates at the right jugulosubclavian junction, the *thoracic duct* at the left jugulosubclavian junction. Besides cranial and cervical tributaries, the lymph from thoracic lymph nodes (mediastinal and tracheobronchial) and from abdominal and caudal lymph nodes may reach the cervical nodes by way of the thoracic duct. As a result, diseases in those organs may lead to cervical lymph node enlargement.

Note: Gastric carcinoma may metastasize to the left supraclavicular group of lymph nodes, producing an enlarged *sentinel node* that suggests an abdominal tumor. Systemic lymphomas may also spread to the cervical lymph nodes by this pathway.

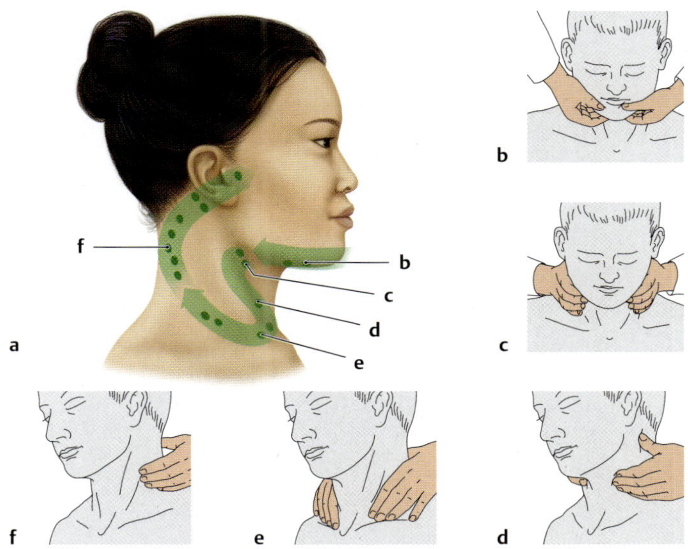

E Systematic palpation of the cervical lymph nodes

The cervical lymph nodes are systematically palpated during the physical examination to ensure the detection of any enlarged nodes (see **D** for the special diagnostic significance of cervical lymph nodes).

a Figure a shows the sequence in which the various nodal groups are successively palpated, **b–f** illustrate how each of the groups are palpated. The examiner usually palpates the submental-submandibular group first (**b**), including the mandibular angle (**c**), then proceeds along the anterior border of the sternocleidomastoid muscle (**d**). The supraclavicular lymph nodes are palpated next (**e**), followed by the lymph nodes along the accessory nerve and the nuchal group of nodes (**f**).

4.10 Overview of the Cranial Nerves

A Functional components of the cranial nerves

The twelve pairs of cranial nerves are designated by Roman numerals according to the order of their emergence from the brain (see topographical organization).

Note: The optic nerve and the olfactory nerve have special status among the cranial nerves. The optic nerve is an extension of the brain enveloped in meninges and containing cells found only in the CNS: oligodendrocytes and microglia cells. Thus, it is actually a component of the CNS and not a peripheral nerve. The olfactory tract and bulb, which together with the olfactory nerve form the externally visible portion of the olfactory system, are also components of the CNS by this definition. However, the olfactory nerve (composed of the filia olfactoria, which themselves are composed of fibers of the olfactory cells) does not belong to the CNS as the olfactory cells develop from the ectodermal olfactory placode and not the neural crest. Its embryologic origin from the placode epithelium gives this structure a special status as well.

Like the spinal nerves, the cranial nerves may contain both *afferent* and *efferent* axons. These axons belong either to the somatic nervous system, which enables the organism to interact with its environment (*somatic fibers*), or to the autonomic nervous system, which regulates the activity of the internal organs (*visceral fibers*). The combinations of these different *general* fiber types in spinal nerves result in four possible compositions that are found chiefly in spinal nerves but also occur in cranial nerves (see functional organization):

General somatic efferents (somatic motor function):
→ E.g., fibers convey impulses from the skin and skeletal muscle spindles

General visceral afferents (visceral sensation):
→ E.g., fibers convey impulses from the viscera and blood vessels

General somatic efferents (somatic motor function):
→ Fibers innervate striated muscles

General visceral efferents (visceral motor function):
→ Fibers (in the cranial nerves only parasympathetic fibers) innervate the smooth muscle of the viscera, intraocular muscles, heart, salivary glands, etc.

Additionally, cranial nerves may contain special fiber types that are associated with particular structures in the head:

Special somatic afferents:
→ E.g., fibers conduct impulses from the retina and from the auditory and vestibular apparatus

Special visceral afferents:
→ E.g., fibers conduct impulses from the taste buds of the tongue and from the olfactory mucosa

Special visceral efferents:
→ E.g., fibers innervate skeletal muscles derived from the branchial arches (*branchiogenic efferents and branchiogenic muscles*)

* *Note:* Cranial nerves with somatic efferent fibers innervating skeletal muscles also have somatic afferent fibers that conduct proprioceptive impulses from the muscle spindles and other structures (for clarity, not listed above).

A characteristic feature of the cranial nerves is that their sensory and motor fibers enter and exit the brainstem at the same sites. This differs from the spinal nerves, in which the sensory fibers enter the spinal cord through the posterior (dorsal) roots while the motor fibers leave the spinal cord through the anterior (ventral) roots.

B Topographical and functional organization of the cranial nerves

Topographical origin	Name	Functional fiber type
Telencephalon	• Olfactory nerve (CN I)	• Special visceral afferent
Diencephalon	• Optic nerve (CN II)	• Special somatic afferent
Mesencephalon	• Oculomotor nerve (CN III)*	• Somatic efferent • Visceral efferent (parasympathetic)
	• Trochlear nerve (CN IV)*	• Somatic efferent
Pons	• Trigeminal nerve (CN V)	• Special visceral efferent (*first branchial arch*) • Somatic afferent
	• Abducent nerve (CN VI)*	• Somatic efferent
	• Facial nerve (CN VII)	• Special visceral efferent (*second branchial arch*) • Special visceral afferent • Visceral efferent (parasympathetic) • Somatic afferent
Medulla oblongata	• Vestibulocochlear nerve (CN VIII)	• Special somatic afferent
	• Glossopharyngeal nerve (CN IX)	• Special visceral efferent (*third branchial arch*) • Special visceral afferent • Visceral afferent (parasympathetic) • Somatic afferent • Visceral efferent
	• Vagus nerve (CN X)	• Special visceral efferent (*fourth and fifth branchial arches*) • Special visceral afferent • Visceral efferent (parasympathetic) • Somatic afferent • Visceral afferent
	• Accessory nerve (CN XI)*	• Somatic efferent
	• Hypoglossal nerve (CN XII)*	• Somatic efferent

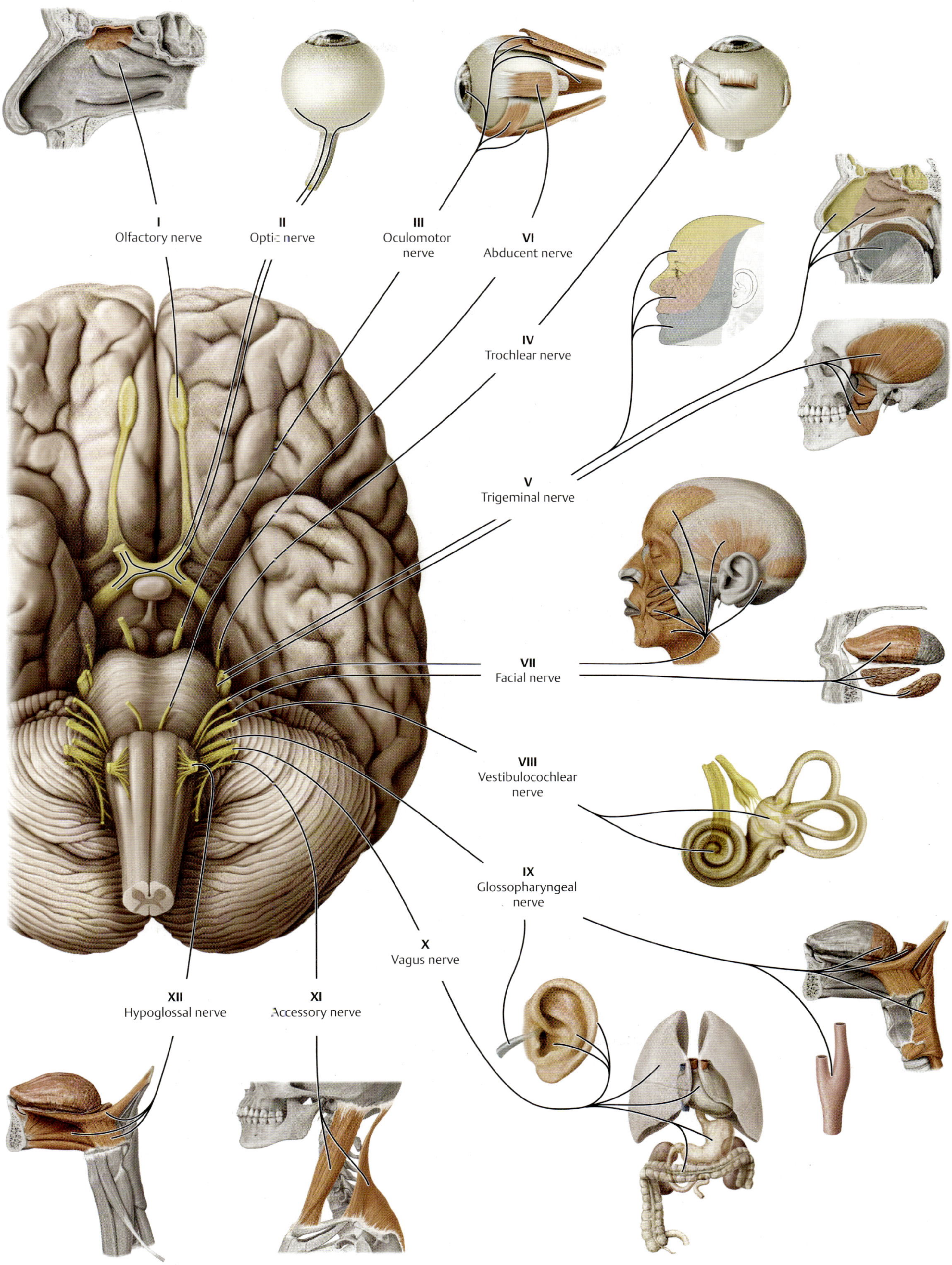
I
Olfactory nerve
II
Optic nerve
III
Oculomotor nerve
VI
Abducent nerve
IV
Trochlear nerve
V
Trigeminal nerve
VII
Facial nerve
VIII
Vestibulocochlear nerve
IX
Glossopharyngeal nerve
X
Vagus nerve
XII
Hypoglossal nerve
XI
Accessory nerve

4.11 Cranial Nerves: Brainstem Nuclei and Peripheral Ganglia

A Overview of the nuclei of cranial nerves III–XII

Just as different fiber types can be distinguished in the cranial nerves (see **B**, p. 112), the nuclei of origin and nuclei of termination of the cranial nerves can also be classified according to different sensory and motor types and modalities. According to this scheme, the nuclei that belong to the parasympathetic nervous system are classified as *general* visceral efferent nuclei, while the nuclei of the branchial arch nerves are classified as *special* visceral efferent nuclei. The visceral afferent nuclei are considered either *general* (lower part of the solitary nuclei) or *special* (upper part, gustatory fibers). The somatic afferent nuclei can be differentiated in a similar way: the principal sensory nucleus of the trigeminal nerve is classified as *general* somatic afferent, while the nucleus of the vestibulocochlear nerve is *special* somatic afferent.

Motor nuclei: (give rise to efferent [motor] fibers, left in **Ca**)

Somatic efferent (somatic motor) nuclei (red):
- Nucleus of oculomotor nerve (CN III: eye muscles)
- Nucleus of trochlear nerve (CN IV: eye muscle)
- Nucleus of abducent nerve (CN VI: eye muscle)
- Nucleus of accessory nerve (CN XI: shoulder and neck muscles)
- Nucleus of hypoglossal nerve (CN XII: lingual muscles)

Visceral efferent (visceral motor) nuclei (blue):

Nuclei associated with the parasympathetic nervous system (light blue):
- Visceral oculomotor (Edinger-Westphal) nucleus (CN III: pupillary sphincter and ciliary muscle)
- Superior salivatory nucleus (CN VII, facial nerve: submandibular and sublingual glands, minor salivary glands, nasal glands, lacrimal gland)
- Inferior salivatory nucleus (CN IX, glossopharyngeal nerve: parotid gland)
- Dorsal vagal nucleus (CN X: viscera)

Nuclei of the branchial arch nerves (dark blue):
- Trigeminal motor nucleus (CN V: muscles of mastication)
- Facial nucleus (CN VII: muscles of facial expression)
- Nucleus ambiguus (CN IX, CN X: pharyngeal and laryngeal muscles)

Sensory nuclei: (where afferent [sensory] fibers terminate, right in **Ca**)

Somatic afferent (somatic sensory) and vestibulocochlear nuclei (light or dark yellow):

Sensory nuclei associated with the trigeminal nerve (CN V, dark yellow):
- Mesencephalic nucleus (proprioceptive afferents from muscles of mastication)
- Principal (pontine) sensory nucleus (touch, vibration, pressure)
- Spinal nucleus (pain and temperature sensation in the head)

Nuclei of the vestibulocochlear nerve (CN VIII, light yellow):
- Vestibular part (sense of balance):
  - Superior vestibular nucleus
  - Lateral vestibular nucleus
  - Medial vestibular nucleus
  - Inferior vestibular nucleus
- Cochlear part (hearing, *light yellow*):
  - Anterior cochlear nucleus
  - Posterior cochlear nucleus

Visceral afferent (visceral sensory) nuclei (light or dark green):
- Nucleus of the solitary tract (nuclear complex):
  - Superior part (special visceral afferents [taste] from CN VII, CN IX, and CN X) (dark green)
  - Inferior part (general visceral afferents from CN IX and CN X) (light green)

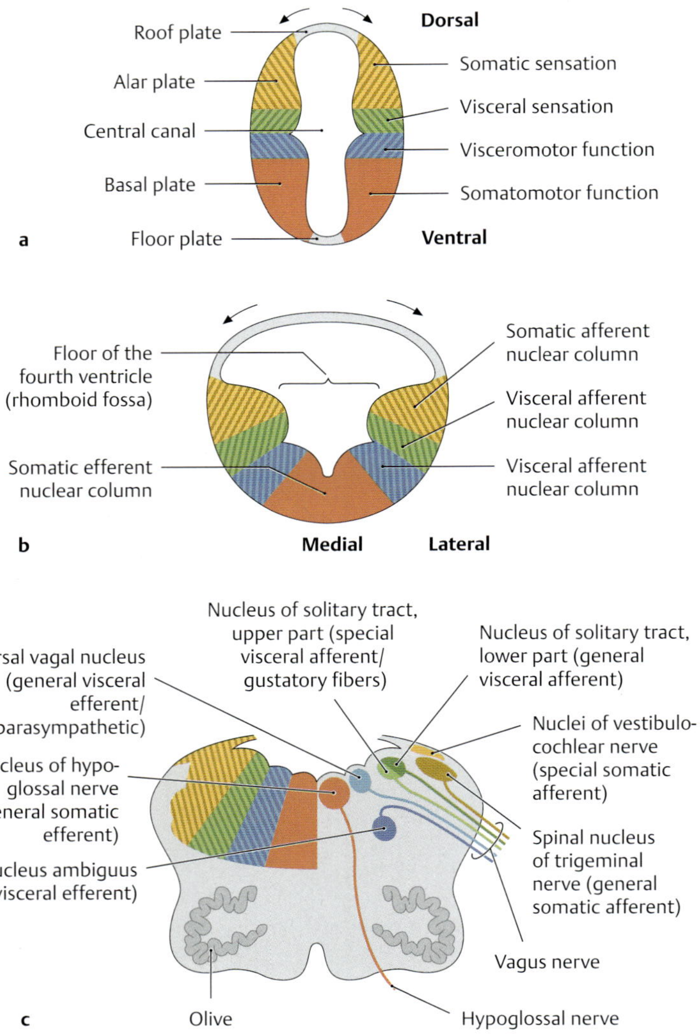

B Arrangement of brainstem nuclear columns during embryonic development

Cross-sections through the spinal cord and brainstem, superior view. The functional organization of the brainstem is determined by the location of the cranial nerve nuclei, which can be explained in terms of the embryonic migration of neuron populations.

a Initial form as seen in the spinal cord: The motor (efferent) neurons are ventral, and the sensory (afferent) neurons are dorsal (= dorsoventral arrangement).

b Early embryonic stage of brainstem development: the neurons of the alar plate (sensory nuclei) migrate laterally while the neurons of the basal plate (motor nuclei) migrate medially. This gives rise to a general mediolateral arrangement of the nuclear columns. The arrows indicate the directions of cell migration.

c Adult brainstem: features a medial to lateral arrangement of four longitudinal nuclear columns (one *somatic efferent*, one *visceral efferent*, one *visceral afferent*, and one *somatic afferent*). In each of these columns, nuclei that have the same function are arranged one above the other in a craniocaudal direction (see **C**). The nuclei in the *somatic afferent* and *visceral afferent* columns are differentiated into general and special afferent nuclei. Similarly, the *visceral efferent nuclear column* is differentiated into general (parasympathetic) and special (branchial) efferent nuclei. This general/special subdivision is not present in the *somatic efferent nuclear column*.

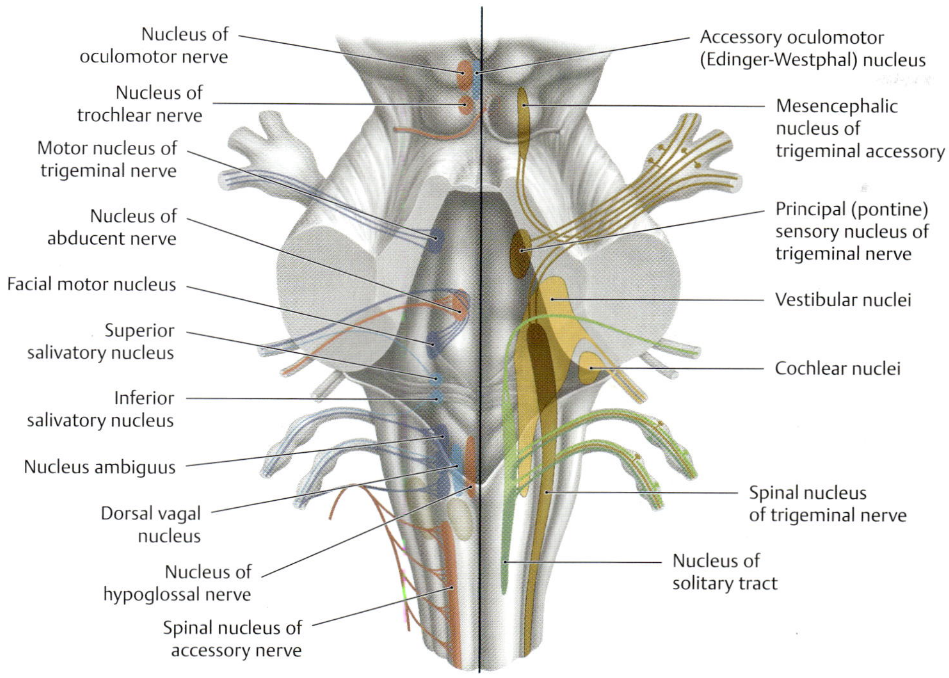

a

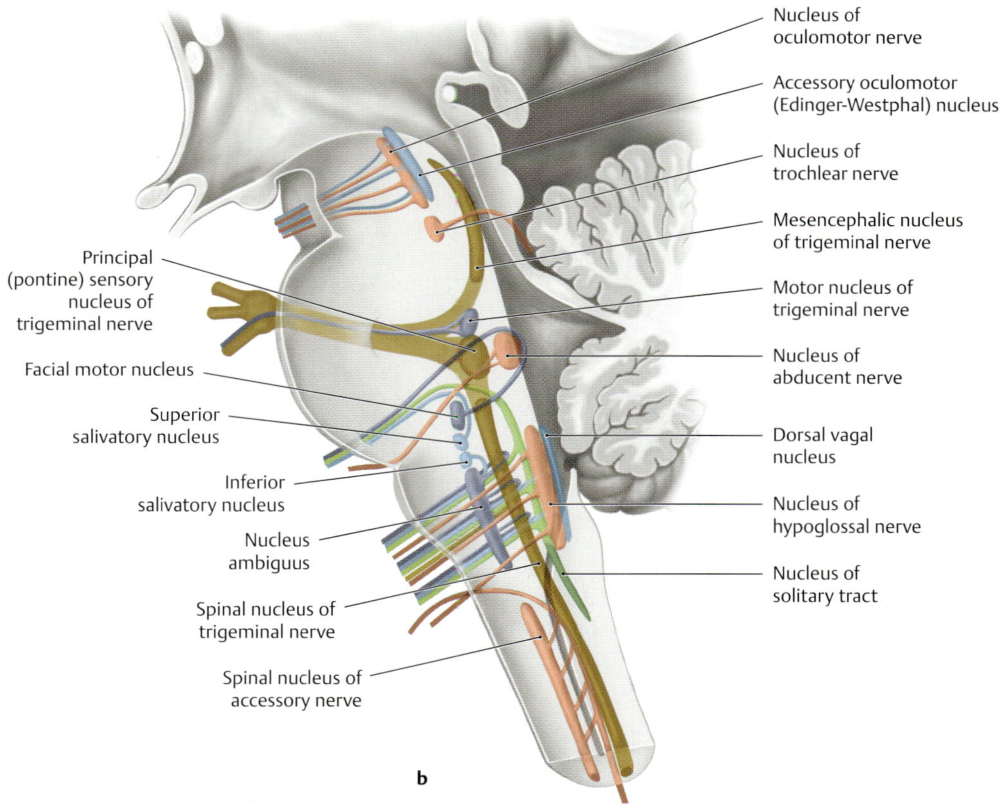

b

- General somatic afferent nuclei
- General visceral afferent nuclei
- General somatic efferent nuclei
- General visceral efferent nuclei
- Special somatic afferent nuclei
- Special visceral afferent nuclei
- Special visceral efferent nuclei

C Location of cranial nerves III–XII in the brainstem

a Posterior view (with cerebellum removed).
b Midsagittal section.

Except for cranial nerves I and II, which are extensions of the brain rather than true nerves, all pairs of cranial nerves are associated with corresponding nuclei in the brainstem. The diagrams show the nerve pathways leading *to* and *from* these nuclei. The arrangement of the cranial nerve nuclei is easier to understand when they are classified into functional nuclear columns (see **B**). The *efferent (motor) nuclei* where the *efferent* fibers arise are shown on the left side in **a**. The *afferent (sensory) nuclei* where the *afferent* fibers end are shown on the right side.

D Ganglia associated with cranial nerves

Ganglia fall into two main categories: sensory and autonomic (parasympathetic). The **sensory ganglia** are analogous to the dorsal root ganglia of the spinal cord. They contain the cell bodies of the *pseudounipolar or bipolar* neurons (= primary afferent neurons). Their peripheral process comes from a receptor, and their central process terminates in the CNS. The mesencephalic nucleus of the trigeminal nerve is an exception to this rule. Synaptic relays do not occur in the sensory ganglia. The **autonomic ganglia** in the head are entirely parasympathetic. They contain the cell bodies of the *multipolar* neurons (= postganglionic neurons). Unlike the sensory ganglia, these ganglia contain synapses between the preganglionic and postganglionic neurons. The parasympathetic preganglionic neurons originate in the brainstem. The fibers of the postganglionic neurons are distributed to the target organs.

Cranial nerves	Sensory ganglia	Autonomic ganglia
Oculomotor nerve (CN III)		• Ciliary ganglion
Trigeminal nerve (CN V)	• Trigeminal ganglion	
Facial nerve (CN VII)	• Geniculate ganglion	• Pterygopalatine ganglion • Submandibular ganglion
Vestibulocochlear nerve (CN VIII)	• Spiral (cochlear) ganglion • Vestibular ganglion	
Glossopharyngeal nerve (CN IX)	• Superior ganglion • Inferior (petrosal) ganglion	• Otic ganglion
Vagus nerve (CN X)	• Superior (jugular) ganglion • Inferior (nodose) ganglion	• Prevertebral and intramural ganglia of thoracic and abdominal viscera

4.12 Cranial Nerves: Olfactory (CN I) and Optic (CN II)

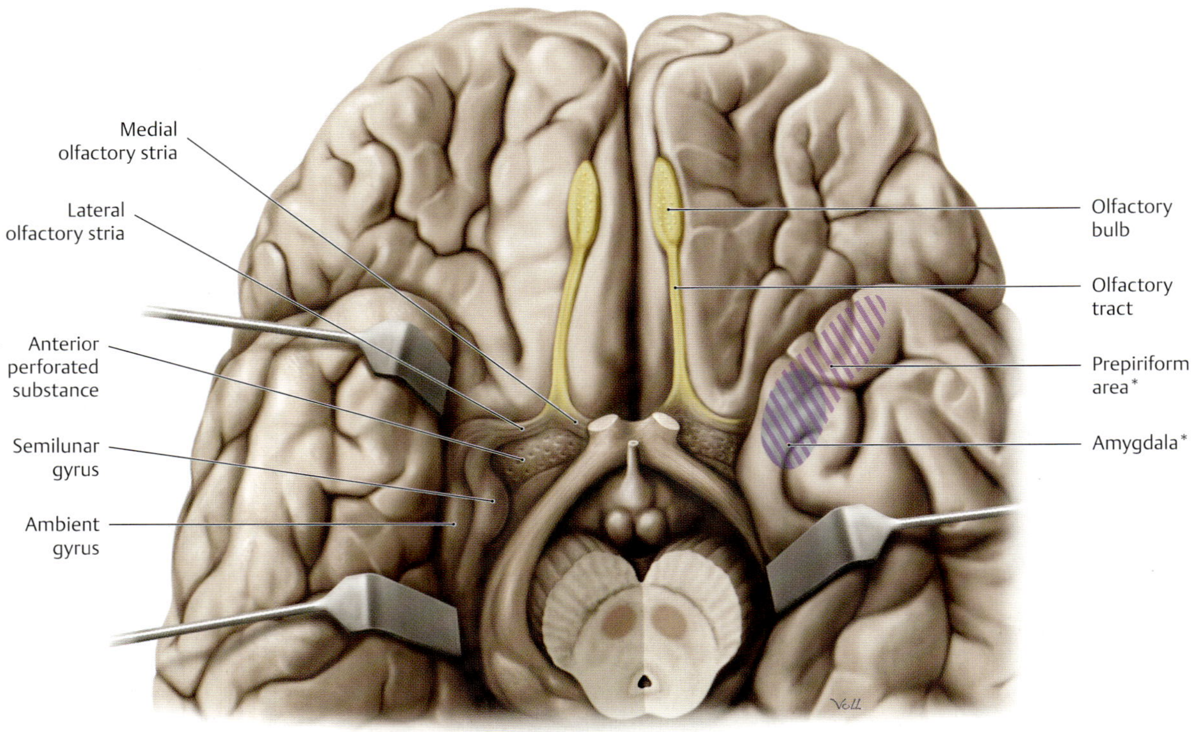

A Olfactory bulb and olfactory tract on the basal surface of the frontal lobes of the brain

The unmyelinated axons of the primary bipolar sensory neurons in the olfactory mucosa are collected into approximately 20 fiber bundles: the filia olfactoria (see **B**), which are referred to collectively as the *olfactory nerve*. These axon bundles pass from the nasal cavity through the cribriform plate of the ethmoid bone into the anterior cranial fossa (see **B**), and synapse in the *olfactory bulb*. The olfactory bulb is a club-like extension on the frontal end of the olfactory tract. Whereas the olfactory bulb has a cortical structure (allocortex, paleocortex), the olfactory tract exhibits the structure of a tract and contains CNS-specific glia such as oligodendrocytes and microglia. The olfactory bulb and tract have a meningeal covering and are components of the central nervous system. In contrast, the olfactory nerve develops from the ectodermal olfactory placode and does not belong to the CNS. Before it enters the telencephalon, the olfactory tract splits into the medial and lateral olfactory striae. Many of the axons of the olfactory tract end directly in the cortex (without joining a nucleus) in the prepiriform area or in the amygdaloid body. The olfactory nerve transmits sensory information from the olfactory mucosa, an area on the roof of the nasal cavity measuring approximately 2–4 cm^2 (superior concha and nasal septum, see **B**). The first neuron of the olfactory tract is the bipolar olfactory cell in the olfactory mucosa.

Note: Injuries to the cribriform plate may damage the meningeal covering of the olfactory fibers, resulting in olfactory disturbances and cerebrospinal fluid leakage from the nose ("runny nose" after head trauma). There is an associated risk of ascending bacterial infection causing meningitis.

Olfactory cells can divide throughout their life. Functionally, they are primary sensory cells. As they have their own axon, they are also neurons. Olfactory cells are thus an example of neurons that can divide throughout their life.

* The shaded structures are deep to the basal surface of the brain.

B Extent of the olfactory mucosa (olfactory region*)

Portion of the left nasal septum and lateral wall of the right nasal cavity, viewed from the left side. The olfactory fibers on the septum and superior concha define the extent of the olfactory region (2–4 cm2). The thin, unmyelinated olfactory fibers enter the skull through the cribriform plate of the ethmoid bone (see p. 25) and pass to the olfactory bulb (see also pp. 182, 330, and 490).

* In the new anatomic nomenclature, the olfactory region is described as the olfactory part of the nasal mucosa.

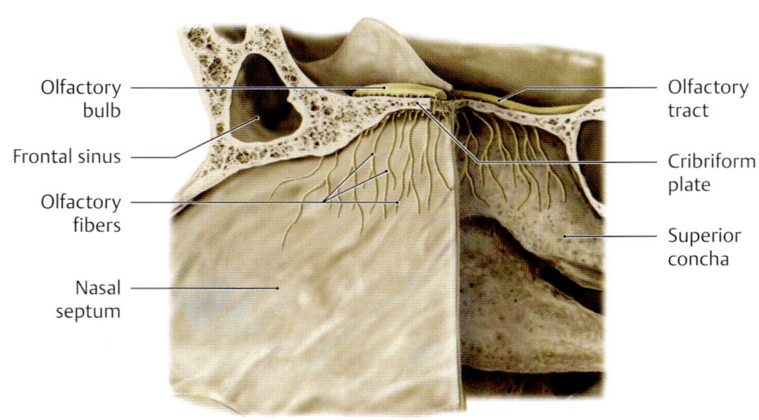

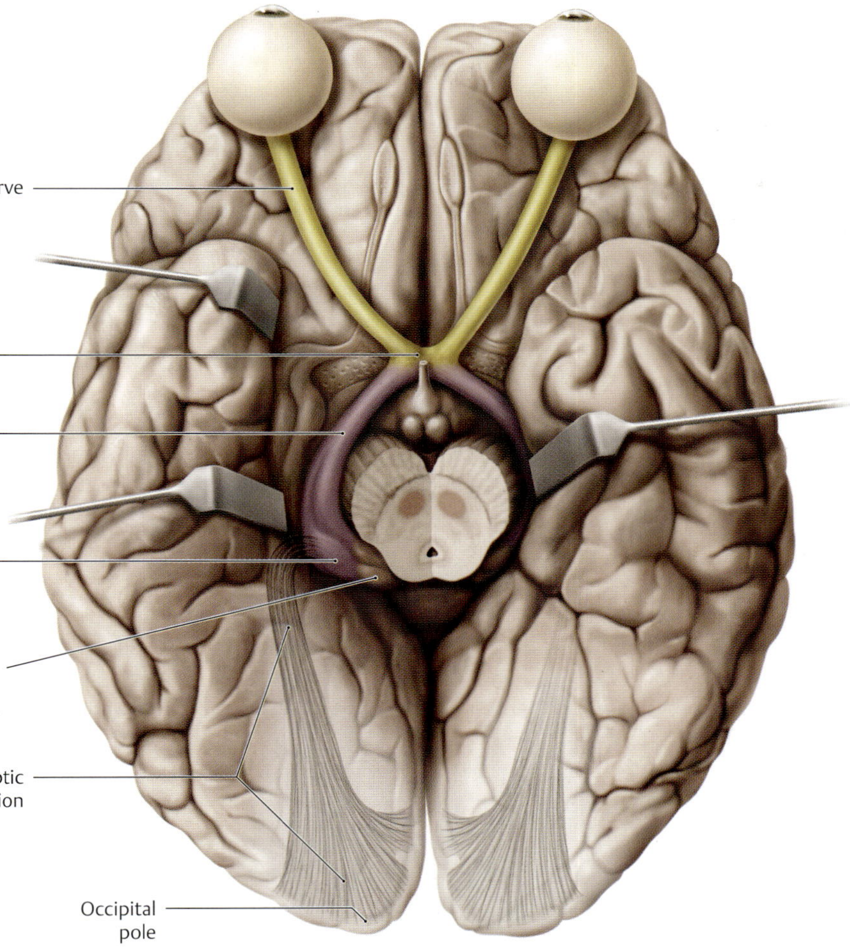

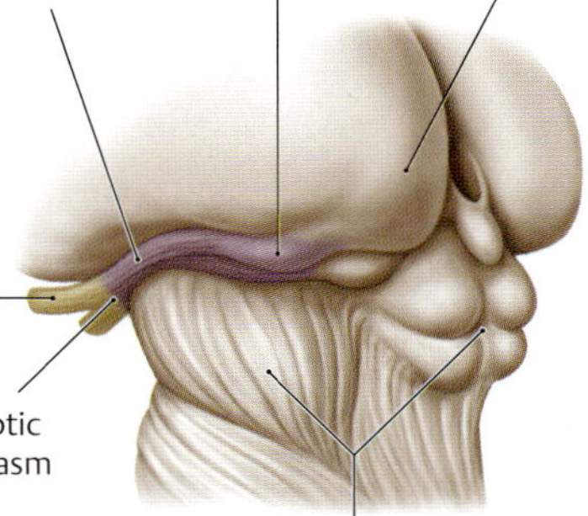

C Eye, optic nerve, optic chiasm, and optic tract

a View of the base of the brain, **b** posterolateral view of the left side of the brainstem. The termination of the optic tract in the lateral geniculate body is shown.

The optic nerve is not a true nerve but an extension of the brain, in this case of the diencephalon. Analogously to the olfactory bulb and tract (see **A**), the optic nerve is sheathed by meninges (removed here) and contains CNS-specific cells (cf. **A**). The optic nerve contains the axons of retinal ganglion cells. These axons terminate mainly in the lateral geniculate body of the diencephalon and in the mesencephalon.

Note: Because the optic nerve is an extension of the brain, the clinician can directly inspect a portion of the brain with an ophthalmoscope. This examination is important in the diagnosis of many neurological diseases (ophthalmoscopy is described on p. 171).

The optic nerve passes from the eyeball through the optic canal into the middle cranial fossa (see **D**). Many, but not all, retinal cell ganglion axons cross the midline to the contralateral side of the brain in the optic chiasm (**a**). The optic tract extends from the optic chiasm to the lateral geniculate body (see also **b**) while some fibers terminate in other destinations.

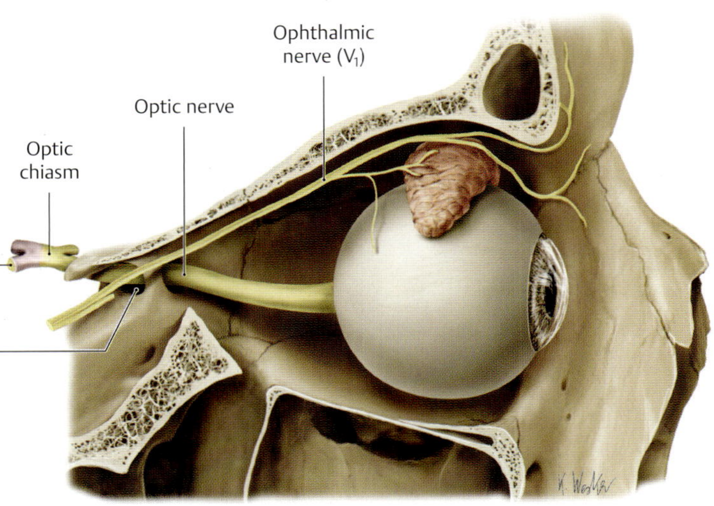

D Course of the optic nerve in the right orbit

Lateral view. The optic nerve extends through the optic canal from the orbit into the middle cranial fossa. It exits the posterior side of the eyeball within the retro-orbital fat (removed here). The other cranial nerves enter the orbit through the superior orbital fissure (only CN V_1 is shown here).

4.13 Cranial Nerves of the Extraocular Muscles: Oculomotor (CN III), Trochlear (CN IV), and Abducent (CN VI)

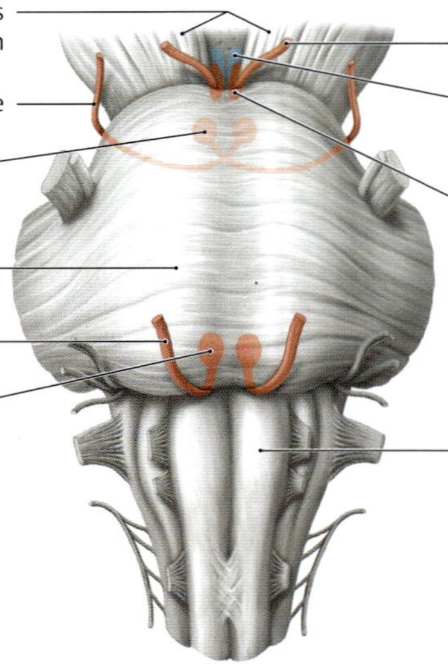

A Emergence of the nerves from the brainstem
Anterior view. All three nerves that supply the extraocular muscles emerge from the brainstem. The nuclei of the oculomotor nerve and trochlear nerve are located in the midbrain (mesencephalon), while the nucleus of the abducent nerve is located in the pons.
Note: Of these three nerves, the oculomotor (CN III) is the only one that contains somatic efferent and visceral efferent fibers and supplies several extraocular muscles (see **C**).

B Overview of the oculomotor nerve (CN III)

The oculomotor nerve contains *somatic efferent* and *visceral efferent* fibers.

Course: The nerve runs anteriorly from the mesencephalon (midbrain = highest level of the brainstem; see pp. 344, 346) and enters the orbit through the superior orbital fissure.

Nuclei and distribution, *ganglia:*
- *Somatic efferents:* Efferents from a nuclear complex (oculomotor nucleus) in the midbrain (see **C**) supply the following muscles:
  - Levator palpebrae superioris (acts on the upper eyelid)
  - Superior, medial, and inferior rectus and inferior oblique (= extraocular muscles, all act on the eyeball).
- *Visceral efferents:* Parasympathetic preganglionic efferents from the visceral oculomotor (Edinger-Westphal) nucleus synapse with neurons in the *ciliary ganglion* that innervate the following intraocular muscles:
  - Pupillary sphincter
  - Ciliary muscle

Effects of oculomotor nerve injury:
Oculomotor palsy, severity depending on the extent of the injury.
- Effects of complete oculomotor palsy (paralysis of the extraocular and intraocular muscles and levator palpebrae):
  - Ptosis (drooping of the eyelid)
  - Downward and lateral gaze deviation in the affected eye
  - Diplopia (in the absence of complete ptosis)
  - Mydriasis (pupil dilated due to sphincter pupillae paralysis)
  - Accommodation difficulties (ciliary paralysis: lens cannot focus).

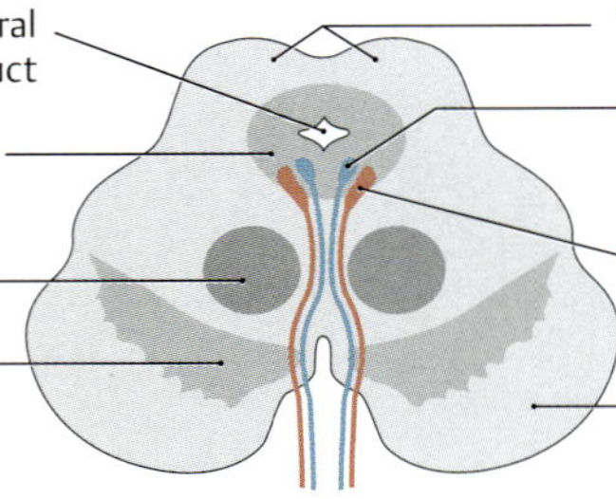

C Topography of the oculomotor nucleus
Cross-section through the brainstem at the level of the oculomotor nucleus, superior view.
Note: The visceral efferent, parasympathetic nuclear complex (accessory oculomotor [Edinger-Westphal] nucleus) can be distinguished from the somatic efferent nuclear complex (nucleus of the oculomotor nerve).

D Overview of the trochlear nerve (CN IV)

The trochlear nerve contains only *somatic efferent fibers.*

Course: The trochlear nerve emerges from the posterior surface of the brainstem near the midline, courses anteriorly around the cerebral peduncle, and enters the orbit through the superior orbital fissure.

Special features:
- The trochlear nerve is the only cranial nerve in which all the fibers cross to the opposite side (see **A**). Consequently, lesions of the nucleus or of nerve fibers very close to the nucleus, before they cross the midline, result in trochlear nerve palsy on the side opposite to the lesion (contralateral palsy). A lesion past the site where the nerve crosses the midline leads to trochlear nerve palsy on the same side as the lesion (ipsilateral palsy).
- The trochlear nerve is the only cranial nerve that emerges from the posterior side of the brainstem.
- It has the longest intracranial course of the three extraocular motor nerves.

Nucleus and distribution: The nucleus of the trochlear nerve is located in the midbrain (mesencephalon). Its efferents supply motor innervation to one extraocular muscle, the superior oblique.

Effects of trochlear nerve injury:
- The affected eye is higher and is also deviated medially because the inferior oblique (responsible for elevation and abduction) becomes dominant due to loss of the superior oblique.
- Diplopia.

E Overview of the abducent nerve (CN VI)

The abducent nerve contains only *somatic efferent fibers.*

Course: The nerve follows a long *extradural* path before entering the orbit through the superior orbital fissure.

Nucleus and distribution:
- The nucleus of the abducent nerve is located in the pons, its fibers emerging at the inferior border of the pons.
- Its efferent fibers supply somatomotor innervation to a single muscle, the lateral rectus.

Effects of abducent nerve injury:
- The affected eye is deviated medially.
- Diplopia.

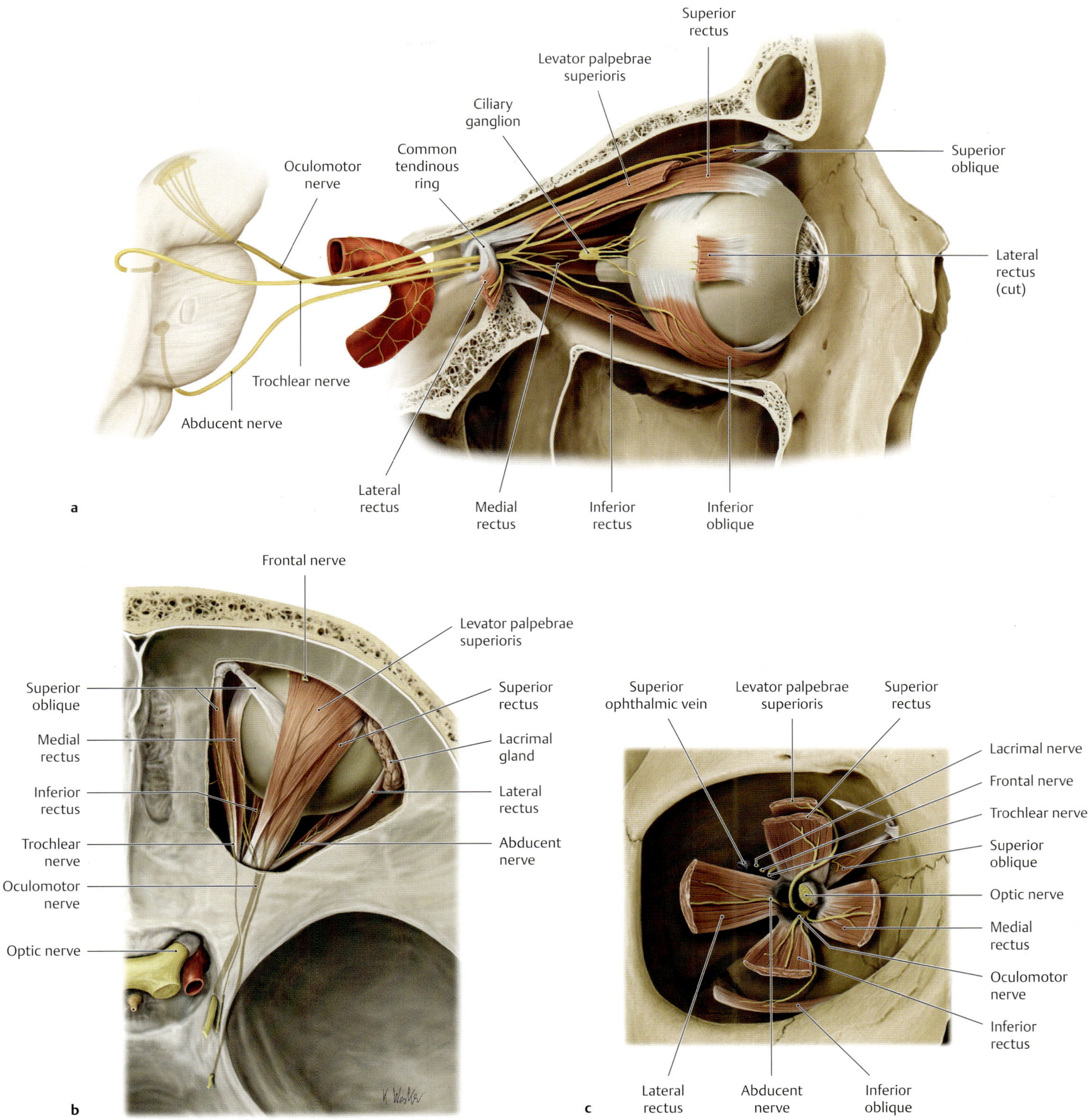

F Course of the nerves supplying the ocular muscles

a Lateral view. Right orbit. **b** superior view (opened), **c** anterior view. All three cranial nerves extend from the brainstem through the superior orbital fissure into the orbit. The oculomotor and abducens nn. pass through the common tendinous ring of the extraocular muscles, while the trochlear n. passes outside the tendinous ring. The *abducent nerve* has the longest *extradural* course. Because of this, abducent nerve palsy may develop in association with meningitis and subarachnoid hemorrhage. Transient palsy may even occur in cases where lumbar puncture has caused an excessive decrease in CSF pressure, with descent of the brainstem exerting traction on the nerve. The *oculomotor nerve* supplies parasympathetic innervation to intraocular muscles (its parasympathetic fibers synapse in the ciliary ganglion) as well as somatic motor innervation to most of the extraocular muscles and the levator palpebrae superioris. Oculomotor nerve palsy may affect the parasympathetic fibers exclusively, the somatic motor fibers exclusively, or both at the same time (see **B** on page 112). Because the preganglionic parasympathetic fibers for the pupil lie directly beneath the epineurium after emerging from the brainstem, they are often the first structures to be affected by pressure due to trauma, tumors, or aneurysms.

4.14 Cranial Nerves: Trigeminal (CN V), Nuclei, and Distribution

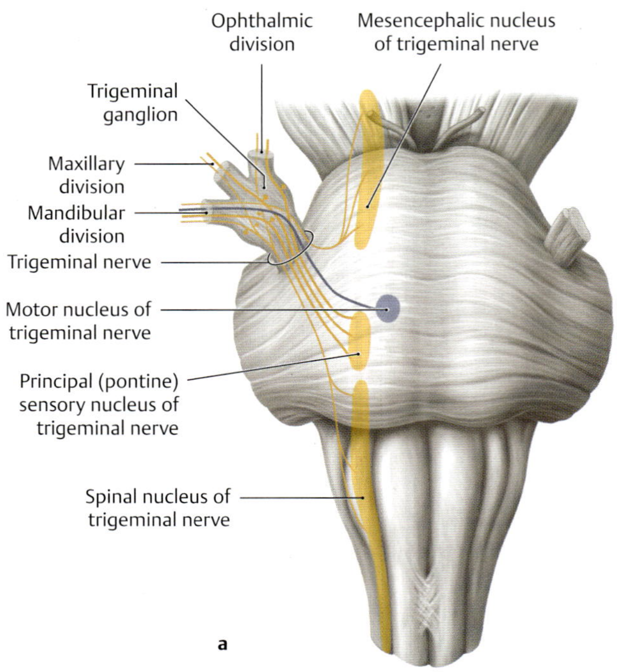

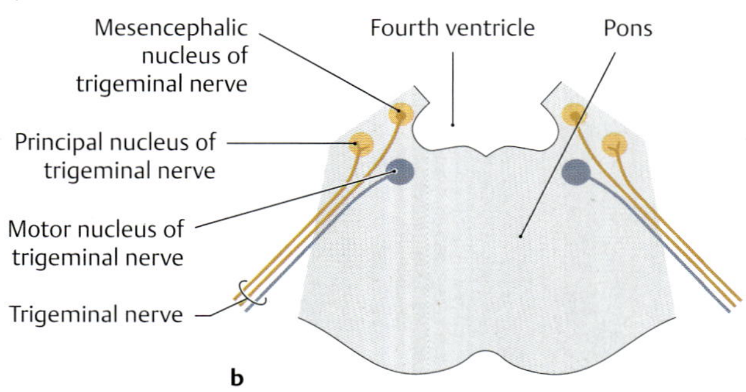

A Nuclei and emergence from the pons

a Anterior view. The larger sensory nuclei of the trigeminal nerve are distributed along the brainstem and extend downward into the spinal cord. The *sensory root* (major part) of the trigeminal nerve forms the bulk of the fibers, while the *motor root* (minor part) is formed by fibers arising from the small motor nucleus in the pons. They supply motor innervation to the muscles of mastication (see **B**). The following *somatic afferent* nuclei are distinguished:

- *Mesencephalic nucleus of the trigeminal nerve:* proprioceptive fibers from the muscles of mastication. Special feature: the neurons of this nucleus are pseudounipolar ganglion cells that have migrated into the brainstem.
- *Principal (pontine) sensory nucleus of the trigeminal nerve:* chiefly mediates touch.
- *Spinal nucleus of the trigeminal nerve:* pain and temperature sensation, also touch. A small, circumscribed lesion of the trigeminal spinal sensory nucleus leads to characteristic sensory disturbances in the face (see **D**).

b Cross-section through the pons at the level of emergence of the trigeminal nerve, superior view (schematic as the three nuclei are located at different levels).

B Overview of the trigeminal nerve (CN V)

The trigeminal nerve, the main sensory nerve of the head, contains mostly *somatic afferent* fibers with a smaller proportion of special visceral *efferent fibers*. Its three major somatic **divisions** have the following **sites of emergence** from the middle cranial fossa:

- *Ophthalmic division (CN V_1):* enters the orbit through the superior orbital fissure.
- *Maxillary division (CN V_2):* enters the pterygopalatine fossa through the foramen rotundum.
- *Mandibular division (CN V_3):* passes through the foramen ovale to the inferior surface of the base of the skull into the infratemporal fossa; this is the only division containing motor fibers.

Nuclei and distribution:

- *Special visceral efferent:* Efferent fibers from the motor nucleus of the trigeminal nerve pass in the mandibular division (CN V_3) to
  - Muscles of mastication (temporalis, masseter, medial and lateral pterygoid)
  - Oral floor muscles: mylohyoid and anterior belly of the digastric
  - Middle ear muscle: tensor tympani
  - Pharyngeal muscle: tensor veli palatini
- *Somatic afferent:* The trigeminal ganglion contains pseudounipolar ganglion cells whose central processes pass to the sensory nuclei of the trigeminal nerve (see **Aa**). Their peripheral processes innervate the facial skin, large portions of the nasopharyngeal mucosa, the surface of the eyeball, the dura of the anterior and middle cranial fossa (see pp. 122–123), and the anterior two-thirds of the tongue (see **C**).
- *"Visceral efferent pathway":* The visceral efferent fibers of some cranial nerves adhere to branches or sub-branches of the trigeminal nerve, by which they travel to their destination:
  - The lacrimal nerve (branch of CN V_1) conveys parasympathetic fibers from the pterygopalatine ganglion that traveled along the zygomatic nerve (branch of CN V_2) to the lacrimal gland.
  - The auriculotemporal nerve (branch of CN V_3) conveys parasympathetic fibers from the otic ganglion to the parotid gland.
  - The lingual nerve (branch of CN V_3) conveys parasympathetic fibers from the chorda tympani of the facial nerve to the submandibular ganglion where they make synapse. The postganglionic fibers innervate the submandibular and sublingual gland.
- *"Visceral afferent pathway":* Gustatory fibers that supply the anterior two-thirds of the tongue travel via the lingual nerve to the chorda tympani and then the facial nerve.

Developmentally,
the trigeminal nerve is the nerve of the first branchial (pharyngeal) arch.

Clinical disorders of the trigeminal nerve:
Sensory disturbances and deficits may arise in various conditions:

- Sensory loss due to traumatic nerve lesions.
- Herpes zoster ophthalmicus (involvement of the territory of the first division of the trigeminal nerve, including the skin and/or the eye, by the varicella-zoster virus); herpes zoster of the face.

The afferent fibers of the trigeminal nerve (together with the facial nerve, see p. 124) are involved in the corneal reflex (reflex closure of the eyelid; see C, p. 479).

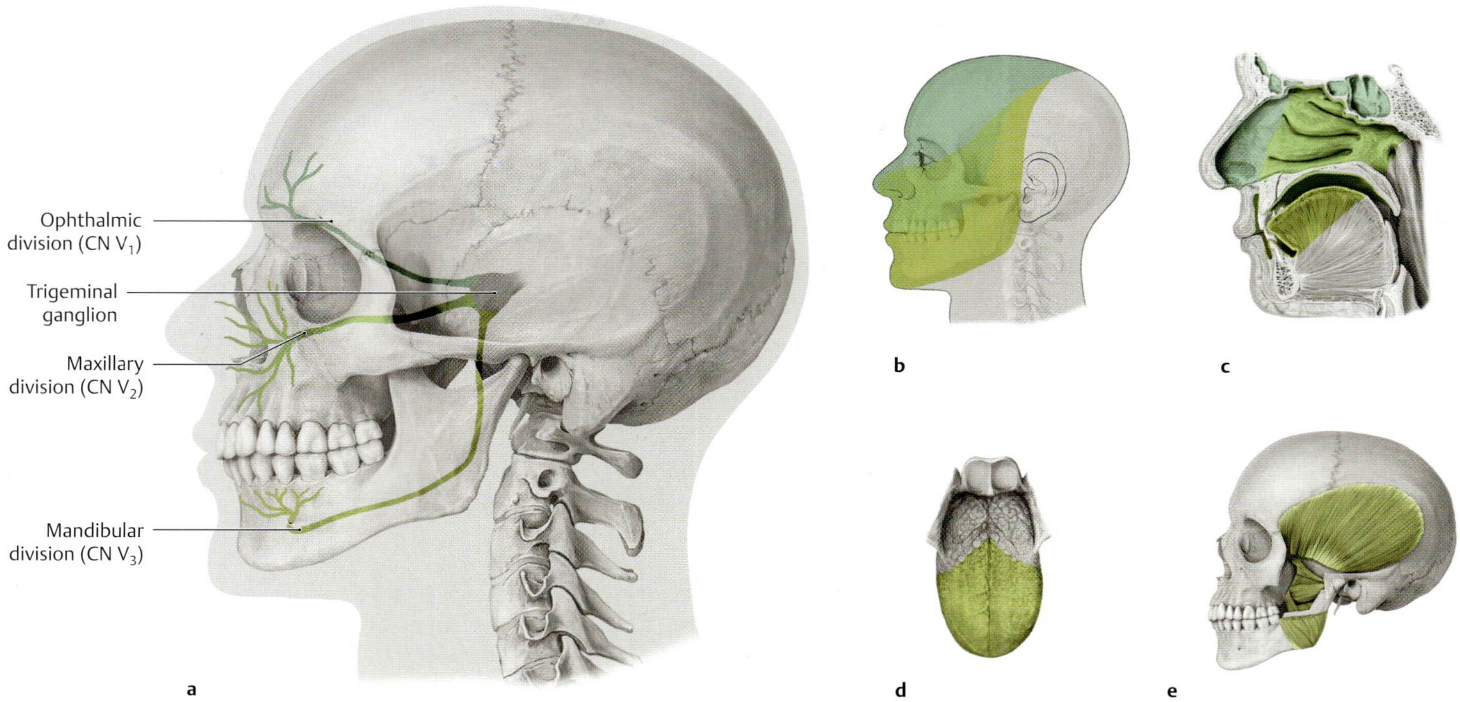

C Course and distribution of the trigeminal nerve

a Left lateral view. The three divisions of the trigeminal nerve and clinically important terminal branches are shown.

All three divisions of the trigeminal nerve supply the skin of the face (**b**) and the mucosa of the nasopharynx (**c**). The anterior two-thirds of the tongue (**d**) receives general sensory innervation (touch, pain and thermal sensation, but not taste) via the lingual nerve, which is a branch of the mandibular division (CN V_3). The taste fibers travel along the lingual nerve to chorda tympani, which is a branch of the facial nerve. The muscles of mastication are supplied by the motor root of the trigeminal nerve. The axons enter the mandibular division (**e**).

Note: The efferent fibers course exclusively in the mandibular division. A peripheral trigeminal nerve lesion involving one of its divisions—ophthalmic (CN V_1), maxillary (CN V_2), or mandibular (CN V_3)—may cause loss of somatic sensation (touch, pain, and temperature) in the area innervated by the afferent nerve (see **b**). This contrasts with the more concentric pattern, and more restricted modality, of sensory deficit produced by a central (CNS) lesion involving trigeminal nuclei and pathways (see **D**).

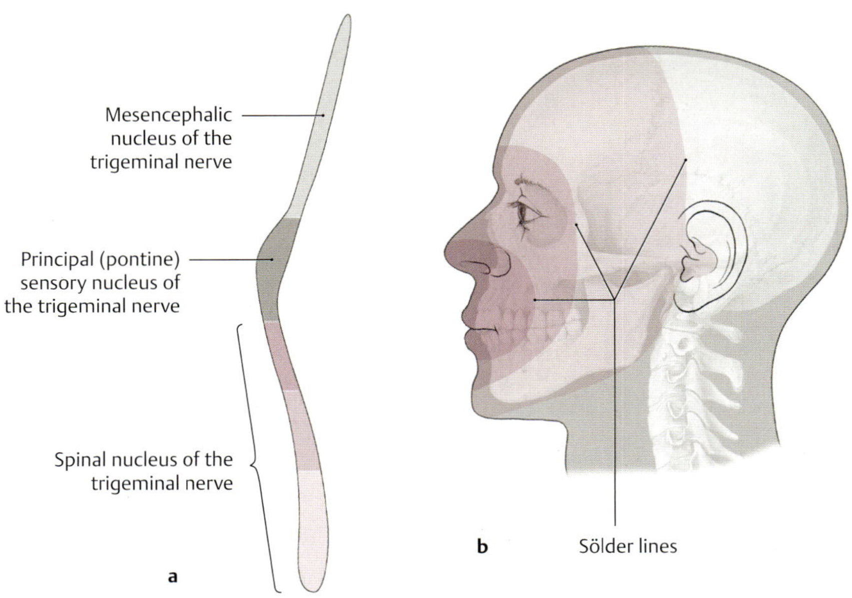

D Central trigeminal lesion

a Somatotopic organization of the spinal nucleus of the trigeminal nerve. **b** Facial zones in which sensory deficits (pain and temperature) arise when certain regions of the trigeminal spinal nucleus are destroyed.

These zones follow the concentric *Sölder lines* in the face. Their pattern indicates the corresponding portion of the trigeminal nucleus in which the lesion is located (matching color shades).

4.15 Cranial Nerves: Trigeminal (CN V), Divisions

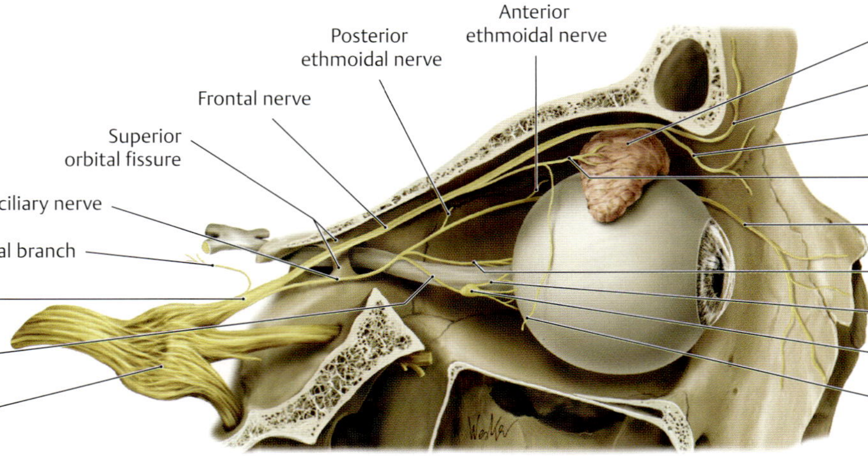

A Branches of the ophthalmic division (= first division of the trigeminal nerve, CN V_1) in the orbital region

Lateral view of the partially opened right orbit. The first small branch arising from the ophthalmic division is the *recurrent meningeal branch*, which supplies sensory innervation to the dura mater. The bulk of the ophthalmic division fibers enter the orbit from the middle cranial fossa by passing through the *superior orbital fissure*. The ophthalmic division divides into three branches the names of which indicate their distribution: the **lacrimal nerve**, **frontal nerve**, and **nasociliary nerve**.

Note: The lacrimal nerve receives postsynaptic, *parasympathetic* secretomotor fibers from the zygomatic nerve (maxillary division of CN V) via a *communicating branch* (branch of the maxillary n., V_2; see **B**). These fibers travel to the lacrimal gland by the lacrimal nerve. *Sympathetic* fibers accompany the long ciliary nerves that arise from the nasociliary nerve, traveling in these nerves to the pupil. The ciliary nerves also contain afferent fibers that mediate the corneal reflex. Sensory fibers from the eyeball course in the nasociliary root, passing through the ciliary ganglion to the nasociliary nerve.

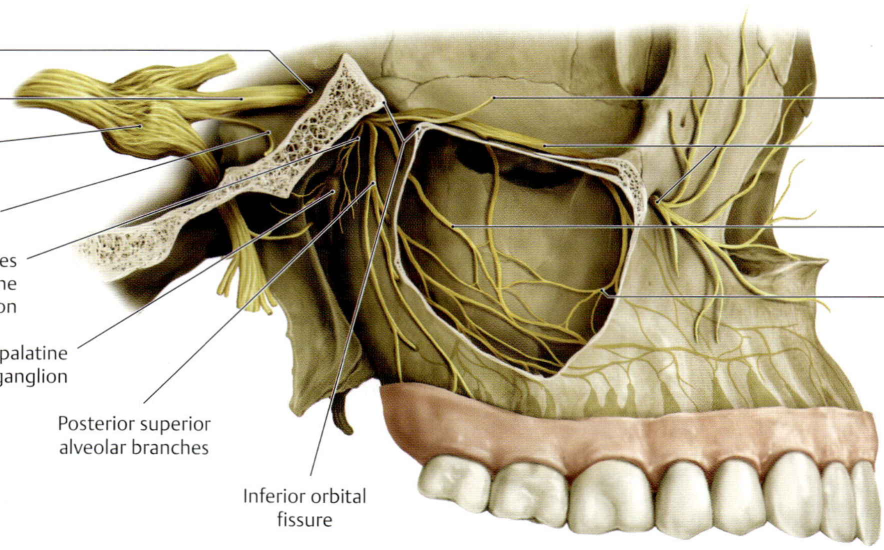

B Branches of the maxillary division (= second division of the trigeminal nerve, CN V2) in the maxillary region

Lateral view of the partially opened right maxillary sinus with the zygomatic arch removed. After giving off a meningeal branch, the maxillary division leaves the middle cranial fossa through the foramen rotundum and enters the pterygopalatine fossa, where it divides into the following branches:

- Zygomatic nerve
- Ganglionic branches to the pterygopalatine ganglion (sensory root of the pterygopalatine ganglion)
- Infraorbital nerve

The **zygomatic nerve** enters the orbit through the *inferior orbital fissure*. Its two terminal branches, the zygomaticofacial branch and zygomaticotemporal branch (not shown here), supply sensory innervation to the skin over the zygomatic arch and temple. Parasympathetic, postsynaptic fibers from the pterygopalatine ganglion are carried to the lacrimal nerve by the communicating branch (see p. 127). The preganglionic fibers originally arise from the facial nerve. The **infraorbital nerve** also passes through the inferior orbital fissure into the orbit, from which it enters the infraorbital canal. Its fine terminal branches supply the skin between the lower eyelid and upper lip. Its other terminal branches form the *superior dental plexus*, which supplies sensory innervation to the maxillary teeth:

- Anterior superior alveolar branches to the incisors
- Middle superior alveolar branch to the premolars
- Posterior superior alveolar branches to the molars

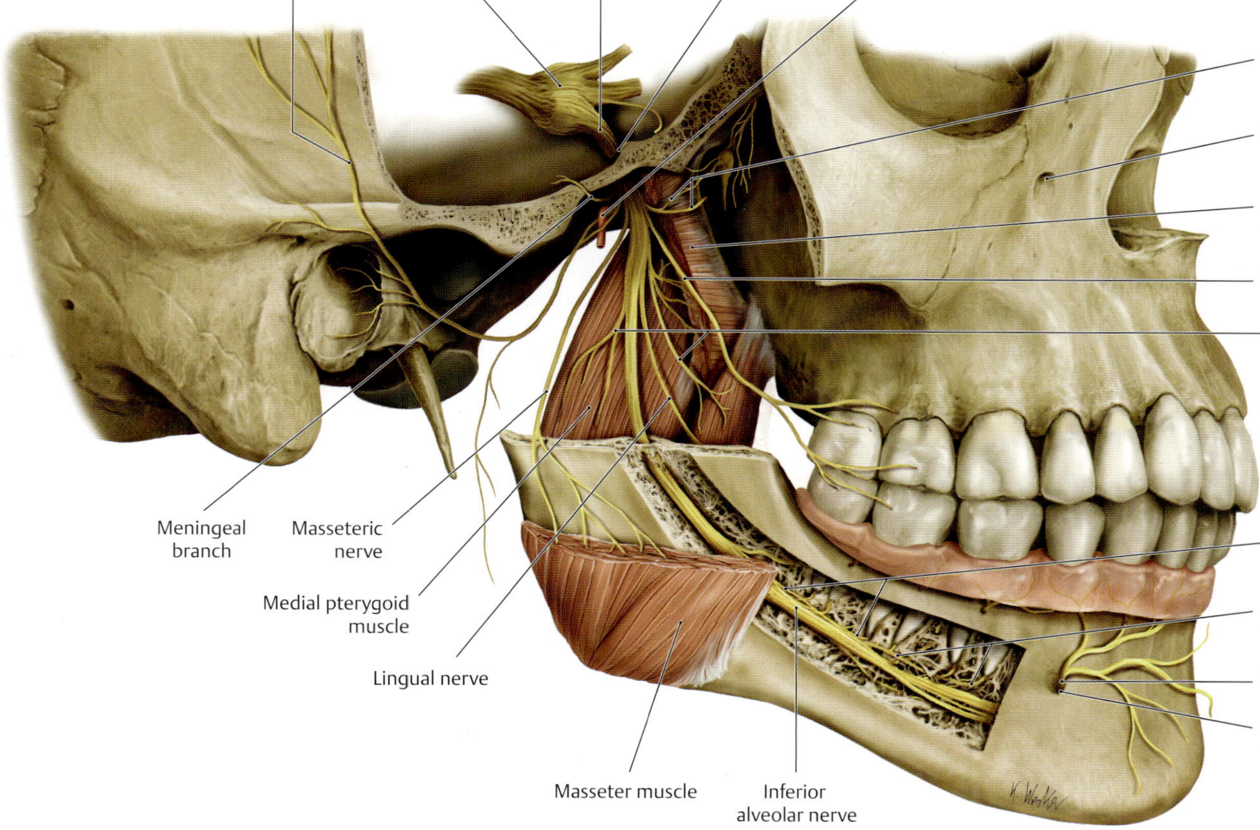

C Branches of the mandibular division (= third division of the trigeminal nerve, CN V3) in the mandibular region

Right lateral view of the partially opened mandible with the zygomatic arch removed. The mixed afferent-efferent mandibular division leaves the middle cranial fossa through the foramen ovale and enters the infratemporal fossa on the external aspect of the base of the skull. Its meningeal branch re-enters the middle cranial fossa to supply sensory innervation to the dura. Its **sensory branches** are as follows:

- Auriculotemporal nerve
- Lingual nerve
- Inferior alveolar nerve (also carries motor fibers, see below)
- Buccal nerve

The branches of the *auriculotemporal nerve* supply the temporal skin, the external auditory canal, and the tympanic membrane. The *lingual nerve* supplies sensory fibers to the anterior two-thirds of the tongue, and gustatory fibers from the chorda tympani (facial nerve branch) travel with it. The *afferent* fibers of the *inferior alveolar nerve* pass through the mandibular foramen into the mandibular canal, where they give off inferior dental branches to the mandibular teeth. The mental nerve is a terminal branch that supplies the skin of the chin, lower lip, and the body of the mandible. The *efferent* fibers that branch from the inferior alveolar nerve supply the mylohyoid muscle and the anterior belly of the digastric (not shown). The *buccal nerve* pierces the buccinator muscle and supplies sensory innervation to the mucous membrane of the cheek. The pure **motor branches** leave the main nerve trunk just distal to the origin of the meningeal branch. They are as follows:

- Masseteric nerve (masseter muscle)
- Deep temporal nerves (temporalis muscle)
- Pterygoid nerves (pterygoid muscles)
- Nerve of the tensor tympani muscle
- Nerve of the tensor veli palatini muscle (not shown here; see **C**, p. 237)

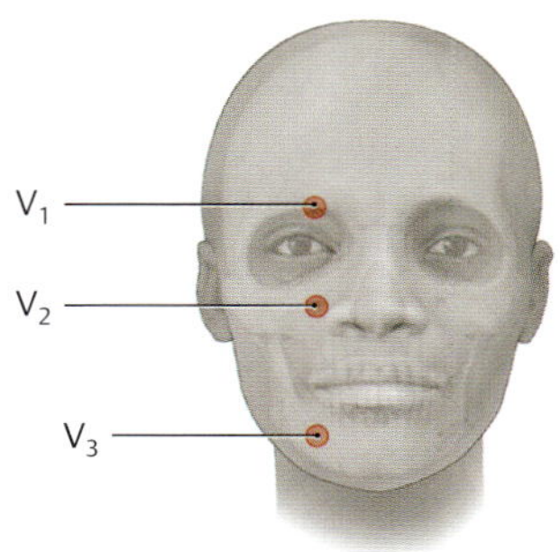

D Clinical assessment of trigeminal nerve function

Each of the three main divisions of the trigeminal nerve is tested separately during the physical examination. This is done by pressing on the nerve exit points with one finger to test the sensation there (local tenderness to pressure). The typical testing of exit point branches of the three divisions are as follows:

- For CN V_1: the supraorbital foramen or supraorbital notch
- For CN V_2: the infraorbital foramen
- For CN V_3: the mental foramen

4.16 Cranial Nerves: Facial (CN VII), Nuclei, and Distribution

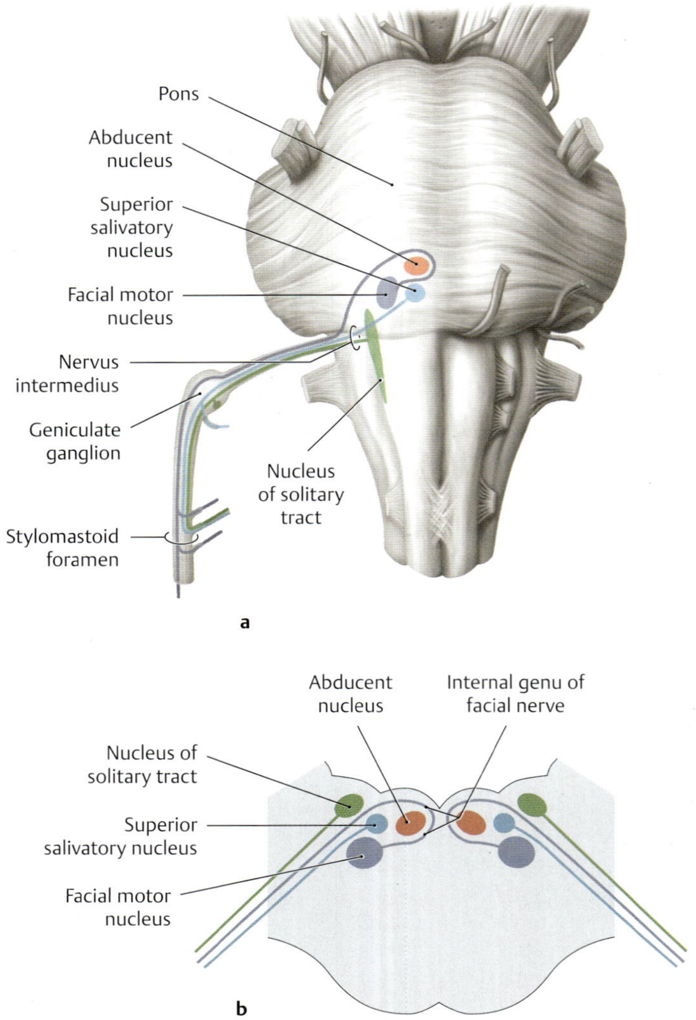

A Nuclei and principal branches of the facial nerve
a Anterior view of the brainstem, showing the site of emergence of the facial nerve from the lower pons. **b** Cross-section through the pons at the level of the internal genu of the facial nerve.
Note: Each of the different fiber types (different sensory modalities) is associated with a particular nucleus.
From the **facial nucleus**, the special visceral efferent axons that innervate the muscles of facial expression first loop backward around the abducent nucleus, where they form the internal genu of the facial nerve. They then pass forward and emerge at the lower border of the pons. The **superior salivatory nucleus** contains *visceromotor*, preganglyonic *parasympathetic* neurons. Together with *viscerosensory* (gustatory) fibers from the nucleus of the solitary tract (superior part), they emerge from the pons as the nervus intermedius and then are bundled with the *visceromotor* axons from the facial motor nucleus to form the facial nerve.

B Overview of the facial nerve (CN VII)

The facial nerve mainly conveys *special visceral efferent* (branchial) fibers from the facial nerve nucleus which innervate the skeletal muscles of facial expression. The other visceral efferent (parasympathetic) fibers from the superior salivatory nucleus are grouped with the *visceral afferent* (gustatory) fibers from the nucleus of the solitary tract to form the *nervus intermedius* and aggregate with the visceral efferent fibers from the facial nerve nucleus.

Sites of emergence: The facial nerve emerges in the cerebellopontine angle between the pons and olive. It exits the cranial cavity through the internal acoustic meatus passing into the petrous part of the temporal bone, where it divides into its branches:
- The special visceral efferent fibers pass through the *stylomastoid foramen* to exit the base of the skull to form the intraparotid plexus (see **C**, exception: stapedius n.).
- The parasympathetic, visceral efferent and visceral afferent fibers, pass through the *sphenopetrosal fissure* to the base of the skull (see **A**, p. 126). While still in the petrous bone, the facial nerve gives off the greater petrosal nerve, stapedial nerve, and chorda tympani.

Nuclei and distribution, *ganglia:*
- *Special visceral efferent:* Efferents from the facial nucleus supply the following muscles:
  - Muscles of facial expression
  - Stylohyoid
  - Posterior belly of the digastric
  - Stapedius (stapedial nerve)
- *Visceral efferent (parasympathetic):* Parasympathetic presynaptic fibers arising from the superior salivatory nucleus synapse with neurons in the *pterygopalatine ganglion* or *submandibular ganglion*. They innervate the following structures:
  - Lacrimal gland
  - Small glands of the nasal mucosa and of the hard and soft palate
  - Submandibular gland
  - Sublingual gland
  - Small salivary glands on the dorsum of the tongue
- *Special visceral afferent:* Central fibers of pseudounipolar ganglion cells from the geniculate ganglion (corresponds to a spinal ganglion) synapse in the nucleus of the solitary tract. The peripheral processes of these neurons form the *chorda tympani* (gustatory fibers from the anterior *two-thirds of the tongue).*
- *Somatic afferent neurons:* Some sensory fibers that supply the auricle, the skin of the auditory canal, and the outer surface of the tympanic membrane travel by the facial nerve and *geniculate ganglion* to the trigeminal sensory nuclei. Their precise course is unknown.

Developmentally, the facial nerve is the nerve of the second branchial (pharyngeal) arch.

Effects of facial nerve injury: A peripheral facial nerve injury is characterized by paralysis of the muscles of facial expression on the affected side of the face (see **D**). Because the facial nerve conveys various fiber components that leave the main trunk of the nerve at different sites, the clinical presentation of facial paralysis is subject to subtle variations marked by associated disturbances of taste, lacrimation, salivation, etc. (see **B**, p. 126).

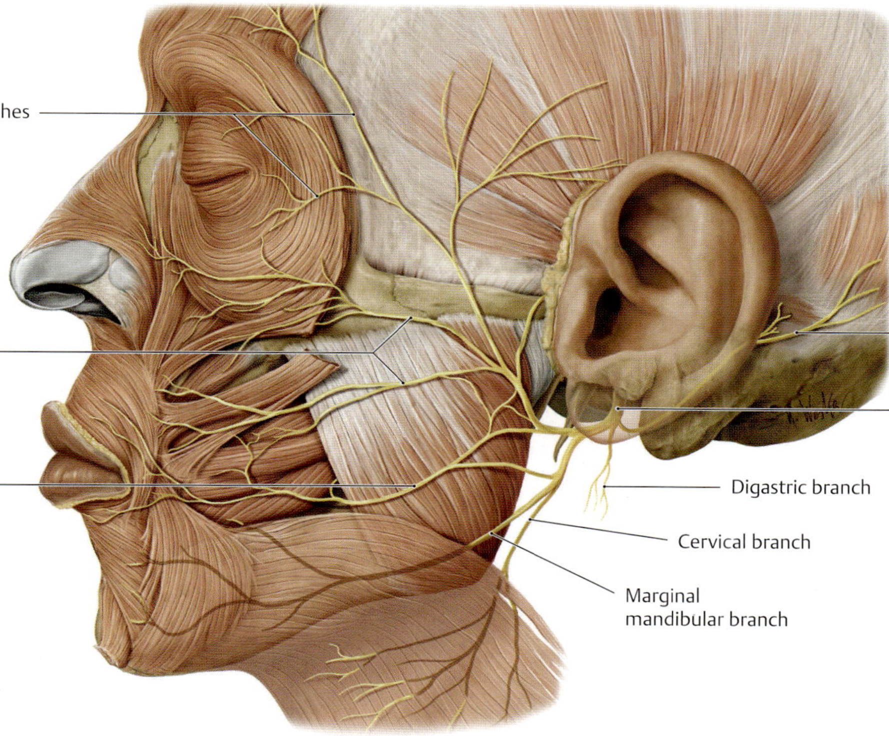

C Facial nerve branches for the muscles of expression
Note the different fiber types. This unit focuses almost exclusively on the *visceral efferent* (branchial) fibers for the muscles of facial expression. (The other fiber types are described on p. 126).
The stapedial nerve (to the stapedius muscle) branches from the facial nerve while still in the petrous part of the temporal bone and is mentioned here only because it also contains visceral efferent fibers (its course is shown on p. 126). The first branch that arises from the facial nerve after its emergence from the stylomastoid foramen is the **posterior auricular nerve**; it supplies *visceral efferent* fibers to the posterior auricular muscles and the posterior belly of the occipitofrontalis. It also conveys *somatosensory* fibers from the external ear, whose pseudounipolar neurons are located in the geniculate ganglion (see p. 126). After leaving the petrous temporal bone, the bulk of the remaining visceral efferent fibers of the facial nerve form the **intraparotid plexus** in the parotid gland, from which successive branches (*temporal*, *zygomatic*, *buccal*, and *marginal mandibular*) are distributed to the muscles of facial expression. These facial nerve branches must be protected during the removal of a benign parotid tumor in order to preserve muscle function. Additionally, there are even smaller branches such as the digastric branch to the posterior belly of the digastric muscle and the stylohyoid branch to the stylohyoid muscle (not shown). The lowest branch arising from the intraparotid plexus is the *cervical branch*. It joins with the transverse cervical nerve, an anterior branch of the C3 spinal nerve.

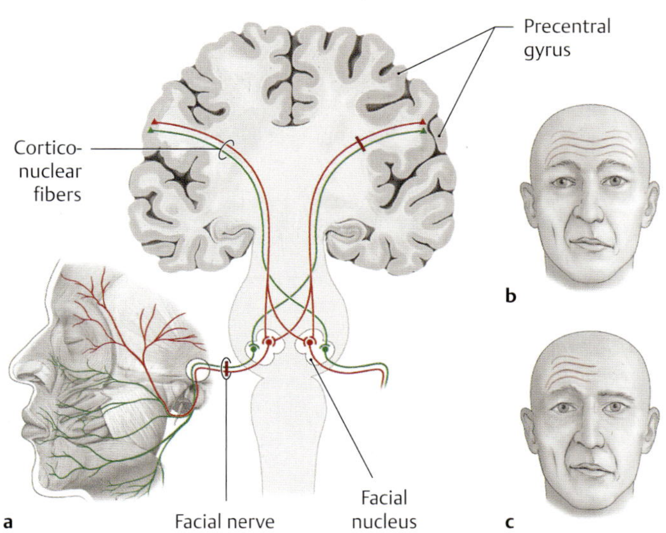

D Paralysis symptoms in case of damage to the facial nucleus
Note for didactic reasons, that an occipital view of the brain is used for the image above when describing the side on which paralysis occurs.
a The facial motor nucleus contains the cell bodies of lower motor neurons which innervate ipsilateral muscles of facial expression. The axons (special visceral efferent) of these neurons reach their muscle targets through the facial nerve. In turn, the lower motor neurons are under the control of upper motor neurons located in the primary somatomotor cortex (precentral gyrus), whose axons enter the corticonuclear tract to reach the facial motor nucleus in the brainstem.
Note: The facial nucleus has a "bipartite" structure, its upper part (posterior part, red neuron) supplying the muscles of the forehead and eyes (temporal branches) while its lower part (anterior part, green neuron) supplying the muscles in the lower half of the face. The upper part of the facial nerve nucleus receives bilateral input from the cerebral cortex, while the lower part of the nucleus receives input only from the contralateral cerebral cortex via upper motor neurons.
b Central (supranuclear) paralysis Loss of the right upper motor neurons. In this case, paralysis affects the muscles of facial expression on the lower side of the face, contralateral to the damaged corticonuclear tract. The muscles of facial expression on the upper part of the face remain unaffected. Thus, the corner of the mouth sags on the left (contralateral) side, but the patient can still wrinkle the forehead and close the eyes on both sides. Speech articulation is impaired.
c Peripheral (infranuclear) paralysis Loss of the left second motor neuron, in this case on the left side, is characterized by complete paralysis of the muscles of facial expression on the entire half of the face ipsilateral to the lesion of the facial nucleus or facial nerve. The patient cannot wrinkle the forehead, the corner of the mouth sags, articulation is impaired, and the eyelid cannot be fully closed. A Bell phenomenon (Bell palsy) is present (the eyeball turns upward and outward, exposing the sclera, when the patient attempts to close the eyelid), and the eyelid closure reflex is abolished. Depending on the site of the lesion, additional deficits may be present such as decreased lacrimation and salivation or loss of taste sensation in the anterior two-thirds of the tongue.

4.17 Cranial Nerves: Facial (CN VII), Branches

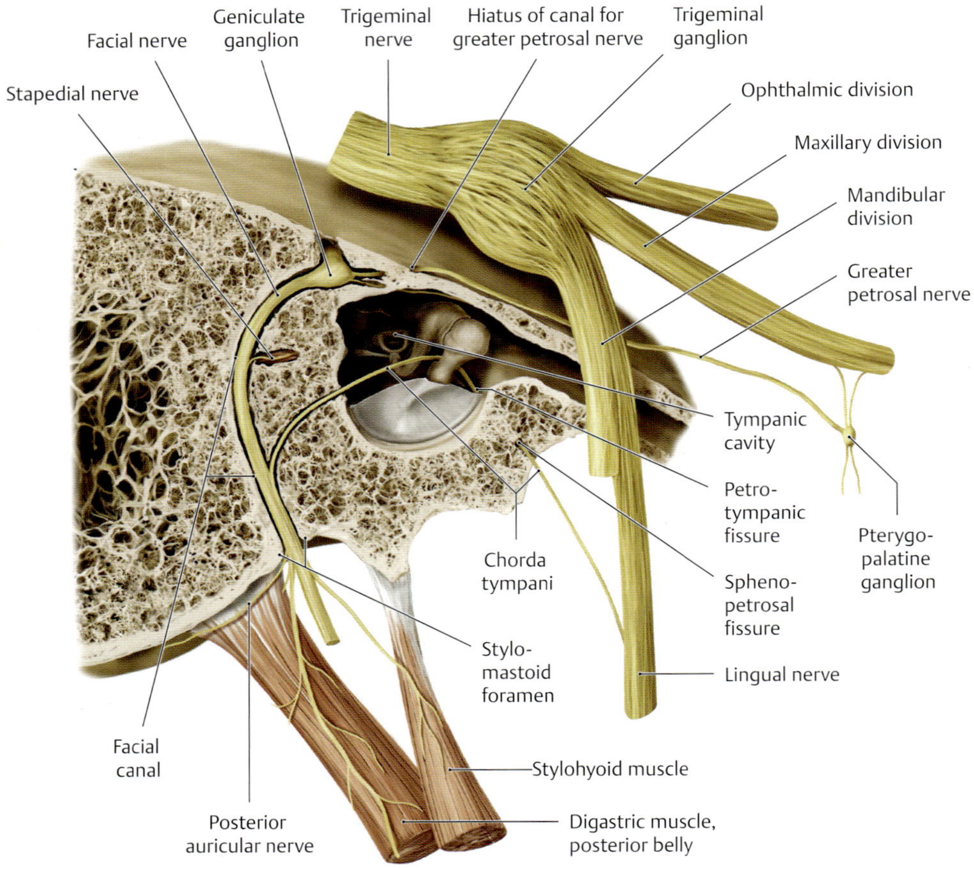

A Facial nerve branches in the temporal bone

Lateral view of the right temporal bone, petrous portion (petrous bone). The facial nerve, accompanied by the vestibulocochlear nerve (CN VIII, not shown), passes through the internal acoustic meatus (not shown) to enter the petrous bone. Shortly thereafter it forms the *external genu* of the facial nerve, which marks the location of the geniculate ganglion. The bulk of the visceral efferent fibers for the muscles of expression pass through the petrous bone and exit onto the base of the skull at the stylomastoid foramen (see p. 125). The facial nerve gives off three branches between the geniculate ganglion and stylomastoid foramen:

- The parasympathetic **greater petrosal nerve** arises directly at the geniculate ganglion. This nerve leaves the anterior surface of the petrous pyramid at the hiatus of the canal for the greater petrosal nerve. It continues through the foramen lacerum (not shown), enters the pterygoid canal (see **C**), and passes to the pterygopalatine ganglion.
- The **stapedial nerve** passes to the stapedius muscle.
- The **chorda tympani** branches from the facial nerve above the stylomastoid foramen. It contains afferent fibers that convey gustatory information, as well as preganglionic parasympathetic fibers. It passes through the tympanic cavity and petrotympanic fissure into the petrous bone and exits at the base of the skull through the sphenopetrosal fissure and then joins the lingual nerve.

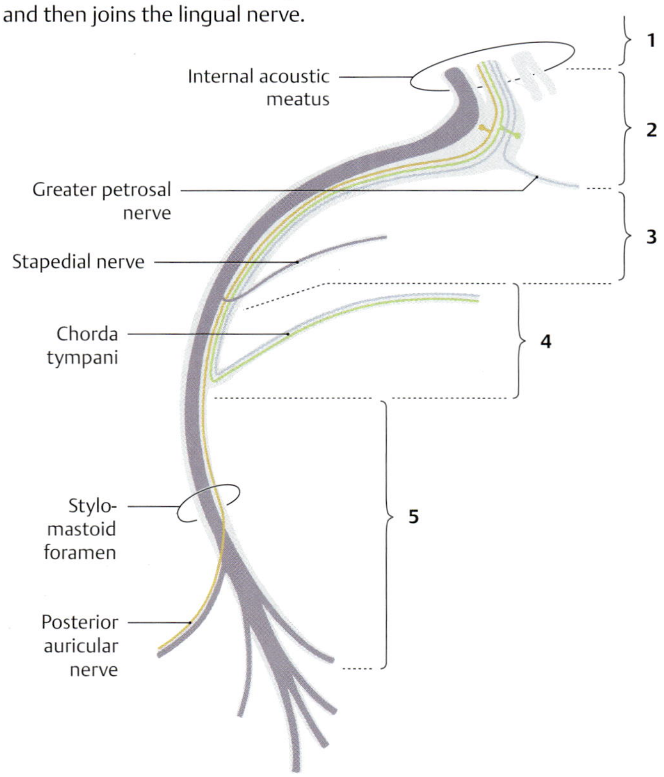

B Branching pattern of the facial nerve: diagnostic significance in temporal bone fractures

The principal signs and symptoms are different depending upon the exact site of the lesion in the course of the facial nerve through the petrous bone.

Note: Only the *principal* signs and symptoms associated with a particular lesion site are described here. The more peripheral the site of the nerve injury, the less diverse the signs and symptoms become.

1 A lesion at this level affects the facial nerve in addition to the vestibulocochlear nerve. As a result, peripheral motor facial paralysis is accompanied by hearing loss (deafness) and vestibular dysfunction (dizziness).
2 Peripheral motor facial paralysis is accompanied by disturbances of taste sensation (chorda tympani), lacrimation, and salivation.
3 Motor paralysis is accompanied by disturbances of salivation and taste. Hyperacusis due to paralysis of the stapedius muscle has little clinical importance.
4 Peripheral motor paralysis is accompanied by disturbances of taste and salivation.
5 Peripheral motor (facial) paralysis is the only manifestation of a lesion at this level.

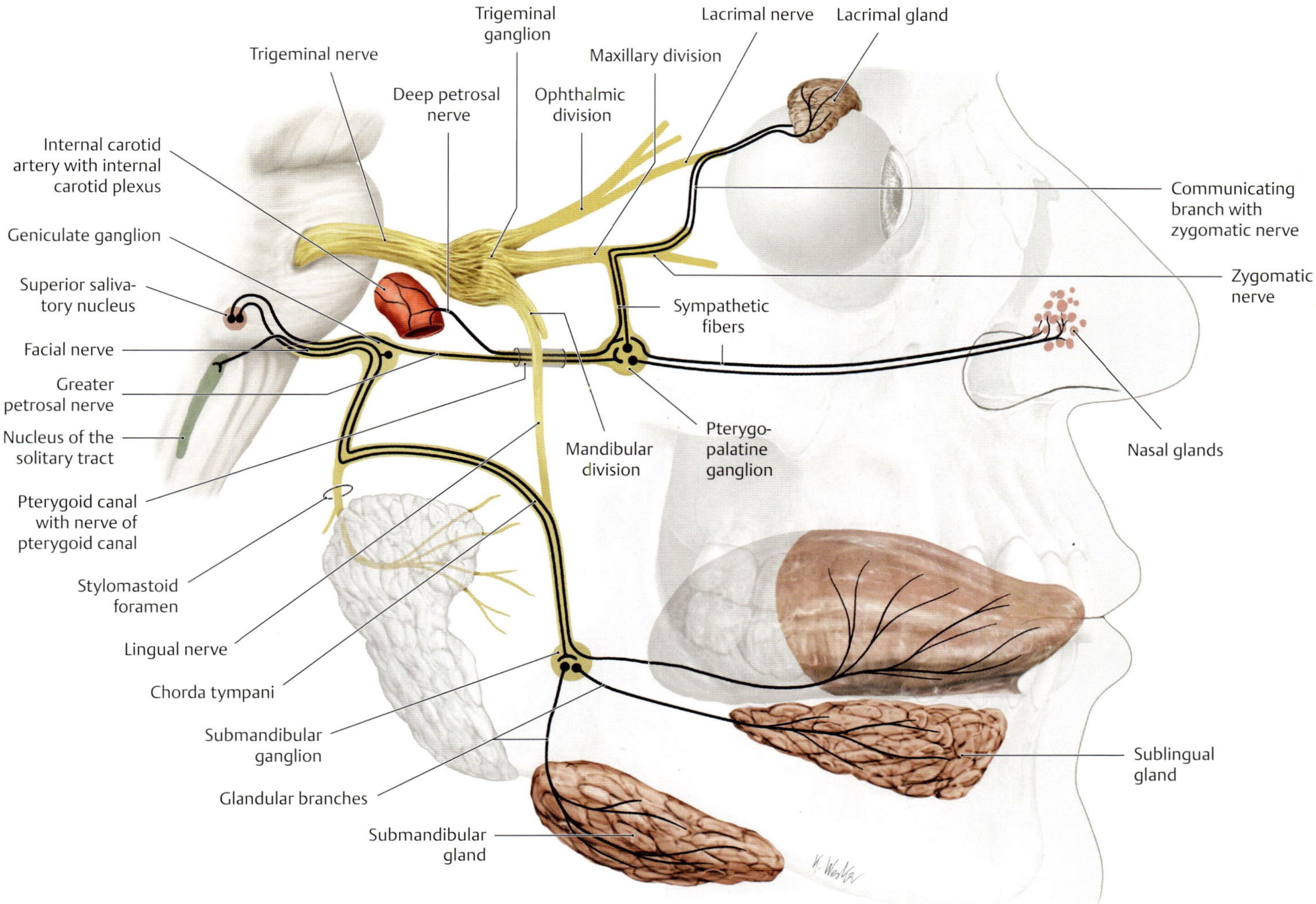

C Parasympathetic visceral efferents and visceral afferents (gustatory fibers) of the facial nerve

The bodies of postganglionic parasympathetic (visceral efferent) neurons are located in the superior salivatory nucleus. Their axons enter and leave the pons with the visceral efferent axons as the nervus intermedius, then travel with the visceral efferent fibers arising from the facial motor nucleus. These preganglionic parasympathetic axons exit the brainstem in the facial nerve and branch from it in the greater petrosal nerve, then mingle with *postganglionic sympathetic axons* (from the superior cervical ganglion, via the deep petrosal nerve) in the nerve of the pterygoid canal. This nerve enters the **pterygopalatine ganglion**, where the preganglionic parasympathetic motor axons synapse; the sympathetic axons pass through uninterrupted to innervate local blood vessels. The pterygopalatine ganglion supplies the lacrimal gland, nasal glands, and nasal, palatine, and pharyngeal mucosa. Fibers from this ganglion enter the maxillary division and travel (via the communicating branch of the zygomatic n.) with it to innervate the lacrimal gland. *Visceral afferent* axons (gustatory fibers) for the anterior two-thirds of the tongue run in the lingual nerve and then chorda tympani. The gustatory fibers originate from pseudounipolar sensory neurons in the **geniculate ganglion**, which corresponds to a spinal sensory (dorsal root) ganglion. The chorda tympani also conveys the presynaptic *parasympathetic visceral efferent fibers* for the submandibular gland, sublingual gland, and small salivary glands in the anterior two-thirds of the tongue. These fibers also travel further with the lingual nerve (branch of CN V3) and synapse in the submandibular ganglion. Glandular postganglionic fibers are then distributed to the respective glands.

D Nerves of the petrous bone

Greater petrosal nerve	Branch of CN VII containing preganglionic parasympathetic fibers to the pterygopalatine ganglion (lacrimal gland, nasal glands)	Lesser petrosal nerve	Branch from CN IX containing preganglionic parasympathetic fibers to the otic ganglion (parotid gland, buccal and labial glands not shown here; see **E**, p. 131)
Deep petrosal nerve	Branch from the internal carotid plexus, containing postganglionic sympathetic fibers; it unites with the greater petrosal nerve to form the nerve of the pterygoid canal, then continues to the pterygopalatine ganglion and supplies the same territory as the greater petrosal nerve (see **C**)		

4.18 Cranial Nerves: Vestibulocochlear (CN VIII)

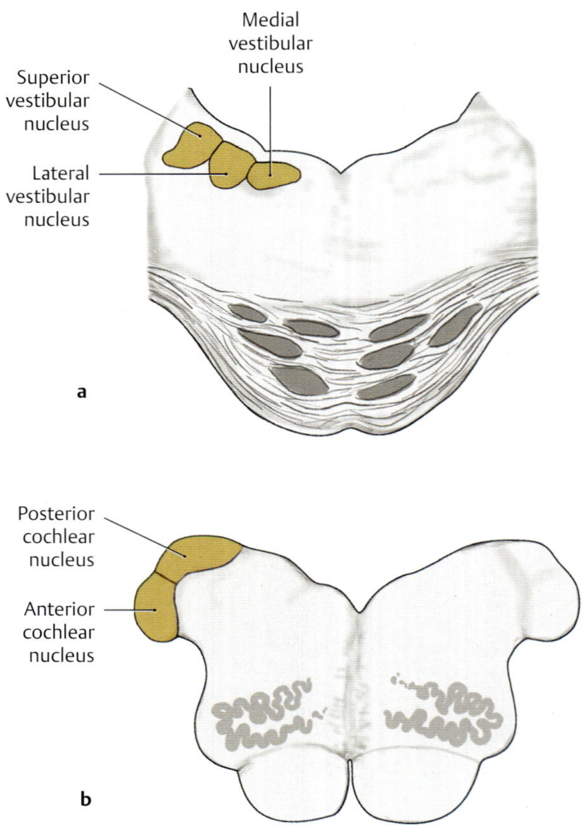

A Nuclei of the vestibulocochlear nerve (CN VIII)
Cross-sections through the upper medulla oblongata.

a Vestibular nuclei. Four nuclear complexes are distinguished:

- Superior vestibular nucleus (of Bechterew)
- Lateral vestibular nucleus (of Deiters)
- Medial vestibular nucleus (Schwalbe) and
- Inferior vestibular nucleus (of Roller)

Note: The inferior vestibular nucleus does not appear in a cross-section at this level (see the location of the cranial nerve nuclei in the brainstem, p. 356).
Most of the axons from the vestibular ganglion terminate in these four nuclei, but a smaller number pass directly through the inferior cerebellar peduncle into the cerebellum (see **Ea**). The vestibular nuclei appear as eminences on the floor of the rhomboid fossa (see **Eb**, p. 355). Their central connections are shown in **Ea**.

b Cochlear nuclei. Two nuclear complexes are distinguished:

- Anterior cochlear nucleus
- Posterior cochlear nucleus

Both nuclei are located lateral and posterior to the vestibular nuclei (see **Aa**, p. 356). Their central connections are shown in **Eb**.

B Overview of the vestibulocochlear nerve (CN VIII)

The vestibulocochlear nerve is a *special somatic afferent* (sensory) nerve that consists anatomically and functionally of two components:

- The *vestibular root* transmits impulses from the vestibular apparatus.
- The *cochlear root* transmits impulses from the auditory apparatus.

These roots are surrounded by a common connective tissue sheath. They pass from the inner ear through the internal acoustic meatus to the cerebellopontine angle, where they enter the brain.

Nuclei and distribution, *ganglia:*

- *Vestibular root:* The vestibular ganglion contains bipolar ganglion cells whose central processes pass to the four vestibular nuclei on the floor of the rhomboid fossa of the medulla oblongata. Their peripheral processes begin at the sensory cells of the semicircular canals, saccule, and utricle.
- *Cochlear root:* The spiral ganglion contains bipolar ganglion cells whose central processes pass to the two cochlear nuclei, which are lateral to the vestibular nuclei in the rhomboid fossa. Their peripheral processes begin at the hair cells of the organ of Corti.

Every thorough physical examination should include a rapid assessment of both nerve components (hearing and balance tests). A lesion of the vestibular root leads to dizziness, while a lesion of the cochlear root leads to hearing loss (ranging to deafness).

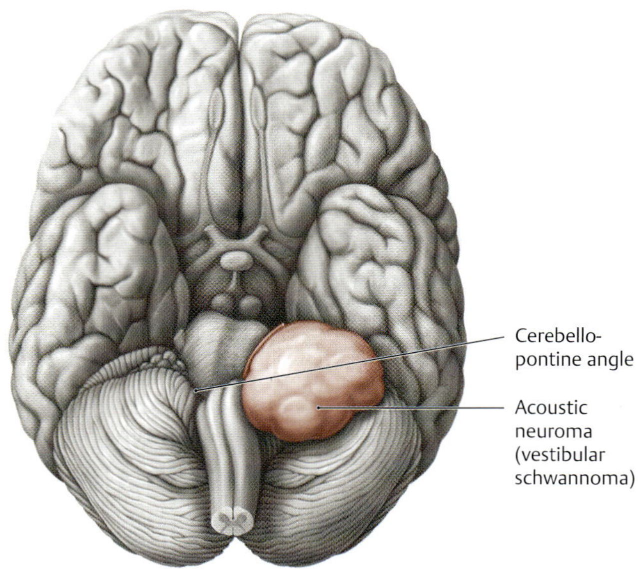

C Acoustic neuroma in the cerebellopontine angle
Acoustic neuromas (more accurately, vestibular schwannomas) are benign tumors of the cerebellopontine angle typically arising from the Schwann cells of the vestibular root of CN VIII. As they grow, they compress and displace the adjacent structures and cause slowly progressive hearing loss and gait ataxia. Large tumors can impair the egress of CSF from the fourth ventricle, causing hydrocephalus and symptomatic intracranial hypertension (vomiting, impairment of consciousness).

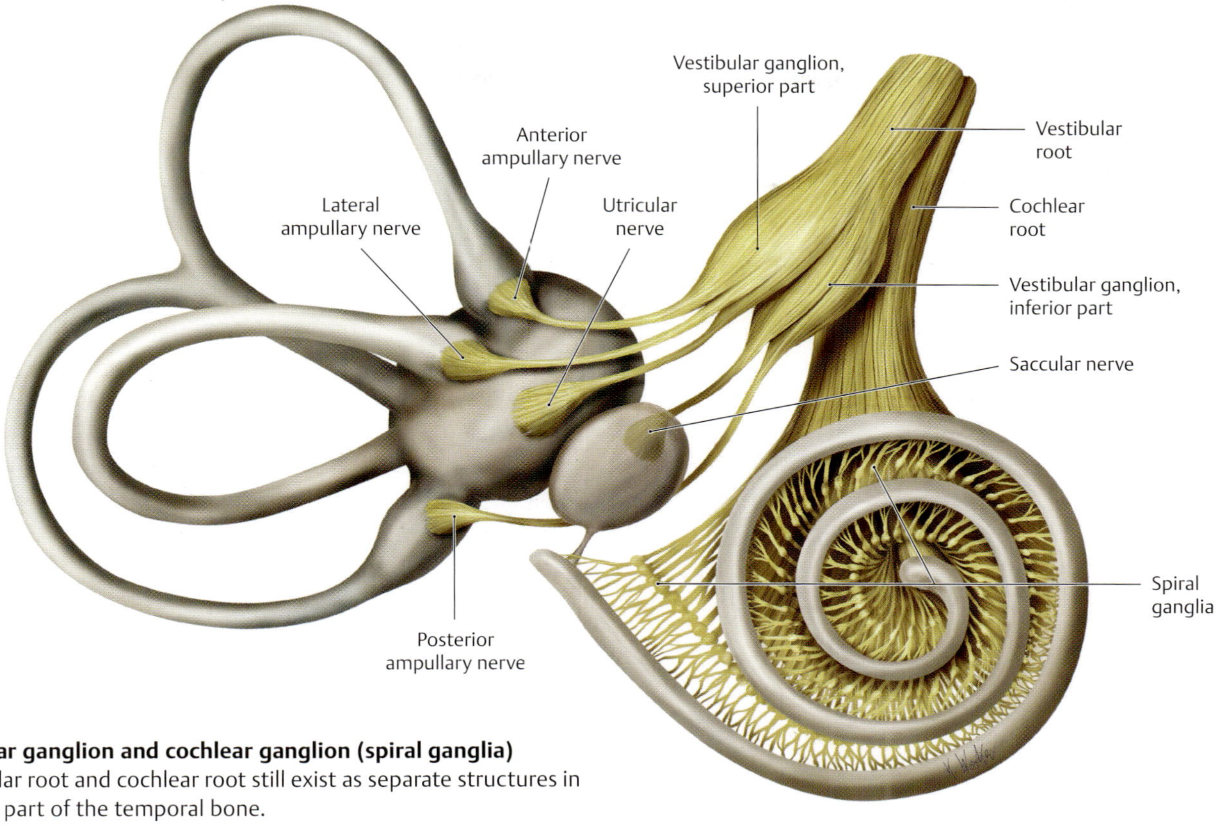

D Vestibular ganglion and cochlear ganglion (spiral ganglia)
The vestibular root and cochlear root still exist as separate structures in the petrous part of the temporal bone.

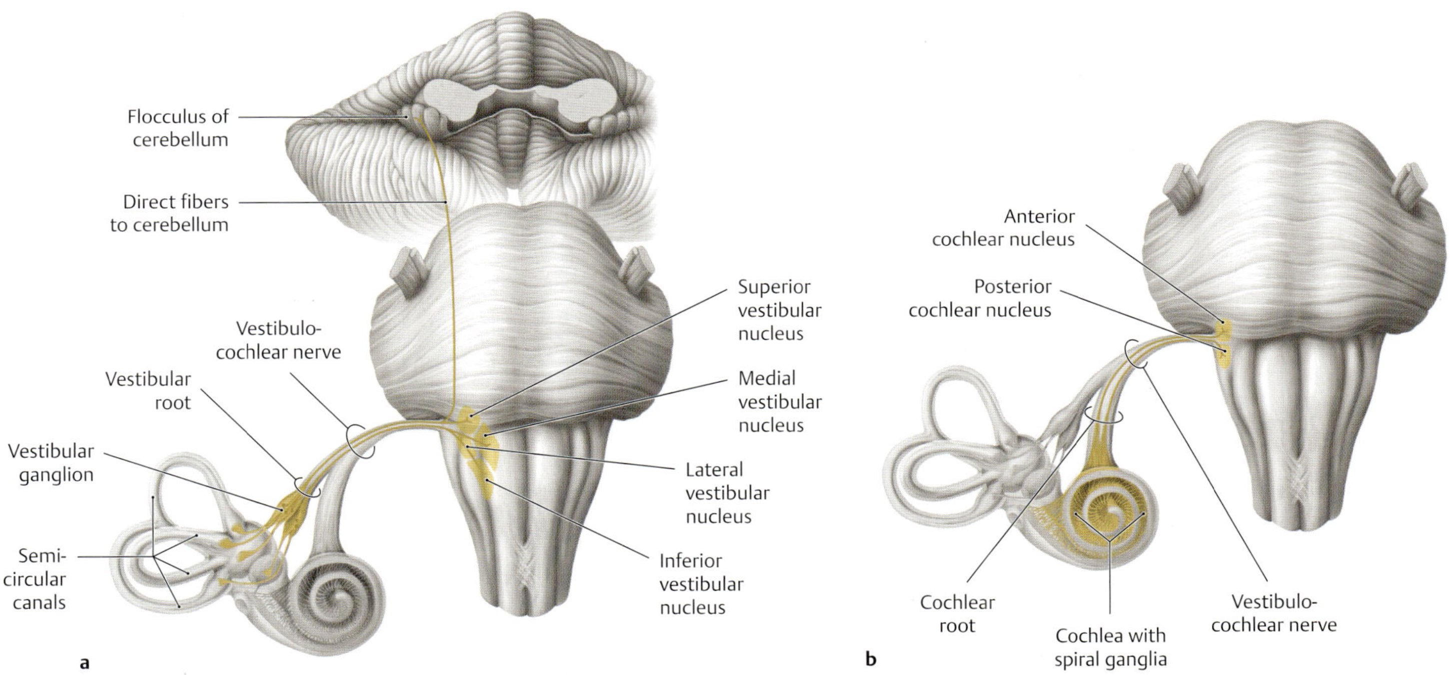

E Nuclei of the vestibulocochlear nerve in the brainstem
Anterior view of the medulla oblongata and pons. The inner ear and its connections with the nuclei are shown schematically.

a Vestibular part: The vestibular ganglion contains bipolar sensory cells whose peripheral processes pass to the semicircular canals, saccule, and utricle. Their axons travel as the vestibular root to the four vestibular nuclei on the floor of the rhomboid fossa (further connections are shown on p. 486). The vestibular organ processes information concerning orientation in space. An acute lesion of the vestibular organ is manifested clinically by dizziness (vertigo).

b Cochlear part: The spiral ganglia form a band of nerve cells that follows the course of the bony core of the cochlea. It contains bipolar sensory cells whose peripheral processes pass to the hair cells of the organ of Corti. Their central processes unite on the floor of the internal auditory canal to form the cochlear root and are distributed to the two nuclei that are lateral and posterior to the vestibular nuclei. Other connections of the nuclei are shown on p. 484.

4.19 Cranial Nerves: Glossopharyngeal (CN IX)

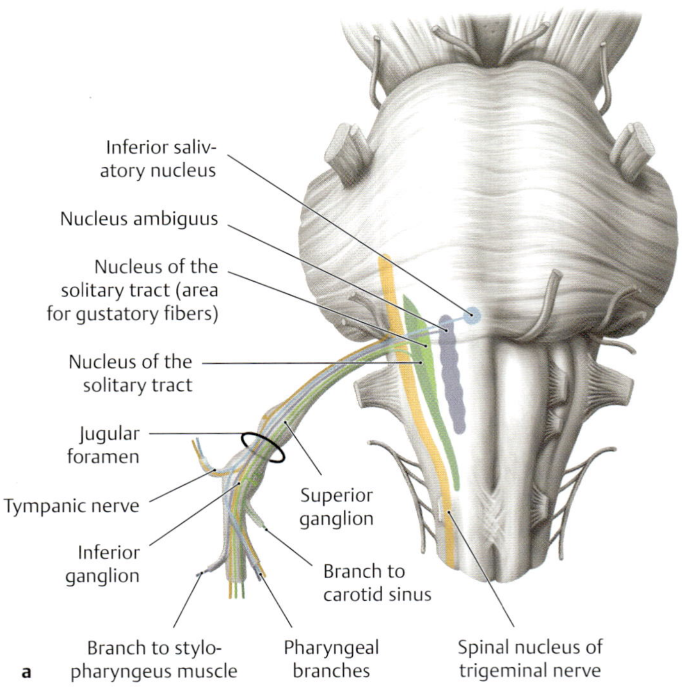

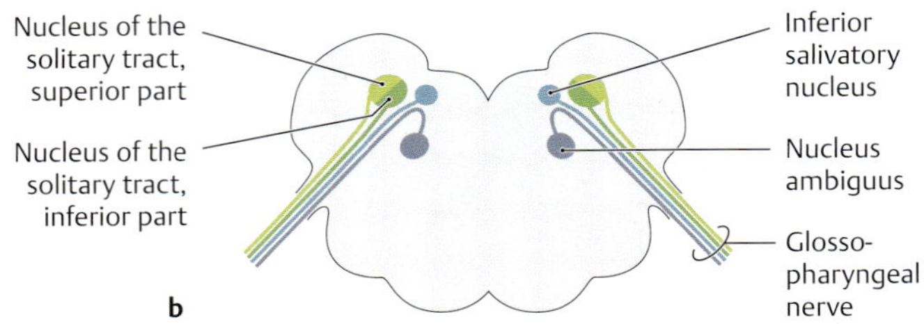

A Nuclei of the glossopharyngeal nerve

a Medulla oblongata, anterior view. **b** Cross-sections through the medulla oblongata at the level of emergence of the glossopharyngeal nerve. For clarity, the nuclei of the trigeminal nerve are not shown (see **B** for further details on the nuclei).

B Overview of the glossopharyngeal nerve (CN IX)

The glossopharyngeal nerve contains *general* and *special visceral efferent* fibers in addition to *visceral afferent* and *somatic afferent fibers*.

Sites of emergence: The glossopharyngeal nerve emerges from the medulla oblongata and leaves the cranial cavity through the jugular foramen.

Nuclei and distribution, *ganglia:*

- *Special visceral efferent (branchial):* The nucleus ambiguus sends its axons to the constrictor muscles of the pharynx (= pharyngeal branches, join with the vagus nerve to form the pharyngeal plexus) and to the stylopharyngeus, palatopharyngeus, salpingopharyngeus, and palatoglossus (see **C**);
- *General visceral efferent (parasympathetic):* The inferior salivatory nucleus sends parasympathetic presynaptic fibers to the otic ganglion. Postsynaptic axons from the otic ganglion are distributed to the parotid gland and to the buccal and labial glands (see **a** and **E**);
- *Somatic afferent:* Central processes of pseudounipolar sensory ganglion cells located in the intracranial superior ganglion or *extracranial inferior ganglion* of the glossopharyngeal nerve terminate in the spinal nucleus of the trigeminal nerve. The peripheral processes of these cells arise from
  - the posterior third of the tongue, soft palate, pharyngeal mucosa, and tonsils (afferent fibers for the gag reflex), see **b** and **c**
  - the mucosa of the tympanic cavity and eustachian tube (tympanic plexus), see **d**
  - the skin of the external ear and auditory canal (blends with the territory supplied by the vagus nerve) and the internal surface of the tympanic membrane (part of the tympanic plexus).
- *Special visceral afferent:* Central processes of pseudounipolar ganglion cells from the inferior ganglion terminate in the superior part of the nucleus of the solitary tract. Their peripheral processes originate in the posterior third of the tongue (gustatory fibers, see **e**).
- *Visceral efferent:* Sensory fibers from the following receptors terminate in the inferior part of the nucleus of the solitary tract:
  - Chemoreceptors in the carotid body
  - Pressure receptors in the carotid sinus (see **f**).

Developmentally, the glossopharyngeal nerve is the nerve of the third branchial arch.

Isolated *lesions* of the glossopharyngeal nerve are rare. Lesions of this nerve are usually accompanied by lesions of CN X and XI (vagus nerve and accessory nerve) because all three nerves emerge jointly from the jugular foramen and are all susceptible to injury in basal skull fractures.

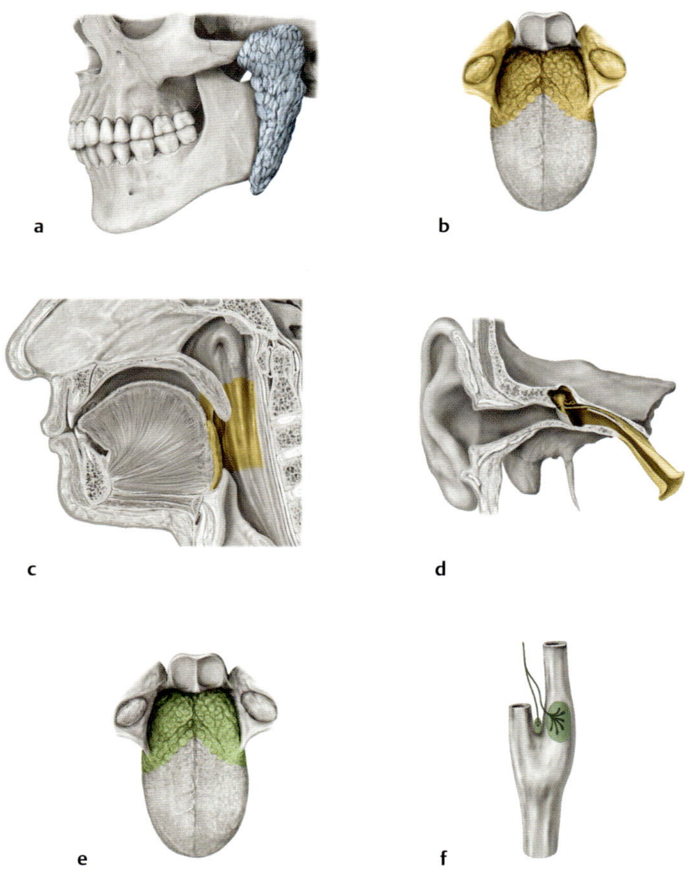

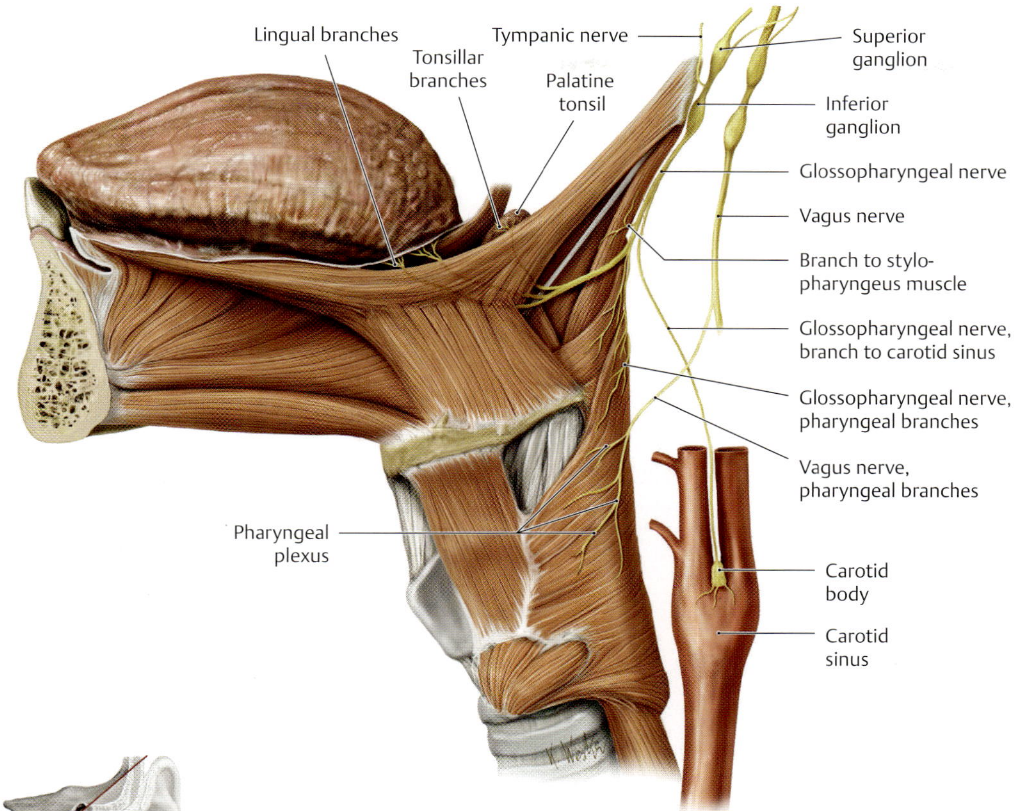

C Branches of the glosso-pharyngeal nerve beyond the skull base
Left lateral view.
Note the close relationship of the glossopharyngeal nerve to the vagus nerve (CN X). The carotid sinus is supplied by both nerves. The most important branches of CN IX seen in the diagram are as follows:

- Pharyngeal branches: three or four branches to the pharyngeal plexus.
- Branch to the stylopharyngeus muscle.
- Branch to the carotid sinus: supplies the carotid sinus and carotid body.
- Tonsillar branches: to the mucosa of the palatine tonsil and its surroundings.
- Lingual branches: somato-sensory and gustatory fibers for the posterior third of the tongue.

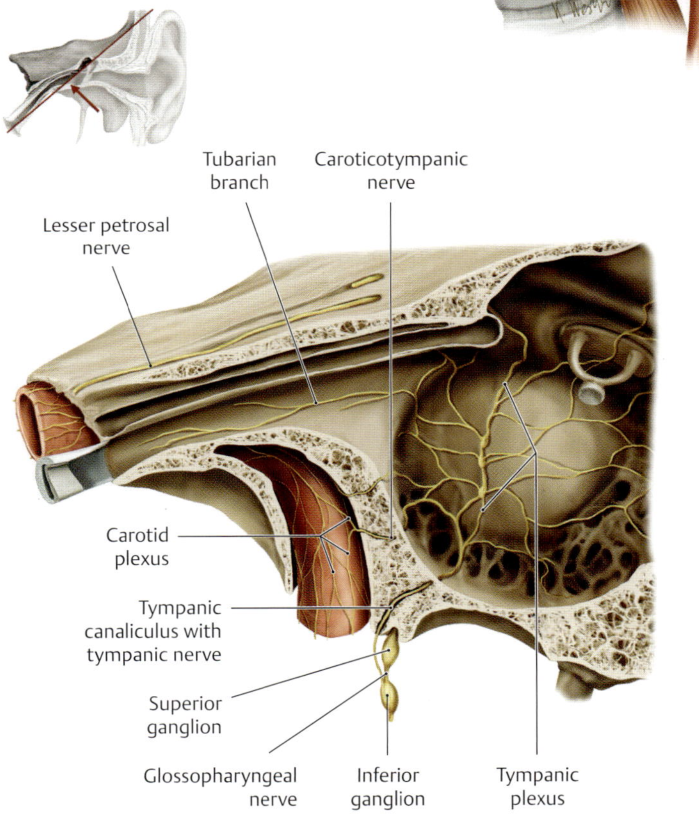

D Branches of the glossopharyngeal nerve in the tympanic cavity
Left petrous portion of the temporal bone, frontal view. The tympanic nerve, which passes through the tympanic canaliculus into the tympanic cavity, is the first branch of the glossopharyngeal nerve. It contains visceral efferent (presynaptic parasympathetic) fibers for the otic ganglion and somatic afferent fibers for the tympanic cavity and pharyngotympanic (eustachian) tube. It joins with sympathetic fibers from the carotid plexus (via the caroticotympanic nerve) to form the tympanic plexus. The parasympathetic fibers travel as the lesser petrosal nerve to the otic ganglion (see p. 237), which provides parasympathetic innervation to the parotid gland.

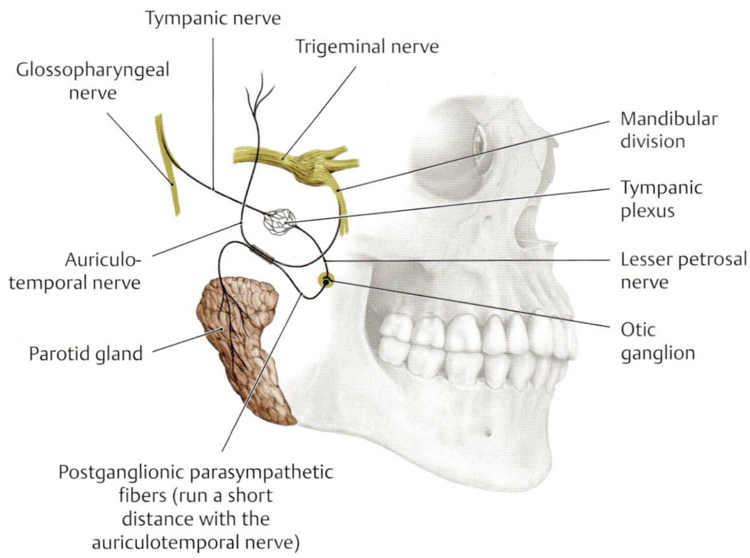

E Visceral efferent (parasympathetic) fibers of the glossopharyngeal nerve
The presynaptic parasympathetic fibers from the inferior salivatory nucleus leave the medulla oblongata with the glossopharyngeal nerve and branch off as the tympanic nerve immediately after emerging from the base of the skull. Within the tympanic cavity, the tympanic n. bifurcates to form the tympanic plexus (see **B**, p. 146), which is joined by postganglionic, sympathetic fibers from the carotid plexus surrounding the middle meningeal a. (not shown here). The tympanic plexus gives rise to the lesser petrosal nerve, which leaves the petrous bone through the hiatus of the canal for the lesser petrosal nerve and enters the middle cranial fossa. Located below the dura, it passes through the spheno-petrosal fissure to the otic ganglion. Its fibers enter the auriculotemporal nerve, pass to the facial nerve, and its autonomic fibers are distributed to the parotid gland via facial nerve branches.

4.20 Cranial Nerves: Vagus (CN X)

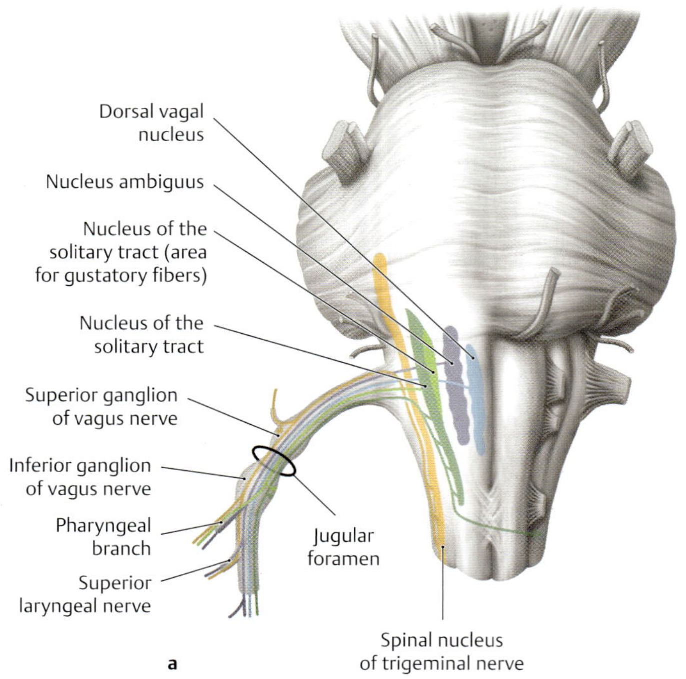

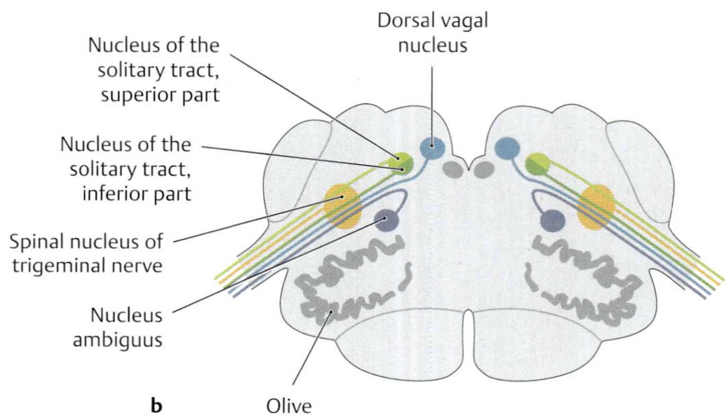

A Nuclei of the vagus nerve

a Medulla oblongata, anterior view showing the site of emergence of the vagus nerve.

b Cross-section through the medulla oblongata at the level of the superior olive. Note the various nuclei of the vagus nerve and their functions.

The *nucleus ambiguus* contains the *somatic efferent* (branchial) fibers for the superior and inferior laryngeal nerves. It has a somatotopic organization (i.e., the neurons for the *superior* laryngeal nerve are above, and those for the *inferior* laryngeal nerve are below). The *dorsal nucleus of the vagus nerve* is located on the floor of the rhomboid fossa and contains presynaptic, parasympathetic visceral efferent neurons. The somatic afferent fibers whose pseudounipolar ganglion cells are located in the superior (jugular) ganglion of the vagus nerve terminate in the *spinal nucleus of the trigeminal nerve*. They use the vagus nerve only as a means of conveyance. The central processes of the pseudounipolar ganglion cells from the inferior (nodose) ganglion are gustatory fibers and visceral afferent fibers. They terminate in the *nucleus of the solitary tract*.

B Overview of the vagus nerve (CN X)

The vagus nerve contains general and special visceral efferent fibers as well as visceral afferent and somatic afferent fibers. It has the most extensive distribution of all the cranial nerves (vagus = "vagabond") and consists of cranial, cervical, thoracic, and abdominal parts. This unit deals mainly with the vagus nerve in the head and neck (its thoracic and abdominal parts are described in the volume on the Internal Organs).

Site of emergence: The vagus nerve emerges from the medulla oblongata and leaves the cranial cavity through the jugular foramen.

Nuclei and distribution, *ganglia:*

- *Special visceral efferent (branchial):* Efferent fibers from the nucleus ambiguus supply the following muscles:
  - Pharyngeal muscles (pharyngeal branch, joins with glossopharyngeal nerve to form the pharyngeal plexus) and muscles of the soft palate (levator veli palatini, muscle of the uvula).
  - All laryngeal muscles: The superior laryngeal nerve supplies the cricothyroid, while the inferior laryngeal nerve supplies the other laryngeal muscles (the origin of the fibers is described on p. 134);
- *General visceral efferent (parasympathetic, see* **Dg***):* Parasympathetic presynaptic efferents from the dorsal vagal nucleus nerve synapse in prevertebral or intramural ganglia with postsynaptic fibers to supply smooth muscle and glands of
  - thoracic viscera and
  - abdominal viscera as far as the left colic flexure (Cannon-Böhm point).
- *Somatic afferent:* Central processes of pseudounipolar ganglion cells located in the superior (jugular) ganglion of the vagus nerve terminate in the spinal nucleus of the trigeminal nerve. The peripheral fibers originate from
  - the dura in the posterior cranial fossa (meningeal branch, see **Df**),
  - the external auditory canal (auricular branch, see **Db**). The auricular branch is the only cutaneous branch of the vagus nerve.
- *Special visceral afferent:* Central processes of pseudounipolar ganglion cells from the inferior nodose ganglion terminate in the superior part of the nucleus of the solitary tract. Their peripheral processes supply the taste buds on the epiglottis (see **Dd**).
- *General visceral afferent:* The cell bodies of these afferents are also located in the inferior ganglion. Their central processes terminate in the inferior part of the nucleus of the solitary tract. Their peripheral processes supply the following areas:
  - Mucosa of the lower pharynx at its junction with the esophagus (see **Da**)
  - Laryngeal mucosa above (superior laryngeal nerve) and below (inferior laryngeal nerve) the glottic aperture (see **Da**)
  - Pressure receptors in the aortic arch (see **De**)
  - Chemoreceptors in the para-aortic body (see **De**)
  - Thoracic and abdominal viscera (see **Dg**)

Developmentally, the vagus nerve is the nerve of the fourth and sixth branchial arches.

A structure of major **clinical** importance is the *recurrent laryngeal nerve*, which supplies visceromotor innervation to the only muscle that abducts the vocal cords, the posterior cricoarytenoid. Unilateral destruction of this nerve leads to hoarseness, and bilateral destruction leads to respiratory distress (dyspnea).

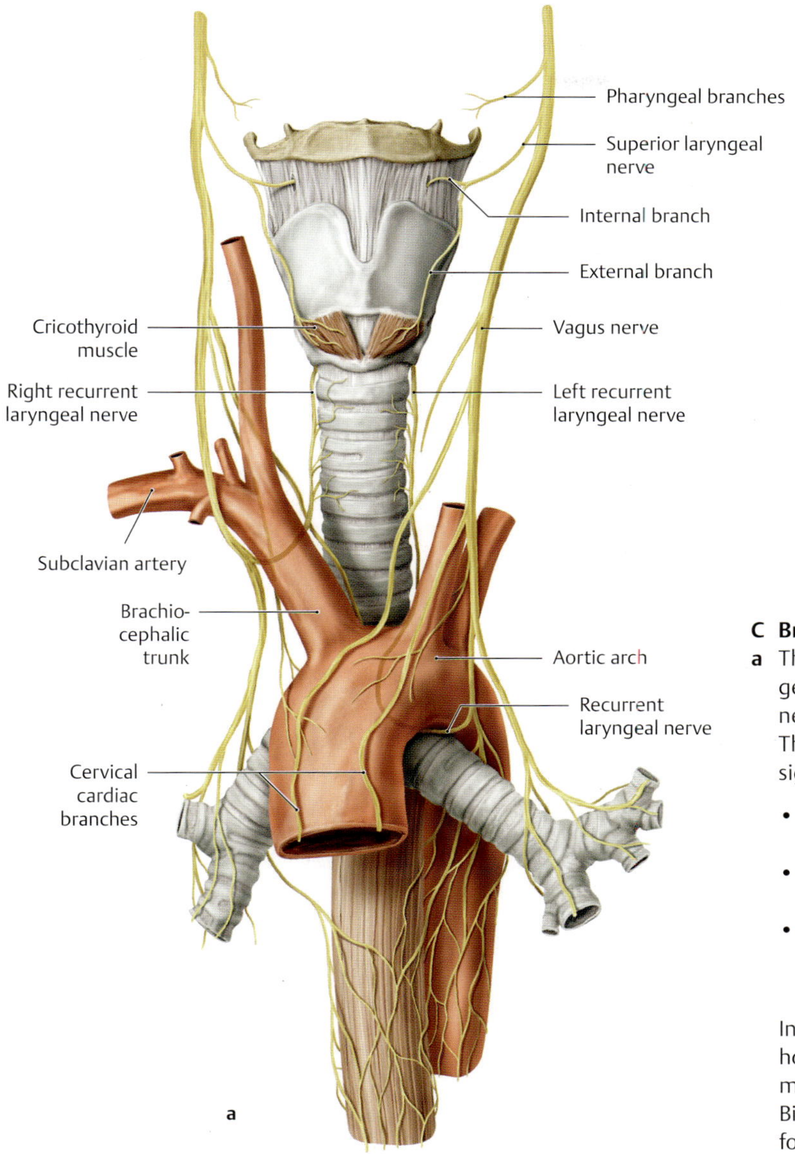

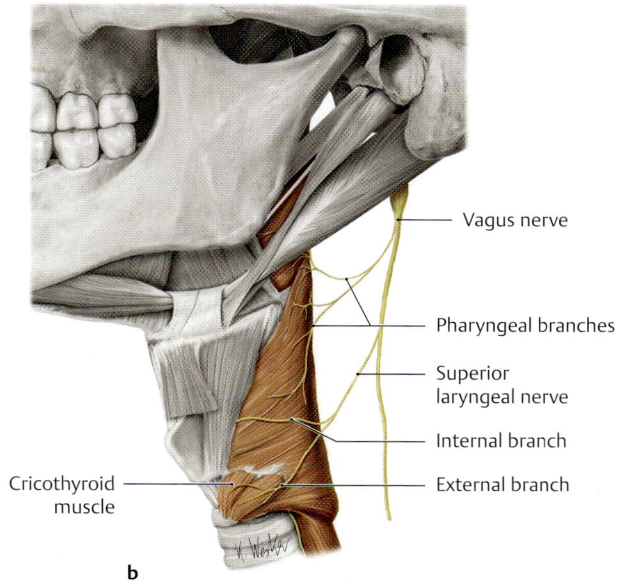

C Branches of the vagus nerve (CN X) in the neck

a The vagus nerve gives off four sets of branches in the neck: pharyngeal branches, the superior laryngeal nerve, the recurrent laryngeal nerve, and the cervical cardiac branches.
The course of the recurrent laryngeal n. gives them particular clinical significance. They get damaged as a result of the following:

- Aortic aneurysm, as the left recurrent laryngeal n. winds around the aortic arch on the left side
- Lymph node metastases of bronchial carcinoma, as the left recurrent laryngeal n. passes close to the left main bronchus
- Thyroid operations, as both right and left recurrent larynegal nn. pass close to the dorsolateral aspects of the thyroid gland on either side

In any case, even unilateral damage to a recurrent laryngeal n. leads to hoarseness given that it supplies visceromotor innervation to the only muscle that abducts the vocal folds, the posterior cricoarytenoid m. Bilateral nerve damage results in breathing difficulties since the vocal folds don't open.

b The superior laryngeal n. divides into an internal larygeal n. that supplies sensory immervation to the mucosa above the vocal fold, and an external laryngeal n. that is motor to only the cricrothyroid m.

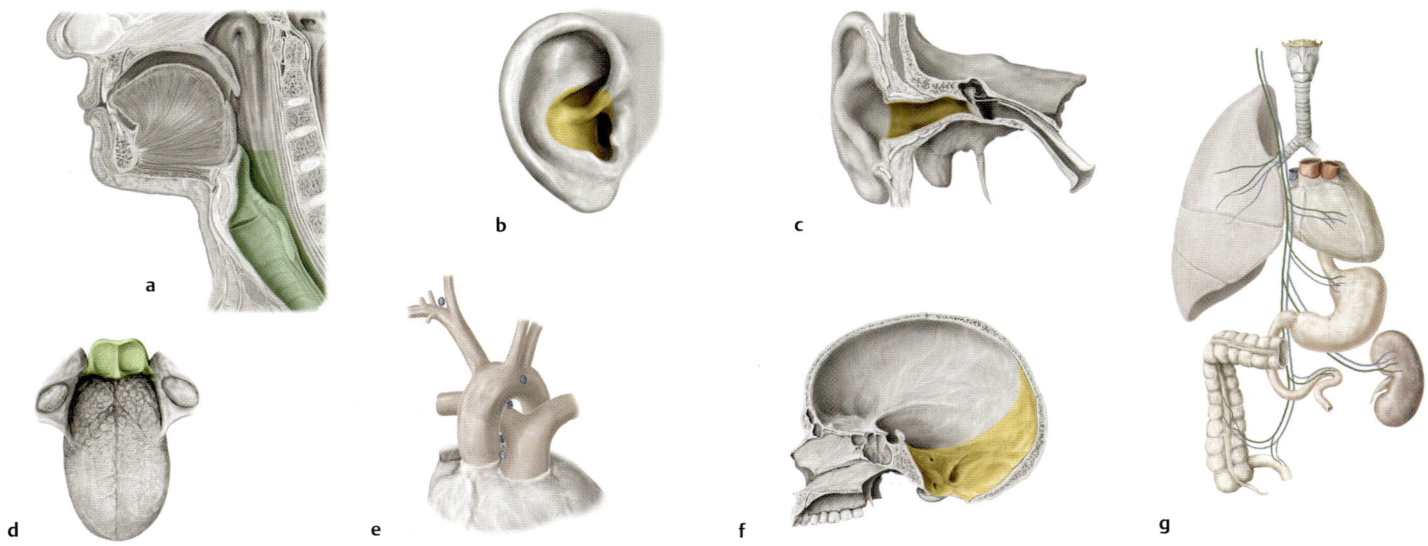

D Visceral and sensory distribution of the vagus nerve (CN X)

4.21 Cranial Nerves: Accessory (CN XI) and Hypoglossal (CN XII)

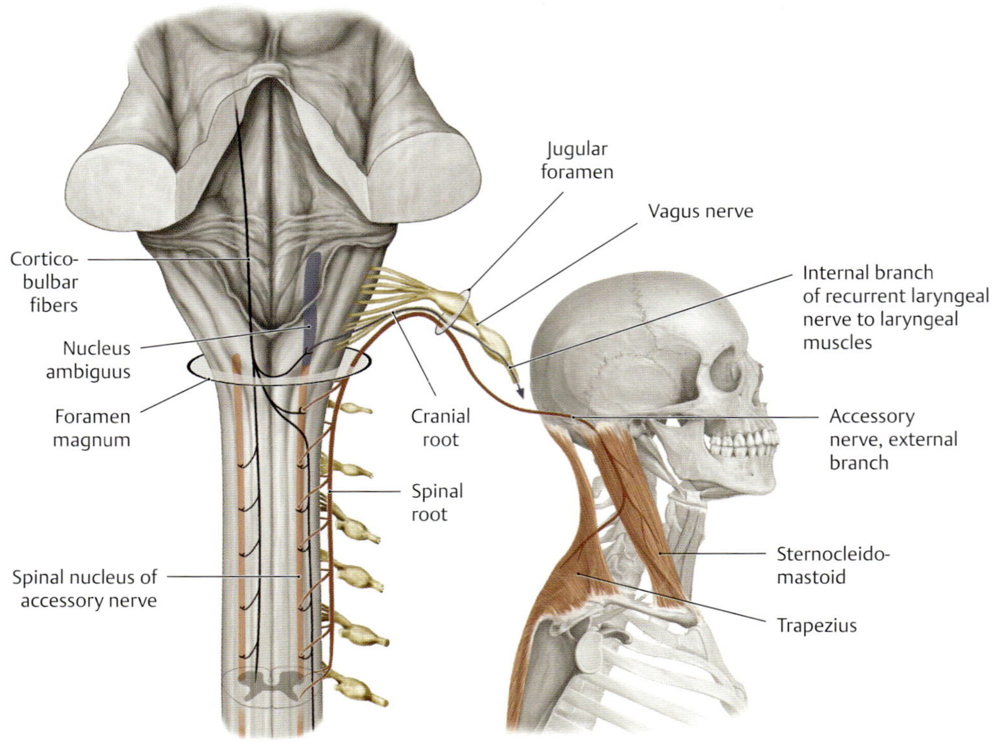

A Nucleus and course of the accessory nerve
Posterior view of the brainstem (with the cerebellum removed). For didactic reasons, the muscles are displayed from the right side (see **C** for further details).

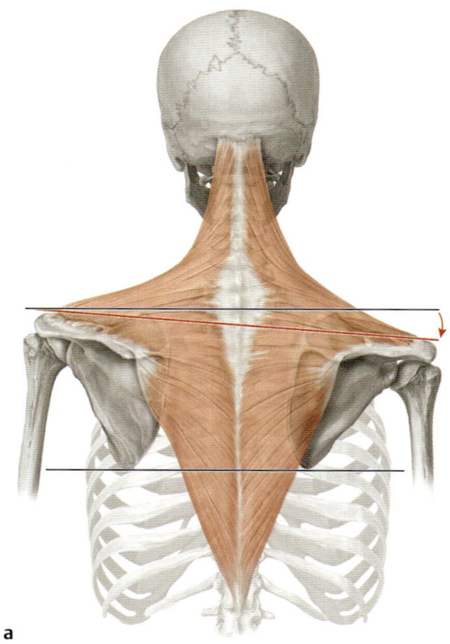
a

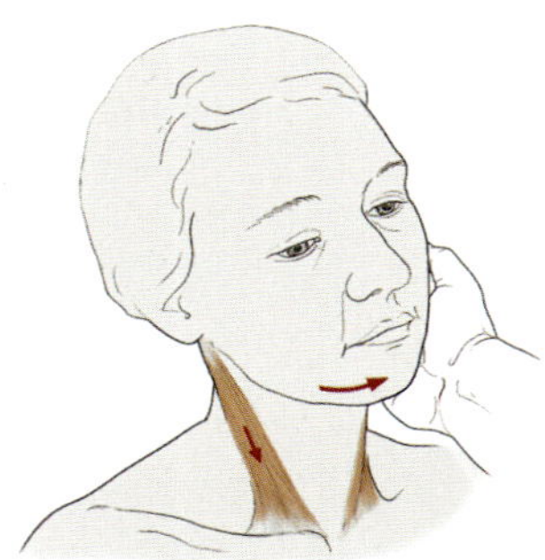
b

B Lesion of the accessory nerve (on the right side)
a Posterior view. Paralysis of the trapezius muscle causes drooping of the shoulder on the affected side.
b Right anterolateral view. With paralysis of the sternocleidomastoid muscle, it is difficult for the patient to turn the head to the opposite side against a resistance.

C Overview of the accessory nerve (CN XI)

The accessory nerve is considered by some authors to be an *independent* part of the vagus nerve (CN X). It contains both visceral and somatic efferent fibers, and has one cranial and one spinal root.

Sites of emergence: The spinal root emerges from the spinal cord, passes superiorly, and enters the skull through the *foramen magnum*, where it joins with the cranial root from the medulla oblongata (which is largely considered now to be in fact a component of CN X). Both roots then leave the skull together through the *jugular foramen*. While still within the jugular foramen, fibers from the cranial root pass to the vagus nerve (internal branch). The spinal portion descends to the nuchal region as the external branch of the accessory nerve.

Nuclei and distribution:

- *Cranial root:* The special visceral efferent fibers of the accessory n. arise from the caudal part of the *Nucleus ambiguus* and form the radix cranialis of the accessory n. which pass to the vagus n. to be distributed by the recurrent laryngeal n. where they innervate all the laryngeal muscles except the cricothyroid. It is largely accepted now to be part of CN X.
- *Spinal root:* The spinal nucleus of the accessory nerve forms a narrow column of cells in the anterior horn of the spinal cord at the level of C2–C5/6. After emerging from the spinal cord, its somatic efferent fibers form the external branch of the accessory nerve, which supplies the trapezius and sternocleidomastoid muscles.

Effects of accessory nerve injury: A unilateral lesion results in the following deficits:

- *Trapezius paralysis:* characterized by drooping of the shoulder and difficulty raising the arm above the horizontal (the trapezius supports the serratus anterior in elevating the arm past 90°). The part of the accessory nerve that supplies the trapezius is vulnerable during operations in the neck (e.g., lymph node biopsies). Since the lower portion of the muscle is also innervated by the C2–4 segments, damage to the accessory n. does not result in complete loss of muscle control.
- *Sternocleidomastoid m.:* torticollis, damage to the accessory n. results in flaccid paralysis. With bilateral lesions it is difficult for patients to hold their head in an upright position.

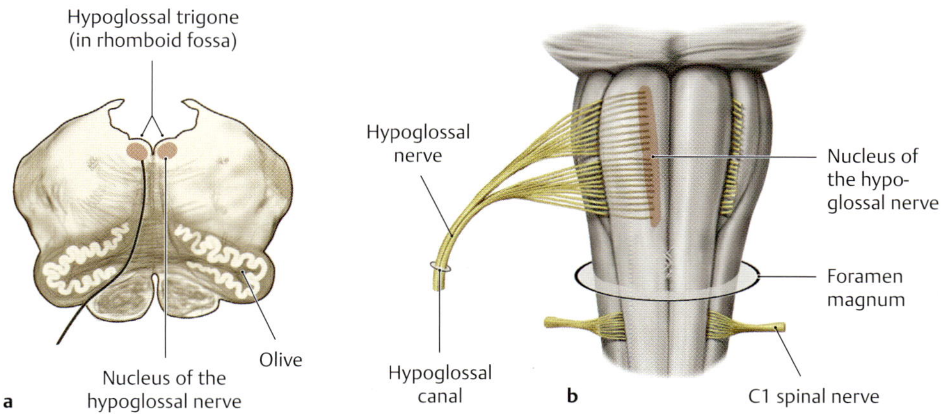

D Nuclei of the hypoglossal nerve

a Cross-section through the medulla oblongata at the level of the olive. This section passes through the nucleus of the hypoglossal nerve. It can be seen that the nucleus lies just beneath the rhomboid fossa and raises the floor of the fossa to form the hypoglossal trigone. Because each nucleus is close to the midline, it is common for more extensive lesions to involve the nuclei on both sides, producing the clinical manifestations of a bilateral nuclear lesion.

b Anterior view. The neurons contained in this nuclear column correspond to the alpha motor neurons of the spinal cord.

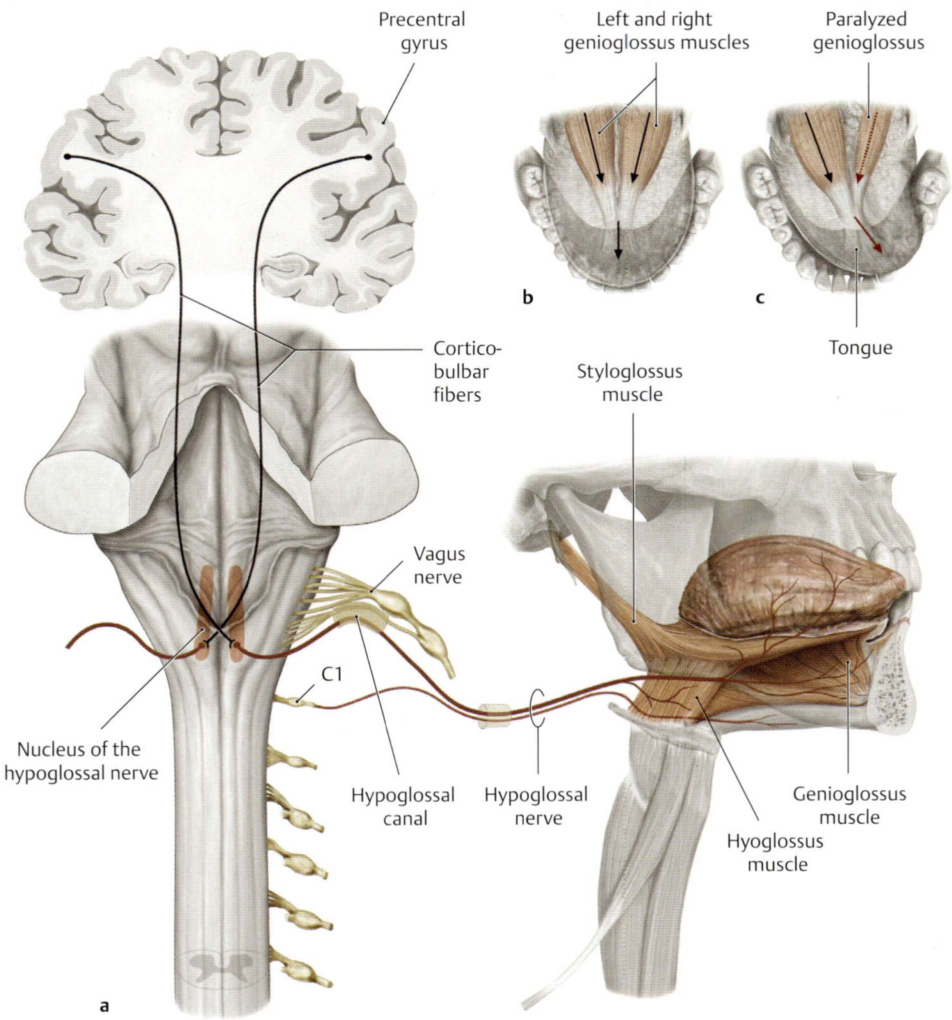

E Overview of the hypoglossal nerve (CN XII)

The hypoglossal nerve is a purely somatic efferent nerve that supplies the musculature of the tongue.

Nucleus and site of emergence: The nucleus of the hypoglossal nerve is located in the floor of the rhomboid fossa. Its somatic efferent fibers emerge from the medulla oblongata, leaving the cranial cavity through the hypoglossal canal and descending lateral to the vagus nerve. The hypoglossal nerve enters the root of the tongue above the hyoid bone and distributes its fibers there.

Distribution: The hypoglossal nerve supplies all intrinsic and extrinsic muscles of the tongue (except for the palatoglossus, CN X). It can be considered a "zeroth" ventral root rather than a true cranial nerve. The ventral fibers of C1 and C2 travel with the hypoglossal nerve but leave it again after a short distance to form the superior root of the ansa cervicalis.

Effects of hypoglossal nerve injury:

- Central hypoglossal paralysis (supranuclear): The tongue deviates away from the side of the lesion, since central fibers cross. Often this manifestation is weak and transient since the hypoglossal nuclei are in general under the influence of both contralateral and ipsilateral cerebral hemispheres.
- Nuclear or peripheral paralysis: The tongue deviates toward the affected side due to a preponderance of muscular action on the healthy side.

F Distribution of the hypoglossal nerve

a Central and peripheral course
b Function of the genioglossus muscle
c Deviation of the tongue toward the paralyzed side

The nucleus of the hypoglossal nerve is innervated (upper motor neurons) by cortical neurons from the contralateral side. With a unilateral *nuclear or peripheral* lesion of the hypoglossal nerve, the tongue deviates toward the side of the lesion when protruded because of the relative dominance of the healthy genioglossus muscle (**c**). When both nuclei are injured, the tongue cannot be protruded (flaccid paralysis).

4.22 Neurovascular Pathways through the Base of the Skull, Synopsis

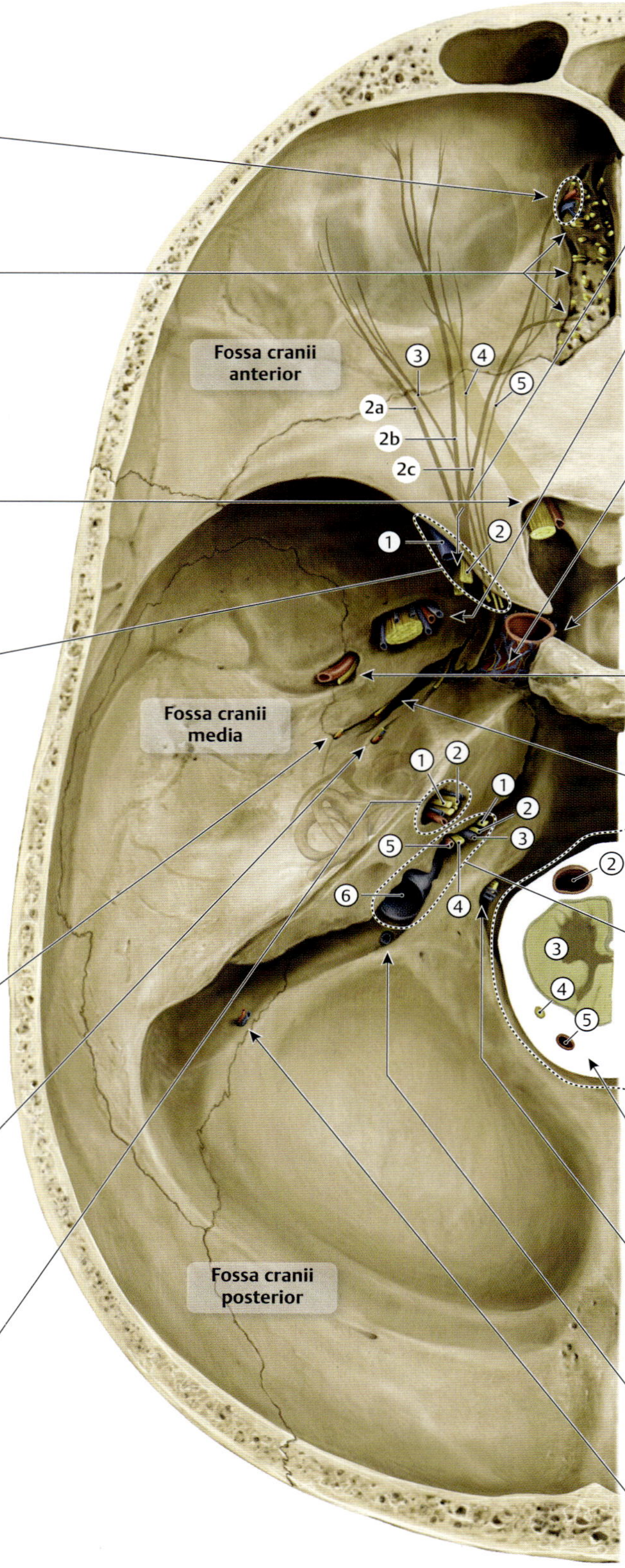

Openings between internal surface of cranial base and other spaces

Anterior cranial fossa

Anterior ethmoidal foramen
- Anterior ethmoidal nerve, artery and vein

→ *Orbit*

Cribriform plate
- Olfactory nerves (I)
- Anterior ethmoidal nerve, artery and vein

→ *Nasal cavity*

Middle cranial fossa

Optic canal
- Optic nerve (II)
- Ophthalmic artery

→ *Orbit*

Superior orbital fissure

① Superior ophthalmic vein
② Ophthalmic nerve (V_1)
  2a Lacrimal nerve
  2b Frontal nerve
  2c Nasociliary nerve
③ Abducens nerve (VI)
④ Oculomotor nerve (III)
⑤ Trochlear nerve (IV)

→ *Orbit*

Hiatus for lesser petrosal nerve
- Greater petrosal nerve (parasympathetic, from IX)
- Superior tympanic artery

→ *Tympanic cavity*

Hiatus for greater petrosal nerve
- Greater petrosal nerve (parasympathetic, from VII)
- Stylomastoid vein and artery

→ *Facial canal*

Posterior cranial fossa

Porus and internal acoustic meatus
- Labyrinthine artery and veins

① Facial nerve (with intermediate nerve) (VII)
② Vestibulocochlear nerve (V_3)

→ *Facial canal, inner ear*

Openings between internal and external surface of cranial base

Middle cranial fossa

Foramen rotundum
- Maxillary nerve (V_2)

Foramen ovale
- Mandibular nerve (V_3)
- Pterygoid meningeal artery
- Venous plexus of foramen ovale

Carotid canal
- Internal carotid artery
- Internal carotid plexus (sympathetic)
- Internal carotid venous plexus

Foramen lacerum

(covered by internal carotid artery)
- Deep petrosal nerve
- Greater petrosal nerve (parasympathetic, from VII)

Foramen spinosum
- Middle meningeal artery
- Meningeal branch of mandibular nerve (V_3)

Petrosphenoidal fissure
- Lesser petrosal nerve (parasympathetic, from IX)

Posterior cranial fossa

Jugular foramen

① Glossopharyngeal nerve (IX)
② Vagus nerve (X)
③ Inferior petrosal sinus
④ Accessory nerve (XI)
⑤ Posterior meningeal artery
⑥ Internal jugular vein

Foramen magnum

See right-hand side

Hypoglossal canal
- Hypoglossal nerve (XII)
- Venous plexus of hypoglossal canal

Condylar canal
- Condylar emissary vein (inconstant)

Mastoid foramen
- Mastoid emissary vein
- Mastoid branch of occipital artery

Openings between external and internal surface of cranial base

Foramen rotundum

(Located in the pterygopalatine fossa and not visible here)

- Maxillary nerve (V_2)

Foramen ovale

- Mandibular nerve (V_3)
- Pterygomeningeal artery
- Venous plexus of foramen ovale

Foramen spinosum

- Middle meningeal artery
- Meningeal branch of mandibular nerve (V_3)

Sphenopetrosal fissure

- Lesser petrosal nerve (parasympathetic, from IX)
- Chorda tympani (parasympathetic and gustatory, from VII)

Foramen lacerum

- Deep petrosal nerve (sympathetic)
- Greater petrosal nerve (parasympathetic and gustatory, from VII)

Carotid canal

- Internal carotid artery
- Internal carotid plexus (sympathetic)
- Internal carotid venous plexus

Hypoglossal canal

- Hypoglossal nerve (XII)
- Venous plexus of hypoglossal canal

Foramen magnum

① Anterior spinal artery
② Vertebral arteries
③ Spinal cord
④ Spinal root of accessory nerve (XI)
⑤ Posterior spinal arteries
⑥ Spinal vein

Condylar canal

- Condylar emissary vein (inconstant)

Jugular foramen

① Glossopharyngeal nerve (IX)
② Vagus nerve (X)
③ Inferior petrosal sinus
④ Posterior meningeal artery
⑤ Accessory nerve (XI)
⑥ Internal jugular vein

Mastoid foramen

- Mastoid emissary vein
- Mastoid branch of the occipital artery

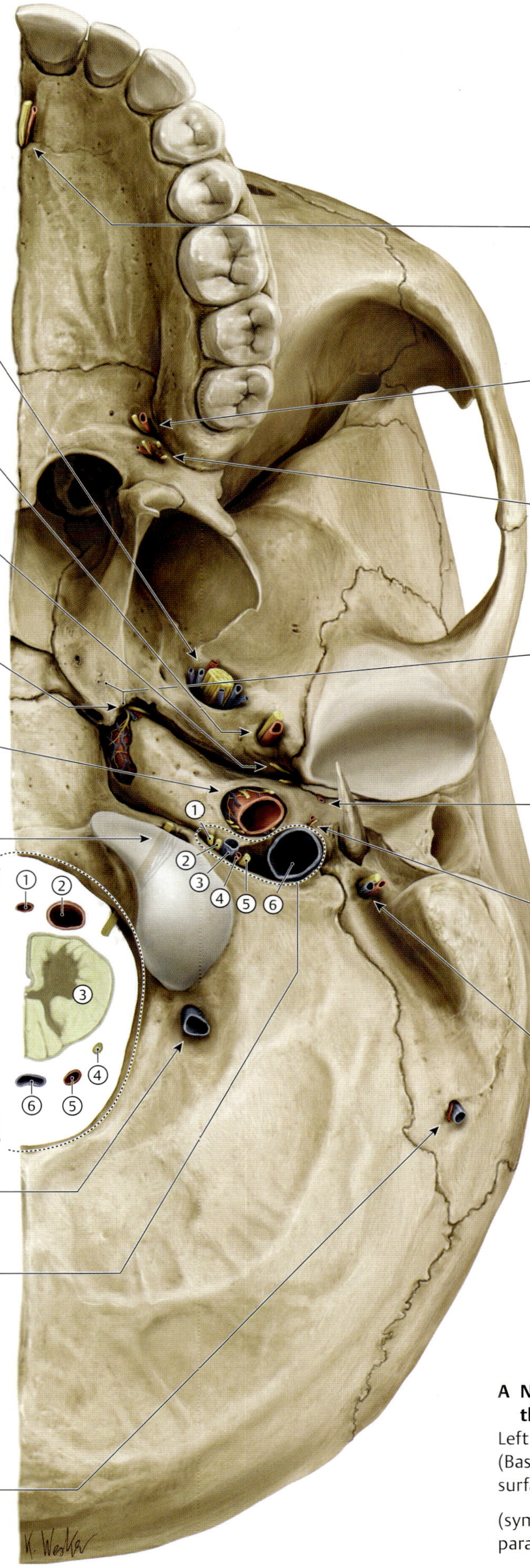

Openings between internal surface of cranial base and other spaces

Incisive fossa with incisive foramen

- Nasopalatine nerve (from V_2)
- Nasopalatine artery

→ *Nasal cavity*

Greater palatine foramen

- Greater palatine nerve
- Greater palatine artery

→ *Pterygopalatine fossa*

Lesser palatine foramen

- Lesser palatine nerves
- Lesser palatine artery

→ *Pterygopalatine fossa*

Pterygoid fossa

- Greater petrosal nerve (parasympathetic, from VII)
- Deep petrosal nerve (sympathetic)
- Artery and vein of pterygoid canal

→ *Pterygopalatine fossa*

Petrotympanic fissure

- Anterior tympanic artery

→ *Tympanic cavity*

Tympanic canaliculus

- Tympanic nerve (parasympathetic and sensory, from IX)
- Inferior tympanic artery

→ *Tympanic cavity*

Stylomastoid foramen

- Facial nerve (VII)
- Stylomastoid artery and vein

→ *Facial canal*

A Neurovascular structures passing through the base of the skull

Left side Internal surface of cranial base (Basis cranii interna); right side external surface of cranial base.

(symp. = sympathetic, parasymp. = parasympathetic)

4.23 Overview of the Nervous System in the Neck and the Distribution of Spinal Nerve Branches

A Overview of the nervous system in the neck

The following structures of the peripheral nervous system are present in the neck: spinal nerves, cranial nerves, and nerves of the autonomic nervous system. The table below reviews the most important structures, following the sequence in which they are discussed in the next sections.

The spinal nerves that supply the neck arise from the C1–C4 segments of the cervical spinal cord. The spinal nerves divide into posterior (dorsal) rami and anterior (ventral) rami:

- The posterior rami of the spinal nerves arising from the C1–C3 spinal cord segments (suboccipital nerve, greater occipital nerve, third occipital nerve) supply motor innervation to the intrinsic nuchal muscles and sensory innervation to the C2 and C3 dermatomes on the back of the neck and occiput (see **B**).
- The anterior rami of the spinal nerves arising from C1–C4 spinal cord segments supply motor innervation to the deep neck muscles (short, direct branches from the anterior rami) and finally unite in the neck to form the cervical plexus (see **C**). This plexus supplies the skin and musculature of the anterior and lateral neck (all but the nuchal region).

The neck contains the following **cranial nerves**, which arise from the brainstem:

- Glossopharyngeal nerve (CN IX)
- Vagus nerve (CN X)
- Accessory nerve (CN XI)
- Hypoglossal nerve (CN XII)

These nerves supply motor and sensory innervation to the pharynx and larynx (CN IX and X) and motor innervation to the trapezius and sternocleidomastoid muscles (CN XI), lingual muscles (CN XII), and floor of the mouth.

The **sympathetic trunk** is part of the autonomic nervous system, consisting of a nerve trunk with three ganglia that extends along the vertebral column on each side. The postganglionic fibers follow the carotid arteries to their territories in the head and neck region.

Another part of the autonomic nervous system, the **parasympathetic system**, is represented in the neck by the vagus nerve.

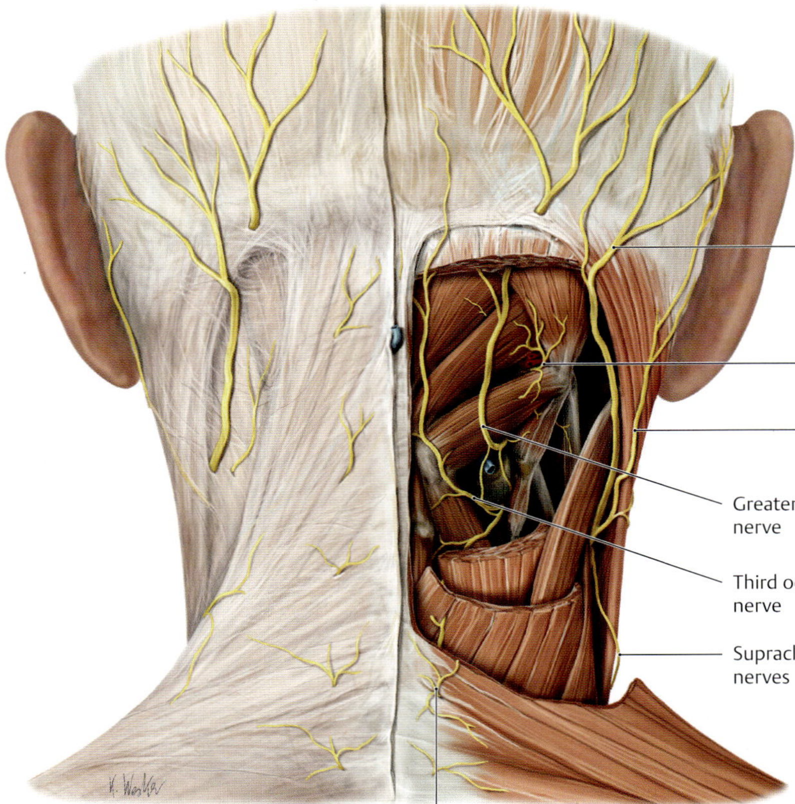

a

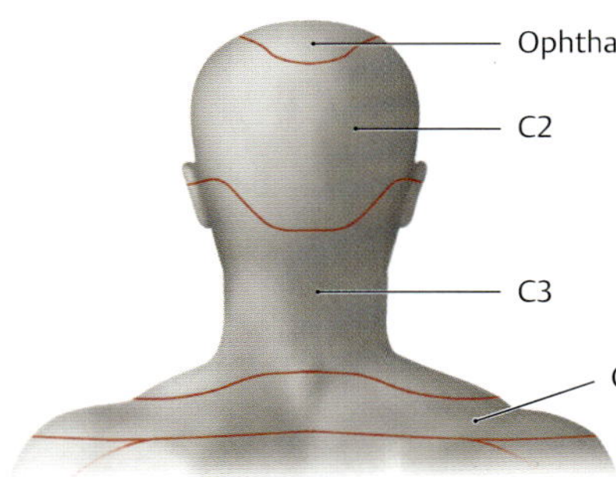

b

B Motor and sensory innervation of the nuchal region

Posterior view. **a** Spinal nerve branches in the nuchal region. **b** Segmental distribution.

The nuchal region receives most of its motor and sensory innervation from *posterior* rami of the cervical spinal nerves arising from the C1–C3 cord segments:

- Suboccipital nerve (C1)
- Greater occipital nerve (C2)
- Third occipital nerve (C3)

Note their subcutaneous course on the left side (**a**). The following nerves are derived from *anterior* rami of the cervical spinal nerves and enter the nuchal region from the lateral side:

- Lesser occipital nerve
- Great auricular nerve

Note: The dorsal ramus of the first cervical spinal nerve (the suboccipital nerve) is purely motor (see **a**), and consequently there is no C1 dermatome.

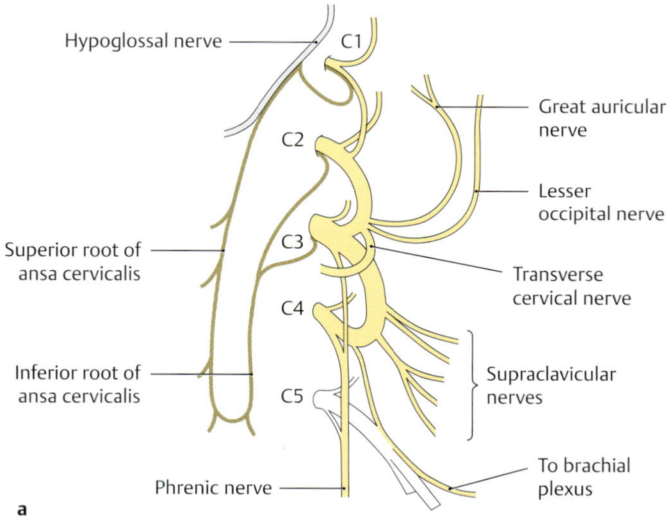

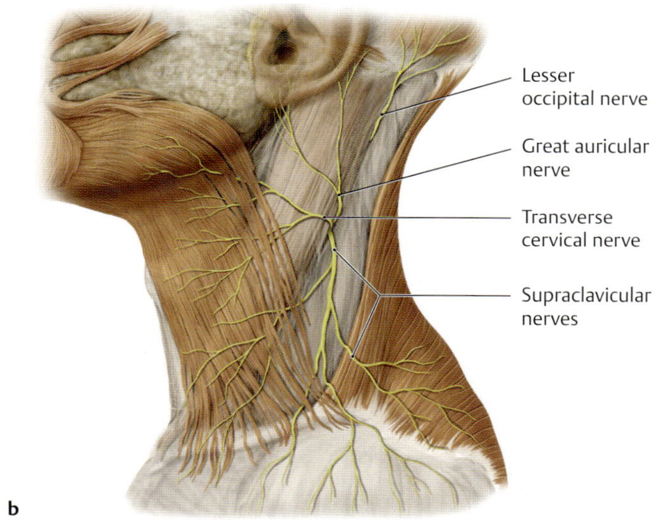

C Motor and sensory innervation of the anterior and lateral neck
The anterolateral portions of the neck, unlike the nuchal region and occiput, are supplied entirely by *anterior* rami of the C1–C4 cervical spinal nerves. These rami distribute short branches to the deep neck muscles (see **c**). They also give off branches that form the cervical plexus, which consists of a sensory part and a motor part supplying the skin and muscles of the neck.

a Branching pattern of the cervical plexus (viewed from the left side). The motor fibers from C1–C3 form the ansa cervicalis*, which innervates the infrahyoid muscles (see **c**). The fibers from C1 course briefly with the hypoglossal nerve, without exchanging fibers with it, before they separate to form the *superior root* of the ansa cervicalis, which supplies the omohyoid, sternothyroid and sternohyoid muscles. Only the fibers for the thyrohyoid and geniohyoid muscles continue to course with the hypoglossal nerve. Other fibers from C2 unite with the fibers from C3 to form the *inferior root* of the ansa cervicalis. The bulk of the fibers from C4 descend in the phrenic nerve to the diaphragm (see D)

b Sensory innervation of the anterior and lateral neck (viewed from the left side). Erb's point is located approximately at the mid-posterior border of the sternocleidomastoid muscle, and is the site where the following nerves of the cervical plexus emerge to supply sensory innervation to the skin of the anterior and lateral neck (the *sensory part* of the cervical plexus):

- Lesser occipital nerve
- Great auricular nerve with its anterior and posterior branches
- Transverse cervical nerve
- Supraclavicular nerves

These nerves course along the surface of the fascia the entire distance (including the descending part of the trapezius, shown here without its fascia for greater clarity). The only muscle they perforate is the platysma, which lacks a fascia.

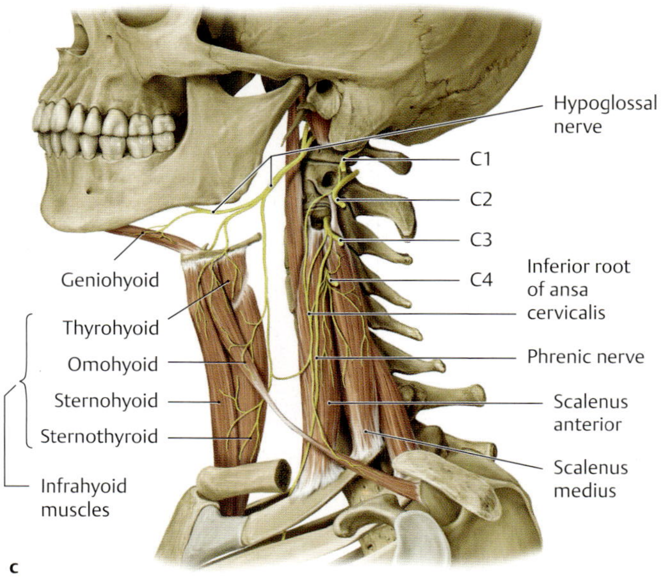

c Motor innervation of the anterior and lateral neck. Most of the anterior and lateral neck muscles are supplied by ventral rami of the spinal nerves. Their motor fibers either pass directly as short fibers from the ventral rami to the deep neck muscles or combine to form the *motor root* of the cervical plexus.

* The deep cervical ansa is the loop of nerves in the cervical plexus shown here. This is distinct from the superficial cervical ansa, which represents an anastomosis between the transverse cervical nerve and the cervical branch of the facial nerve (see p. 241).

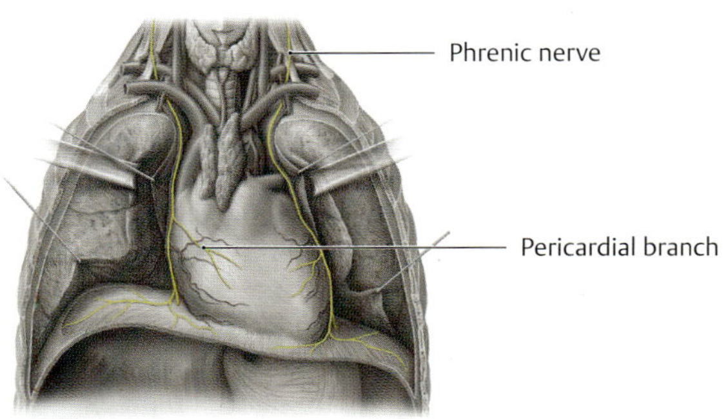

D Phrenic nerve
Anterior view. The phrenic nerve arises from the C3, 4, and 5 anterior roots ("C3, 4, and 5 keep the diaphragm alive"), with the major contribution from C4. It descends through the cervical region in front of the scalenus anterior, behind the sternocleidomastoid, through the thoracic inlet to the diaphragm, which it provides with motor innervation. Although this is an unusual anatomical relation between nerve origin and target location in the adult, the embryonic diaphragm develops from a precursor (the septum transversum) at the cervical level, and carries its innervation with it as it migrates inferiorly. If the C4 segment of the spinal cord (the main root of the phrenic nerve) sustains bilateral injury in an accident, the victim will usually die at the scene from asphyxiation brought on by paralysis of the diaphragm.

4.24 Cranial Nerves and Autonomic Nervous System in the Neck

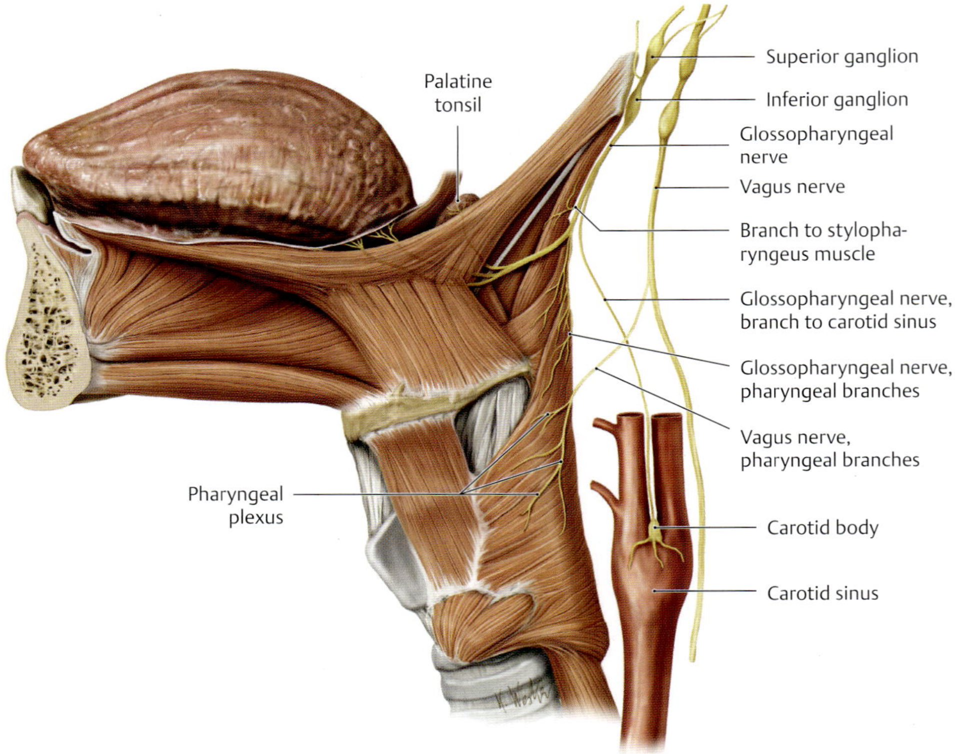

A Glossopharyngeal nerve
Left lateral view. The glossopharyngeal nerve (CN IX) carries the motor fibers for the stylopharyngeus as well as sensory fibers for the pharyngeal mucosa, the tonsils, and the posterior third of the tongue including the gustatory fibers. It sends small branches to anastomose with both the sympathetic trunk and the vagus nerve. It also sends nerve fibers (carotid sinus branch) to the bifurcation of the common carotid artery, which contains specialized collections of cells that are important in autonomic control of the circulatory system. Mechanoreceptors in the carotid sinus sense blood pressure, and chemoreceptors in the carotid body monitor blood pH and carbon dioxide and oxygen levels. This information is relayed by the glossopharyngeal nerve to the centers regulating breathing and heart rate in the brainstem.

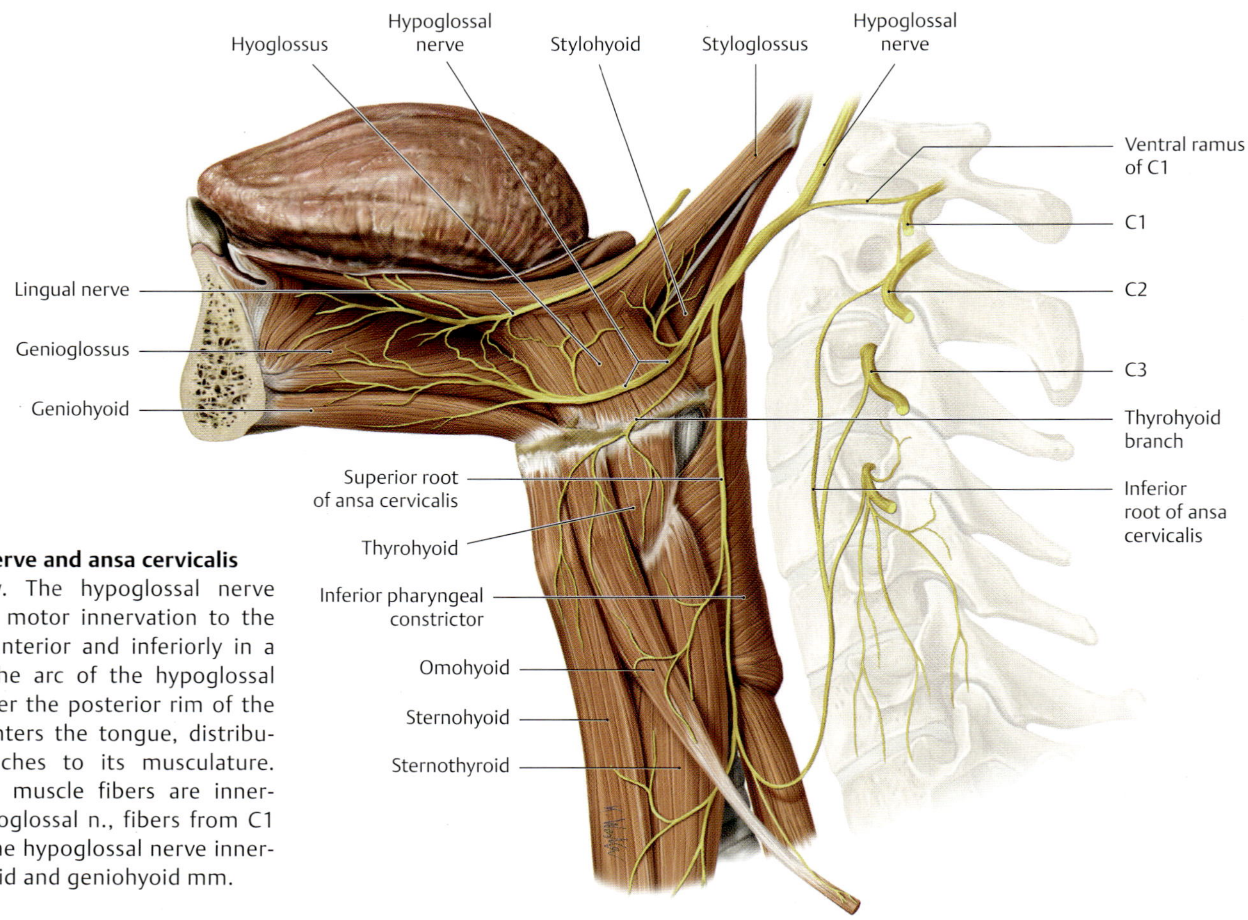

B Hypoglossal nerve and ansa cervicalis
Left lateral view. The hypoglossal nerve (CN XII) supplies motor innervation to the tongue. It runs anterior and inferiorly in a curved course (the arc of the hypoglossal nerve), passes over the posterior rim of the oral floor, and enters the tongue, distributing motor branches to its musculature. While all tongue muscle fibers are innervated by the hypoglossal n., fibers from C1 that travel with the hypoglossal nerve innervate the thyrohyoid and geniohyoid mm.

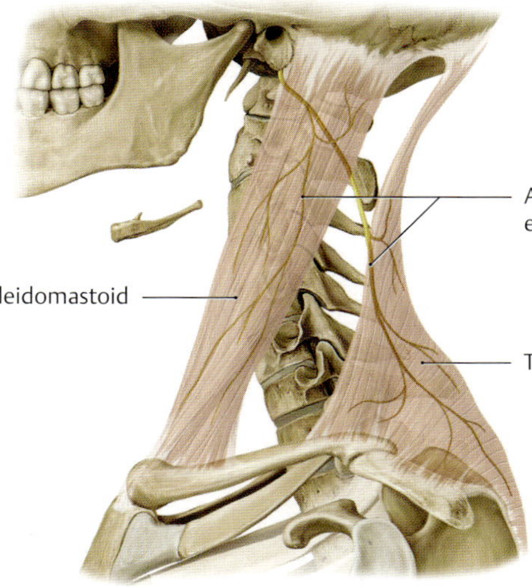

C Accessory nerve in the neck

Left lateral view. The accessory nerve (CN XI) is purely motor. Some of its fibers enter the sternocleidomastoid muscle from behind while others continue on to the trapezius. A deep (prescalene) lymph node biopsy may injure the accessory nerve in the neck. Damage to the fibers supplying the trapezius results in lateral rotation of the scapula and some shoulder drop. Damage to the fibers supplying the sternocleidomastoid leads to weakness in turning the head to the opposite side.

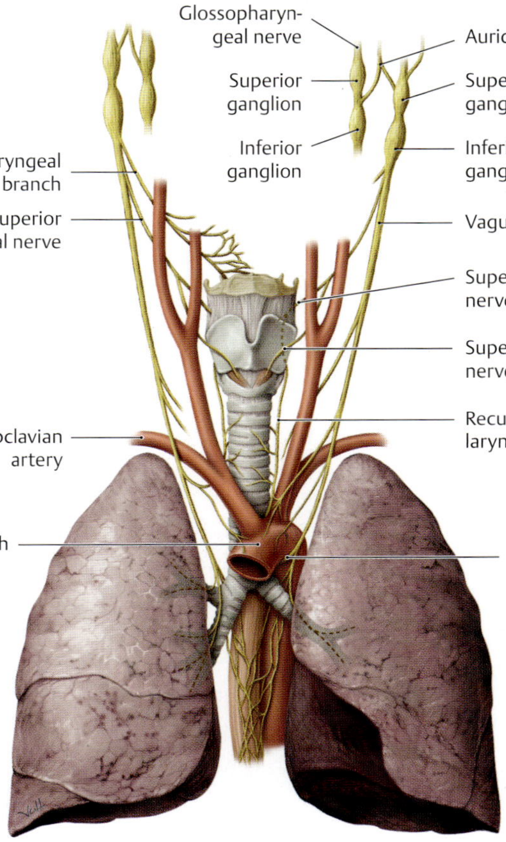

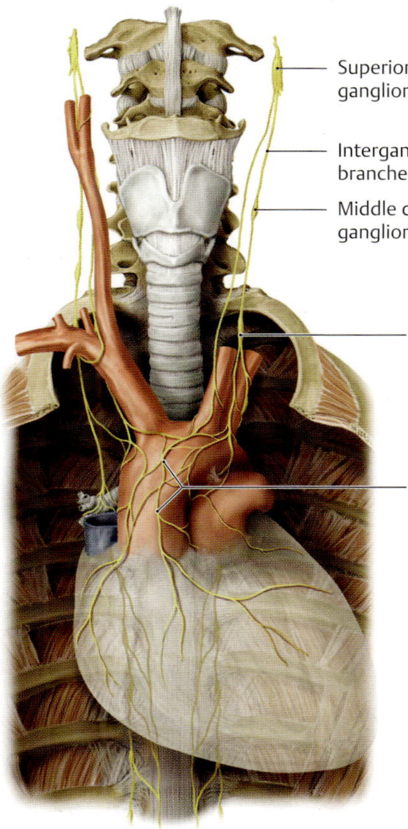

D Vagus nerve in the neck and the cervical sympathetic trunk

a Anterior view. The vagus nerve (CN X) conveys the fibers of the cranial portion of the parasympathetic nervous system (part of the autonomic nervous system) that supply the neck, thorax, and parts of the abdominal cavity. It passes down the neck in the carotid sheath (see topographical anatomy, p. 242), giving off only a few branches in the head and neck:

- The auricular branch, a somatic afferent branch that supplies the back surface of the ear and the external auditory canal
- The pharyngeal branch, special visceral efferent fibers for supplying muscles of the pharynx and soft palate
- The superior laryngeal n., a mixed nerve with sensory and special visceral efferent fibers, that
- The recurrent laryngeal n., which supplies the skeletal laryngeal muscles and the mucosa surrounding them (see p. 218). The recurrent laryngeal n. winds around the subclavian a. on the right side and the aortic arch on the left side.

b Anterior view. The paravertebral chain of sympathetic ganglia terminates in the cervical region at the superior cervical ganglion, approximately 2 cm below the base of the skull. Postganglionic fibers from this ganglion follow both the internal and external carotid arteries to provide sympathetic innervation to the entire cranial vasculature, to the iris, and to glands and mucosa in the head. The lowest of the cervical ganglia in the paravertebral chain is often fused with the first thoracic sympathetic ganglion to form the stellate ganglion.

5.1 Ear: Overview and Supply to the External Ear

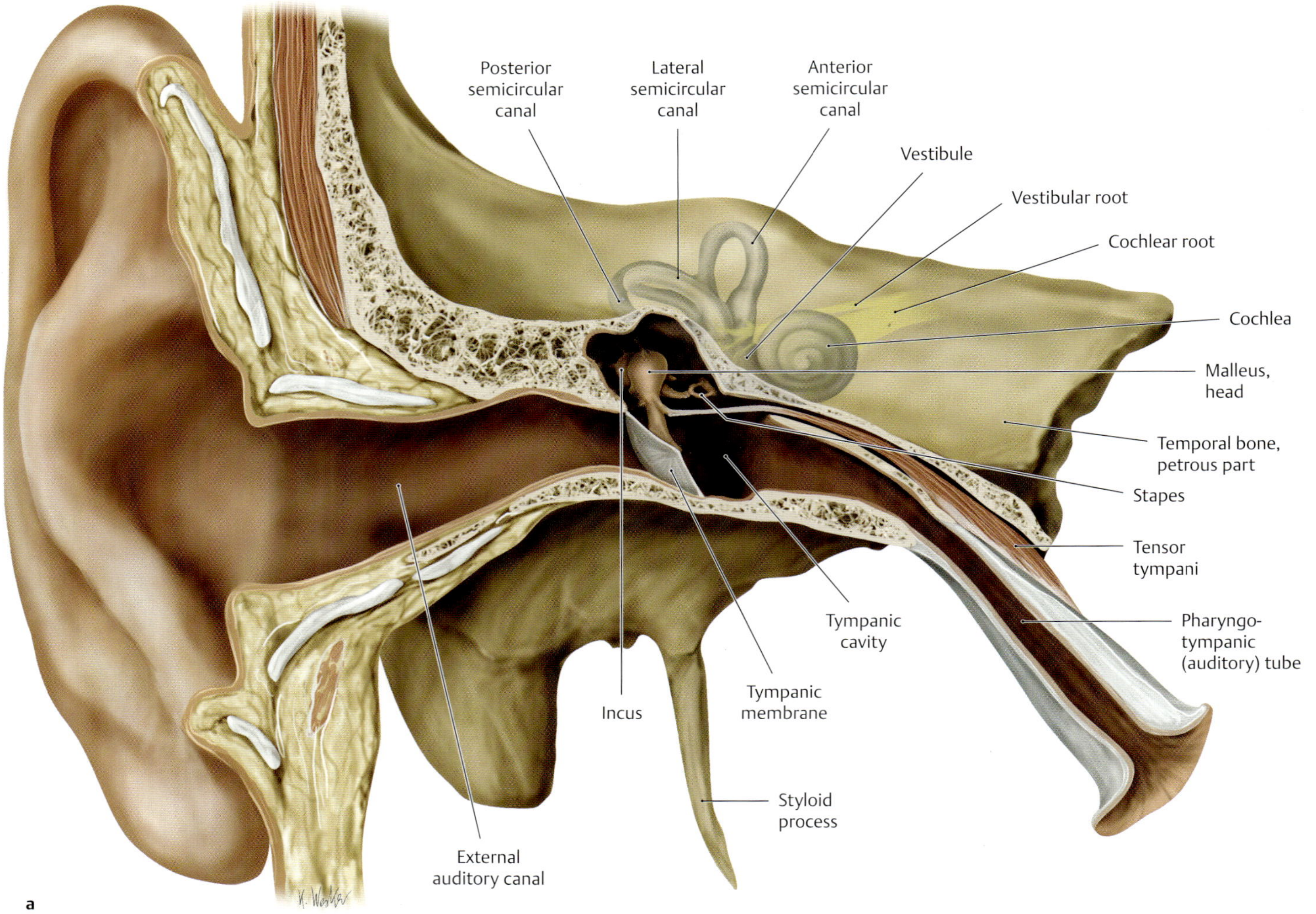

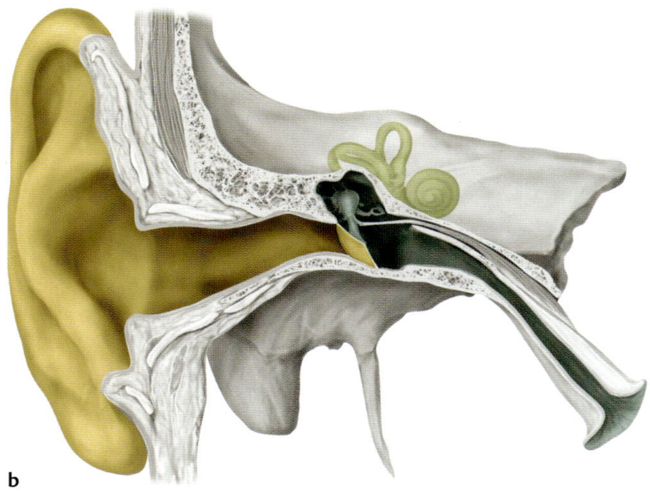

A Auditory and vestibular apparatus in situ

a Coronal section through the right ear, anterior view. **b** Main parts of the auditory apparatus: external ear (yellow), middle ear (blue), and inner ear (green).

The auditory and vestibular apparatus are located deep in the petrous part of the temporal bone (petrous bone). The **auditory apparatus** consists of the external ear, middle ear, and inner ear (see **b**). Sound waves are captured by the *external* ear (auricle, see **B**) and travel through the external auditory canal to the tympanic membrane, which marks the lateral boundary of the *middle* ear. The sound waves set the tympanic membrane into motion, and these mechanical vibrations are transmitted by the chain of auditory ossicles in the middle ear to the oval window, which leads into the *inner* ear (see p. 146). The ossicular chain induces vibrations in the membrane covering the oval window, and these in turn cause a fluid column in the inner ear to vibrate, setting receptor cells in motion (see p. 153). The transformation of sound waves into electrical impulses takes place in the inner ear, which is the actual organ of hearing. The external ear and middle ear, on the other hand, constitute the *sound conduction apparatus*. The organ of balance is the **vestibular apparatus**, which is also located in the auditory apparatus and will be described after the units that deal with the auditory apparatus. It contains the *semicircular canals* for the perception of angular acceleration (rotational head movements) and the *saccule* and *utricle* for the perception of linear acceleration. Diseases of the vestibular apparatus produce dizziness (vertigo).

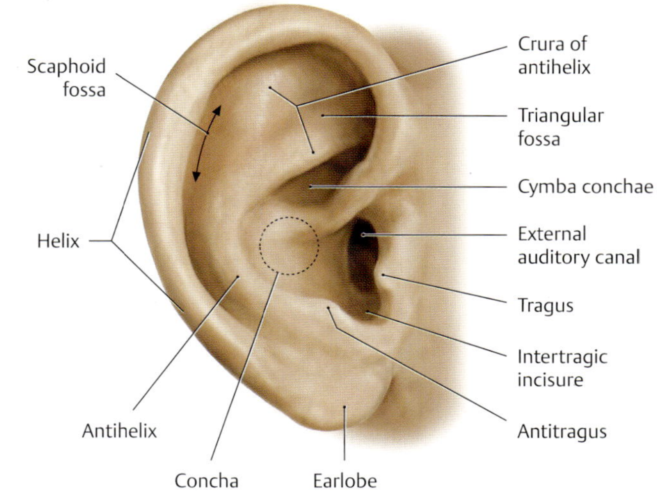

B Right auricle
The auricle of the ear encloses a cartilaginous framework (auricular cartilage) that forms a funnel-shaped receptor for acoustic vibrations.

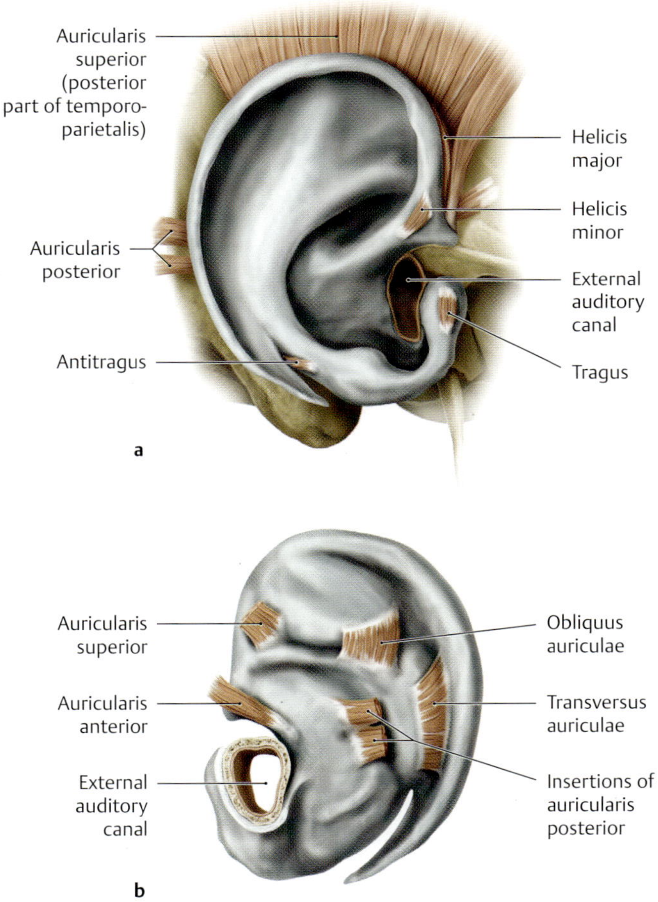

C Cartilage and muscles of the auricle
a Lateral view of the external surface. **b** Medial view of the posterior surface of the right ear.
The skin (removed here) is closely applied to the elastic cartilage of the auricle (shown in light blue). The muscles of the ear are classified as muscles of facial expression and, like the other members of this group, are supplied by the facial nerve. Prominent in other mammals, the auricular muscles are vestigial in humans, with no significant function.

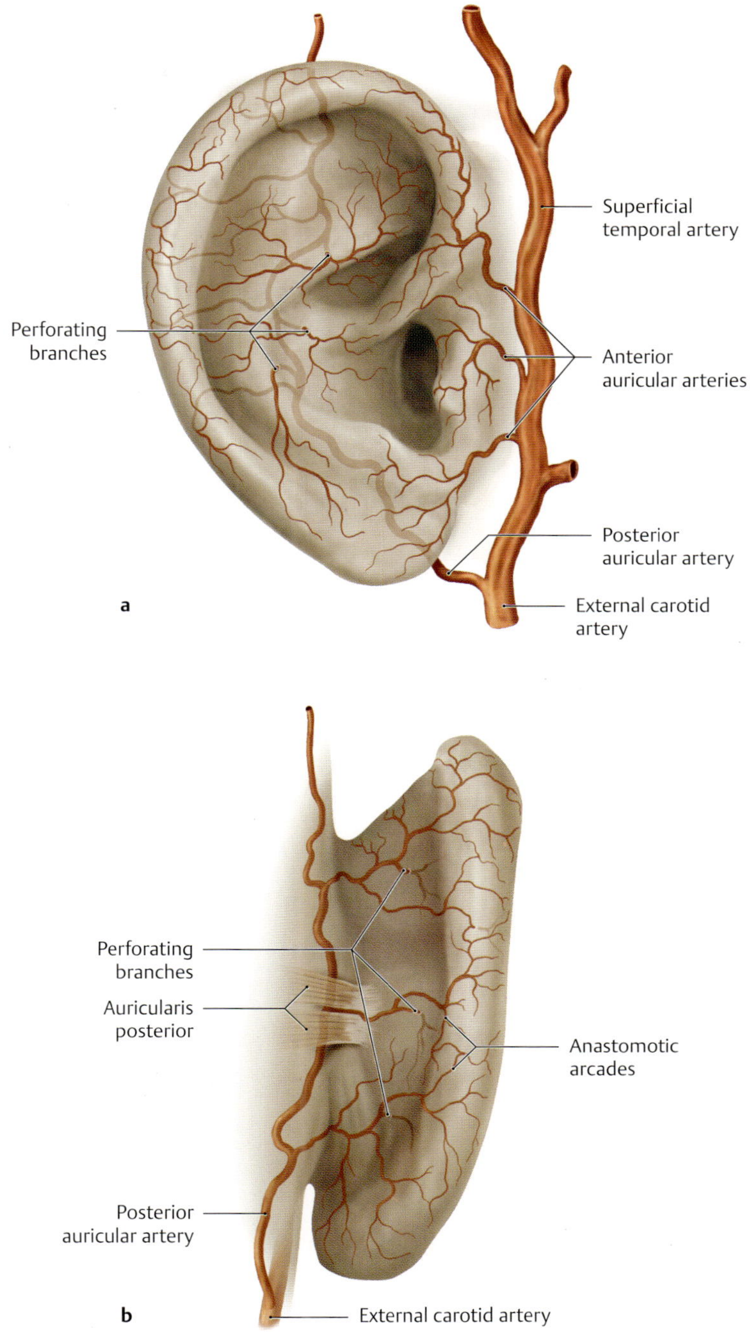

D Arterial supply of the right auricle
Lateral view (**a**) and posterior view (**b**).
The proximal and medial portions of the laterally directed anterior surface of the ear are supplied by the anterior auricular arteries, which arise from the superficial temporal artery (see p. 101). The other parts of the ear are supplied by branches of the posterior auricular artery, which arises from the external carotid artery. These vessels are linked by extensive anastomoses, so operations on the external ear are unlikely to compromise the auricular blood supply. The copious blood flow through the auricle contributes to temperature regulation: dilation of the vessels helps dissipate heat through the skin. The lack of insulating fat predisposes the ear to frostbite, which is particularly common in the upper third of the auricle. The lymphatic drainage and innervation of the auricle are covered in the next unit.

5.2 External Ear: Auricle, Auditory Canal, and Tympanic Membrane

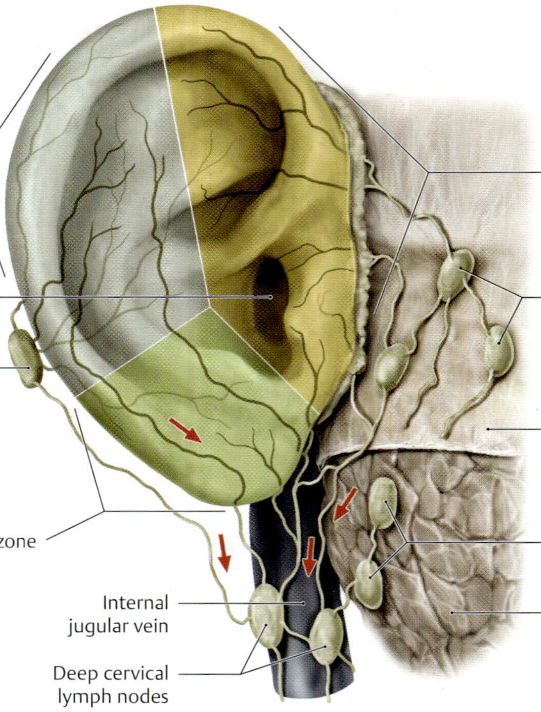

A Auricle and external auditory canal: lymphatic drainage and regional groups of lymph nodes

Right ear, oblique lateral view. The cartilaginous framework and blood supply of the ear were described in the previous unit. The lymphatic drainage of the ear is divided into three zones, all of which drain directly or indirectly into the deep cervical lymph nodes along the internal jugular vein. The lower zone drains directly into the deep cervical lymph nodes. The anterior zone first drains into the parotid lymph nodes, the posterior zone into the mastoid lymph nodes.

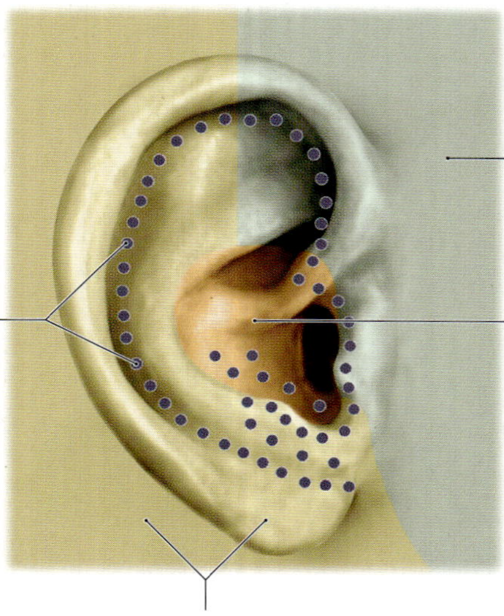

a

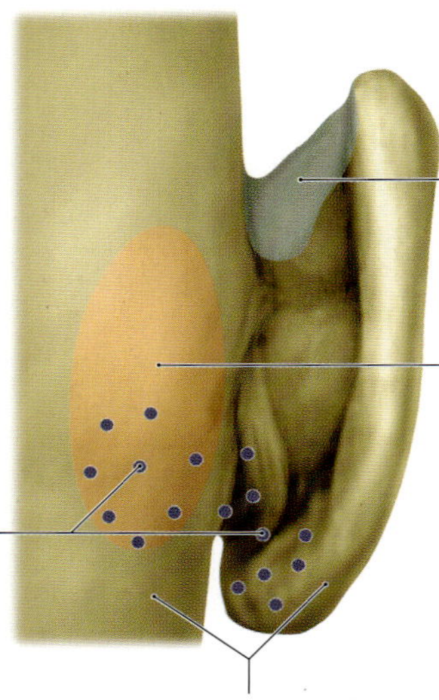

b

B Sensory innervation of the auricle

Right ear, lateral view (**a**) and posterior view (**b**). The auricular region has a complex nerve supply because, developmentally, it is located at the boundary between cranial nerves (pharyngeal arch nerves) and branches of the cervical plexus. Four **cranial nerves** contribute to the innervation of the auricle:

- Trigeminal nerve (CN V),
- Facial nerve (CN VII; the skin area that receives sensory innervation from the facial nerve is not precisely known)
- Glossopharyngeal nerve (CN IX) and vagus nerve (CN X)

Two branches of the **cervical plexus** are involved:

- Lesser occipital nerve (C_2)
- Great auricular nerve (C_2, C_3)

Note: Because the vagus nerve (see pp. 132 and 141) contributes to the innervation of the external auditory canal (auricular branch, see below), mechanical cleaning of the ear canal (by inserting an aural speculum or by irrigating the ear) may evoke coughing and nausea. The auricular branch of the vagus nerve passes through the mastoid canaliculus and through a space between the mastoid process and the tympanic part of the temporal bone (tympanomastoid fissure, see p. 29) to the external ear and external auditory canal. The ear canal receives sensory fibers from the glossopharyngeal nerve through its communicating branch with the vagus nerve.

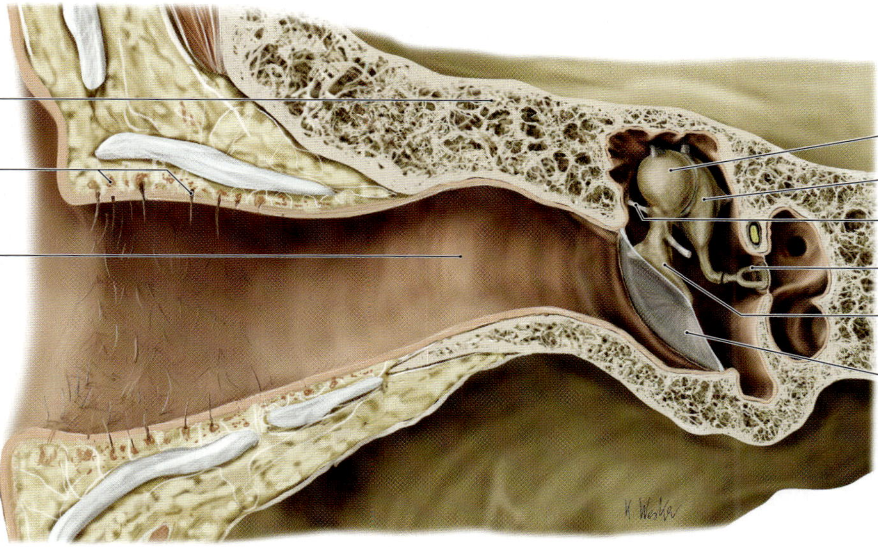

C External auditory canal, tympanic membrane, and tympanic cavity

Right ear, coronal section, anterior view. The tympanic membrane (eardrum, see **E**) separates the external auditory canal from the tympanic cavity, which is part of the middle ear (see p. 146). The external auditory canal is an S-shaped tunnel (see **D**) that is approximately 3 cm long with an average diameter of 0.6 cm. The outer third of the ear canal is cartilaginous. The inner two-thirds of the canal are osseous, the wall being formed by the tympanic part of the temporal bone. The cartilaginous part in particular bears numerous sebaceous and cerumen glands beneath the keratinized stratified squamous epithelium. The cerumen glands produce a watery secretion that combines with the sebum and sloughed epithelial cells to form a protective barrier (cerumen, "earwax") that screens out foreign bodies and keeps the epithelium from drying out. If the cerumen absorbs water (e.g., water in the ear canal after swimming), it may obstruct the ear canal (cerumen impaction), temporarily causing a partial loss of hearing.

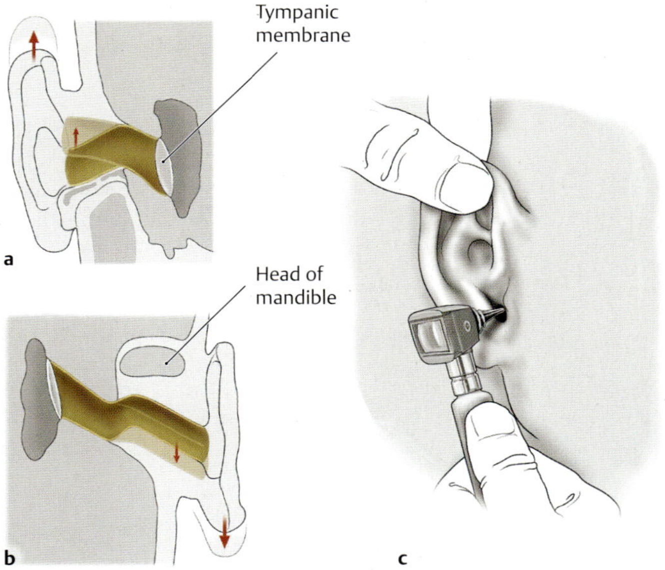

D Curvature of the external auditory canal

Right ear, anterior view (**a**) and transverse section (**b**).

The external auditory canal is most curved in its cartilaginous portion. It is important for the clinician to know how the ear canal is curved. When the tympanic membrane is inspected with an otoscope, the auricle should be pulled backward and upward in order to straighten the cartilaginous part of the ear canal so that the speculum of the otoscope can be introduced (**c**).

Note the proximity of the cartilaginous anterior wall of the external auditory canal to the temporomandibular joint. This allows the examiner to palpate movements of the mandibular head by inserting the small finger into the outer part of the ear canal.

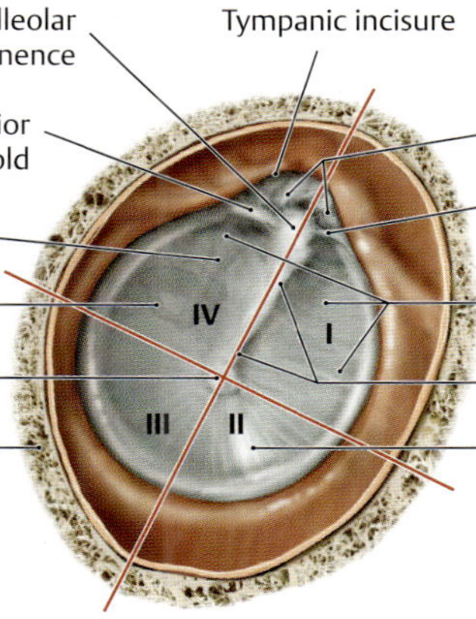

E Tympanic membrane

Right tympanic membrane, external view. The healthy tympanic membrane has a pearly gray color and an oval shape with an average surface area of approximately 75 mm^2. It consists of a lax portion, the *pars flaccida* (Shrapnell membrane), and a larger taut portion, the *pars tensa*, which is drawn inward at its center to form the umbo ("navel"). The umbo marks the lower tip of the handle (manubrium) of the malleus, which is attached to the tympanic membrane all along its length. It is visible through the pars tensa as a light-colored streak (malleolar stria). The anterior and posterior malleolar fold contains the chorda tympani and is referred to by ear, nose, and throat specialists as the anterior and posterior stria of the tympanic membrane. The tympanic membrane is divided into four quadrants along the malleolar stria and a line intersecting it perpendicularly at the umbo. The quadrants of the tympanic membrane are clinically important because they are used in describing the location of lesions. The function of the tympanic membrane is reviewed on pp. 142 and 148. A triangular area of reflected light can be seen in the anteroinferior quadrant of a normal tympanic membrane.

5.3 Middle Ear: Tympanic Cavity and Pharyngotympanic Tube

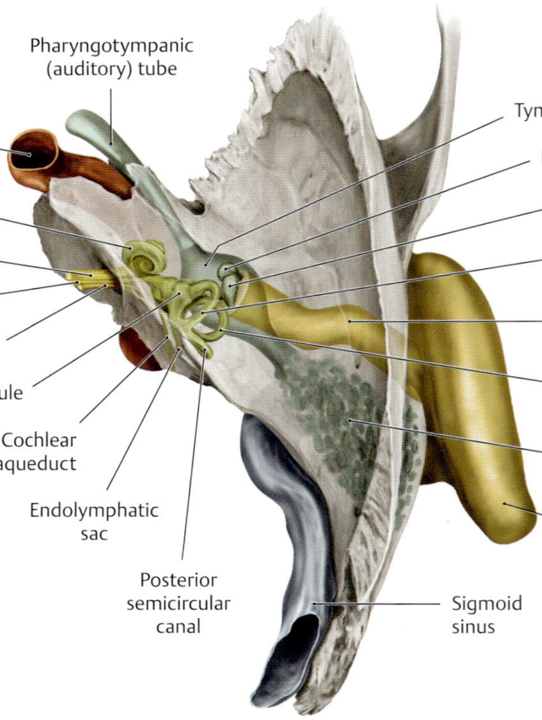

A The middle ear and associated structures
Right petrous bone, superior view. The middle ear (light blue) is located within the petrous part of the temporal bone between the external ear (yellow) and inner ear (green). The tympanic cavity of the middle ear contains the chain of auditory ossicles, of which the malleus (hammer) and incus (anvil) are visible here. The tympanic cavity communicates anteriorly with the pharynx via the pharyngotympanic (auditory) tube, and it communicates posteriorly with the mastoid air cells. Infections can spread from the pharynx to the mastoid cells by this route (see **C**).

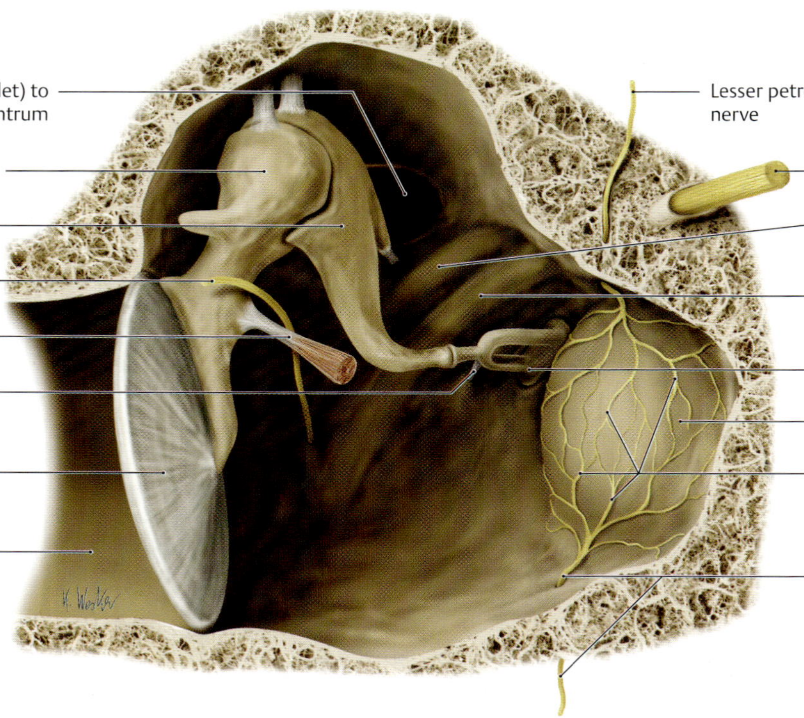

B Walls of the tympanic cavity
Anterior view with the anterior wall removed. The tympanic cavity is a slightly oblique space that is bounded by six walls:

- Lateral (membranous) wall: boundary with the external ear; formed largely by the tympanic membrane.
- Medial (labyrinthine) wall: boundary with the inner ear; formed largely by the promontory, or the bony eminence, overlying the basal turn of the cochlea.
- Inferior (jugular) wall: forms the floor of the tympanic cavity and borders on the bulb of the jugular vein.
- Posterior (mastoid) wall: borders on the air cells of the mastoid process, communicating with the cells through the aditus (inlet) of the mastoid antrum.
- Superior (tegmental) wall: forms the roof of the tympanic cavity.
- Anterior (carotid) wall (removed here): includes the opening to the pharyngotympanic (auditory) tube and borders on the carotid canal.

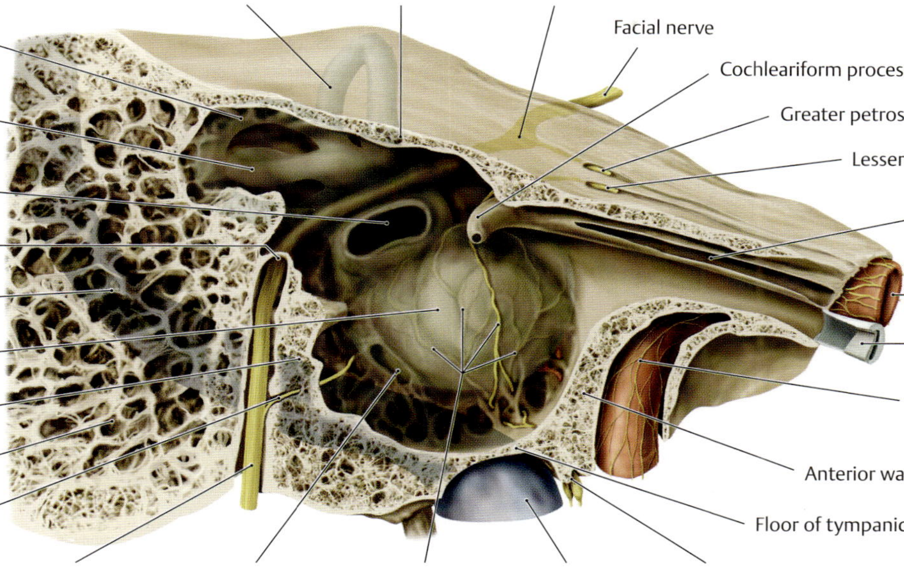

C Tympanic cavity: clinically important anatomical relationships
Oblique sagittal section through the right tympanic cavity, lateral view of the posterior wall (cf. **B**). The anatomical relationships of the tympanic cavity are particularly important in treating chronic suppurative otitis media. During this inflammation of the middle ear, pathogenic bacteria may spread upward to adjacent regions. For example, bacteria may spread upward through the roof of the tympanic cavity into the middle cranial fossa (inciting meningitis or a cerebral abscess, especially of the temporal lobe); they may invade the mastoid air cells (mastoiditis) or sigmoid sinus (sinus thrombosis); they may pass through the air cells of the petrous apex and enter the CSF space, causing abducent paralysis, trigeminal nerve irritation, or visual disturbances (Gradenigo syndrome); or they may invade the facial nerve canal, resulting in facial paralysis.

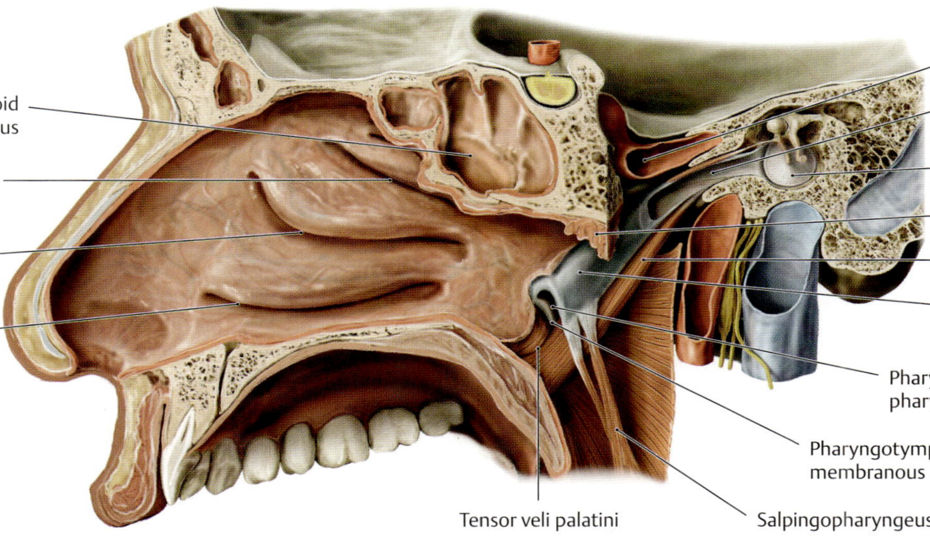

D Pharyngotympanic (auditory) tube
Medial view of the right half of the head. The pharyngotympanic tube (auditory tube) creates an open channel between the middle ear and pharynx. One-third of the tube is bony and two-thirds are cartilaginous. The bony part of the tube is located in the petrous bone, and the cartilaginous part continues onward to the pharynx, where it expands into a funnel-shaped orifice. As it expands, it forms a hook (hamulus) which is attached to a membranous part (membranous lamina) that enlarges toward the pharynx. The pharyngotympanic tube also opens during swallowing. Air passing through the tube serves to equalize the air pressure on the two sides of the tympanic membrane. This equalization is essential for maintaining normal tympanic membrane mobility, which, in turn, is necessary for normal hearing. The pharyngotympanic tube is opened by the muscles of the soft palate (tensor veli palatini and levator veli palatini) and by the salpingopharyngeus, which is part of the superior pharyngeal constrictor. The fibers of the tensor veli palatini arising from the membranous lamina of the pharyngotympanic tube are of special significance: When the tensor veli palatini tenses the soft palate during swallowing, its fibers attached to the membranous lamina simultaneously open the pharyngotympanic tube. The tube is lined with ciliated respiratory epithelium whose cilia beat toward the pharynx, thus inhibiting the passage of microorganisms into the middle ear. If this nonspecific protective mechanism fails, bacteria may migrate up the tube and incite a purulent middle ear infection (cf. **C**).

5.4 Middle Ear: Auditory Ossicles and Tympanic Cavity

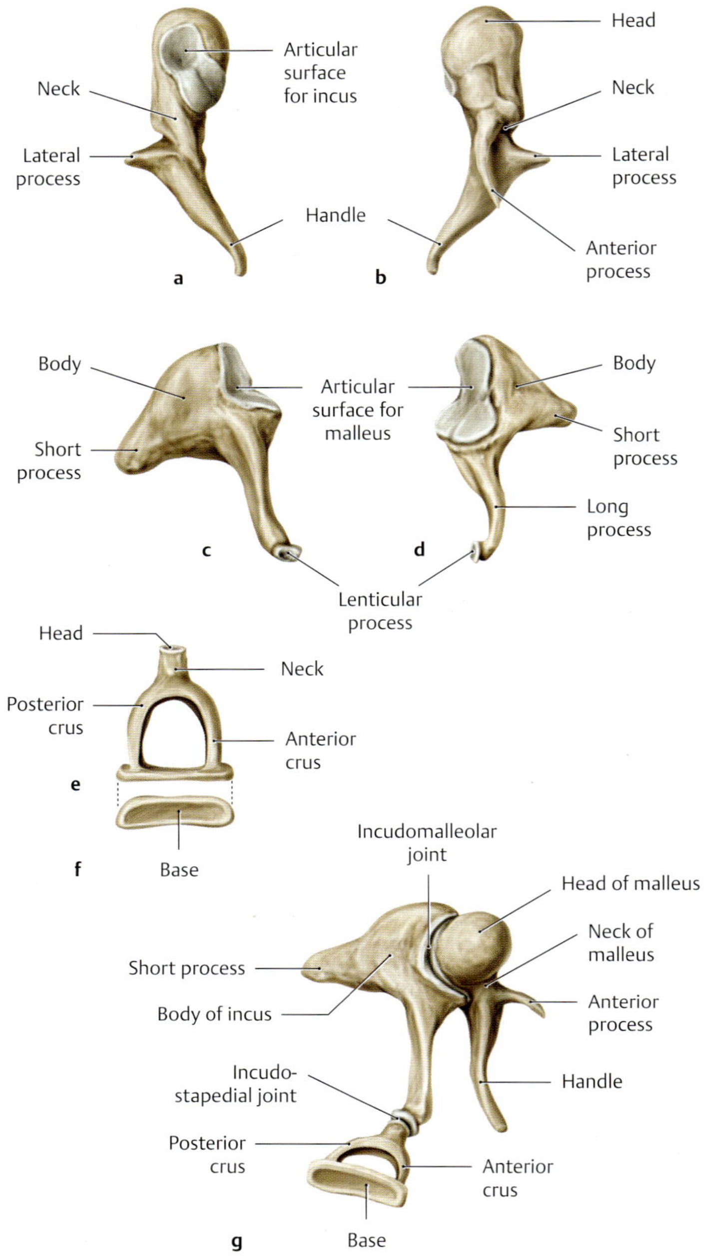

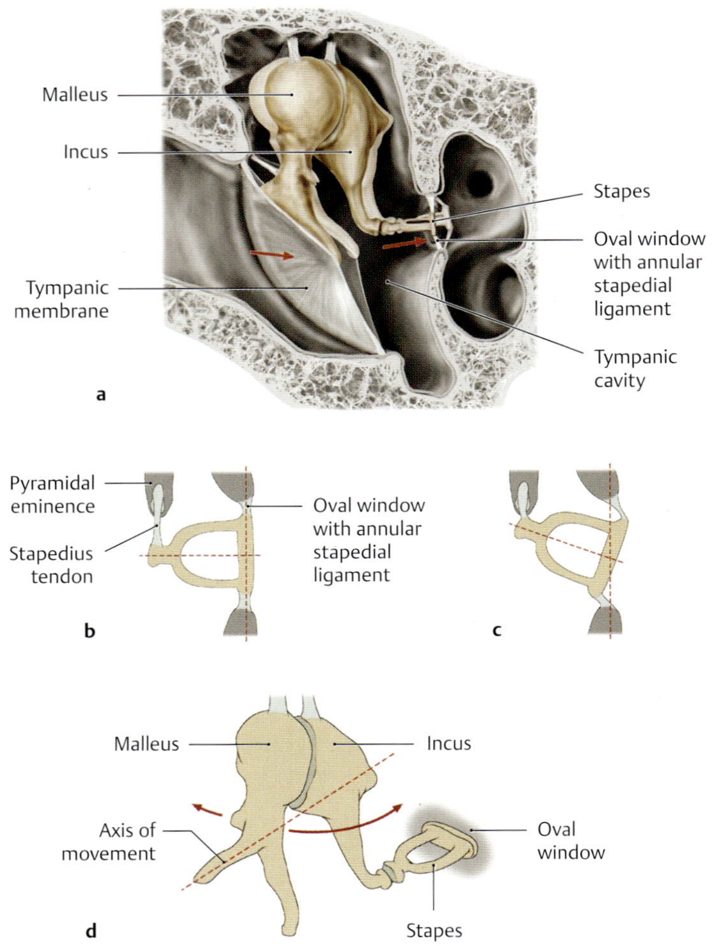

A Auditory ossicles

The auditory ossicles of the left ear. The ossicular chain consists of three small bones in the middle ear (chain function is described in **B**). It establishes an articular connection from the tympanic membrane to the oval window and consists of the following bones:

- Malleus ("hammer")
- Incus ("anvil")
- Stapes ("stirrup")

a, b Malleus: posterior view and anterior view
c, d Incus: medial view and anterolateral view
e, f Stapes: superior view and medial view
g Medial view of the ossicular chain

Note the articulations between the malleus and incus (incudomalleolar joint) and between the incus and stapes (incudostapedial joint).

B Function of the ossicular chain

Anterior view.

a Sound waves (periodic pressure fluctuations in the air) set the tympanic membrane into vibration. The ossicular chain transmits the vibrations of the tympanic membrane (and thus the sound waves) to the oval window, which in turn communicates them to an aqueous medium, the perilymph. While sound waves encounter very little resistance in air, they encounter considerably higher impedance when they reach the fluid interface of the inner ear (perilymph). The sound waves must therefore be amplified ("impedance matching"). The difference in surface area between the tympanic membrane and oval window increases the sound pressure by a factor of 17, and this is augmented by the 1.3-fold mechanical advantage of the lever action of the ossicular chain. Thus, in passing from the tympanic membrane to the inner ear, the sound pressure is amplified by a factor of 22. If the ossicular chain fails to transform the sound pressure between the tympanic membrane and stapes base (footplate), the patient will experience conductive hearing loss of magnitude approximately 20 dB.

b, c Sound waves impinging on the tympanic membrane induce motion in the ossicular chain, causing a tilting movement of the stapes (**b** normal position, **c** tilted position). The annular ligament of the stapes forms a mobile connection between the borders of the oval window and the stapes. The movements of the stapes base then induce corresponding waves in the fluid column in the inner ear.

d The movements of the ossicular chain are essentially rocking movements (the dashed line indicates the axis of the movements, the arrows indicate their direction). Two muscles affect the mobility of the ossicular chain: the tensor tympani and the stapedius (see **C**).

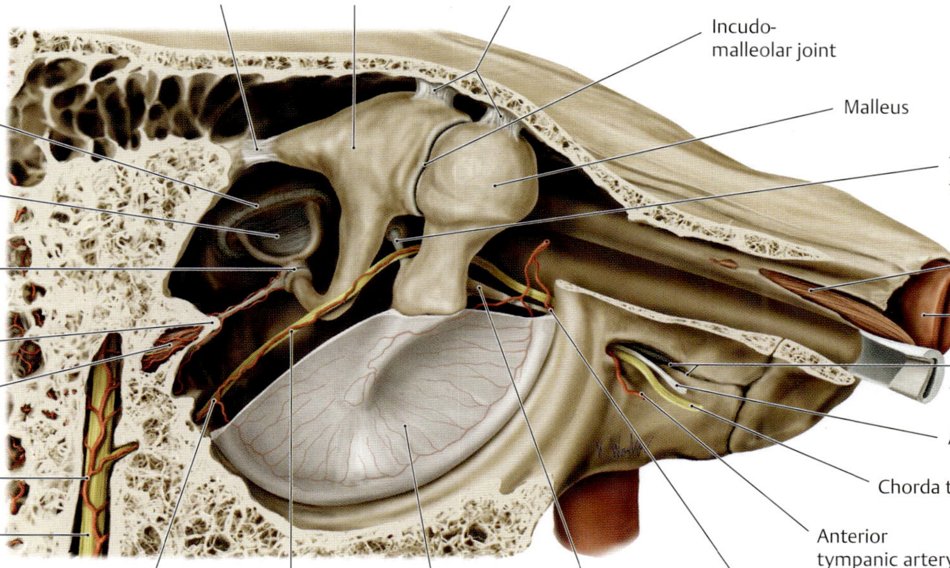

C Ossicular chain in the tympanic cavity
Lateral view of the right ear. The joints and their stabilizing ligaments can be seen. The two muscles of the middle ear—the stapedius and tensor tympani—can also be identified. The *stapedius* (innervated by the stapedial branch of the facial nerve) inserts on the stapes. When it contracts, it stiffens the sound conduction apparatus and decreases sound transmission to the inner ear. This filtering function is believed to be particularly important at high sound frequencies ("high-pass filter"). When sound is transmitted into the middle ear through a probe placed in the external ear canal, one can measure the action of the stapedius (stapedius reflex test) by measuring the change in acoustic impedance (i.e., the amplification of the sound waves). Contraction of the *tensor tympani* (Innervation: tensor tympani n., V_3) stiffens the tympanic membrane, thereby reducing the transmission of sound. Both muscles undergo a reflex contraction in response to loud acoustic stimuli.
Note: The chorda tympani, which contains gustatory fibers for the anterior two-thirds of the tongue, passes through the middle ear without a bony covering (making it susceptible to injury during otological surgery).

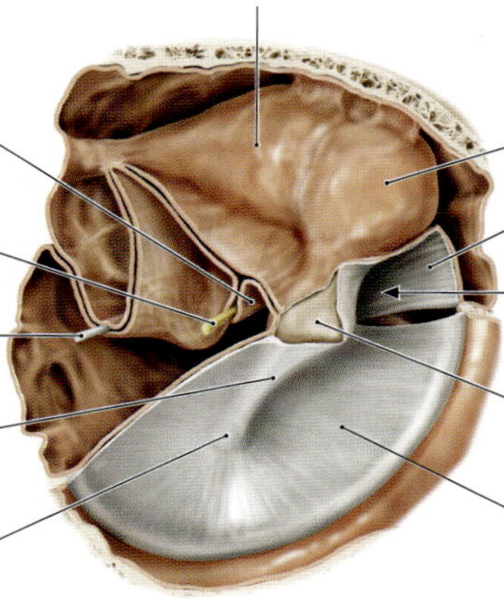

D Mucosal lining of the tympanic cavity
Posterolateral view with the tympanic membrane partially removed. The tympanic cavity and the structures it contains (ossicular chain, tendons, nerves) are covered with mucosa that is raised into folds and deepened into depressions conforming to the covered surfaces. The epithelium consists mainly of a simple squamous type, with areas of ciliated columnar cells and goblet cells. Because the tympanic cavity communicates directly with the respiratory tract through the pharyngotympanic tube, it can also be interpreted as a specialized paranasal sinus. Like the sinuses, it is susceptible to frequent infections (otitis media).

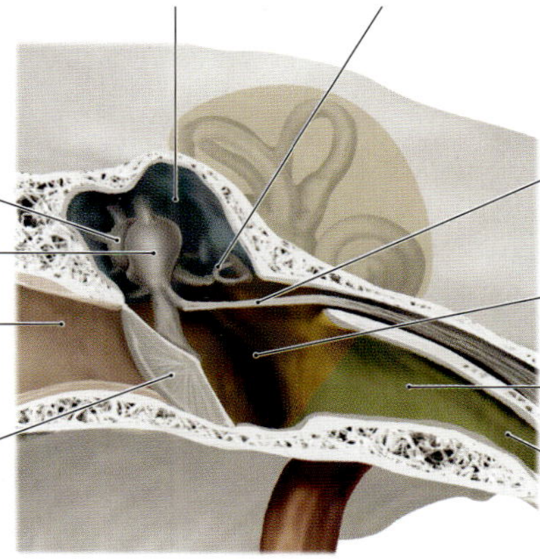

E Clinically important levels of the tympanic cavity
The tympanic cavity is divided into three levels in relation to the tympanic membrane:

- The epitympanum (epitympanic recess, attic) above the tympanic membrane
- The mesotympanum medial to the tympanic membrane
- The hypotympanum (hypotympanic recess) below the tympanic membrane

The epitympanum communicates with the mastoid air cells, and the hypotympanum communicates with the pharyngotympanic tube.

5.5 Inner Ear: Overview

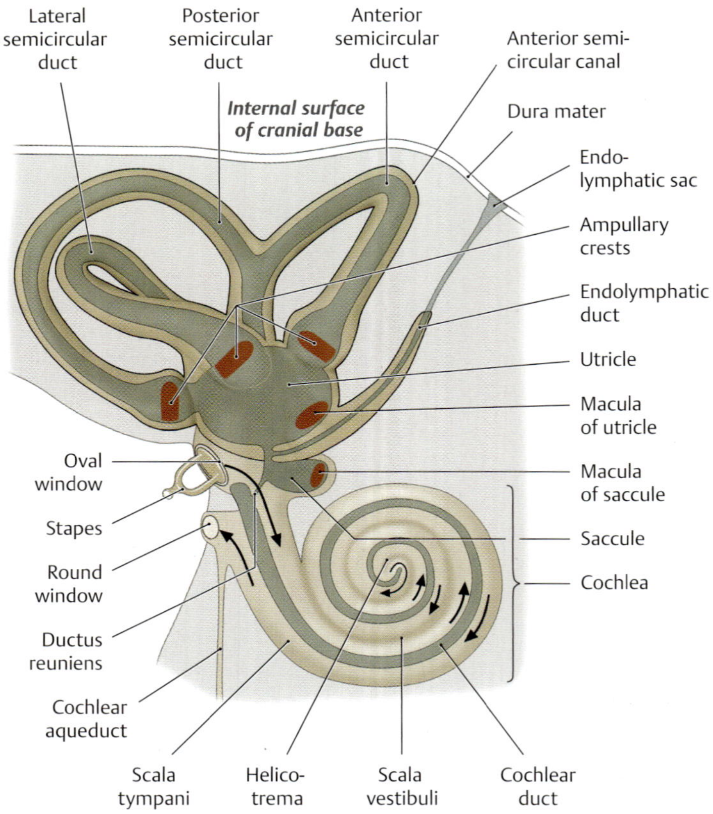

A Schematic diagram of the inner ear

The inner ear is embedded within the petrous part of the temporal bone (see **B**) and contains the auditory and vestibular apparatus for hearing and balance (see p. 146 ff). It comprises a *membranous labyrinth* contained within a similarly shaped *bony labyrinth*. The **auditory apparatus** consists of the cochlear labyrinth with the membranous *cochlear duct*. The membranous duct and its bony shell make up *the cochlea*, which contains the sensory epithelium of the auditory apparatus (*organ of Corti*). The **vestibular apparatus** includes the vestibular labyrinth with three *semicircular canals* (semicircular ducts), a *saccule*, and a *utricle*, each of which contains sensory epithelium. While each of the membranous semicircular ducts is encased in its own bony shell (semicircular canal), the utricle and saccule are contained in a common bony capsule, the *vestibule*. The cavity of the *bony labyrinth* is filled with perilymph (*perilymphatic space*, beige), whose composition reflects its being an ultrafiltrate of blood. The perilymphatic space is connected to the subarachnoid space by the cochlear aqueduct (= perilymphatic duct). It ends at the external skull base medial to the jugular fossa. The *membranous labyrinth* "floats" in the bony labyrinth, being loosely attached to it by connective-tissue fibers. It is filled with endolymph (*endolymphatic space*, blue-green), whose ionic composition of which corresponds to that of intracellular fluid. The endolymphatic spaces of the auditory and vestibular apparatus communicate with each other through the *ductus reuniens* and are connected by the *endolymphatic duct* to the endolymphatic sac, an epidural sac at the outer surface of the petrous bone between internal acoustic opening and sigmoidal sinus sulcus in which the endolymph is absorbed.

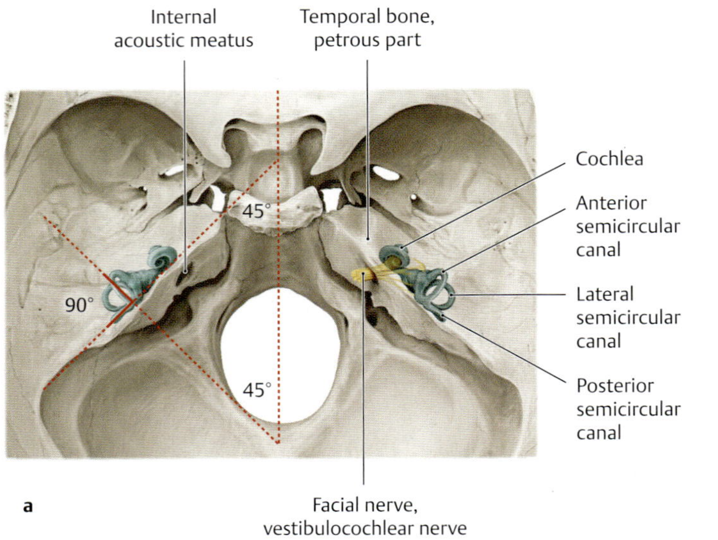

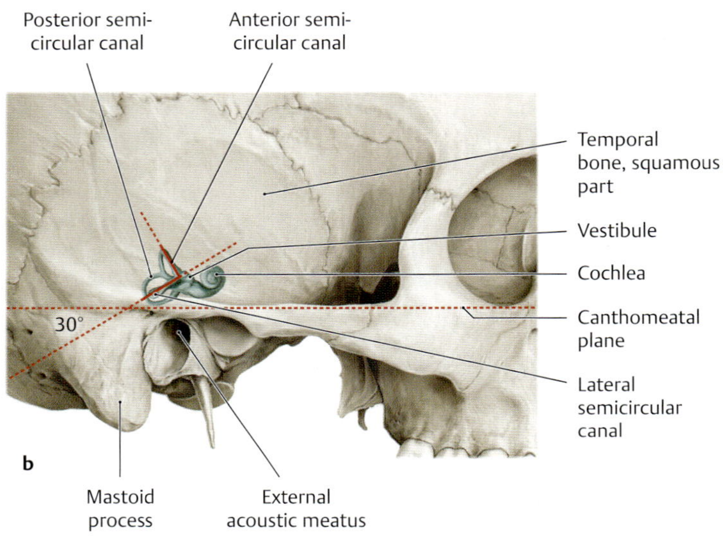

B Projection of the inner ear onto the bony skull

a Superior view of the petrous part of the temporal bone. **b** Right lateral view of the squamous part of the temporal bone.

The apex of the cochlea is directed anteriorly and laterally—not upward as might be intuitively expected. The bony semicircular canals are oriented at an approximately 45° angle to the cardinal body planes (coronal, transverse, and sagittal). It is important to know this arrangement when interpreting thin-slice CT scans of the petrous bone.

Note: The location of the semicircular canals is of clinical importance in thermal function tests of the vestibular apparatus. The lateral (horizontal) semicircular canal is directed 30° forward and upward (see **b**). If the head of the supine patient is elevated by 30°, the horizontal semicircular canal will assume a vertical alignment. Since warm fluids tend to rise, irrigating the auditory canal with warm (44° C) or cool (30° C) water (relative to the normal body temperature) can induce a thermal current in the endolymph of the semicircular canal, causing the patient to manifest vestibular nystagmus (jerky eye movements, vestibulo-ocular reflex). Because head movements always stimulate both vestibular apparatuses, caloric testing is the only method of *separately* testing the function of each vestibular apparatus (important in the diagnosis of unexplained vertigo).

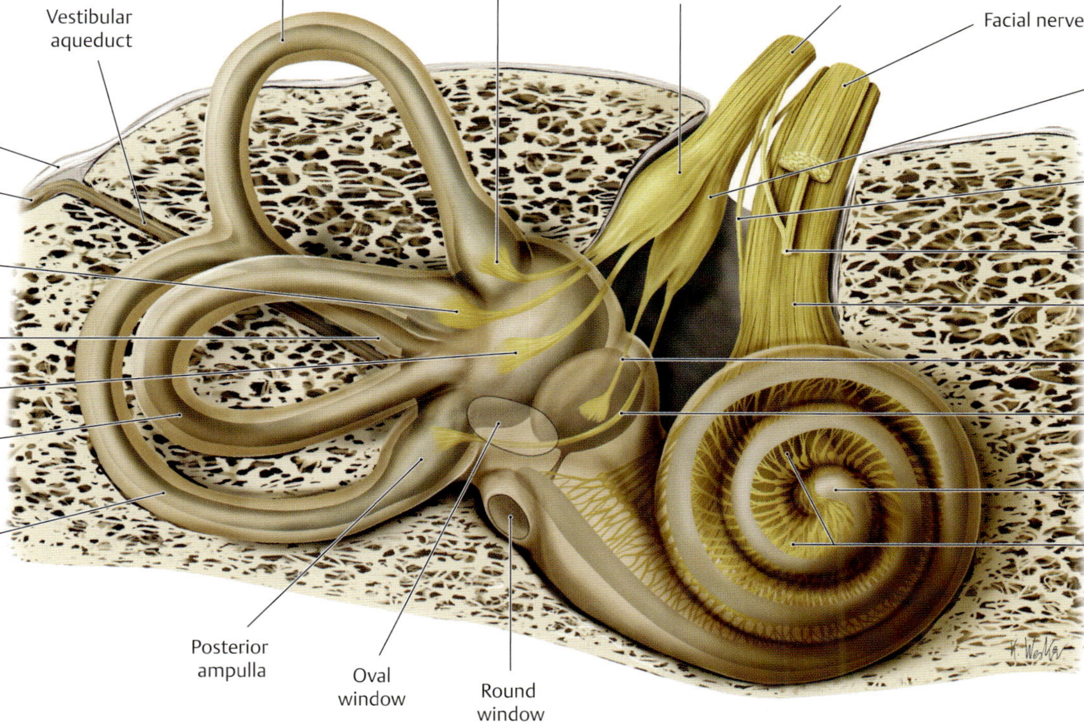

C Innervation of the membranous labyrinth

Right ear, anterior view. **Afferent impulses** from the receptor organs of the utricle, saccule, and semicircular canals (i.e., the **vestibular apparatus**) are first relayed by dendritic (peripheral) processes to the two-part *vestibular ganglion* (superior and inferior parts), which contains the cell bodies of the afferent neurons (bipolar ganglion cells). Their central processes form the *vestibular part* of the *vestibulocochlear nerve* through the internal acoustic meatus and the cerebellopontine angle to the brainstem. **Afferent impulses** from the receptor organs of the cochlea (i.e., the **auditory apparatus**) are first transmitted by dendritic (peripheral) processes to the *spiral ganglia,* which contain the cell bodies of the bipolar ganglion cells. They are located in the central bony core of the cochlea (modiolus). Their central processes form the *cochlear* part of the *vestibulocochlear nerve*.

Note also the section of the facial nerve with its parasympathetic fibers (nervus intermedius) within the internal auditory canal (see **D**).

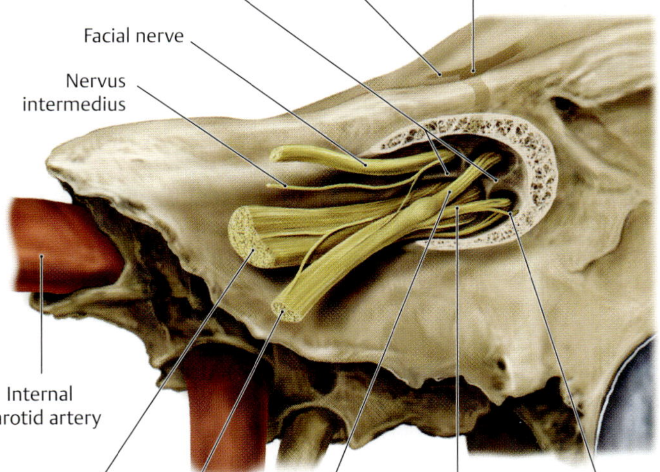

D Passage of cranial nerves through the right internal acoustic meatus

Posterior oblique view of the fundus of the internal acoustic meatus. The approximately 1 cm long internal auditory canal begins at the internal acoustic meatus on the posterior wall of the petrous bone. It contains

- the vestibulocochlear nerve with its cochlear and vestibular parts,
- the markedly thinner facial nerve with its parasympathetic fibers (nervus intermedius), and
- the labyrinthine artery and vein (not shown).

Given the close proximity of the vestibulocochlear nerve and facial nerve in the bony canal, a tumor of the vestibulocochlear nerve (*acoustic neuroma*) may exert pressure on the facial nerve, leading to peripheral facial paralysis (see also p. 125). Acoustic neuroma is a benign tumor that originates from the Schwann cells of vestibular fibers, and so it would be more accurate to call it a *vestibular schwannoma* (see also p. 128). Tumor growth always begins in the internal auditory canal; as the tumor enlarges it may grow into the cerebellopontine angle. Acute, unilateral inner ear dysfunction with hearing loss (sudden sensorineural hearing loss), often accompanied by tinnitus, typically reflects an underlying vascular disturbance (vasospasm of the labyrinthine artery causing decreased blood flow).

5.6 Ear: Auditory Apparatus

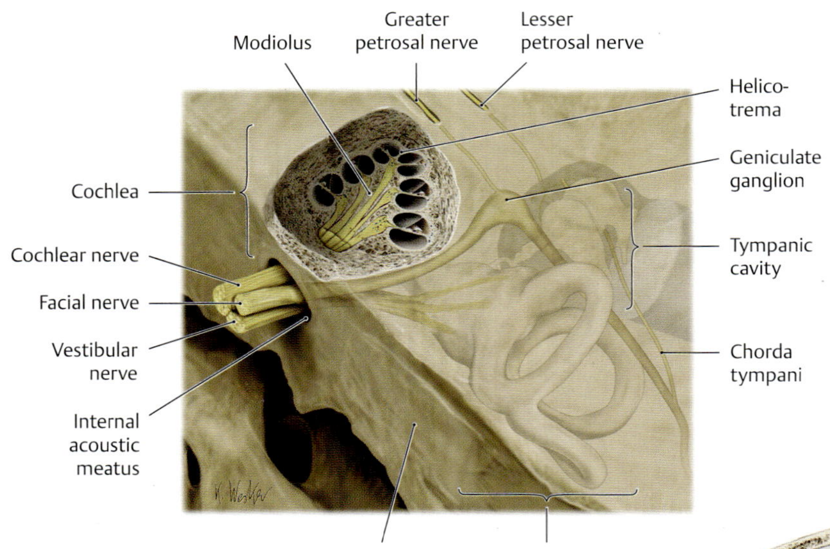

a

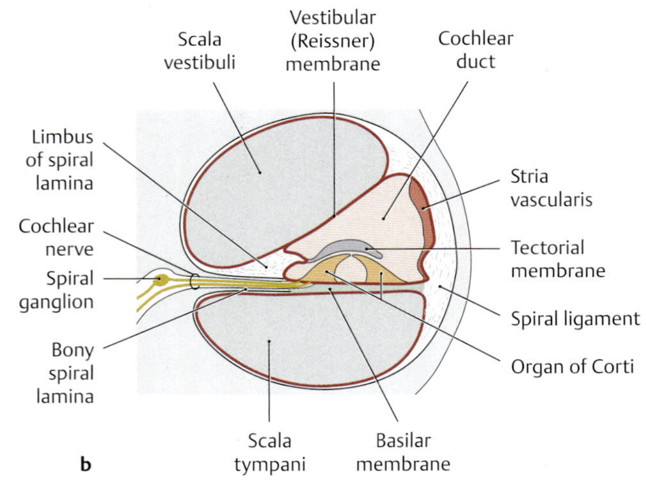

b

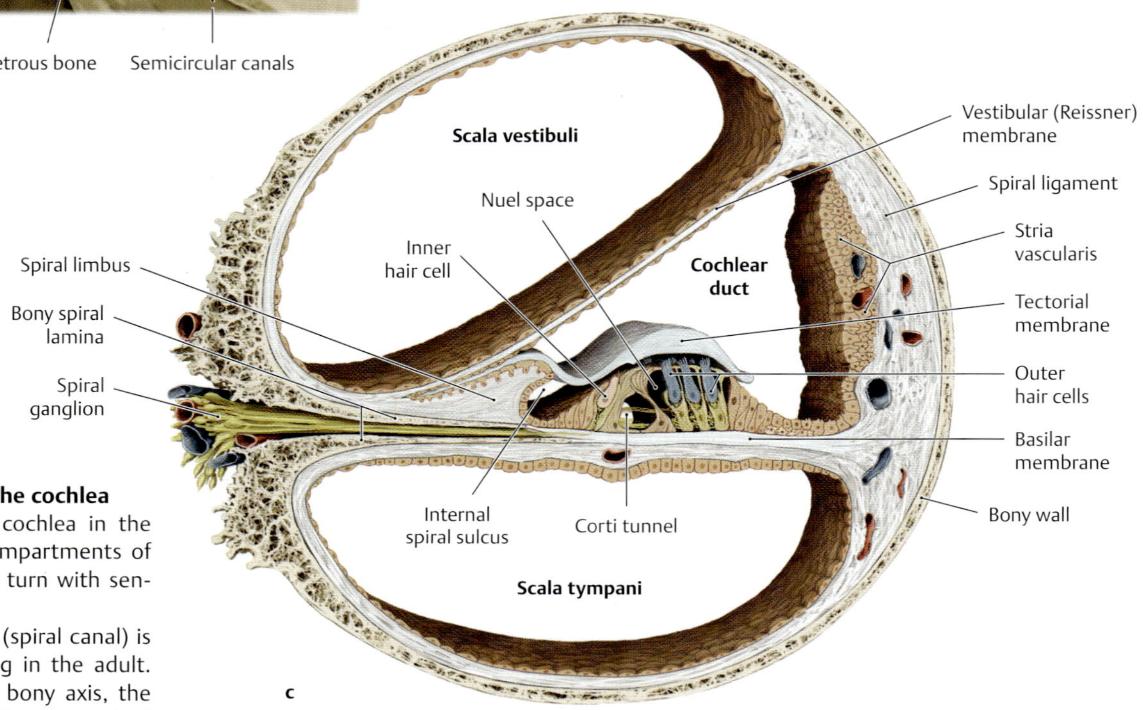

c

A Location and structure of the cochlea
a Cross-section through the cochlea in the petrous bone. **b** The three compartments of the cochlear canal. **c** Cochlear turn with sensory apparatus.

The bony canal of the cochlea (spiral canal) is approximately 30–35 mm long in the adult. It makes 2½ turns around its bony axis, the *modiolus,* which is permeated by branched cavities and contains the spiral ganglion (cell bodies of the afferent neurons). The base of the cochlea is directed toward the internal acoustic meatus (**a**). A cross-section through the cochlear canal displays three membranous compartments arranged in three levels (**b**). The upper and lower compartments, the *scala vestibuli and scala tympani,* each contain perilymph, while the middle level, the *cochlear duct* (scala media), contains endolymph. The perilymphatic spaces are interconnected at the apex by the *helicotrema,* while the endolymphatic space ends blindly at the apex. The cochlear duct, which is triangular in cross-section, is separated from the scala vestibuli by the *vestibular (Reissner) membrane* and from the scala tympani by the *basilar membrane.* The basilar membrane represents a bony projection of the modiolus (*spiral lamina*) and widens steadily from the base of the cochlea to the apex. High frequencies (up to 20,000 Hz) are perceived by the narrow portions of the basilar membrane while low frequencies (down to about 200 Hz) are perceived by its broader portions (*tonotopic organization*). The basilar membrane and bony spiral lamina form the floor of the cochlear duct, upon which the actual organ of hearing, the organ of Corti, is located. This organ consists of a system of sensory cells and supporting cells covered by an acellular gelatinous flap, the *tectorial membrane.* The sensory cells (inner and outer hair cells) are the receptors of the organ of Corti (**c**). These cells bear approximately 50–100 stereocilia, and on their apical surface synapse on their basal side with the endings of afferent and efferent neurons. They have the ability to transform mechanical energy into electrochemical potentials (see below). A magnified cross-sectional view of a cochlear turn (**c**) also reveals the stria *vascularis,* a layer of vascularized epithelium in which the endolymph is formed. This endolymph fills the membranous labyrinth (appearing here as the cochlear duct, which is part of the labyrinth). The organ of Corti is located on the basilar membrane. It transforms the energy of the acoustic traveling wave into electrical impulses, which are then carried to the brain by the cochlear nerve. The principal cell of signal transduction is the inner hair cell. The function of the basilar membrane is to transmit acoustic waves to the inner hair cell, which transforms them into impulses that are received and relayed by the cochlear ganglion.

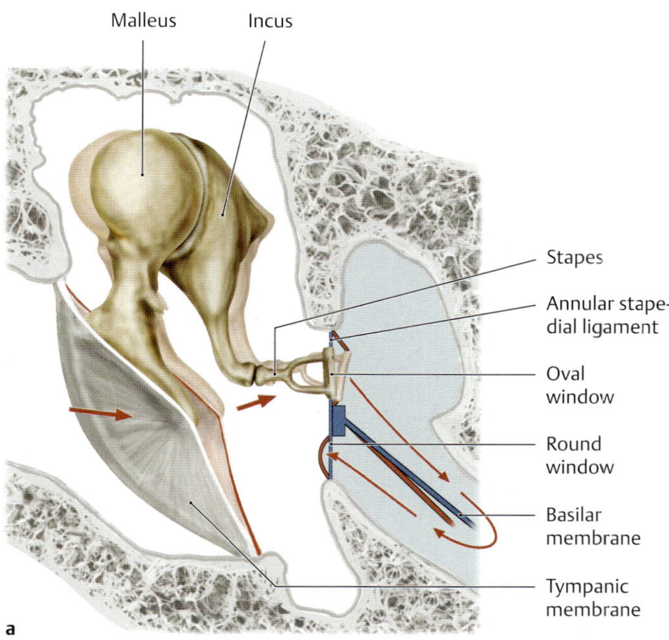

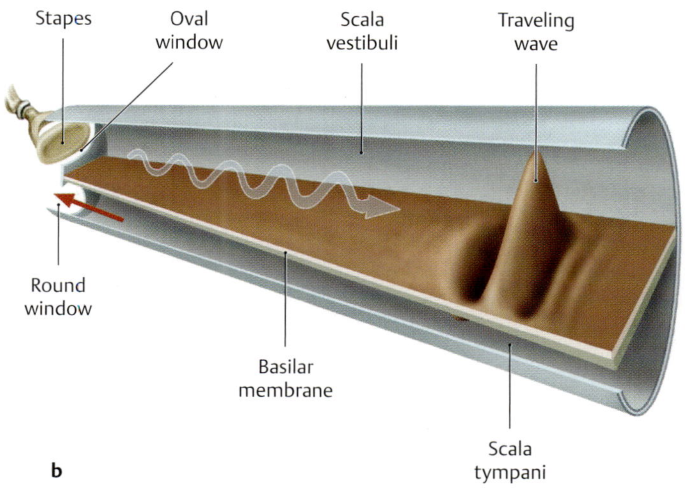

B Sound conduction during hearing

a Sound conduction from the middle ear to the inner ear: Sound waves in the air deflect the tympanic membrane, whose vibrations are conducted by the ossicular chain to the oval window. The sound pressure induces motion of the oval window membrane, whose vibrations are in turn, transmitted through the perilymph to the basilar membrane of the inner ear (see **b**). The round window equalizes pressures between the middle and inner ear.

b Formation of a traveling wave in the cochlea: The sound wave begins at the oval window and travels up the scala vestibuli to the apex of the cochlea ("traveling wave"). The amplitude of the traveling wave gradually increases as a function of the sound frequency and reaches a maximum value at particular sites (shown greatly exaggerated in the drawing). These are the sites where the receptors of the organ of Corti are stimulated and signal transduction occurs. To understand this process, one must first grasp the structure of the organ of Corti (the actual organ of hearing), which is depicted in **C**.

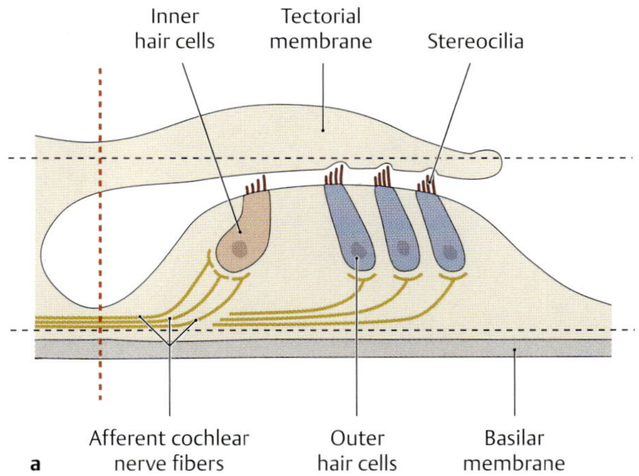

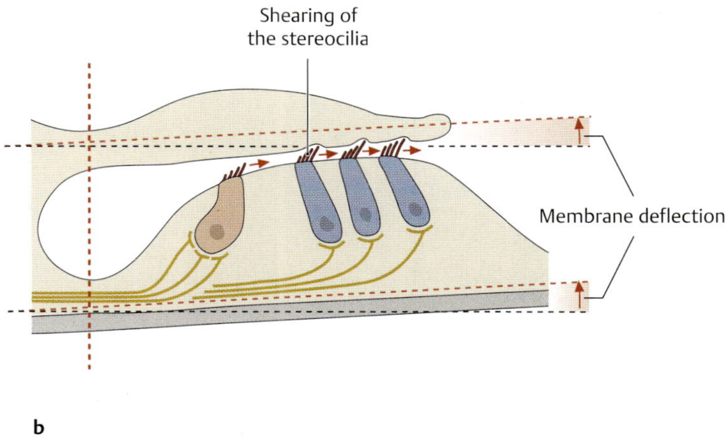

C Organ of Corti at rest (a) and deflected by a traveling wave (b)
The traveling wave is generated by vibrations of the oval window membrane (cf. **Bb**). At each site that is associated with a particular sound frequency, the traveling wave causes a maximum deflection of the basilar membrane and in turn of the tectorial membrane, setting up shearing movements between the two membranes. These shearing movements cause the stereocilia on the *outer* hair cells to bend. In response, the hair cells actively change their length, thereby increasing the local amplitude of the traveling wave. This additionally bends the stereocilia of the *inner* hair cells, stimulating the release of glutamate at their basal pole. The release of this substance generates an excitatory potential on the afferent nerve fibers, which is transmitted to the brain.

5.7 Inner Ear: Vestibular Apparatus

A Structure of the vestibular apparatus

The vestibular apparatus is the organ of balance. It consists of the membranous semicircular ducts, which contain sensory ridges (ampullary crests) in their dilated portions (ampullae), and of the saccule and utricle with their macular organs (their location in the petrous bone is shown in **B**, p. 150). The sensory organs in the semicircular ducts respond to *angular acceleration* while the macular organs, which have an approximately vertical and horizontal orientation, respond to horizontal (utricular macula) and vertical (saccular macula) *linear acceleration*, as well as to gravitational forces.

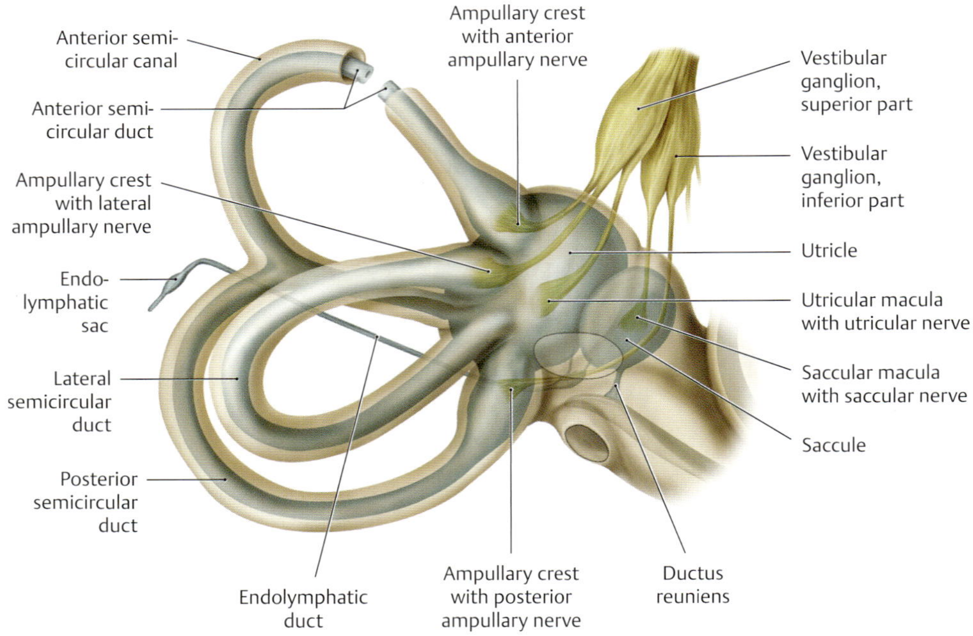

B Structure of the ampulla and ampullary crest

Cross-section through the ampulla of a semicircular canal. Each canal has a bulbous expansion at one end (ampulla) that is traversed by a connective tissue ridge with sensory epithelium (ampullary crest). Extending above the ampullary crest is a gelatinous cupula, which is attached to the roof of the ampulla. Each of the sensory cells of the ampullary crest (approximately 7,000 in all) exhibits one long kinocilium and approximately 80 shorter stereocilia on their apical pole, which project into the cupula. When the head is rotated in the plane of a particular semicircular canal, the inertial lag of the endolymph causes a deflection of the cupula, which in turn causes a bowing of the stereocilia. The sensory cells are either depolarized (excitation) or hyperpolarized (inhibition), depending on the direction of ciliary displacement (see details in **E**).

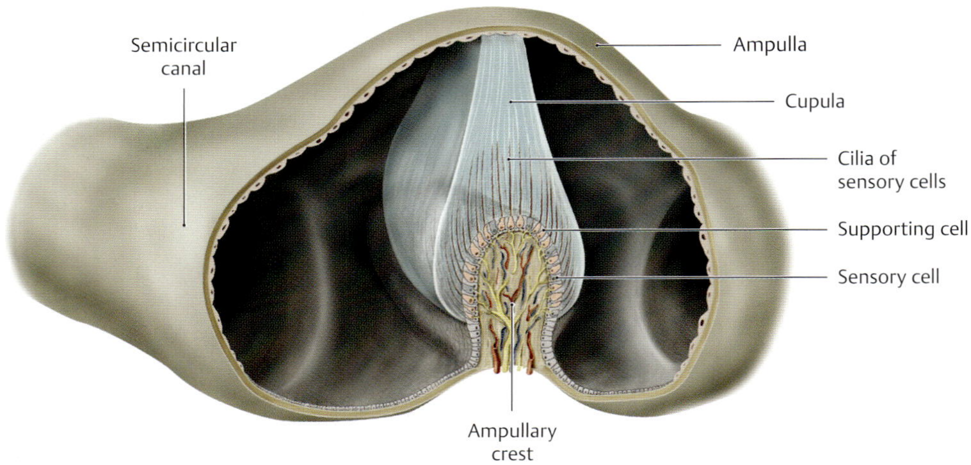

C Structure of the utricular and saccular maculae

The maculae are thickened oval areas in the epithelial lining of the utricle and saccule, each averaging 2 mm in diameter and containing arrays of sensory and supporting cells. Like the sensory cells of the ampullary crest, those of the macular organs bear specialized stereocilia, which project into an otolithic membrane. The latter consists of a gelatinous layer, similar to the cupula, but it has calcium carbonate crystals or otoliths (*statoliths*) embedded in its surface. With their high specific gravity, these crystals exert traction on the gelatinous mass in response to linear acceleration, and this induces shearing movements of the cilia. The sensory cells are either depolarized or hyperpolarized by the movement, depending on the orientation of the cilia. There are two distinct categories of vestibular hair cells (type I and type II); type I cells (light red) are goblet-shaped.

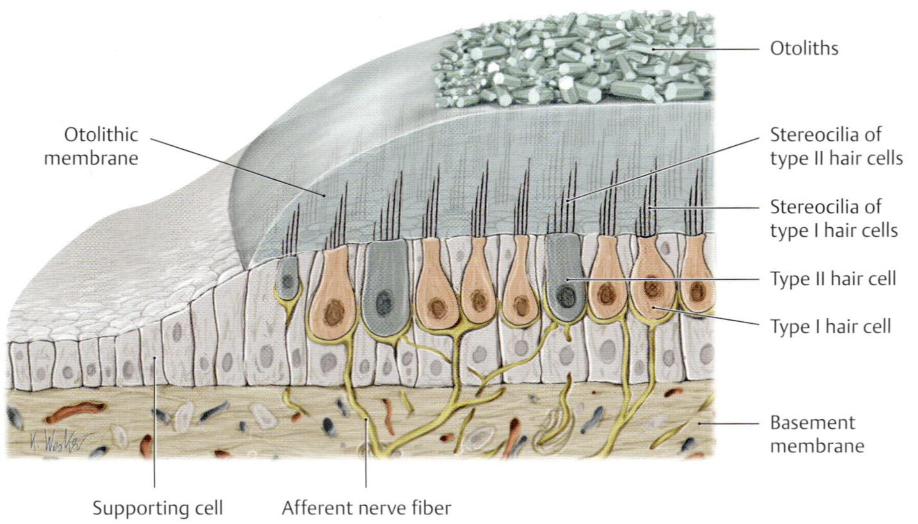

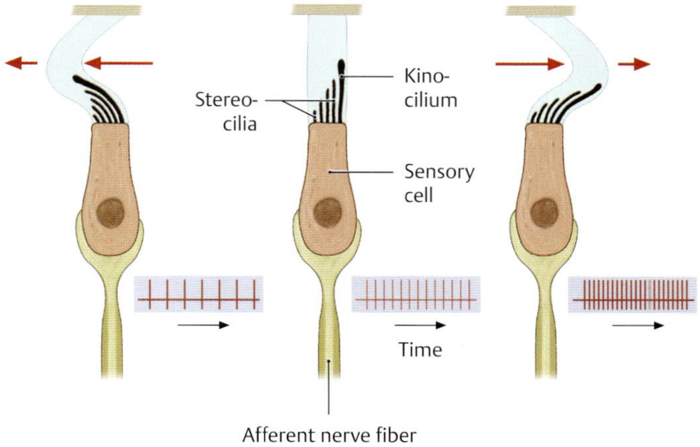

D Stimulus transduction in the vestibular sensory cells

Each of the sensory cells of the maculae and ampullary crest bears on its apical surface one long kinocilium and approximately 80 stereocilia of graduated lengths, forming an array that resembles a pipe organ. This arrangement results in a polar differentiation of the sensory cells. The cilia are straight while in a resting state. When the stereocilia are deflected toward the kinocilium, the sensory cell depolarizes and the frequency of action potentials (discharge rate of impulses) is increased (right side of diagram). When the stereocilia are deflected away from the kinocilium, the cell hyperpolarizes and the discharge rate is decreased (left side of diagram). This mechanism regulates the release of the transmitter glutamate at the basal pole of the sensory cell, thereby controlling the activation of the afferent nerve fiber (depolarization stimulates glutamate release, and hyperpolarization inhibits it). In this way the brain receives information on the magnitude and direction of movements and changes of position.

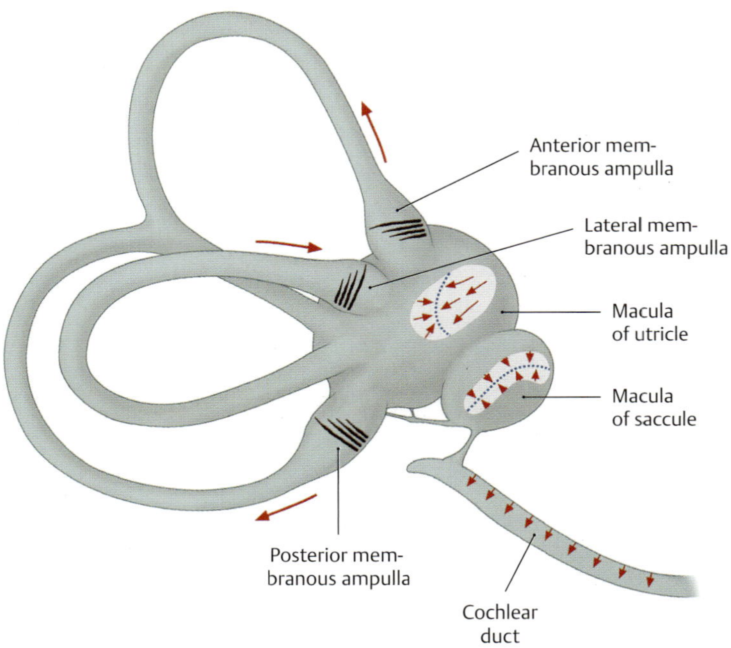

E Specialized orientations of the stereocilia in the vestibular apparatus (ampullary crest and maculae)

Because the stimulation of the sensory cells by deflection of the stereocilia *away from* or *toward* the kinocilium is what initiates signal transduction, the spatial orientation of the cilia must be specialized to ensure that every position in space and every movement of the head stimulates or inhibits certain receptors. The ciliary arrangement shown here ensures that every direction in space will correlate with the maximum sensitivity of a particular receptor field. The arrows indicate the polarity of the cilia (i.e., each of the arrowheads points in the direction of the kinocilium in that particular field).

Note that the sensory cells show an opposite, reciprocal arrangement in the sensory fields of the utricle and saccule.

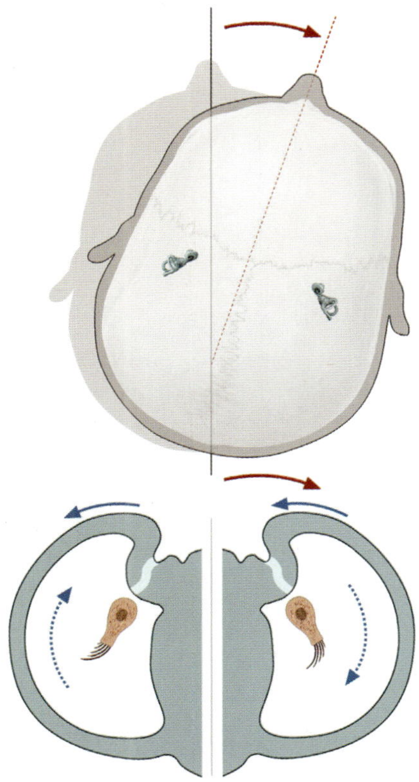

F Interaction of contralateral semicircular canals during head rotation

When the head rotates to the right (red arrow), the endolymph flows to the left because of its inertial mass (solid blue arrow, taking the head as the reference point). Owing to the alignment of the stereocilia, the left and right semicircular ducts are stimulated in opposite fashion. On the right side, the stereocilia are deflected toward the kinocilium (dotted arrow; the discharge rate increases). On the left side, the stereocilia are deflected away from the kinocilium (dotted arrow; the discharge rate decreases). This arrangement heightens the sensitivity to stimuli by increasing the stimulus contrast between the two sides. The difference between the decreased firing rate on one side and the increased firing rate on the other side enhances the perception of the kinetic stimulus.

5.8 Ear: Blood Supply

A Origin of the principal arteries of the tympanic cavity

Except for the caroticotympanic arteries, which arise from the petrous part of the internal carotid artery, all of the vessels that supply blood to the tympanic cavity arise from the external carotid artery. The vessels have many anastomoses with one another and reach the auditory ossicles, for example, through folds of mucosa. The ossicles are also traversed by intraosseous vessels.

Artery	Origin	Distribution
Caroticotympanic arteries	Internal carotid artery	Pharyngotympanic (auditory) tube and anterior wall of the tympanic cavity
Stylomastoid artery	Posterior auricular artery	Posterior wall of the tympanic cavity, mastoid air cells, stapedius muscle, stapes
Inferior tympanic artery	Ascending pharyngeal artery	Floor of the tympanic cavity, promontory
Deep auricular artery	Maxillary artery	Tympanic membrane, floor of the tympanic cavity
Posterior tympanic artery	Stylomastoid artery (alternatively: posterior auricular artery, see **Ab**, p. 98)	Chorda tympani, tympanic membrane, malleus
Superior tympanic artery	Middle meningeal artery	Tensor tympani, roof of the tympanic cavity, stapes
Anterior tympanic artery	Maxillary artery	Tympanic membrane, mastoid antrum, malleus, incus

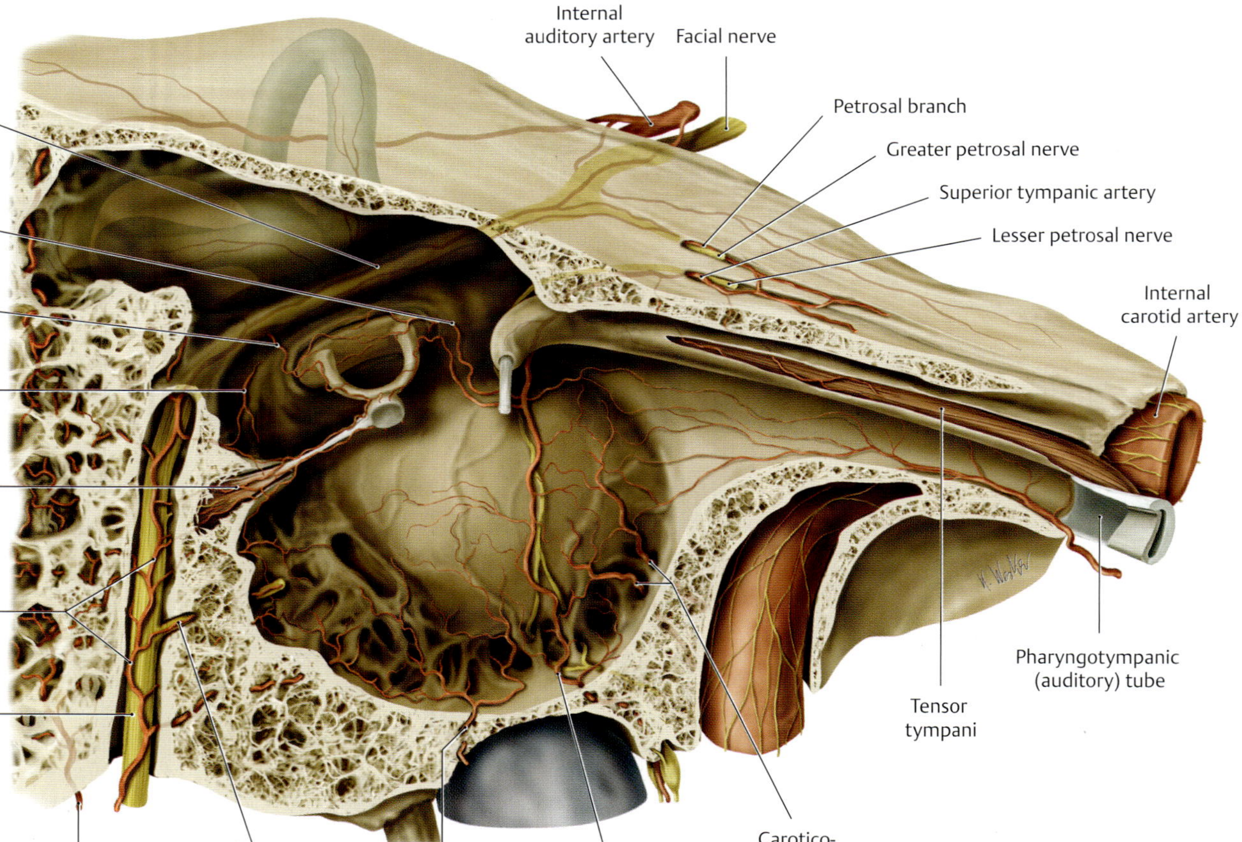

B Arteries of the tympanic cavity and mastoid air cells

Petrous portion of the right temporal bone, lateral oblique view. The malleus, incus, portions of the chorda tympani, and the anterior tympanic artery have been removed.

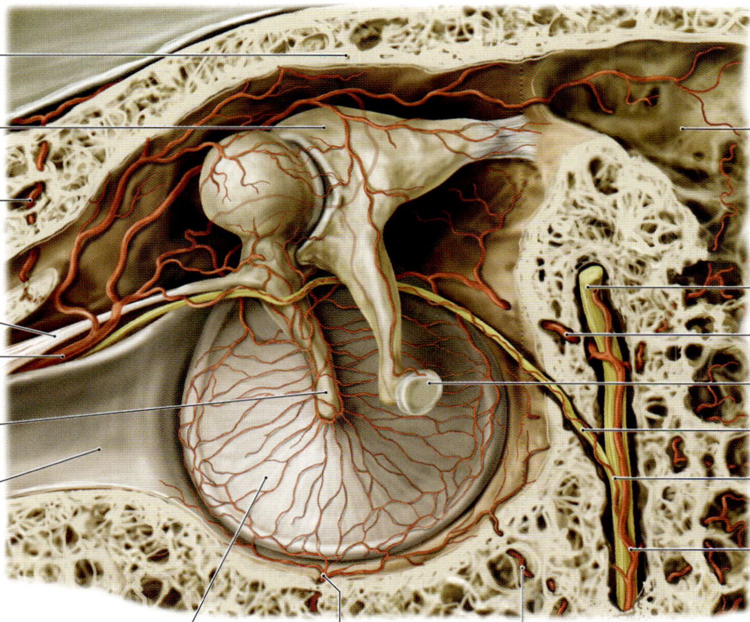

C Vascular supply of the ossicular chain and tympanic membrane
Medial view of the right tympanic membrane. This region receives most of its blood supply from the anterior tympanic artery. With inflammation of the tympanic membrane, the arteries may become so dilated that their course in the tympanic membrane can be seen, as illustrated here.

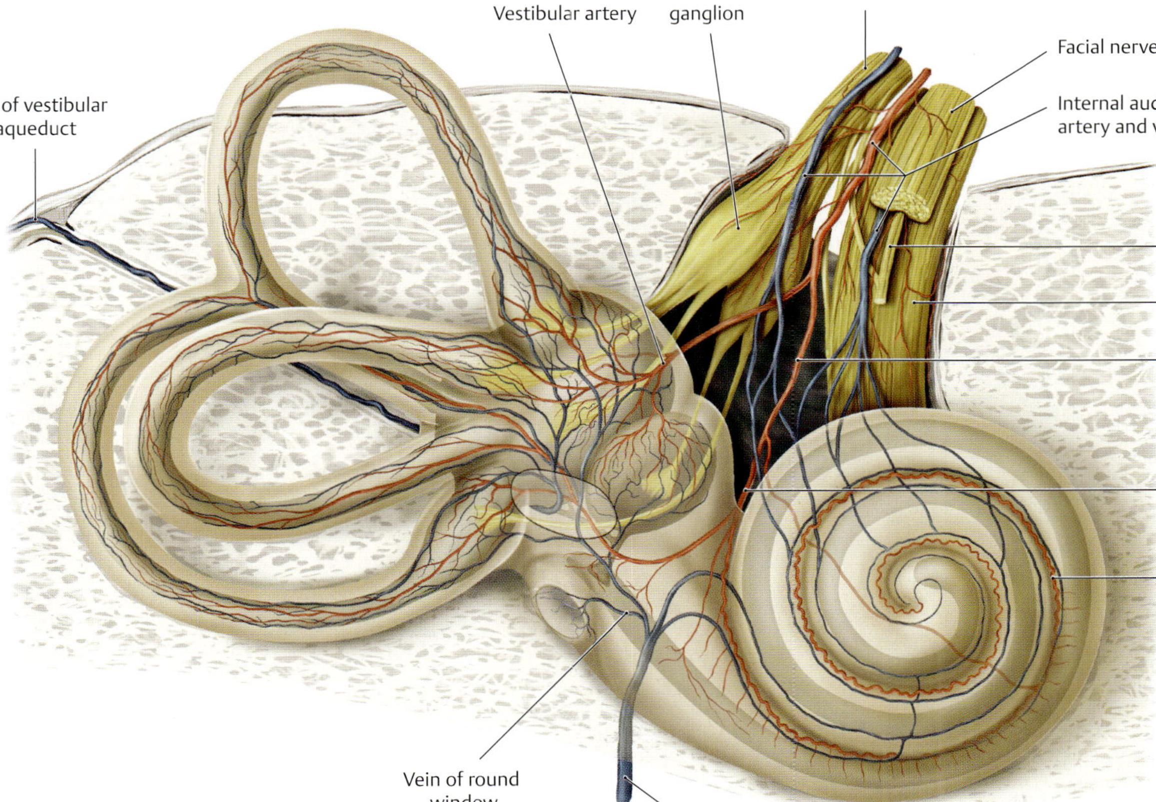

D Blood supply of the labyrinth
Right anterior view. The labyrinth receives all of its arterial blood supply from the internal auditory artery, a branch of the anterior inferior cerebellar artery. The labyrinthine artery occasionally arises directly from the basilar artery.

5.9 Eye: Orbital Region, Eyelids, and Conjunctiva

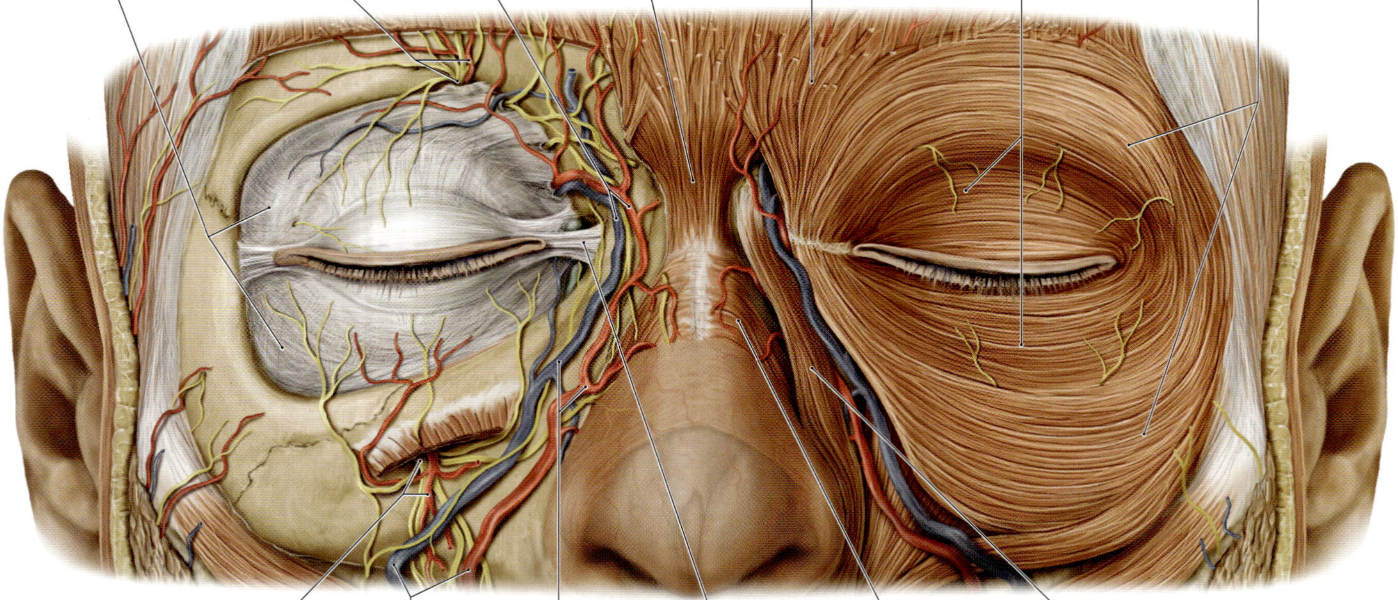

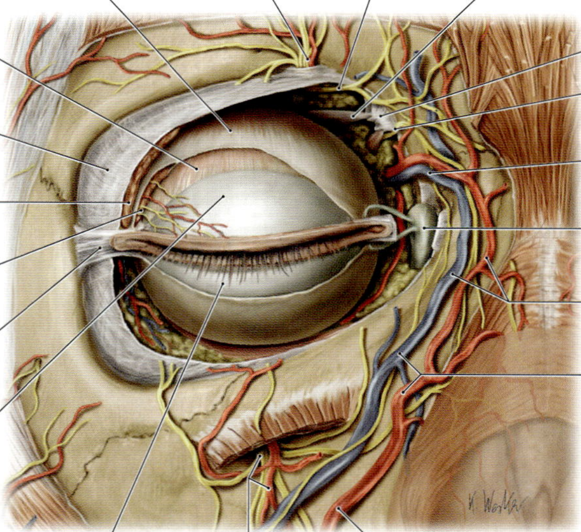

A Superficial and deep neurovascular structures of the orbital region

Right eye, anterior view.

a Superficial layer. The orbital septum on the right side has been exposed by removal of the orbicularis oculi. **b** Deep layer. Anterior orbital structures have been exposed by partial removal of the orbital septum.

The regions supplied by the *internal* carotid artery (supraorbital artery) and *external* carotid artery (infraorbital artery, facial artery) meet in this region. The anastomosis between the angular vein (extracranial) and superior ophthalmic veins (intracranial) creates a portal of entry by which microorganisms may reach the cavernous sinus (risk of sinus thrombosis, meningitis); therefore it is sometimes necessary to ligate this anastomosis in the orbital region, in patients with extensive infections of the external facial region (see p. 227).

Note the passage of the supra- and infraorbital nerves (branches of CN V1 and CN V2) through the foramina of the same name. The sensory function of these two trigeminal nerve divisions can be tested at these nerve exit points.

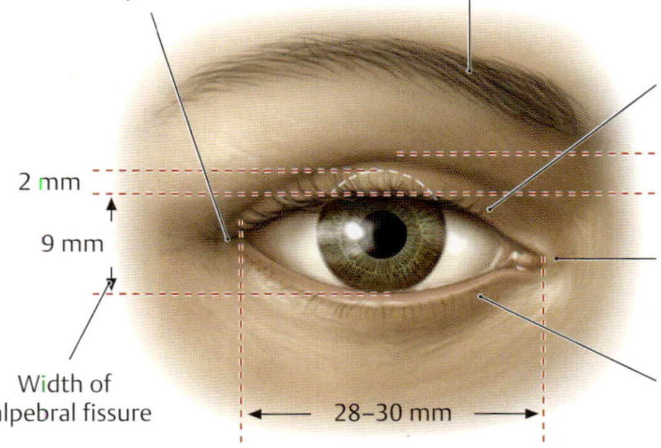

B Surface anatomy of the eye

Right eye, anterior view. The measurements indicate the width of the normal palpebral fissure. It is important to know these measurements because there are a number of diseases in which they are altered. For example, the palpebral fissure may be widened in peripheral facial paralysis or narrowed in ptosis (drooping of the eyelid) due to oculomotor palsy.

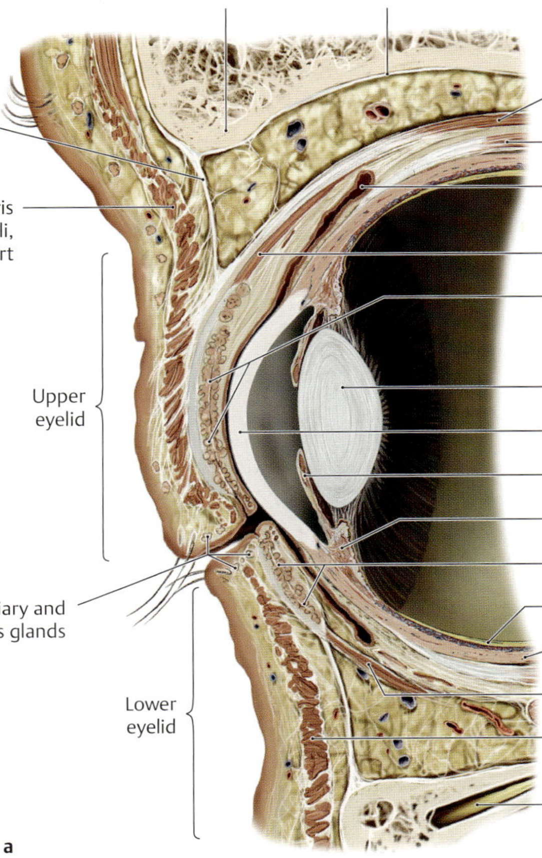

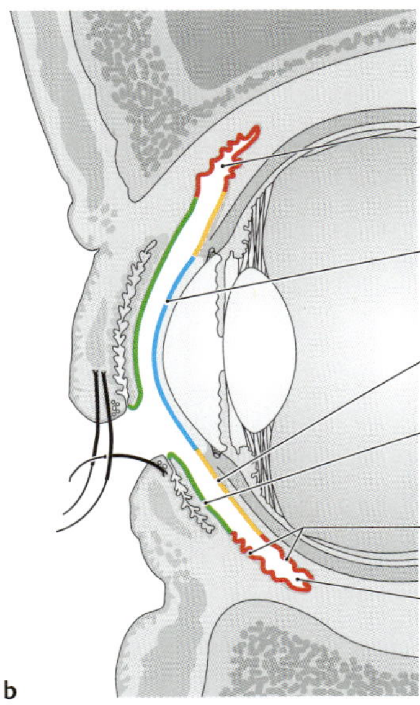

C Structure of the eyelids and conjunctiva

a Sagittal section through the anterior orbital cavity. **b** Anatomy of the conjunctiva.

The **eyelid** consists clinically of an outer and an inner layer with the following components:

- Outer layer: palpebral skin, sweat glands, ciliary glands (modified sweat glands, Moll glands), sebaceous glands (Zeis glands), and two skeletal muscles, the orbicularis oculi and levator palpebrae (upper eyelid only), innervated by the facial nerve and the oculomotor nerve, respectively.
- Inner layer: the tarsus (fibrous connective tissue plate), the superior and inferior tarsal muscles (of Müller; *smooth* muscle innervated by sympathetic fibers), the tarsal or palpebral conjunctiva, and the tarsal glands (Meibomian glands).

Regular blinking (20–30 times per minute) keeps the eyes from drying out by evenly distributing the lacrimal fluid and glandular secretions (see p. 161). Mechanical irritants (e.g., grains of sand) evoke the *blink reflex*, which also serves to protect the cornea and **conjunctiva**. The conjunctiva (tunica conjunctiva) is a vascularized, thin, serous mucous membrane that is subdivided into the *palpebral conjunctiva* (see above), *fornical conjunctiva*, and *ocular conjunctiva*. The ocular conjunctiva borders directly on the corneal surface and combines with it to form the **conjunctival sac**, whose functions include

- facilitating ocular movements,
- enabling painless motion of the palpebral conjunctiva and ocular conjunctiva relative to each other (lubricated by lacrimal fluid), and
- protecting against infectious pathogens (collections of lymphocytes along the fornices).

The superior and inferior fornices are the sites where the conjunctiva is reflected from the upper and lower eyelid, respectively, onto the eyeball. They are convenient sites for the instillation of ophthalmic medications. *Inflammation of the conjunctiva* is common and causes a dilation of the conjunctival vessels resulting in "pink eye." Conversely, a deficiency of red blood cells (anemia) may lessen the prominence of vascular markings in the conjunctiva. This is why the conjunctiva should be routinely inspected in every clinical examination.

5.10 Eye: Lacrimal Apparatus

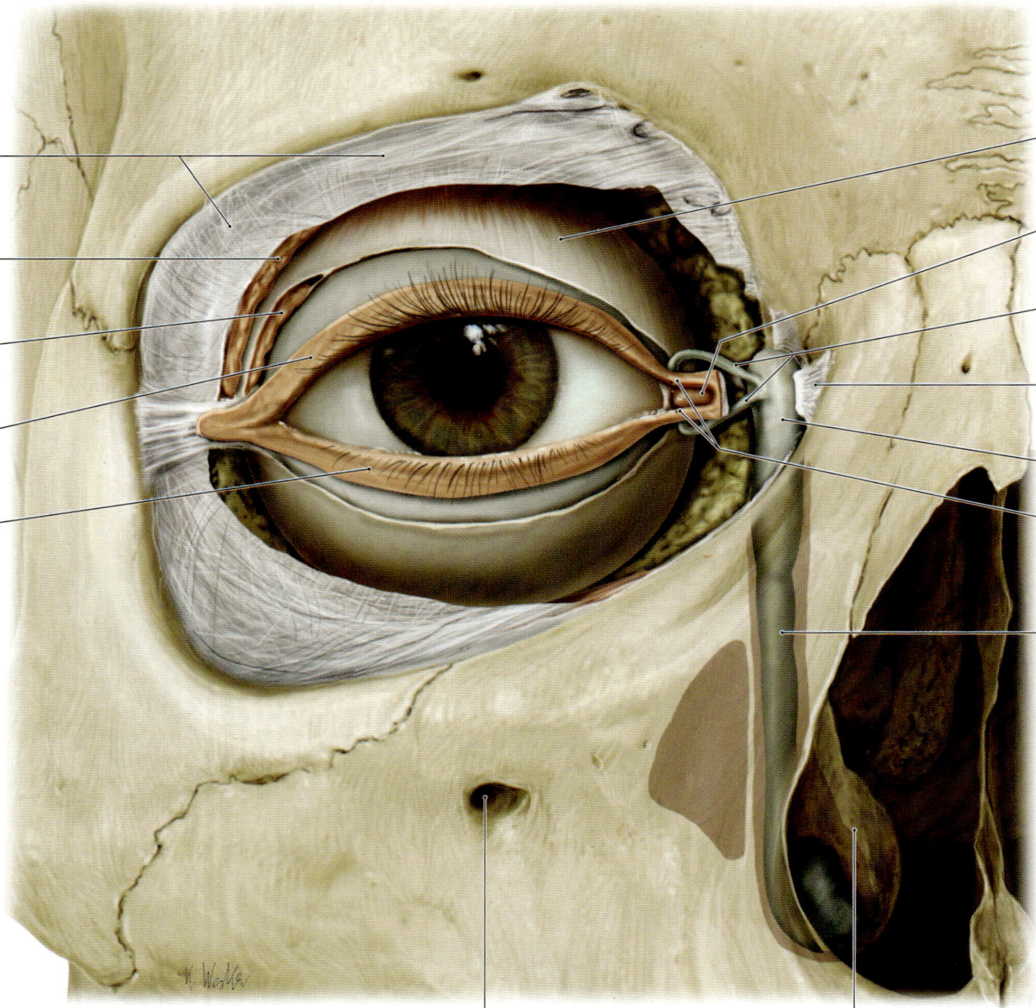

A Lacrimal apparatus

Right eye, anterior view. The orbital septum has been partially removed, and the tendon of insertion of the levator palpebrae superioris has been divided. The hazelnut-sized **lacrimal gland** is located in the lacrimal fossa of the frontal bone and produces most of the lacrimal fluid. Smaller *accessory lacrimal glands* (Krause or Wolfring glands) are also present. The tendon of levator palpebrae superioris subdivides the lacrimal gland, which normally is not visible or palpable, into an *orbital lobe* (two-thirds of gland) and a *palpebral lobe* (one-third). The sympathetic fibers innervating the lacrimal gland originate from the superior cervical ganglion and travel along arteries to reach the lacrimal gland. The parasympathetic innervation of the lacrimal gland is complex (see p. 127). The function of the **lacrimal apparatus** can be understood by tracing the flow of lacrimal fluid obliquely from upper temporal (or lateral) to lower nasal (or medial). From the superior and inferior *puncta,* the lacrimal fluid enters the superior and inferior *lacrimal canaliculi,* which direct the fluid into the *lacrimal sac.* Finally it drains through the *nasolacrimal duct* to an outlet below the inferior concha of the nose. "Watery eyes" are a typical cold symptom caused by obstruction of the inferior opening of the nasolacrimal duct.

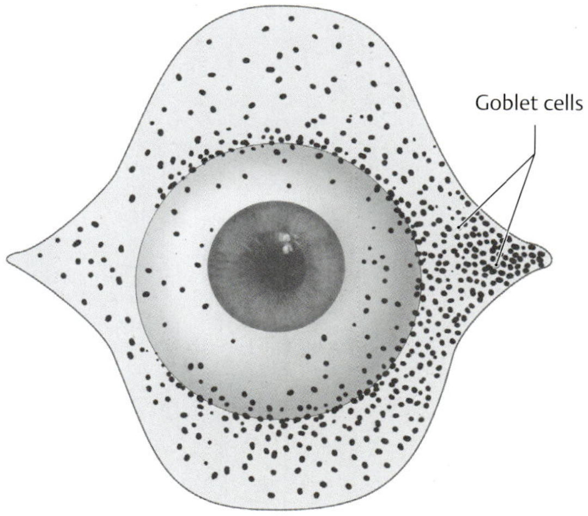

B Distribution of goblet cells in the conjunctiva
Goblet cells are mucous-secreting cells with an epithelial covering. Their secretions (mucins) are an important constituent of the lacrimal fluid (see **C**). Besides the goblet cells, mucins are also secreted by the main lacrimal gland.

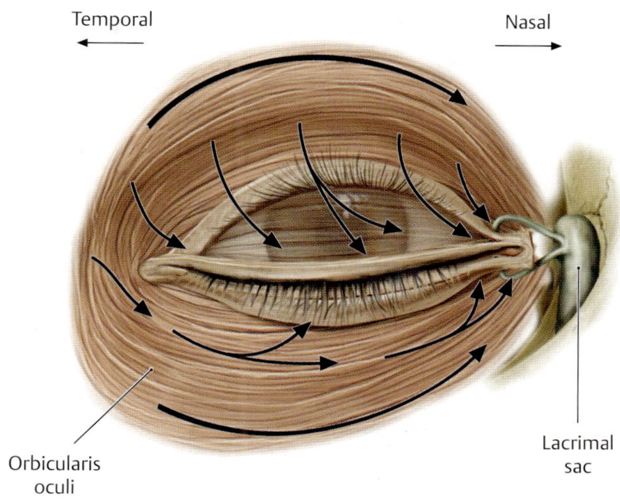

D Mechanical propulsion of the lacrimal fluid
During closure of the eyelids, contraction of the orbicularis oculi proceeds in a temporal-to-nasal direction. The successive contraction of these muscle fibers propels the lacrimal fluid toward the lacrimal passages.
Note: Facial paralysis prevents closure of the eyelids, causing the eye to dry out.

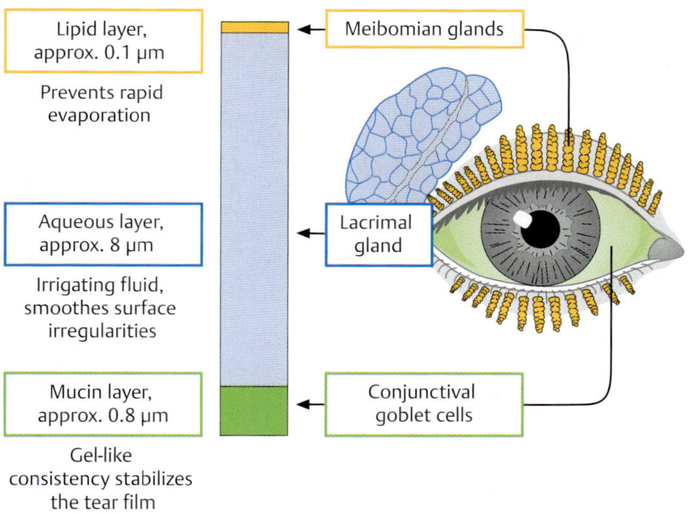

C Structure of the tear film (after Lang)
The tear film is a complex fluid with several morphologically distinct layers, whose components are produced by individual glands. The outer lipid layer, produced by the Meibomian glands, protects the aqueous middle layer of the tear film from evaporating.

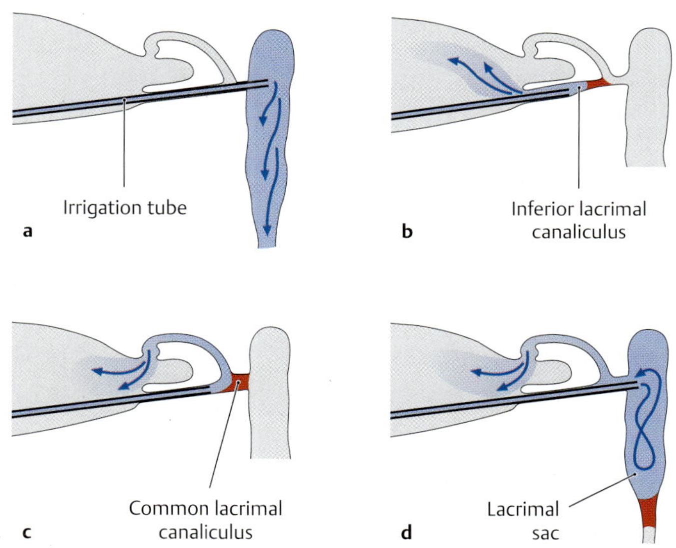

E Obstructions to lacrimal drainage (after Lang)
Sites of obstruction in the lacrimal drainage system can be located by irrigating the system with a special fluid. To make this determination, the examiner must be familiar with the anatomy of the lacrimal apparatus and the normal drainage pathways for lacrimal fluid (see **A**).

a No obstruction to lacrimal drainage (cf. **A**).
b, c Stenosis in the inferior or common lacrimal canaliculus. The stenosis causes a damming back of lacrimal fluid behind the obstructed site. In **b** the fluid refluxes through the inferior lacrimal canaliculus, and in **c** it flows through the superior lacrimal canaliculus.
d Stenosis below the level of the lacrimal sac (postlacrimal sac stenosis). When the entire lacrimal sac has filled with fluid, the fluid begins to reflux into the superior lacrimal canaliculus. In such cases, the lacrimal fluid often has a purulent, gelatinous appearance.

5.11 Eyeball

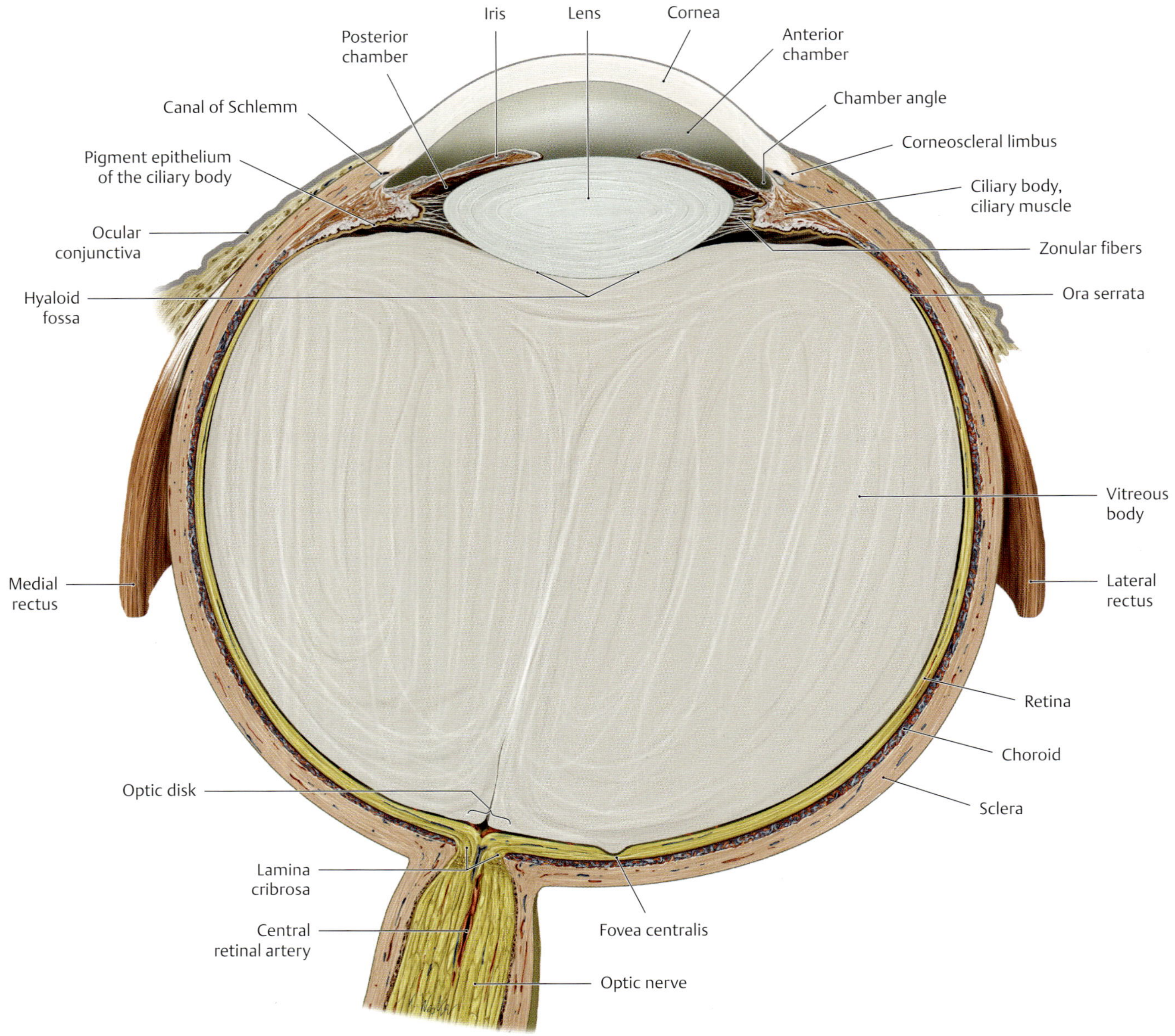

A Transverse section through the eyeball

Right eye, superior view. Most of the eyeball is composed of three concentric layers (from outside to inside): the sclera, choroid, and retina. The anterior portion of the eyeball has a different structure, however. The **outer coat** of the eye in this region is formed by the **cornea** (anterior portion of the fibrous coat). As the "window of the eye," it bulges forward while covering the structures behind it. At the corneoscleral limbus, the cornea is continuous with the less convex **sclera**, which is the posterior portion of the outer coat of the eyeball. It is a firm layer of connective tissue that gives attachment to the tendons of all the extraocular muscles. Anteriorly, the sclera in the angle of the anterior chamber forms the trabecular meshwork (see p. 167), which is connected to the canal of Schlemm. On the posterior side of the eyeball, the axons of the optic nerve pierce the lamina cribrosa of the sclera. Beneath the sclera is the **vascular coat** of the eye, also called the **uveal tract**. It consists of three parts in the anterior portion of the eye: the iris, ciliary body, and choroid, the latter being distributed over the entire eyeball. The iris shields the eye from excessive light (see p. 167) and covers the lens. Its root is continuous with the ciliary body, which contains the ciliary muscle for visual accommodation (alters the refractive power of the lens, see p. 165). The epithelium of the ciliary body produces the aqueous humor. The *ciliary body* is continuous at the ora serrata with the middle layer of the eye, the **choroid**. The choroid organ is the most highly vascularized region in the body and serves to regulate the temperature of the eye and to supply blood to the outer layers of the retina. The **inner layer** of the eye is the **retina**, which includes an inner layer of photosensitive cells (the sensory retina) and an outer layer of retinal pigment epithelium. The latter is continued forward as the pigment epithelium of the ciliary body and the epithelium of the iris. The *fovea centralis* is a depressed area in the central retina that is approximately 4 mm temporal to the optic disk. Incident light is normally focused onto the fovea centralis, which is the site of greatest visual acuity. The interior of the eyeball is occupied by the **vitreous humor** (**vitreous body**, see **C**).

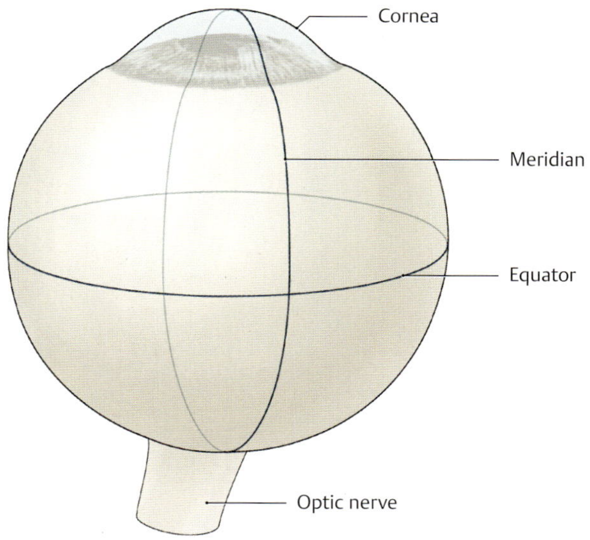

B Reference lines and points on the eye

The line marking the greatest circumference of the eyeball is the *equator.* Lines perpendicular to the equator are called *meridians.*

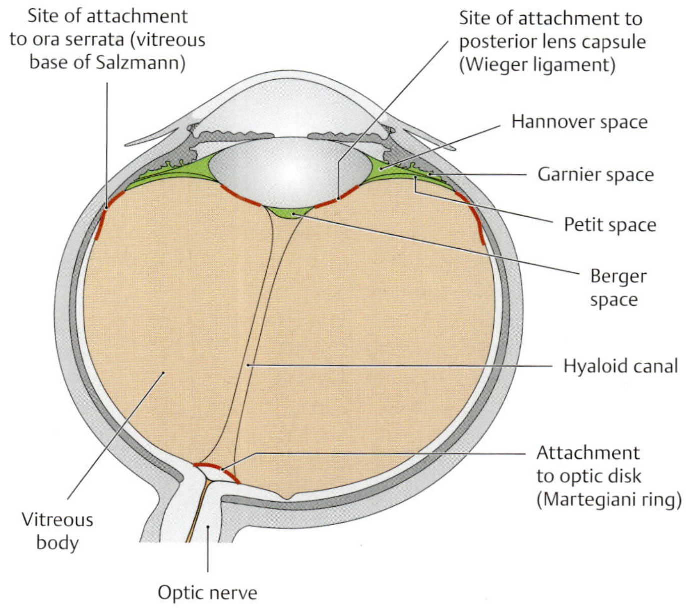

C Vitreous body (vitreous humor) (after Lang)

Right eye, transverse section viewed from above. Sites where the vitreous body is attached to other ocular structures are shown in red, and adjacent spaces are shown in green. The vitreous body stabilizes the eyeball and protects against retinal detachment. Devoid of nerves and vessels, it consists of 98% water and 2% hyaluronic acid and collagen. The "hyaloid canal" is an embryological remnant of the hyaloid artery. For the treatment of some diseases, the vitreous body may be surgically removed (vitrectomy) and the resulting cavity filled with physiological saline solution.

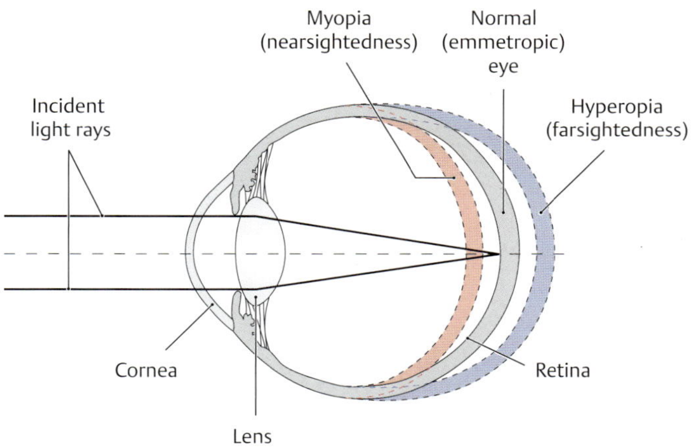

D Light refraction in a normal (emmetropic) eye and in myopia and hyperopia

Parallel rays from a distant light source are normally refracted by the cornea and lens to a focal point on the retinal surface.

- Shortsightedness (myopia, blue): eyeball is too long, the light is focused in front of the retina.
- Farsightedness (hyperopia, red): the eyeball is too short, the light is focused behind the retina

In addition to the ocular anomalies discussed here, myopia and hyperopia can also be the result of other rare causes such as refractive anomalies.

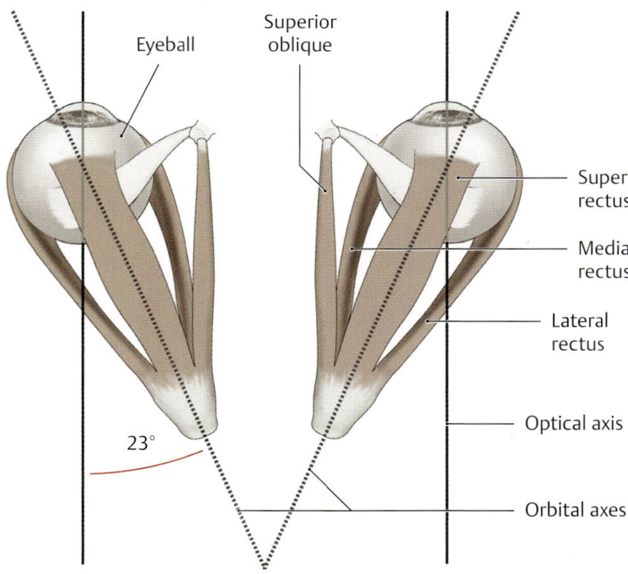

E Optical axis and orbital axis

Superior view of both eyes showing the medial, lateral and superior recti and the superior oblique. The optical axis deviates from the orbital axis by 23°. Because of this disparity, the point of maximum visual acuity, the fovea centralis, is lateral to the "blind spot" of the optic disk (see **A**).

5.12 Eye: Lens and Cornea

A Overview: Position of the lens and cornea in the eyeball
Histological section through the cornea, lens, and suspensory apparatus of the lens. The normal lens is clear and transparent and is only 4 mm thick. It is suspended in the hyaloid fossa of the vitreous body (see p. 162). The lens is attached by rows of fibrils (zonular fibers) to the ciliary muscle, whose contractions alter the shape and focal length of the lens (the structure of the ciliary body is shown in **B**). The lens is a dynamic structure that can change its shape in response to visual requirements (see **Cb**). The anterior chamber of the eye is situated in front of the lens, and the posterior chamber is located between the iris and the anterior epithelium of the lens (see p. 166). The lens, like the vitreous body, is devoid of nerves and blood vessels and is composed of elongated epithelial cells: the lens fibers.

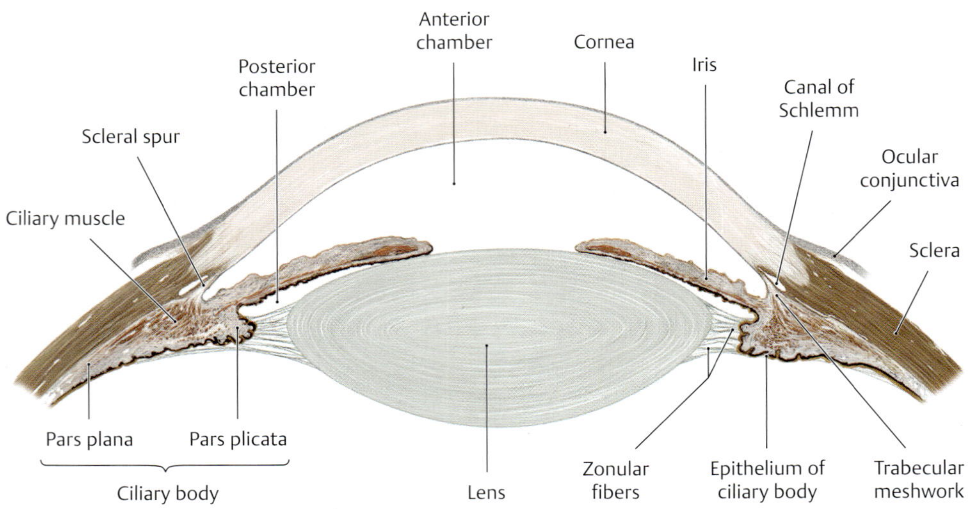

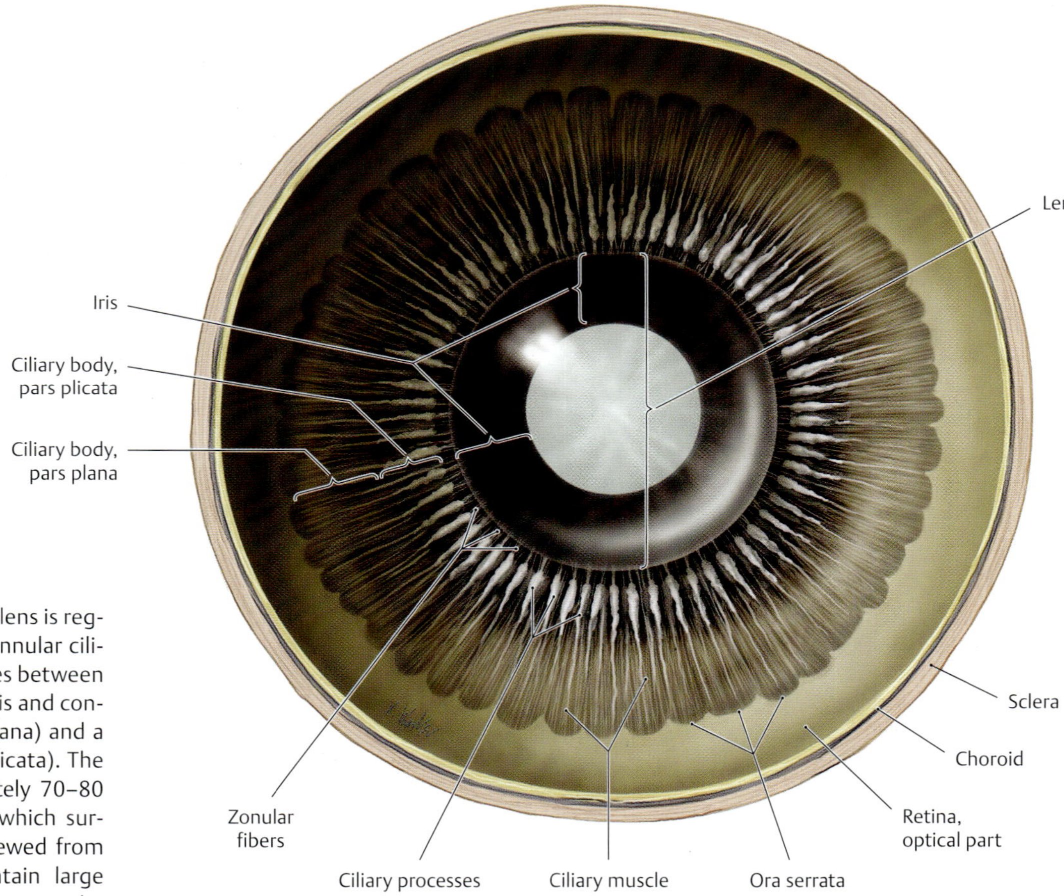

B The lens and ciliary body
Posterior view. The curvature of the lens is regulated by the muscle fibers of the annular ciliary body (see **Cb**). The *ciliary body* lies between the ora serrata and the root of the iris and consists of a relatively flat part (pars plana) and a part that is raised into folds (pars plicata). The latter part is ridged by approximately 70–80 radially oriented ciliary processes, which surround the lens like a halo when viewed from behind. The ciliary processes contain large capillaries, and their epithelium secretes the aqueous humor (see p. 167). Very fine *zonular fibers* extend from the basal layer of the ciliary processes to the equator of the lens. These fibers and the spaces between them constitute the suspensory apparatus of the lens, called the *zonule.* Most of the ciliary body is occupied by the ciliary muscle, a smooth muscle composed of meridional, radial, and circular fibers. It arises mainly from the scleral spur (a reinforcing ring of sclera just below the canal of Schlemm), and it attaches to structures including the Bruch membrane of the choroid and the inner surface of the sclera. When the ciliary muscle contracts, it pulls the choroid forward and relaxes the zonular fibers. As these fibers become lax, the intrinsic resilience of the lens causes it to assume the more convex relaxed shape that is necessary for near vision (see **Cb**). This is the basic mechanism of visual accommodation.

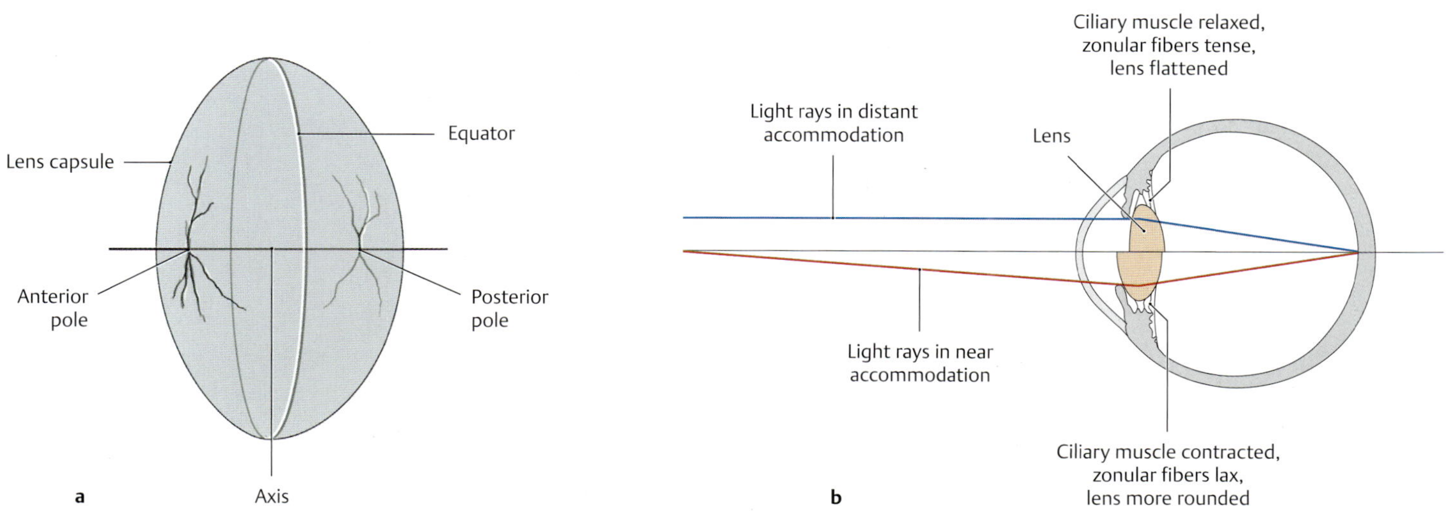

C Reference lines and dynamics of the lens

a Principal reference lines of the lens: Ahe lens has an *anterior* and *posterior pole,* an axis passing between the poles, and an equator. The lens has a biconvex shape with a greater radius of curvature posteriorly (16 mm) than anteriorly (10 mm). Its function is to transmit light rays and make fine adjustments in refraction. Its refractive power ranges from 10 to 20 diopters, depending on the state of accommodation. The cornea has a considerably higher refractive power of 43 diopters.

b Light refraction and dynamics of the lens:

- Upper half of diagram: fine adjustment of the eye for *far vision.* Parallel light rays arrive from a distant source, and the lens is flattened.
- Lower half of diagram: For *near vision* (accommodation to objects less than 5 m from the eye), the lens assumes a more rounded shape (see **B**). This is effected by contraction of the ciliary muscle (parasympathetic innervation from the oculomotor nerve), causing the zonular fibers to relax and allowing the lens to assume a more rounded shape because of its intrinsic resilience.

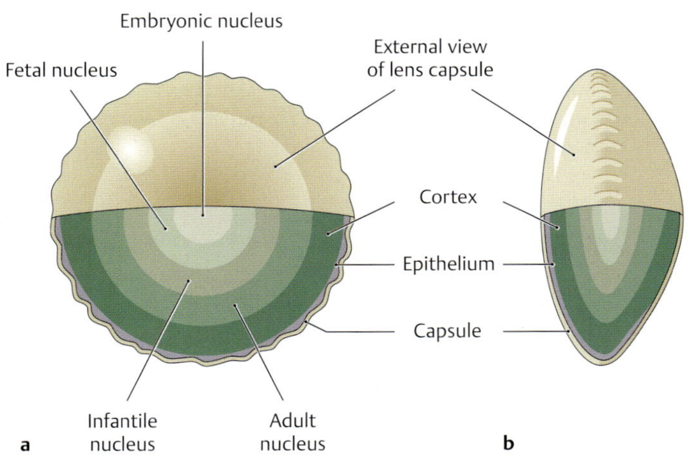

D Growth of the lens and zones of discontinuity (after Lang)

a Anterior view, **b** lateral view.

The lens continues to grow throughout life, doing so in a manner opposite to that of other epithelial structures, i.e., the youngest cells are at the surface of the lens while the oldest cells are deeper. Due to the constant proliferation of epithelial cells, which are all firmly incorporated in the lens capsule, the tissue of the lens becomes increasingly dense with age. A slit-lamp examination will demonstrate zones of varying cell density (zones of discontinuity). The zone of highest cell density, the *embryonic nucleus,* is at the center of the lens. With further growth, it becomes surrounded by the *fetal nucleus.* The *infantile nucleus* develops after birth, and finally the *adult nucleus* begins to form during the third decade of life. These zones are the basis for the morphological classification of cataracts, a structural alteration in the lens, causing opacity, that is more or less normal in old age (present in 10% of all 80-year-olds).

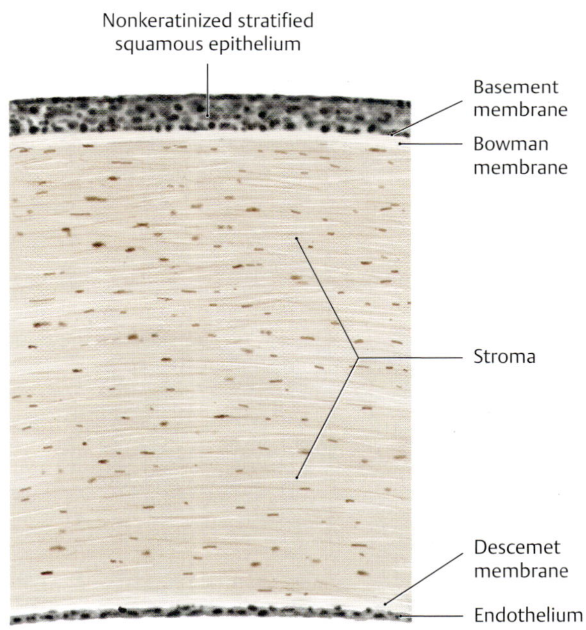

E Structure of the cornea

The cornea is covered externally by nonkeratinized stratified squamous epithelium whose basal membrane borders on the anterior limiting lamina (Bowman membrane). The stroma (substantia propria) makes up approximately 90% of the corneal thickness and is bounded on its deep surface by the posterior limiting lamina (Descemet membrane). Beneath is a single layer of corneal endothelium. The cornea does have a nerve supply (for corneal reflexes) but it is not vascularized and therefore has an immunologically privileged status: normally, a corneal transplant can be performed without fear of a host rejection response.

5.13 Eye: Iris and Ocular Chambers

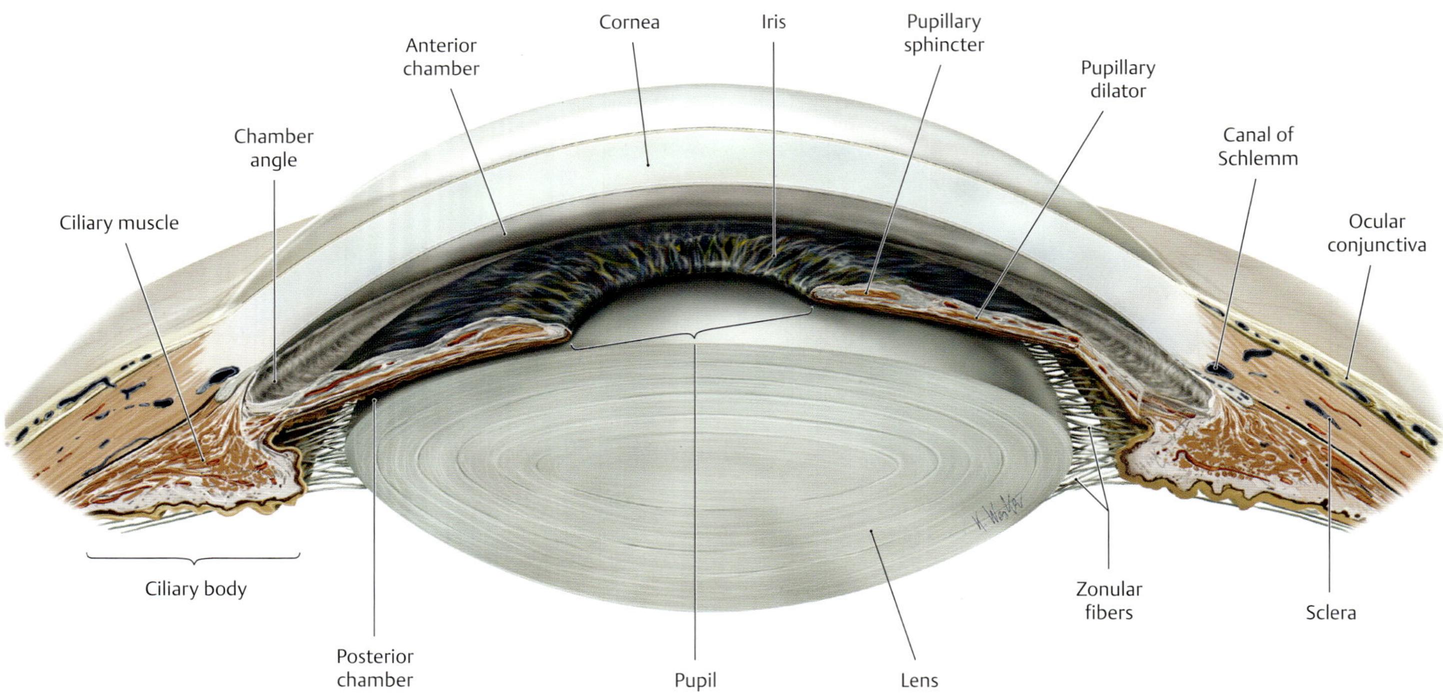

A Location of the iris and the anterior and posterior chambers
Transverse section through the anterior segment of the eye, superior view. The iris, the choroid, and the ciliary body at the periphery of the iris are part of the uveal tract. In the iris, the pigments are formed that determine eye color (see **D**). The iris is an optical diaphragm with a central aperture, the pupil, placed in front of the lens. The pupil is 1–8 mm in diameter; it constricts on contraction of the pupillary sphincter (*parasympathetic* innervation via the oculomotor nerve and ciliary ganglion) and dilates on contraction of the pupillary dilator (*sympathetic* innervation from the superior cervical ganglion via the internal carotid plexus). Together, the iris and lens separate the anterior chamber of the eye from the posterior chamber. The posterior chamber behind the iris is bounded posteriorly by the vitreous body, centrally by the lens, and laterally by the ciliary body. The anterior chamber is bounded anteriorly by the cornea and posteriorly by the iris and lens.

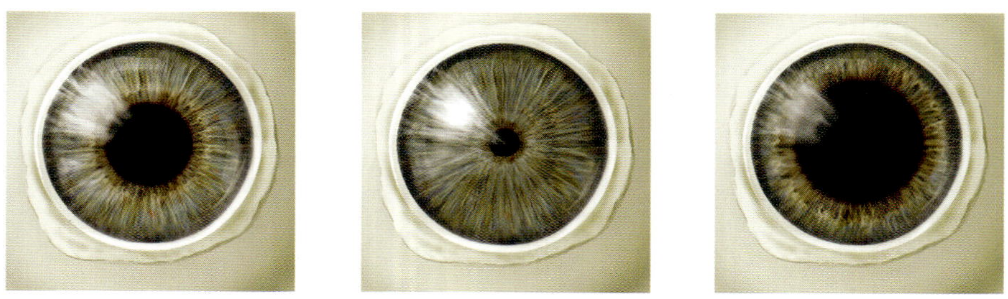

B Pupil size
a Normal pupil size, **b** maximum constriction (miosis), **c** maximum dilation (mydriasis).
The regulation of pupil size is aided by the two intraocular muscles, the pupillary sphincter and pupillary dilator (see **D**). The pupillary sphincter, which receives parasympathetic innervation, narrows the pupil while the pupillary dilator, which receives sympathetic innervation, enlarges the pupil. Pupil size is normally adjusted in response to incident light and serves mainly to optimize visual acuity. Normally, the pupils are circular in shape and equal in size (3–5 mm). Various influences (listed in **C**) may cause the pupil size to vary over a range from 1.5 mm (miosis) to 8 mm (mydriasis). The condition of unequal pupil size is called *anisocoria.* Mild anisocoria is physiological in some individuals. Pupillary reflexes such as convergence and the consensual light response are described on p. 480.

C Causes of miosis and mydriasis

Miosis (Bb)	Mydriasis (Bc)
Light	Darkness
Sleep, fatigue	Pain, excitement
Miotics (parasympathomimetics, e.g. pilocarpine and sympatholytics)	Mydriatics (parasympatholytics, e.g. atropine and sympathomimetics, e.g. adrenaline)
Horner syndrome (including ptosis and a narrow palpebral fissure)	Oculomotor palsy
Morphine abuse	Migraine, glaucoma
Pontine lesion, meningitis	Mesencepahlic lesion
Anesthesia	Cocaine

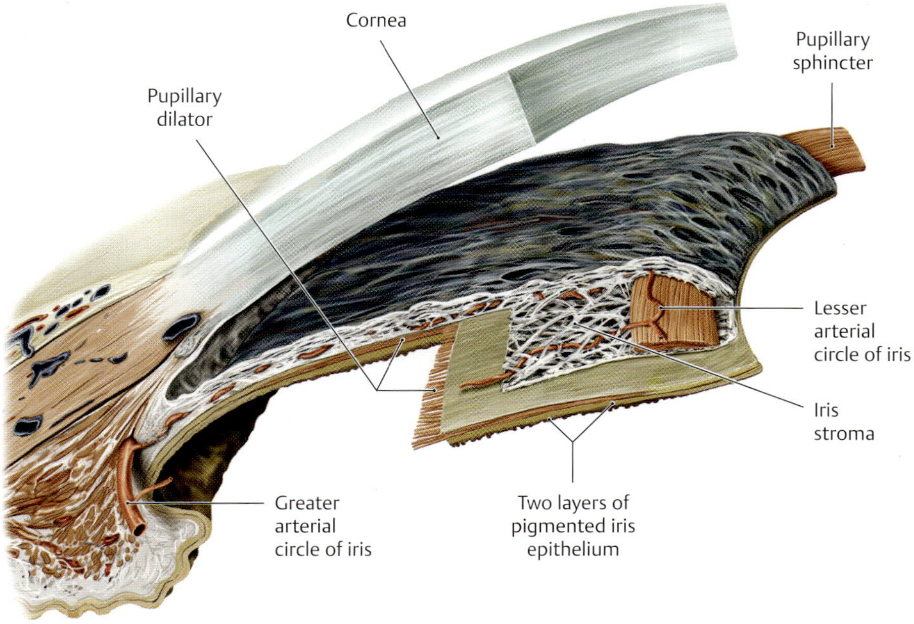

D Structure of the iris

The basic structural framework of the iris is the vascularized stroma, which is bounded on its deep surface by two layers of pigmented iris epithelium. The loose, collagen-containing stroma of the iris contains outer and inner vascular circles (greater and lesser arterial circles), which are interconnected by small anastomotic arteries. The pupillary sphincter is an annular muscle located in the stroma bordering the pupil. The radially disposed pupillary dilator is not located in the stroma; rather it is composed of numerous myofibrils in the iris epithelium (myoepithelium). The stroma of the iris is permeated by pigmented connective tissue cells (melanocytes). When heavily pigmented, these melanocytes of the anterior border zone of the stroma render the iris brown or "black." Otherwise, the characteristics of the underlying stroma and epithelium determine eye color, in a manner that is not fully understood.

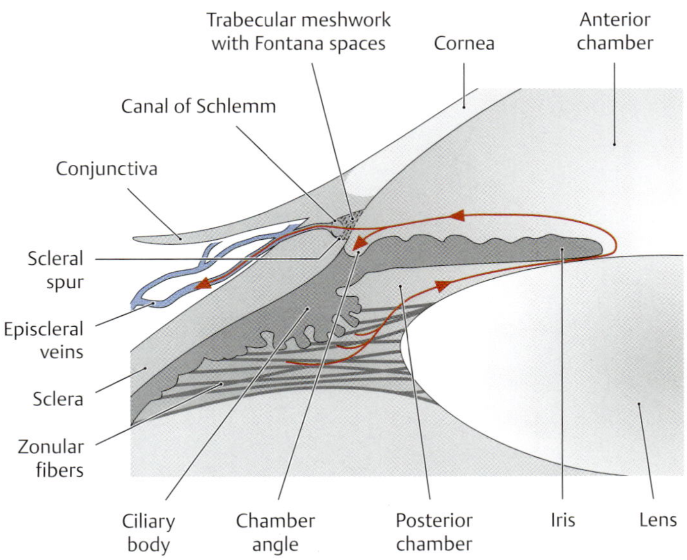

E Normal drainage of aqueous humor

The aqueous humor (approximately 0.3 ml per eye) is an important determinant of the intraocular pressure (see **F**). It is produced by the nonpigmented ciliary epithelium of the ciliary processes in the *posterior* chamber (approximately 0.15 ml/hour) and passes through the pupil into the *anterior* chamber of the eye. The aqueous humor seeps through the spaces of the trabecular meshwork (Fontana spaces) in the chamber angle and enters the canal of Schlemm (venous sinus of the sclera), through which it drains to the episcleral veins. The draining aqueous humor flows toward the chamber angle along a pressure gradient (intra-ocular pressure = 15 mm Hg, pressure in the episcleral veins = 9 mm Hg) and must surmount a physiological resistance at two sites:

- the *pupillary resistance* (between the iris and lens) and
- the *trabecular resistance* (narrow spaces in the trabecular meshwork).

Approximately 85% of the aqueous humor flows through the trabecular meshwork into the canal of Schlemm. Only 15% drains through the uveoscleral vascular system into the vortical veins (uveoscleral drainage route).

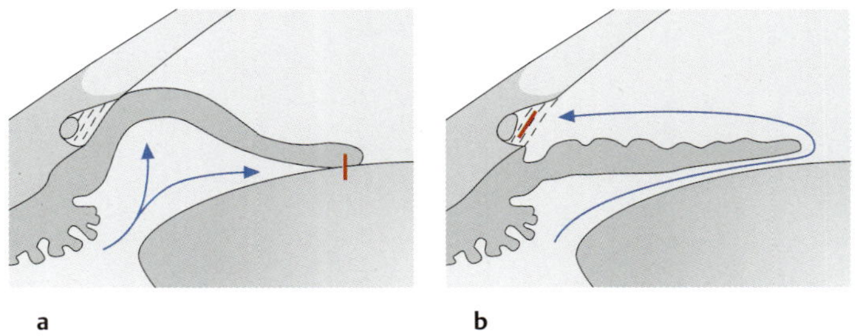

F Obstruction of aqueous drainage and glaucoma

The normal intraocular pressure in adults (15 mm Hg) is necessary for a functioning optical system, partly because it maintains a smooth curvature of the corneal surface and helps keep the photoreceptor cells in contact with the pigment epithelium. When *glaucoma* is present (see **D**, p. 159), the intraocular pressure is elevated and the optic nerve becomes constricted at the lamina cribrosa, where it emerges from the eyeball through the sclera. This constriction of the optic nerve eventually leads to blindness. The elevated pressure is caused by an obstruction that hampers the normal drainage of aqueous humor, which can no longer overcome the pupillary or trabecular resistance (see **E**). One of two conditions may develop:

- *Acute or angle-closure glaucoma* (**a**), in which the chamber angle is obstructed by iris tissue. The aqueous fluid cannot drain into the anterior chamber and pushes portions of the iris upward, blocking the chamber angle.
- *Chronic or open-angle glaucoma* (**b**), in which the chamber angle is open but drainage through the trabecular meshwork is impaired (the red bar marks the location of each type of obstruction).

By far the most common form (approximately 90% of all glaucomas) is primary chronic open-angle glaucoma (**b**), which becomes more prevalent after 40 years of age. The primary goal of treatment is to improve the drainage of aqueous humor (e.g., with parasympathomimetics that induce sustained contraction of the ciliary muscle and pupillary sphincter) or decrease its production.

5.14 Eye: Retina

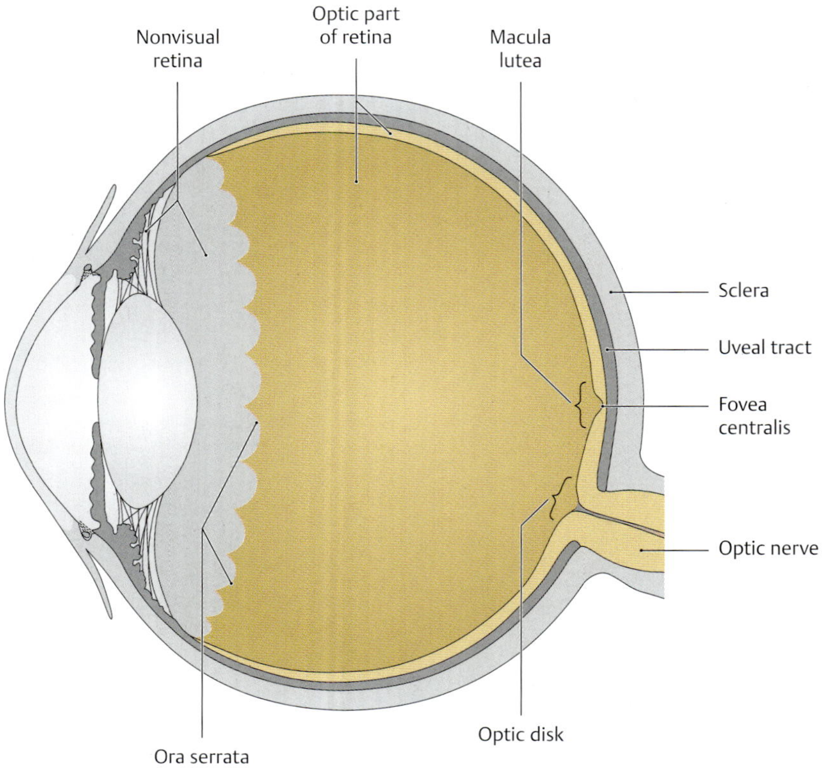

A Overview of the retina
The retina is the third, innermost layer of the eyeball. It consists mainly of a photosensitive *optic part* and a smaller, non-photosensitive forward prolongation called the *nonvisual retina.* The optic part of the retina, shown here in yellow, varies in thickness at different locations. It overlies the pigment epithelium of the uveal tract and is pressed against it by intraocular pressure. The pars optica merges with the pars caeca at a jagged margin—the ora serrata (cf. **B**). The site on the retina where visual acuity is highest is the *fovea centralis,* a small depression at the center of a yellowish area, the *macula lutea.* The optic part of the retina is particularly thin at this site; it is thickest at the point where the optic nerve emerges from the eyeball at the lamina cribrosa.

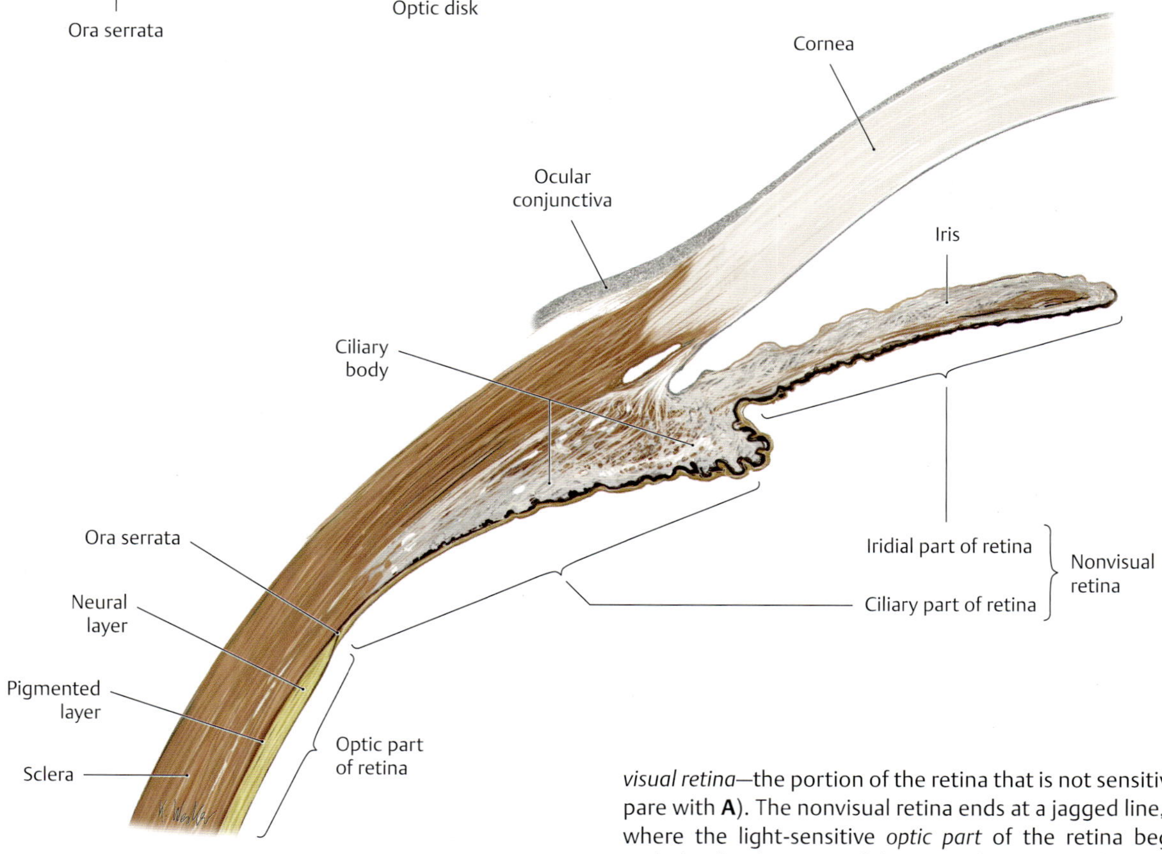

B Parts of the retina
The posterior surface of the iris bears a double layer of pigment epithelium, the *iridial* part of the retina. Just peripheral to it is the *ciliary part* of the retina, also formed by a double layer of epithelium (one of which is pigmented) and covering the posterior surface of the ciliary body. The iridial and ciliary parts of the retina together constitute the *nonvisual retina*—the portion of the retina that is not sensitive to light (compare with **A**). The nonvisual retina ends at a jagged line, the ora serrata, where the light-sensitive *optic part* of the retina begins. Consistent with the development of the retina from the embryonic optic cup, two layers can be distinguished within the optic part:

- An outer layer nearer the sclera: the *pigmented layer,* consisting of a single layer of pigmented retinal epithelium (cf. **Ca**).
- An inner layer nearer the vitreous body: the *neural layer,* comprising a system of receptor cells, interneurons, and ganglion cells (see **Cb**).

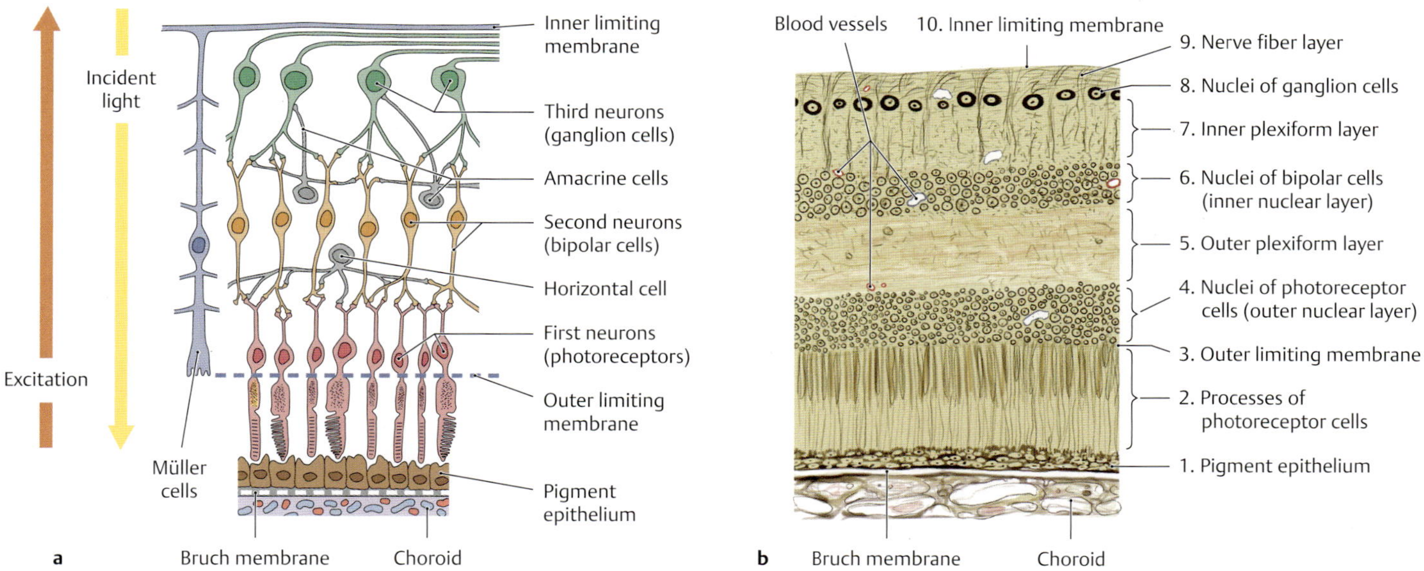

C Structure of the retina

a Schematic diagram of the first three neurons in the visual pathway and their connections. **b** The ten anatomical layers of the retina.

Light must pass through all the inner layers of the retina (the layers nearest the vitreous body) before reaching the photosensitive elements of the photoreceptors. The direction of transmission of sensory information, however, is inward, opposite to the direction of the incoming light. The first three neurons of the visual pathway are located within the retina. Starting with the outermost neuron, they are as follows (**a**):

- First neuron: Photoreceptor cells (rods and cones) are light-sensitive sensory cells that transform light stimuli into electrochemical signals. The two types of *photoreceptors* are rods and cones, named for the shape of their receptor segment. The retina contains 100–125 million rods, which are responsible for twilight and night vision, but only about 6–7 million cones. Different cones are specialized for the perception of red, green, and blue.
- Second neuron: bipolar cells that receive impulses from the photoreceptors and relay them to the ganglion cells
- Third neuron: retinal ganglion cells whose axons converge at the optic disk to form the optic nerve and reach the lateral geniculate and superior colliculus

In addition to these largely "vertical" connections, there are also horizontal cells and amacrine cells that function as *interneurons* to establish lateral connections. In this way the impulses transmitted by the receptor cells are processed and organized while still within the retina (signal convergence). The retinal *Müller cells* are glial cells that span the neural layer radially from the inner to outer limiting membranes and create a supporting framework for the neurons. External to these cells is the *pigment epithelium,* whose basement membrane is attached to the Bruch membrane (contains elastic fibers and collagen fibrils) and mediates the exchange of substances between the adjacent choroid (choriocapillaris) and the photoreceptor cells.

Note: The outer segments of the photoreceptors are in contact with the pigment epithelium but are not attached to it. The intraocular pressure alone pushes the retina against the pigment epithelium. This explains why the retina may become separated from the pigment epithelium (retinal detachment; untreated, leads to blindness). Traditionally, a histological section of the retina consists of ten layers (**b**) that are formed by elements of the three neurons (e.g., nuclei or cellular processes) that occupy a consistent level within any given layer.

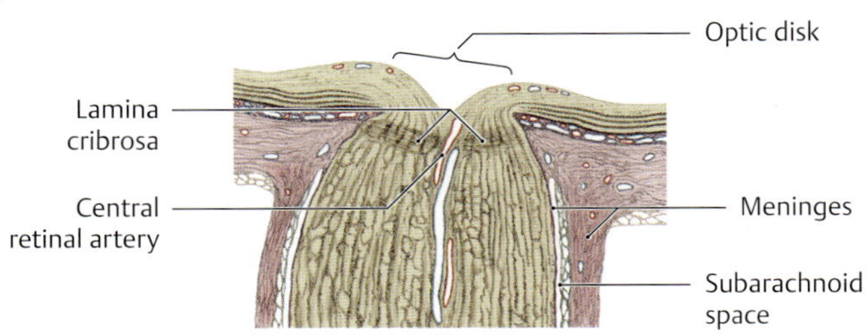

D Optic disk ("blind spot") and lamina cribrosa

The unmyelinated axons of the retinal ganglion cells (approximately 1 million axons per eye) pass to a collecting point at the posterior pole of the eye, the optic disk. There they unite to form the optic nerve and leave the retina through numerous perforations in the sclera (lamina cribrosa). In the optic nerve, these axons are myelinated by oligodendrocytes.

Note the central retinal artery entering the eye at this location (see p. 171) and the coverings of the optic nerve. Because the optic nerve is a forward prolongation of the diencephalon, it has all the coverings of the brain (dura mater, arachnoid, and pia mater). It is surrounded by a subarachnoid space that contains cerebrospinal fluid and communicates with the subarachnoid spaces of the brain and spinal cord.

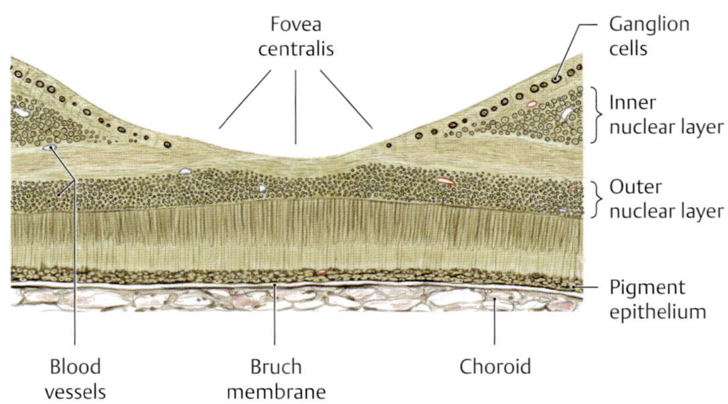

E Macula lutea and fovea centralis

Temporal to the optic disk is the macula lutea. At its center is a funnel-shaped depression approximately 1.5 mm in diameter, the fovea centralis, which is the site of maximum visual acuity. At this site the inner retinal layers are heaped toward the margin of the depression, so that the cells of the photoreceptors (just cones, no rods) are directly exposed to the incident light. This arrangement significantly reduces scattering of the light rays.

5.15 Eye: Blood Supply

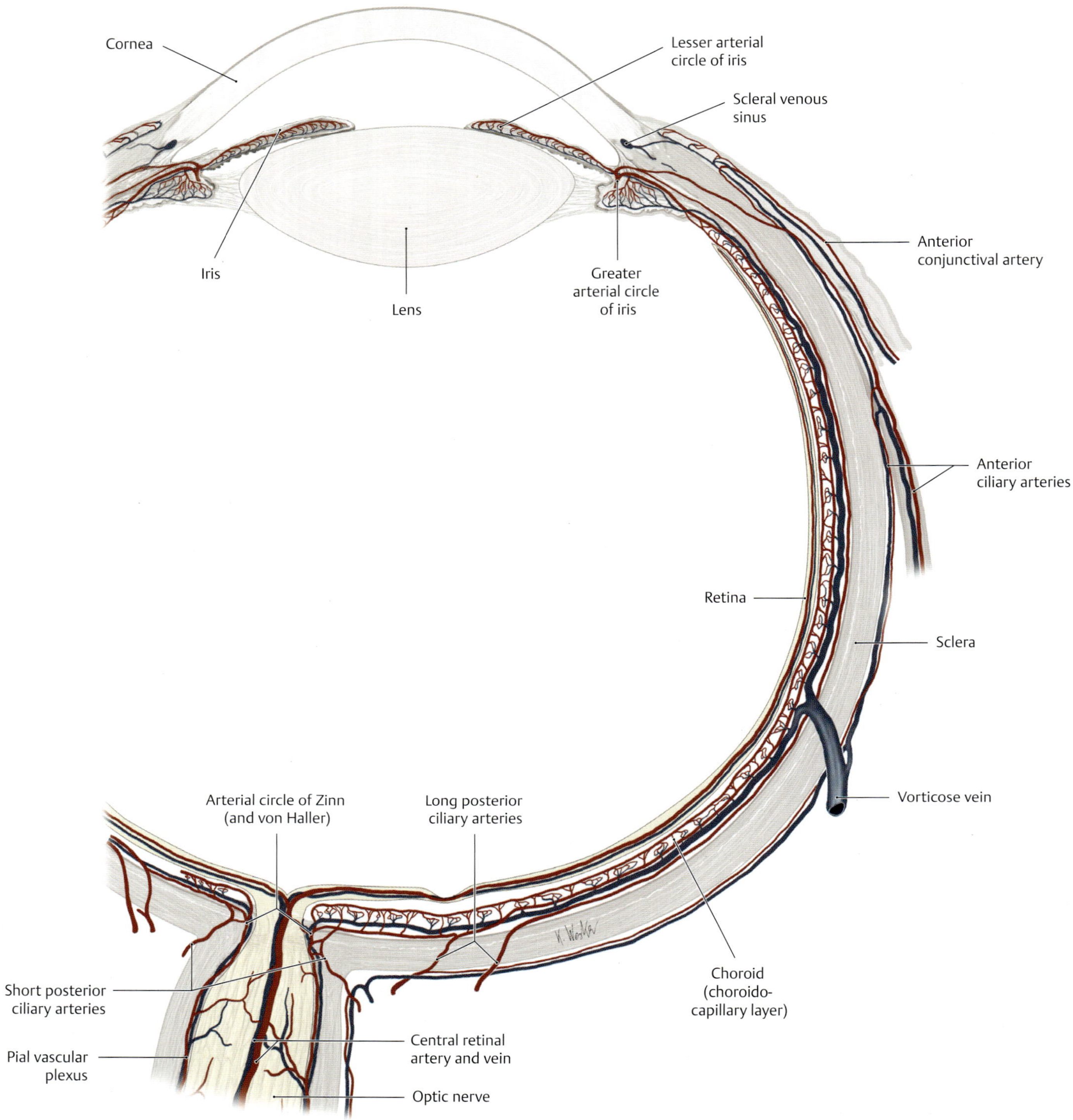

A Blood supply of the eye
Horizontal section through the right eye at the level of the optic nerve, viewed from above. All of the arteries that supply the eye arise from the *ophthalmic artery,* a terminal branch of the internal carotid artery (see p. 103). Its ocular branches are as follows:

- Central retinal artery to the retina (see **B**)
- Short posterior ciliary arteries to the choroid
- Long posterior ciliary arteries to the ciliary body and iris, where they supply the greater and lesser arterial circles of the iris (see **D**, p. 167)
- Anterior ciliary arteries, which arise from the vessels of the rectus muscles of the eye and anastomose with the posterior ciliary vessels

Blood is drained from the eyeball by 4 to 8 vorticose veins, which pierce the sclera behind the equator and open into the superior or inferior ophthalmic vein.

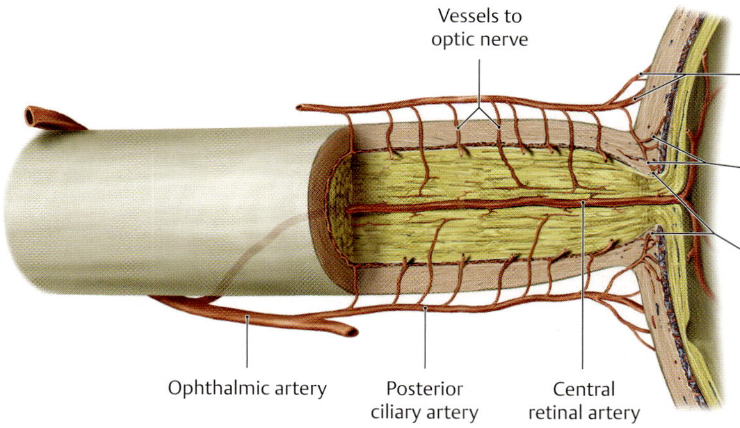

B Arterial blood supply of the optic nerve and optic nerve head

Lateral view. The central retinal artery, the first branch of the ophthalmic artery, enters the optic nerve from below approximately 1 cm behind the eyeball and courses with it to the retina while giving off multiple small branches. The posterior ciliary artery also gives off several small branches that supply the optic nerve. The optic nerve head receives its arterial blood supply from an arterial ring (circle of Zinn and von Haller) formed by anastomoses among the side branches of the short posterior ciliary arteries and central retinal artery.

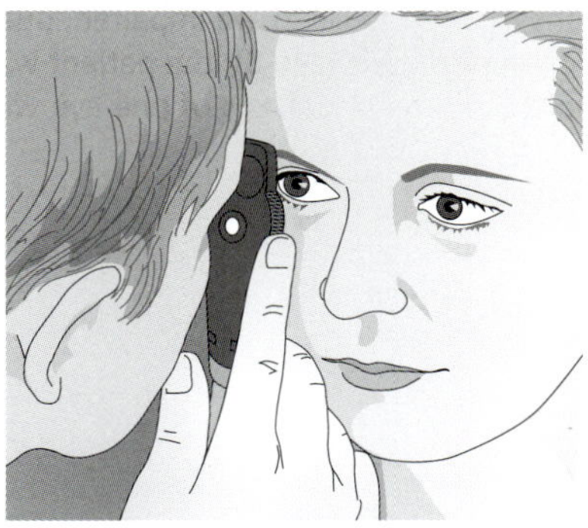

a

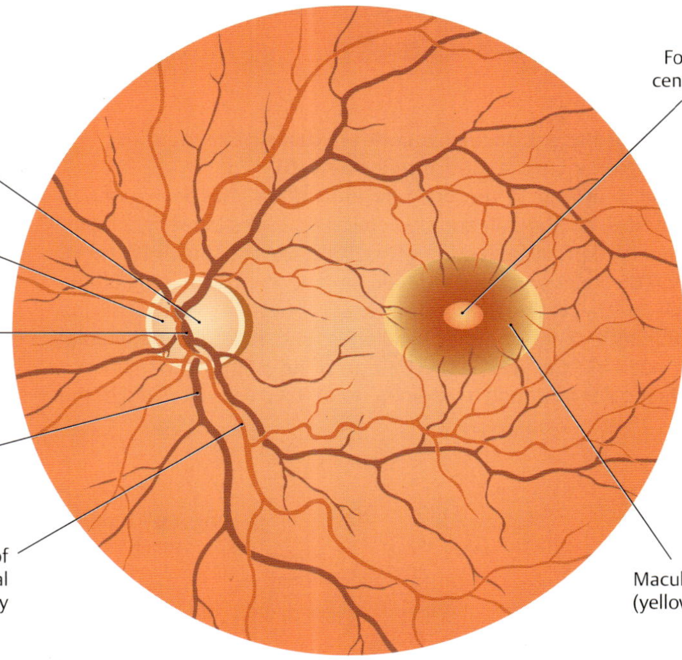

b

C Ophthalmoscopic examination of the optic fundus

a Examination technique (direct ophthalmoscopy). **b** Normal appearance of the optic fundus.

In direct ophthalmoscopy, the following structures of the optic fundus can be directly evaluated at approximately 16x magnification:

- The condition of the retina
- The blood vessels (particularly the central retinal artery)
- The optic disk (where the optic nerve emerges from the eyeball)
- The macula lutea and fovea centralis

Because the retina is transparent, the color of the optic fundus is determined chiefly by the pigment epithelium and the blood vessels of the choroid. It is uniformly pale red in light-skinned persons and is considerably browner in dark-skinned persons. Abnormal detachment of the retina is usually associated with a loss of retinal transparency, and the retina assumes a yellowish-white color. The central retinal artery and vein can be distinguished from each other by their color and caliber: arteries have a brighter red color and a smaller caliber than the veins. This provides a means for the early detection of vascular changes (e.g., stenosis, wall thickening, microaneurysms), such as those occurring in diabetes mellitus (diabetic retinopathy) or hypertension. The *optic disk* normally has sharp margins, a yellow-orange color, and a central depression, the physiological cup. The disk is subject to changes in pathological conditions such as elevated intracranial pressure (papilledema with ill-defined disk margins). On examination of the *macula lutea,* which is 3–4 mm temporal to the optic disk, it can be seen that numerous branches of the central retinal artery radiate toward the macula but do not reach its center, the fovea centralis (the fovea receives its blood supply from the choroid). A common age-related disease of the macula lutea is macular degeneration, which may gradually lead to blindness.

5.16 Orbit: Extraocular Muscles

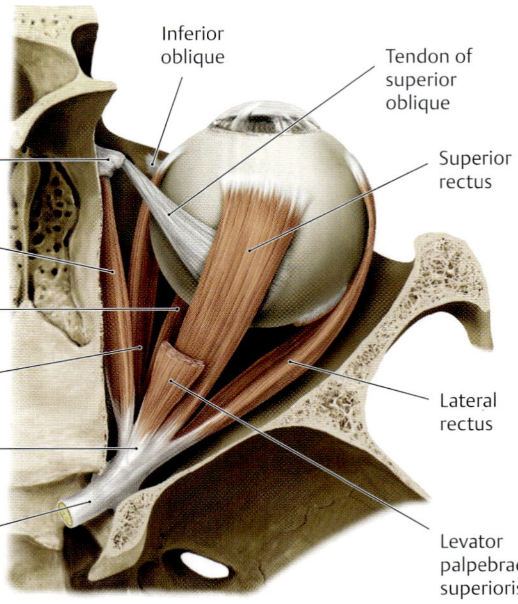

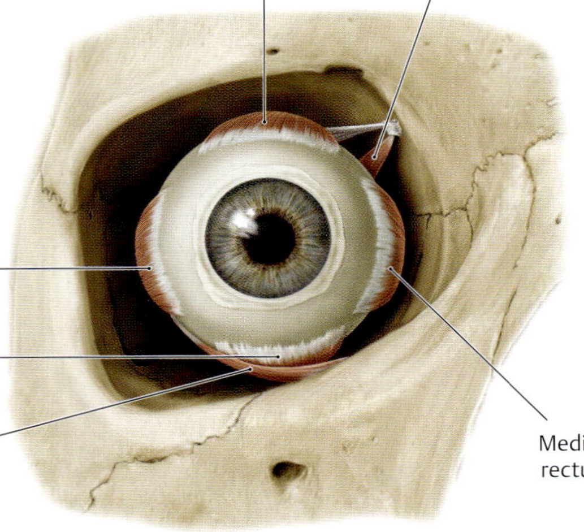

A Location of the extraocular muscles (extrinsic eye muscles)
Right eye, superior view (**a**) and anterior view (**b**).
The eyeball is moved in the orbit by four rectus muscles (superior, inferior, medial, and lateral) and two oblique muscles (superior and inferior); innervation and direction of movements are shown **B** and **D**. Except for the inferior oblique (origin on the medial margin of the orbit), all of the extraocular muscles arise from a tendinous ring around the optic canal (common tendinous ring). All of the extraocular muscles insert on the sclera. The tendon of insertion of the superior oblique first passes through a tendinous loop (trochlea) attached to the superomedial orbital margin, which redirects it posteriorly at an acute angle to its insertion on the temporal aspect of the superior surface of the eyeball. The functional competence of all six extraocular muscles and their coordinated interaction are essential in directing both eyes toward the visual target. It is the task of the brain to process the two perceived retinal images in a way that provides binocular visual perception. If the coordinated actions of these muscles are impaired, due, for example, to the paralysis of one eye muscle (see **E**), the patient will perceive a double image (diplopia), i.e., the visual axis of one eye will deviate from its normal position.

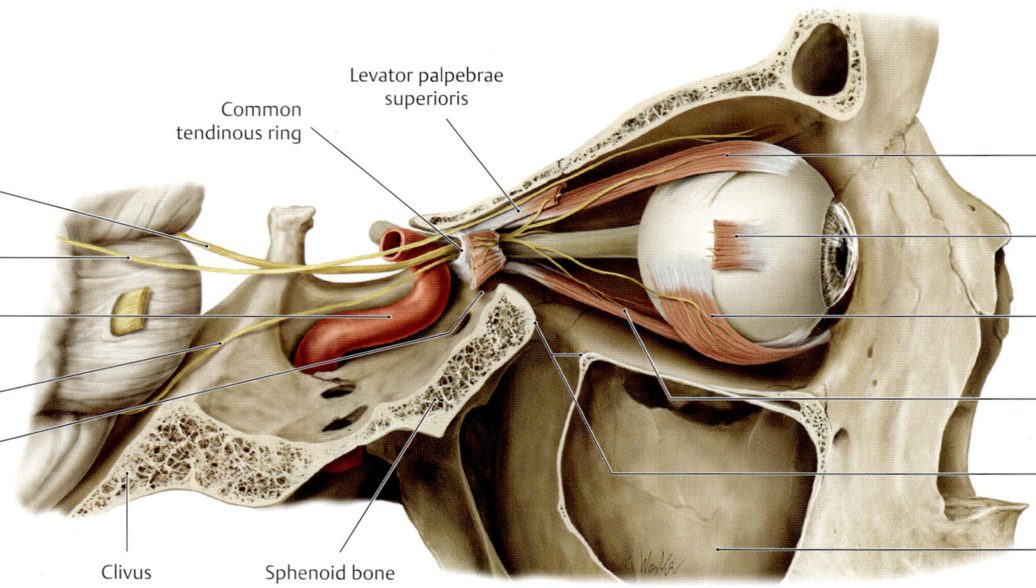

B Innervation of the extraocular muscles
Right eye, lateral view with the temporal wall of the orbit removed. Except for the superior oblique (trochlear nerve) and lateral rectus (abducent nerve), the ocular muscles (superior, medial and inferior rectus and inferior oblique) are supplied by the oculomotor nerve. Its superior branch supplies the superior rectus and the levator palpebrae superioris, which is not one of the extraocular muscles. Its inferior branch supplies the inferior rectus, medial rectus, and inferior oblique.
After emerging from the brainstem, cranial nerves III, IV, and VI first pass through the cavernous sinus (or its lateral wall, see **A**, p. 176), where they are in close proximity to the internal carotid artery. From there they traverse the superior orbital fissure (see **B**, p. 176) to enter the orbit and supply their respective muscles.

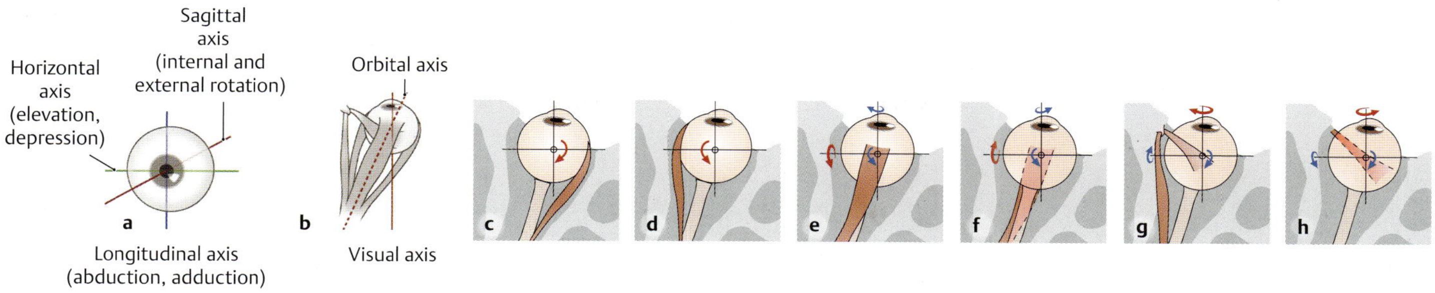

	Muscle	Primary action	Secondary action	Innervation
Horizontal extraocular muscles	• Lateral rectus • Medial rectus	• Abduction • Adduction	• None • None	• Abducent nerve (VI) • Oculomotor nerve (III), inferior branch
Straight vertical extraocular muscles	• Inferior rectus • Superior rectus	• Depression • Elevation	• External rotation and adduction • Internal rotation and adduction	• Oculomotor nerve (III), inferior branch • Oculomotor nerve (III), superior branch
Oblique vertical extraocular muscles	• Inferior oblique • Superior oblique	• External rotation (excycloduction) • Internal rotation (incycloduction)	• Elevation and abduction • Depression and abduction	• Oculomotor nerve (III), inferior branch • Trochlear nerve (IV)

C Ocular axes; function and innervation of the extraocular muscles
Right eye. Except for **a**, superior view. Longitudinal axis is visible only as a point in **b–h**.

a and **b** Eye movements occur around three perpendicular axes. In primary position, the eye is turned slightly inward, i.e., the orbital axis is not identical to the visual axis or, respectively, the visual axis is externally rotated about 23°. To evaluate the mobility of individual ocular muscles, the eye must be brought into a specific cardinal direction of gaze (see E).
c–h The six extraocular muscles are thus considered in pairs. See table.
The two **straight vertical extraocular muscles** are the most important elevators and depressors over their entire range of eye motion. These primary actions are more pronounced in abduction than in adduction (direction of pull of the muscle corresponds to the orbital axis, see **b**). The two muscles also have secondary actions: The superior rectus internally rotates the eye (incycloduction), the inferior rectus externally rotates it (excycloduction). Both also have a slight adductive effect. Note that both secondary actions are strongest in maximum adduction and decrease as the eye moves through the primary position toward abduction.
Oblique vertical extraocular muscles: The main action of the superior oblique is incycloduction, which can be expected to be strongest in abduction. The most important secondary action is depression. In contrast to incycloduction, it is strongest in adduction. The main action of the inferior oblique is excycloduction, whereas its most important secondary action is elevation. As with the superior oblique, the muscle's main action is strongest in abduction and its secondary action is strongest in adduction. Both oblique vertical extraocular muscles also have a slight abductive effect.

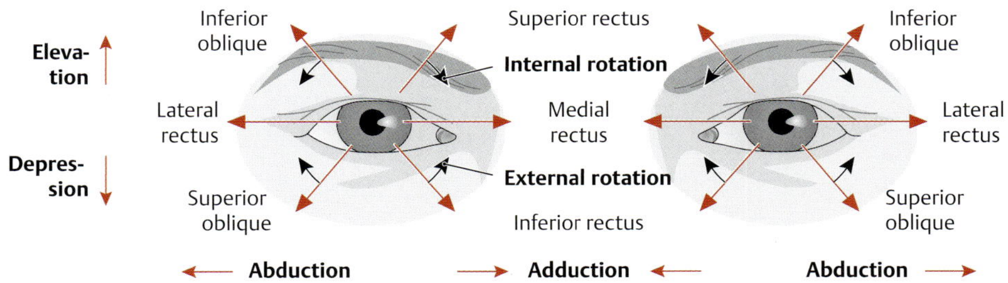

D Primary action of the extraocular muscles on the eyeball in primary position
In primary position (looking straight ahead) the maximum combined effect of all ocular muscles occurs, i.e., all primary and secondary actions are performed, yet none of them to the full extent (red arrows; linear effect, black arrows: rotational effect).

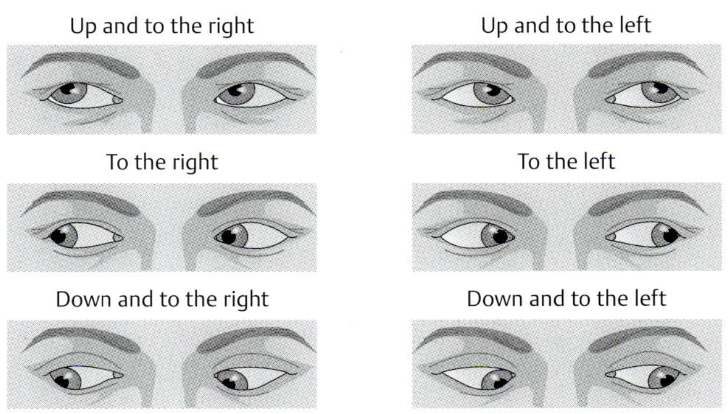

E The six cardinal directions of gaze
(schematic diagram after Hering)
Displayed here are the directions of gaze in which the function of individual ocular muscles is evaluation or which are most heavily affected when a primary ocular muscle is paralyzed (increasing condition of double vision).
Note: The rotational effect cannot be identified without additional methods of testing.

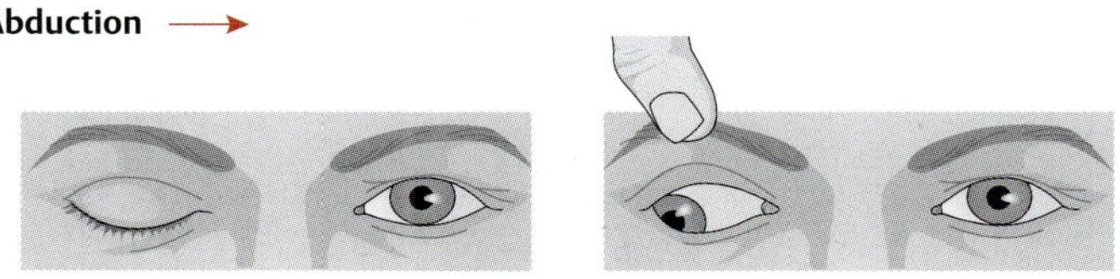

F Oculomotor palsy
Complete oculomotor palsy involves the failure of both the extraocular muscles (superior, inferior, medial rectus and the inferior oblique; see **C**) as well as the intrinsic ciliary and sphincter pupillae muscles and the eyelid elevators, which also receive their parasympathetic supply from the oculomotor nerve. The result is impaired bulbar motility and pupil motor function: The affected eye is depressed and externally rotated, the pupil is dilated (mydriasis due to failure of the sphincter pupillae). Loss of near-field accommodation (failure of the ciliary muscle) occurs, and the eyelid is more or less closed (ptosis) due to failure of the levator palpebrae superioris. In complete ptosis as shown here, the patient does not have diplopia because only one eye is functional. Intrinsic and extraocular oculomotor palsies, in which only the intrinsic or only the extraocular muscles are paralyzed, are discussed on p. 118.

5.17 Orbit: Subdivisions and Neurovascular Structures

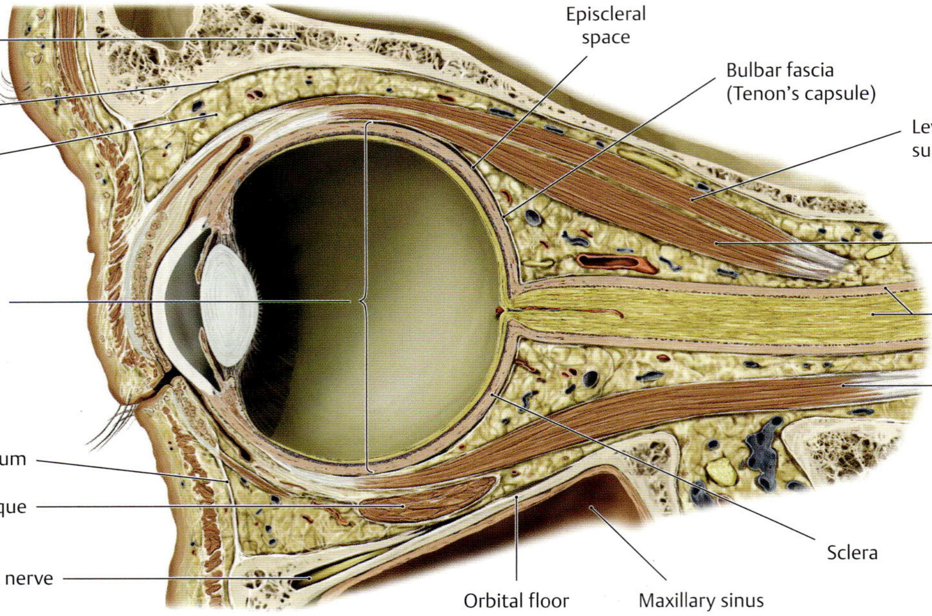

A Subdivision of the orbit into upper, middle, and lower levels
Sagittal section through the right orbit viewed from the medial side. The orbit is lined by periosteum (periorbita) and contains the following structures, which are embedded within the retro-orbital fat: eyeball, optic nerve, lacrimal gland (not visible in this plane of section), extra-ocular muscles, and the neurovascular structures that supply them. The retro-orbital fat is bounded anteriorly by the orbital septum and toward the eyeball by a mobile sheath of connective tissue (bulbar fascia,Tenon's capsule). The narrow space between the bulbar fascia and sclera is called the episcleral space. Topographically, the orbit is divided into three levels with the following boundaries:

- *Upper level:* between orbital roof and the superior rectus
- *Middle level:* between superior rectus and inferior rectus
- *Lower level:* between inferior rectus m. and orbital floor

The contents of the different levels are listed in **B**.

B The three upper orbital levels and their main neurovascular structures

The lacrimal gland is the dominant structure in the upper level, whereas the eyeball is the landmark in the middle level. (The sites of entry of neurovascular structures into the orbit are described on p. 36.)

Level	Contents	Source/associated structures
Upper level	• Lacrimal nerve • Lacrimal artery • Lacrimal vein • Frontal nerve • Supraorbital nerve and supratrochlear nerve • Supraorbital artery • Supraorbital vein • Trochlear nerve • Infratrochlear nerve	• Branch of ophthalmic nerve (CN V_1) • Branch of ophthalmic artery (from internal carotid artery) • Passes to superior ophthalmic vein • Branch of ophthalmic nerve (CN V_1) • Terminal branches of frontal nerve • Terminal branch of ophthalmic artery • Unites with supratrochlear veins to form angular vein • Nucleus of trochlear nerve in mesencephalon • Branch of nasociliary nerve (subbranch of ophthalmic nerve [V_1])
Middle level	• Ophthalmic artery • Central retinal artery • Posterior ciliary arteries • Nasociliary nerve • Abducent nerve • Oculomotor nerve, superior branch • Optic nerve • Short ciliary nerves • Ciliary ganglion • Parasympathetic root • Sympathetic root • Nasociliary root • Superior ophthalmic veint	• Branch of internal carotid artery • Branch of ophthalmic artery • Branches of ophthalmic artery • Branch of ophthalmic nerve (CN V_1) • Abducent nucleus in pons • Oculomotor nucleus in mesencephalon • Retina (retinal ganglion cells) • Postsynaptic autonomic fibers to the eyeball • Parasympathetic ganglion for ciliary muscle and pupillary sphincter • Presynaptic autonomic fibers of oculomotor nerve • Postsynaptic fibers from the superior cervical ganglion • Sensory fibers from eyeball through ciliary ganglion to nasociliary nerve • Passes into cavernous sinus
Lower level	• Oculomotor nerve, inferior branch • Inferior ophthalmic vein • Infraorbital nerve • Infraorbital artery	• Oculomotor nucleus in mesencephalon • Passes into cavernous sinus • Branch of maxillary nerve (CN V_2) • Terminal branch of maxillary artery (external carotid artery)

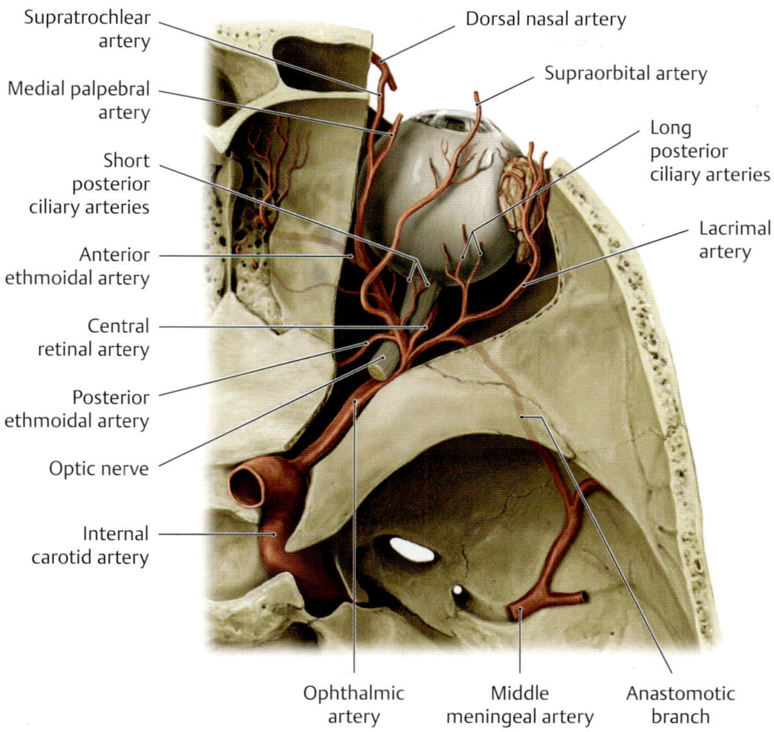

C Branches of ophthalmic artery
Right orbit, superior view after opening of the optic canal and orbital roof. The ophthalmic artery is a branch of the internal carotid artery. It runs below the optic nerve through the optic canal into the orbit and supplies the intraorbital structures including the eyeball.

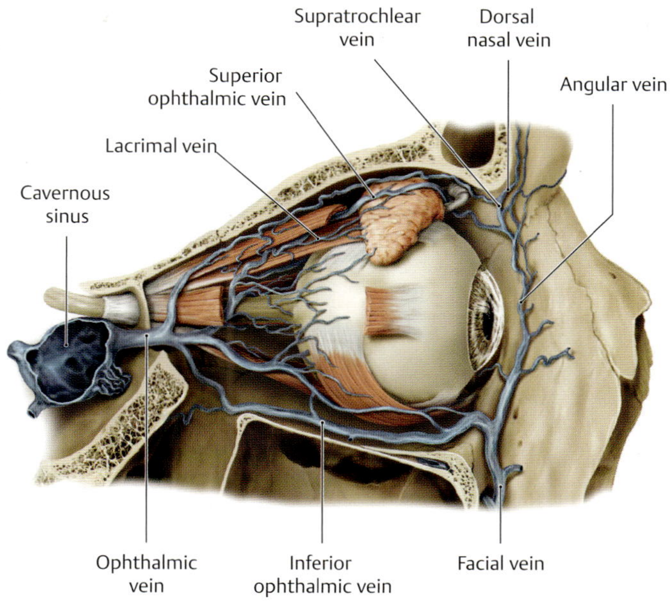

D Veins of the orbit
Right orbit, lateral view with the lateral orbital wall removed and the maxillary sinus opened. The veins of the orbit communicate with the veins of the superficial and deep facial region and with the cavernous sinus in the middle cranial fossa (potential spread of infectious pathogens).

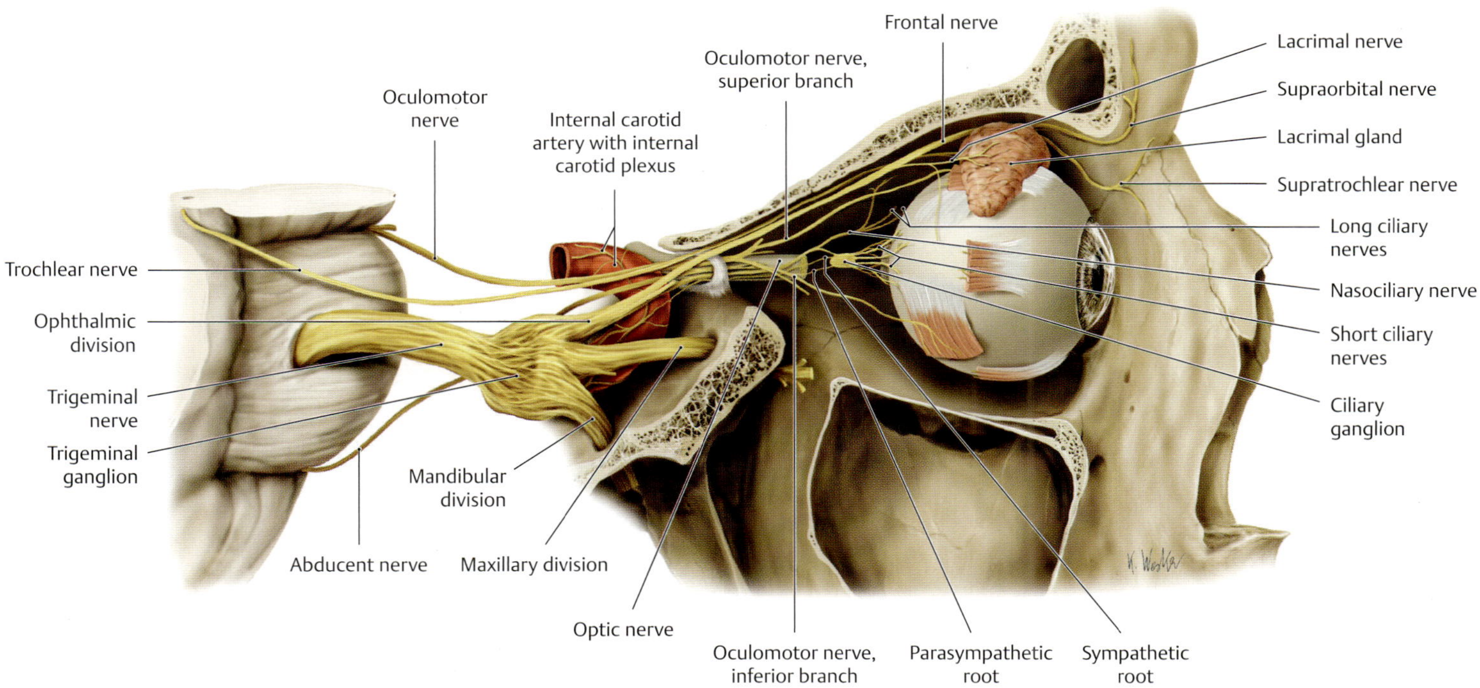

E Innervation of the orbit
Right orbit, lateral view with the temporal bony wall removed. The orbit receives motor, sensory and autonomic innervation from four cranial nerves: the oculomotor nerve (CN III), the trochlear nerve (CN IV), the abducent nerve (CN VI), and the ophthalmic division of the trigeminal nerve (CN V_1). The oculomotor nerve also conveys presynaptic parasympathetic fibers to the ciliary ganglion. Postsynaptic sympathetic fibers pass into the orbit by way of the internal carotid plexus and ophthalmic plexus.

5.18 Orbit: Topographical Anatomy

A Topography of the right orbit: contents of the upper level
Superior view.

a The bony roof of the orbit has been removed and the periorbita partially cut away. Dissection of the contents of the orbit with careful removal of the retrobulbar fatty tissue.

b The periorbita of the entire orbital roof and the retrobulbar fatty tissue have been completely removed.

Note in **a** the course of the frontal nerve on the levator palpebrae superioris. The frontal nerve is the first nerve that one sees after opening the periorbita from a superior approach.

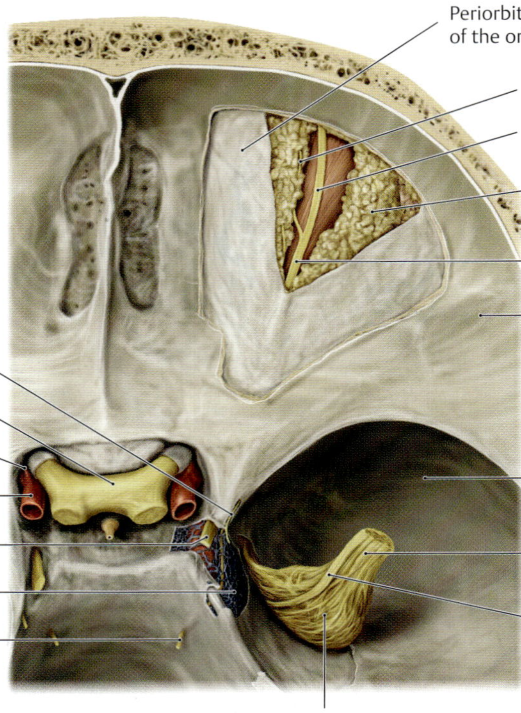

a

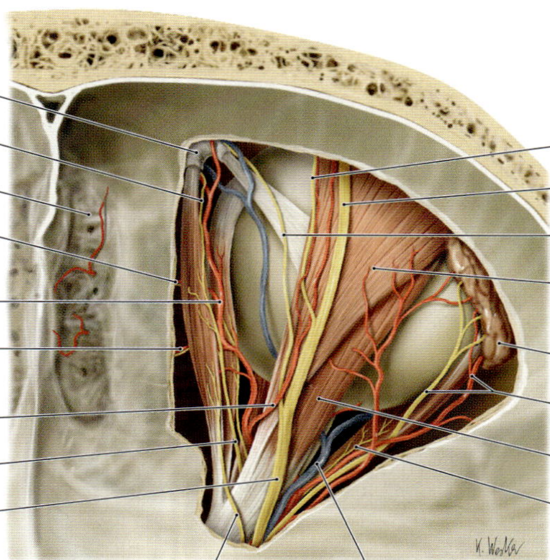

b

B Topography of the right orbit: contents of the middle level
Superior view. The levator palpebrae superioris and the superior rectus have been divided and reflected posteriorly, and all fatty tissue has been removed to better expose the optic nerve.
Note: The ciliary ganglion is approximately 2 mm in diameter and lies lateral to the optic nerve approximately 2 cm behind the eyeball. The parasympathetic innervation for the intraocular muscles (ciliary muscle and pupillary sphincter) is relayed through the ciliary ganglion where they synapse. The postsynaptic sympathetic fibers for the pupillary dilator, from the superior cervical ganglion, also pass through this ganglion.

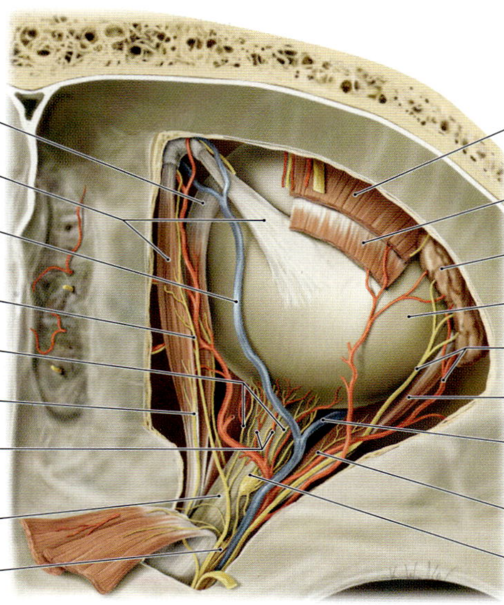

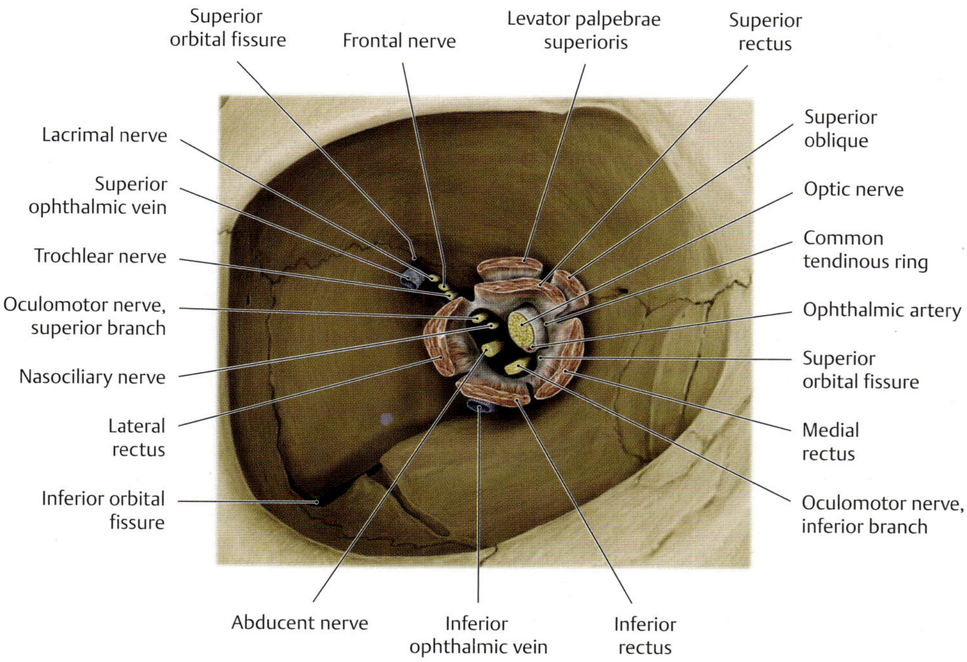

C Topography of the right orbit: contents of the upper level

Superior view. The bony roof of the orbit, the periorbita, and the retro-orbital fat have been removed. The optic nerve and ophthalmic artery enter the eye socket through the optic canal. Of the neurovascular structures that enter the eye socket via the superior orbital fissure, some run inside and some outside the common tendinous ring:

- inside: superior and inferior branches of the oculomotor nerve, abducent nerve, and nasociliary nerve,
- outside: superior and inferior ophthalmic veins, frontal nerve, lacrimal nerve, and trochlear nerve.

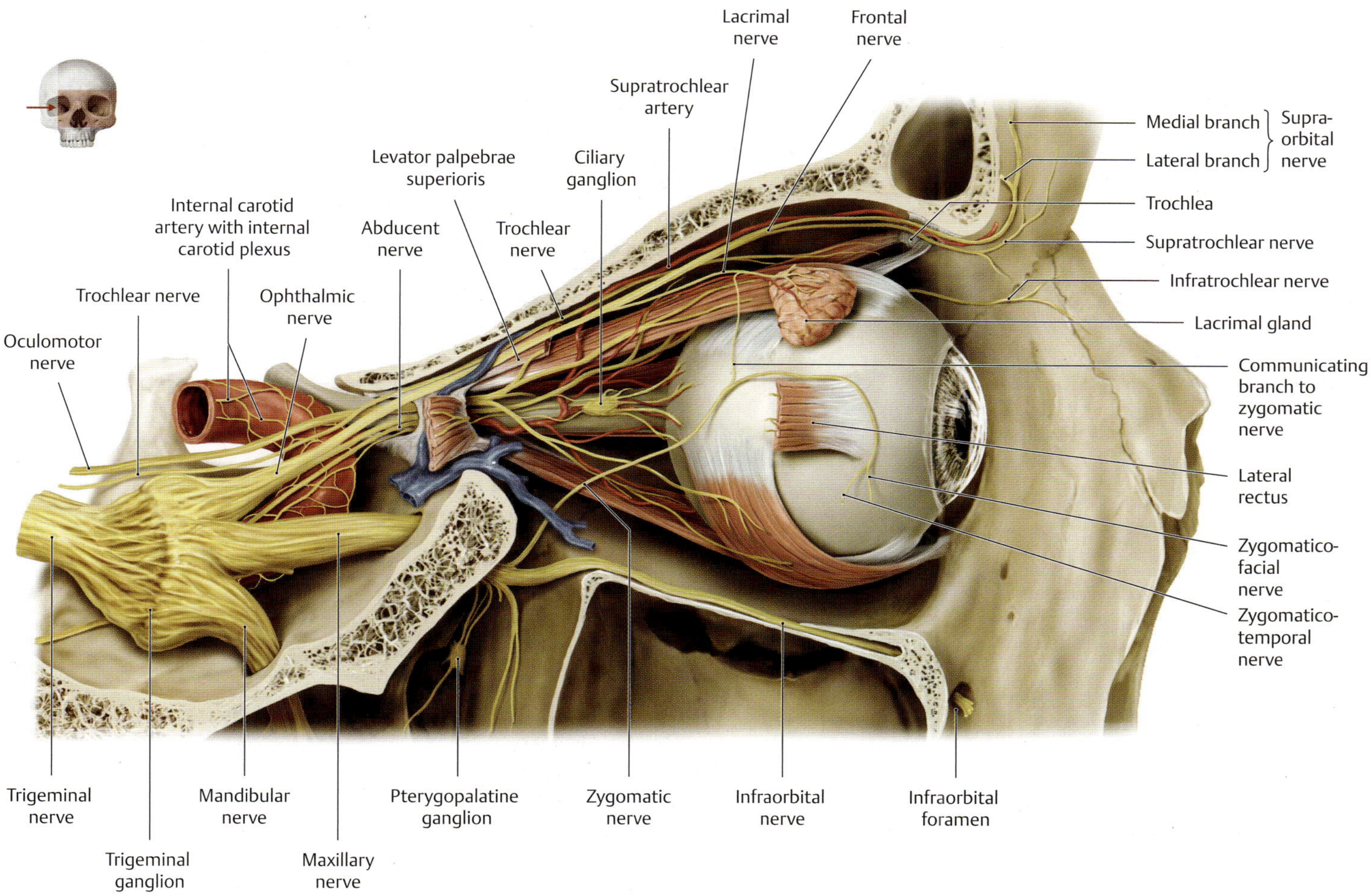

D Right orbit

Lateral view.

The following structures have been removed: lateral orbital wall as far as the inferior orbital fissure (see navigator), lateral portions of the orbital roof as well as retrobulbar fatty tissue and the anterior two-thirds of the levator palpebrae superioris. The lateral rectus has been divided. The entire orbital contents can now be easily dissected, especially the ciliary ganglion and the communicating branch to the zygomatic nerve (parasympathetic fibers from the pterygopalatine ganglion for the lacrimal gland). If one also removes the greater wing of the sphenoid bone, one will also see the trigeminal ganglion and the opened cavernous sinus.

Note that the removed orbital surface of the zygomatic bone contains the points of entry of the zygomaticofacial and zygomaticotemporal branches, the sensory terminal branches of the zygomatic nerve supplying the skin over the zygomatic bone and temple.

5.19 Topography of the Cavernous Sinus

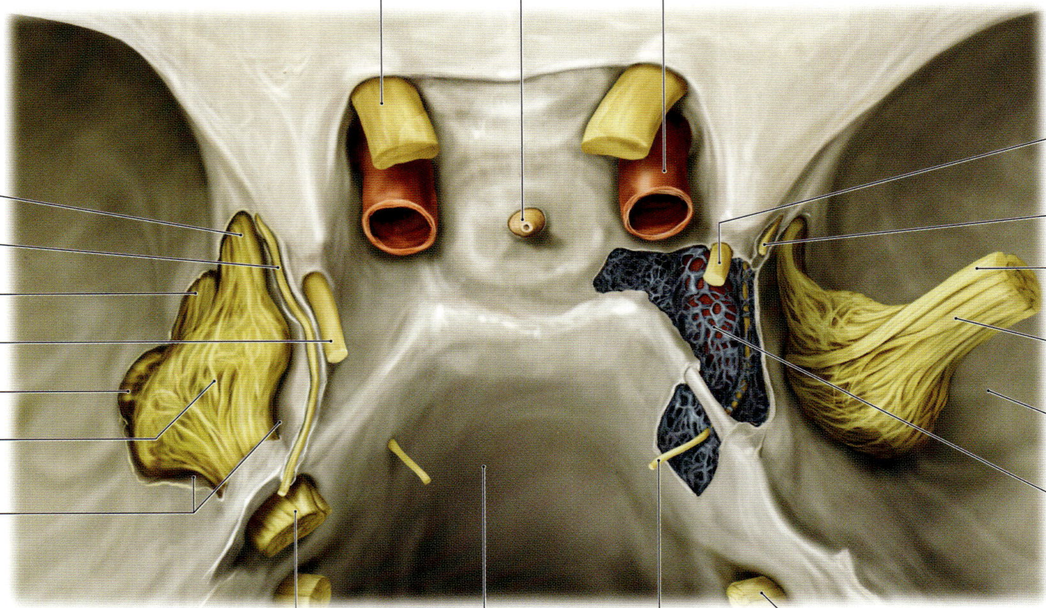

A Course of the cranial nerves supplying the orbit through the cavernous sinus

Sella turcica with partially opened cavernous sinus on the right side, superior view. The two trigeminal ganglia are exposed. The right ganglion has also been retracted laterally (thus opening the trigeminal cave) to demonstrate the open cavernous sinus with the cavernous part of the internal carotid artery coursing within it.

Note the abducent nerve which also courses within the cavernous sinus immediately adjacent to the carotid. All the other nerves coursing here (oculomotor, trochlear, and trigeminal nerves) course in a rostral or inferior direction in the lateral wall of the dura mater of the cavernous sinus. A carotid artery aneurysm within the cavernous sinus therefore most often affects the abducent nerve, and often that nerve alone. The expanding aneurysm compresses the nerve, causing loss of function. Therefore, one should always consider a carotid artery aneurysm as a possible cause of a sudden isolated abducent nerve palsy (see **D**). In contrast, an isolated *trochlear nerve* palsy is very rare. The trochlear nerve tends to be affected *secondarily,* for example in the setting of cavernous sinus thrombosis, which then affects all nerves passing through the cavernous sinus, often including the first two branches of the trigeminal nerve.

B Coronal section through the cavernous sinus at the level of the pituitary gland

Rostral view.

Note the structures coursing within the lateral wall and within the cavernous sinus.

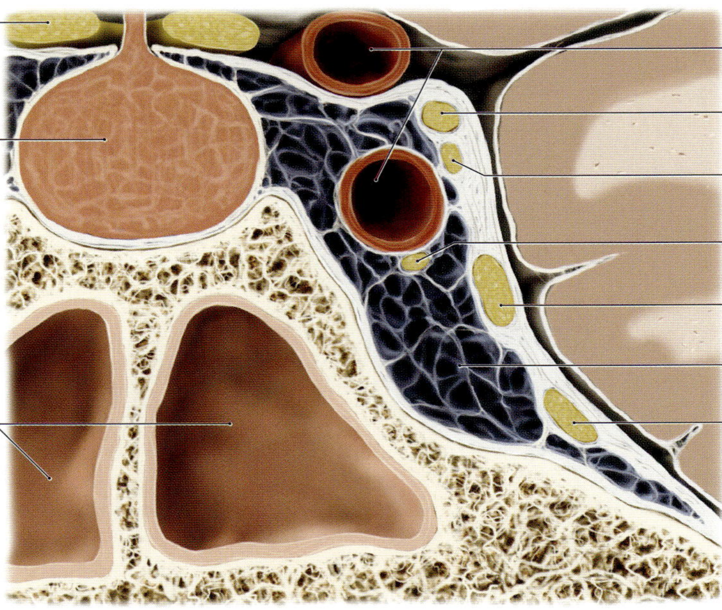

C Topography of the extradural course of the abducent nerve on the clivus after removal of the right cavernous sinus

Right view; the oculomotor and trochlear nerves have been retracted laterally for clarity. *Note* the long extradural course of the abducent nerve. This begins as it exits from the dura mater in the superior third of the clivus (before which its subarachnoid segment lies at the level of the prepontine cistern) over the "abducent bridge" (deep to the ligament of Gruber through the canal of Dorello) at the level of tip of the pyramid of the petrous bone (passing from the posterior cranial fossa to the middle cranial fossa). It continues through the cavernous sinus immediately adjacent to the internal carotid artery, finally entering the orbit through the superior orbital fissure.

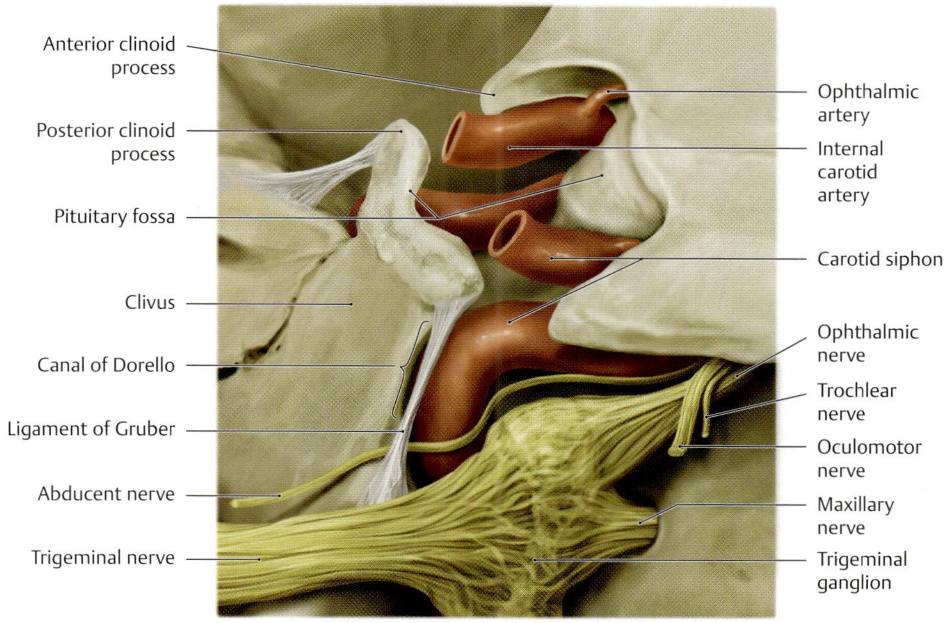

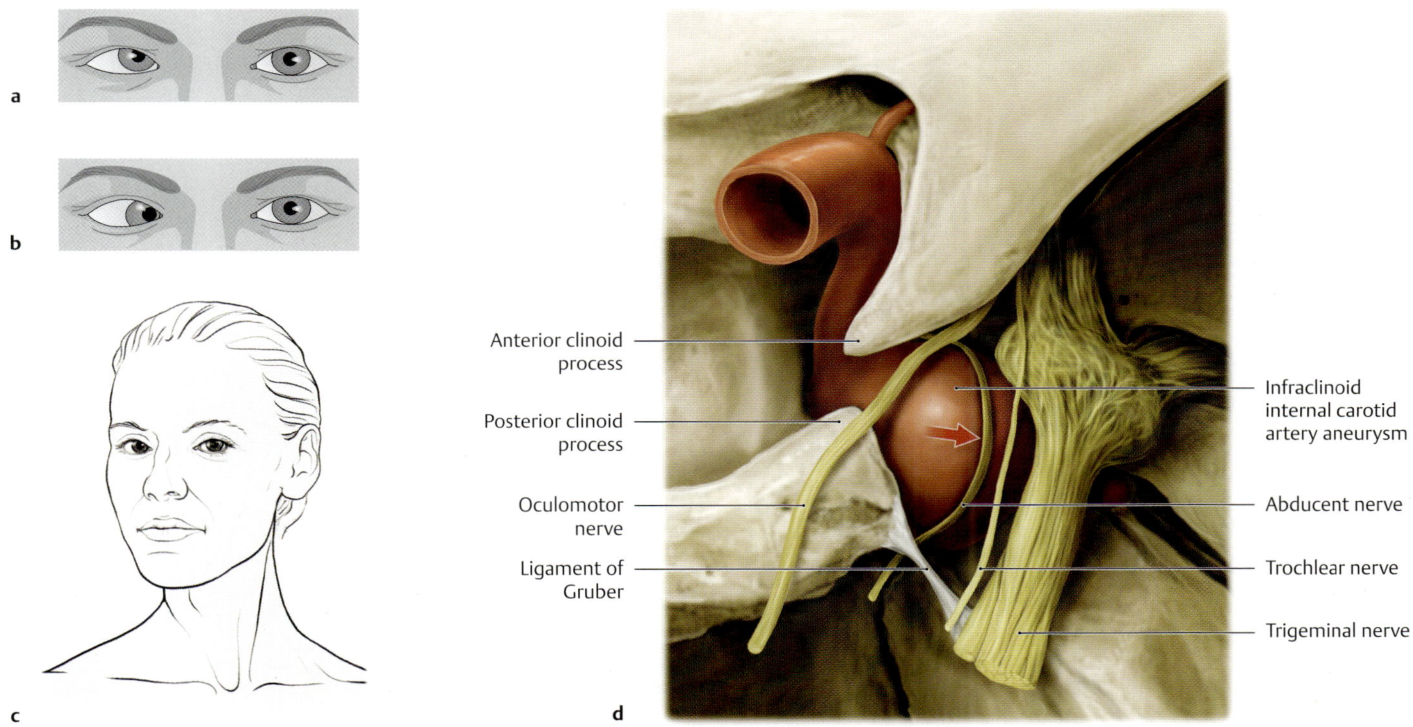

D Trochlear and abducent nerve palsies

a Right trochlear nerve palsy; **b** right abducent nerve palsy (patient looking straight ahead in each case); **c** compensatory head posture in right abducent nerve palsy; **d** infraclinoid carotid artery aneurysm within the cavernous sinus compressing the abducent nerve. Posterosuperior view.

Ophthalmoplegia can result from a lesion in the nucleus, along the course of the respective cranial nerve, or within the ocular muscle itself (see p. 173). Sequelae include an abnormal gaze of the affected eye that varies according to the muscle involved and the occurrence of diplopia, which the patient attempts to avoid with a compensatory head posture. For example, loss of the abducent nerve (at 47% of all cases, abducent nerve palsies are the most common peripheral neurogenic disturbance of ocular motility) causes the affected eye to deviate medially even in primary position due to the isolated loss of the lateral rectus (esotropia). The disturbing diplopia induces a compensatory head posture (**c**), that is a head posture in which diplopia does not occur or is greatly reduced. The patient turns the head laterally towards the side of the affected muscle (a position in which the paretic muscle has no effect anyway). Internal carotid artery aneurysms within the cavernous sinus can lie in a supraclinoid or infraclinoid position, whereby the infraclinoid aneurysms (**d**) in particular exhibit a slowly progressive mass effect leading to isolated compression of the abducent nerve (red arrow = compression site).

5.20 Nose: Overview

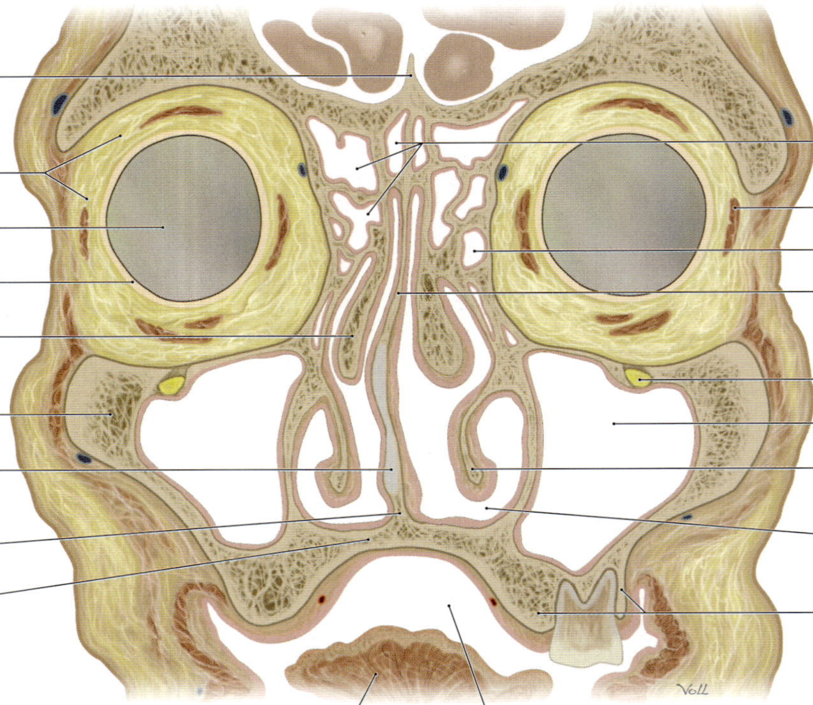

a

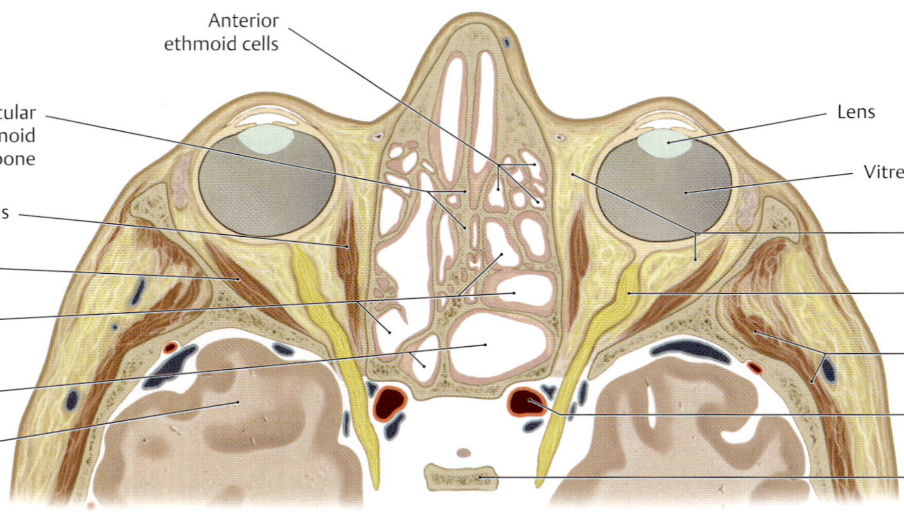

b

A Overview of the nose and paranasal sinuses

a Coronal section, anterior view. **b** Transverse section, superior view. The reader is assumed to be familiar with the bony anatomy of the nasal cavity (especially the openings of the various passages below the nasal conchae, see p. 42 f). The nasal cavities and paranasal sinuses are arranged in pairs. The left and right nasal cavities are separated by the nasal septum and have an approximately triangular shape. Below the base of the triangle is the oral cavity. The following paired paranasal sinuses are shown in the drawings:

- Ethmoid cells (ethmoid sinus*)
- Maxillary sinus
- Sphenoid sinus

The interior of each sinus is lined with ciliated pseudostratified columnar epithelium with goblet cells (respiratory epithelium) (see p. 184).

* The term "ethmoid sinus" has been dropped from the latest anatomical nomenclature, although it is still widely used by medical practitioners.

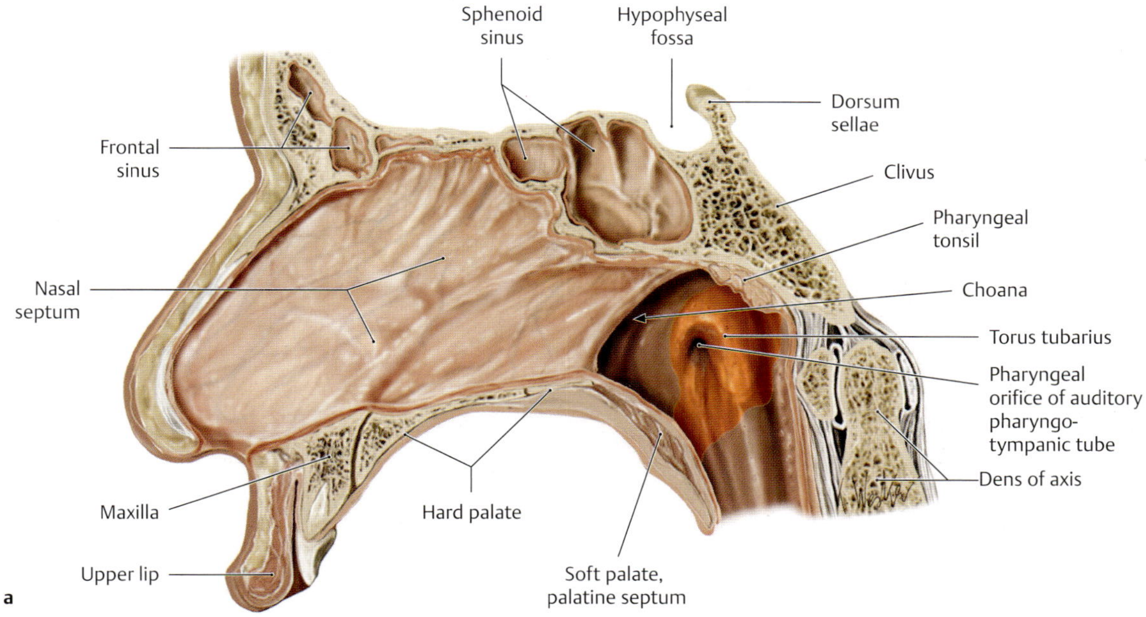

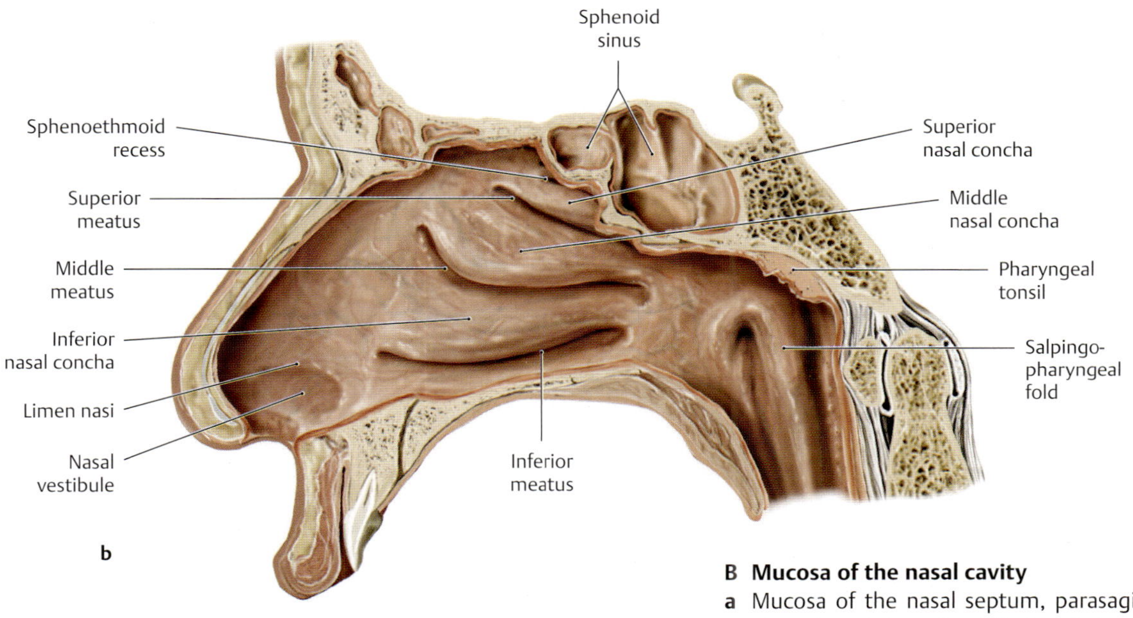

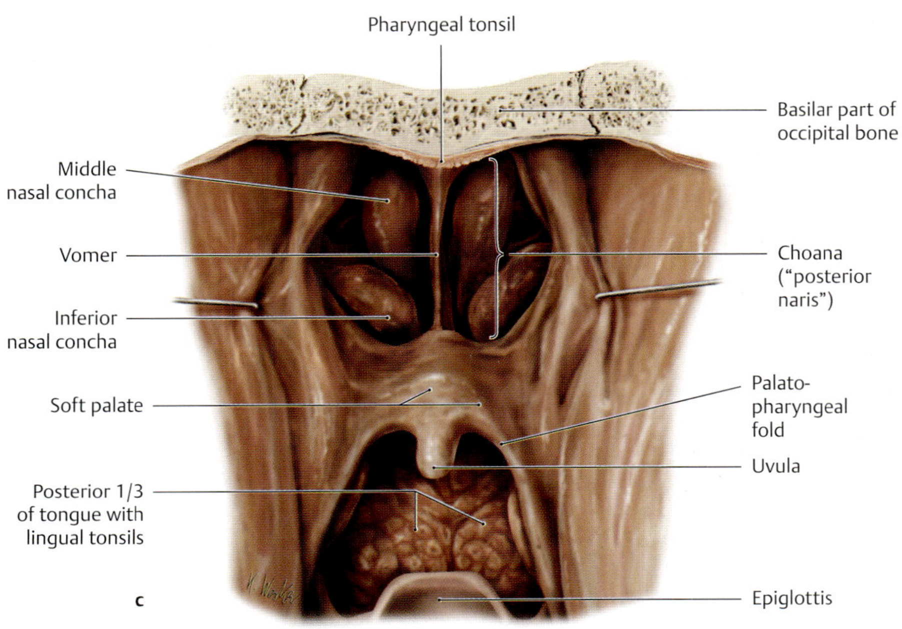

B Mucosa of the nasal cavity

a Mucosa of the nasal septum, parasagittal section viewed from the left side. **b** Mucosa of the right lateral nasal wall, viewed from the left side. **c** Posterior view through the choanae into the nasal cavity.

Note: The mucous membrane around the torus tubarius (orange colored region in **a**) is contoured by the small, primarily mucosal salivary glands deep to the mucous membrane (for the importance of the small salivary glands see p. 211**B**).

While the medial wall of the nasal cavity is smooth, its lateral wall is raised into folds by the three conchae (superior, middle, and inferior concha). These increase the surface area of the nasal cavity, enabling it to warm and humidify the inspired air more efficiently (cf. p. 184). A section of the right sphenoid sinus is shown in **b**. The choanae (**c**) are the posterior openings by which the nasal cavity communicates with the nasopharynx. Note the close proximity of the choanae to the pharyngotympanic (auditory) tube and pharyngeal tonsil (see p. 197).

5.21 Nasal Cavity: Neurovascular Supply

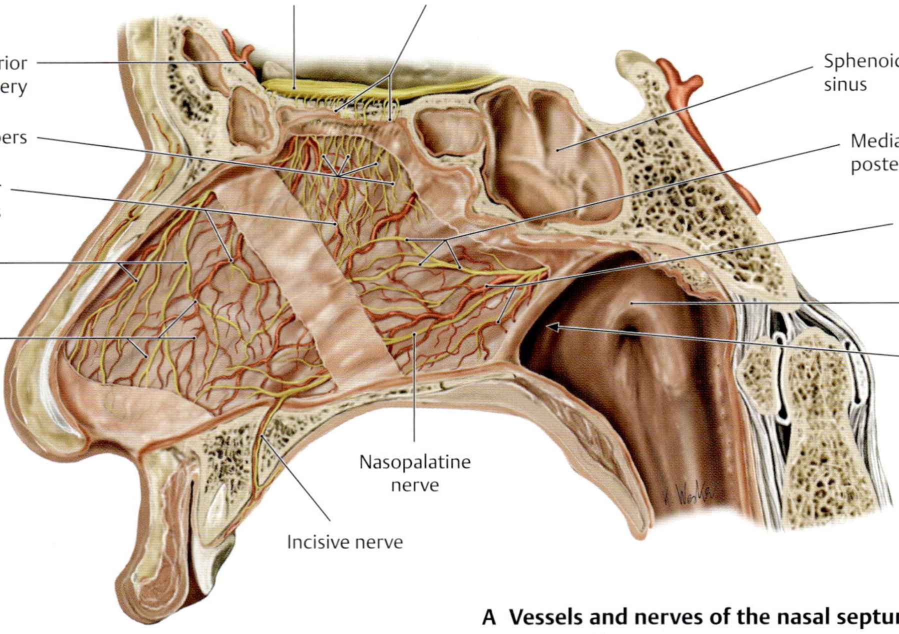

A Vessels and nerves of the nasal septum with the mucosa removed

Parasagittal section, viewed from the left side. The arterial supply of the nasal septum is of particular clinical interest in the diagnosis and treatment of nosebleed (see **C**).

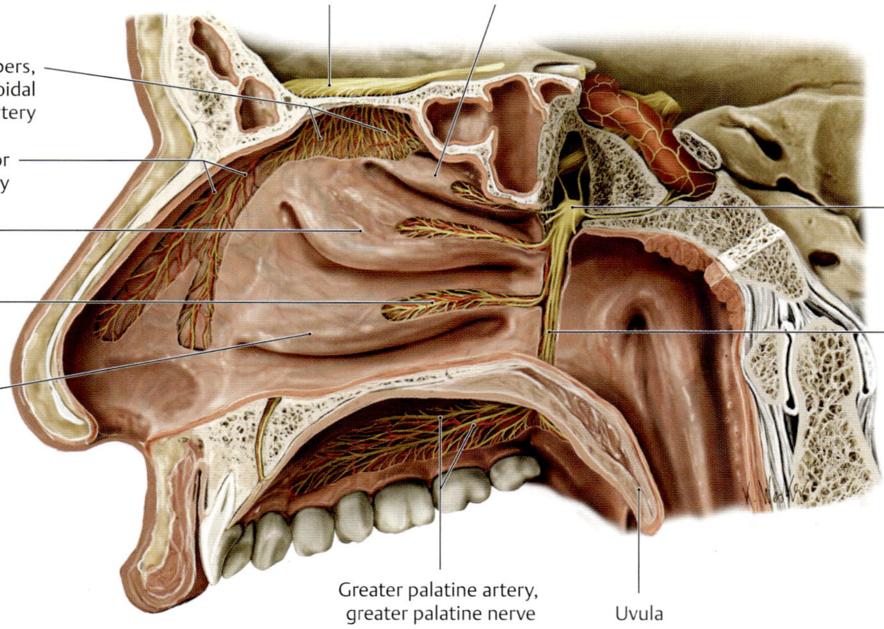

B Vessels and nerves of the right lateral nasal wall

Left lateral view. The pterygopalatine ganglion, an important relay in the parasympathetic nervous system (see pp. 127 and 239), has been exposed here by partial resection of the sphenoid bone. The nerve arising from it pass to the small nasal glands of the nasal conchae, entering the conchae from the posterior side with the blood vessels. At the level of the superior concha, the olfactory fibers pass through the cribriform plate to the olfactory mucosa. The nasal wall is supplied from above by the two ethmoidal arteries, which arise from the ophthalmic artery. It is supplied from behind by the lateral posterior nasal arteries, which arise from the sphenopalatine artery.

The figures below depict the functional groups of arteries and nerves supplying the nasal cavity. As in a dissection, the septum is displayed first, followed by the lateral wall.

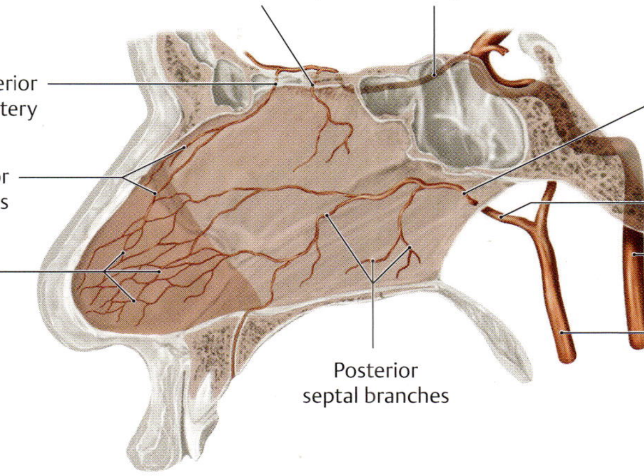

C Arteries of the nasal septum
Left lateral view. The vessels of the nasal septum arise from branches of the external and internal carotid arteries. The anterior part of the septum contains a highly vascularized area called Kiesselbach's area (indicated by color shading), which is supplied by vessels from both major arteries. This area is the most common site of significant nosebleed.

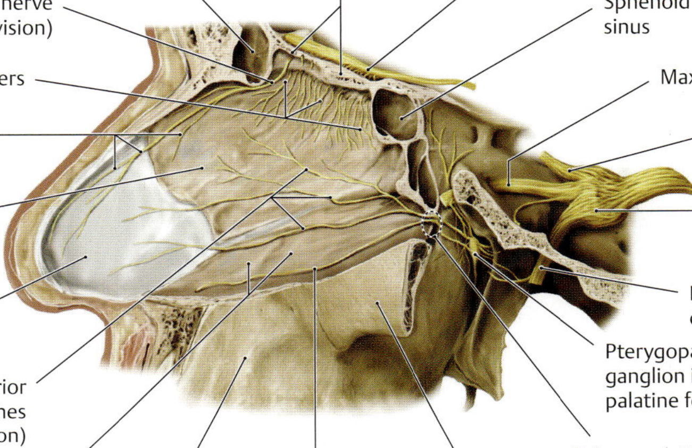

D Nerves of the nasal septum
Left lateral view. The nasal septum receives its sensory innervation from branches of the trigeminal nerve (CN V). The anterosuperior part of the septum is supplied by branches of the ophthalmic division (CN V_1), and the rest by branches of the maxillary division (CN V_2). Bundles of olfactory nerve fibers (CN I) arise from receptors in the olfactory mucosa.

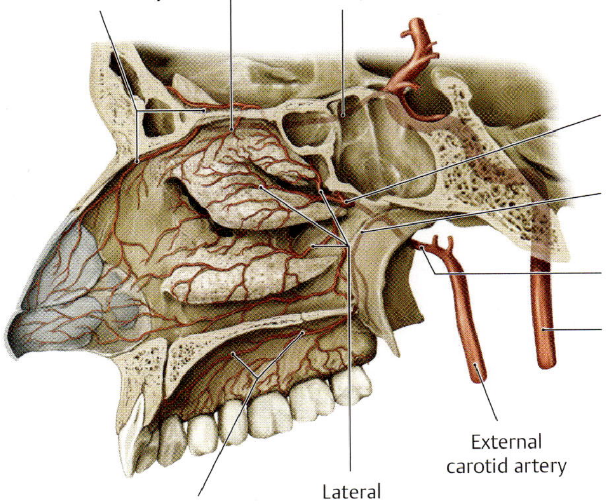

E Arteries of the right lateral nasal wall
Left lateral view.
Note the vascular supply from the branches of the internal carotid artery (from above) and the external carotid artery (from behind).

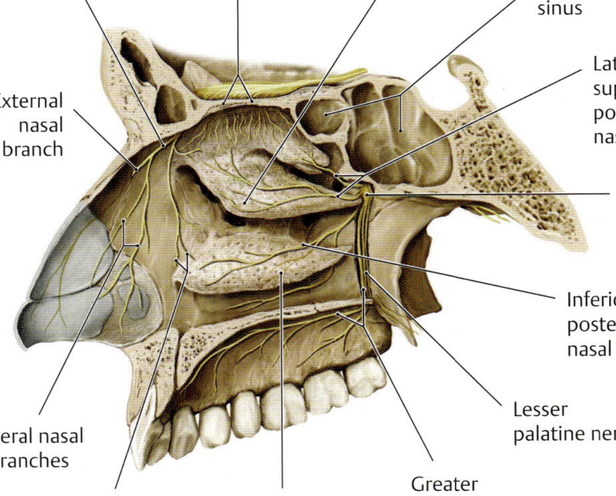

F Nerves of the right lateral nasal wall
Left lateral view. The lateral nasal wall derives its sensory innervation from branches of the ophthalmic division (CN V_1) and the maxillary division (CN V_2 of the trigeminal n.). Receptor neurons in the olfactory mucosa send their axons in the olfactory nerve (CN I) to the olfactory bulb.

5.22 Nose and Paranasal Sinuses: Histology and Clinical Anatomy

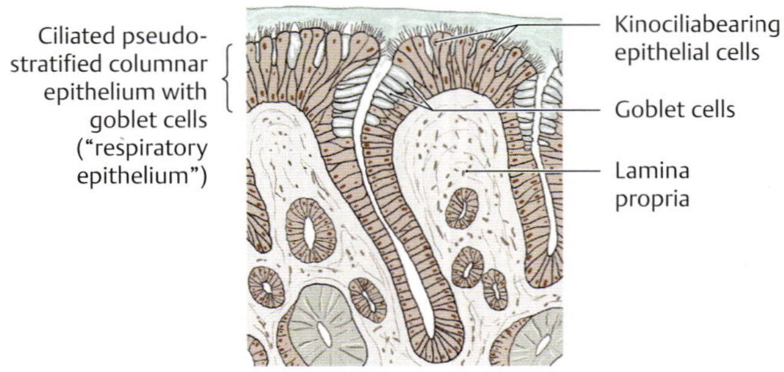

A Histology of the nasal mucosa
The surface of the respiratory epithelium of the nasal mucosa consists of kinocilia-bearing cells and goblet cells, the latter secreting their mucous into a watery film on the epithelial surface. Serous and seromucous glands are embedded in the lamina propria and also release secretions into the superficial fluid film. The directional fluid flow produced by the cilia (see **C** and **D**) is an important component of the nonspecific immune response. If coordinated beating of the cilia is impaired, the patient will suffer chronic recurring infections of the respiratory tract.

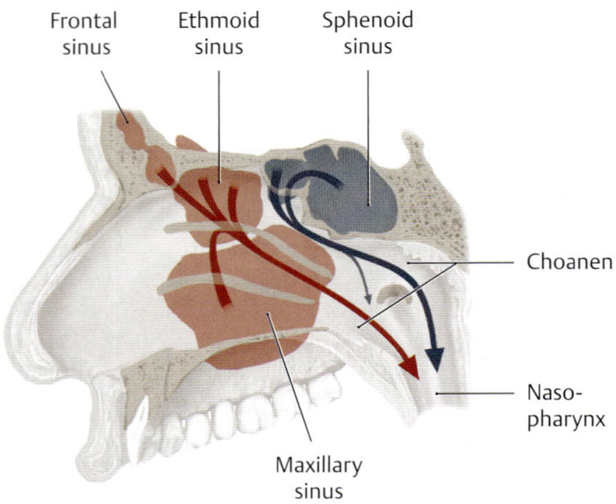

B Normal drainage of secretions from the paranasal sinus
Left lateral view. The beating cilia propel the mucous blanket over the cilia (see **D**) and through the choana into the nasopharynx, where it is swallowed.

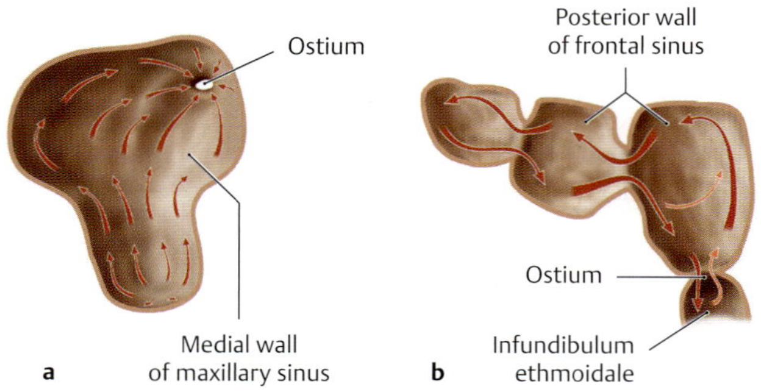

C Direction of ciliary beating and fluid flow in the right maxillary sinus and frontal sinus
Schematic coronal sections of the right maxillary sinus (**a**) and frontal sinus (**b**), anterior view. The location of the sinuses is shown in **B**.
Beating of the cilia produces a flow of fluid in the paranasal sinuses that is always directed toward the sinus ostium. This clears the sinus of particles and microorganisms that are trapped in the mucous layer. If the ostium is obstructed due to swelling of the mucosa, inflammation may develop in the affected sinus (*sinusitis*). This occurs most commonly in the ostiomeatal unit of the maxillary sinus—ethmoid ostium (see p. 42 f).

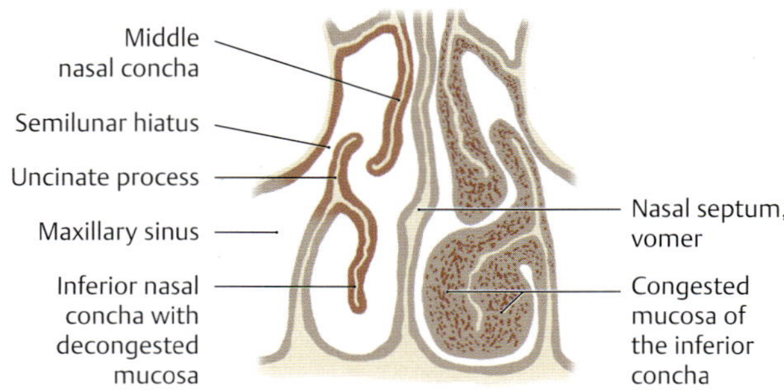

D Functional states of the mucosa in the nasal cavity
Coronal section, anterior view.
The function of the nasal mucosa is to warm and humidify the inspired air. This is accomplished by an increase of blood flow through the mucosa (see pp. 101 and 103), placing it in a congested (swollen) state. The mucous membranes are not simultaneously congested on both sides, however, but undergo a normal cycle of congestion and decongestion that lasts approximately 6 hours (the right side is decongested in the drawing). Examination of the nasal cavity can be facilitated by first administering a decongestant to shrink the mucosa, roughly as it appears here on the right side.

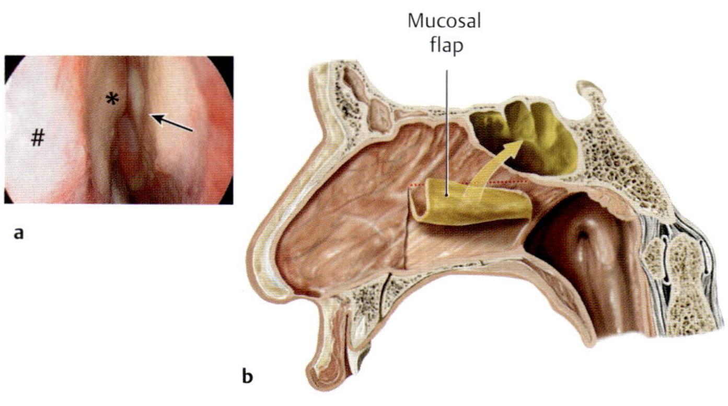

E Sparing the olfactory mucosa in operations on the sphenoid sinus

a Endoscopic image of the olfactory mucosa (from: Simmen-Kistler D, Jones N, editors. *Chirurgie der Nasennebenhöhlen*. Stuttgart: Thieme; 2013). The endoscope is in the left nostril, placed approximately as in anterior rhinoscopy in position II (see **Ga**). The olfactory mucosa (arrow) is the lighter, less well perfused region (*, superior nasal concha; #, middle nasal concha). This region should be spared in operations on the sphenoid sinus.

b Nasal septum. Left view. The mucosal region deep to the olfactory mucosa can be grafted as a mucosal flap.

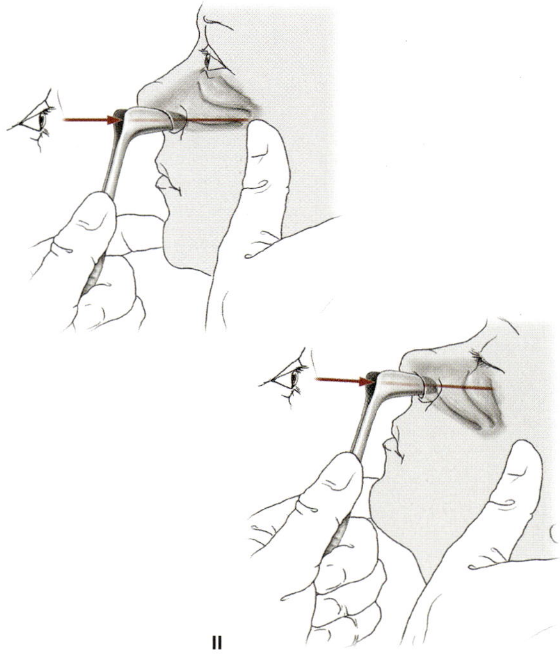

I

a II

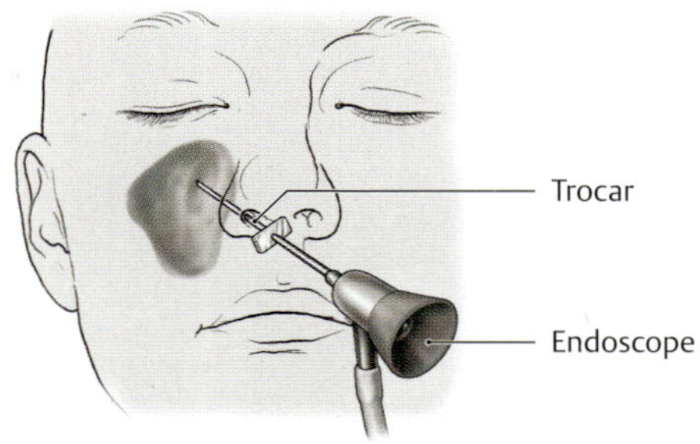

F Endoscopy of the maxillary sinus
Anterior view. The maxillary sinus is not accessible to direct inspection and must therefore be examined with an endoscope. To enter the maxillary sinus, the examiner pierces the thin bony wall below the inferior concha with a trocar and advances the endoscope through the opening. The scope can then be angled and rotated to inspect all of the mucosal surfaces.

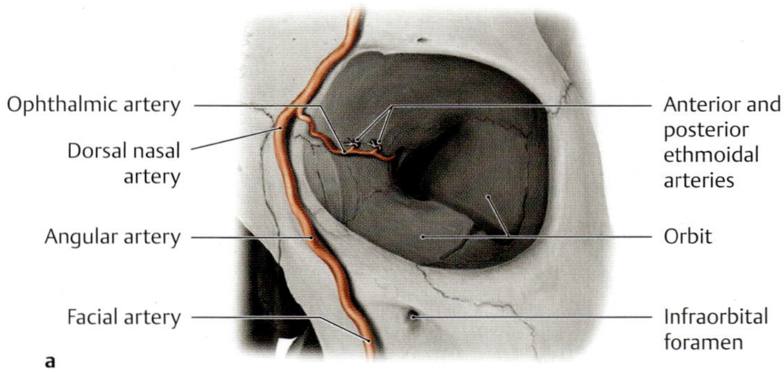

a

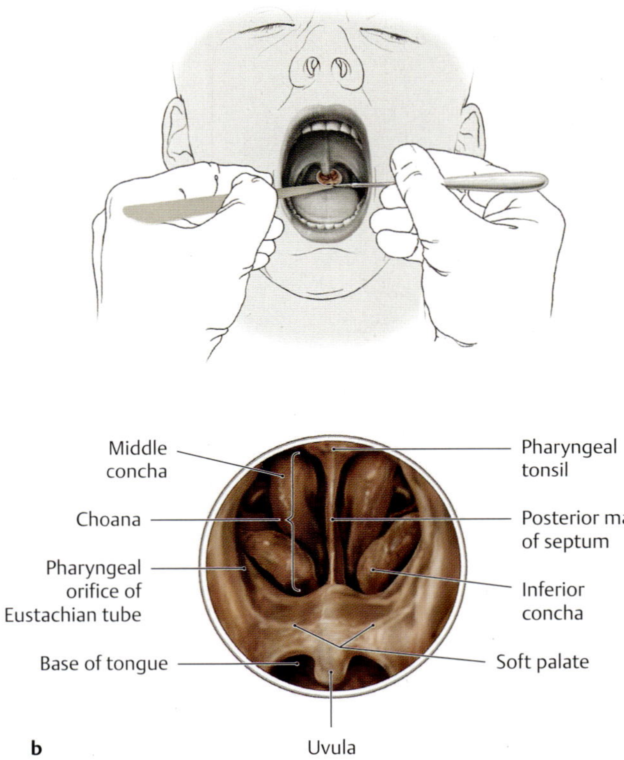

b

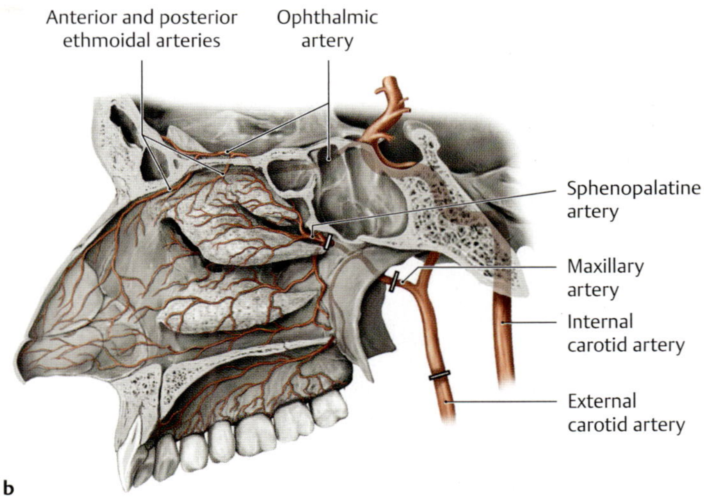

b

G Anterior and posterior rhinoscopy

a Anterior rhinoscopy is a procedure for inspection of the nasal cavity. Two different positions (I, II) are used to ensure that all of the anterior nasal cavity is examined.

b In posterior rhinoscopy, the choanae and pharyngeal tonsil are accessible to clinical examination. The rhinoscope can be angled and rotated to demonstrate the structures shown in the composite image. Today the rhinoscope is frequently replaced by an endoscope.

H Sites of arterial ligation for the treatment of severe nosebleed
If a severe nosebleed cannot be controlled with ordinary intranasal packing, it may be necessary to ligate relatively large arterial vessels. The following arteries may be ligated:

- In the case of anterior nasal bleeding, the anterior and posterior ethmoidal arteries (**a**)
- In the case of posterior nasal bleeding, the sphenopalatine artery or the maxillary artery (**b**)
- In very severe cases, the external carotid artery (**b**)

5.23 Oral Cavity: Overview; Hard and Soft Palate

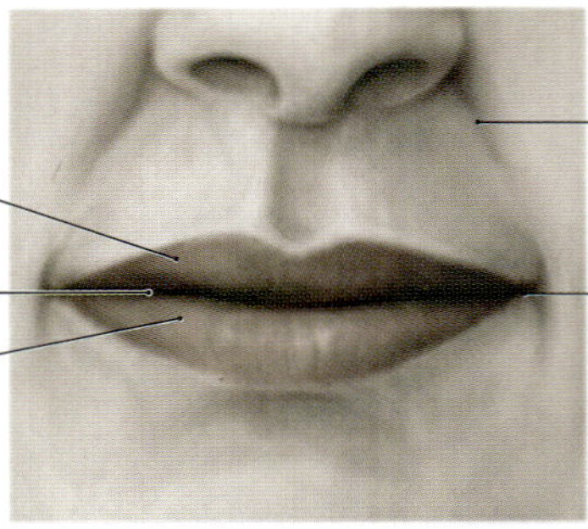

A Lips and labial creases
Anterior view. The upper and lower lips meet at the angle of the mouth. The oral fissure opens into the oral cavity. Changes in the lips noted on visual inspection may yield important diagnostic clues: Blue lips (cyanosis) suggest a disease of the heart, lung, or both, while deep nasolabial creases may reflect chronic diseases of the digestive tract.

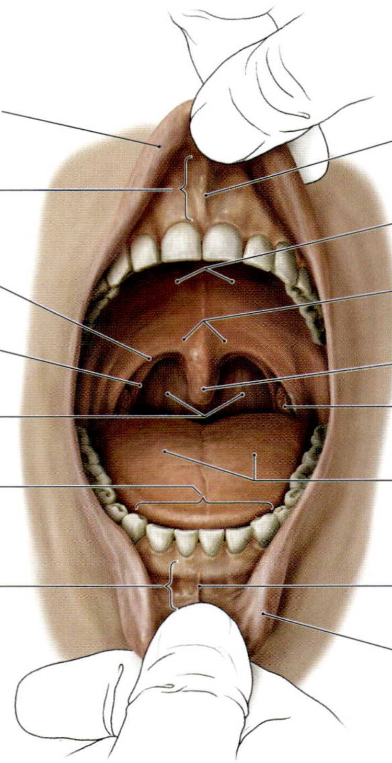

B Oral cavity
Anterior view. The dental arches with the alveolar processes of the maxilla and mandible subdivide the oral cavity into several parts (see also **C**):

- Oral vestibule: the part of the oral cavity bounded on one side by the teeth and on the other side by the lips or cheeks
- Oral cavity proper: the cavity of the mouth in the strict sense (within the dental arches, bounded posteriorly by the palatoglossal arch)
- Fauces: the throat (boundary with the pharynx: palatopharyngeal arch)

The fauces communicate with the pharynx through the faucial isthmus. The oral cavity is lined with nonkeratinized, stratified squamous epithelium which is moistened by secretions from the salivary glands (see p. 211). Squamous cell carcinomas of the oral cavity are particularly common in smokers and heavy drinkers.

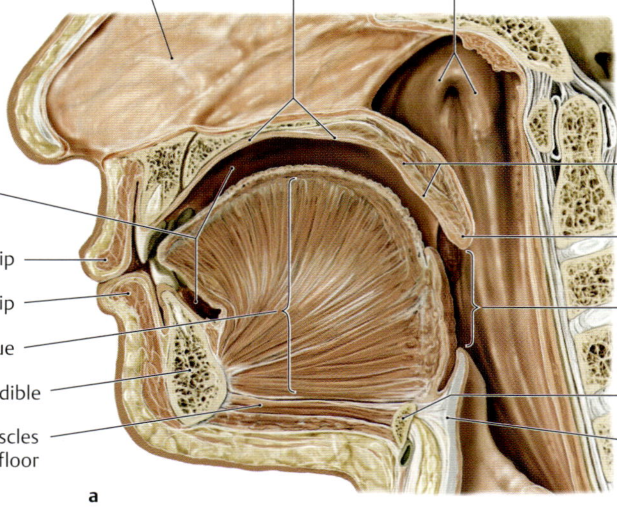

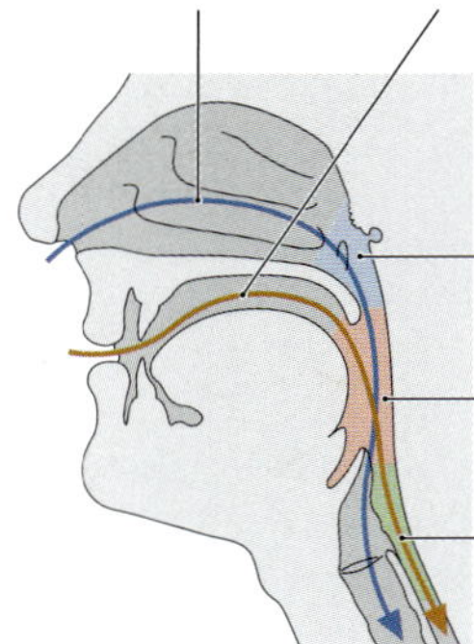

C Organization and boundaries of the oral cavity
Midsagittal section, left lateral view. The muscles of the oral floor and the adjacent tongue together constitute the inferior boundary of the oral cavity proper. The roof of the oral cavity is formed by the hard palate in its anterior two-thirds and by the soft palate (velum) in its posterior third (see **F**). The uvula hangs from the soft palate between the oral cavity and pharynx. The keratinized stratified squamous epithelium of the skin blends with the nonkeratinized stratified squamous epithelium of the oral cavity at the vermilion border of the lip. The oral cavity is located below the nasal cavity and anterior to the pharynx. The midportion of the pharynx, called the oropharynx, is the area in which the airway and foodway intersect (**b**).

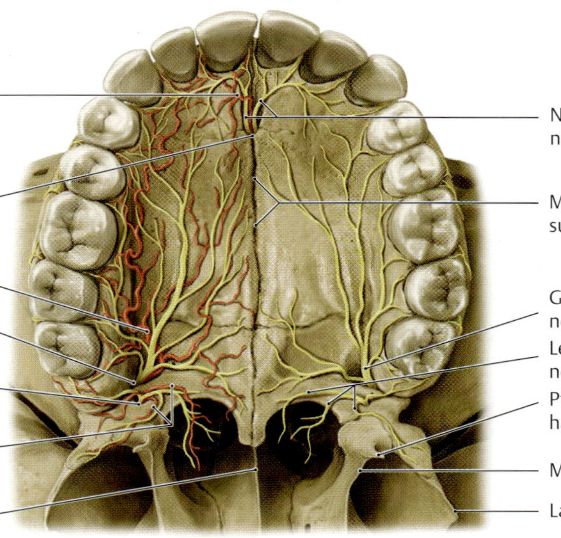

D Neurovascular structures of the hard palate

Inferior view. The arteries and nerves of the hard palate (skeletal anatomy is shown on p. 44) pass downward through the incisive foramen and the greater and lesser palatine foramina into the oral cavity. The nerves are terminal branches of the trigeminal nerve's maxillary division (CN V_2), and the arteries arise from the territory of the maxillary artery off the external carotid a. (neither are shown here).

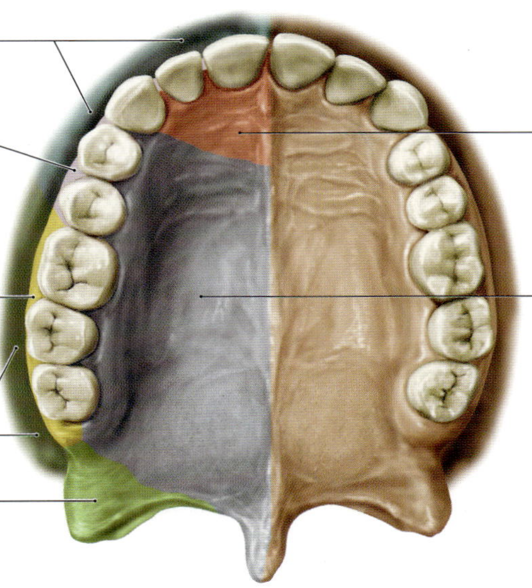

E Sensory innervation of the palatal mucosa, upper lip, cheeks, and gingiva

Inferior view.

Note that the region shown in the drawing receives sensory innervation from different branches of the trigeminal nerve (buccal nerve from the mandibular division (CN V_3, all other branches are from the maxillary division, CN V_2).

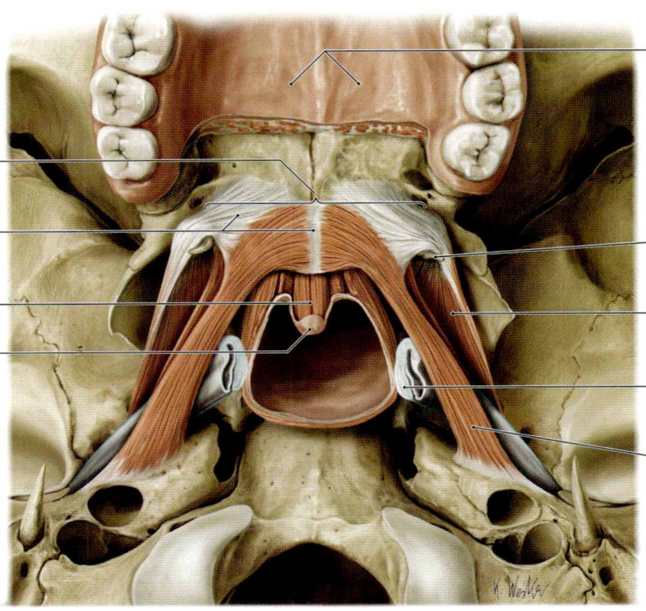

F Muscles of the soft palate

Inferior view. The soft palate forms the posterior boundary of the oral cavity, separating it from the oropharynx. The muscles are attached at the midline to the palatine aponeurosis, which forms the connective tissue foundation of the soft palate. The tensor veli palatini, levator veli palatini, and musculus uvulae can be identified in this dissection. While the tensor veli palatini tightens the soft palate, simultaneously opening the inlet to the pharyngotympanic (auditory) tube, the levator veli palatini raises the soft palate to a horizontal position. Both of these muscles, but not the musculus uvulae, also contribute structurally to the lateral pharyngeal wall.

5.24 Tongue: Muscles and Mucosa

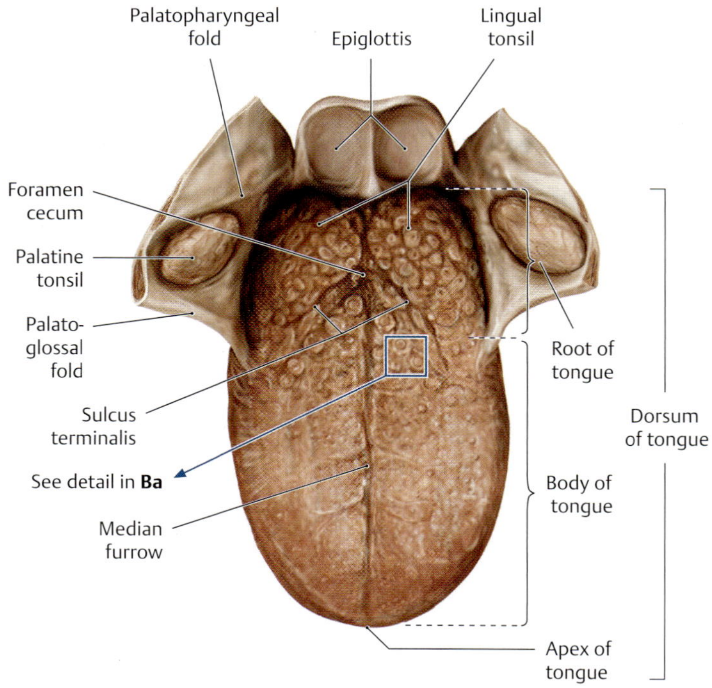

A Surface anatomy of the lingual mucosa
Superior view. While the motor properties of the tongue are functionally important during mastication, swallowing, and speaking, its equally important sensory functions include taste and fine tactile discrimination. The tongue is endowed with a very powerful muscular body (see **Ca**). The upper surface (dorsum) of the tongue is covered by a highly specialized mucosal coat and consists, from front to back, of an apex (tip), body, and root.
The V-shaped furrow on the dorsal surface (the sulcus terminalis) further divides the tongue into an anterior (oral, presulcal) part and a posterior (pharyngeal, postsulcal) part. The anterior part comprises the anterior two-thirds of the tongue, and the posterior part comprises the posterior third. At the tip of the "V" is the foramen cecum (vestige of embryological migration of the thyroid gland). This subdivision is a result of embryological development and explains why each part has a different nerve supply (see p. 191). The mucosa of the anterior part is composed of numerous papillae (see **B**), and the connective tissue between the mucosal surface and musculature contains many small salivary glands. The physician should be familiar with them because they may give rise to tumors (usually malignant).
The taste buds are bordered by serous glands (see **Bb–e**) that are known also as *von Ebner glands*; they produce a watery secretion that keeps the taste buds clean.

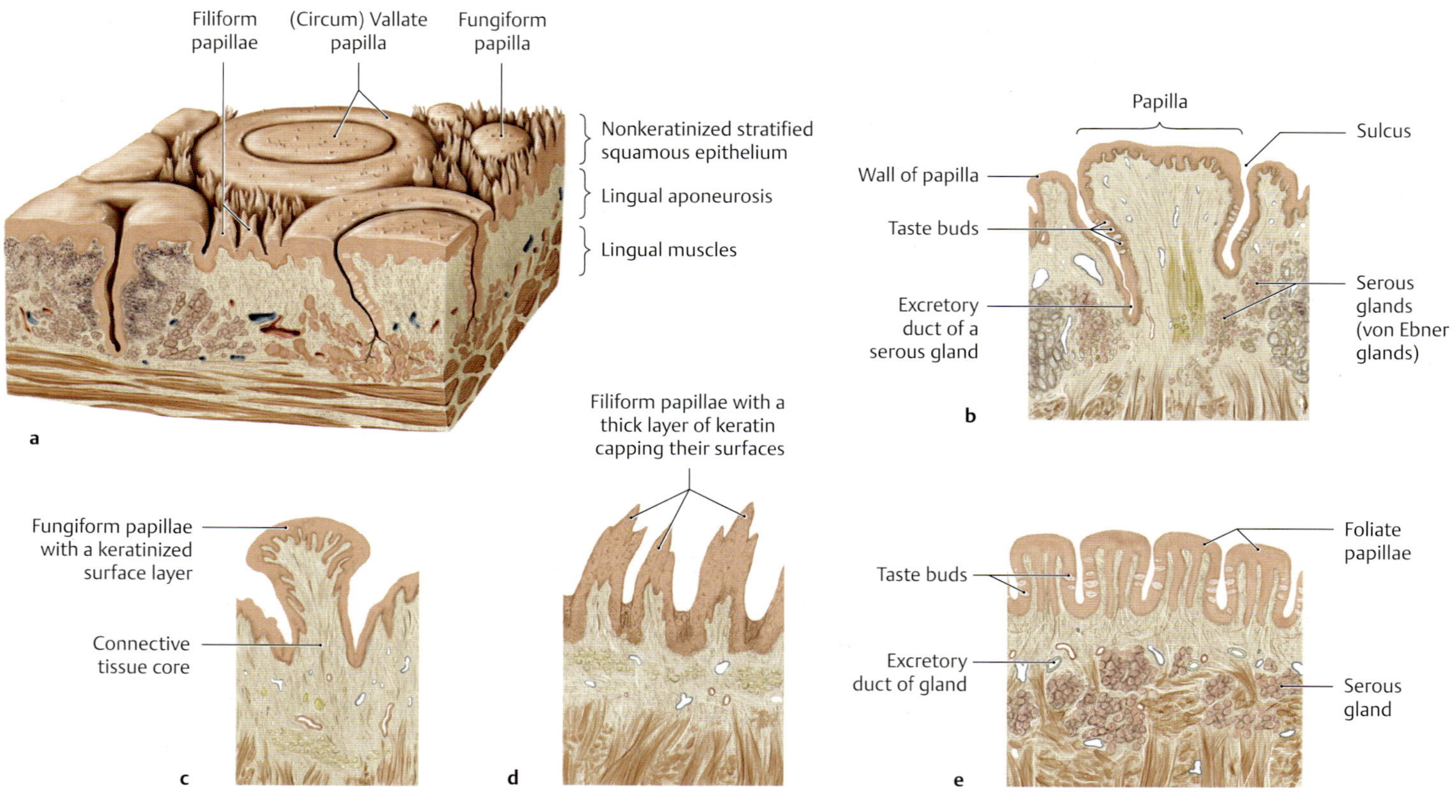

B The papillae of the tongue
a Sectional block diagram of the lingual papillae. **b–e** Types of papillae.

The papillae are divided into four morphologically distinct types:

b (Circum) Vallate papillae: encircled by a depression and containing abundant taste buds on their lateral surfaces
c Fungiform papillae: mushroom-shaped, located at the sides of the tongue (they exhibit mechanical receptors, thermal receptors, and taste buds)
d Filiform papillae: rasp-like papillae with a thick cap of keratin that are sensitive to tactile stimuli
e Foliate papillae: located on the posterior sides of the tongue, containing numerous taste buds

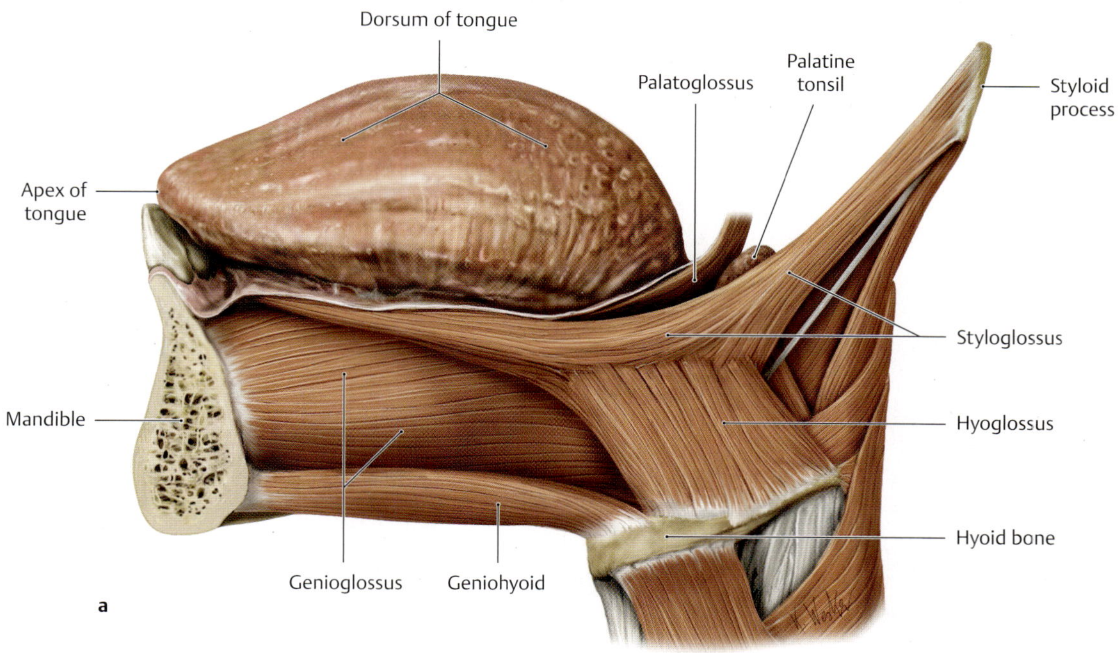

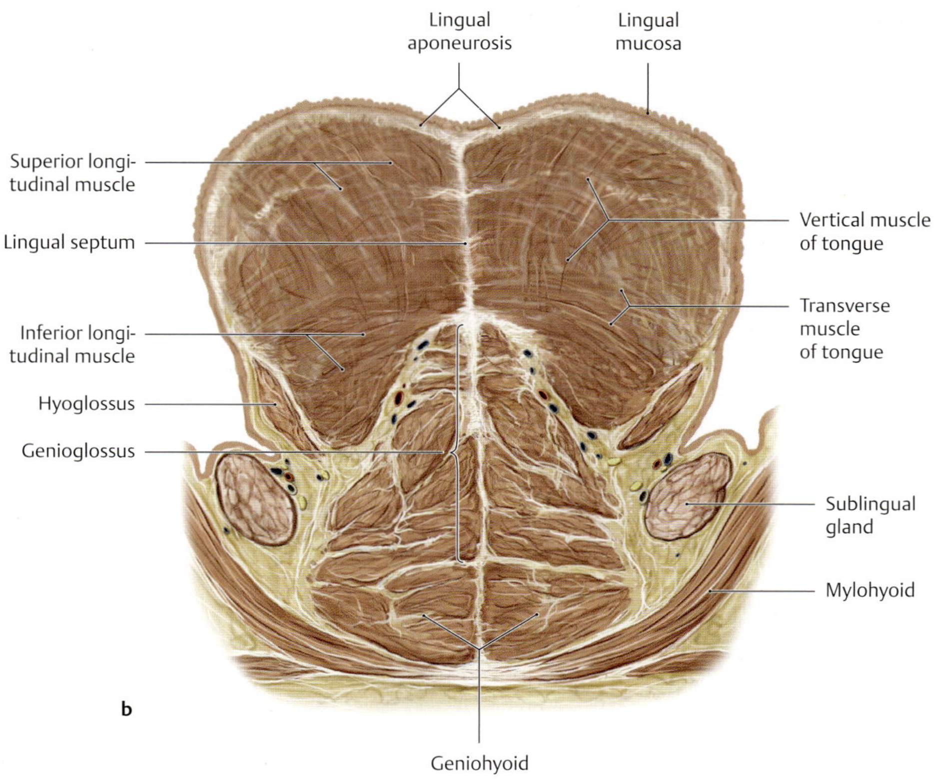

C Muscles of the tongue
b Left lateral view, **b** anterior view of a coronal section.
There are two sets of lingual muscles: extrinsic and intrinsic. The extrinsic muscles are attached to specific bony sites outside the tongue, while the intrinsic muscles have no attachments to skeletal structures. The extrinsic lingual muscles include the

- genioglossus,
- hyoglossus,
- styloglossus.

The *intrinsic* lingual muscles include the

- superior longitudinal muscle,
- inferior longitudinal muscle,
- transverse muscle,
- vertical muscle.

The extrinsic muscles move the tongue as a whole, while the intrinsic muscles alter its shape. All of the true lingual muscles mentioned here are innervated by the hypoglossal nerve (CN XII). Although the palatoglossus (see **a**) acts on the tongue, it is in fact a muscle of the palate or fauces, belonging to the palatine and faucial muscles and not to the lingual muscles. Accordingly, it is still supplied by the vagus nerve.

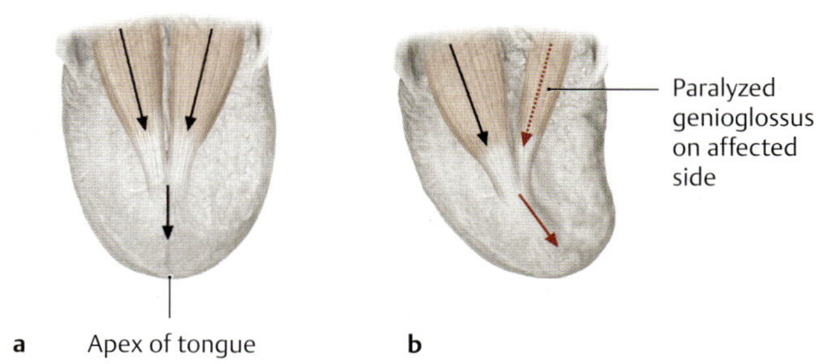

D Unilateral hypoglossal nerve palsy
Active protrusion of the tongue with an intact hypoglossal nerve (***a***) and with a unilateral hypoglossal nerve lesion (**b**).
When the hypoglossal nerve is damaged on one side, the genioglossus muscle is paralyzed on the affected side. As a result, the healthy (innervated) genioglossus on the opposite side dominates the tongue across the midline toward the affected side. When the tongue is protruded, it deviates toward the paralyzed side.

5.25 Tongue: Neurovascular Structures and Lymphatic Drainage

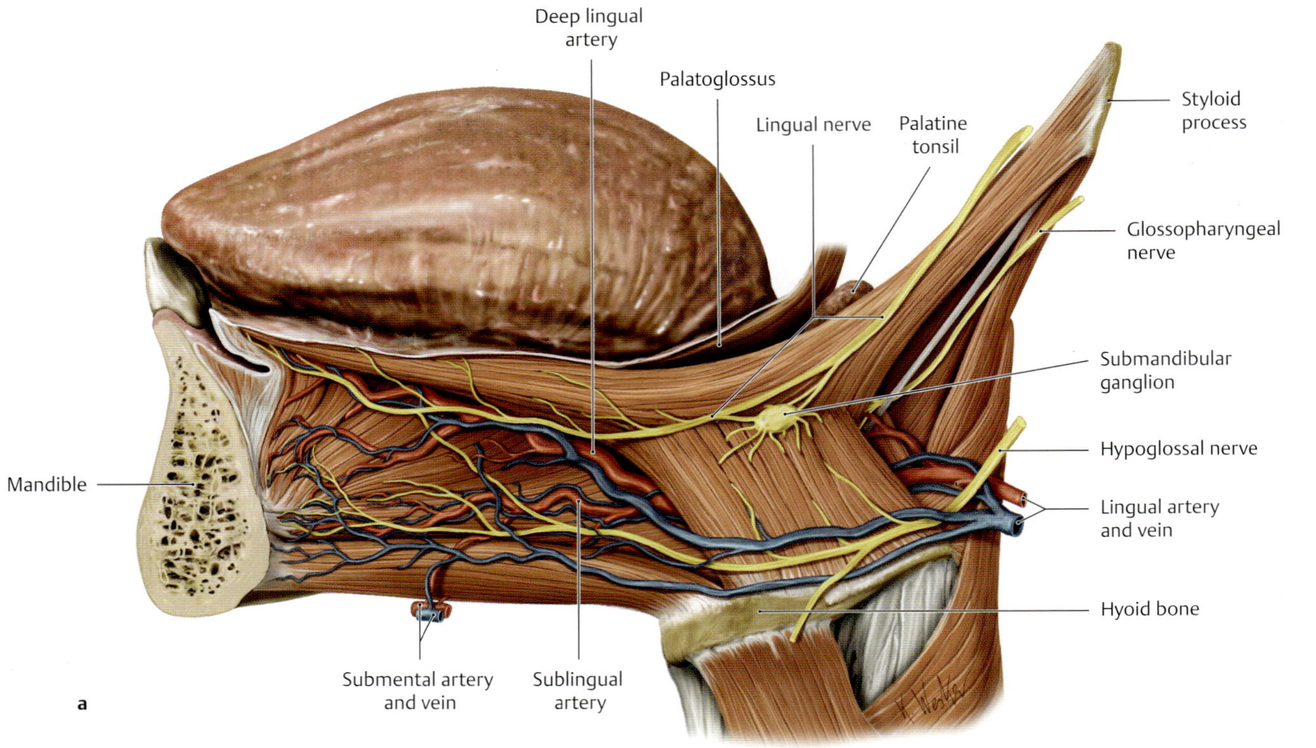

a

A Nerves and vessels of the tongue

a Left lateral view, **b** view of the inferior surface of the tongue.

The tongue is supplied by the *lingual artery* (from the external carotid a.), which divides into its terminal branches, the deep lingual artery and the sublingual artery. The lingual vein usually runs parallel to the artery and drains into the *internal jugular vein*. The lingual mucosa receives its somatosensory innervation (sensitivity to thermal and tactile stimuli) from the *lingual nerve*, which is a branch of the trigeminal nerve's mandibular division (CN V_3). The lingual nerve transmits fibers from the chorda tympani of the facial nerve (CN VII), among them the afferent taste fibers for the anterior two-thirds of the tongue. The chorda tympani also contains presynaptic, parasympathetic visceromotor axons which synapse in the submandibular ganglion, whose neurons in turn innervate the submandibular and sublingual glands (see p. 127 for further details). The palatoglossal m. receives its motor innervation by the vagus n. (CN X). The hypoglossal n. (CN XII) provides motor innervation to the remaining tongue muscles.

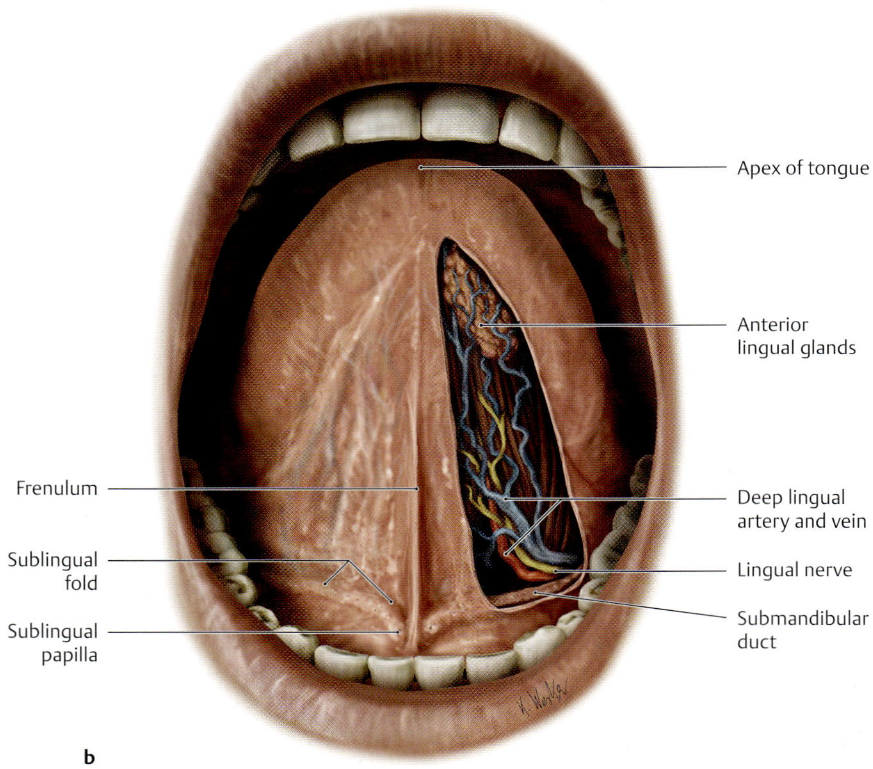

b

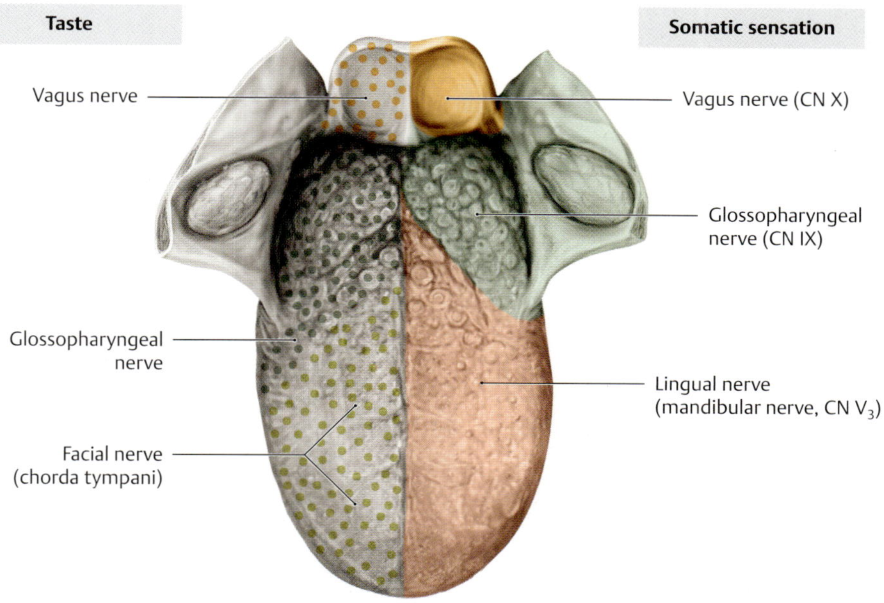

B Somatosensory innervation (left side) and taste innervation (right side) of the tongue

Anterior view. The tongue receives its *somatosensory* innervation (e.g., touch, pain, thermal sensation) from three cranial nerve branches:

- Lingual nerve (branch of mandibular nerve CN V_3),
- Glossopharyngeal nerve (CN IX)
- Vagus nerve (CN X)

Three cranial nerves also convey the *taste* fibers: CN VII (facial nerve, chorda tympani), CN IX (glossopharyngeal nerve), and CN X (vagus nerve). Thus, a disturbance of taste sensation involving the anterior two-thirds of the tongue indicates the presence of a facial nerve lesion, whereas a disturbance of tactile, pain, or thermal sensation indicates a trigeminal nerve lesion (see also pp. 121 and 127).

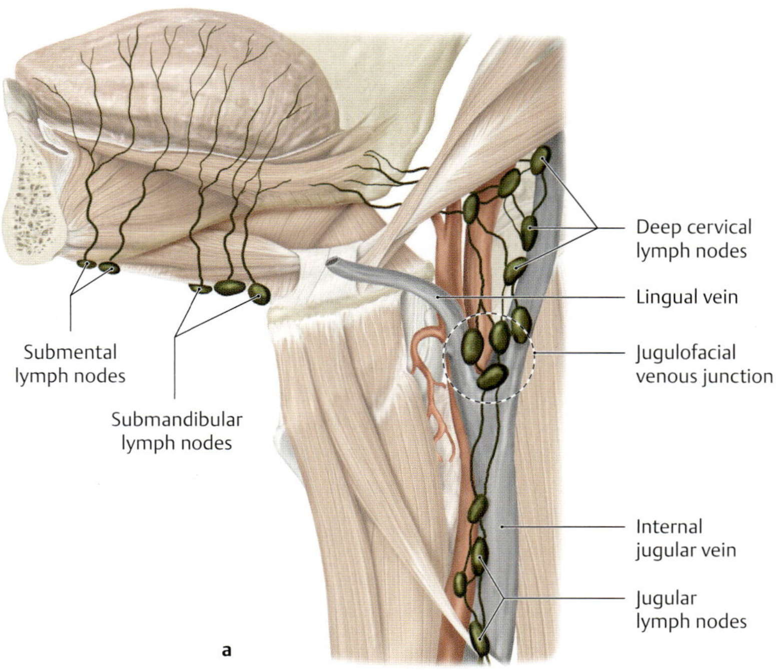

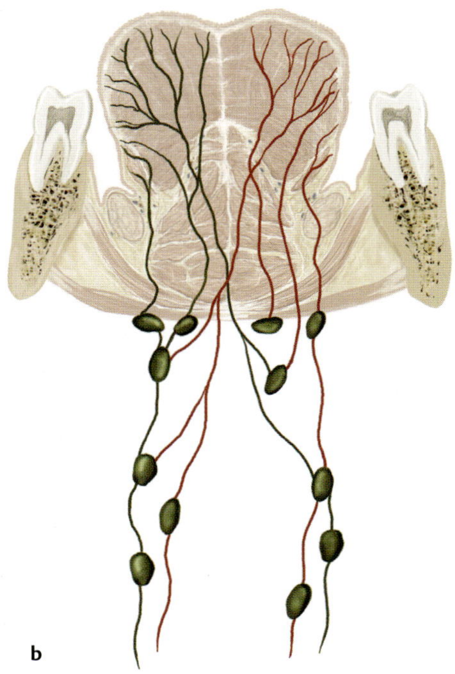

C Lymphatic drainage of the tongue and oral floor

Left lateral view (**a**) and anterior view (**b**).

The lymphatic drainage of the tongue and oral floor is mediated by submental and submandibular groups of lymph nodes that ultimately drain into the lymph nodes along the internal jugular vein (**a**, jugular lymph nodes). Because the lymph nodes receive drainage from both the ipsilateral and contralateral sides (**b**), tumor cells may become widely disseminated in this region (for example, metastatic squamous cell carcinoma, especially on the lateral border of the tongue, frequently metastasizes to the opposite side).

5.26 Topography of the Open Oral Cavity

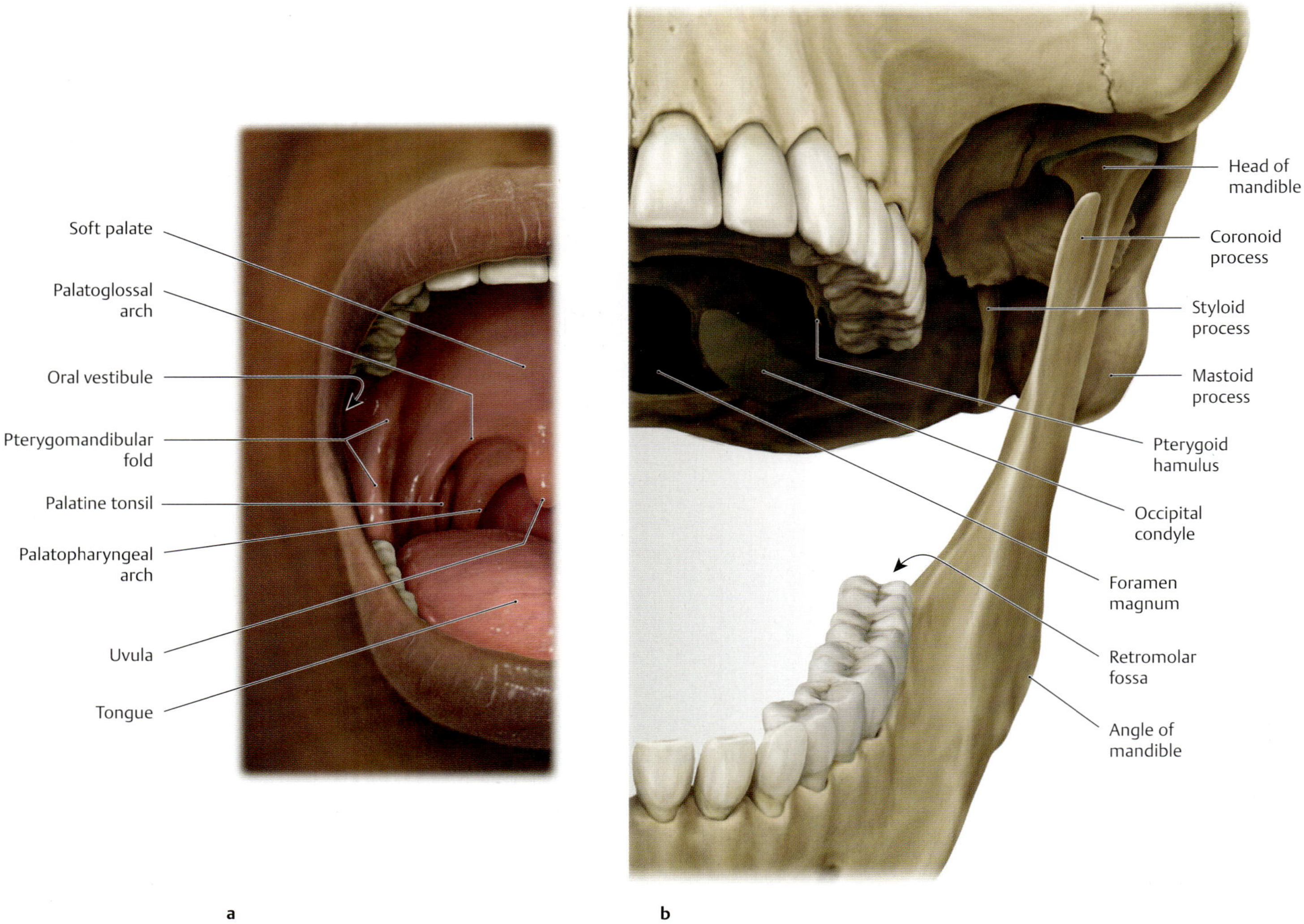

A Mucosal structures versus bony architecture of the upper and lower jaw

Anterior view with the mouth fully open.

The comparison shows where which **bony structures** (**b**) lie under the **oral mucosa** (**a**). Here one is looking past the isthmus of the fauces at the posterior wall of the pharynx. Anterior to the lateral border of the fauces, i.e., anterior to the palatopharyngeal arch, palatoglossal arch, and palatine tonsil between them, there is a readily visible mucosal fold on both sides that extends in a medial arch. This is the pterygomandibular fold. This thick ridge defines the posterior border of the oral vestibule. It extends from the retromolar fossa of the lower jaw (posterior to the last molar and part of the retromolar trigone, see p. 48) in the direction of the hard palate to the pterygoid hamulus. The base of the pterygomandibular fold is a well-defined tendinous strip (pterygomandibular raphe) between fossa and hamulus. Inserting into it are both the superior pharyngeal constrictor (buccopharyngeal part) and buccinator, occasionally referred to as the "trumpeter's muscle." It represents an important landmark for administering a nerve block of the inferior alveolar nerve (see **Bb**). A fully open oral cavity is practically never seen in an **anatomy lab** as the donor cadavers are usually fixed with the mouth shut so that the tongue more or less completely fills the oral cavity. There are also often only a few teeth or even none. The oral cavity is usually dissected in half a head divided by a median sagittal section. The anatomy student never sees the entire, fully open oral cavity. Yet in **clinical reality**, inspection of the open oral cavity and the pharyngeal ring (lips, oral mucosa, tongue, tonsils, and pharynx as well as teeth and gums) is an integral part of the even the most cursory physical examination. This is because the oral cavity reflects habits (such as whether a person smokes), indicates the extent of personal care (condition of the teeth), and shows signs of disorders of internal organs (such as atrophic glossitis or "bald tongue," atrophy of the papillae in iron-deficiency anemia or Crohn's disease) and of the oral cavity itself. Thus, every irregularity (leukoplakia, nodes, ulceration, etc.) in the mucosa should be evaluated as a suspected malignancy. In addition to inspection, palpation plays an important role, as one can obtain information about the consistency and extent of irregularities and changes in coloration within the oral mucosa. Findings in the floor of the oral cavity or the cheek region are palpated with both hands from inside and outside the oral cavity (see p. 211). Finally, familiarity with the topography of the open oral cavity is an important requirement for properly administering local anesthesia, for example in dental procedures.

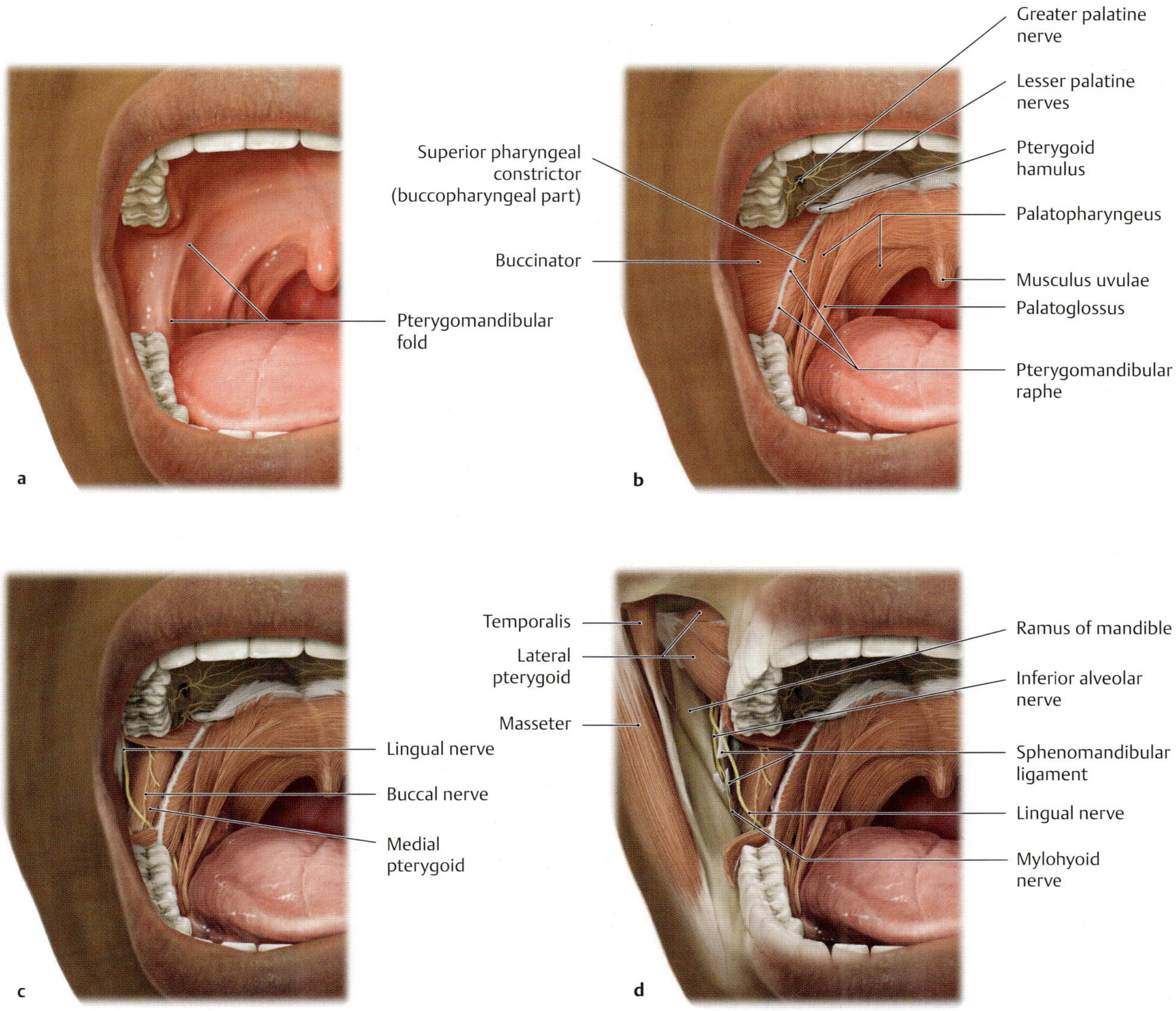

B Course of the inferior alveolar nerve, lingual nerve, and mylohyoid nerve in the region of the medial ramus of the mandible (pterygomandibular space)

a–d Anterolateral views of various layers of the lower jaw. In these views, the neurovascular structures, muscles, and pterygomandibular fold lie in different positions relative to one another than they do in the anterior view (see **A**). As one invariably approaches the most frequently anesthetized nerve, the inferior alveolar nerve, from the contralateral premolar region, this lateral view is extremely important for orientation. The lower jaw is in focus here as that is where not only the inferior alveolar nerve courses, but also the lingual nerve and mylohyoid nerve. These latter structures can be easily injured if the wrong approach is chosen. The various layers also convey an impression of the size of the pterygomandibular space.

a View of the oral mucosa in the region of the right pterygomandibular fold; **b** the oral mucosa has been completely removed and the pterygomandibular raphe is exposed; **c** the buccinator has been cut away or reflected, exposing the pterygoideus medialis and the pterygomandibular space, through which the inferior alveolar nerve as well as the lingual and mylohyoid nerves course; **d** the skin of the cheek has been cut away, revealing the sphenomandibular ligament. It courses on the medial aspect of the ramus of the mandible from the sphenoidal spine to the lingula of the mandibular foramen and covers the inferior alveolar nerve immediately before its point of entry into the mandibular foramen. With the distal ligament cut away, one can see the bifurcation of the mylohyoid nerve at the level of the lingula of the mandible.

Note: Injuries to the lingual nerve can occur in the setting of facial trauma as well as in dental procedures (for example surgical removal of wisdom teeth or administration of an inferior alveolar nerve block).

5.27 Oral Floor

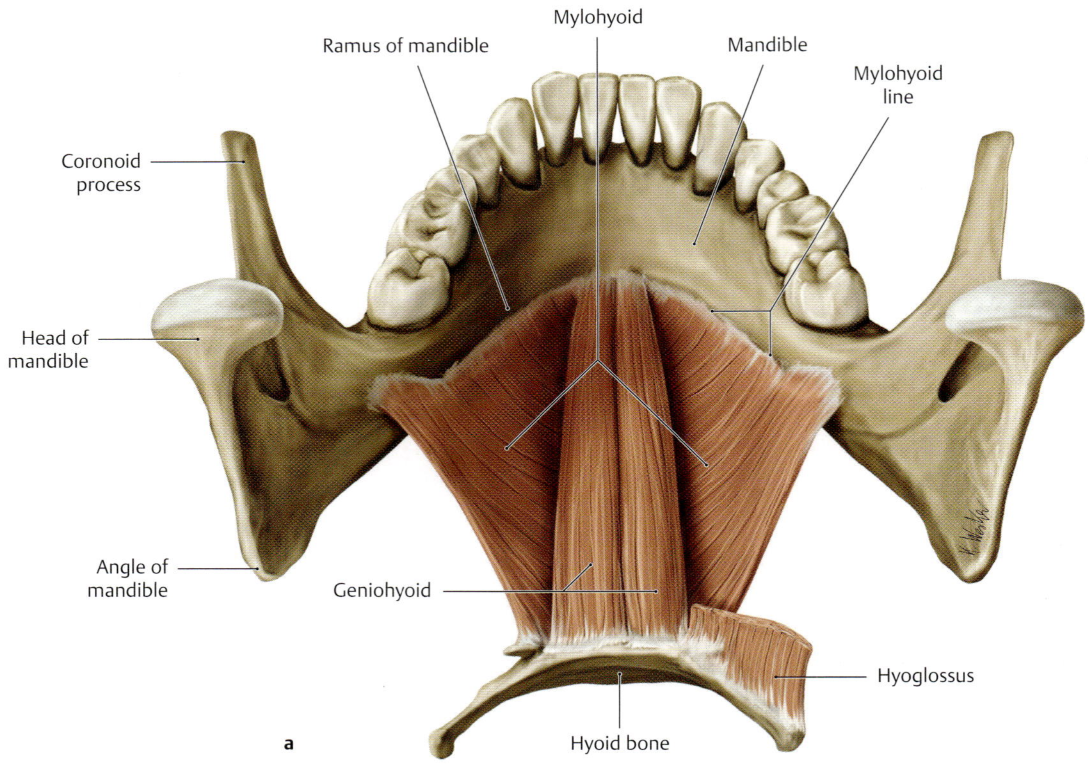

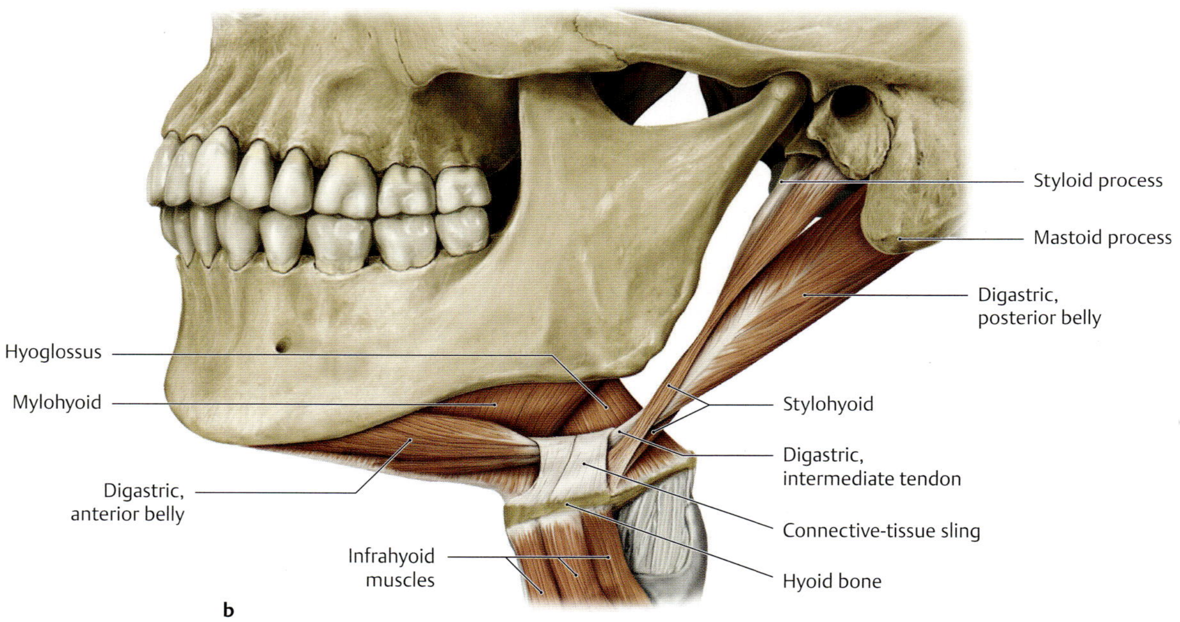

A Muscles of the oral floor
Superior view (**a**) and left lateral view (**b**).
The oral floor is formed by a muscular sheet that stretches between the two rami of the mandible. This sheet consists of four muscles, all of which are located above the hyoid bone and are thus collectively known as the suprahyoid muscles (for details see **A**, p. 90):

1. Mylohyoid: The muscle fibers from each side fuse in a median raphe (covered superiorly by the geniohyoid).
2. Geniohyoid: strengthens the central portion of the oral floor.
3. Digastric: The anterior belly of the digastric is located in the oral floor region; its posterior belly arises from the mastoid process.
4. Stylohyoid: arises from the styloid process. Its tendon is perforated by the intermediate tendon of the digastric.

All four muscles participate in active opening of the mouth. They also elevate the hyoid bone and move it forward during swallowing.

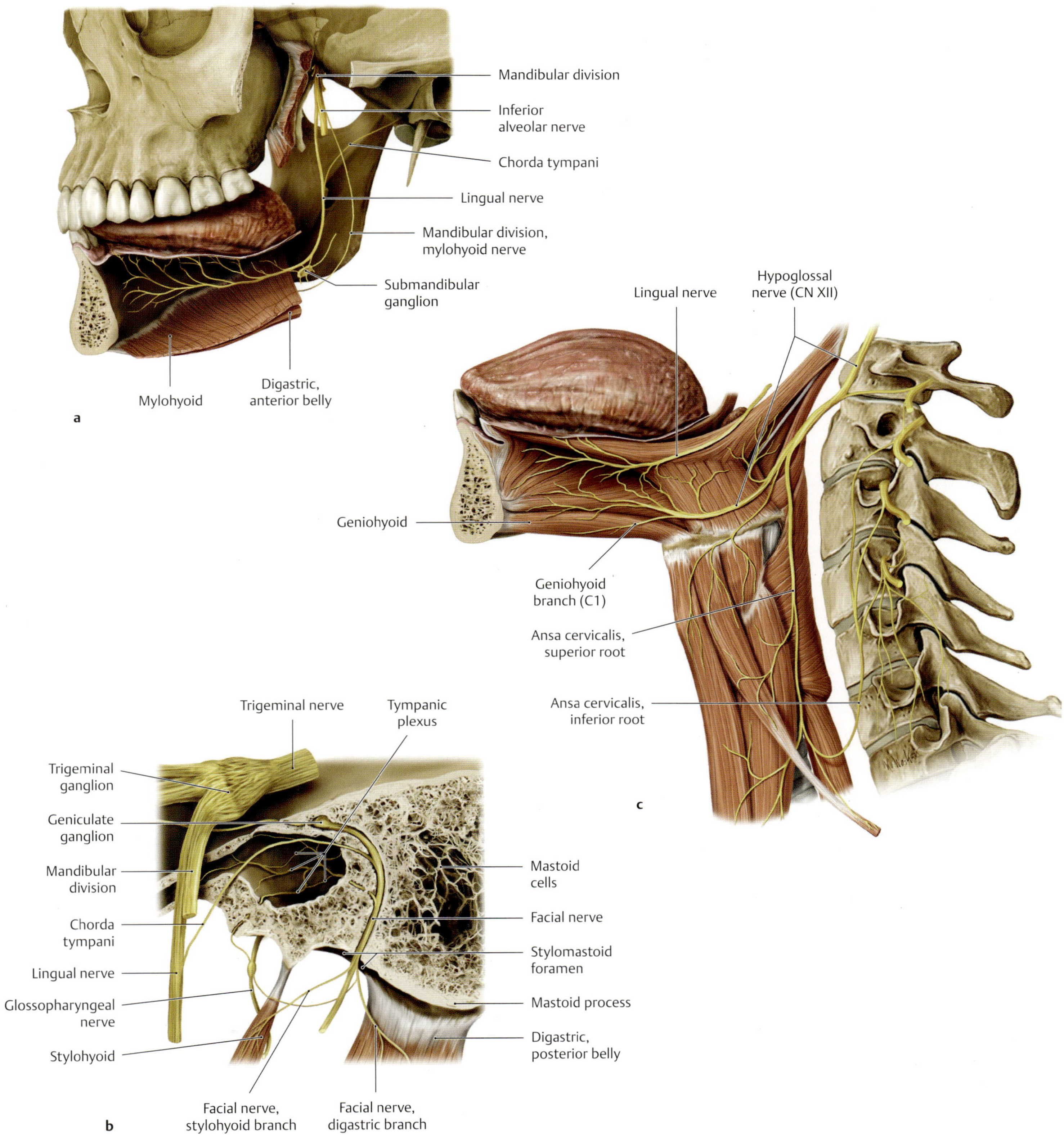

B Innervation of the oral floor muscles

a Left lateral view (right half of the mandible viewed from the medial side). **b** Sagittal section through the right petrous bone at the level of the mastoid process and mastoid air cells, viewed from the medial side. **c** Left lateral view.

The muscles of the oral floor have a complex nerve supply due to different branchial arch derivations, with contributions from three different nerves:

- **a** The derivatives of the mandibular arch (mylohyoid, anterior belly of the digastric) are supplied by the mylohyoid nerve, a branch of the mandibular division (CN V_3).
- **b** The derivatives of the second branchial arch (posterior belly of the digastric, stylohyoid) are supplied by the facial nerve.
- **c** The geniohyoid (and the thyrohyoid) muscles are supplied by the ventral ramus of C1 spinal nerve, which travels with the hypoglossal nerve.

5.28 Oral Cavity: Pharynx and Tonsils

A Waldeyer's ring
Posterior view of the opened pharynx. All the components of Waldeyer's ring can be seen in this view. Waldeyer's ring is composed of immunocompetent lymphatic tissue (tonsils and lymph follicles). The tonsils are "immunological sentinels" surrounding the passageways from the mouth and nasal cavity to the pharynx. The lymph follicles are distributed over all of the epithelium, showing marked regional variations. Waldeyer's ring consists of the following structures:

- The unpaired pharyngeal tonsil on the roof of the pharynx
- The paired palatine tonsils
- The lingual tonsil
- The paired tubal tonsils (tonsillae tubariae), which may be thought of as lateral extensions of the pharyngeal tonsil
- The paired lateral bands.

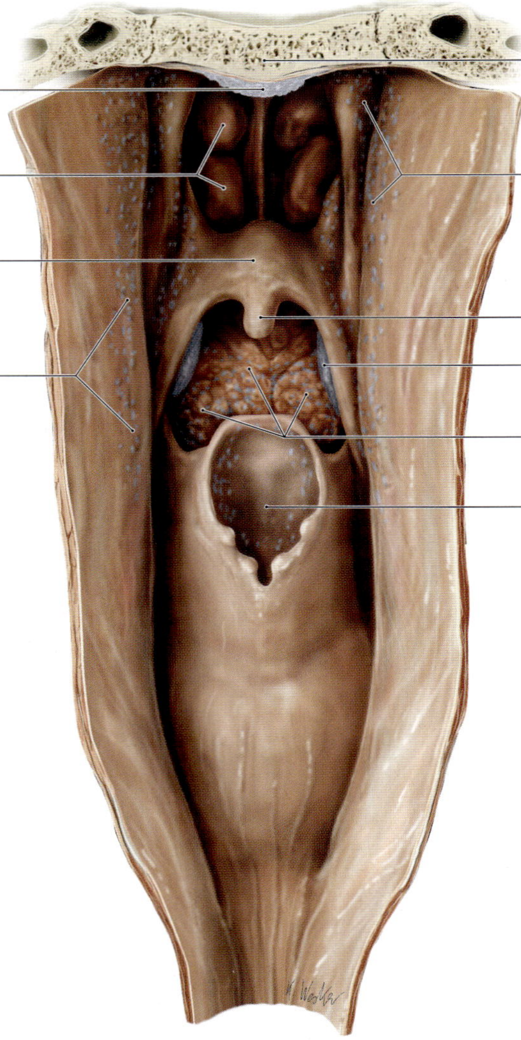

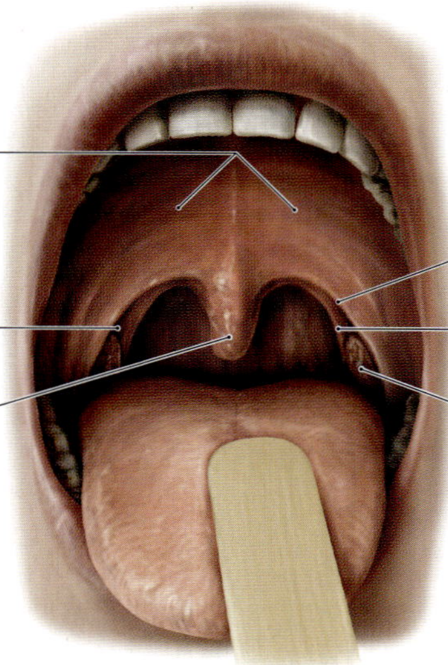

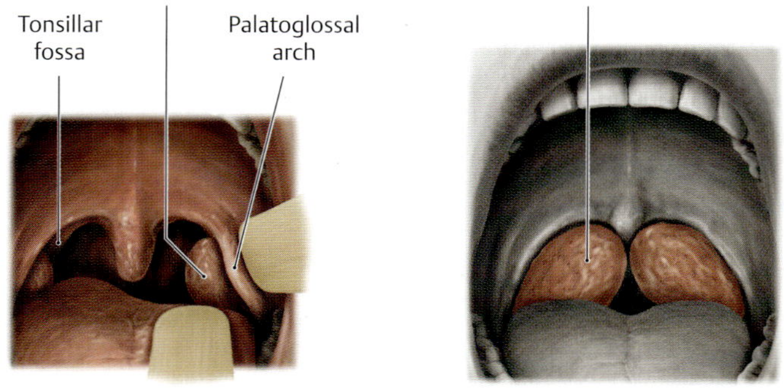

B Palatine tonsils: location and abnormal enlargement
Anterior view of the oral cavity.

a The palatine tonsils occupy a shallow recess on each side, the tonsillar fossa, which is located between the anterior and posterior pillars (palatoglossal and palatopharyngeal folds which together comprise the arch of the same name).

b and **c** The palatine tonsil is examined clinically by placing a tongue depressor on the anterior pillar and displacing the tonsil from its fossa while a second instrument depresses the tongue. Severe enlargement of the palatine tonsil (due to viral or bacterial infection, as in tonsillitis) may significantly narrow the outlet of the oral cavity, causing difficulty in swallowing (dysphagia).

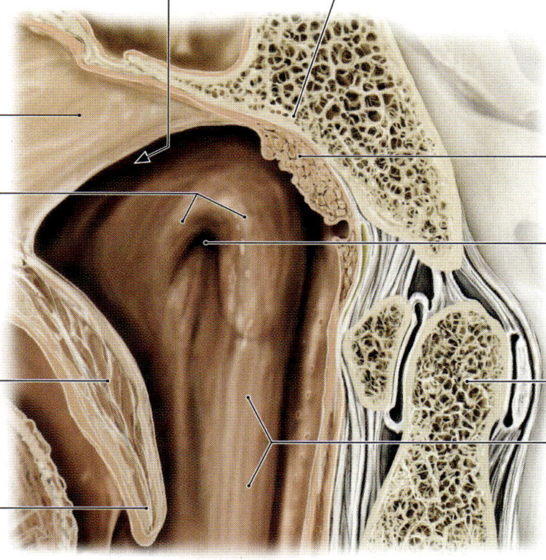

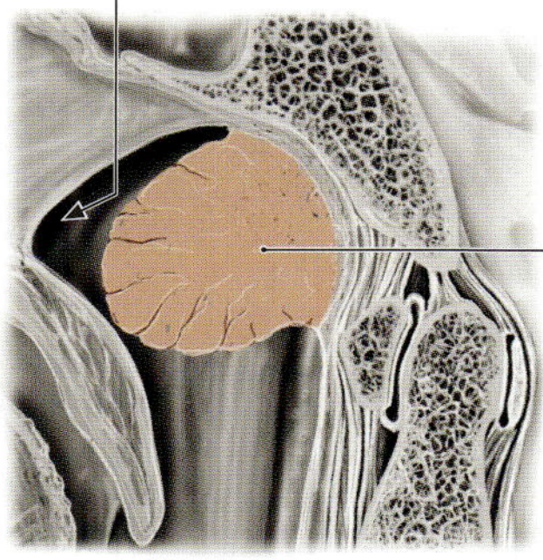

C Pharyngeal tonsil: location and abnormal enlargement
Sagittal section through the roof of the pharynx.

- **a** Located on the roof of the pharynx, the unpaired pharyngeal tonsil can be examined by means of posterior rhinoscopy (see p. 185). It is particularly well developed in (small) children and begins to regress at 6 or 7 years of age.
- **b** An enlarged pharyngeal tonsil is very common in preschool-age children. (Chronic recurrent nasopharyngeal infections at this age often evoke a heightened immune response in the lymphatic tissue, causing “adenoids” or “polyps.”) The enlarged pharyngeal tonsil blocks the choanae, obstructing the nasal airway and forcing the child to breathe through the mouth. Since the mouth is then constantly open during respiration at rest, an experienced examiner can quickly diagnose the adenoidal condition by visual inspection.

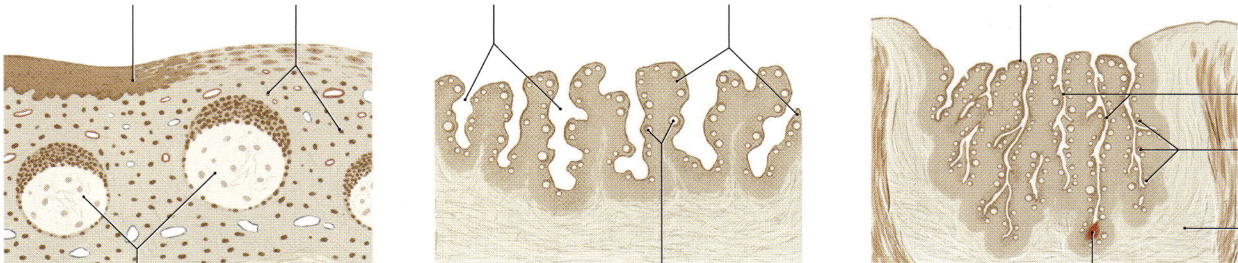

D Histology of the lymphatic tissue of the oral cavity and pharynx
Due to the close anatomical relationship between the epithelium and lymphatic tissue, the lymphatic tissue of Waldeyer’s ring is also designated lymphoepithelial tissue.

- **a Lymphoepithelial tissue.** Lymphatic tissue, both organized and diffusely distributed, is found in the lamina propria of all mucous membranes and is known as mucosa-associated lymphatic tissue (MALT). The epithelium acquires a looser texture, with abundant lymphocytes and macrophages. Besides the well-defined tonsils, smaller collections of lymph follicles may be found in the lateral bands (salpingopharyngeal folds). They extend almost vertically from the lateral wall to the posterior wall of the oropharynx and nasopharynx.
- **b Structure of the pharyngeal tonsil.** The mucosal surface of the pharyngeal tonsil is raised into ridges that greatly increase its surface area. The ridges and intervening crypts are lined by ciliated respiratory epithelium.
- **c Structure of the palatine tonsil.** The surface area of the palatine tonsil is increased by deep depressions (crypts) in the mucosal surface (creating an active surface area as large as 300 cm2). The mucosa is covered by nonkeratinized stratified squamous epithelium.

5.29 Pharynx: Muscles

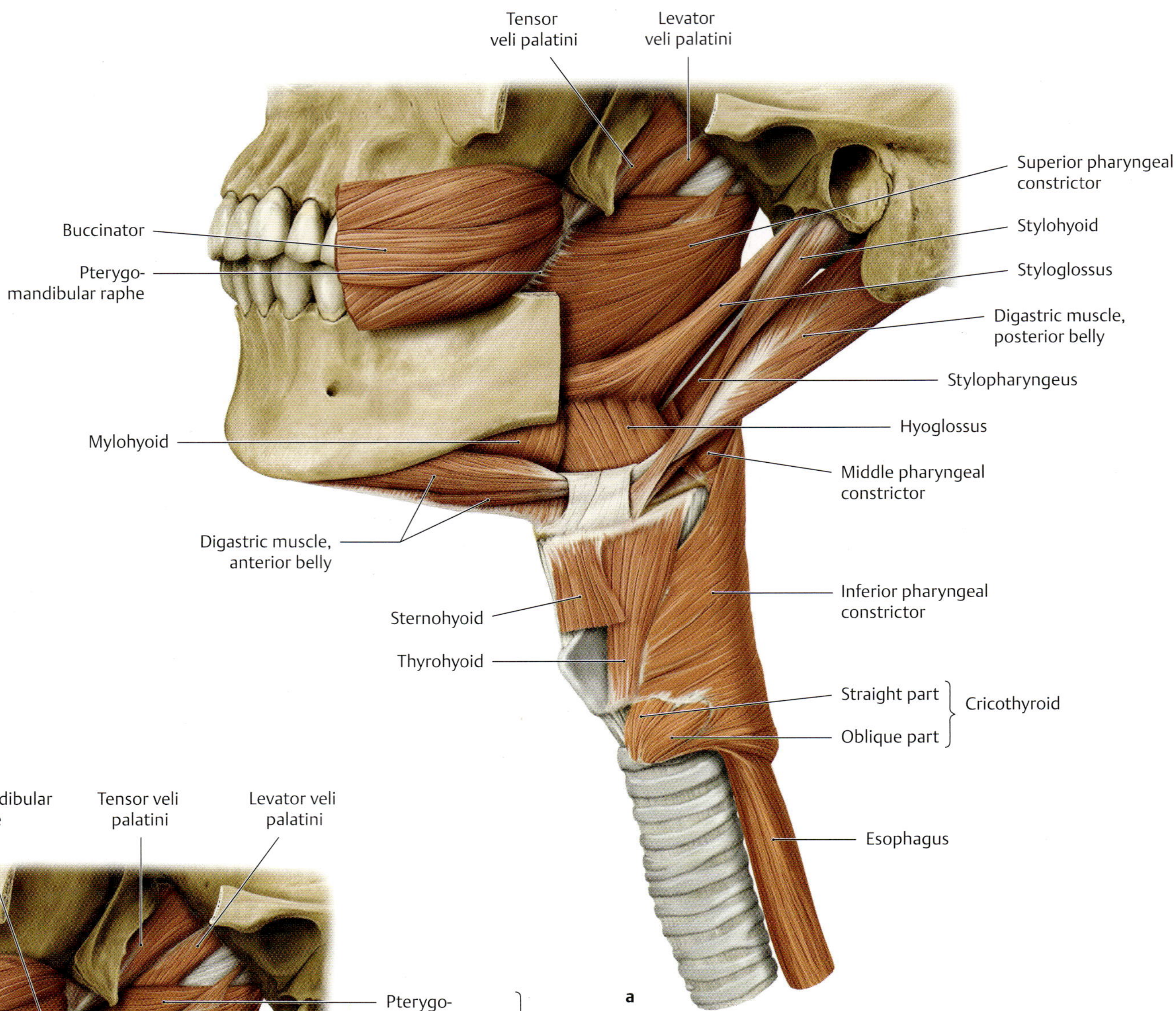

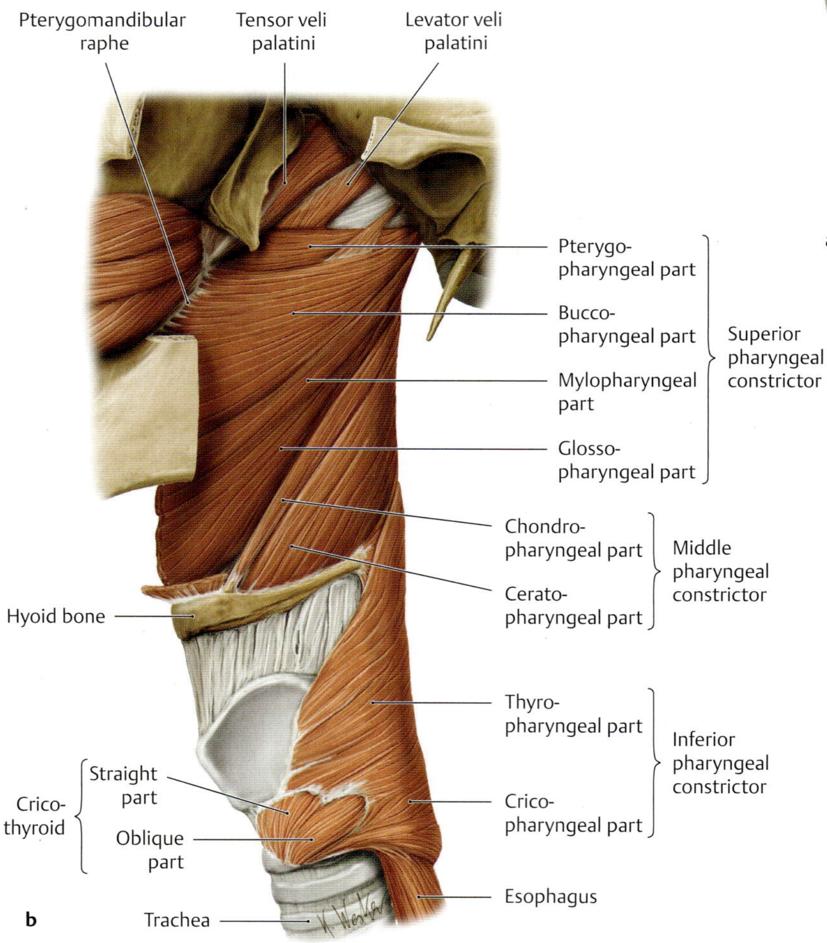

A Muscles of the pharynx viewed from the left side

a Overview of the pharyngeal muscles, left lateral view. The pharynx is a muscular tube whose skeletal muscles are attached to the base of the skull and are continuous with the esophagus at the level of the cricoid cartilage (opposite the C6 vertebral body). Although the pharynx looks like a continuous muscular tube externally, it is divided internally into three levels (see p. 202). The pharyngeal musculature consists of the *pharyngeal constrictors* (details in **b**) and the relatively weak *pharyngeal elevators*.

b **Subdivision of the constrictors:** The muscular wall of the pharynx is formed by a trio of constrictor muscles on each side: the superior, middle, and inferior pharyngeal constrictors. Each of these muscles consists of several parts.

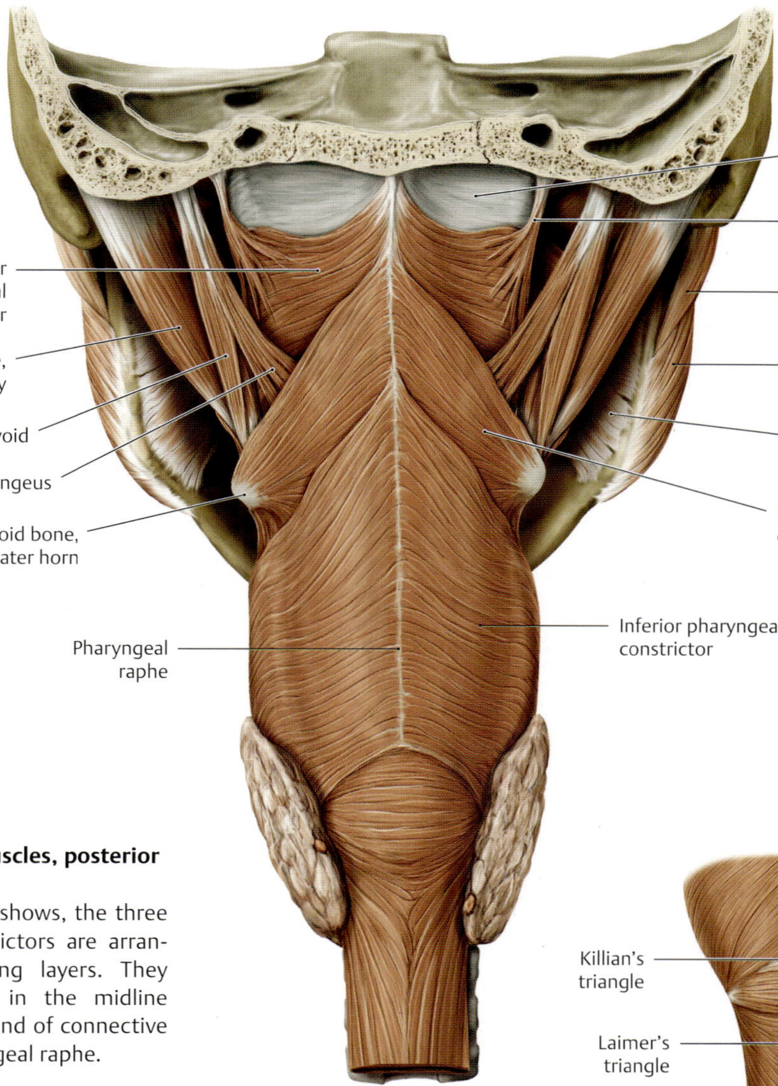

B Pharyngeal muscles, posterior view

As this dissection shows, the three pharyngeal constrictors are arranged in overlapping layers. They meet posteriorly in the midline along a vertical band of connective tissue, the pharyngeal raphe.

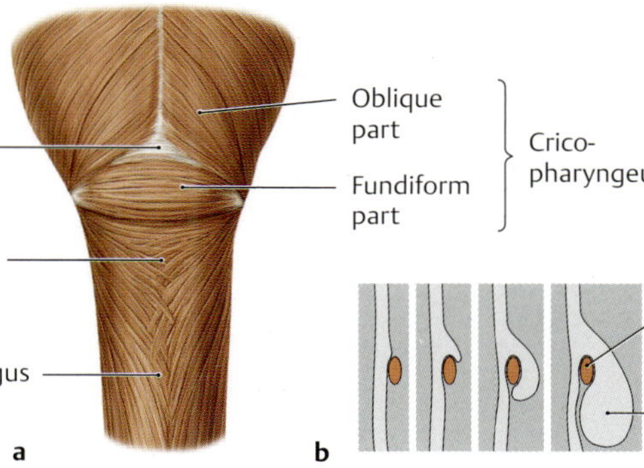

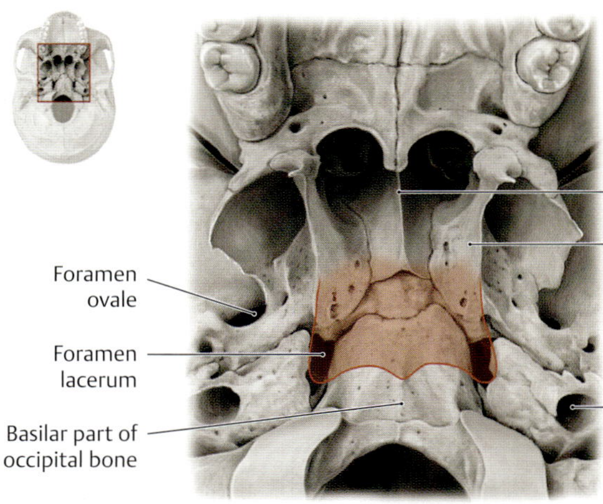

C Pharyngobasilar fascia at the base of the skull

Inferior view. The pharyngeal muscles originate from the base of the skull with a dense connective tissue membrane, the pharyngobasilar fascia. Their insertion is projected onto the base of the skull and marked as a red line. The U-shaped area surrounded by fascia and muscles is part of the bony roof of the pharynx (light red).

D Junction of the pharyngeal and esophageal musculature and the development of Zenker diverticula

a Posterior view, **b** left lateral view.

The cricopharyngeal part of the inferior pharyngeal constrictor muscle is further subdivided into an oblique part and a fundiform part. Between these two parts is an area of muscular weakness known as the *Killian triangle*. At the inferior border of the fundiform part, the muscle fibers form a V-shaped area called the *Laimer triangle*. The weak spot at Killian's triangle may allow the mucosa of the hypopharynx to bulge outward through the fundiform part of the cricopharyngeus muscle (**b**). *Note:* Killian's triangle and Laimer's triangle are often used synonymously.

This can result in a *Zenker diverticulum*, a sac-like protrusion in which food residues may collect and gradually expand the sac (with risk of obstructing the esophageal lumen by extrinsic pressure from the diverticulum). The diagnosis is suggested by the regurgitation of trapped food residues. Zenker diverticula are most common in middle-aged and elderly individuals. In elderly patients, who can undergo surgeries only to a limited extent, the fundiform part of the inferior pharyngeal constrictor m. is cut endoscopically.

Note: Because a Zenker diverticulum is located at the junction of the hypopharynx with the esophagus, it is known also as a pharyngoesophageal diverticulum (the term "esophageal diverticulum," while common, is incorrect).

5.30 Pharynx: Surface Anatomy of the Mucosa and Its Connections with the Skull Base

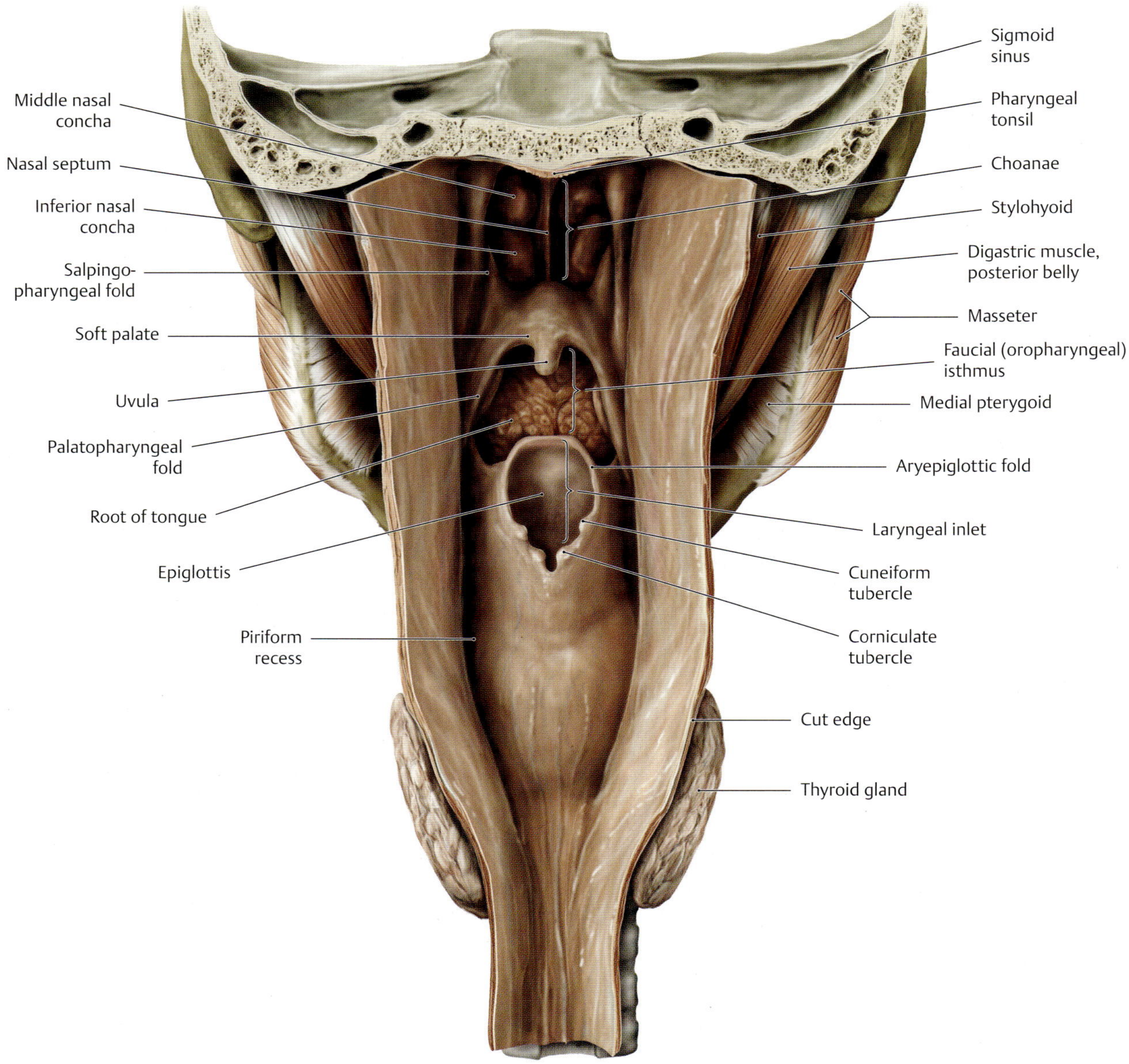

A Surface anatomy of the pharyngeal mucosa

Posterior view. The muscular posterior wall of the pharynx is opened along its midline. The anterior part of the pharyngeal wall is interrupted by three openings:

- To the nasal cavity (choanae)
- To the oral cavity (faucial [oropharyngeal] isthmus)
- To the laryngeal inlet (aditus)

The pharynx is divided accordingly into a naso-, ovo-, and laryngopharynx (see p. 202).

B Posterior rhinoscopy

The nasopharynx can be visually inspected by posterior rhinoscopy.

a Technique of holding the tongue blade and mirror. The angulation of the mirror is continually adjusted to permit complete inspection of the nasopharynx (see **b**).

b Composite posterior rhinoscopic image acquired at various mirror angles. The orifice of the auditory (pharyngotympanic) tube and pharyngeal tonsil can be identified (see p. 196).

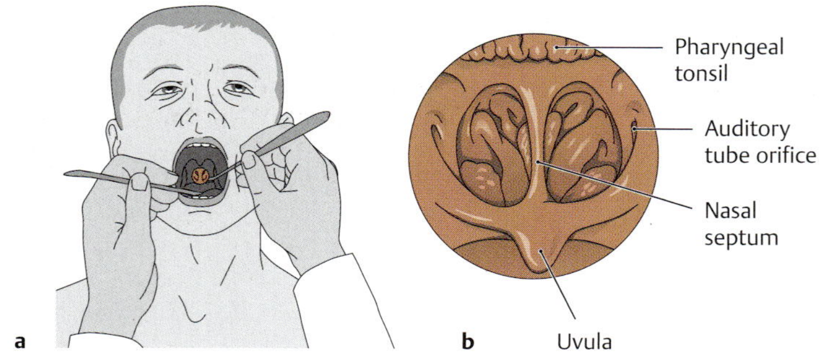

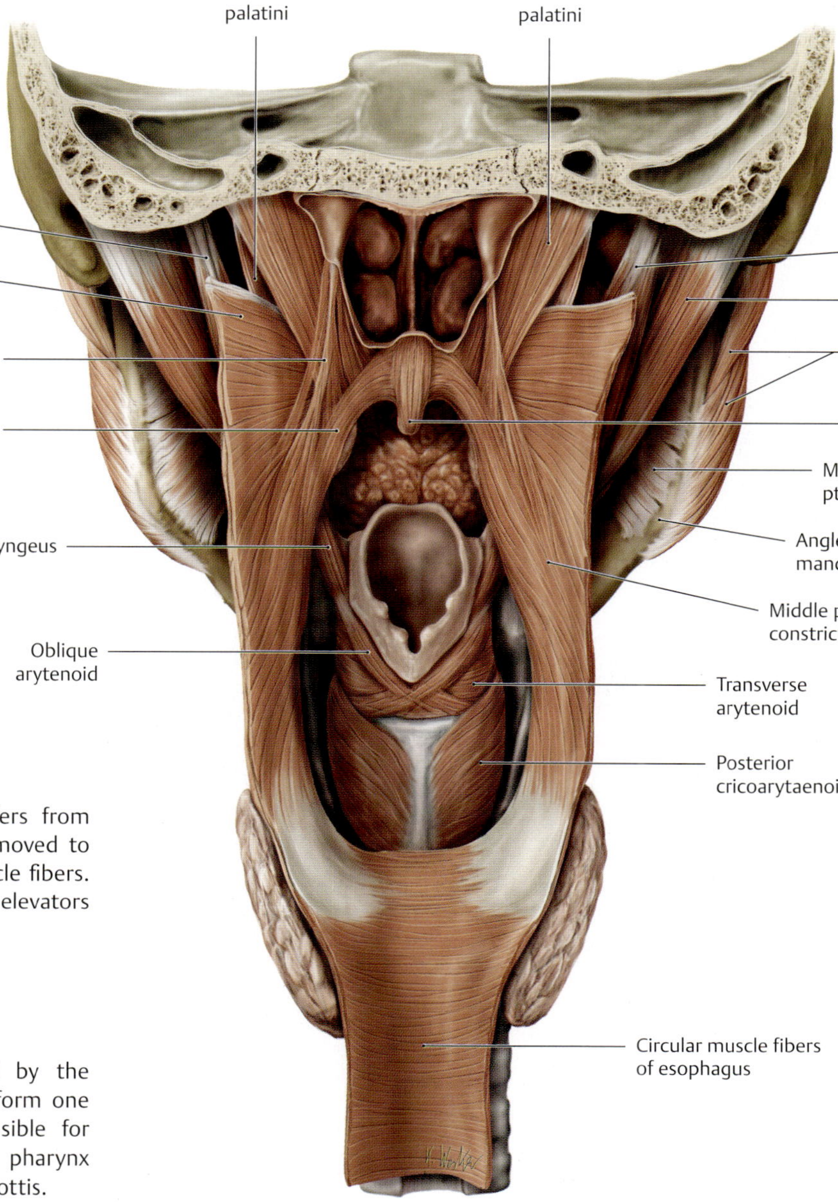

C Pharyngeal musculature

Posterior view. This dissection differs from **A** in that the mucosa has been removed to demonstrate the course of the muscle fibers. Posterior view. The pharyngeal elevators consist of three muscles:

- salpingopharyngeus m.
- palatopharyngeus m., and
- stylopharyngeus m.

All three muscles are innervated by the glossopharyngeal n. (CN IX). They form one functional group, which is responsible for shortening (lifting/elevating) the pharynx when swallowing or closing the epiglottis.

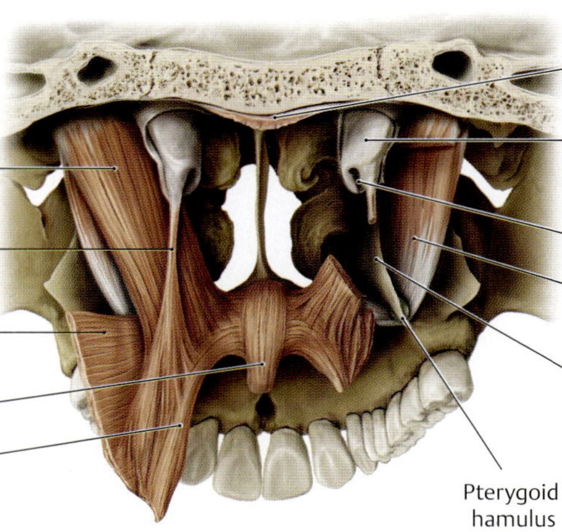

D Muscles of the soft palate and eustachian tube

Posterior view. The sphenoid bone has been sectioned posterior to the choanal opening in the coronal plane, and the following muscles have been resected on the right side: levator veli palatini, salpingopharyngeus, palatopharyngeus, and superior pharyngeal constrictor. These muscles are part of the pharynx (space between the soft palate, palatine arches, and lingual dorsum) that forms the posterior boundary of the oral cavity.

5.31 Pharynx: Topographical Anatomy and Innervation

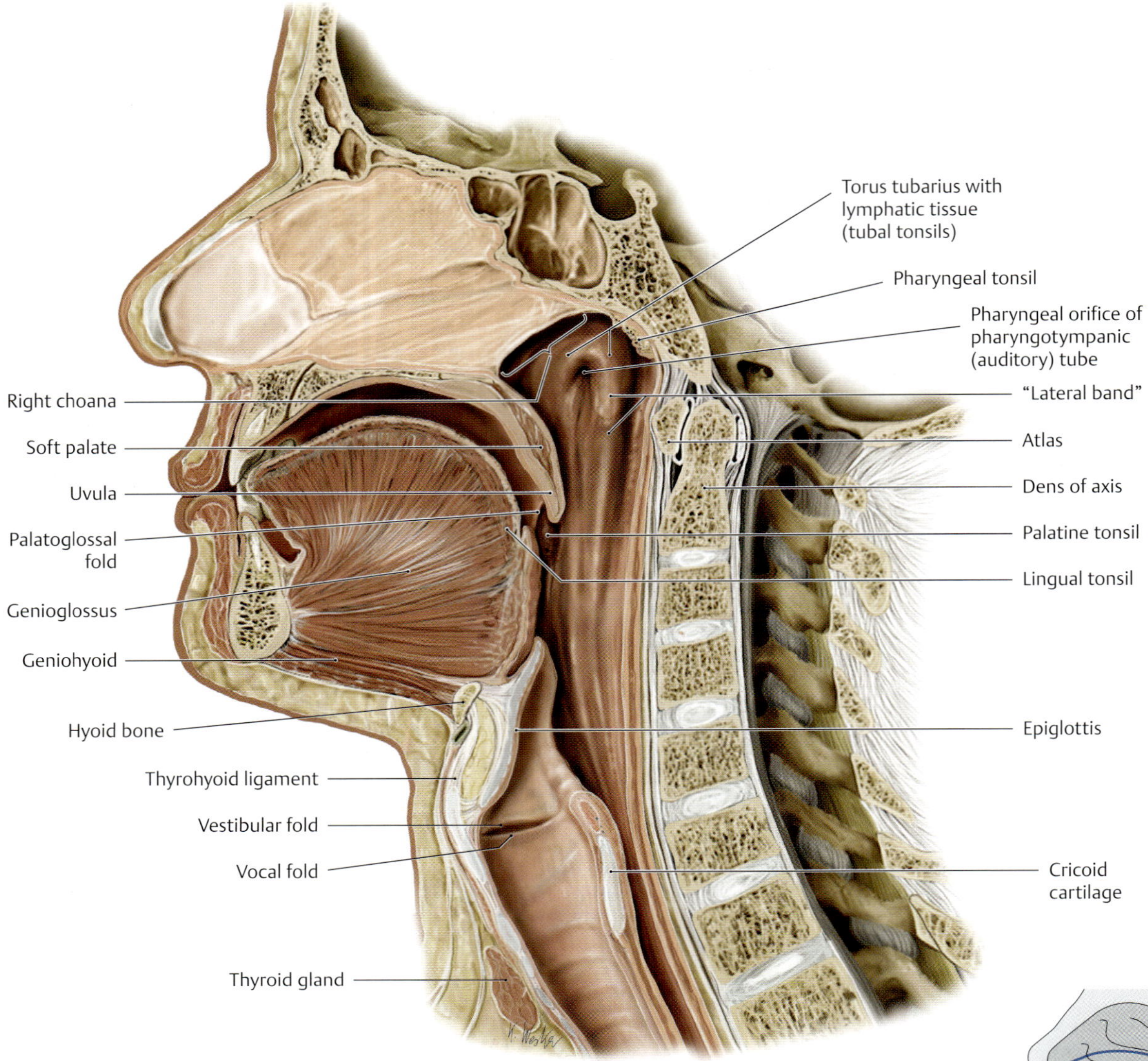

A Midsagittal section

Left lateral view. The nasal septum, oral cavity, pharynx, trachea, and esophagus can be identified in this dissection. The lymphatic tissues of "Waldeyer's ring" are located at the junction of the nasal and oral cavities with the pharynx. A prominent part of this defensive ring is the array of tonsils that play an important role in the early recognition of pathogenic microorganisms and the initiation of an immune response (more complex infections spread to the peripharyngeal space, see p. 204). This array consists of the single *pharyngeal tonsil* (on the roof of the pharynx), the paired *palatine tonsils* (between the palatal folds), and the paired *lingual tonsils* (at the base of the tongue). Additional masses of lymphatic tissue are located around the pharyngeal orifice of each pharyngotympanic (auditory) tube (tubal tonsils) and are continued inferiorly as the "lateral bands."

The pharyngotympanic tube connects the pharynx with the tympanic cavity and serves to equalize the air pressure in the middle ear. Swelling around the pharyngotympanic tube orifice (tubal tonsils), which may occur even with a mild inflammation, and may occlude the orifice and prevent pressure equalization in the middle ear. This restricts the mobility of the tympanic membrane, causing a mild degree of hearing loss. Enlargement of the pharyngeal tonsil (e. g., polyps in small children) may also obstruct the lumen of the pharyngotympanic tube.

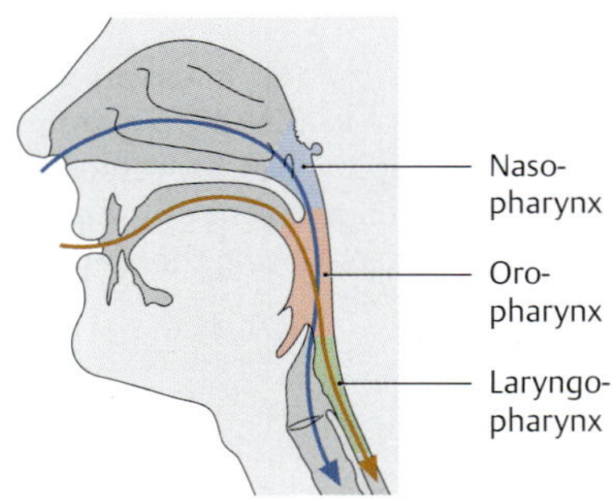

B Levels of the pharyngeal cavity

Left lateral view. The pharyngeal cavity is divided into the *nasopharynx*, *oropharynx*, and *laryngopharynx*. The upper airway and lower foodway intersect in the oropharynx. The following synonyms for the three pharyngeal levels are in common use:

Upper level:	Nasal part of pharynx	Nasopharynx	Epipharynx
Middle level:	Oral part of pharynx	Oropharynx	Mesopharynx
Lower level:	Laryngeal part of pharynx	Laryngopharynx	Hypopharynx

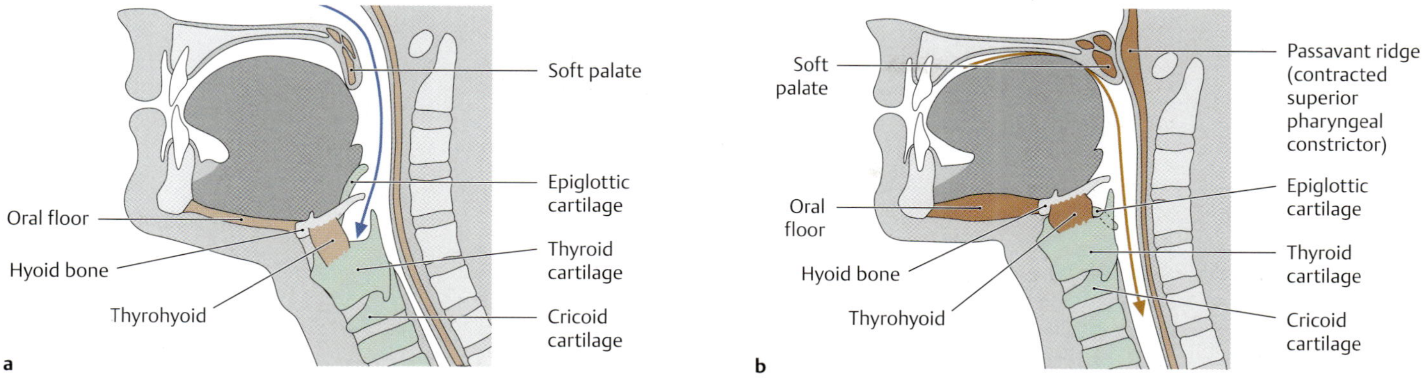

C Anatomy of swallowing

As part of the airway, the larynx in the adult is located at the inlet to the digestive tract (**a**). During swallowing (**b**), therefore, the airway must be briefly occluded to keep food from entering the trachea. The act of swallowing consists of three phases:

1. Voluntary initiation of swallowing
2. Reflex closure of the airway
3. Reflex transport of the food bolus down the pharynx and esophagus

During the second phase of swallowing, the oral floor muscles (mylohyoid and digastric) and the thyrohyoid muscles elevate the larynx and the epiglottis covers the laryngeal inlet, sealing off the lower airway. Meanwhile the soft palate is tightened, elevated, and apposed to the posterior pharyngeal wall, sealing off the upper airway.

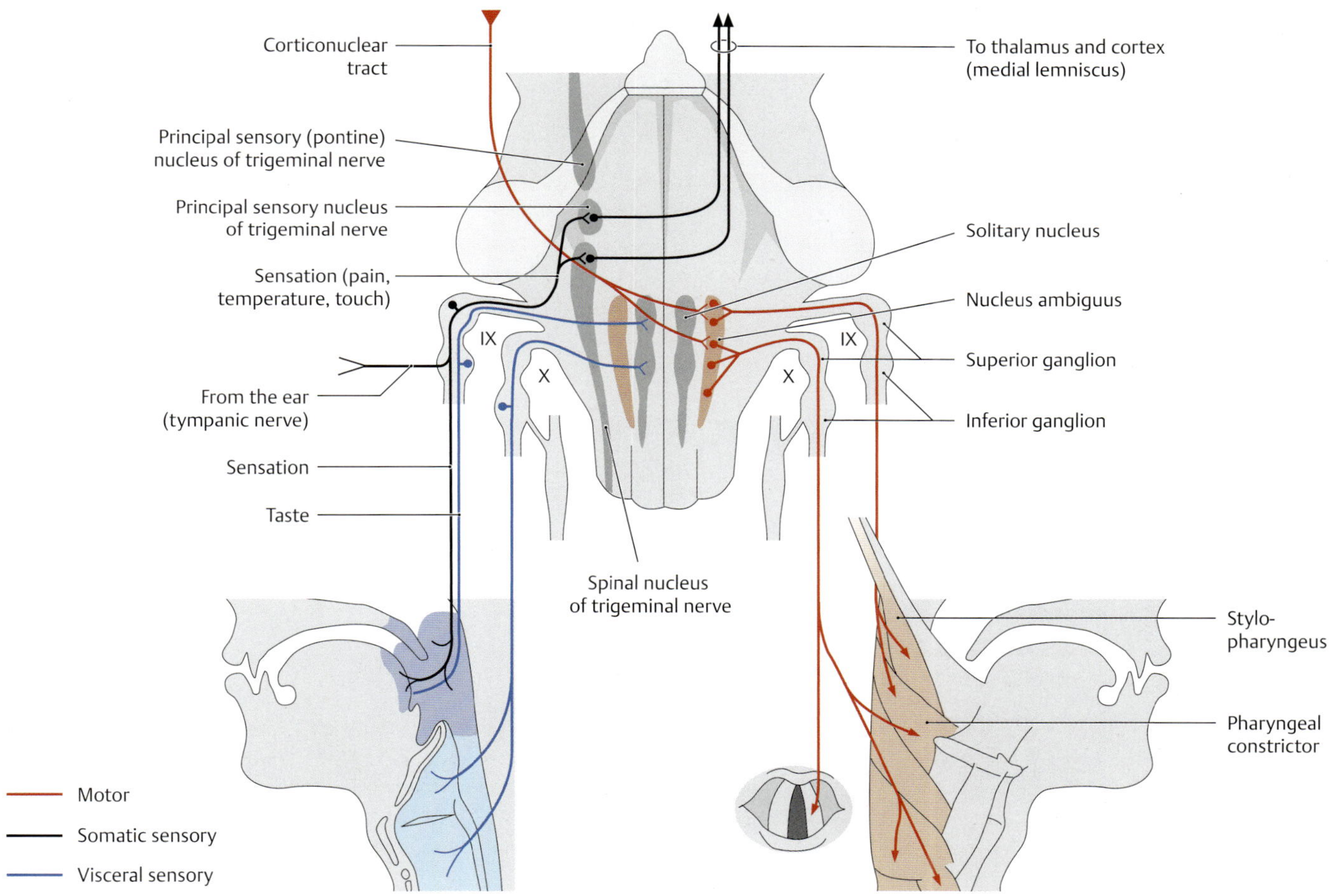

D Vagus nerve and glossopharyngeal nerve: their peripheral distribution and brainstem nuclei (after Duus)

Posterior view. Both the glossopharyngeal nerve (CN IX) and the vagus nerve (CN X) originate from nuclei in the brainstem. In this simplified schematic, motor pathways are depicted on the right and sensory pathways on the left.

Note that both nerves contribute to the sensory and motor supply of the pharynx. Together they form the pharyngeal plexus.

5.32 Pharynx: The Parapharyngeal Space and Its Clinical Significance

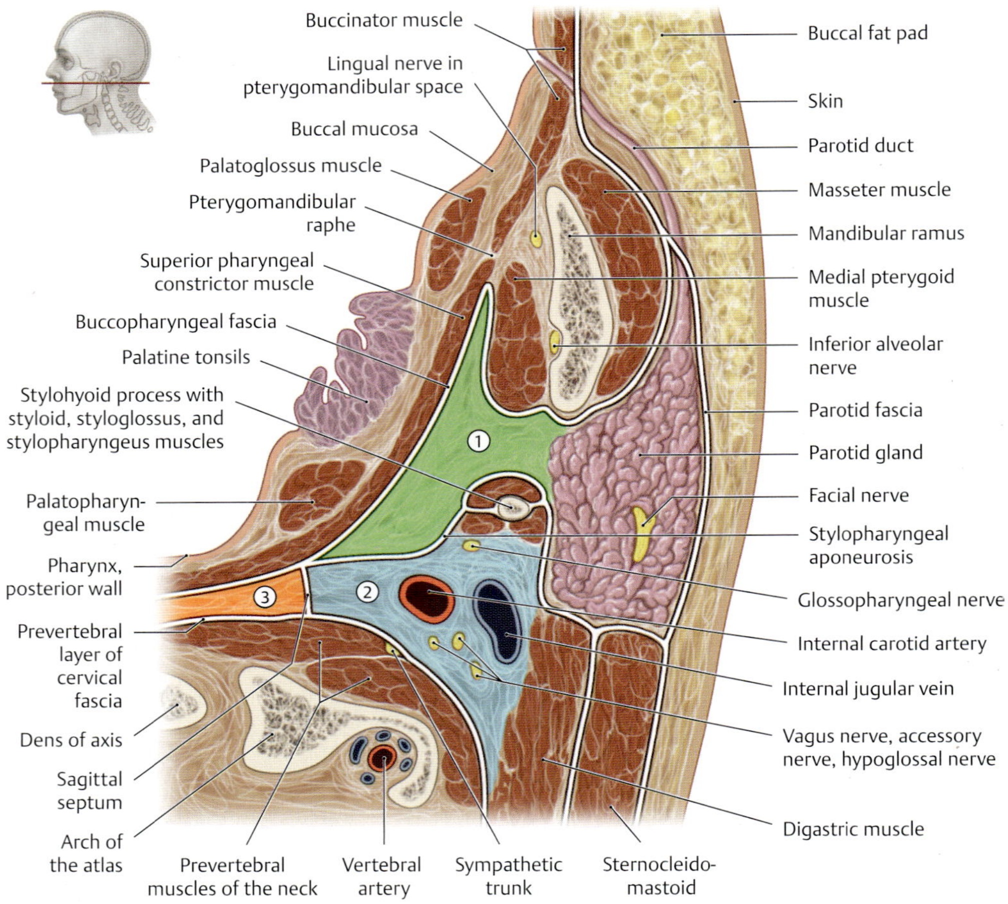

A Parapharyngeal space
Horizontal section, at the level of dens axis and tonsillar fossa.

The peripharyngeal space is an area of connective tissue, which extends from the base of the skull to the mediastinum. Topographically, it is divided into a *parapharyngeal (lateral) space* (①+②) on either side of the pharynx and a *retropharyngeal space* (③) posterior to the pharynx. The border separating the two is the *sagittal septum* made of connective tissue that extends between the prevertebral cervical fascia and the posterior pharyngeal wall.

- The unpaired **retropharyngeal space** is a thin gap between the posterior wall of the pharynx and the prevertebral cervical fascia which covers the prevertebral neck muscles. The space includes branches of the ascending pharyngeal a. and veins of the pharyngeal venous plexus.
- The paired **lateral pharyngeal spaces** contain loose connective tissue and are divided by the stylopharyngeal aponeurosis (the common connective tissue sheath of muscles which arise from the styloid process) into an anterior part (prestyloid) and posterior part (*retrostyloid*).
  - ① *Anterior part:* communicates with the retromandibular fossa and contains all the structures which run from the infratemporal fossa to the face (e.g. medial pterygoid m., inferior alveolar n., lingual n., auriculotemporal n., otic ganglion, as well as the maxillary a. and its branches).
  - ② *Posterior part:* includes the internal carotid a., internal jugular v., cranial nn. IX–XII as well as the sympathetic trunk, which runs below or along the layer of prevertebral cervical fascia.

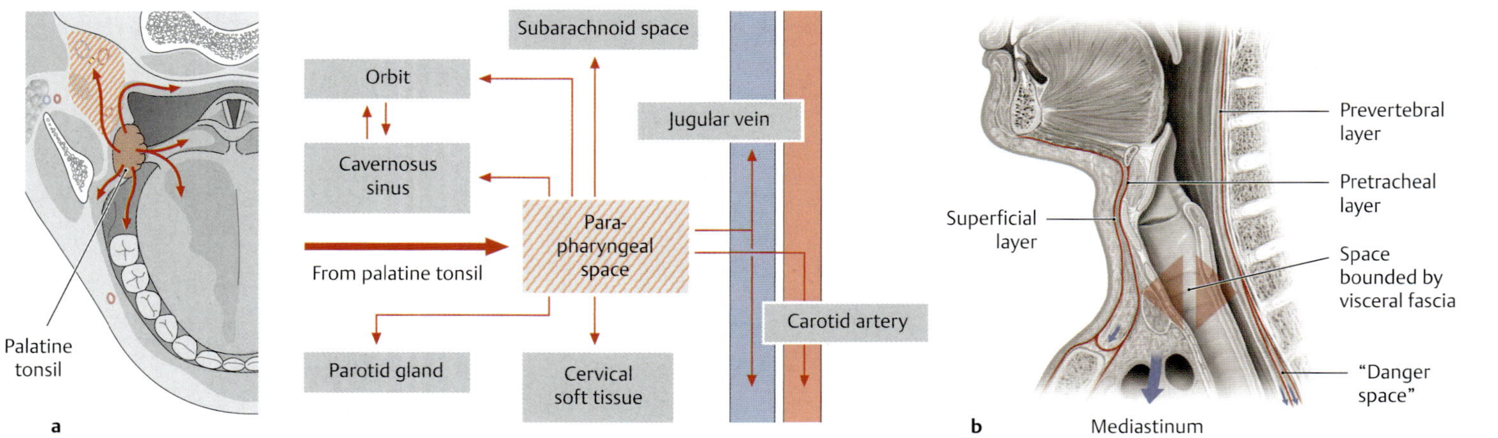

B Clinical significance of the parapharyngeal space
(after Becker, Naumann, and Pfaltz)

a Bacteria and inflammatory cells in the palatine tonsil can infiltrate into the parapharyngeal space from where they can spread

- into the internal jugular v.: risk of sepsis
- into the subarachnoid space: risk of meningitis

b Additional complications include sinking abscesses (the inflammation spreads between the superficial and medial layers of the cervical fascia or along the carotid sheath into the mediastinum causing mediastinitis). From the "danger space" (a cleft-like divided space of the prevertebral fascia) infections can directly reach the posterior mediastinum. By administering modern antibiotics early and broadly, these complications now rarely occur.

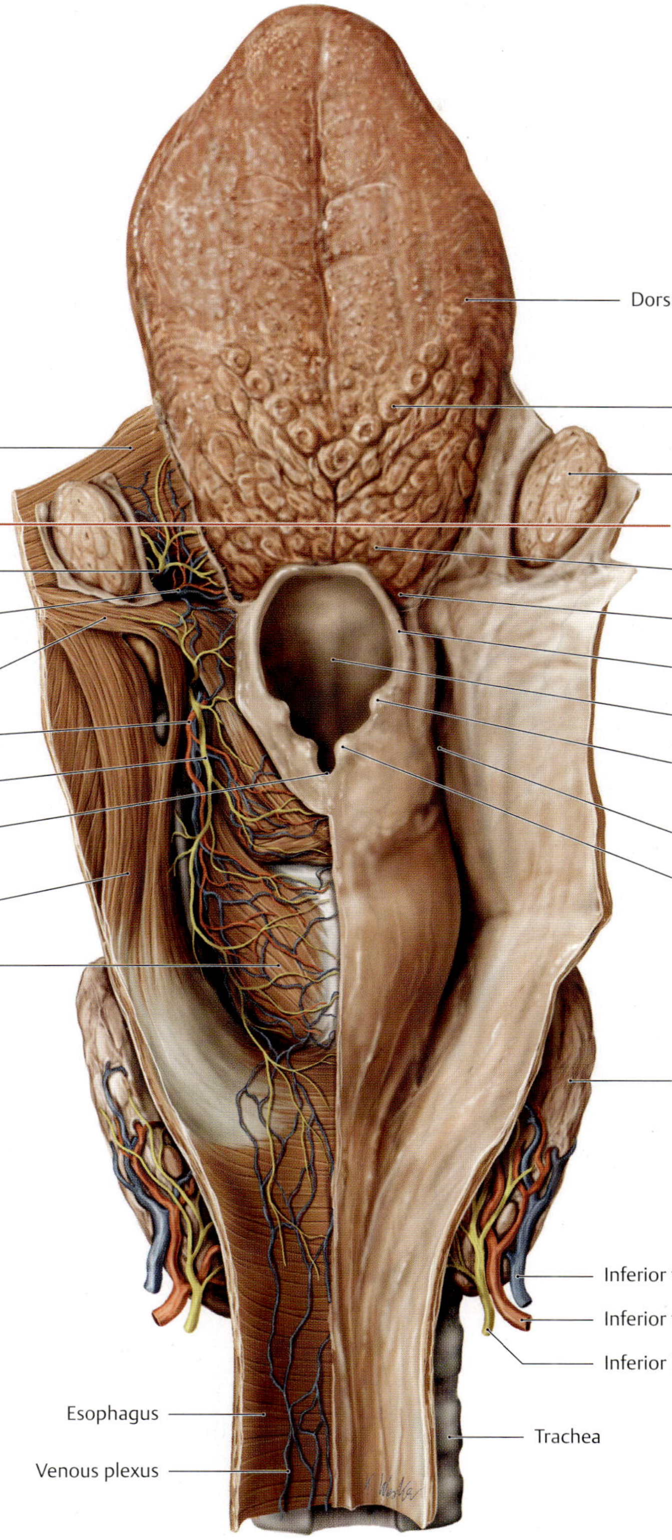

C Neurovascular structures of the parapharyngeal space

Posterior view of a specimen composed of the tongue, larynx, esophagus, and thyroid gland, as it would be resected at autopsy for pathologic evaluation of the neck. This dissection clearly demonstrates the branching pattern of the neurovascular structures that occupy the plane between the pharyngeal muscles. The large neck pathways and their organ-supplying vessels and nerves (see p. 230 f.) are embedded in an area of connective tissue, the peripharyngeal space (cf. **A**). This allows for their mobility during neck movement. The bifurcation of the pathways in the layer between the pharyngeal muscles is clearly identifiable. The tonsillar branches arise from the ascending palatine artery as shown here but occasionally directly from the facial artery as well. *Note* the vascular supply to the palatine tonsil and its proximity to the neurovascular bundle, which creates a risk of hemorrhage during tonsillectomy.

5.33 Pharynx: Neurovascular Structures in the Parapharyngeal Space (Superficial Layer)

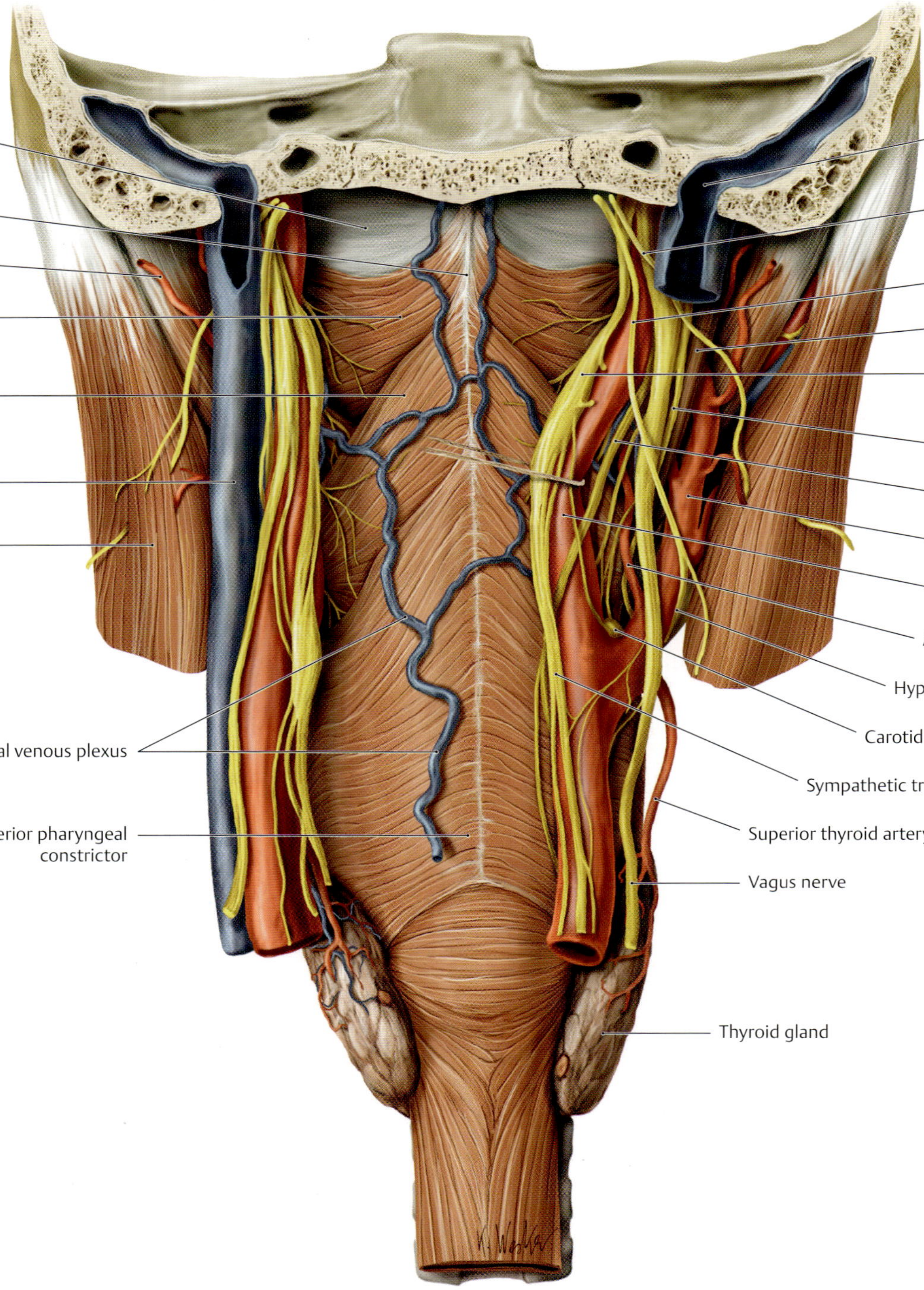

A Parapharyngeal space, posterior view

The vertebral column and all structures posterior to it have been completely removed to display the posterior wall of the pharynx from the posterior aspect. The neurovascular structures on the left side are intact, while the right internal jugular vein has been removed to demonstrate neurovascular structures lying anterior to the vein. After passing through the base of the skull, the internal carotid a., vagus n., and sympathetic trunk are shifted medially to the para- and lateral pharyngeal spaces.

Note the exposed carotid body, which is innervated by the vagus nerve, glossopharyngeal nerve, and sympathetic trunk.

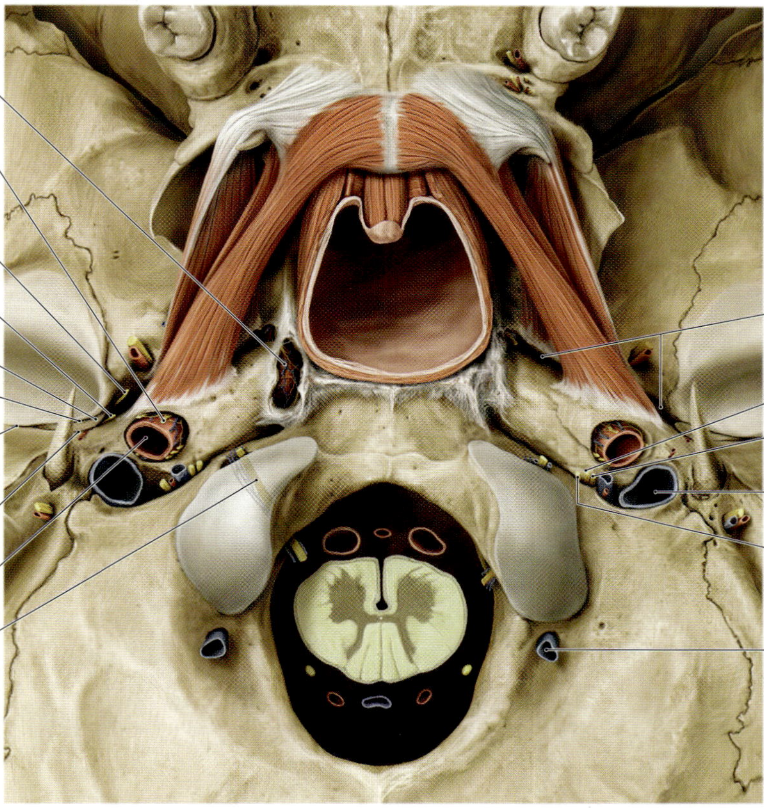

B Neurovascular structures in the peripharyngeal space: points of emergence from the base of the skull.

The neurovascular structures pass through the following openings:

- **Petrotympanic fissure (Glaserian fissure)**
  - Anterior tympanic a.
  - Chorda tympani
- **Tympanosquamous fissure**
- **Sphenopetrosal fissure;** its wide extension forms the foramen lacerum
  - Lesser petrosal n.
  - Chorda tympani
- **Foramen lacerum**
  - Greater petrosal n.
  - Deep petrosal n.
- **Jugular foramen**
  - Internal jugular v.
  - Glossopharyngeal n. (CN IX)
  - Vagus n. (CN X)
  - Accessory n. (CN XI)
- **Hypoglossal canal**
  - Hypoglossal n. (CN XII)
- **Condylar canal**
  - Condylar emissary v.
- **Carotid canal**
  - Internal carotid a., Internal carotid sympathetic plexus

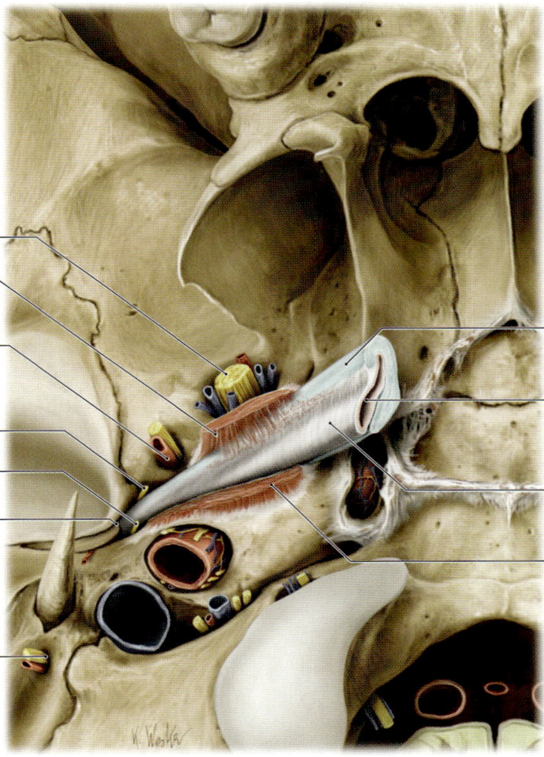

C Course of the auditory tube at the base of the skull

Detail of **B**. Directly below the base of the skull, in the cranial aspect of the lateral pharyngeal space lies the **cartilaginous part** of the auditory tube. When projected onto the base of the skull, it lies in the *sphenopetrosal fissure*, an extension of the petrosquamous fissure (the exit point of the *lesser* petrosal n., see **B**). Medially, the sphenopetrosal fissure widens toward the *foramen lacerum* (exit point of the greater petrosal n.), which is covered by fibrocartilagious tissue. The cartilaginous portion of the auditory tube begins at the funnel-shaped opening (opening of the auditory tube) lateral to the superior margin of the pharyngeal wall close to the choanae and runs obliquely in a lateral-posterior direction (at a 45° angle to the mid-sagittal plane). The auditory tube cartilage creates a channel which is open at its lateral and inferior margin, where the tubal mucosa is located. In cross-section it appears hook-shaped. The lateral wall is composed of connective tissue and forms the membranous lamina.

The **bony part** of the auditory tube represents around one-third of the auditory tube's entire length and runs together with the tensor tympani m. in the musculotubarus canal to the tympanic cavity. Its opening is located between the carotid canal and the foramen spinosum (at the level of the petrosquamous fissure). The narrowest part of the auditory tube (the isthmus) is between the cartilaginous and osseous parts. For functions of the levator and tensor veli palatini mm. see p. 147.

5.34 Pharynx: Neurovascular Structures in the Parapharyngeal Space (Deep Layer)

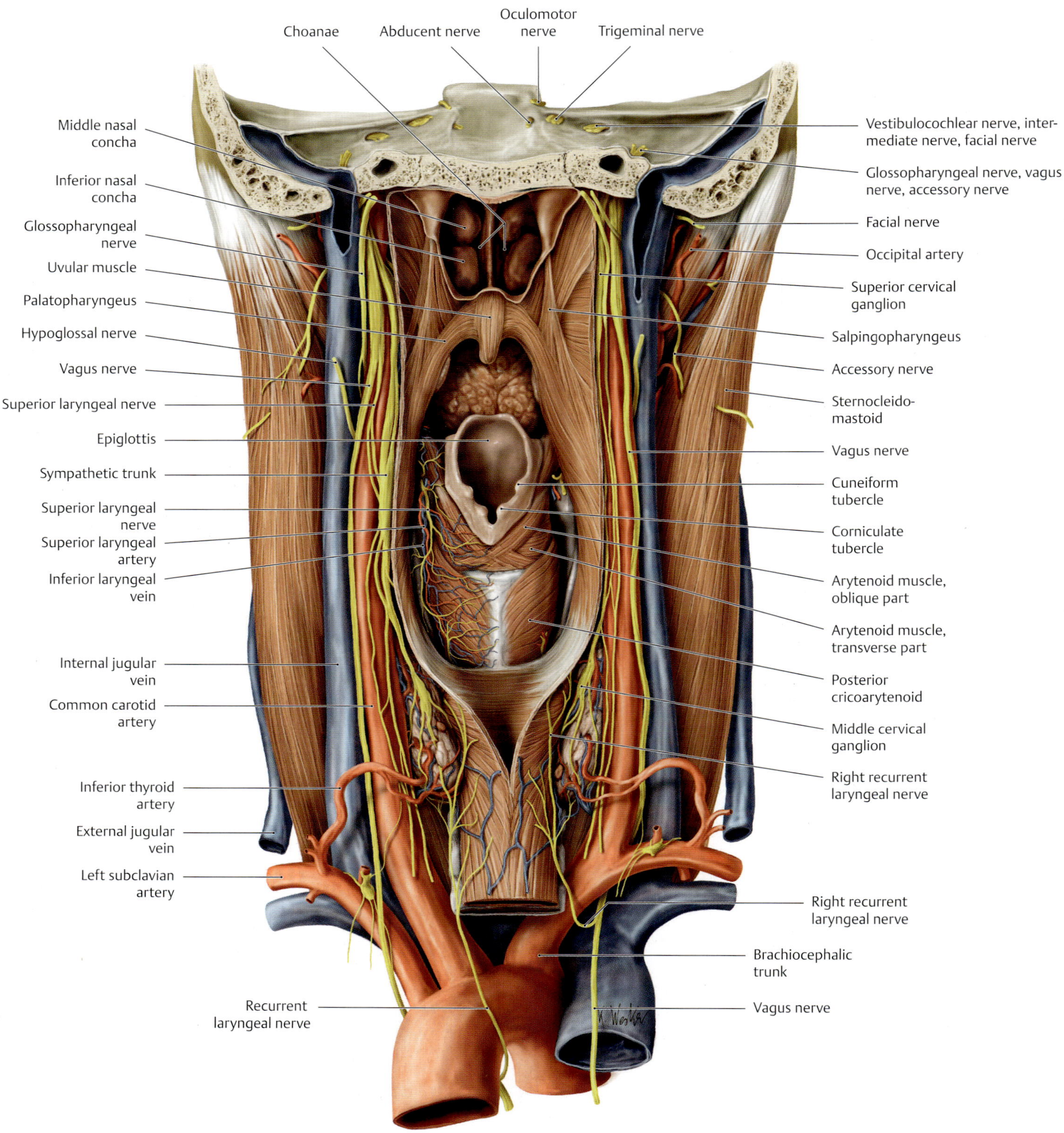

A Parapharyngeal space
Posterior view. The neurovascular structures in the parapharyngeal space are fully displayed from the posterior cranial fossa to the thoracic inlet. Also, the posterior wall of the pharynx has been longitudinally incised and spread open to demonstrate the cavity of the pharynx from the choanae down to the esophagus.

Note: The major neurovascular structures in the neck course along the pharynx in a tightly clustered configuration. Stab injuries that perforate the lumen (from accidentally ingested bones, for example) may lead to inflammation of the parapharyngeal space, causing significant damage (see p. 204). Even minor injuries may incite a purulent bacterial inflammation that spreads rapidly within this connective tissue space (cellulitis).

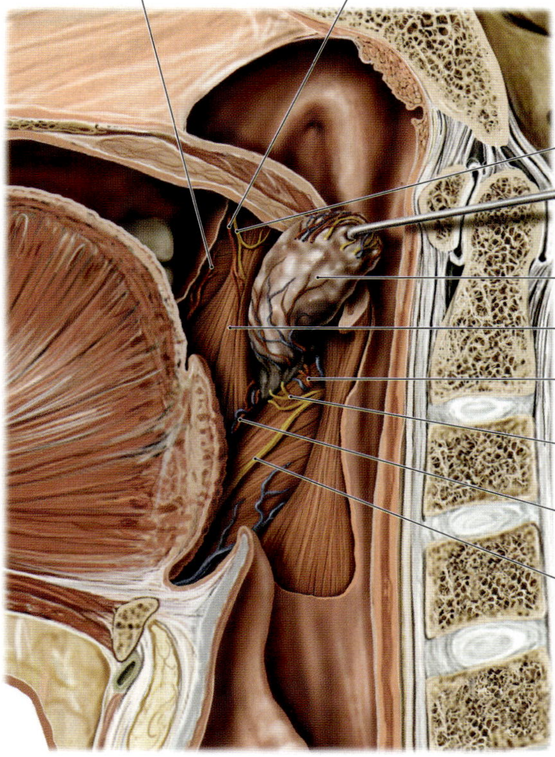

B Vascular and nerve supply of the palatine tonsil

Median sagittal section, medial view. The palatine tonsil lies between the palatoglossal and palatopharyngeal folds. For a better illustration of its pathways, the tonsil was detached from the tonsillar bed and tilted cranially. The pathways originate from, or extend to, the peripharyngeal space.

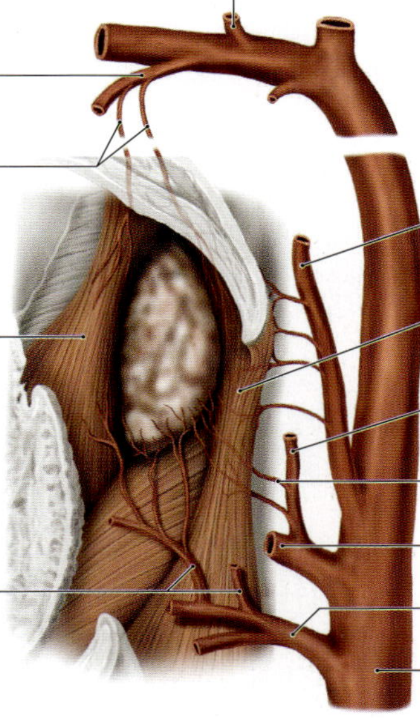

C Arterial supply of the palatine tonsil

During tonsillectomies, branches of those arteries must be cauterized or ligated to prevent them from bleeding.

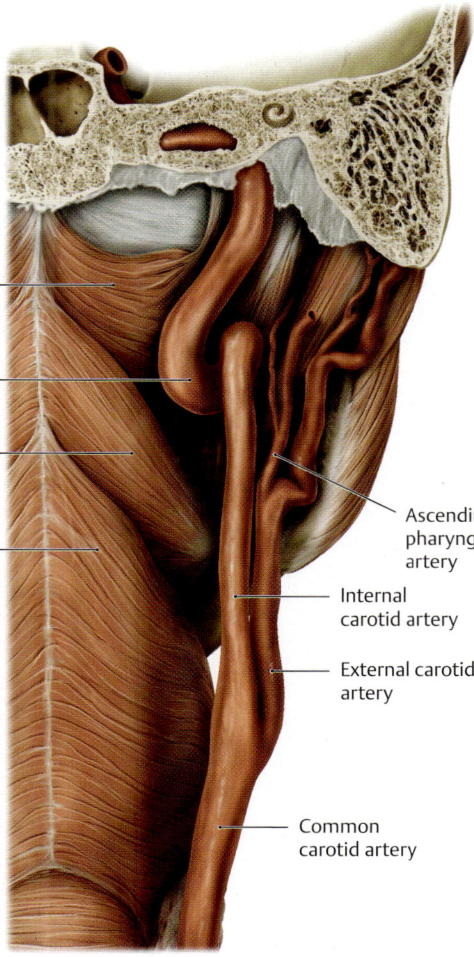

D Dangerous loop of the internal carotid a.

(based on a specimen that is part of the anatomical collection of the University in Kiel)

Dorsal view. A siphon-shaped loop of the carotid a. on the pharyngeal constrictor m. in the area around the tonsillar bed can be found in approximately 5% of the population. Damaging this loop during a tonsillectomy is dangerous and can result in severe arterial bleeding.

5.35 Salivary Glands

A Major salivary glands
Lateral view (**a**) and superior view (**b**).
Three large, paired sets of glands are distinguished:

1. Parotid glands
2. Submandibular glands
3. Sublingual glands

The parotid gland is a purely serous gland (watery secretions). The submandibular gland is a mixed seromucous gland, and the sublingual gland is a predominantly mucous-secreting (mucoserous) gland. The glands produce approximately 0.5–2 liters of saliva per day. Their excretory ducts open into the oral cavity. The excretory duct of the parotid gland (the parotid duct) crosses over the masseter muscle, pierces the buccinator, and opens in the oral vestibule opposite the second upper molar. The excretory duct of the submandibular gland (submandibular duct) opens on the sublingual papilla behind the lower incisor teeth. The sublingual gland has many smaller excretory ducts that open on the sublingual fold, or into the submandibular duct. The saliva keeps the oral mucosa moist, and it contains the starch-splitting enzyme amylase and the bactericidal enzyme lysozyme. The presynaptic *parasympathetic* fibers (not shown here) for autonomic control of the salivary glands arise from the superior and inferior salivatory nuclei and are distributed to the glands in various nerves (see pp. 124, 127, and 130), where they synapse with clusters of local ganglion cells, or in the submandibular ganglion. *Sympathetic fibers* are distributed to the ducts along vascular pathways. The long winding duct of the submandibular gland has a tendency to become obstructed by salivary calculi.

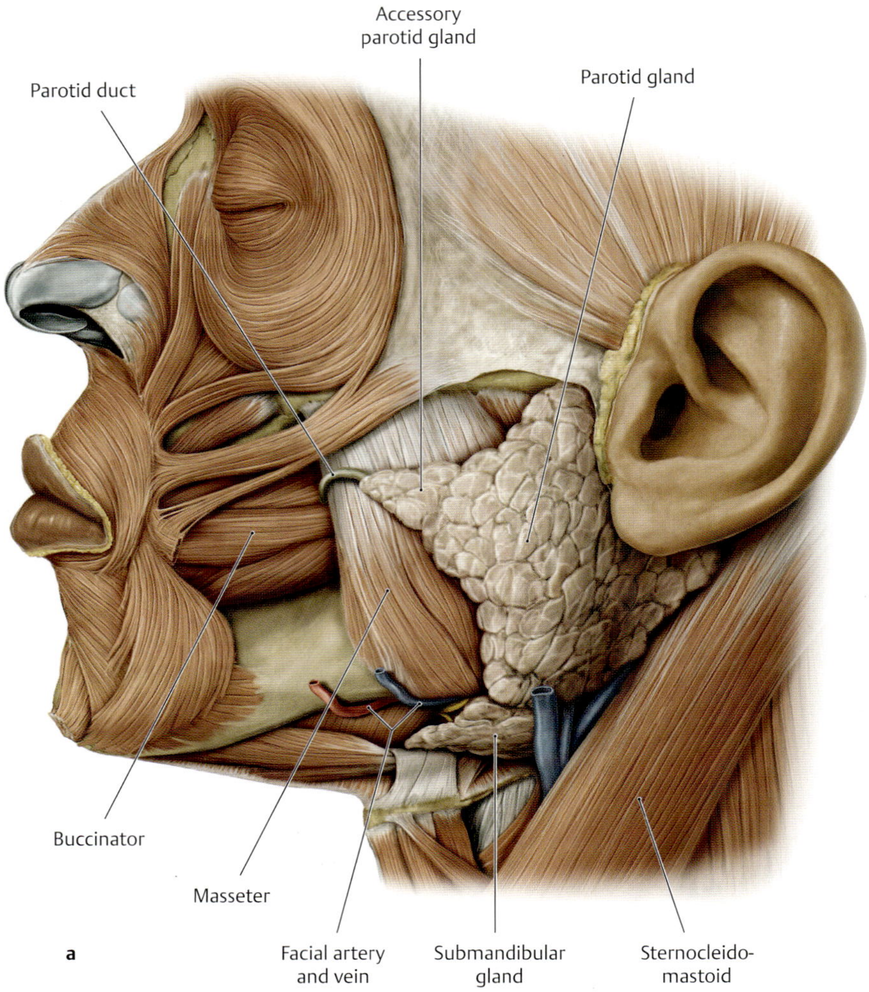

a

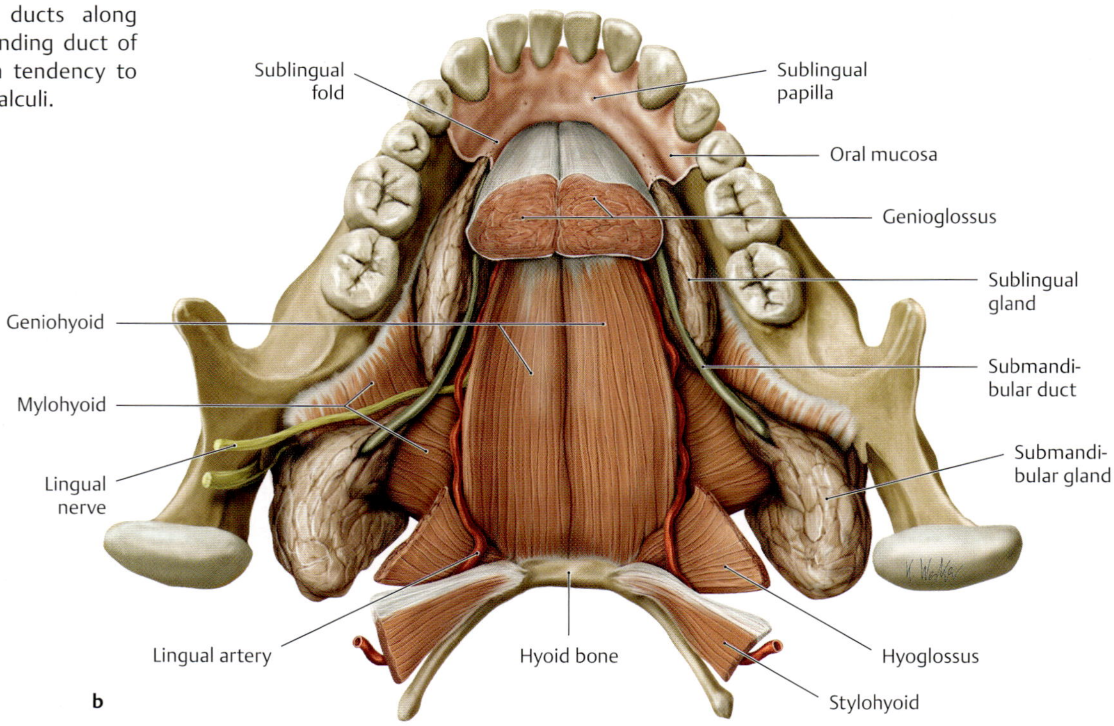

b

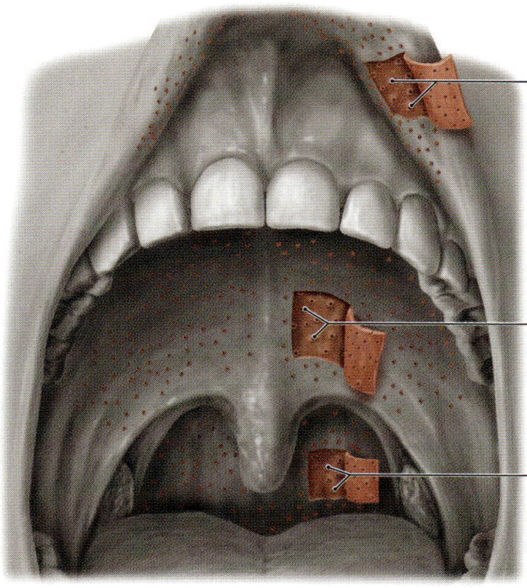

B Minor salivary glands
In addition to the three major paired glands, 700–1000 minor glands also secrete saliva into the oral cavity. They produce only 5–8% of the total output but this amount keeps the mouth moist when the major salivary glands secrete only during mastication.
Note: Tumors originating in the minor salivary glands are more often malignant than those originating in the major salivary glands. This is another reason for the clinical significance of these glands.

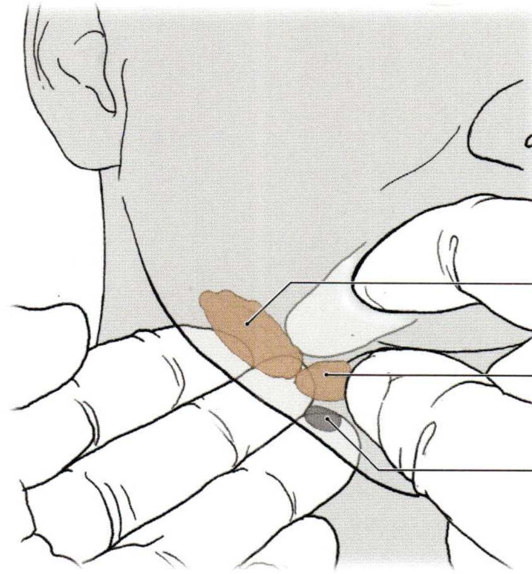

C Bimanual examination of the salivary glands
The submandibular and sublingual glands, as well as the adjacent lymph nodes, are located around the mobile oral floor, and so they must be palpated against resistance. This is done with bimanual examination.

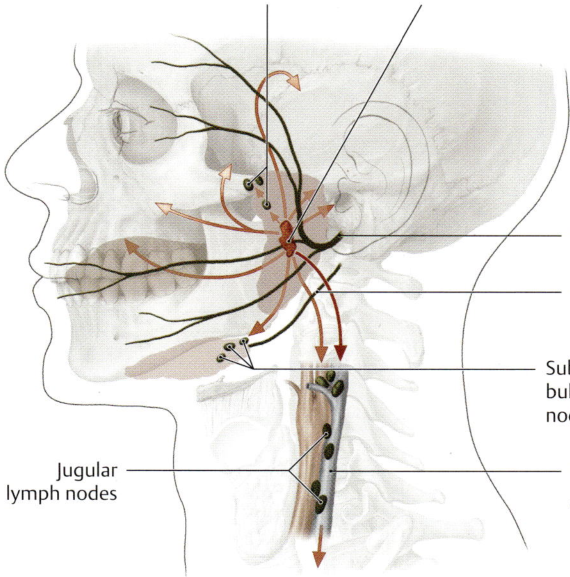

D Spread of malignant parotid tumors along anatomical pathways
Malignant tumors of the parotid gland may directly invade surrounding structures (open arrows); they may also spread via regional lymph nodes (solid arrows), or spread systemically (metastasize) through the vascular system.

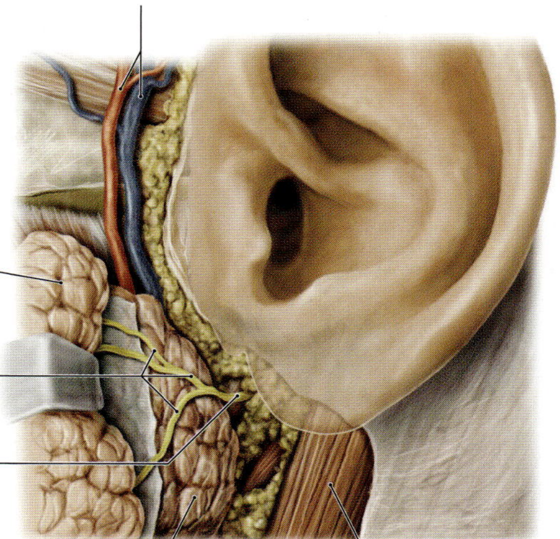

E Intraglandular course of the facial nerve in the parotid gland
The facial nerve divides into branches within the parotid gland (the parotid plexus separates the gland into a superficial part and deep part) and is vulnerable during the surgical removal of parotid tumors. To preserve the facial nerve during parotidectomy, it is first necessary to locate and identify the facial nerve trunk. The best landmark for locating the nerve trunk is the tip of the cartilaginous auditory canal.

5.36 Larynx: Location, Shape, and Laryngeal Cartilages

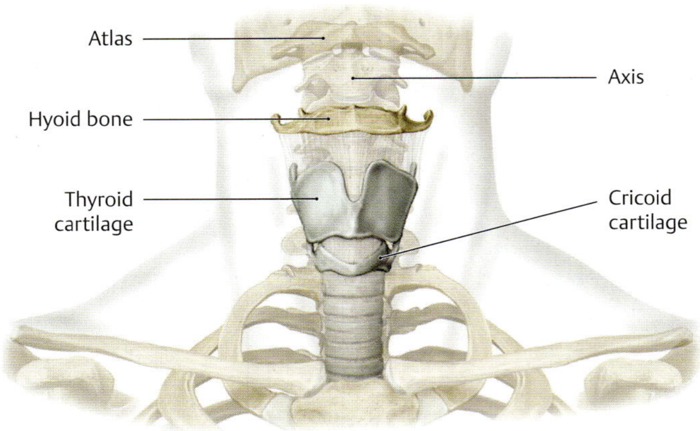

A Location of the larynx in the neck
Anterior view. In the adult male, when the head is upright and the larynx is centered in the neck:

- The hyoid bone is at the level of the C3 vertebra.
- The superior border of the thyroid cartilage is at the C 4 level.
- The laryngotracheal junction is at the C6–C7 level.

These structures are located approximately one-half vertebra higher in women and children. The upper part of the larynx (the thyroid cartilage, see **B**) is especially prominent in the male, forming the laryngeal prominence or "Adam's apple."

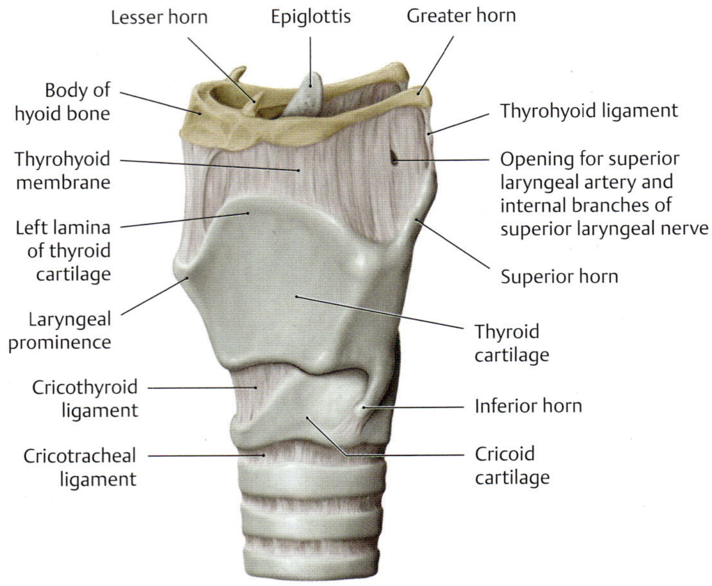

B General features of the larynx
Left anterior oblique view. The following cartilaginous structures of the larynx can be identified in this view:

- Epiglottis (see **D**)
- Thyroid cartilage (see **E**)
- Cricoid cartilage (see **F**)

These cartilages are connected to one another and to the trachea and hyoid bone by elastic ligaments, which allow some degree of laryngeal motion during swallowing (see p. 203). The arytenoid cartilages and corniculate cartilage are not visible in this view (see **G**).

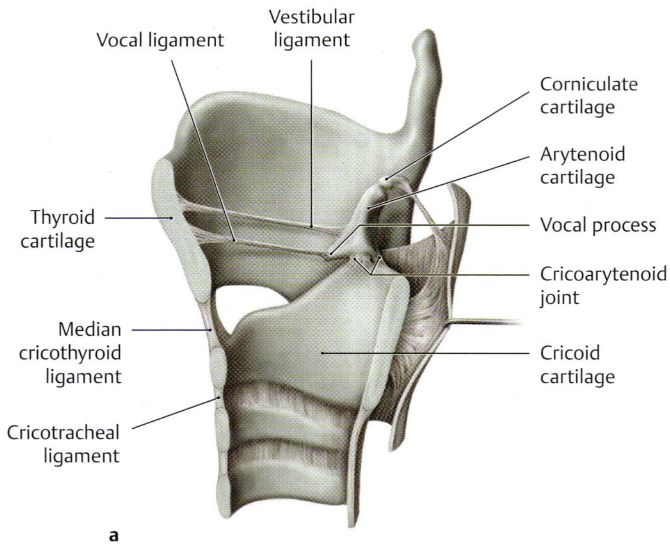

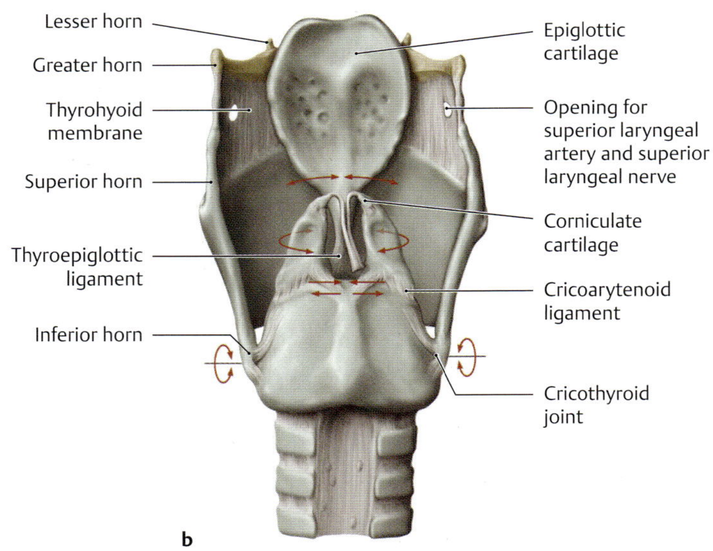

C Laryngeal cartilages and ligaments

a Sagittal section, viewed from the left medial aspect. The thyroid cartilage encloses most of the laryngeal cartilages, its inferior part articulating with the cricoid cartilage (cricothyroid joint).

b Posterior view. Arrows indicate the directions of movement in the various joints. The thyroid cartilage can tilt relative to the cricoid cartilage in the cricothyroid joint. The base of the arytenoid cartilage on each side can translate or rotate relative to the upper edge of the cricoid cartilage at the cricoarytenoid joint. The arytenoid cartilages move during phonation.

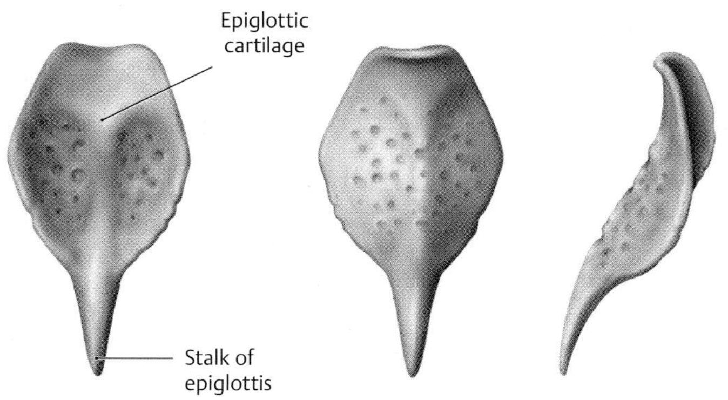

D Epiglottic cartilage

Laryngeal, lingual, and left lateral views. The internal skeleton of the epiglottis is composed of elastic cartilage shown here (the epiglottic cartilage). This cartilage enables the epiglottis to return spontaneously to its initial position at the end of swallowing (when muscular traction is lost). If the epiglottis is removed as part of a tumor resection, the patient must go through an arduous process of learning how to swallow effectively without an epiglottis, avoiding aspiration of ingested material into the trachea.

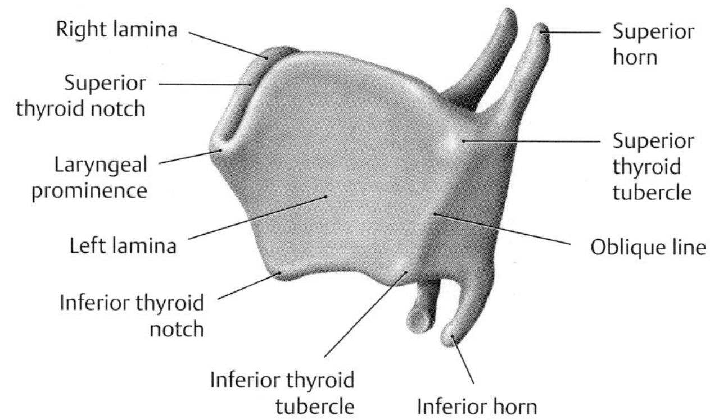

E Thyroid cartilage

Left oblique view. This hyaline cartilage consists of two quadrilateral plates, the right and left laminae, which are joined in the midline to form a keel-shaped projection. At the upper end of this junction is the laryngeal prominence, called the "Adam's apple" in the male. The posterior ends of the laminae are prolonged to form the superior and inferior horns, which serve as anchors for ligaments (see **B**).

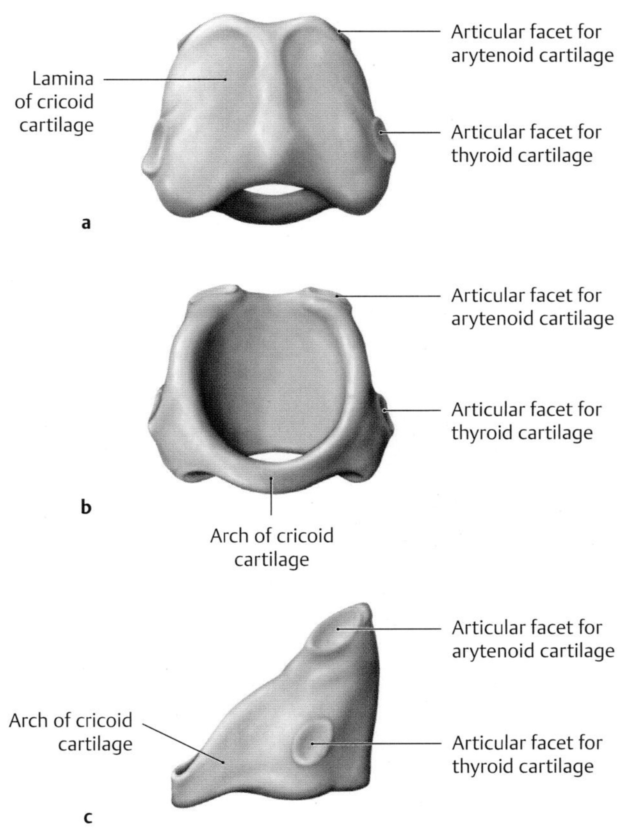

F Cricoid cartilage

Posterior view (**a**), anterior view (**b**), left lateral view (**c**). This hyaline cartilage is shaped like a signet ring. It consists posteriorly of an expanded cartilaginous plate, the lamina of the cricoid cartilage. The upper end of the plate bears an articular facet for the arytenoid cartilage, and the lower end bears a facet for the thyroid cartilage. The inferior border of the cricoid cartilage is connected to the highest tracheal cartilage by the cricotracheal ligament (see **B** and **C**).

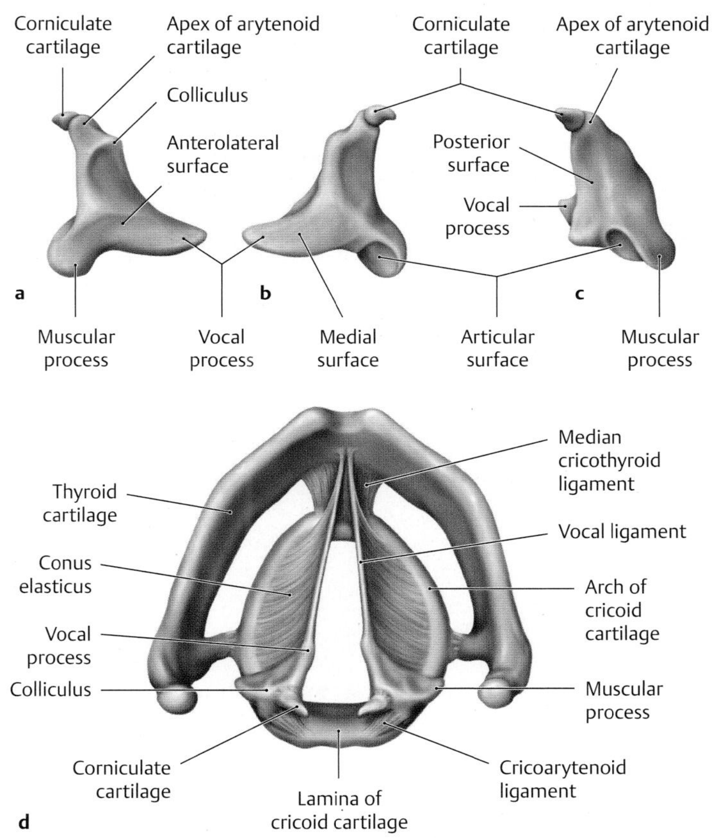

G Arytenoid cartilage and corniculate cartilage

Right cartilages, viewed from the lateral (**a**), medial (**b**), posterior (**c**), and superior (**d**) aspects. The function of the arytenoid cartilage ("arytenoid" literally means "ladle-shaped") is to alter the position of the vocal cords during phonation (see p. 207). The pyramid-shaped, hyaline arytenoid cartilage has three surfaces (anterolateral, medial, and posterior), a base with two processes (vocal and muscular), and an apex. The apex articulates with the tiny corniculate cartilage, which is composed of elastic fibrocartilage.

5.37 Larynx: Internal Features and Neurovascular Structures

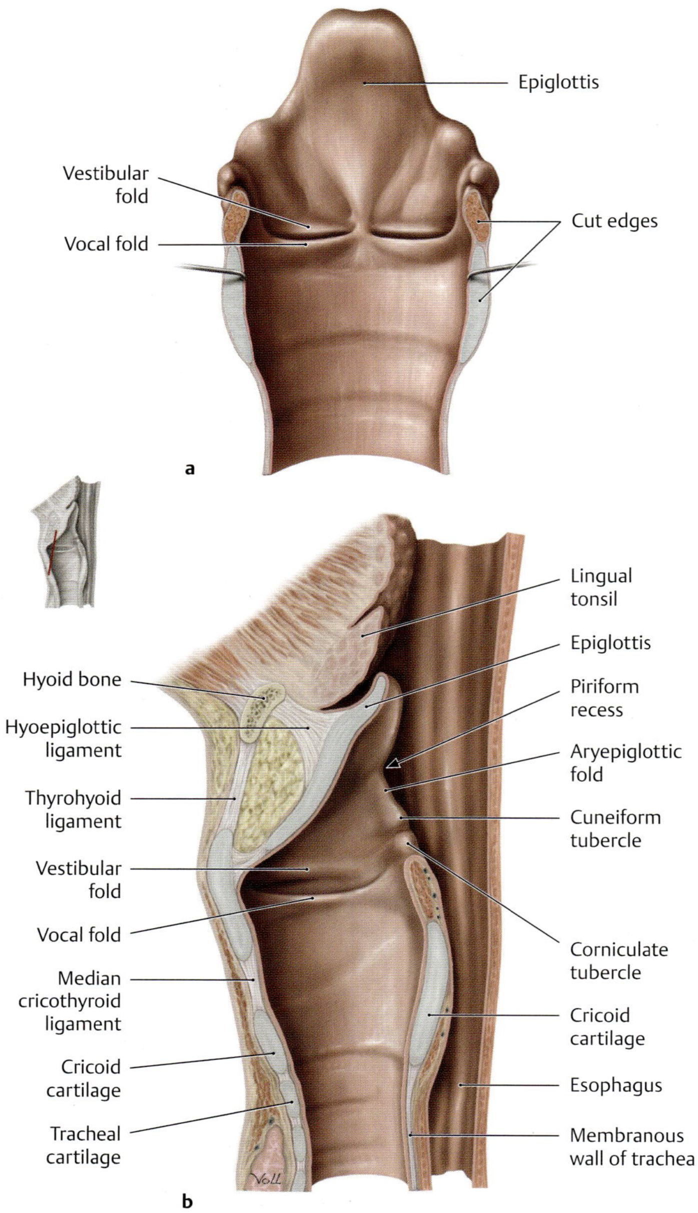

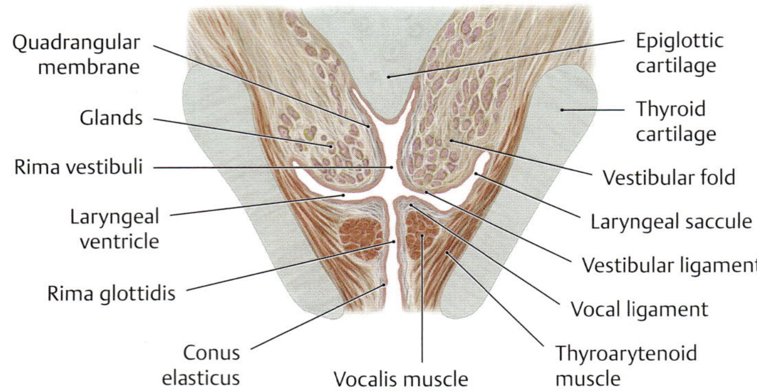

B Vestibular folds and vocal folds

The vestibular folds ("false vocal cords") are clearly displayed in this coronal section. They contain the vestibular ligament, which is the free inferior end of the quadrangular membrane. The fissure between the vestibular folds is the rima vestibuli. Below the vestibular folds are the vocal folds (also called the true vocal folds), which contain the vocal ligament and the vocalis muscle. The fissure between the vocal folds is the rima glottidis (glottis), which is narrower than the rima vestibuli.
Note: The loose connective tissue of the laryngeal inlet may become markedly swollen in response to an insect bite or inflammatory process, obstructing the rima vestibuli. This laryngeal edema (often incorrectly called "glottic edema") presents clinically with dyspnea and a risk of asphyxiation.

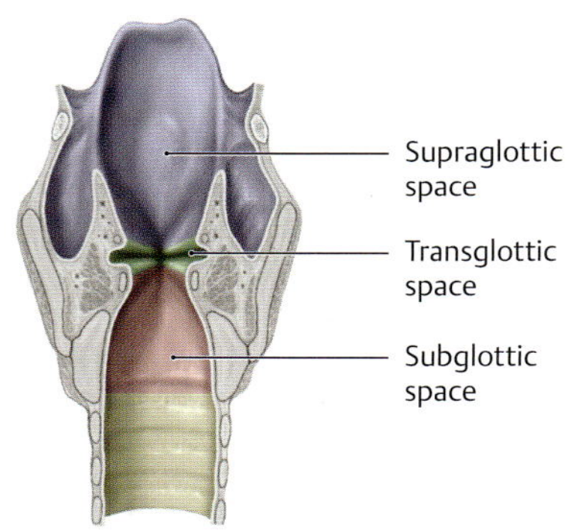

A Cavity of the larynx: mucosal surface anatomy and division into levels

a **Posterior view.** The muscular tube of the pharynx and esophagus has been incised posteriorly and spread open (cut edges). Mucous membrane completely lines the interior of the larynx and, except at the vocal folds, is loosely applied to its underlying tissue (creating the potential for laryngeal edema, see **B**). The aryepiglottic folds are located on each side of the laryngeal cavity between the arytenoid cartilages and epiglottis, and lateral to those folds are pear-shaped mucosal fossae, the piriform recesses.
Note: These recesses have an important role in food transport. The airway and foodway intersect in this region, and the piriform recesses channel food past the larynx and into the esophagus. The epiglottis seals off the laryngeal inlet during swallowing (see p. 203).

b **Midsagittal section viewed from the left side.** The cavity of the larynx can be divided into three levels or spaces to aid in describing the precise location of a laryngeal lesion (cf. **C**).

C Clinical classification of the major laryngeal regions and their borders

Posterior view. The larynx is divided into three levels from above downward to aid in describing the precise location of abnormalities. These three levels are also important in terms of lymphatic drainage.

Levels of the larynx	Extent
Level I: supraglottic space (laryngeal vestibule)	From the laryngeal inlet to the vestibular folds
Level II: transglottic space (intermediate laryngeal cavity)	From the vestibular folds across the laryngeal ventricle (lateral evagination of mucosa) to the vocal folds
Level III: subglottic space (infraglottic cavity)	From the vocal folds to the inferior margin of the cricoid cartilage

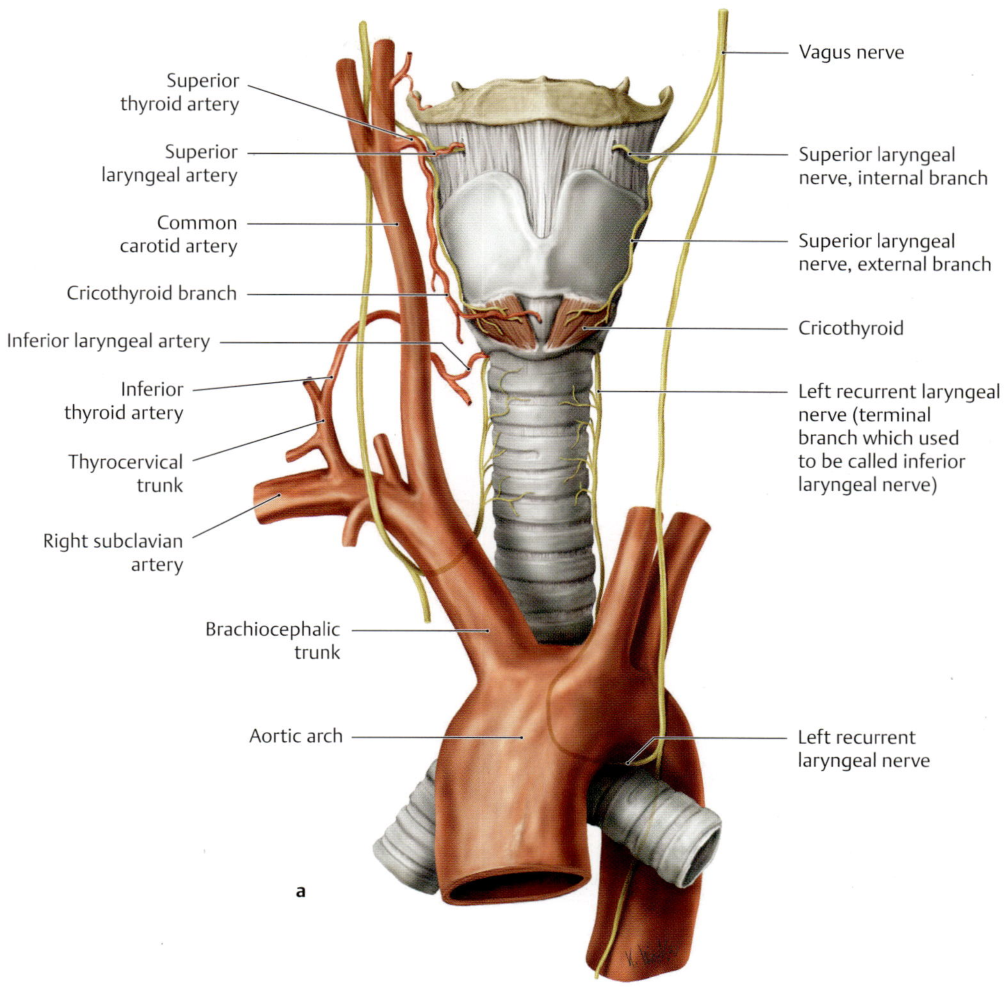

a

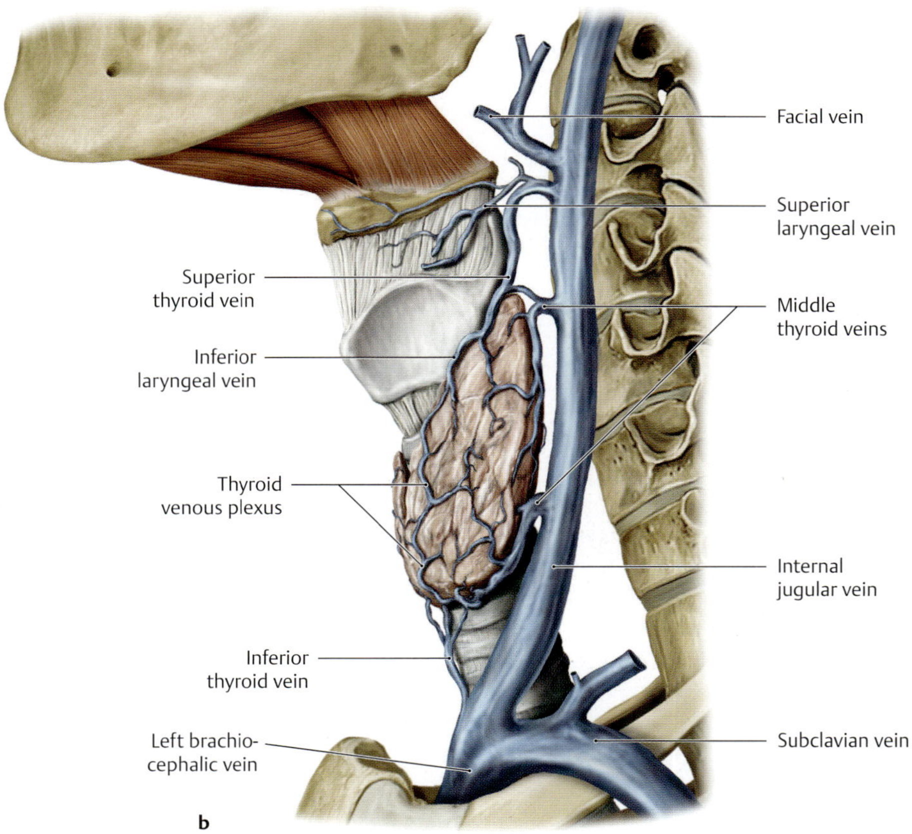

b

D Blood supply and innervation

a Arterial and nerve supply. Anterior view. The larynx derives its *blood supply* from two major arteries: (1) the superior laryngeal artery from superior thyroid branches of the external carotid artery and (2) the inferior laryngeal artery from the inferior thyroid artery off the subclavian artery. Thus the arterial supply of the larynx is analogous to that of the thyroid gland. Responsible for the *innervation* are the superior laryngeal and recurrent laryngeal nn. (both from the vagus n., see p. 141).
Note: Owing to the close proximity of the nerves and arteries, a left-sided aortic aneurysm may cause left recurrent laryngeal nerve palsy resulting in hoarseness (the pathophysiology is explored more fully on p. 219).

b Venous drainage. Left lateral view. The superior laryngeal vein drains into the superior thyroid vein, which terminates at the internal jugular vein. The inferior laryngeal vein drains into the thyroid venous plexus, which usually drains into the left brachiocephalic vein via the inferior thyroid vein.

5.38 Larynx: Muscles

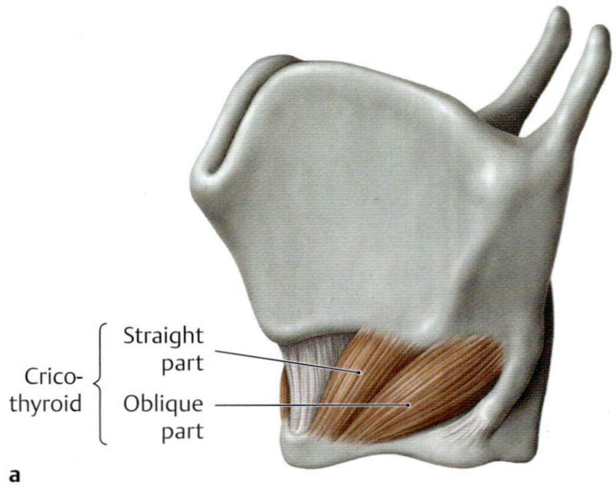

a Left lateral oblique view

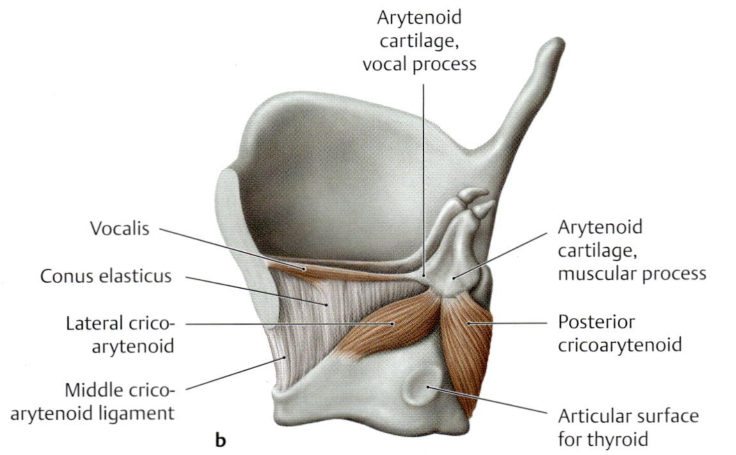

b Left lateral view with the left half of the thyroid cartilage removed

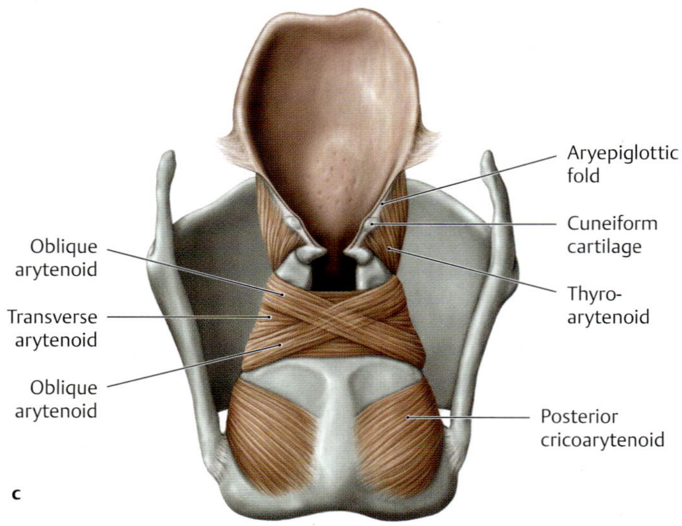

c Posterior view

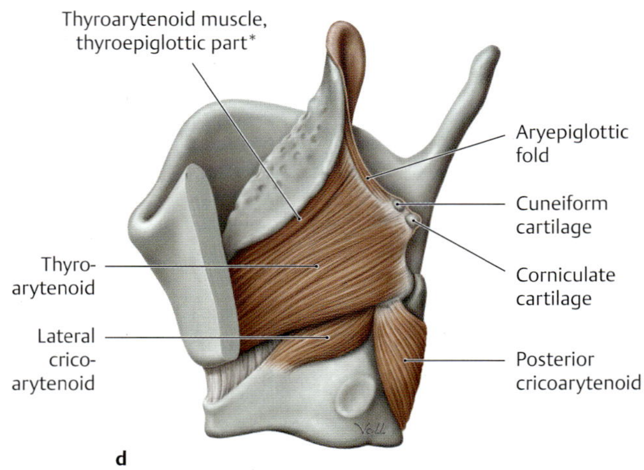

d Left lateral view with the left half of the thyroid cartilage almost completely removed to view the epiglottis and the thyroidarytenoid m., external part*

A Laryngeal muscles

a Extrinsic laryngeal muscles. The cricothyroid (or anterior cricothyroid) is the only laryngeal muscle that attaches to the external surface of the larynx. Contraction of the cricothyroid muscle tilts the cricoid cartilage posteriorly, acting with the *vocalis muscle* (see **b**) to increase tension on the vocal folds. The cricothyroid is the only muscle innervated by the external branch of the superior laryngeal nerve.

b–d Intrinsic laryngeal muscles (the posterior and lateral cricoarytenoids and the thyroarytenoid). These muscles insert on the arytenoid cartilage and can alter the position of the vocal folds. Contraction of the *posterior cricoarytenoid* rotates the arytenoid cartilage outward and slightly to the side; thus it is the only laryngeal muscle that abducts the vocal cords. The *lateral cricoarytenoid* adducts the cords. It opens the intercartilaginous portion (part of glottis located between the arytenoid cartilages) and closes the intermembranous portion (part of the glottis located between the thyroid cartilage and the tip of the vocal process, see **B**) which brings the tips of the vocal processes close to each other. Because this mechanism initiates speech production, this intrinsic laryngeal muscle is also called the *muscle of phonation*. Besides the vocalis muscle, the *transverse arytenoid* and *thyroarytenoid* muscles produce *complete* closure of the rima glottidis (see **c**).

Note: All *intrinsic* laryngeal muscles receive their motor innervation via the recurrent laryngeal n. Unilateral loss of the recurrent laryngeal nerve (e. g., on the left side due to nodal metastases from a hilar bronchial carcinoma) leads to ipsilateral palsy of the posterior cricoarytenoid muscle. This prevents complete abduction of the vocal folds, resulting in hoarseness. Bilateral loss of the recurrent laryngeal nerve (e.g., due to thyroid surgery) leads to dominance of the muscles that close the rima glottidis, causing adduction of the vocal folds with a risk of asphyxiation, but speech is not completely lost (see p. 132).

The muscles described here move the laryngeal cartilages relative to one another and affect the tension and/or position of the vocal folds. The muscles that move the larynx as a whole (infra and suprahyoid muscles as well as inferior pharyngeal constrictor m.) are described on p. 90.

* In older nomenclature, the thyroepiglottic portion of the thyroarytenoid m. was called the thyroepiglottic m. and the band of muscle fibers below the aryepiglottic fold was the aryepiglottic m.

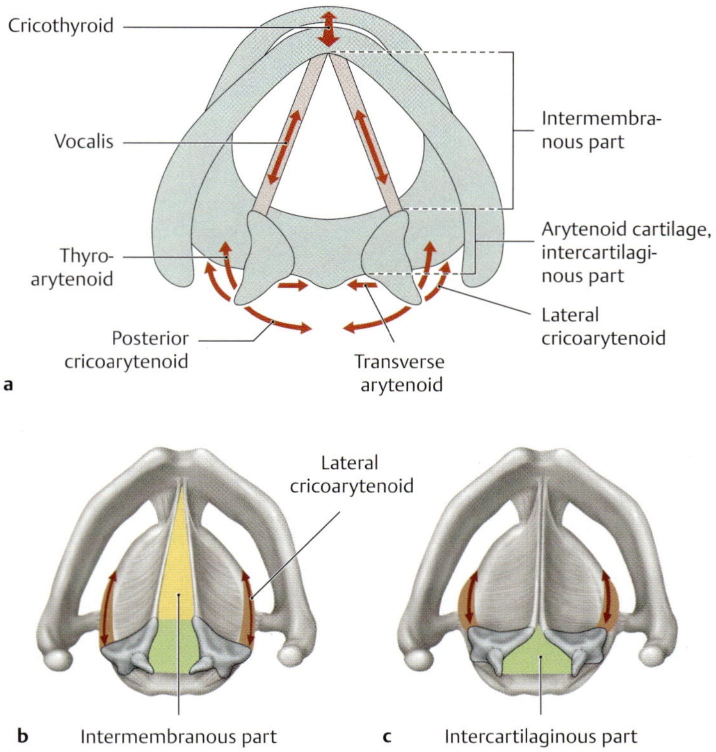

B The laryngeal muscles and their actions (arrows indicate directions of pull)

Posterior cricoarytenoid muscle	Abduct the vocal folds (open the rima glottidis)
Lateral cricoarytenoid muscle (see **b** and **c**)	Adduct the vocal folds (close the rima glottidis)
Transverse arytenoid muscle, thyroarytenoid muscle	Adduct the vocal folds (close the rima glottidis)
Cricothyroid muscle, vocalis muscle	Tighten the vocal folds

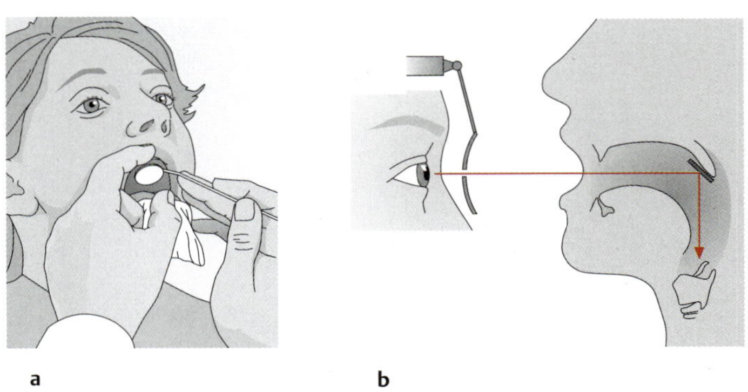

C Indirect laryngoscopy

a From the perspective of the examiner: The larynx—without anesthesia—can only be viewed indirectly with the aid of a mirror (laryngoscope, alternatively endoscope) (cf. **Da**). The examiner holds the patient's tongue while introducing the mirror with the other hand.

b Optical path in laryngoscopy: The mirror directs the light—from the uvula—in a caudal direction to the larynx (findings see **D**).

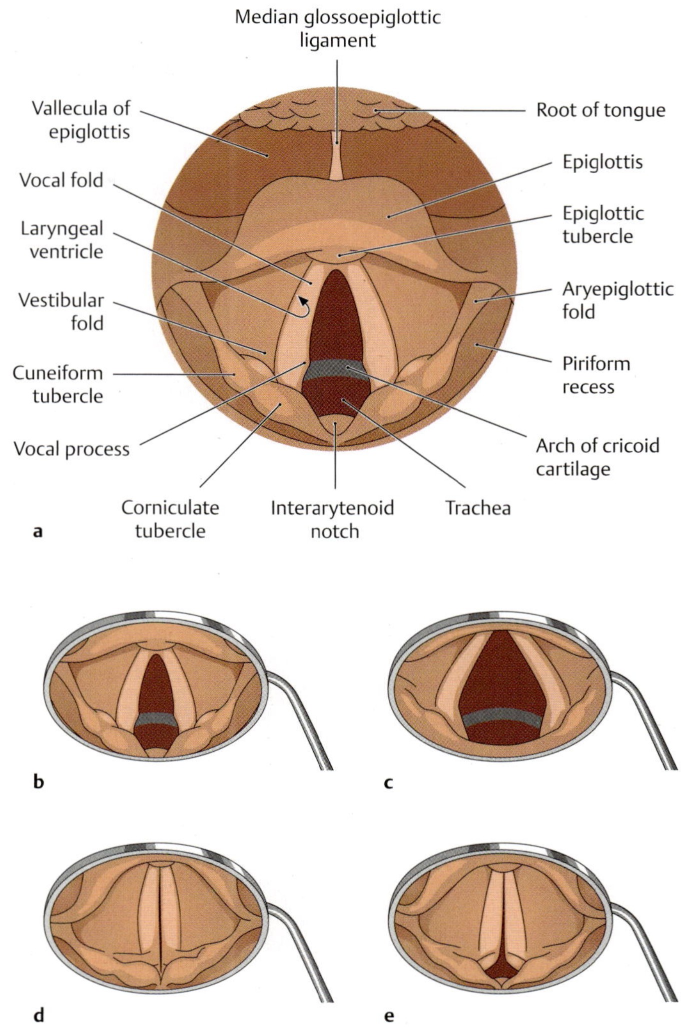

D Mirror image seen by laryngoscopy

a The **mirror image** is a virtual image that shows an anatomically correct portrayal of the left and right side: The right vocal fold appears on the right side of the mirror image. However, anatomically anterior and posterior structures appear at the top or at the bottom of the image: that is tongue base, valleculae or epiglottis (all anterior) at the top, the interarytenoid incisure (posterior) at the bottom. The vocal folds appear as smooth-edged bands. Unlike the surrounding mucosa, the vocal folds do not have blood vessels and are thus markedly lighter in color. The glottis is evaluated in both the respiratory (open) and phonation (closed) positions by having the patient alternately breathe and sing "hiii." The evaluation is based on pathoanatomical (redness, swelling, ulceration) as well as functional changes (e.g., abnormal vocal fold position).

b–e Physiological findings: *Respiratory positions:* opening of the rima glottidis during normal (**b**) and vigorous respiration (**c**). Phonation position with the vocal folds completely adducted (**d**). During whispered speech, the vocal folds are slightly abducted in their posterior third (**e**).

5.39 Larynx: Topographical and Clinical Anatomy

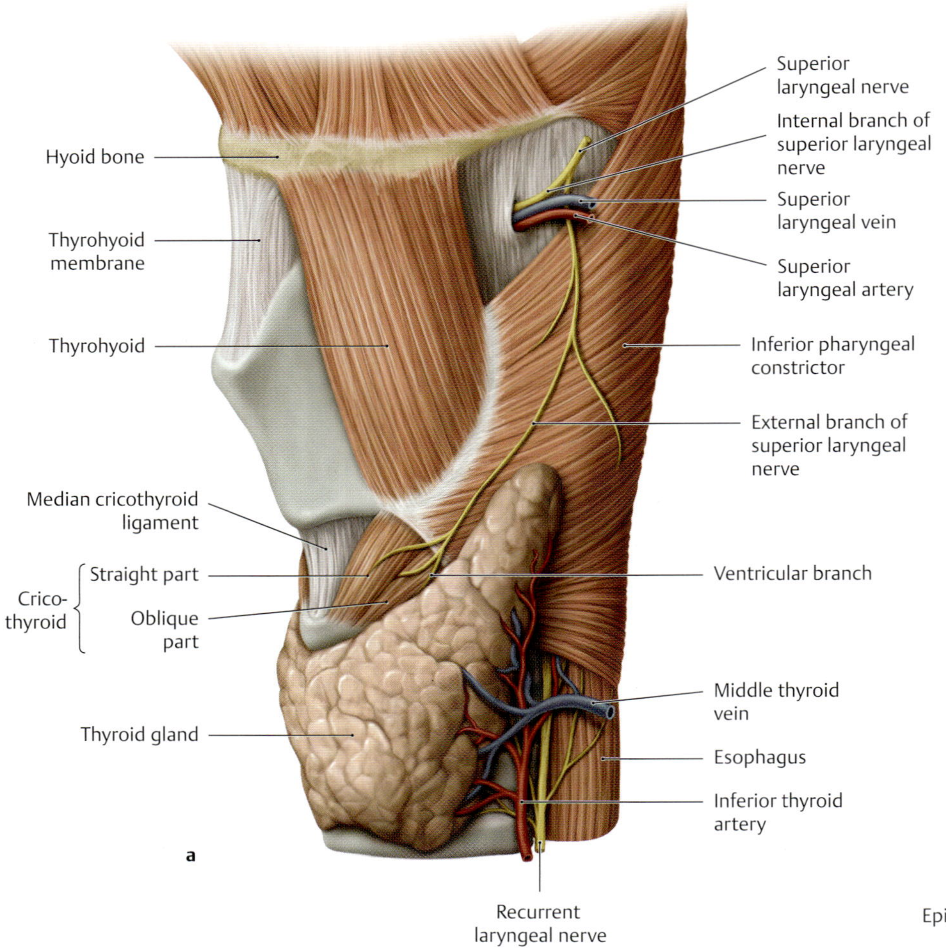

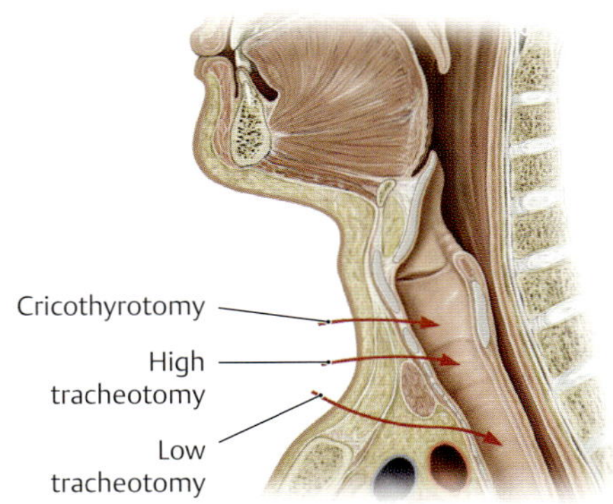

B Approaches to the larynx and trachea
Midsagittal section, left lateral view. When an acute edematous obstruction of the larynx (e.g., due to an allergic reaction) poses an acute risk of asphyxiation, the following surgical approaches are available for creating an emergency airway:

- Division of the median cricothyroid ligament (cricothyrotomy)
- Incision of the trachea (tracheotomy) at a level just below the cricoid cartilage (high tracheostomy) or just superior to the jugular notch (low tracheostomy).

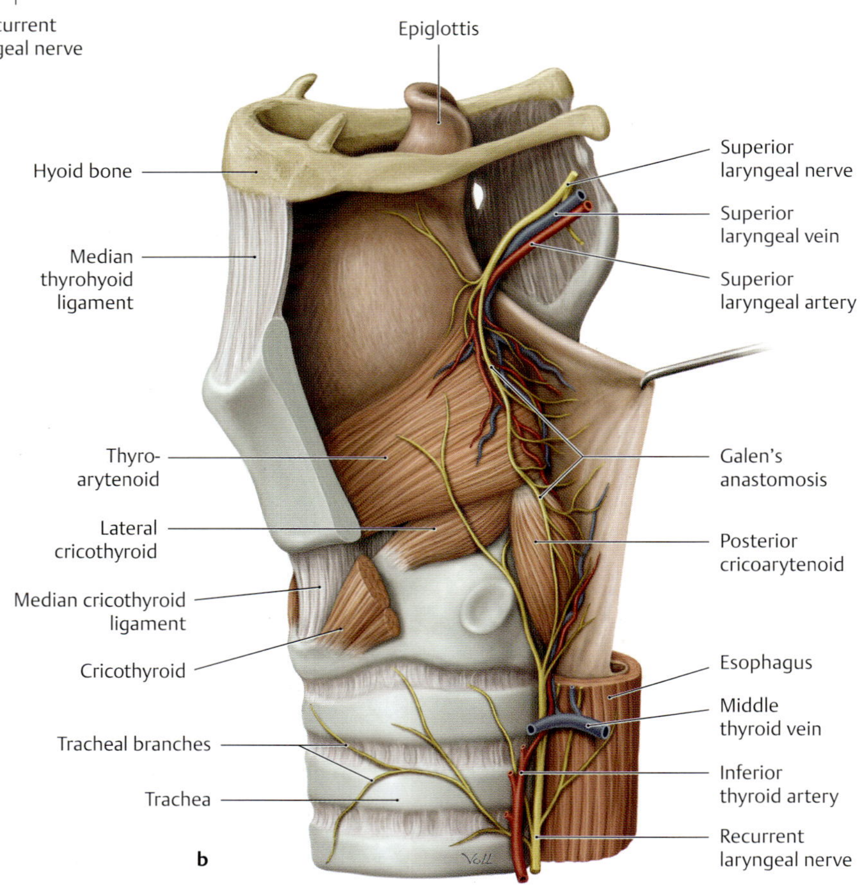

A Topographical anatomy of the larynx: blood supply and innervation
Left lateral view. **a** Superficial layer, **b** deep layer. The cricothyroid muscle and left lamina of the thyroid cartilage have been removed, and the pharyngeal mucosa has been mobilized and retracted. Arteries and veins enter the larynx mainly from the posterior side.
Note: The motor (external) branch of the superior laryngeal nerve supplies the cricothyroid muscle, and its sensory (internal) branch supplies the laryngeal mucosa down to the level of the vocal folds. The recurrent laryngeal n., supplies motor innervation to *all* other (intrinsic) larynx muscles as well as sensory innervation to the laryngeal mucosa below the vocal folds.
The external branch of the superior laryngeal n. gives off an endolaryngeal branch, the ventricular branch. It runs in a cranial direction along the interior surface of the larynx and ends at the level of the vestibular folds. It probably innervates the ventricular m. but is not yet included in the Nomina anatomica.

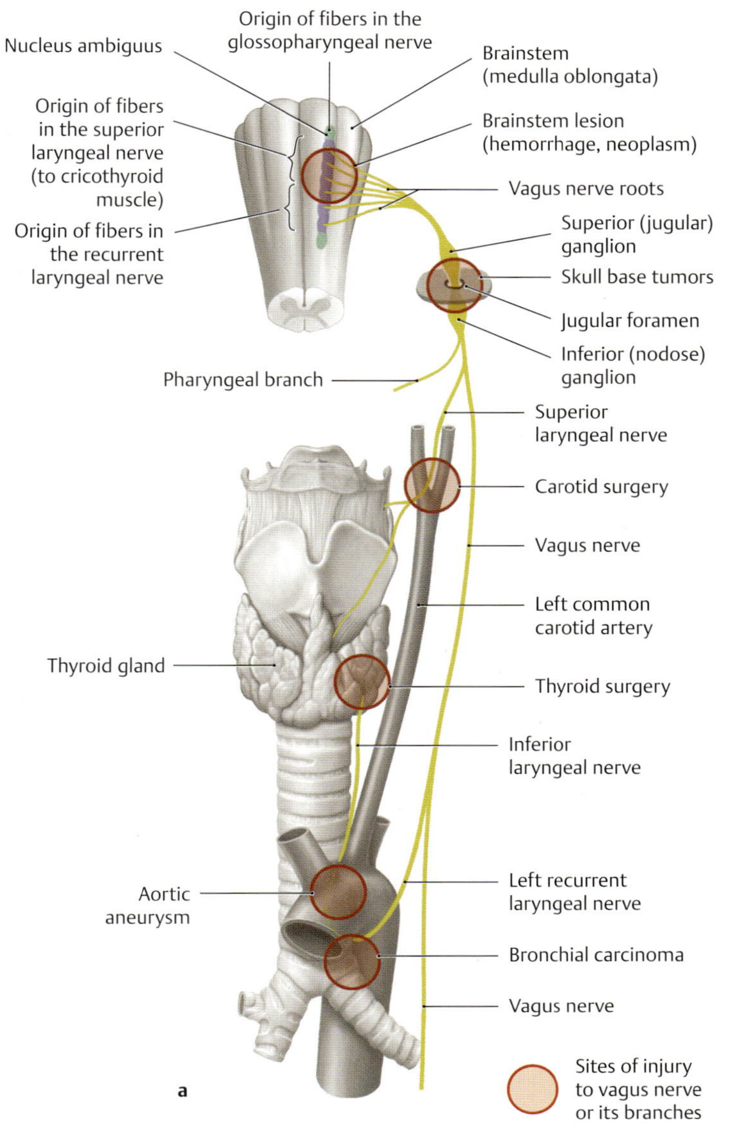

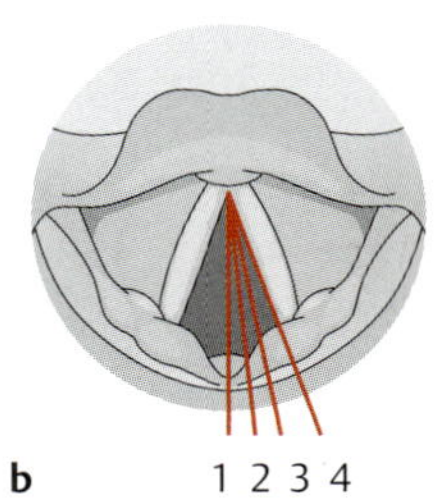

Positions of the vocal folds
1. Median or phonation position
2. Paramedian position
3. Intermediate position
4. Lateral or respiratory position

C Vagus nerve and the position of the vocal folds
The motor fibers of the vagus n. innervate the pharyngeal and laryngeal muscles. They originate in the brainstem in the nucleus ambiguus, the cell groups of which are arranged in somatic order: Between the fibers of the glossopharyngeal n. (cranial origin) and Accessory n. (caudal origin) lie the original neurons of the superior and recurrent laryngeal nn. as well as the motor fibers for the muscles of the soft palate and pharynx. Central or high peripheral vagal lesions lead to pharyngeal or laryngeal muscle palsy and thereby influence the positions of the vocal folds:

- *Central lesions in the brainstem or higher* involving the nucleus ambiguus (e. g., caused by a tumor or hemorrhage) → an intermediate or paramedian position of the vocal fold on the affected side (see **b**).
- *Peripheral lesions of the vagus nerve* have variable effects, depending on the site of the lesion:
  - Skull base lesions at the level of the jugular foramen (e.g., caused by a nasopharyngeal tumor) → an intermediate or paramedian position of the affected vocal fold due to a flaccid paralysis of all intrinsic and extrinsic laryngeal muscles (see **b**) → inability to close the glottis with severe hoarseness. Sensation is lost in the larynx on the affected side.
  - Superior laryngeal nerve in the midcervical region (e.g., as a complication of carotid surgery) → hypotonicity of the cricothyroid muscle → mild hoarseness with a weak voice, especially at higher frequencies. Sensation is lost above the vocal fold.
  - Inferior (recurrent) laryngeal nerve in the lower neck (e.g., lesion caused by thyroid surgery, bronchial carcinoma, or an aortic aneurysm) → paralysis of all intrinsic laryngeal muscles on the affected side → a median or paramedian position of the vocal fold, mild hoarseness, poor tonal control, rapid voice fatigue, no dyspnea. Sensation is lost below the vocal fold.

Note: Bilateral lesions usually worsen the symptoms; e.g., recurrent laryngeal nerve palsy results in the vocal cord being in the paramedian position, significant dyspnea and inspiratory stridor (necessitating tracheotomy in acute cases, see **B**). In addition to motor deficits, sensation is lost at various sites in the laryngeal mucosa depending on the location of the lesion (see **Ab**). Moreover, vagus nerve lesions lead to diminished gag reflexes, swallowing difficulty, foreign-body sensation, coughing and hypernasal speech (deficient closure of the oronasal cavity); usually drooping of the soft palate on the affected side (dysfunction of the levator veli palatini) and deviation of the uvula to the unaffected side.

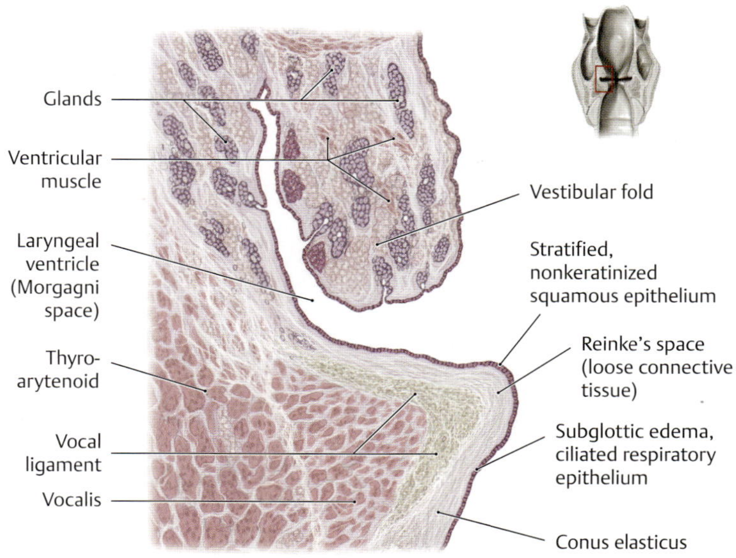

D Structure of the vocal fold
Schematic coronal histologic section, posterior view.
Subjected to severe mechanical stress, the vocal folds are covered by nonkeratinized stratified squamous epithelium (degenerative changes may lead to squamous cell carcinoma). Respiratory (ciliated) epithelium is located in the adjacent subglottic space. The muscoa sits on loose connective tissue. Chronic irritation from smoking may cause chronic edema in Reinke's space which can result in a hoarse voice ("smoker's voice").
Particularly at the base of the vestibular folds, but also occasionally at the fold itself, exist bands of skeletal muscle, referred to as the ventricular m. The official nomenclature does not list this muscle any longer, yet several authors have described it. Functionally, every voice pathologist is familiar with it, because the vestibular folds contract with the help of this muscle.

5.40 Endotracheal Intubation

a
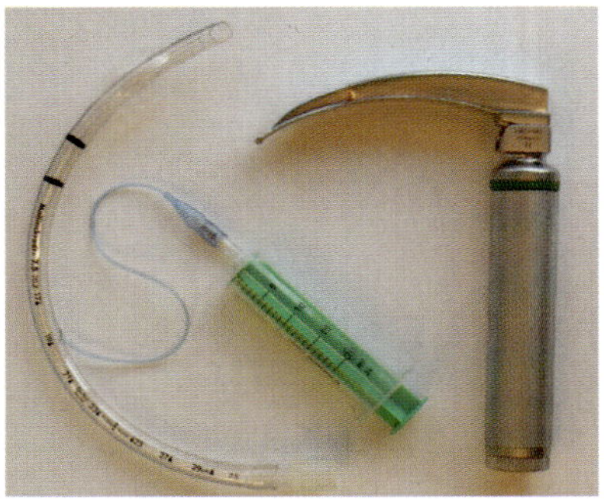

b
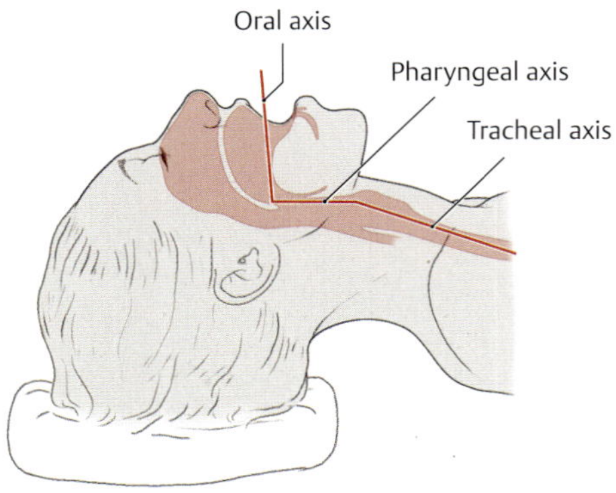

c
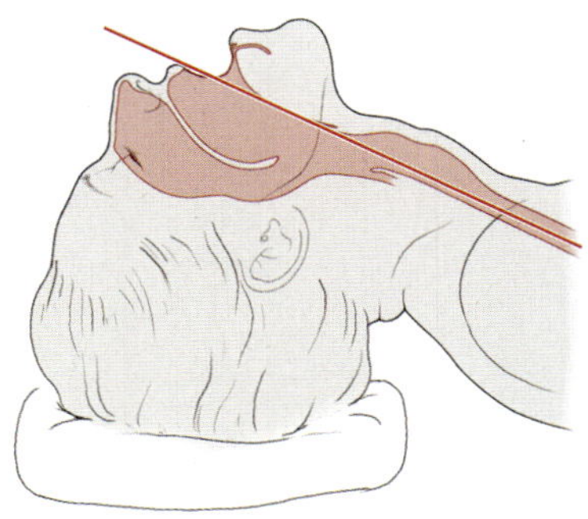

A Equipment and positioning of the head for endotracheal intubation

a Endotracheal (ET) tube with an inflatable cuff (left) and laryngoscope with handle and curved spatula (right).

b, **c** Unfavorable and optimal positioning of the head for endotracheal intubation. *Endotracheal intubation*, inserting a tube into the trachea of a patient, is the *safest* way to keep the airways clear to allow for *effective* ventilation. Depending on access there are four ways to achieve endotracheal intubation:

- orotracheal = via the mouth (gold standard),
- nasotracheal = via the nose (performed if orotracheal intubation is not possible), and
- pertracheal = intubation through tracheostomy (used for long-term ventilation), and
- cricothyrotomy (used only in an emergencies when there is the threat of impending suffocation).

Endotracheal intubation requires the use of a laryngoscope and an ET tube (**a**). The tubes are available in different sizes (10–22 cm) and diameters (2.5–8 mm). They have a circular cross piece that has a proximal connector for a ventilation hose and a beveled distal end. An inflatable cuff on the ET ensures that the trachea is hermetically sealed (see **Cb**). With orotracheal intubation, the oral, pharyngeal, and tracheal axes should lie in a straight line (the "sniffing position," see **c**).This facilitates direct visualization of the laryngeal inlet (see **B**) and shortens the distance between the teeth and glottis in young adults (13–16 cm).
Note: In patients with suspected cervical spine injury, manipulation of the head position without maintaining the stability of the cervical spine is contraindicated.

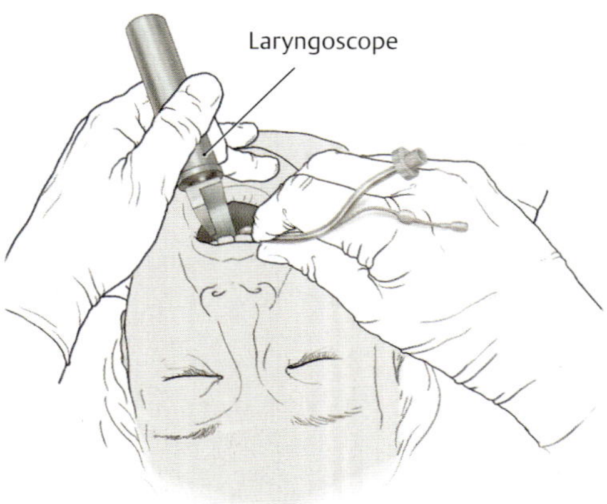

a

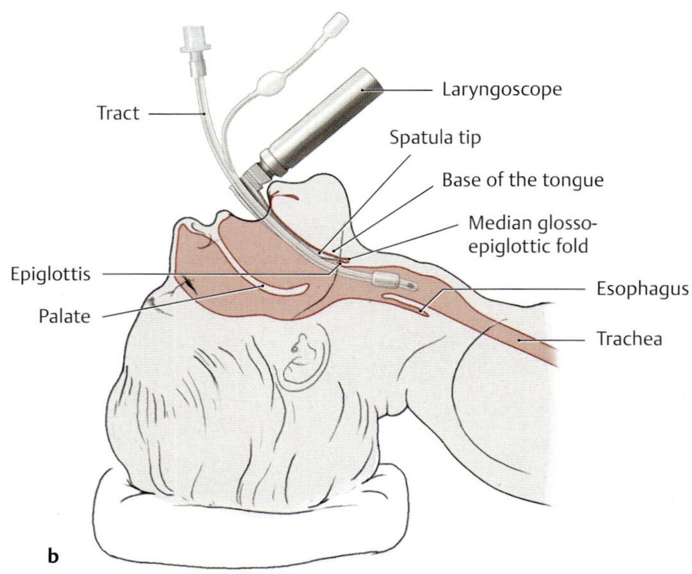

b

B Placement of the laryngoscope and the endotracheal tube (ET)

a Handling and placement of the laryngoscope from the perspective of the physician. **b** Placement of the ET tube.

To place the ET tube, the physician stands at the head of the patient and introduces the spatula of the laryngoscope into the patient's mouth. The spatula is then used to push the patient's tongue to the left to get a clear view of the larynx.

Under direct visualization, the spatula tip is then advanced until it lies in the vallecula.

Note: If the spatula is introduced too deep, its tip reaches behind the epiglottis, and orientation is difficult.

The physician then pulls the spatula in the direction of the floor of mouth without using the upper teeth as a fulcrum. This elevates the epiglottis and the base of the tongue such that the physician now has an unobstructed view of the laryngeal inlet (see **Ca**). The physician then pushes the ET tube through the rima glottis into the trachea (see **b**). Placement under laryngoscopic control ensures that the ET tube is placed in the trachea and does not accidentally enter the esophagus.

Note: The ET tube has markings in centimeter increments that serve as an orientation aid to the physician. The distance from the upper teeth to the center of the trachea in the adult is about 22 cm and in newborns is about 11 cm. Distances greater than these might be an indicator that the tube is inserted too deeply and is in the right main bronchus.

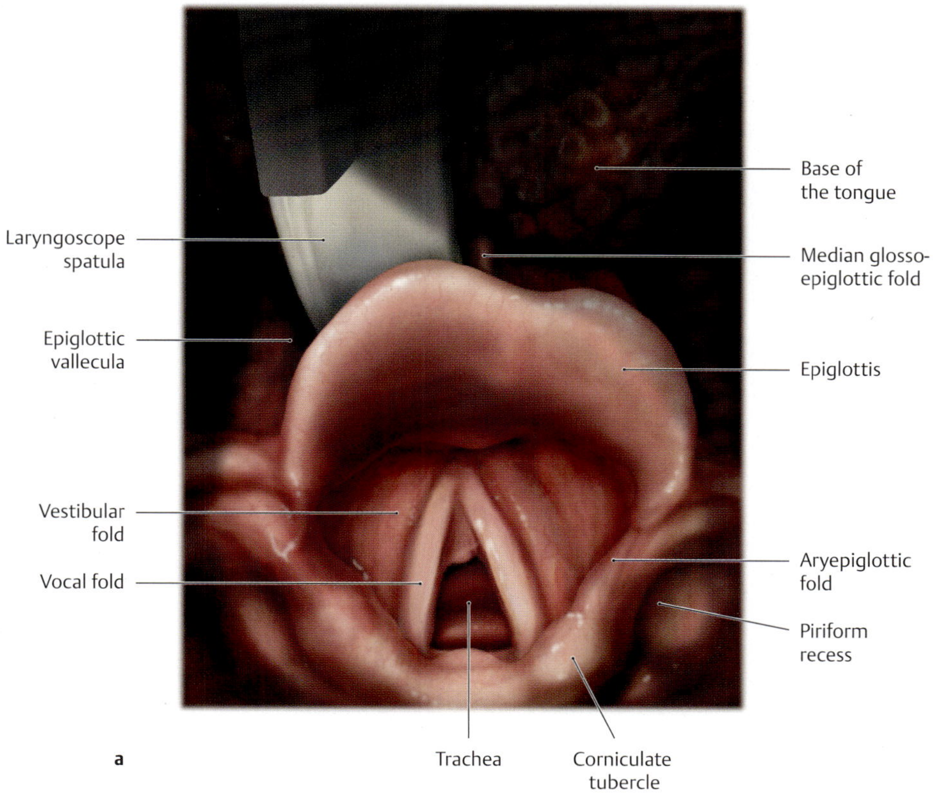

C View of the laryngeal inlet and location of the endotracheal tube after intubation

a Laryngoscopic view of larynx, epiglottis, and median glossoepiglottic fold. **b** Median sagittal section viewed from the right of an ET tube in situ with its cuff inflated.

a shows the entrance to the trachea after placement of the laryngoscope (cf. **Ba**). **b** depicts the ET tube in situ in the trachea. The inflatable cuff seals the trachea in all directions and eliminates leakage during ventilation and prevents aspiration of foreign bodies, mucus, or gastric juice.

To check if the ET tube has been placed correctly, the physician looks at the patient's chest to evaluate if chest movement is symmetrical, he auscultates for equal breath sounds over both lung fields and the absence of breath sounds over the stomach. Further indicators that the ET tube is placed correctly include vapor condensation on the inside of the ET tube with exhalation and measurement of end-tidal carbon dioxide. If there is any doubt as to the positioning of the tube, it should be removed.

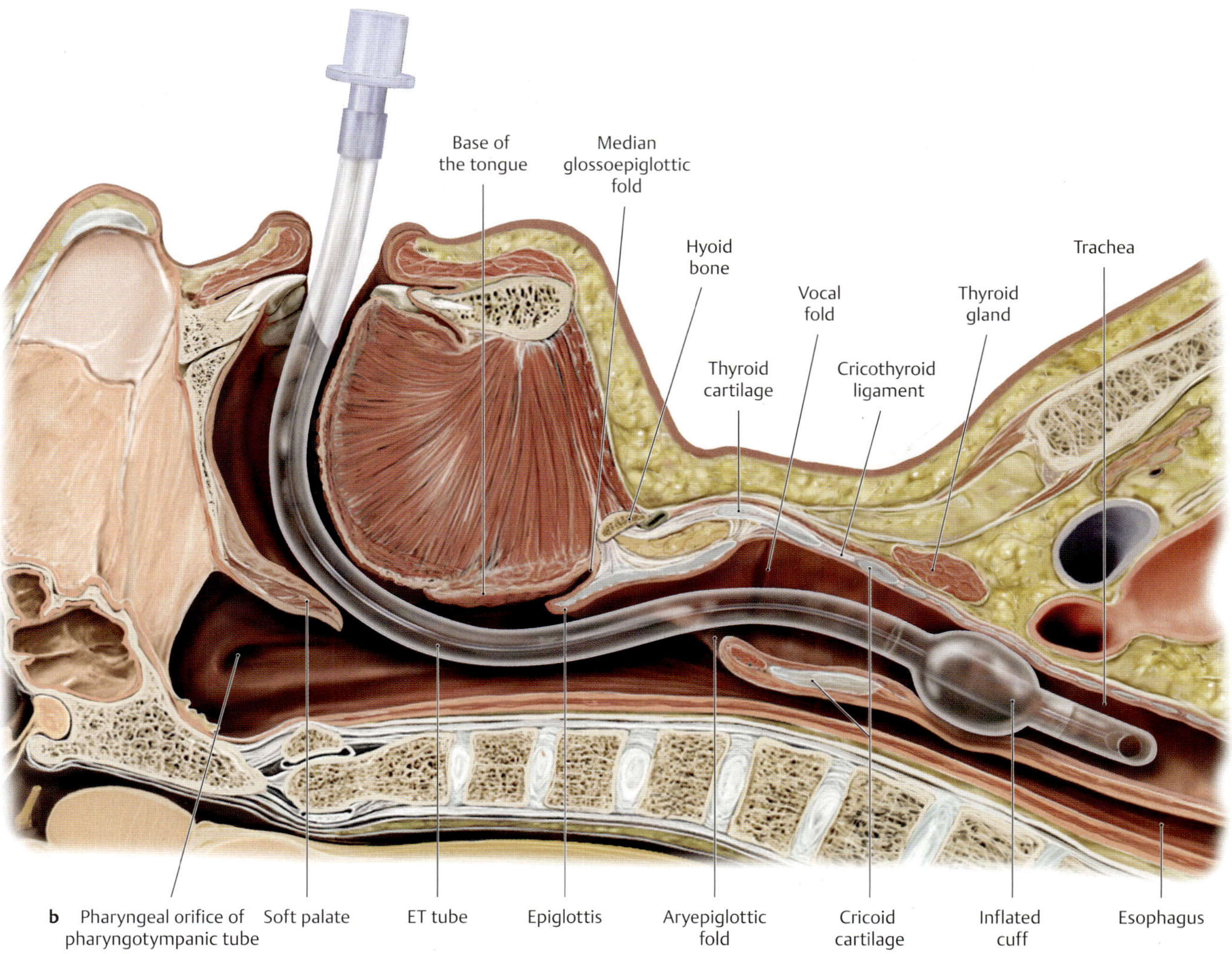

5.41 Thyroid Gland and Parathyroid Glands

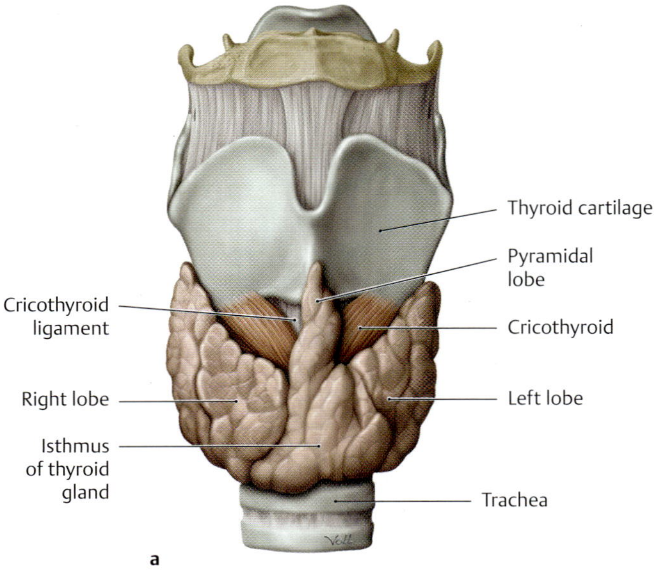

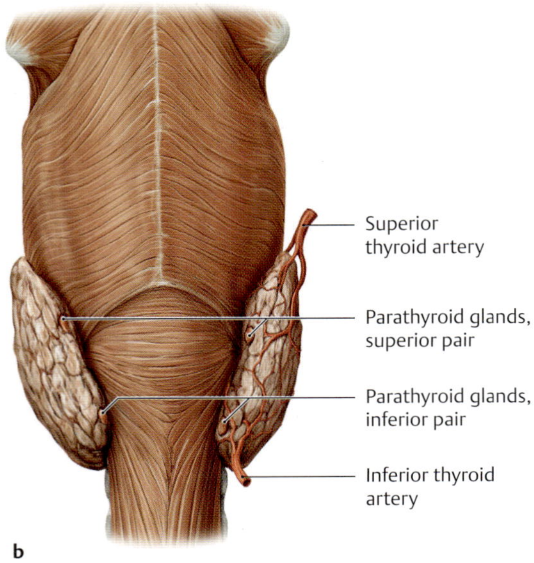

A Thyroid gland and parathyroid glands

a Thyroid gland, anterior view. The thyroid gland consists of two laterally situated lobes and a central narrowing or isthmus. In place of the isthmus there is often a pyramidal lobe, whose apex points cranially to the embryonic origin of the thyroid at the base of the tongue (see p. 11).

b Thyroid gland and parathyroid glands, posterior view. The parathyroid glands may show considerable variation in their number (generally four) and location.

Note: Because the parathyroid glands are usually contained within the capsule of the thyroid gland, there is a considerable risk of removing them during thyroid surgery (see **B**).

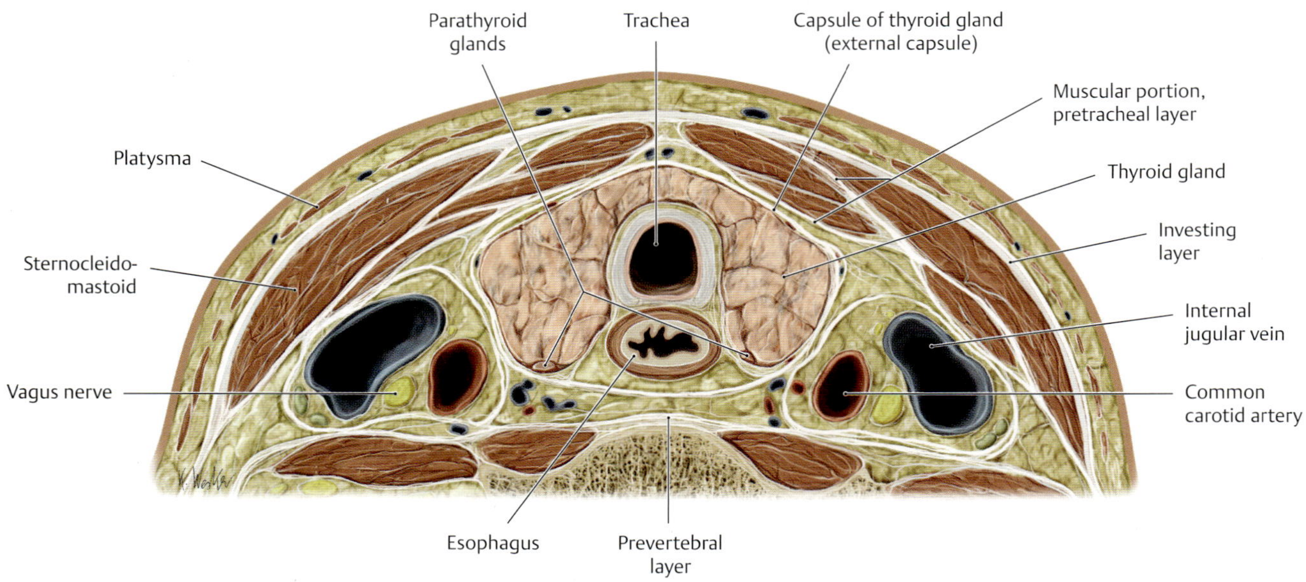

B Relationship of the thyroid gland to the trachea and neurovascular structures

Transverse section through the neck at the level of T1 superior view. The thyroid gland partially surrounds the trachea and is bordered posterolaterally by the neurovascular bundle within the carotid sheath. When the thyroid gland is pathologically enlarged (e.g., due to iodine-deficiency goiter), it may gradually compress and narrow the tracheal lumen, causing respiratory distress.

Note the arrangement of the fasciae: The thyroid gland is surrounded by a fibrous capsule composed of an internal and external layer. The delicate internal layer (*internal capsule*, not shown here) directly invests the thyroid gland and is fused with its glandular parenchyma. Vascularized fibrous slips extend from the internal capsule into the substance of the gland, subdividing it into lobules. The internal capsule is covered by the tough *external capsule*, which is part of the pretracheal layer of the deep cervical fascia. This capsule invests the thyroid gland and parathyroid glands and is also called the "surgical capsule" because it must be opened to gain surgical access to the thyroid gland. Between the external and internal capsules is a potential space that is traversed by vascular branches and is occupied by the parathyroid glands.

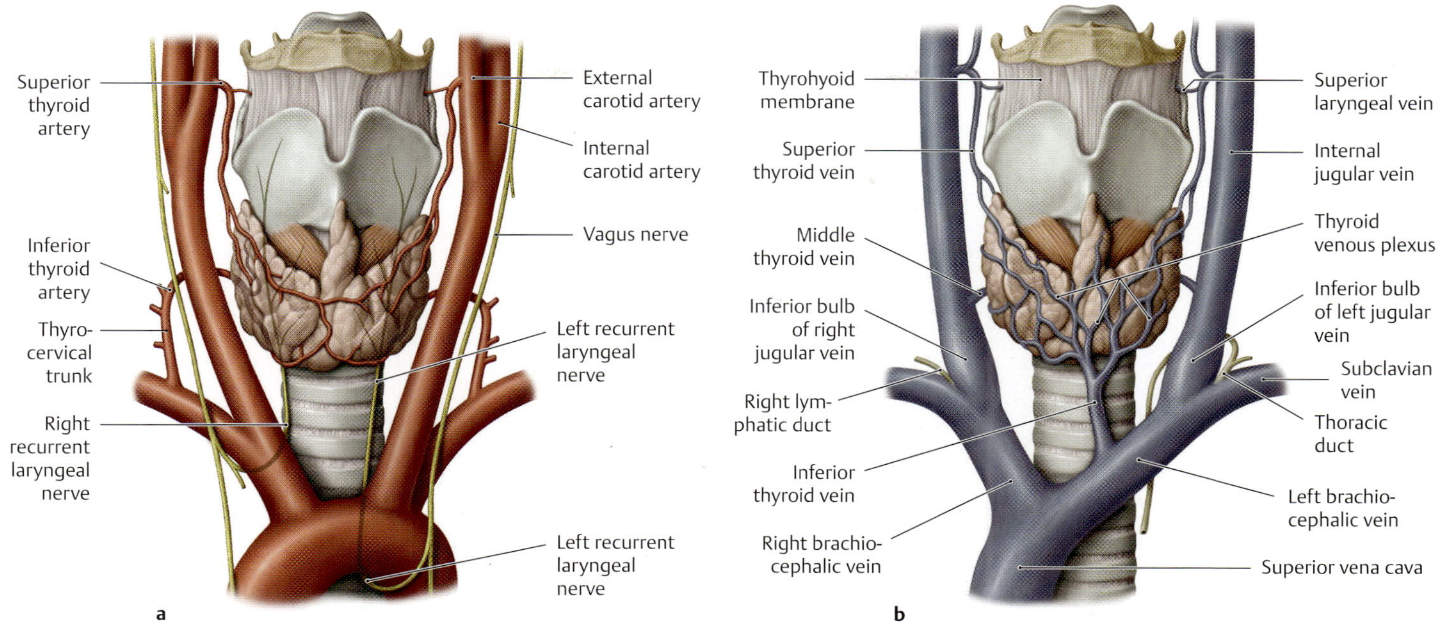

C Blood supply and innervation of the thyroid gland
Anterior view.

a Arterial supply: The thyroid gland derives most of its arterial blood supply from the superior thyroid artery (the first branch of the external carotid artery), which runs forward and downward to supply the gland. It is supplied from below by the inferior thyroid artery, which branches from the thyrocervical trunk (see p. 224). All of these arteries, which course on the right and left sides of the organ, must be ligated during surgical removal of the thyroid gland.
Note: Operations on the thyroid gland carry a risk of injury to the recurrent (inferior) laryngeal nerve, which is closely related to the posterior surface of the gland. Because it supplies important laryngeal muscles, unilateral injury to the nerve will cause postoperative hoarseness while bilateral injury may additionally result in dyspnea (difficulty in breathing). Prior to thyroid surgery, therefore, an otolaryngologist should confirm the integrity of the nerve supply to the laryngeal muscles and exclude any preexisting nerve lesion.

b Venous drainage: The thyroid gland is drained anteroinferiorly by a well-developed *thyroid venous plexus*, which usually drains through the inferior thyroid vein to the left brachiocephalic vein. Blood from the thyroid gland also drains to the internal jugular vein via the superior and middle thyroid veins.

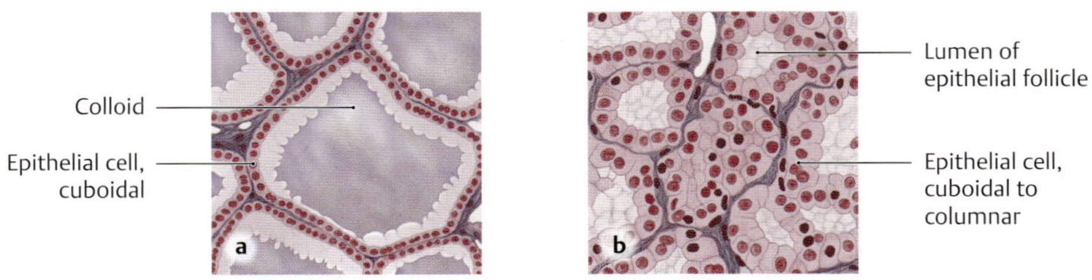

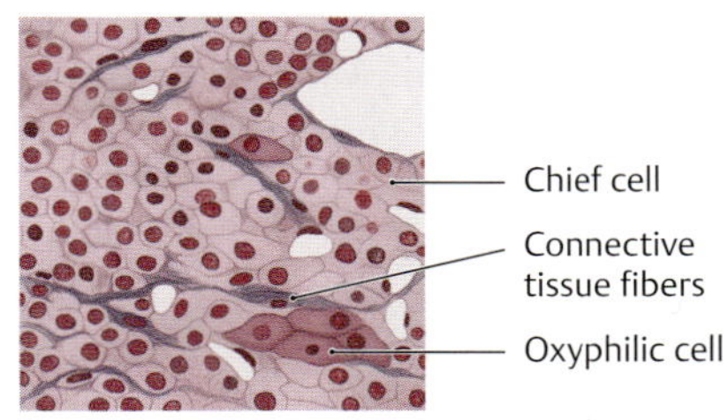

D Histology of the thyroid gland
The follicular cells of the thyroid gland uptake iodide from the blood and use it to make the thyroid hormones: T4 (thyroxine or tetraiodothyronine), T3 (triiodothyronine), and reverse T3. These hormones are stored in the gland and secreted by the parafollicular cells into the bloodstream, where they are bound to proteins in circulation. A special feature of the thyroid gland is the appearance of its epithelium, which varies depending on whether it is storing hormones or releasing them into the blood. The epithelial cells are low cuboidal in shape when in their resting or "storage state" (**a**), but they are columnar in shape when in their active or "secretory state" (**b**). The epithelial morphology thus indicates the current functional state of the cells. Iodine deficiency causes an enlargement of the colloidal follicular lumen, which eventually results in a gross increase in the size of the thyroid (goiter). With prolonged iodine deficiency there is a reduction in body metabolism, and concomitant lethargy, fatigue, and mental depression. Conversely, hyperactivity of the thyroid, as in Graves' disease (an autoimmune disorder), causes a generalized metabolic acceleration, with irritability and weight loss. Scattered between follicles, there are parafollicular cells (C cells), which secrete calcitonin. Calcitonin inhibits bone resorption and reduces the calcium concentration in the blood.

E Histology of the parathyroid gland
The chief cells of the parathyroid gland secrete parathormone which indirectly stimulates osteoclasts (via the osteoblasts) leading to increased bone resorption. As a result of bone resorption, the calcium concentration in the blood increases. Inadvertent removal of the parathyroid glands can lead to *hyoparathyroidism*. The body produces so little parathormone, the calcium concentration in the blood decreases which causes *hypocalcemia*, resulting in tetanic seizures involving skeletal muscle. Benign parathyroid tumors (adenoma) are associated with unregulated, excessive parathormone production resulting in increased calcium concentration in the blood (*hypercalcemia*) and excessive urinary calcium excretion (*hypercalciuria*). At the same time, phosphate metabolism is also affected given that parathormone stimulates renal phosphate excretion, resulting in a very low level of phosphate in the blood (*hypophosphatemia*) and very high levels of phosphate in the urine (*hypophosphaturia*). Clinical symptoms of hyperparathyroidism include muscle weakness, lethargy, small intestinal ulcers and pancreatitis.

5.42 Topography and Imaging of the Thyroid Gland

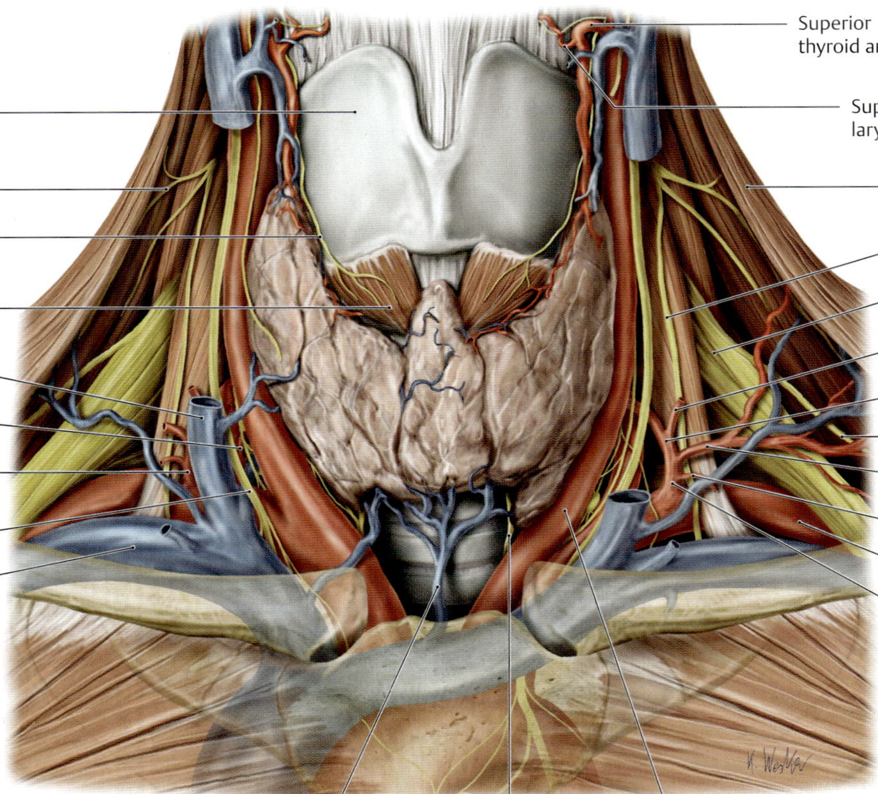

A Deep anterior cervical region with the thyroid gland
Anterior view. The following neurovascular structures are clearly visible in their course through the thoracic inlet: the common carotid artery, subclavian artery, subclavian vein, internal jugular vein, inferior thyroid vein, vagus nerve, phrenic nerve, and recurrent laryngeal nerve. It can be seen that a retrosternal goiter enlarging the inferior pole of the thyroid gland can easily compress neurovascular structures at the thoracic inlet (see Fig. **E**, p. 7).

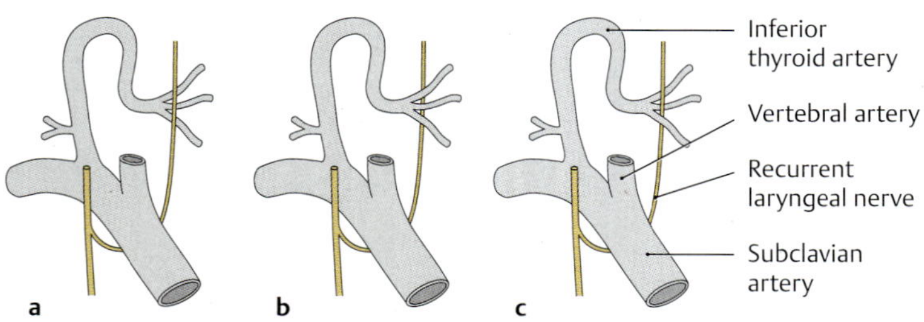

B Course of the right recurrent laryngeal nerve (after von Lanz and Wachsmuth)
Anterior view. The recurrent laryngeal n. is a special visceral efferent and sensory branch of the vagus n., which among others innervates the posterior cricoarytenoid m. This is the only muscle to fully open the glottis (see p. 217). Unilateral damage to this nerve supply results in hoarseness, while bilateral damage leads to a closed glottis with severe dyspnea. The recurrent laryngeal nerve may pass in front of (**a**), behind (**b**), or between (**c**) the branches of the inferior thyroid artery. Its course should be noted during operative procedures on the thyroid gland.

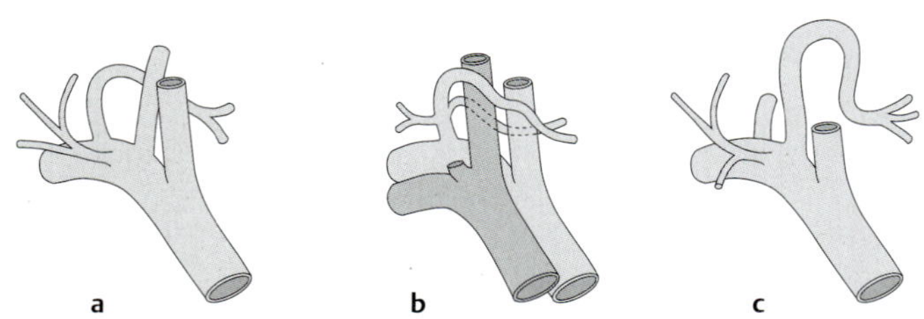

C Variations in the branching pattern of the right inferior thyroid artery (after Platzer)
The course of the inferior thyroid a. is highly variable. It can run medially behind the vertebral a. (**a**), divide immediately after arising from the thyrocervical trunk (sometimes, **b**) or it may arise as the first branch of the subclavian a. (**c**).

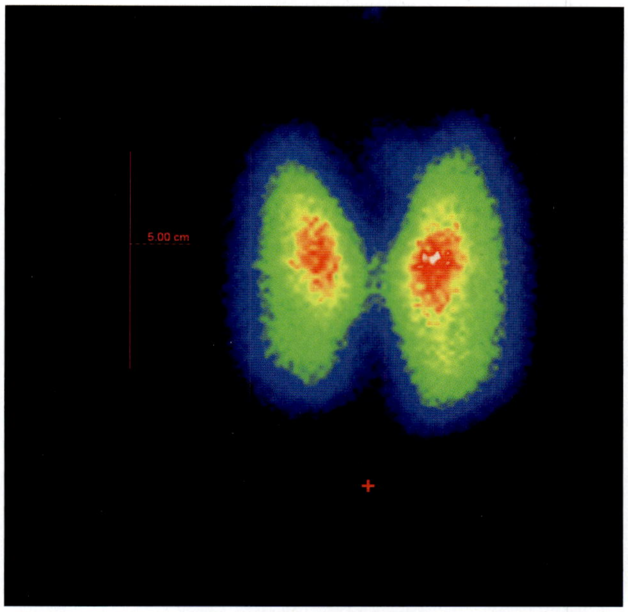

a

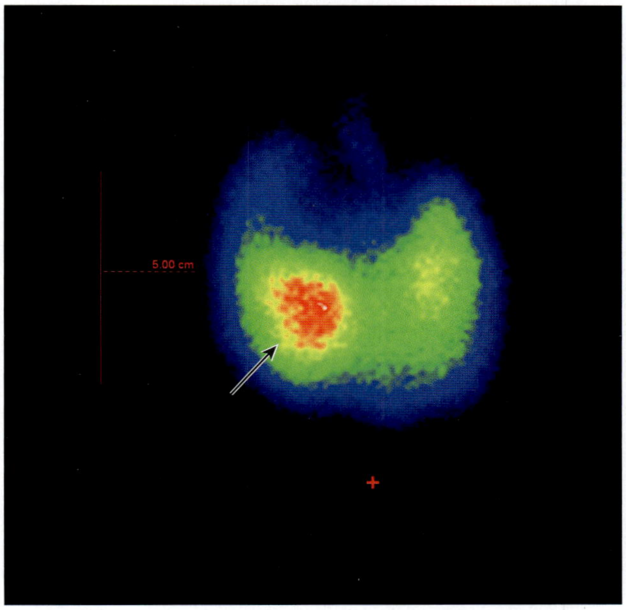

b

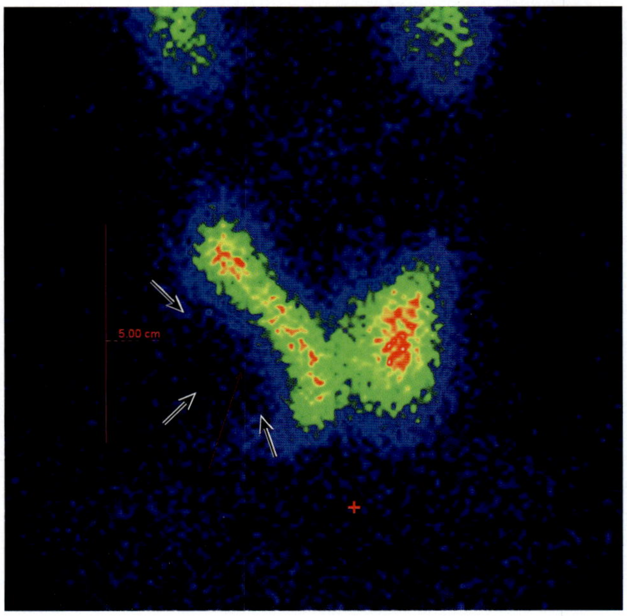

c

D Scintigrams of the thyroid gland

Frontal views. To perform thyroid gland scintigraphy, ^{99m}Tc pertechnetate (TcO_4) is injected intravenously. It is absorbed by the sodium-iodide symporter, which are characteristic to the thyroid gland, located in the principal cells. This uptake is visualized with the aid of a special thyroid gland camera (producing a thyroid gland scintigram). It forms the basis for evaluation of, position, shape, size and storage capacity of the thyroid gland.

a $^{99m}TcO_4$ uptake in the normally functioning thyroid gland

b warm nodule in the right lobe of the thyroid gland. The presence of a warm nodule means higher absorption of $^{99m}TcO_4$, the technetium uptake is identifiable by the larger red-shaded area on the right lobe; the findings can indicate thyroid hyperfunction.

c cold nodule in the right lobe of the thyroid gland. The presence of a cold nodule means that less radioactive material is taken up, identifiable by the lack of a red-shaded areas on the right. The findings can indicate a benign tumor or thyroid carcinoma.

(Images used with the kind permission of Prof. S. Klutmann, M.D., Klinik für Nuklearmedizin, Universitätskrankenhaus Hamburg-Eppendorf.)

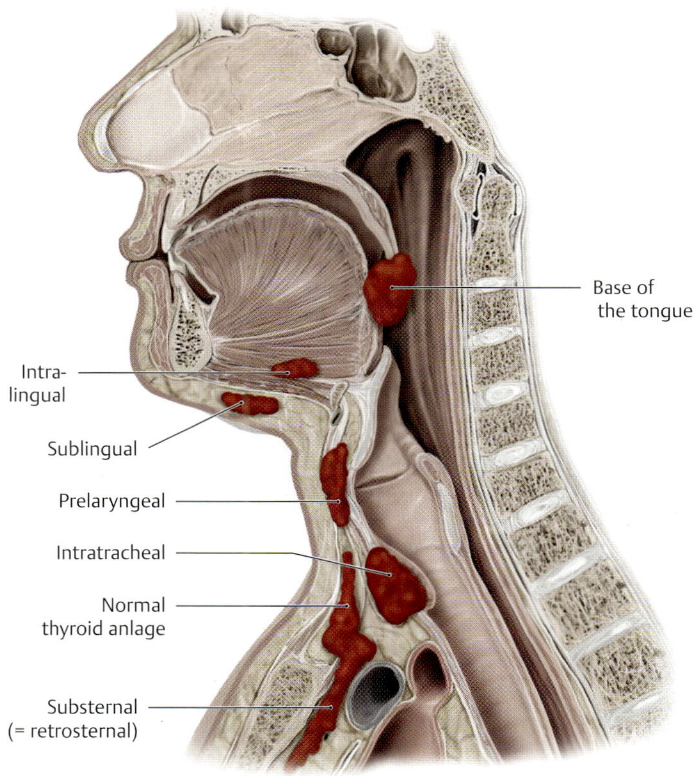

E Thyroid gland ectopias

Median sagittal section, left lateral view. Thyroid gland ectopia describes the location of the thyroid gland other than the normal position. It is the result of an abnormal descent during its embryological development (see p. 11). These position anomalies can be visualized with the help of thyroid gland scintigraphy so that they can be surgically corrected if necessary.

6.1 Face: Nerves and Vessels

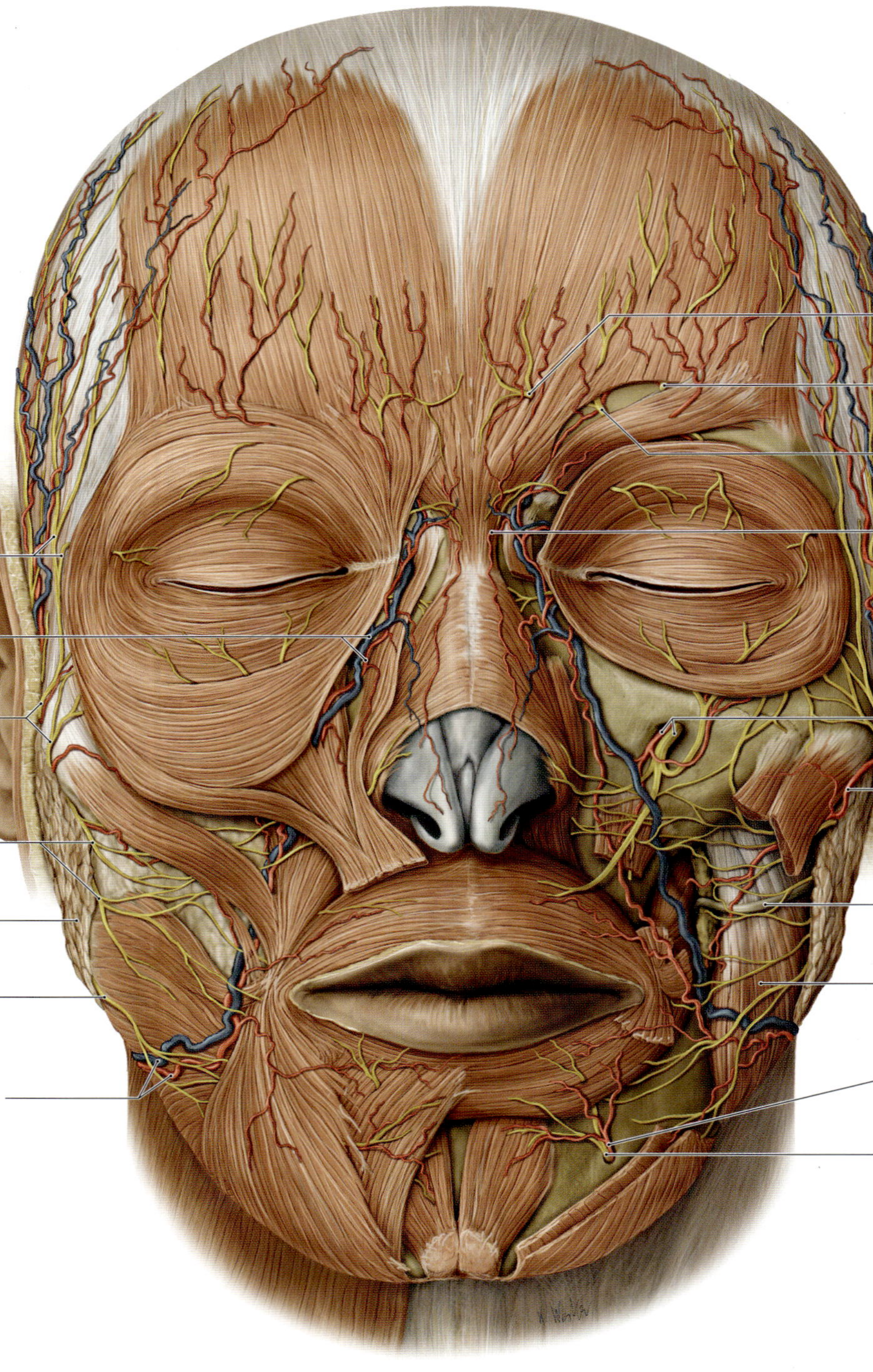

A Superficial nerves and vessels of the anterior facial region
The skin and fatty tissue have been removed to demonstrate the superficial muscular layer—the muscles of facial expression. This layer has been partially removed on the left side of the face to display underlying portions of the muscles of mastication. The muscles of facial expression receive their motor innervation from the *facial nerve*, which emerges laterally from the parotid gland. The face receives its sensory innervation from the *trigeminal nerve*, whose three terminal branches are shown here (see **E**). Branches from the third division of the trigeminal nerve additionally supply motor innervation to the muscles of mastication. The face receives most of its blood supply from the *external carotid artery*. Only small areas around the medial and lateral canthi of the eyes and in the forehead are supplied by the *internal carotid artery* (see **B**).

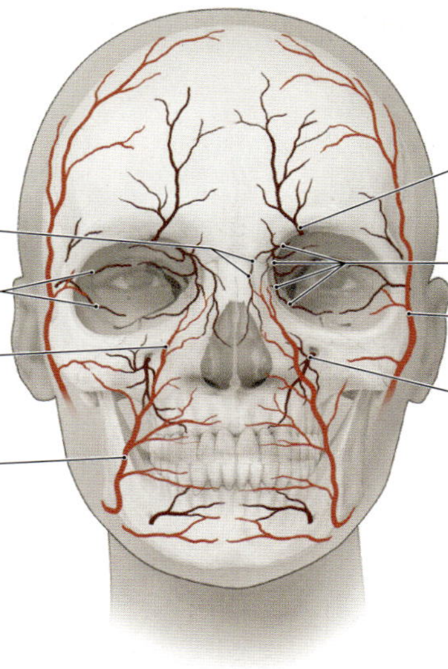

B Distribution of the external carotid artery (red) and internal carotid artery (brown) in the face

Hemodynamically significant anastomoses may develop between these two arterial territories. Even a marked reduction of flow in the internal carotid artery by atherosclerosis may not lead to cerebral ischemia, as long as there is adequate compensatory flow through the superficial temporal artery. If this is the case, then ligation of the superficial temporal artery is contraindicated (the artery might otherwise be ligated, for example, in a biopsy to confirm the diagnosis of temporal arteritis; see p. 101).

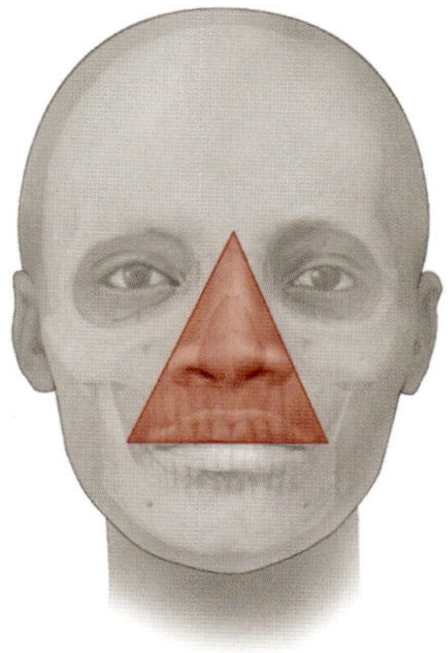

C Triangular danger zone in the face

This zone is marked by the presence of venous connections from the face to the dural venous sinuses. Because the veins in this region are valveless, there is a particularly high risk of bacterial dissemination into the cranial cavity. A furuncle (boil) may lead to propagation of infection inside the cranial cavity—see p. 107.

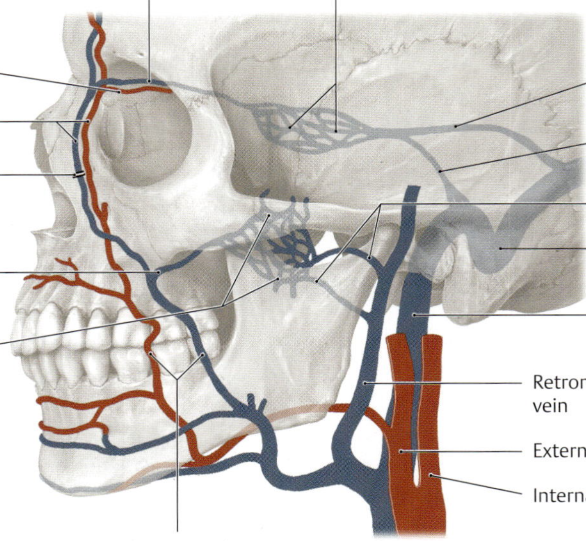

D Clinically important vascular relationships in the face

Note the connections between the exterior of the face and the dural sinuses.

If a purulent inflammation develops in the "danger zone" (see **C**), the angular vein can be ligated at a standard site to prevent the transmission of infectious organisms to the cavernous sinus.

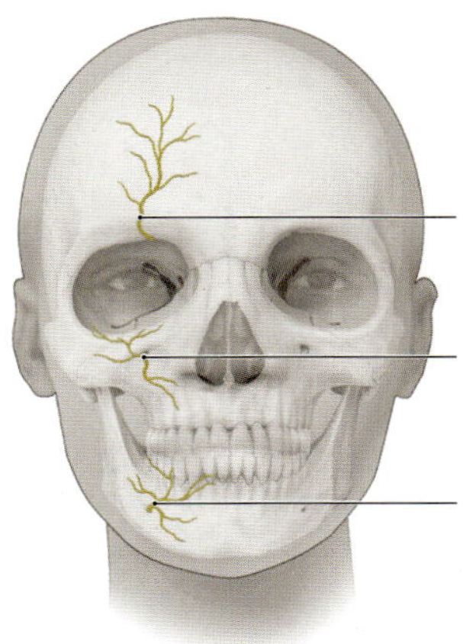

E Nerve exit point of the three trigeminal branches

The trigeminal nerve (CN V) is the major somatic sensory nerve of the head. The diagram shows the sites of emergence of its three large sensory branches:

- branch of CN V_1: supraorbital nerve (supraorbital foramen)
- branch of CN V_2: infraorbital nerve (infraorbital foramen)
- branch of CN V_3: mental nerve (mental foramen); see also p. 123.

6.2 Neck, Ventral View: Superficial Layers

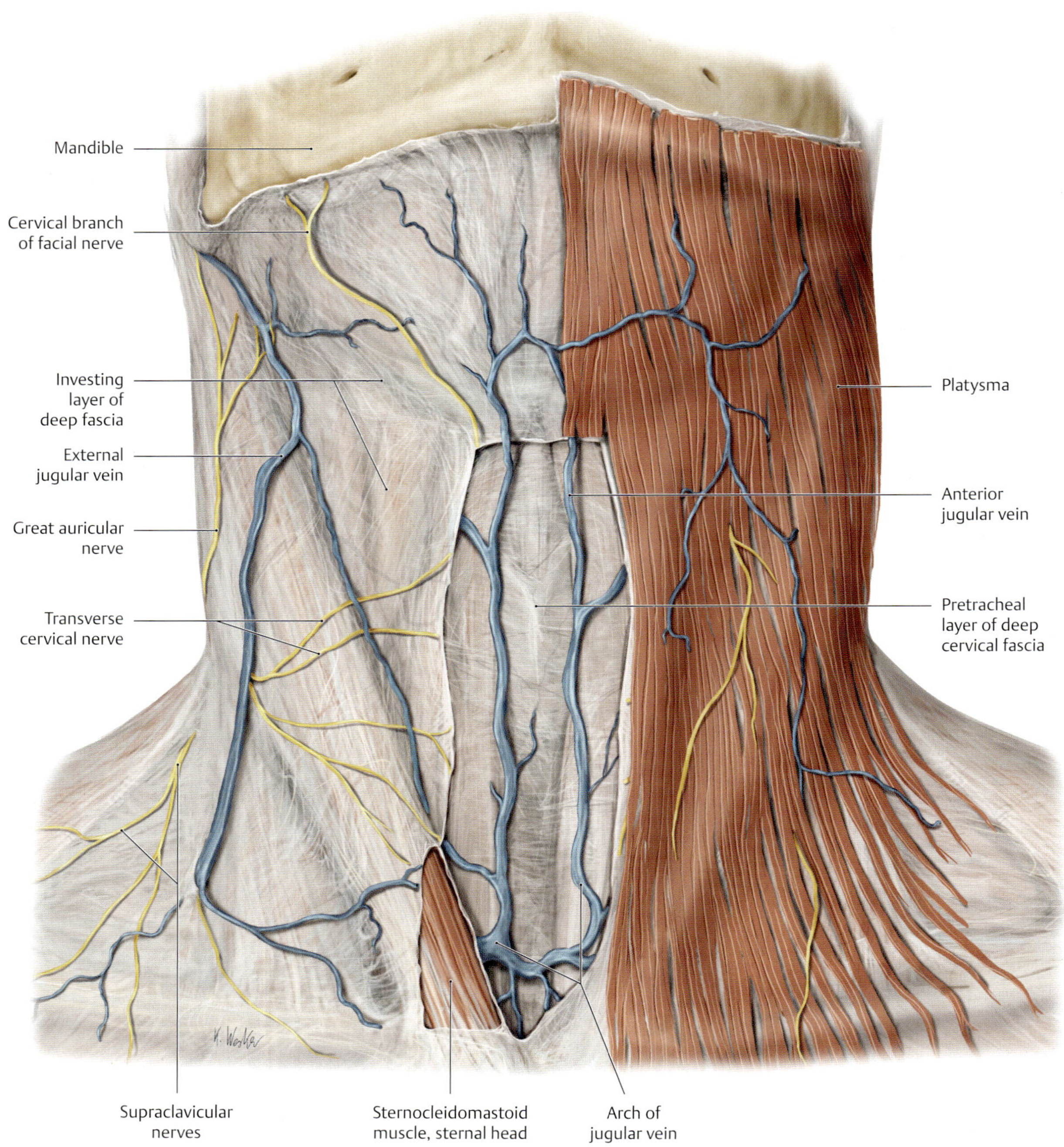

A The neck, superficial layer
Anterior view. The subcutaneous platysma has been removed on the right side, and the investing layer of the deep cervical fascia (see p. 4 for cervical fascial structure) has been split in the midline and partially removed, exposing the sternal head of the right sternocleidomastoid muscle. The anterior cervical triangle, which is bounded posteriorly by the sternocleidomastoid muscle and superiorly by the lower border of the mandible, is particularly well delineated on the right side. The anterior jugular vein and arch of the jugular vein can be identified.
Note also the cutaneous nerves of the cervical plexus (great auricular, transverse cervical, supraclavicular), which radiate from Erb's point (see p. 240).

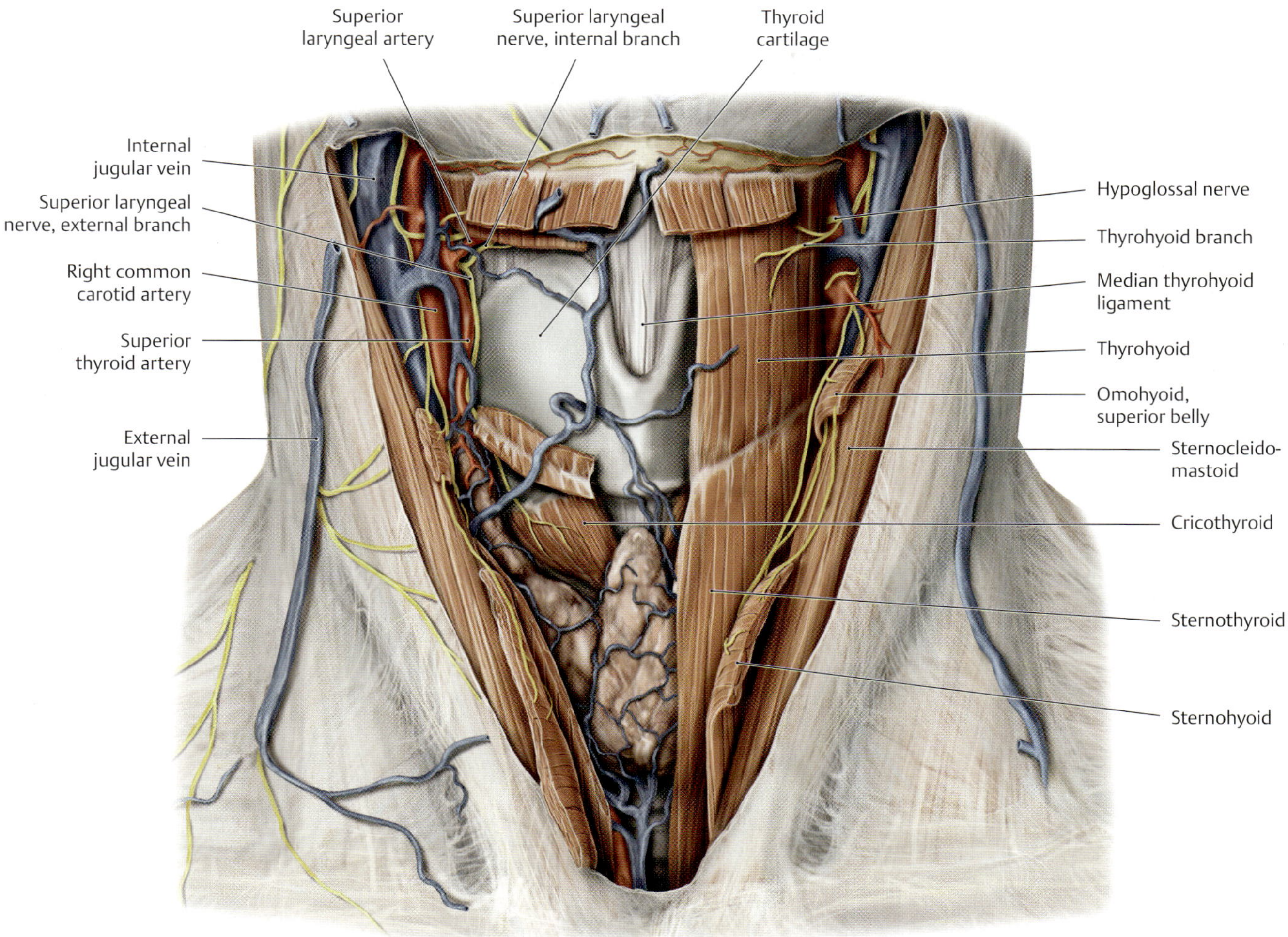

B Neck, middle layer
Anterior view. The pretracheal lamina (middle layer of cervical fascia) has been removed. The infrahyoid muscles inserting on the pretracheal lamina have been resected and the visceral fascia has been removed to expose the thyroid gland, which is posterior to the infrahyoid muscles. The superior thyroid artery, the first branch of the external carotid artery, can be identified. The external branch of the superior laryngeal nerve, a branch of the vagus nerve, courses with the superior thyroid artery to the cricothyroid muscle. The internal branch of the superior laryngeal nerve passes through the thyrohyoid membrane with the superior laryngeal artery to supply the larynx.

6.3 Neck, Ventral View: Deep Layers

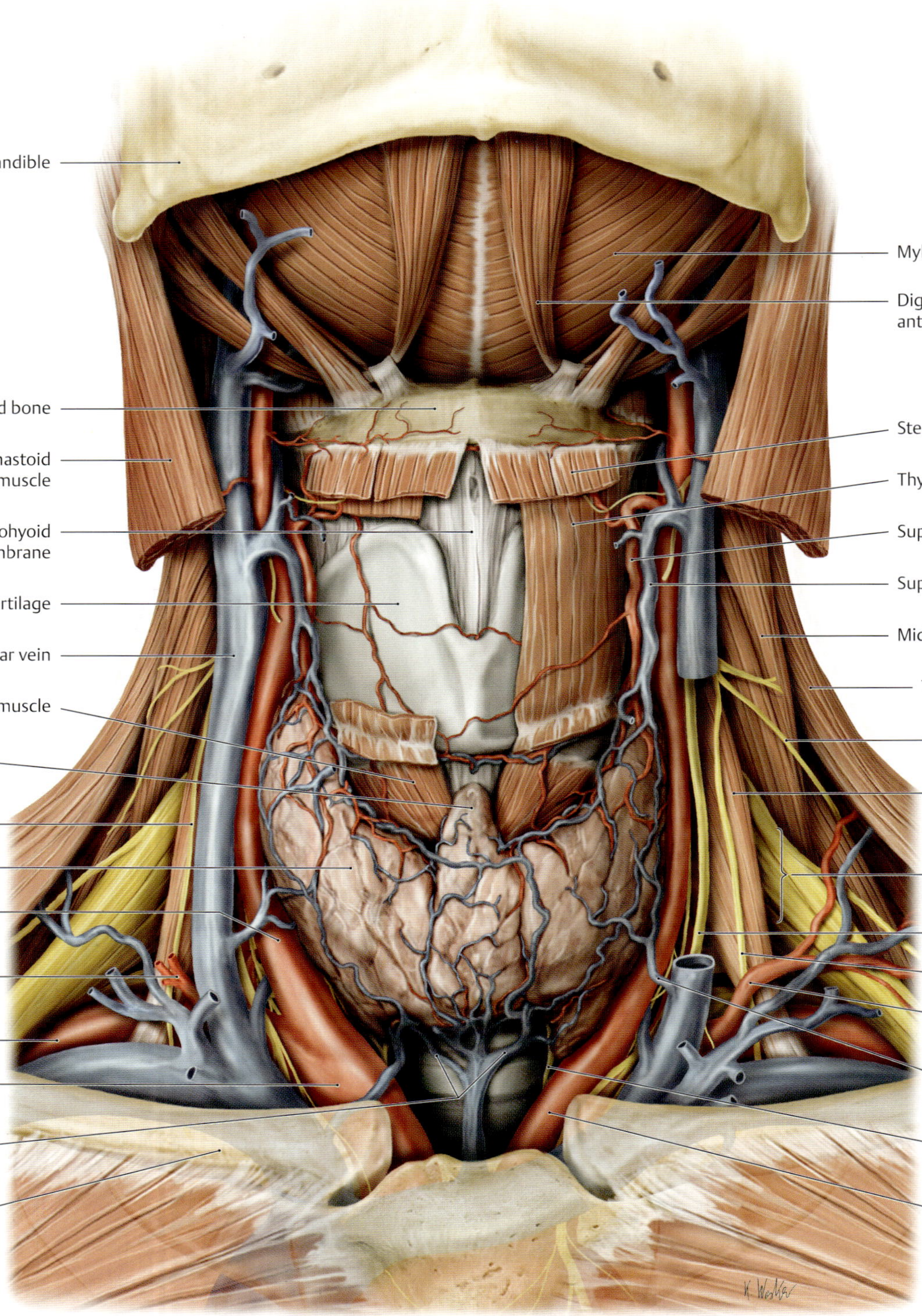

A Deep cervical fascia, ventral view

Identifiable are the viscera of the neck, larynx, and thyroid gland, located along and around the midline. Lateral to both, vertical pathways run to and from the head. The arterial blood supply to the thyroid gland is provided primarily by the cranially and posteriorly located superior thyroid a. Its venous drainage is carried out primarily by the caudally and anteriorly located thyroid venous plexus. The discernible nerves include the vagus n. (CN X) and the phrenic n. The recurrent laryngeal n. comes from the superior thoracic aperture and runs lateral to the trachea behind the thyroid gland to the larynx, the muscles of which it innervates.

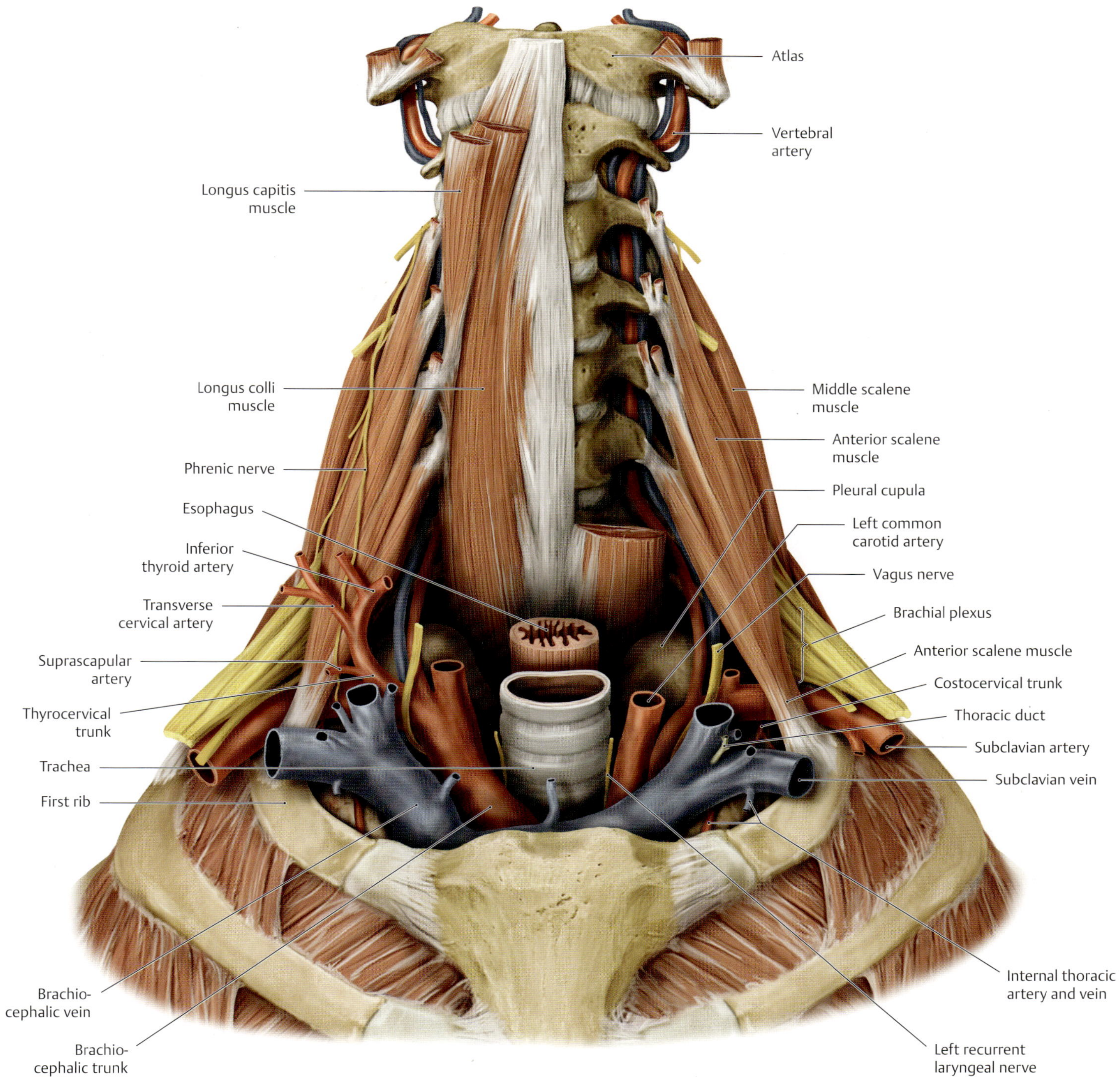

B Deepest layer of deep cervical fascia

The viscera of the neck, larynx and thyroid gland, have been removed, also the trachea and esophagus. The two large cervical vessels (common carotid a. and internal jugular v.) have been dissected on both sides. The deeper-lying vertebral a. is now visible on the left side. On the right side, it is still covered by prevertebral muscles. The vertebral a. runs through the transverse foramen of the cervical vertebrae and travels across the arch of the atlas (C1) to the inside of the skull (via the foramen magnum) where in particular it supplies the brainstem. The cervical plexus and phrenic n., is identifiable. It runs from the anterior scalene m. in a caudal direction to the diaphragm, which it innervates. In this layer, two arterial trunks along with their branches are identifiable:

- on the right thyrocervical trunk with
  - Inferior thyroid a.
  - Transverse cervical a. with its deep and superficial branches, and
  - Suprascapular a.
- on the left costcocervical trunk with
  - Deep cervical a.
  - Supreme intercostal a.

In the scalene gap between the anterior and middle scalene m. runs the brachial plexus and the subclavian a., whereas the subclavian v. runs in front of the the anterior scalene m. The thoracic duct, which drains the lymph from ¾ of the body, empties into the left venous angle—the junction of left subclavian v. and left internal jugular v.

6.4 Head, Lateral View: Superficial Layer

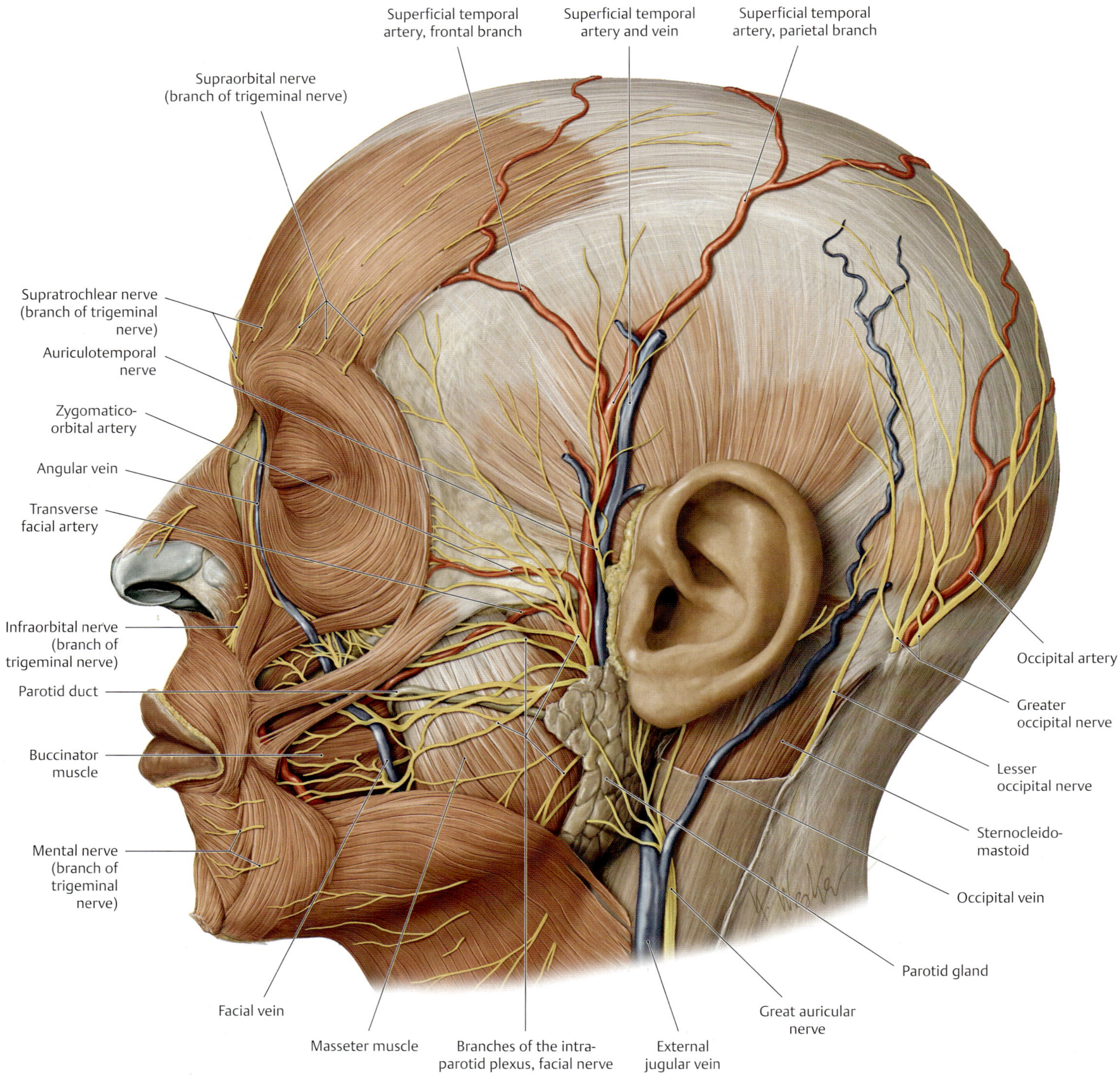

A Superficial vessels and nerves of the head

Left lateral view. All the arteries visible in this diagram arise from the *external carotid artery*, which is too deep to be visible in this superficial dissection. The lateral head region is drained by the *external jugular vein*. The facial vein, however, drains into the deeper internal jugular vein (not shown here). The *facial nerve* has divided in the parotid gland to form the parotid plexus, whose branches leave the parotid gland at its anterior border and are distributed to the facial muscles (see **C**). This lateral head region also receives sensory innervation from branches of the *trigeminal nerve* (see **D**), while the portion of the occiput visible in the figure is supplied by the *greater* and *lesser occipital nerves*. Unlike the trigeminal nerve, the occipital nerves originate from the spinal nerves of the cervical plexus (see **E**). The secretory duct of the parotid gland (the parotid duct) is easy to identify at dissection. It passes forward on the surface of the masseter muscle, pierces the buccinator, and terminates in the oral vestibule opposite the second upper molar (not shown).

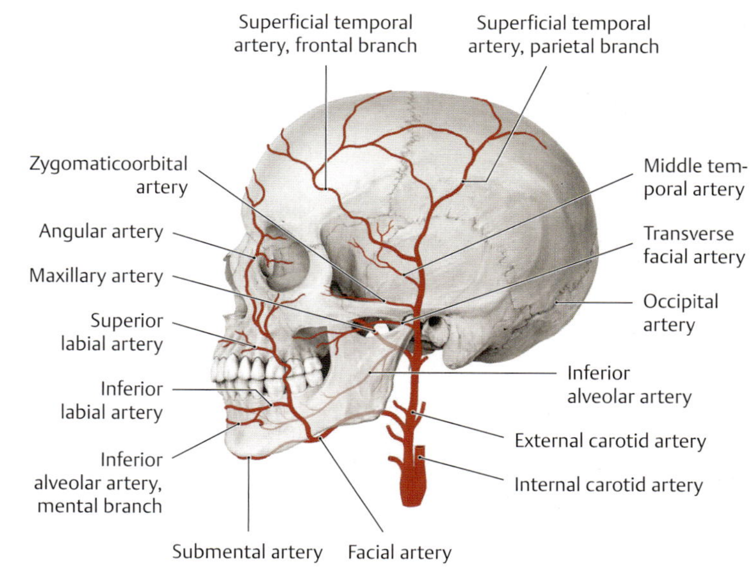

B Superficial branches of the external carotid artery
Left lateral view. This diagram shows the arteries in isolation to demonstrate their branches and their relationships to one another (cf. **A**; details see p. 94).

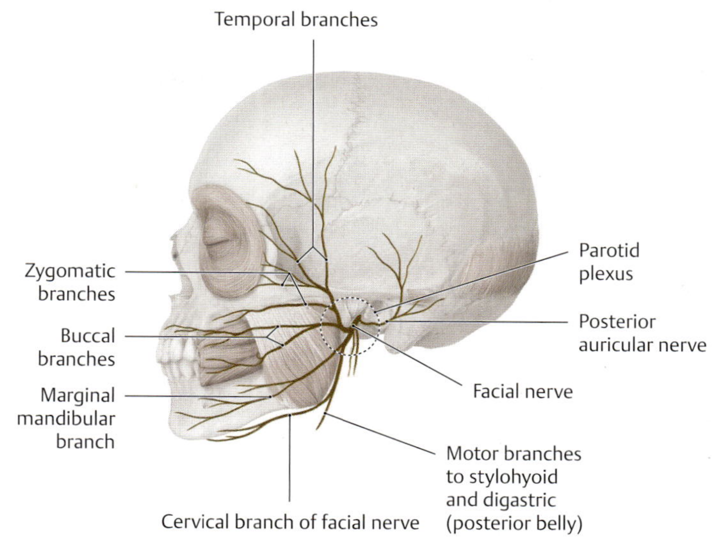

C Facial nerve (CN VII)
Left lateral view. The muscles of facial expression receive all of their motor innervation from the seventh cranial nerve (see p. 119).

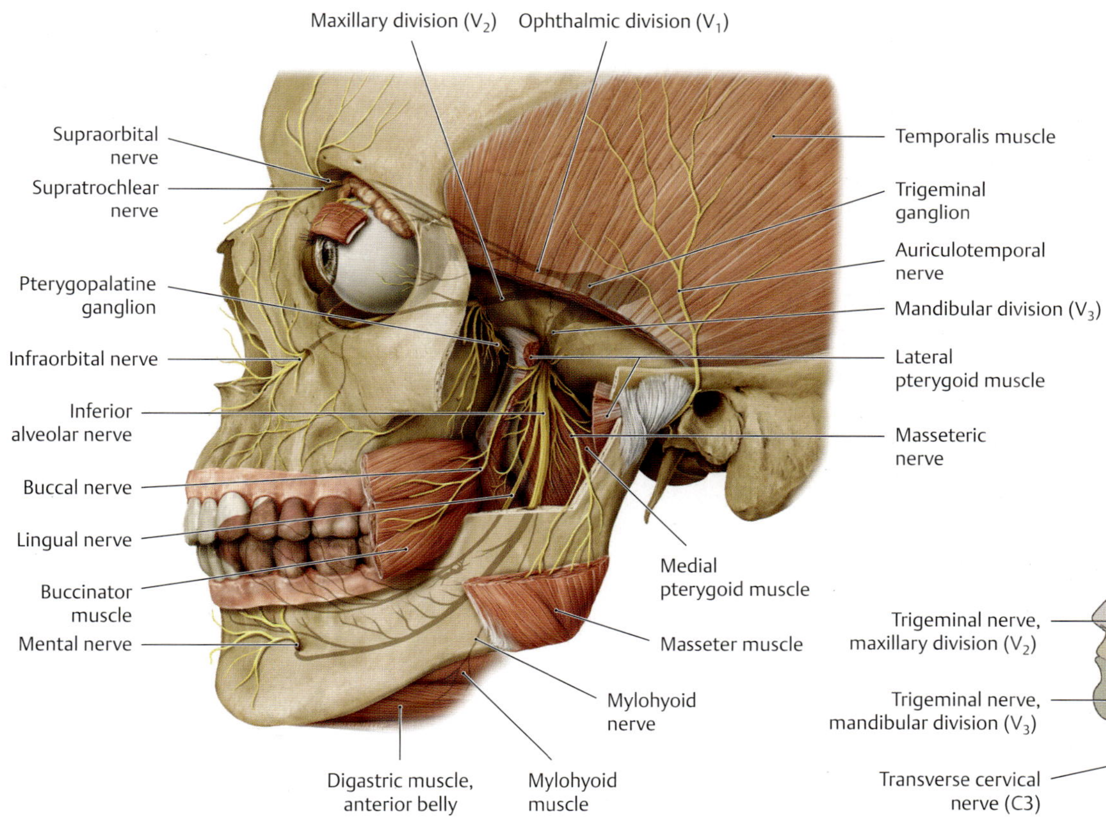

D Trigeminal nerve (CN V)
Left lateral view. In the region shown here, the head derives its somatic sensory supply from three large branches of the trigeminal nerve (supraorbital nerve, infraorbital nerve, and mental nerve). The diagram illustrates their course in the skull and their sites of emergence in the anterior facial region (see the anterior view on p. 226). The trigeminal nerve is partly a mixed nerve because motor fibers travel with the mandibular nerve (= third division of the trigeminal nerve) to supply the muscles of mastication.

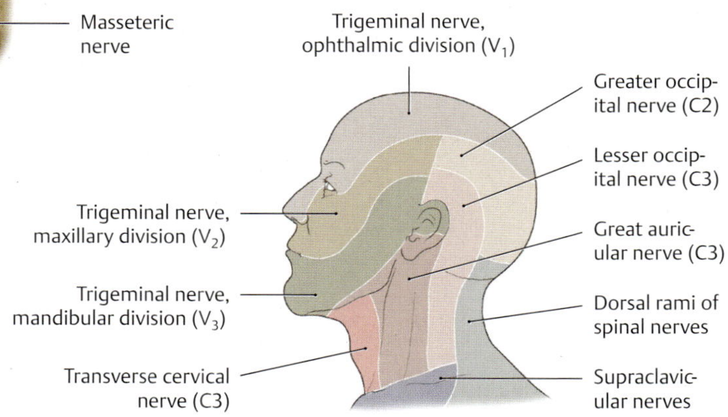

E Nerve territories of the lateral head and neck
Left lateral view.
Note: The lateral head and neck region receives its sensory supply from one cranial nerve (trigeminal nerve and its branches), and from the dorsal rami (greater occipital nerve) and ventral rami (lesser occipital nerve, great auricular nerve, transverse cervical nerve) of spinal nerves. The C1 spinal nerve has only motor neurons; it therefore provides no sensory innervation to the skin (i.e., it has no dermatome).

6.5 Head, Lateral View: Middle and Deep Layers

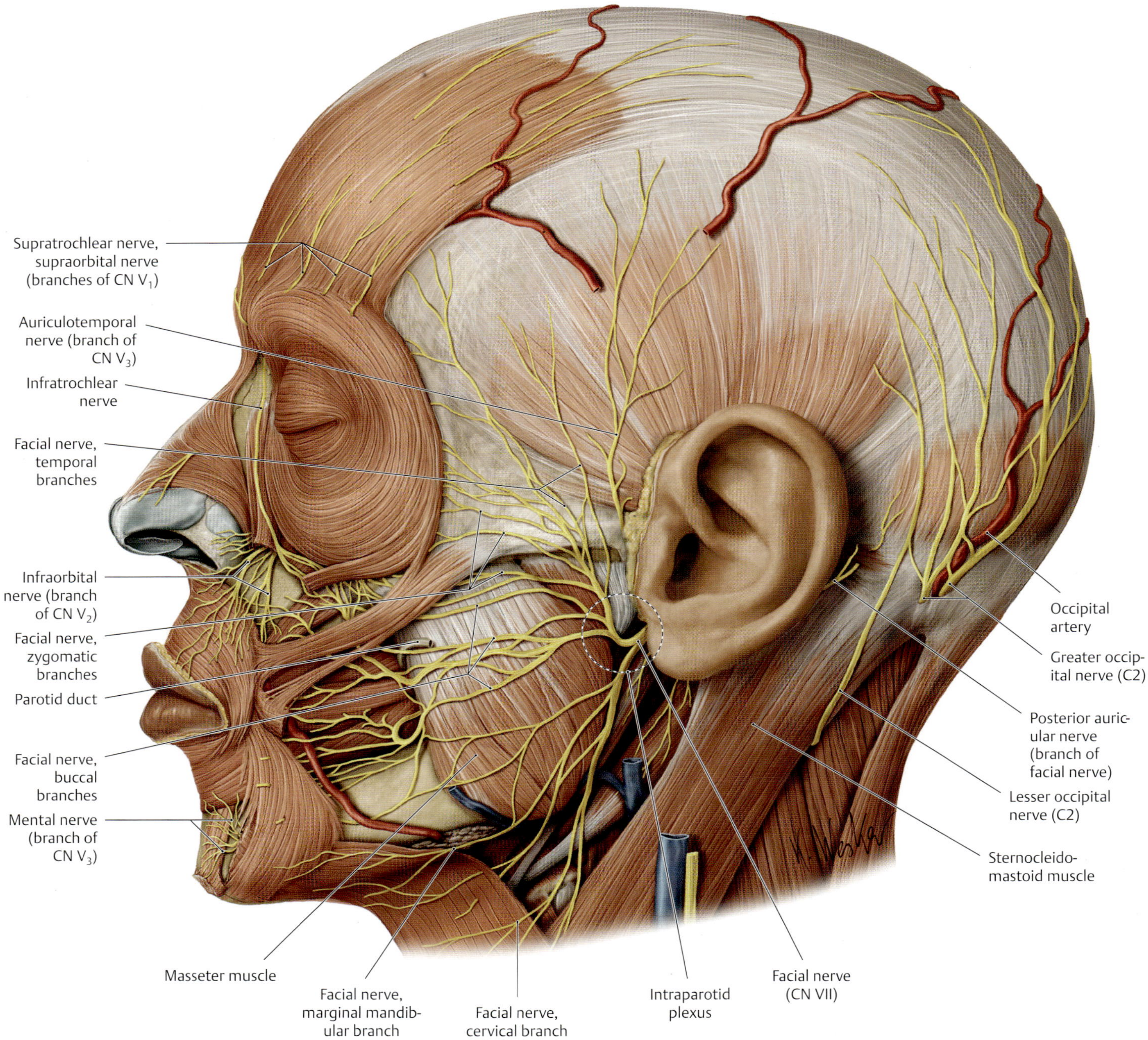

A Vessels and nerves of the intermediate layer
Left lateral view. The parotid gland has been removed to demonstrate the structure of the intraparotid plexus of the facial nerve.
Note certain nerves have been described in previous units. The veins have been removed for clarity.

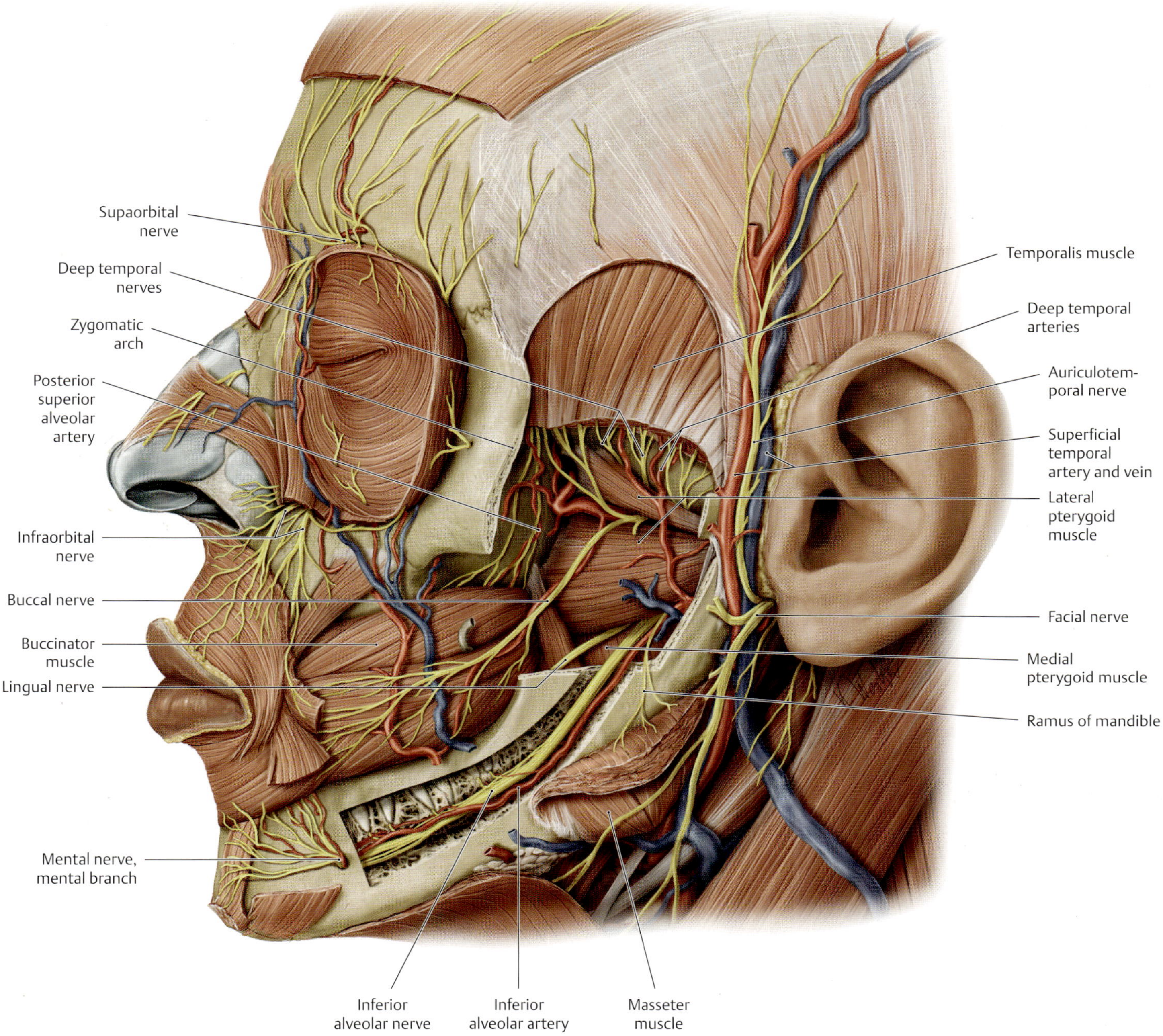

B Vessels and nerves of the deep layer

Left lateral view. The masseter muscle and zygomatic arch have been divided to gain access to the deep structures. Also, the ramus of the mandible has been opened to demonstrate the neurovascular structures that traverse it.

6.6 Infratemporal Fossa

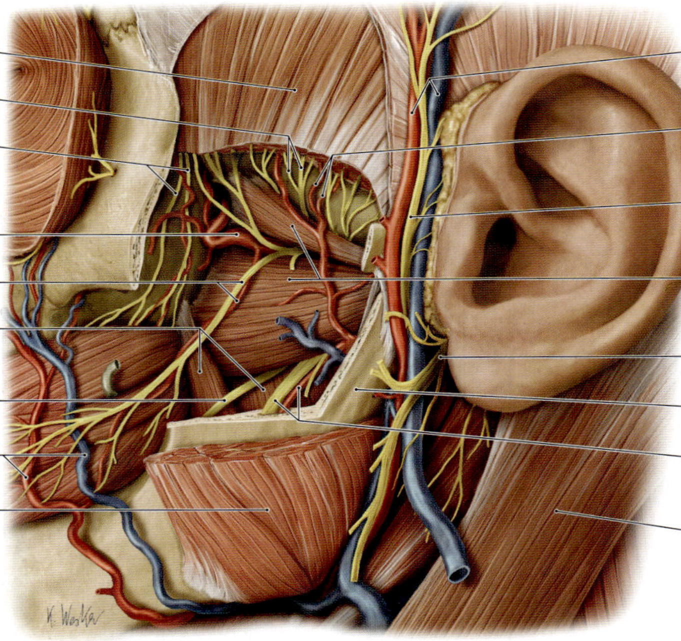

A Left infratemporal fossa, superficial layer

Lateral view. A separate unit is devoted to the infratemporal fossa because of the many structures that it contains. The zygomatic arch and the anterior half of the mandibular ramus have been removed in this dissection to gain access to the infratemporal fossa. The mandibular canal has been opened, and the inferior alveolar artery and nerve can be seen entering the canal (the accompanying vein has been removed). The maxillary artery divides into its terminal branches deep within the infratemporal fossa (see **B**).

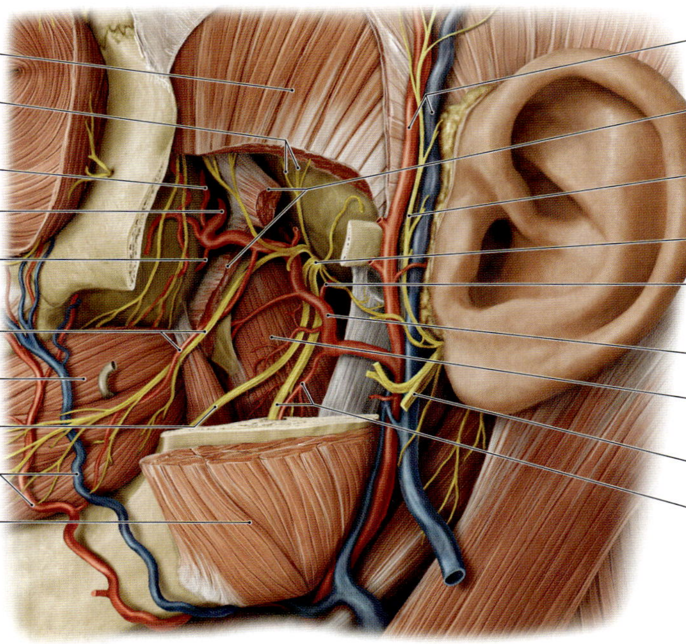

B Left infratemporal fossa, deep layer

Lateral view. This differs from the previous dissection in that both heads of the lateral pterygoid muscle have been partially removed, so that only their stumps are visible. The branches of the maxillary artery and mandibular division of the trigeminal nerve (CN V) can be identified. By careful dissection, it is possible to define the site where the auriculotemporal nerve (branch of the mandibular division) splits around the middle meningeal artery before entering the middle cranial fossa through the foramen spinosum (see p. 123).

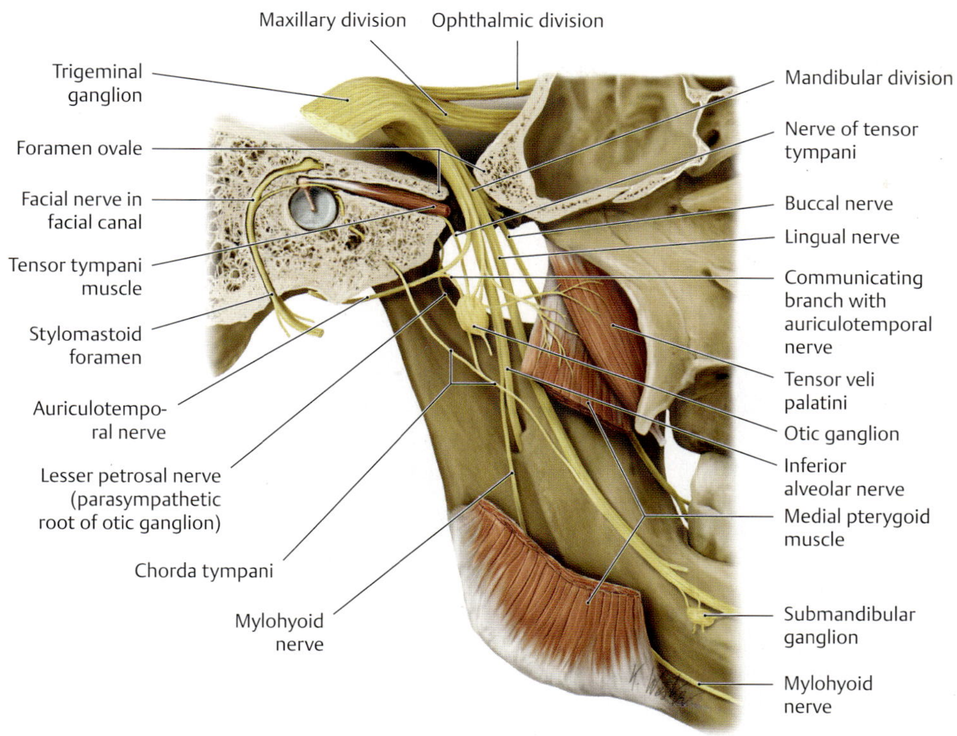

C Left otic ganglion and its roots located deep in the infratemporal fossa

Medial view. The small, flat otic ganglion is located medial to the mandibular nerve just inferior to the foramen ovale. The parasympathetic fibers for the parotid gland are relayed in the ganglion.

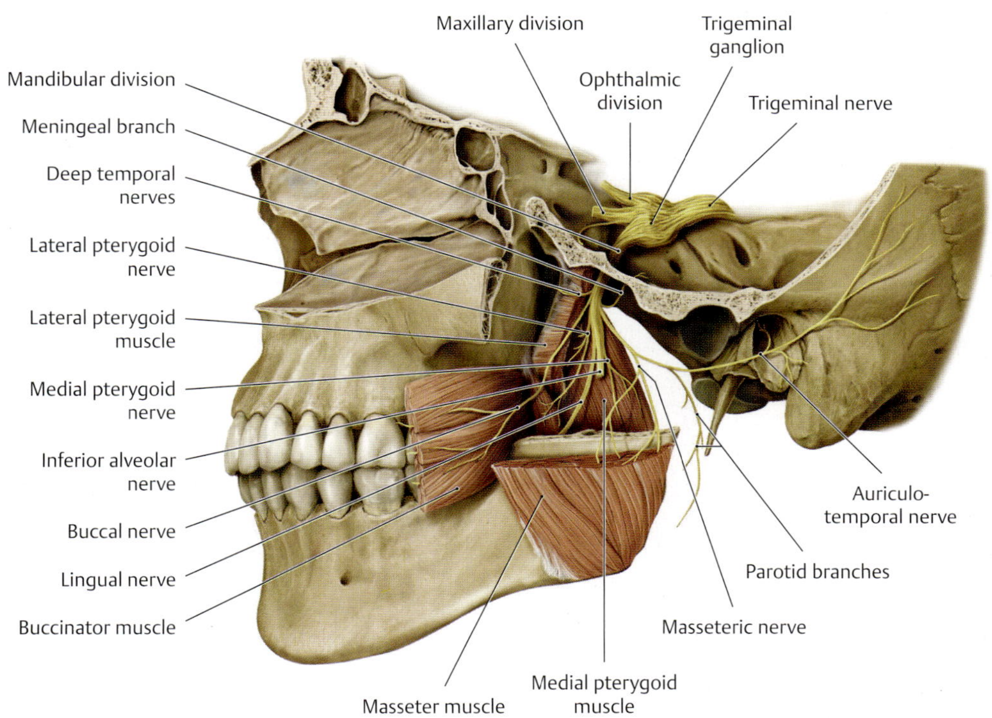

D Branches of the mandibular division in the infratemporal fossa

Left lateral view. The medial pterygoid muscle can be identified deep within the fossa. The third division of the trigeminal nerve passes through the foramen ovale from the middle cranial fossa to enter the infratemporal fossa. Traveling with it are motor fibers (motor root) that supply the muscles of mastication (only a few of the fibers are illustrated here).

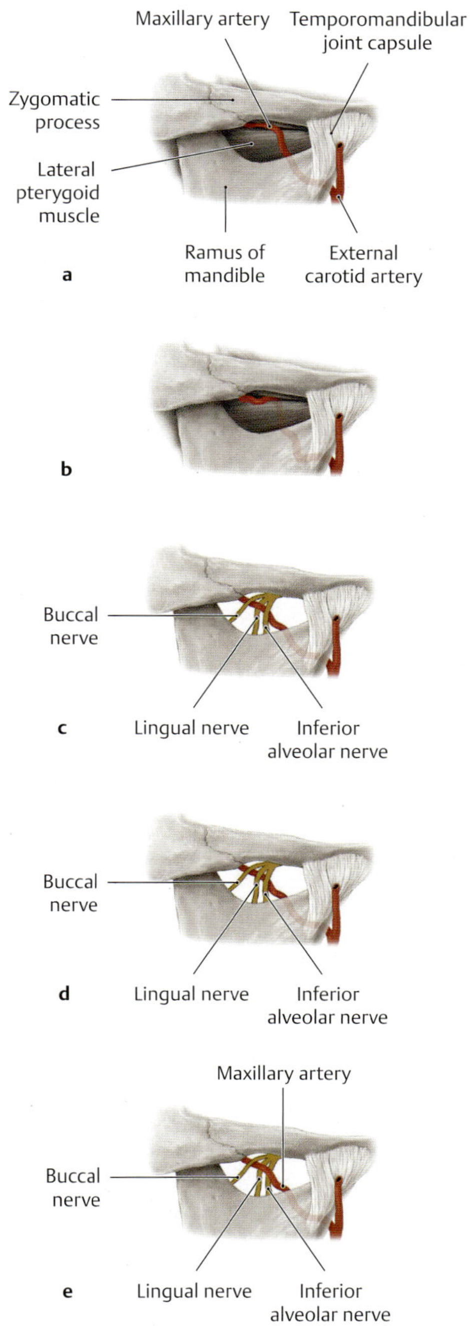

E Variants of the left maxillary artery

Lateral view. The course of the maxillary artery exhibits numerous variations. The most common variants are listed below:

- **a** Runs lateral to the lateral pterygoid muscle (common).
- **b** Runs medial to the lateral pterygoid muscle.
- **c** Runs in medial direction from the trunk of the mandibular n.
- **d** Runs medial to the buccal nerve but lateral to the lingual nerve and inferior alveolar nerve.
- **e** Runs lateral to the inferior alveolar n. and medial to the buccal and lingual nn.

6.7 Pterygopalatine Fossa

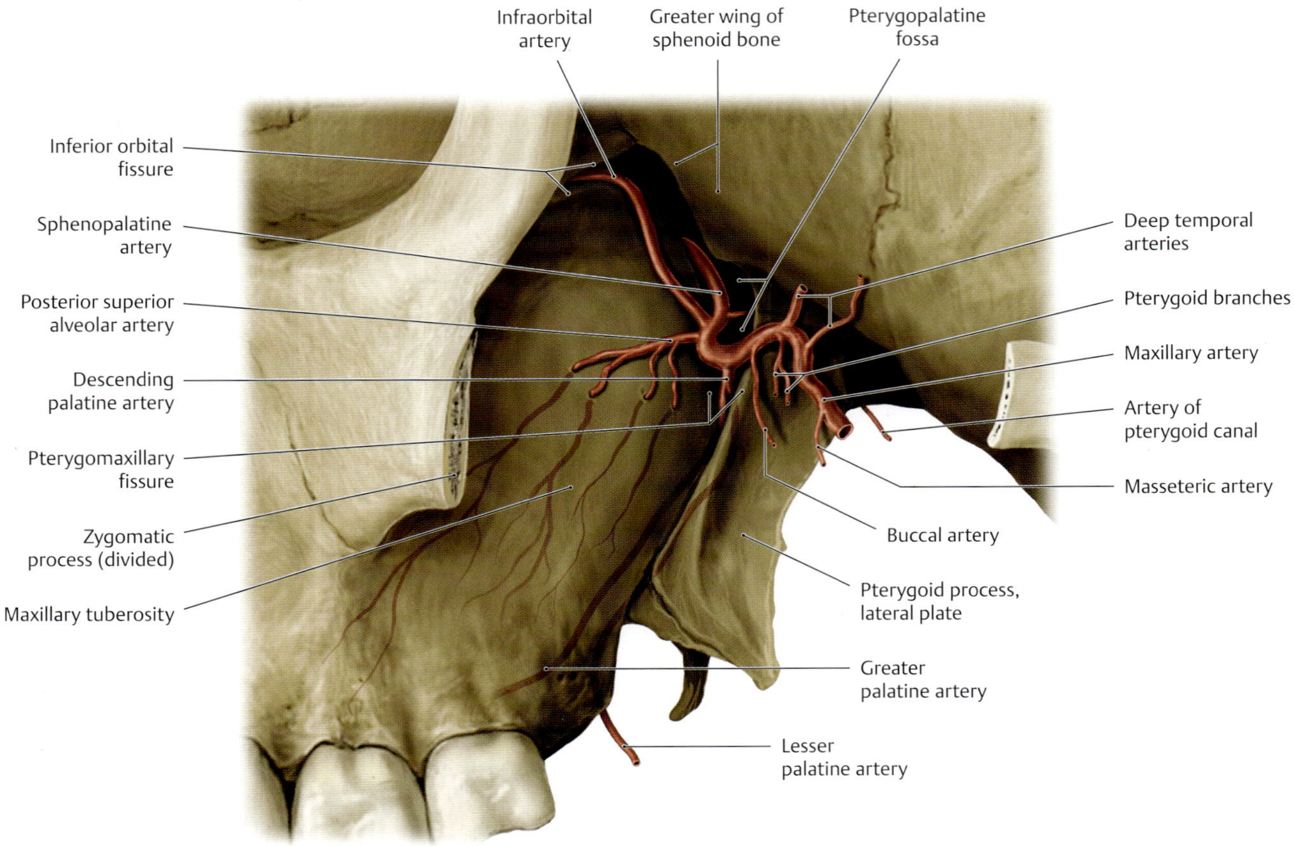

A Course of the arteries in the left pterygopalatine fossa
Lateral view. The infratemporal fossa (see previous unit, p. 236) is continuous with the pterygopalatine fossa shown here, with no clear line of demarcation between them. The anatomical boundaries of the pterygopalatine fossa are listed in **B** (cf. p. 39). The pterygopalatine fossa is a crossroad for neurovascular structures traveling between the middle cranial fossa, orbit, nasal cavity, and oral cavity (see the passageways in **E**). Because so many small arterial branches arise here, the arteries and veins have been shown separately for better clarity. The maxillary artery divides into its terminal branches in the pterygopalatine fossa (see p. 100). The maxillary artery can be ligated within the fossa for the control of severe nosebleed (epistaxis, see p. 185).

B Structures bordering the pterygopalatine fossa

Direction	Bordering structure
Anterior	Maxillary tuberosity
Posterior	Pterygoid process (lateral plate)
Medial	Perpendicular plate of the palatine bone
Lateral	Communicates with the infratemporal fossa via the pterygomaxillary fissure
Superior	Greater wing of the sphenoid bone, junction with the inferior orbital fissure
Inferior	Opens into the retropharyngeal space

C Larger branches of the maxillary artery
The maxillary artery consists of a mandibular part, pterygoid part, and pterygopalatine part. Because the vessels of the mandibular part lie outside the area of the dissection, they are not listed in the table below (see p. 100).

Branch	Distribution
Pterygoid part:	
• Masseteric artery	• Masseter muscle
• Deep temporal arteries	• Temporalis muscle
• Pterygoid branches	• Pterygoid muscles
• Buccal artery	• Buccal mucosa
Pterygopalatine part:	
• Posterior superior alveolar artery	• Maxillary molars, maxillary sinus, gingiva
• Infraorbital artery	• Maxillary alveolae
• Descending palatine artery	
– Greater palatine artery	• Hard palate
– Lesser palatine artery	• Soft palate, palatine tonsil, pharyngeal wall
• Sphenopalatine artery	
– Lateral posterior nasal arteries	• Lateral wall of nasal cavity, choanae
– Posterior septal branches	• Nasal septum

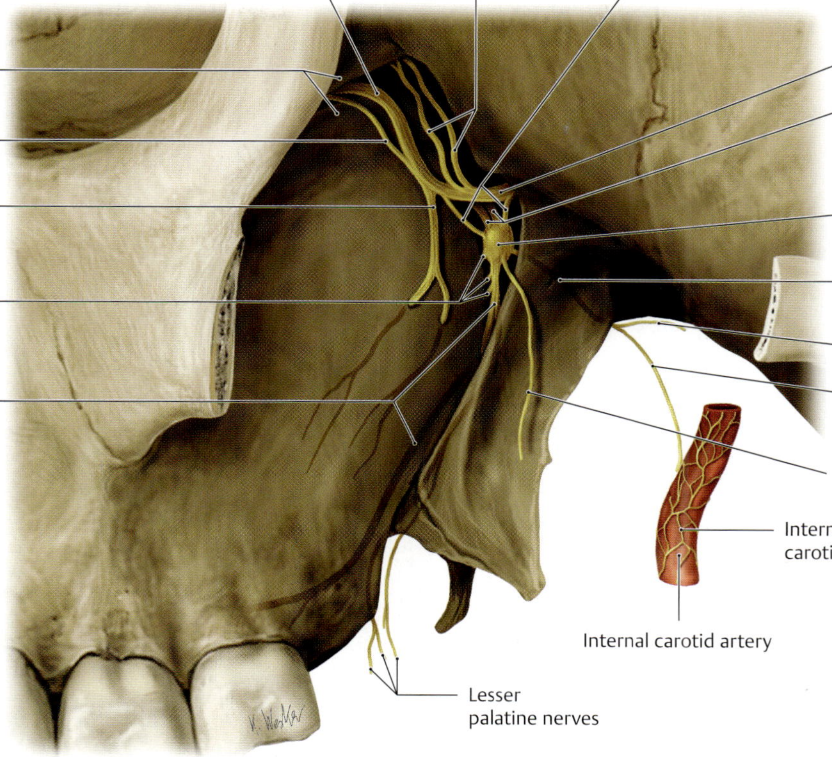

D Course of the nerves in the left pterygopalatine fossa

Lateral view. The maxillary division, the second division of CN V, passes from the middle cranial fossa through the foramen rotundum into the pterygopalatine fossa. Closely related to the maxillary nerve is the parasympathetic pterygopalatine ganglion, in which preganglionic fibers synapse with postganglionic neurons that, in turn, innervate the lacrimal glands and the small palatal and nasal glands. The pterygopalatine ganglion receives its presynaptic fibers from the greater petrosal nerve. This nerve is the parasympathetic root of the nervus intermedius branch of the facial nerve. The sympathetic fibers of the deep petrosal nerve (sympathetic root), like the sensory fibers of the maxillary nerve (sensory root), pass through the ganglion without synapsing.

E Passageways to the pterygopalatine fossa and transmitted neurovascular structures

Passageway	Connection with ...	Transmitted structures
Foramen rotundum	Middle cranial fossa	• Maxillary nerve (CN V_2)
Pterygoid canal	Base of the skull (inferior aspect)	• Artery of the pterygoid canal with accompanying veins • Nerve of the pterygoid canal (comes from the parasympathetic branch of the facial nerve—the great petrosal n. and sympathetic deep petrosal n. in the canal)
Greater palatine canal/foramen	Palate	• Greater palatine a. (from descending palatine a.) • Greater palatine n.
Lesser palatine canals	Palate	• Lesser palatine aa. (terminal branches of the descending palatine nn.) • Lesser palatine nn.
Sphenopalatine foramen	Nasal cavity	• Sphenopalatine artery (and accompanying veins) • Medial and lateral superior and inferior posterior nasal branches (from nasopalatine nerve, CN V_2)
Inferior orbital fissure	Orbit	• Infraorbital artery (and accompanying veins) • Inferior ophthalmic vein • Infraorbital nerve (plus accompanying veins) • Zygomatic nerve (from CN V_2) • Orbital branches (from CN V_2)
Pterygomaxillary fissure	Infratemporal fossa	• Maxillary a.

6.8 Posterior Cervical Triangle

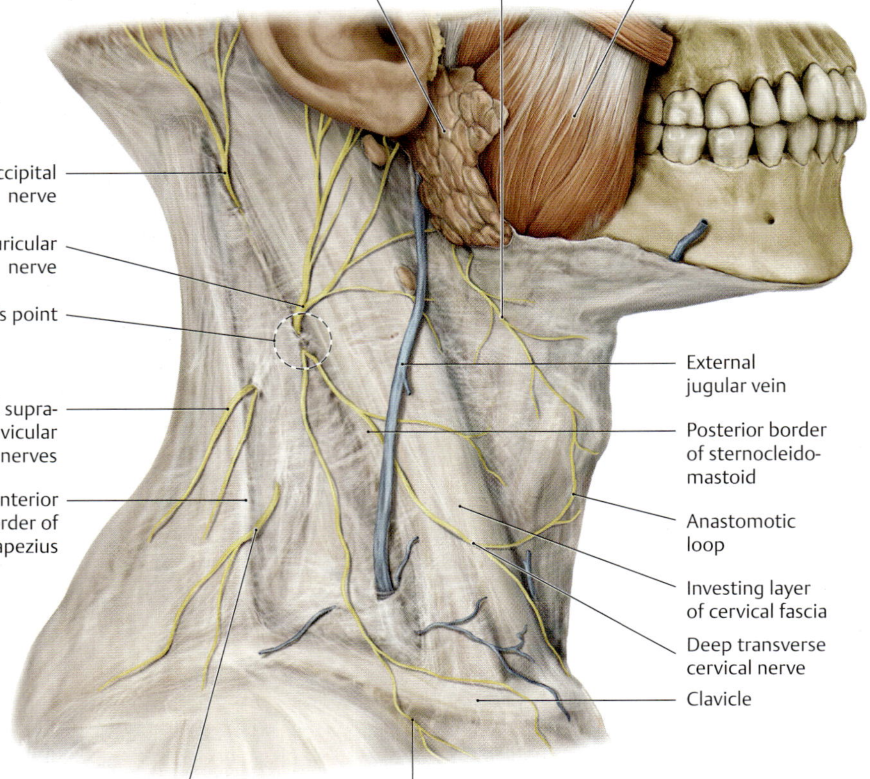

A Lateral view of the neck, subcutaneous layer

The posterior cervical triangle is a topographically important region bounded by the clavicle, the anterior border of the trapezius, and the posterior border of the sternocleidomastoid muscle.

This and the following figures show progressively deeper dissections of the lateral cervical region. The adjacent sternocleidomastoid region and the anterior cervical region are also exposed. The skin and subcutaneous fat have been removed to display the subcutaneous, purely sensory cutaneous nerves from the cervical plexus in the lateral cervical region. They perforate the investing layer of the deep cervical fascia at the Erb's point to supply the anterior and lateral neck. Specifically these nerves are the lesser occipital, great auricular, transverse cervical, and supraclavicular nn. (medial, intermediate, and lateral).

Note: The transverse cervical nerve passes beneath the external jugular vein and forms an anastomosis with the cervical branch of the facial nerve. This mixed loop contains motor fibers from the facial nerve and sensory fibers for the neck from the transverse cervical nerve.

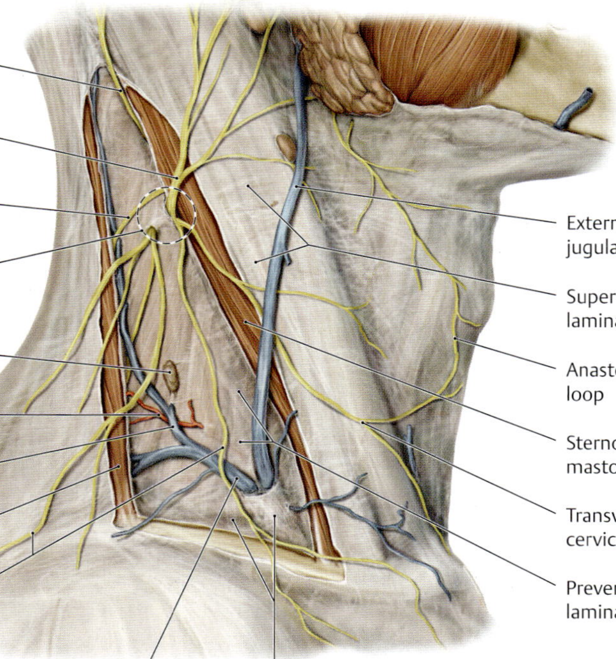

B Lateral cervical region (posterior cervical triangle), subfascial layer

Right lateral view. The investing layer of the deep cervical fascia has been removed over the posterior cervical triangle to expose the prevertebral layer of the cervical fascia, which is fused to the pretracheal lamina at the level of omohyoid muscle (see p. 5). The cutaneous nerves from the cervical plexus perforate the investing layer of the deep cervical fascia at approximately the mid-posterior border of the sternocleidomastoid muscle (Erb's point) and are distributed in the subcutaneous plane.

Note the external branch of the accessory nerve, which passes to the trapezius muscle. A surgeon taking a lymph node biopsy may accidentally sever the external branch. This injury restricts the mobility of the scapula, and the patient may be unable to elevate the upper limb beyond 90°.

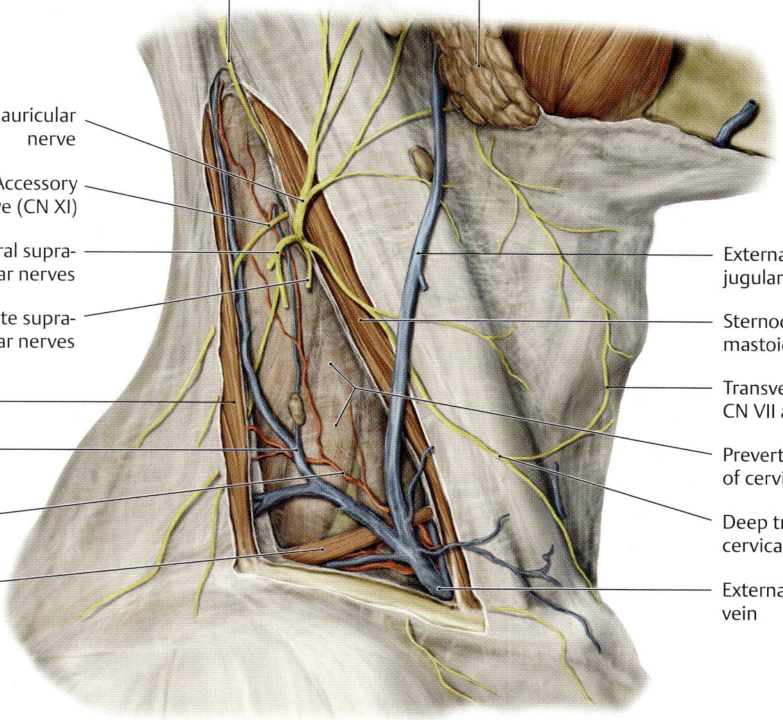

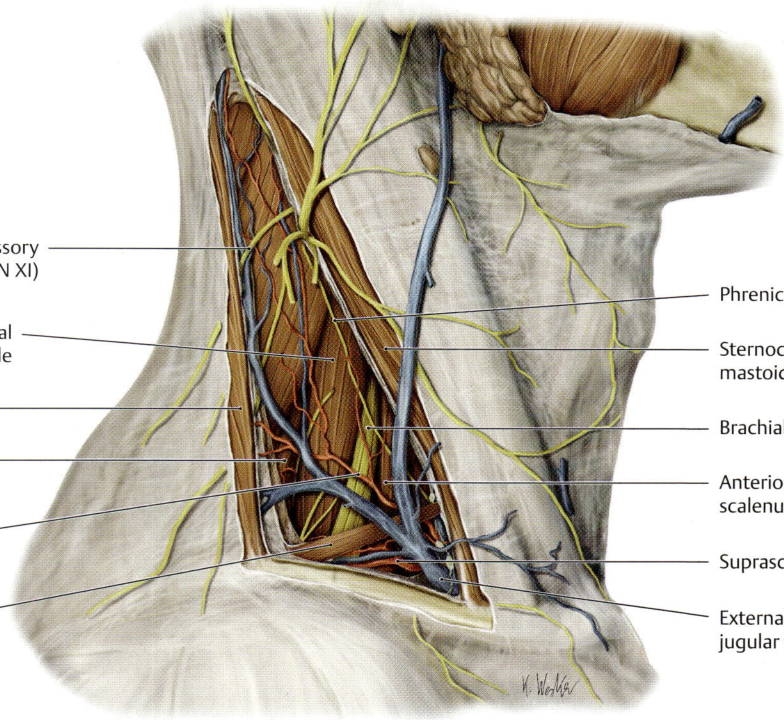

C Posterior cervical triangle

a Deeper layer, right lateral view. In this dissection, the pretracheal layer of the deep cervical fascia has additionally been removed to display the omohyoid muscle, which is enveloped by that fascia.

b Deepest layer with a view of the brachial plexus. The prevertebral layer has been removed to expose the scalene muscles.
Note the phrenic nerve, which runs obliquely over the scalenus anterior muscle to the thoracic inlet.

6.9 Deep Lateral Cervical Region, Carotid Triangle, and Thoracic Inlet

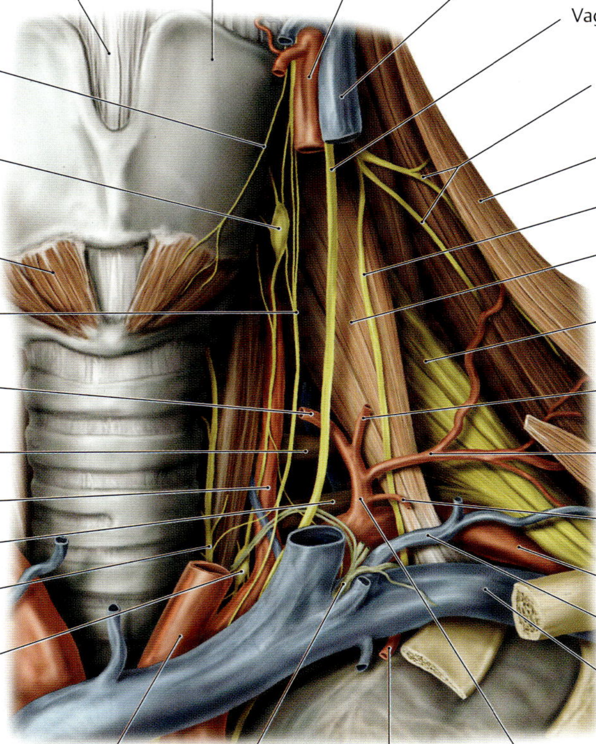

A Base of neck and thoracic inlet on the left side

Anterior view. The sternal end of the clavicle, the anterior end of the first rib, the manubrium sterni, and the thyroid gland have been removed to expose the thoracic inlet. The subclavian artery and thyrocervical trunk can be identified.

Note the course of the following structures: The internal thoracic artery descends parallel to the sternum. It is of special clinical interest. In patients with coronary heart disease, the internal thoracic artery can be mobilized and anastomosed to the coronary artery past the point of the stenosis. The sympathetic trunk, vagus nerve, phrenic nerve, and portions of the brachial plexus are visible, the latter passing through the interscalene space (see **C**). *Note* also the termination of the thoracic duct at the jugulosubclavian venous junction and the left recurrent laryngeal nerve. This branch of the vagus nerve winds around the aortic arch and ascends to the larynx.

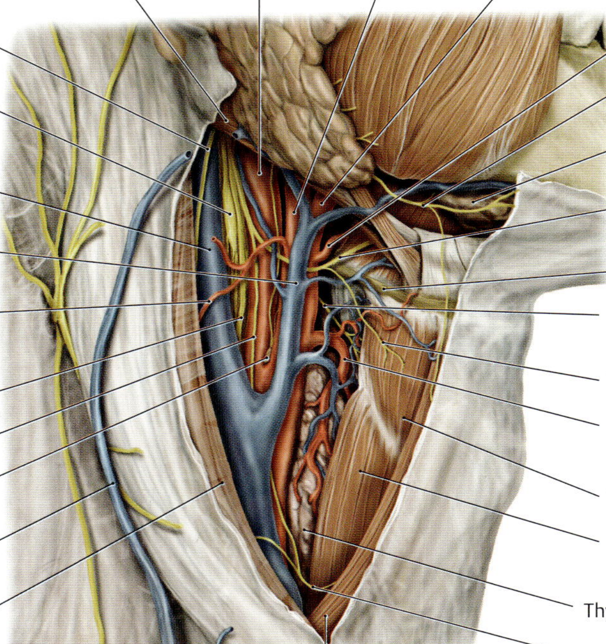

B Carotid triangle

Right lateral view. The carotid triangle is a subregion of the anterior cervical triangle. It is bounded by the sternocleidomastoid muscle, the posterior belly of the digastric muscle, and the superior belly of the omohyoid muscle. The submandibular gland can be seen at the inferior border of the mandible and the sternocleidomastoid muscle has been retracted posterolaterally. The following structures are located in the carotid triangle:

- Internal and external carotid arteries (the superior thyroid and lingual arteries branch from the latter)
- Hypoglossal nerve (CN XII)
- Vagus nerve (CN X)
- Accessory nerve (CN XI)
- Sympathetic trunk with associated ganglia.

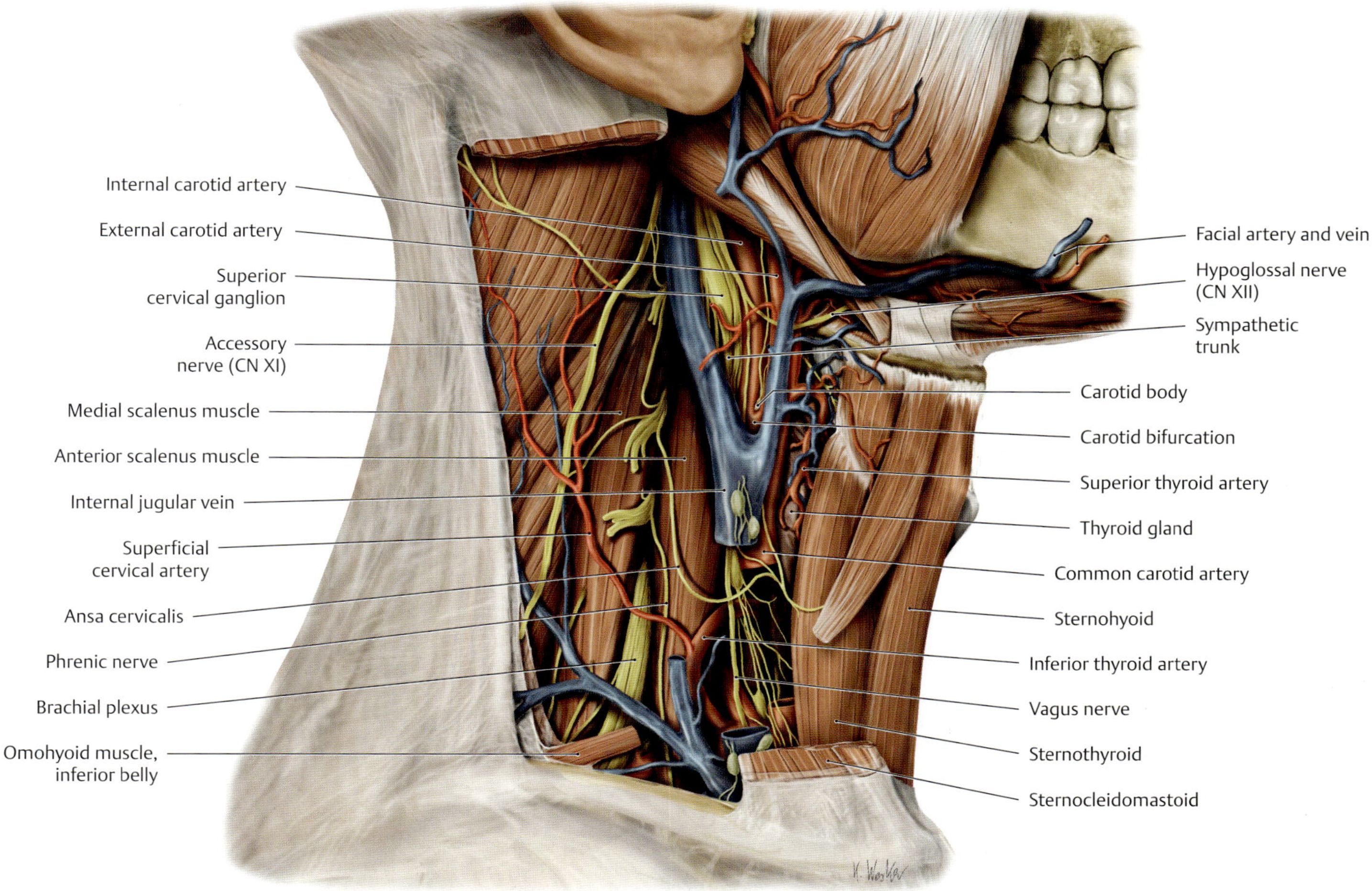

C Deep lateral cervical region
Right lateral view. The sternocleidomastoid region and carotid triangle have been dissected along with adjacent portions of the posterior and anterior cervical triangles. The carotid sheath has been removed in this dissection along with the cervical fasciae, sternocleidomastoid muscle, and omohyoid muscle to demonstrate all important neurovascular structures in the neck:

- Common carotid artery with its division into the internal and external carotid arteries
- Superior and inferior thyroid arteries
- Internal jugular vein
- Deep cervical lymph nodes along the internal jugular vein
- Sympathetic trunk including its ganglia
- Vagus nerve
- Hypoglossal nerve
- Accessory nerve
- Brachial plexus
- Phrenic nerve

The phrenic nerve originates from the C3–C5 segments and therefore is part of the cervical plexus. The muscular landmark for locating the phrenic nerve is the scalenus anterior, along which the nerve descends in the neck. The (posterior) interscalene space is located between the scalenus anterior and medius and the first rib and is traversed by the brachial plexus and subclavian artery. The subclavian vein passes deeply through the interval formed by the scalenus anterior, the sternocleidomastoid muscle (resected), and the first rib (the anterior interscalene space).

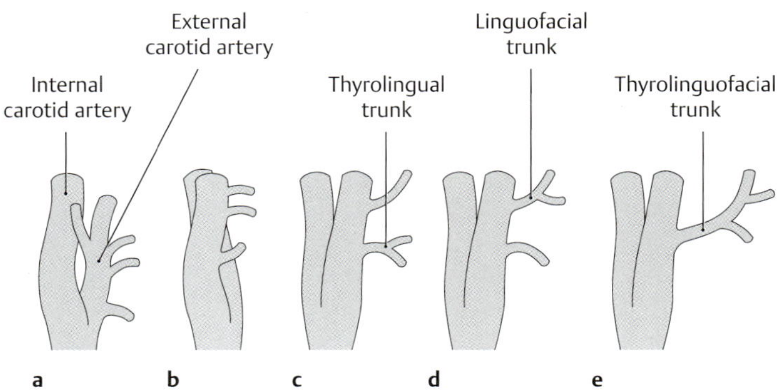

D Variable position of the external and internal carotid arteries and variants in the anterior branches of the external carotid artery (after Faller and Poisel-Golth)

a, b The internal carotid artery may arise from the common carotid artery posterolateral (49%) or anteromedial (9%) to the external carotid artery, or at other intermediate sites.

c–e The external carotid artery may give origin to a thyrolingual trunk (4%), linguofacial trunk (23%), or thyrolinguofacial trunk (0.6%).

6.10 Posterior Cervical and Occipital Regions

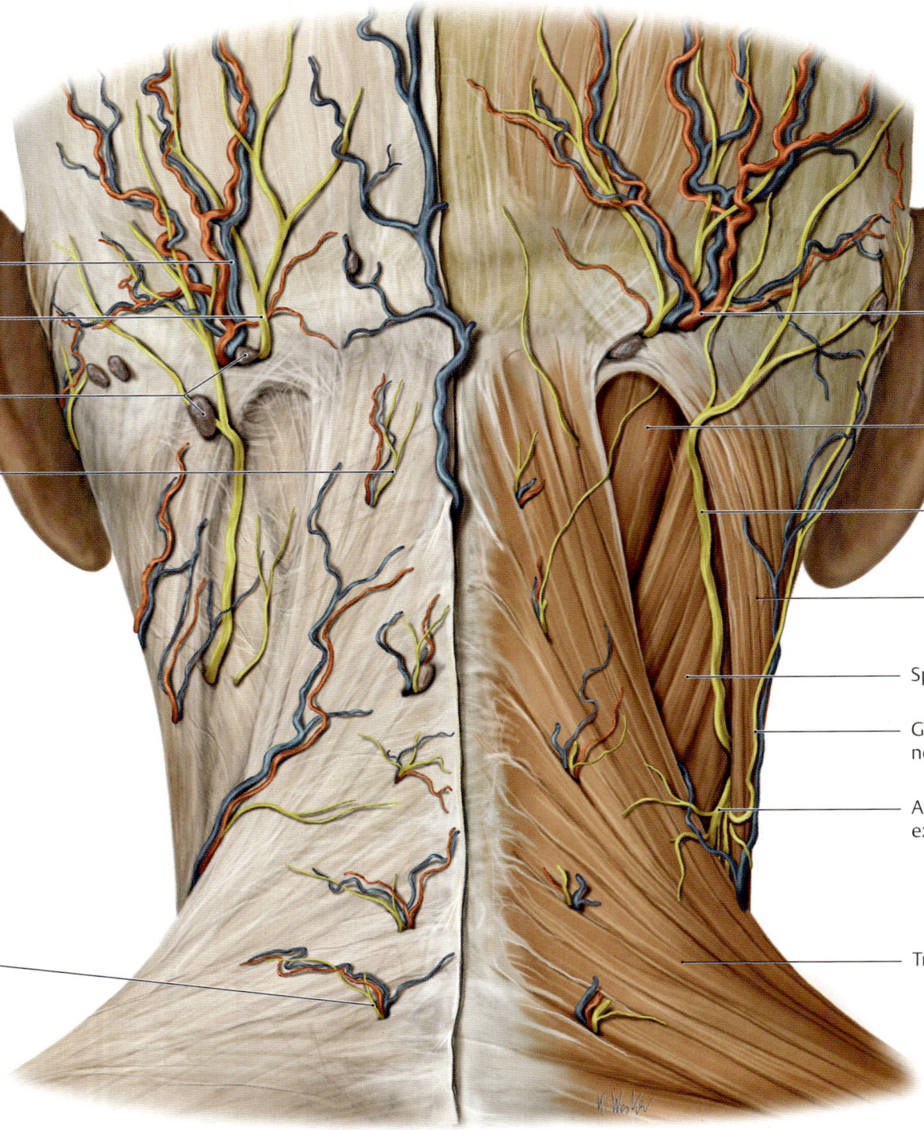

A Posterior cervical region and occipital region
Posterior view of the subcutaneous layer on the left side and the subfascial layer on the right side. Although the occipital region is part of the head, it is discussed here because it borders on the posterior cervical region. The principal arterial vessel in this region is the occipital artery, the second branch arising from the posterior side of the external carotid artery. The medially situated greater occipital nerve is a dorsal ramus of the C2 spinal nerve, while the laterally situated lesser occipital nerve is a *ventral* ramus of C2 that arises from the cervical plexus (see p. 139). The lymph nodes are located at the sites where the nerves and veins emerge through the cervical fascia.
Note the accessory nerve, which crosses the lateral cervical triangle at a relatively superficial level.

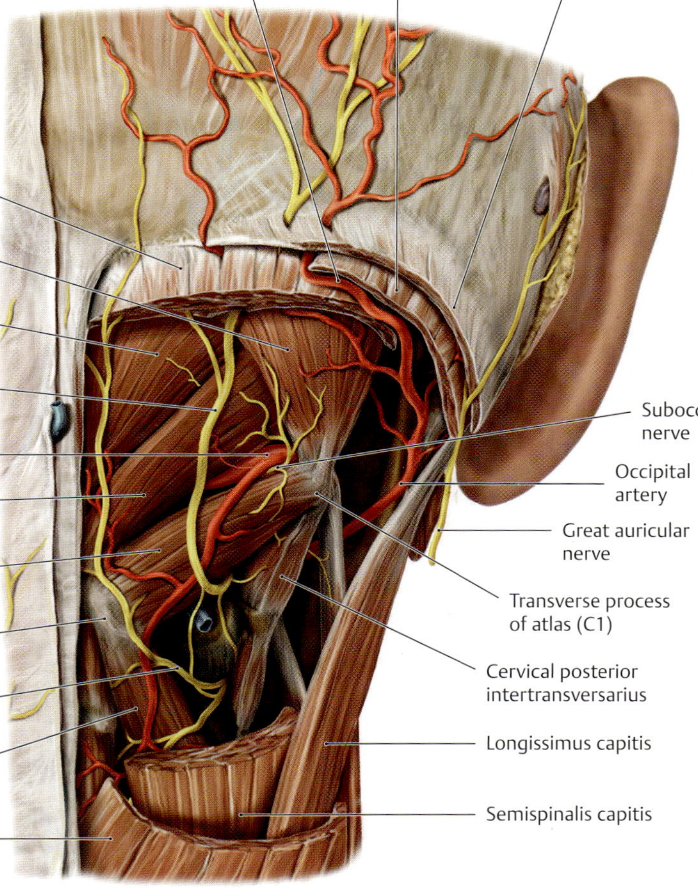

B Right suboccipital triangle

Posterior view. The suboccipital triangle is bounded superiorly by the rectus capitis posterior major, laterally by the obliquus capitis superior, and inferiorly by the obliquus capitis inferior. This muscular triangle can be seen only after the trapezius, splenius capitis, and semispinalis capitis muscles have been removed. A short, free segment of the vertebral artery runs through the deep part of the triangle after leaving the transverse foramen and before exiting the triangle by perforating the atlanto-occipital membrane (not visible here). That segment of the vertebral artery gives off branches to the surrounding short nuchal muscles. Both vertebral arteries unite intracranially to form the basilar artery, which is a major contributor to cerebral blood flow.

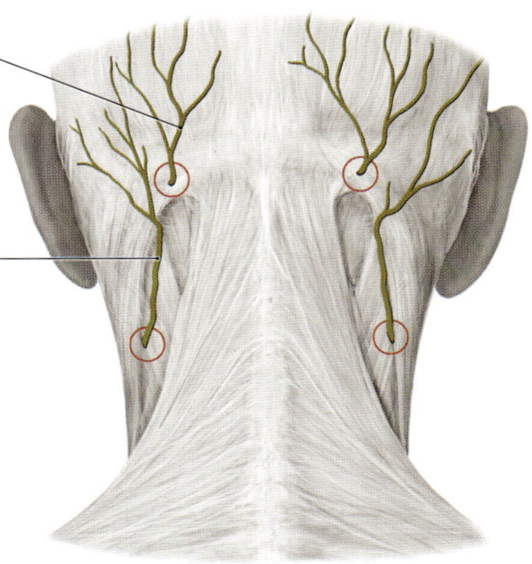

C Clinically important sites of emergence of the occipital nerves

Posterior view. The sites where the lesser and greater occipital nerves emerge from the fascia into the subcutaneous connective tissue are clinically important because they are tender to palpation in certain diseases (e.g., meningitis). The examiner tests the sensation of these nerves by pressing lightly on the circled points with the thumb. If these points (but not their surroundings) are painful, the finding is described, logically, as "tenderness over the occipital nerves."

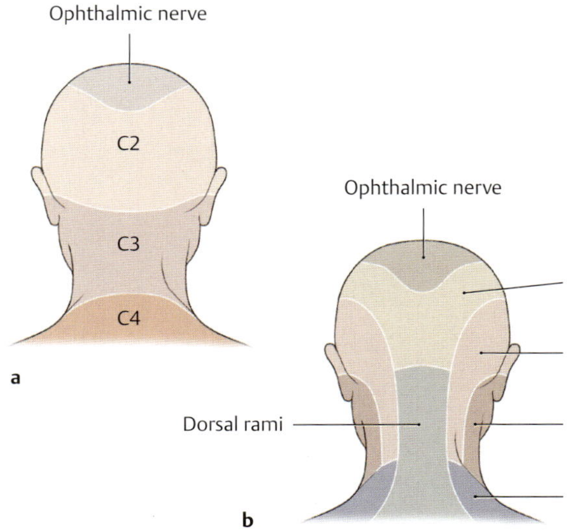

D Cutaneous innervation of the neck

Posterior view. The pattern of segmental innervation is illustrated on the left, and the territorial assignments of specific cutaneous nerves on the right. The occiput and neck derive most of their segmental innervation from the second and third cervical segments. The ophthalmic nerve supplying the area above the C2 level is the first branch of the trigeminal nerve (CN V).

Note that in the peripheral innervation pattern, the greater occipital nerve is a dorsal *spinal* nerve ramus while the lesser occipital nerve is a *ventral* ramus (see p. 22).

7.1 Coronal Sections: Anterior Orbital Margin and Retrobulbar Space

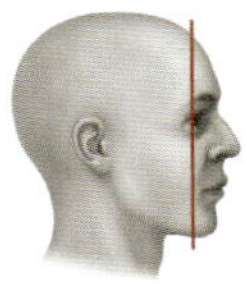

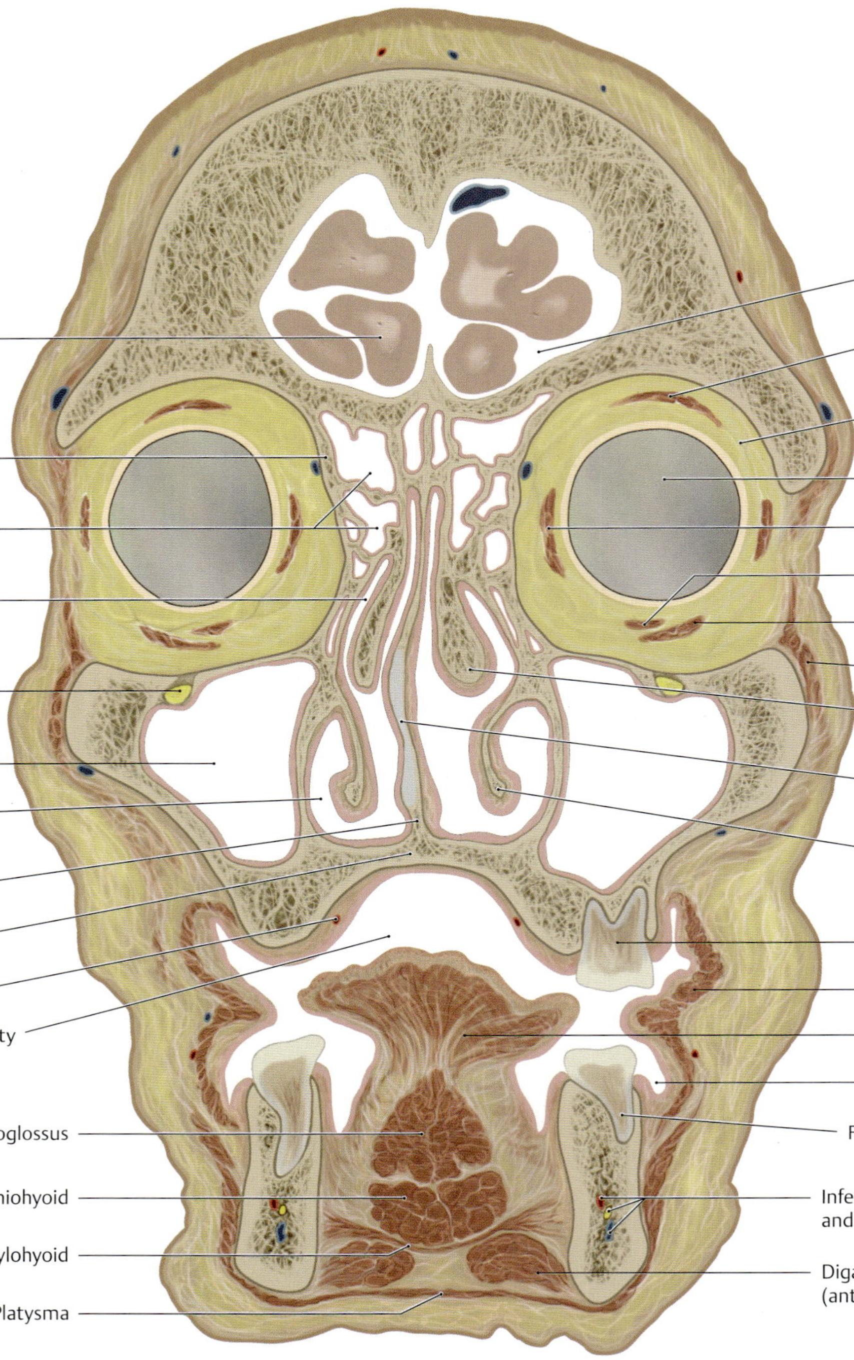

A Coronal section through the anterior orbital margin

Anterior view. This section of the skull can be roughly subdivided into four regions: the oral cavity, the nasal cavity and sinus, the orbit, and the anterior cranial fossa.

Inspecting the region in and around the **oral cavity**, we observe the muscles of the oral floor, the apex of the tongue, the neurovascular structures in the mandibular canal, and the first molar. The hard palate separates the oral cavity from the **nasal cavity**, which is divided into left and right halves by the nasal septum. The inferior and middle nasal conchae can be identified along with the laterally situated maxillary sinus. The structure bulging down into the roof of the sinus is the infraorbital canal, which transmits the infraorbital nerve (branch of the maxillary division of the trigeminal nerve, CN V_2). The plane of section is so far anterior that it does not cut the lateral bony walls of the **orbits** because of the lateral curvature of the skull. The section passes through the transparent vitreous body, and three of the six extraocular muscles can be identified in the retro-orbital fat. Two additional muscles can be seen in the next deeper plane of section (see **B**). The space between the two orbits is occupied by the ethmoid cells.

Note: The bony orbital plate (medial wall of the orbit) is very thin (lamina papyracea) and may be penetrated by infection, trauma, and neoplasms.

In the **anterior cranial fossa**, the section passes through both frontal lobes of the brain in the most anterior portions of the cerebral gray matter. Very little white matter is visible at this level.

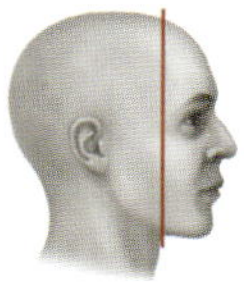

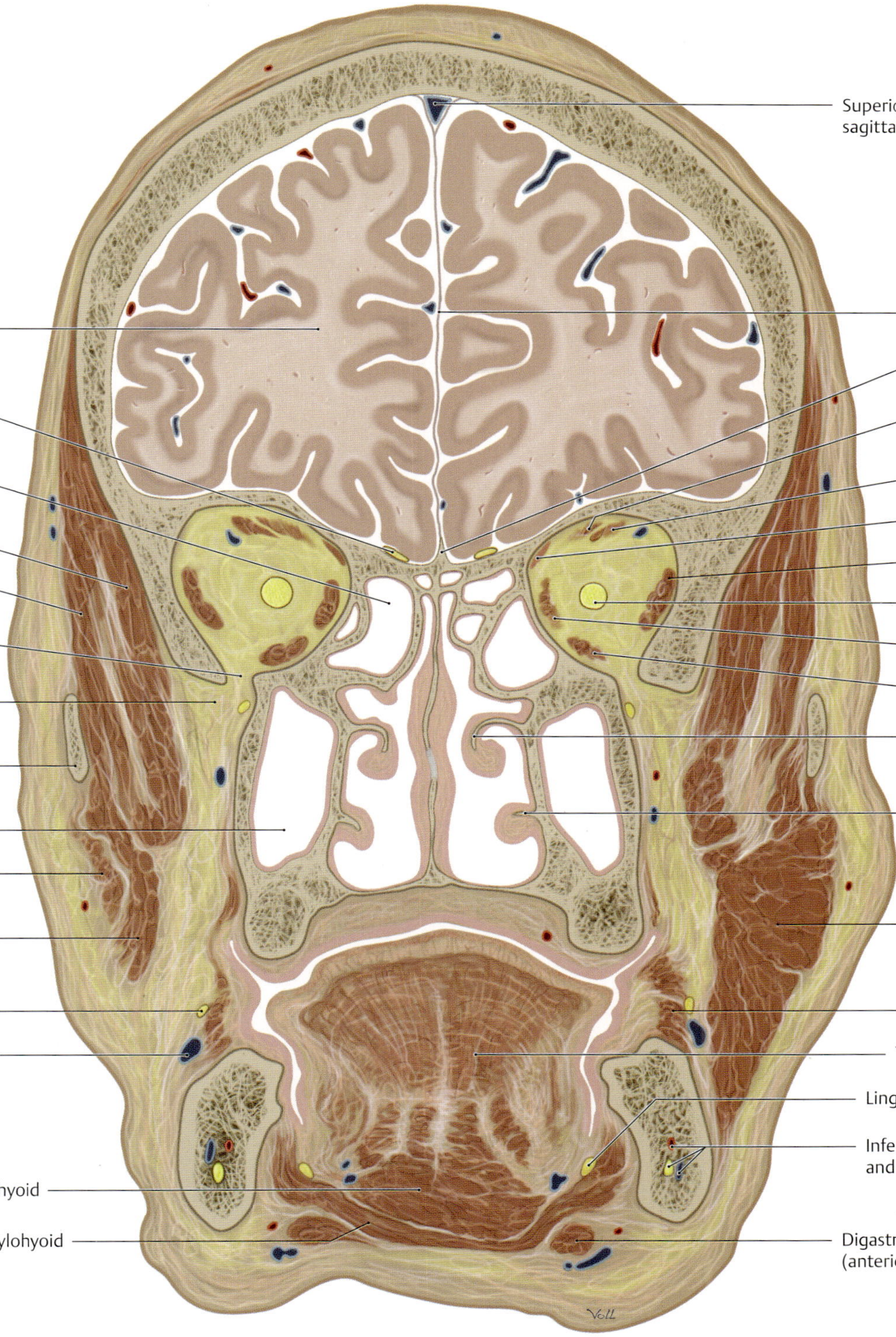

B Coronal section through the retrobulbar space

Anterior view. Here, the tongue is cut at a more posterior level than in **A** and therefore appears broader. In addition to the oral floor muscles, we see the muscles of mastication on the sides of the skull. In the orbital region we can identify the retrobulbar space with its fatty tissue, the extraocular muscles, and the optic nerve. The orbit communicates laterally with the infratemporal fossa through the inferior orbital fissure. This section cuts through both olfactory bulbs in the anterior cranial fossa, and the superior sagittal sinus can be recognized in the midline.

7.2 Coronal Sections: Orbital Apex and Hypophysis

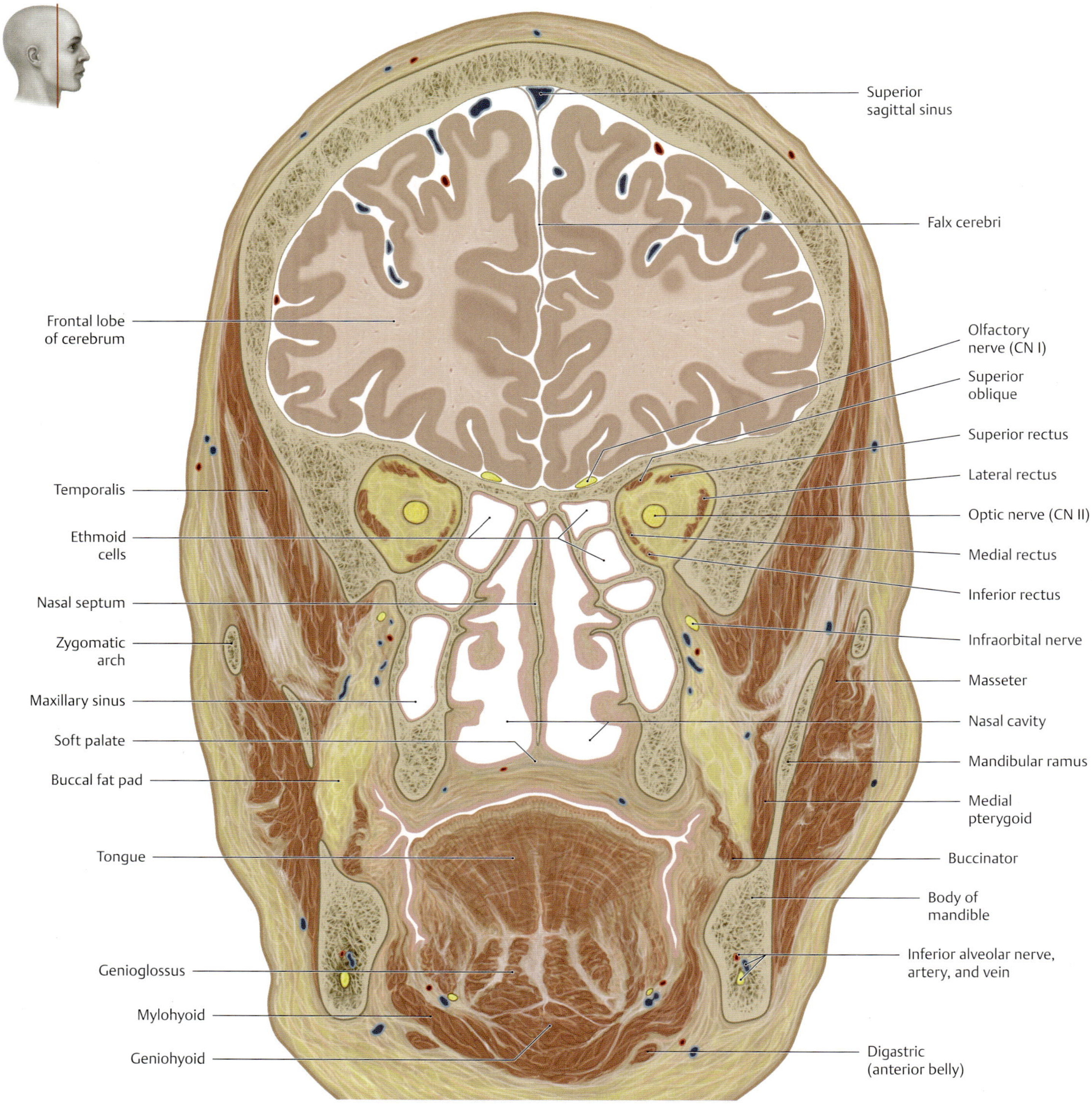

A Coronal section through the orbital apex

Anterior view. The soft palate replaces the hard palate in this plane of section, and the nasal septum becomes osseous at this level. The buccal fat pad is also visible in this plane. Because the buccal pad is composed of fat, it is attenuated in wasting diseases; this is why the cheeks are sunken in patients with end-stage cancer. This coronal section is slightly angled, producing an apparent discontinuity in the mandibular ramus on the left side of the figure (compare with the continuous ramus on the right side).

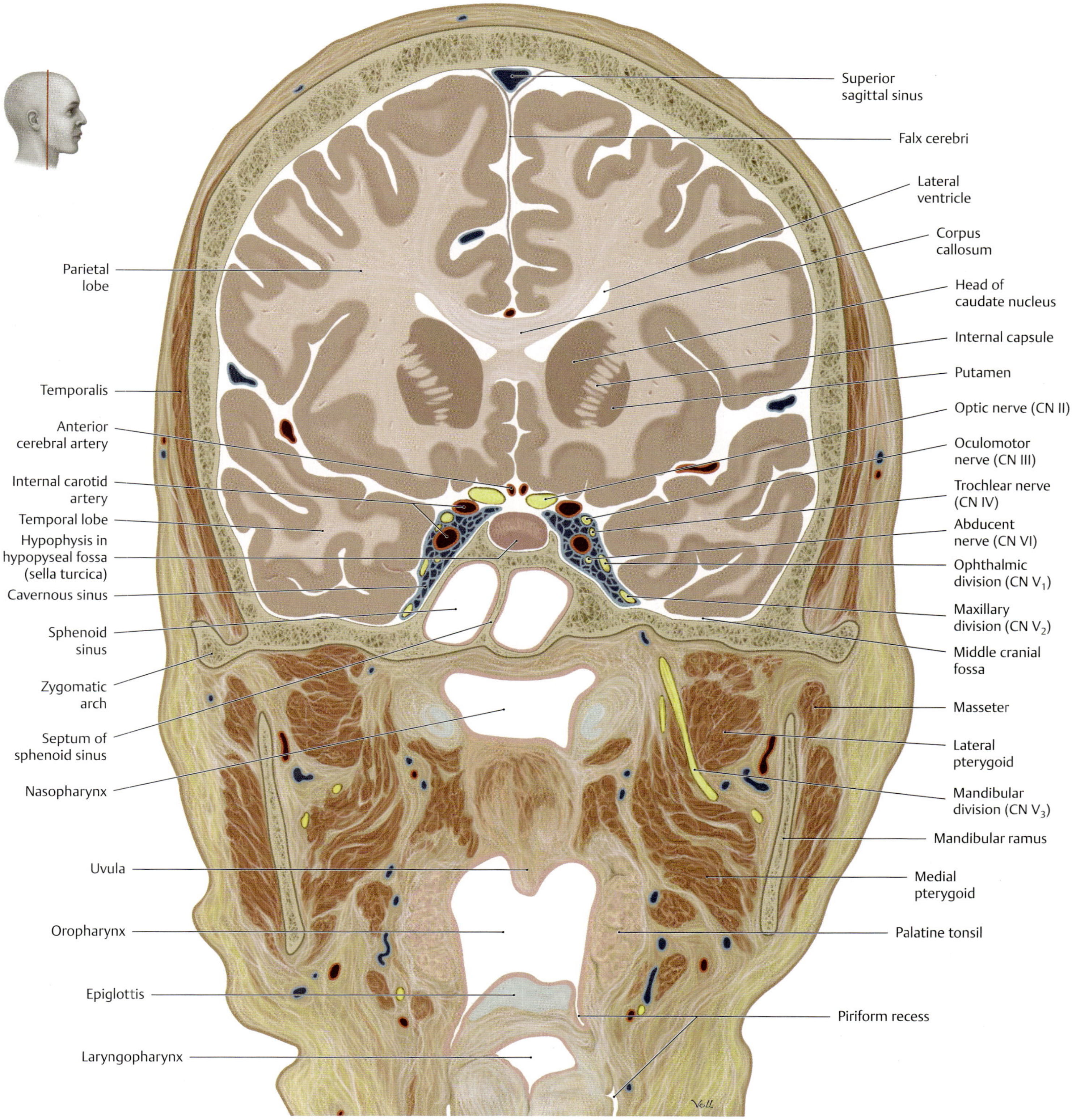

B Coronal section through the pituitary
Anterior view. The nasopharynx, oropharynx, and laryngopharynx can now be identified. This section cuts the epiglottis, below which is the supraglottic space. The plane cuts the mandibular ramus on both sides, and a relatively long segment of the mandibular division (CN V_3) can be identified on the left side. The paired sphenoid sinuses are visible, separated by a median septum. Above the roof of the sphenoid sinuses is the hypophysis (pituitary), which lies in the hypophyseal fossa. In the cranial cavity, the plane of section passes through the middle cranial fossa. Due to the presence of the carotid siphon (a 180° bend in the cavernous part of the internal carotid artery), the section cuts the internal carotid artery twice on each side. Cranial nerves can be seen passing through the cavernous sinus on their way from the middle cranial fossa to the orbit. The superior sagittal sinus appears in cross-section at the attachment of the falx cerebri. At the level of the cerebrum, the plane of section passes through the parietal and temporal lobes. Intracerebral structures appearing in this section include the caudate nucleus, the putamen, the internal capsule, and the anterior horn of each lateral ventricle.

7.3 Transverse Sections: Orbits and Optic Nerve

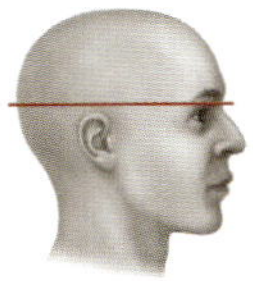

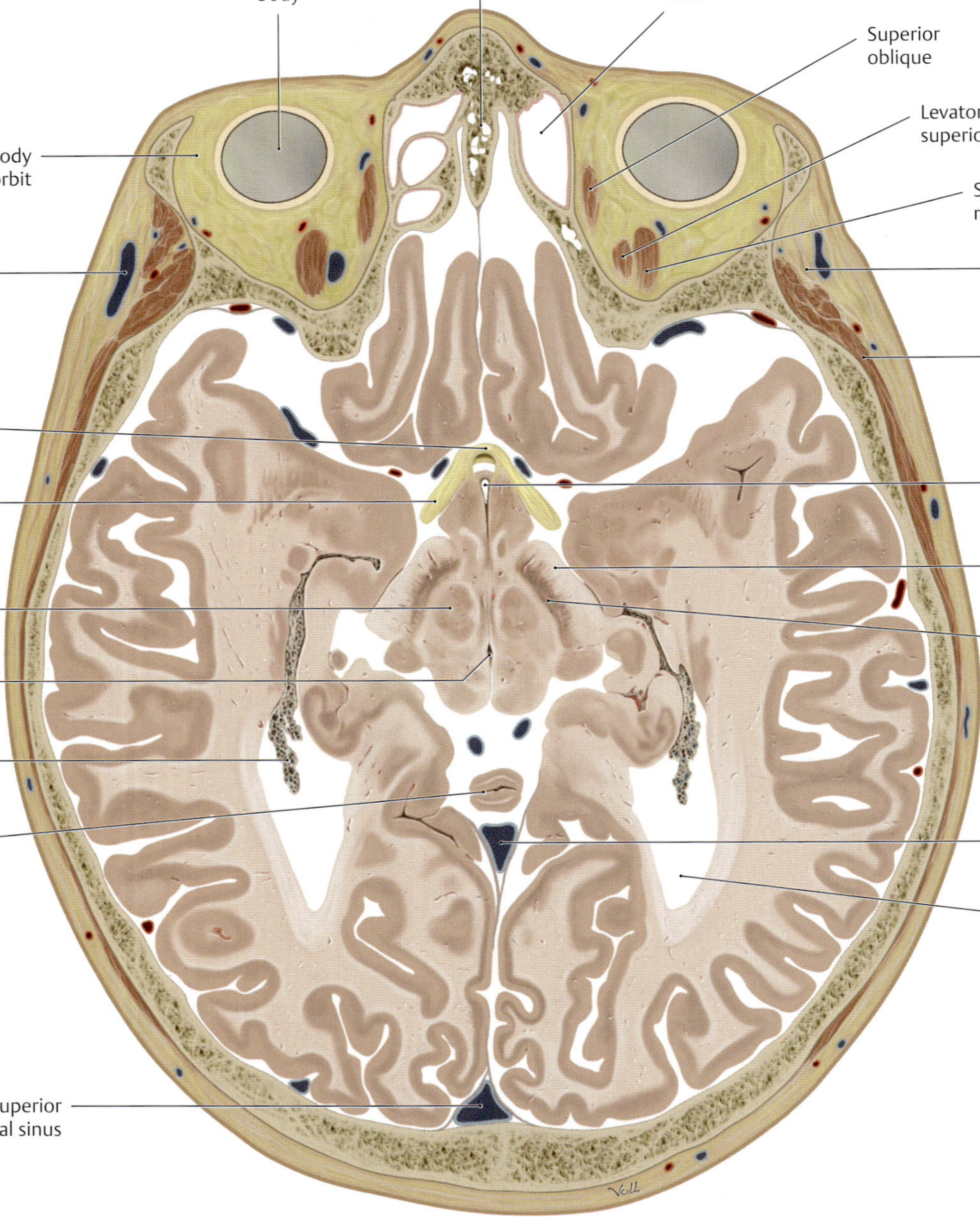

A Transverse section through the upper level of the orbits
Superior view. The highest section in this series displays the muscles in the upper level of the orbit (the orbital levels are described on p. 176 ff). The section cuts the bony crista galli in the anterior cranial fossa, flanked on each side by cells of the ethmoid sinus. The sections of the optic chiasm and adjacent optic tract are parts of the diencephalon, which surrounds the third ventricle at the center of the section. The red nucleus and substantia nigra are visible in the mesencephalon. The pyramidal tract descends in the cerebral peduncles. The section passes through the posterior (occipital) horns of the lateral ventricles and barely cuts the vermis of the cerebellum in the midline.

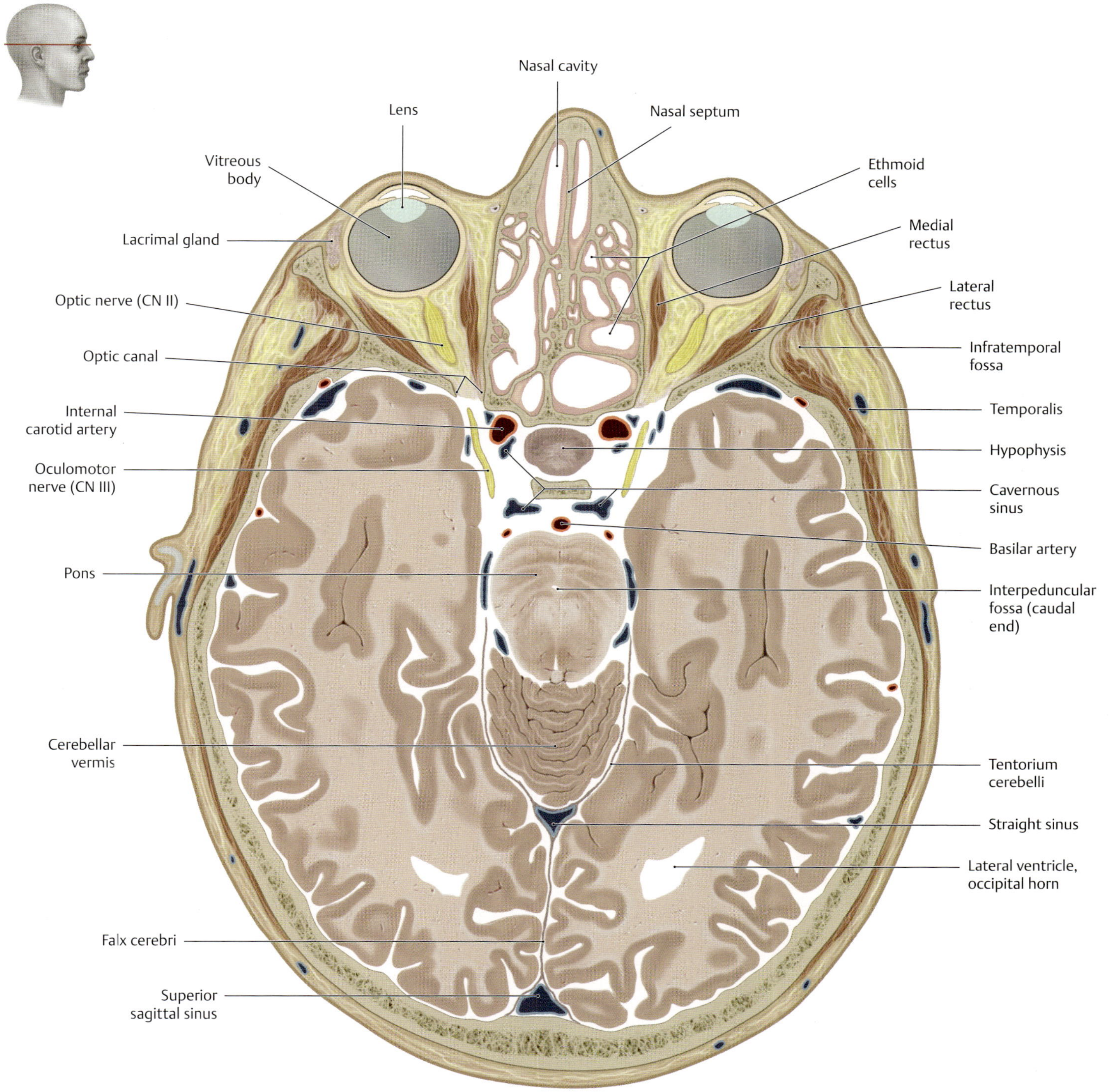

B Transverse section through the optic nerve and pituitary
Superior view. The optic nerve is seen just before its entry into the optic canal, indicating that the plane of section passes through the middle level of the orbit. Because the nerve completely fills the canal, growth disturbances of the bone at this level may cause pressure injury to the nerve. This plane cuts the ocular lenses and the cells of the ethmoid labyrinth. The internal carotid artery can be identified in the middle cranial fossa, embedded in the cavernous sinus. The section cuts the oculomotor nerve on either side, which courses in the lateral wall of the cavernous sinus. The pons and cerebellar vermis are also seen. The falx cerebri and tentorium cerebelli appear as thin lines that come together at the straight sinus.

7.4 Transverse Sections: Sphenoid Sinus and Middle Nasal Concha

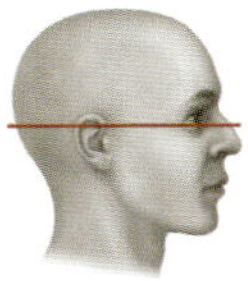

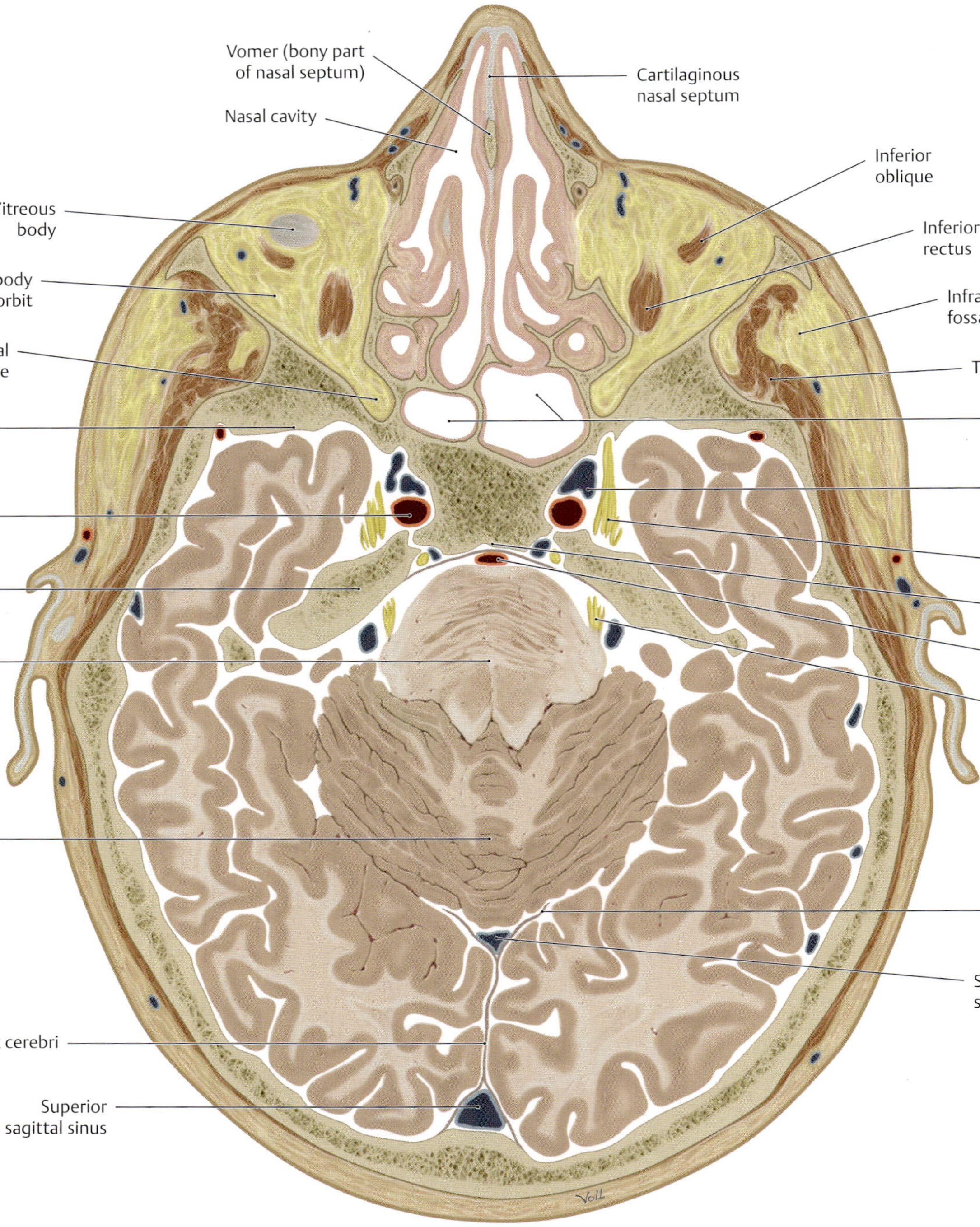

A Transverse section through the sphenoid sinus
Superior view. This section cuts the infratemporal fossa on the lateral aspect of the skull and the temporalis muscle that lies within it. The plane passes through the lower level of the orbit, and a small portion of the eyeball is visible on the left side. The orbit is continuous posteriorly with the inferior orbital fissure. This section displays the anterior extension of the two greater wings of the sphenoid bone and the posterior extension of the two "petrous bones" (petrous parts of the temporal bones), which mark the boundary between the middle and posterior cranial fossae (see p. 22 f). The clivus is part of the posterior cranial fossa and lies in contact with the basilar artery. The pontine origin of the trigeminal nerve and its intracranial course are clearly demonstrated.

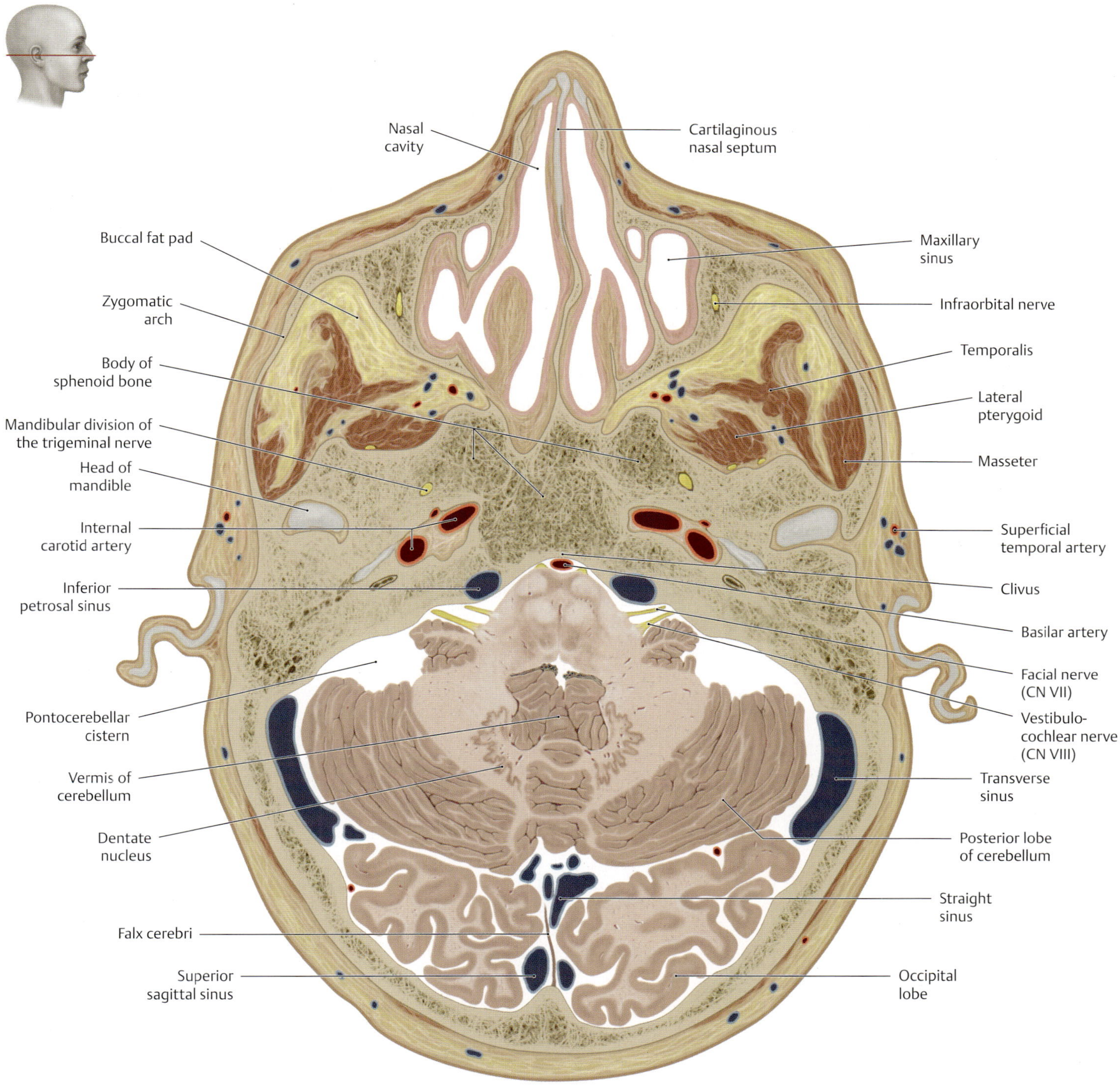

B Transverse section through the middle nasal concha

Superior view. This section below the orbit passes through the infraorbital nerve in the accordingly named canal. Medial to the infraorbital nerve is the roof of the maxillary sinus. The zygomatic arch is visible in its entirety, and portions of the muscles of mastication medial to the zygomatic arch (masseter, temporalis, and lateral pterygoid) can be seen. The plane of section passes through the upper part of the head of the mandible. The mandibular division (CN V_3) appears in cross-section in its bony canal, the foramen ovale. It is evident that the body of the sphenoid bone forms the bony center of the base of the skull. The facial nerve and vestibulocochlear nerve emerge from the brainstem. The dentate nucleus lies within the white matter of the cerebellum. The space around the anterior part of the cerebellum, the pontocerebellar cistern, is filled with cerebrospinal fluid in the living individual. The transverse sinus is prominent among the dural sinuses of the brain.

7.5 Transverse Sections: Nasopharynx and Median Atlantoaxial Joint

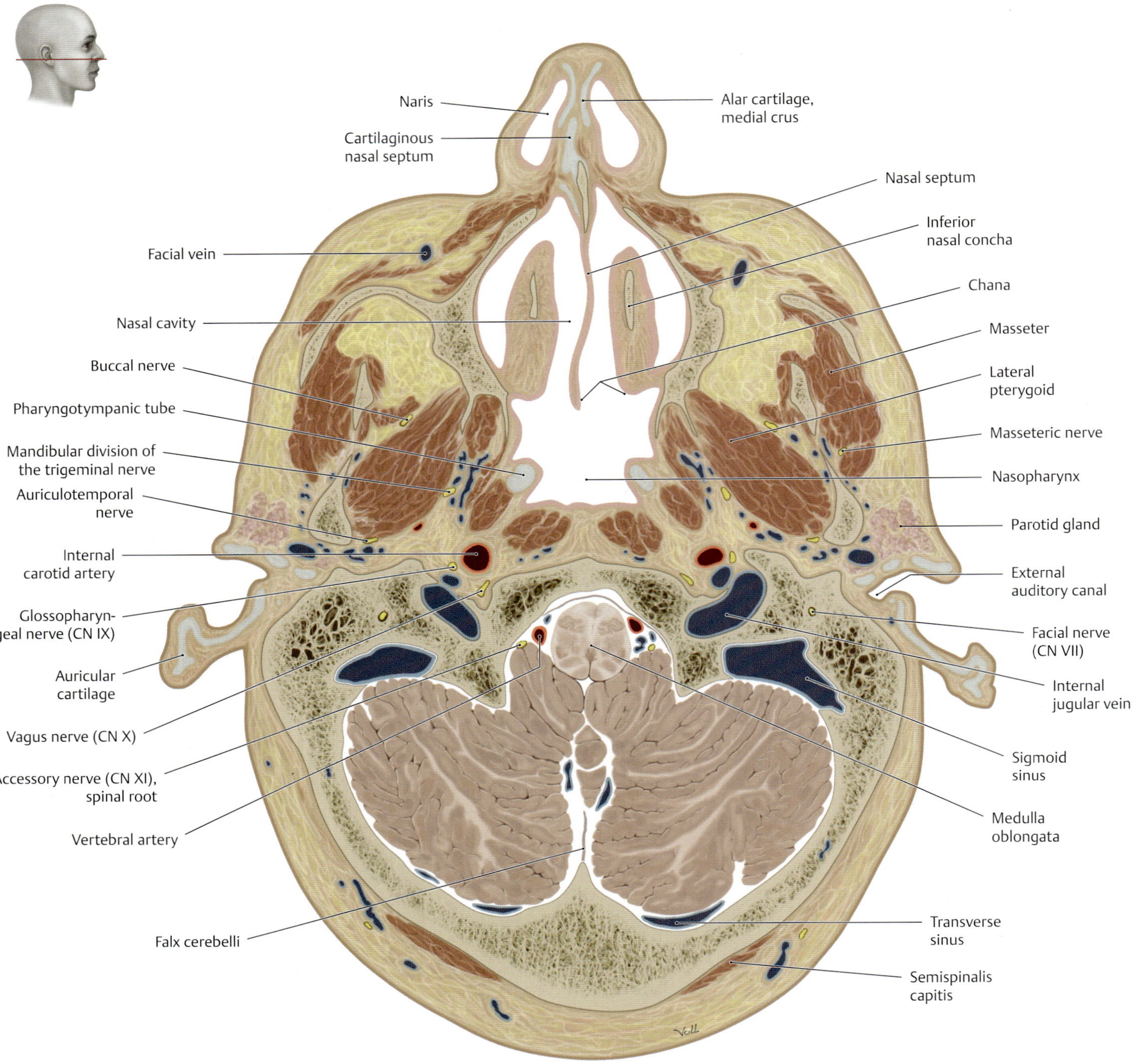

A Transverse section through the nasopharynx
Superior view. This section passes through the external nose and portions of the cartilaginous nasal skeleton. The nasal cavities communicate with the nasopharynx through the choanae. Cartilaginous portions of the pharyngotympanic tube project into the nasopharynx. The arterial blood vessels that supply the brain can also be seen: the internal carotid artery and vertebral artery.

Note the internal jugular vein and vagus nerve, which pass through the carotid sheath in company with the internal carotid artery.
A number of cranial nerves that emerge from the skull base are displayed in cross-section, such as the facial nerve coursing in the facial canal. This section also cuts the auricle and portions of the external auditory canal.

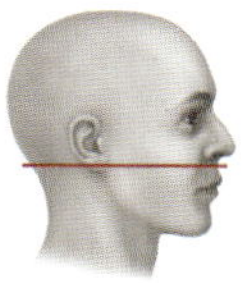

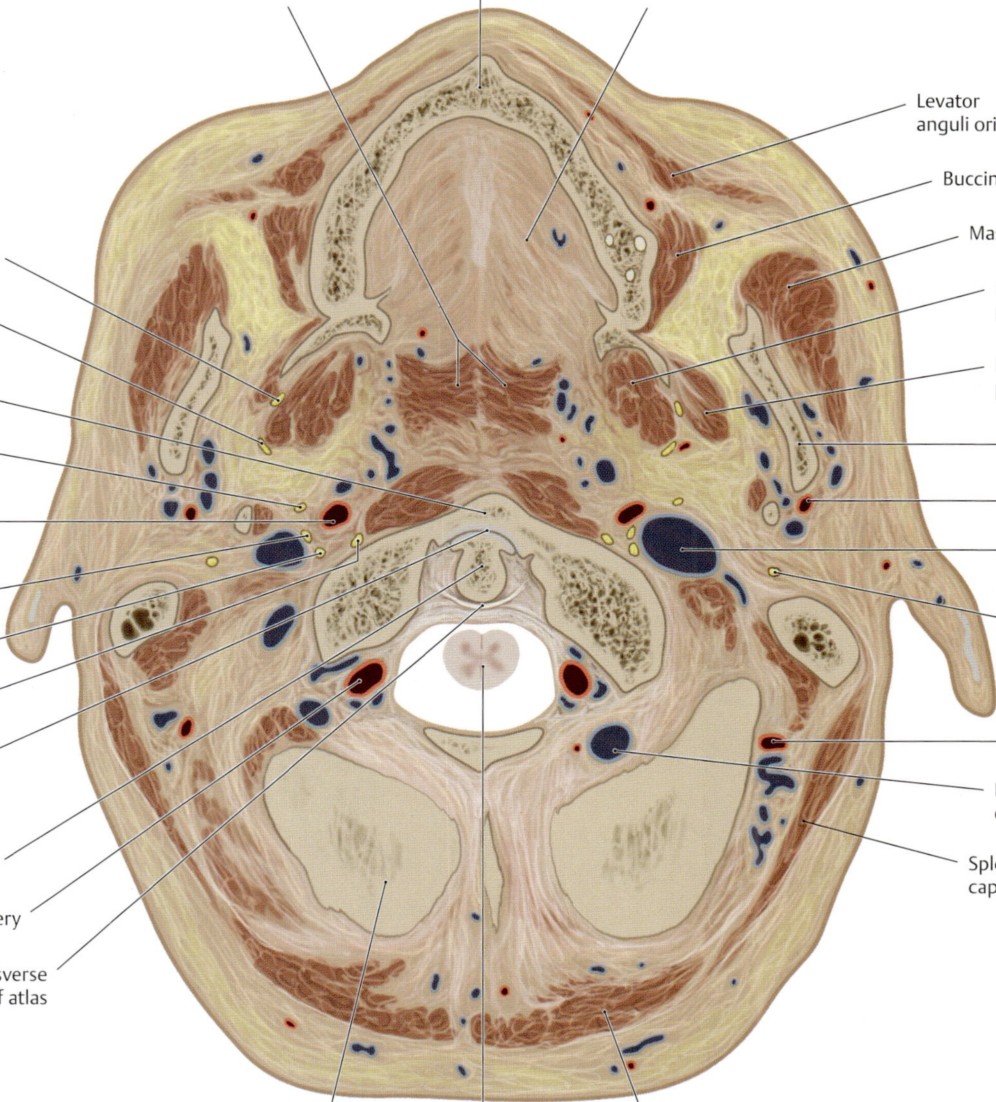

B Transverse section through the median atlantoaxial joint
Superior view. The section at this level passes through the connective-tissue sheet that stretches over the bone of the hard palate. Portions of the upper pharyngeal muscles are sectioned close to their origin. The neurovascular structures in the carotid sheath are also well displayed. The dens of the axis articulates in the median atlantoaxial joint with the facet for the dens on the posterior surface of the anterior arch of the atlas. The transverse ligament of the atlas that helps to stabilize this joint can also be identified. The vertebral artery and its accompanying veins are displayed in cross-section, as is the spinal cord. In the occipital region, the section passes through the upper portion of the posterior neck muscles.

7.6 Transverse Sections: C5–C6

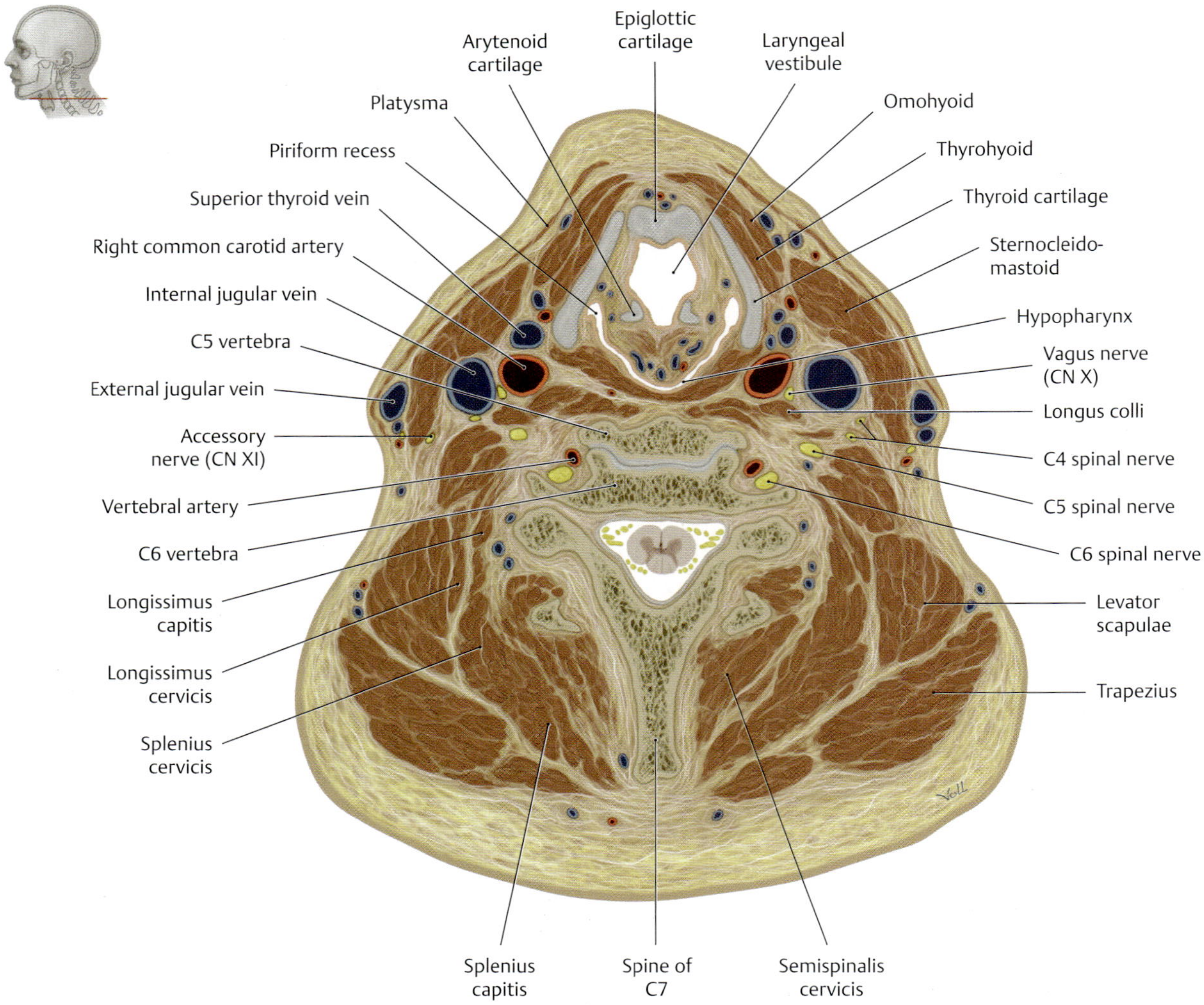

A Transverse cross-section at the level of the C5 vertebral body
Caudal view. The elongated spinous process of the C7 vertebra (vertebra prominens) is also visible at this level owing to the lordotic curvature of the neck. The triangular shape of the arytenoid cartilage is clearly demonstrated in the laryngeal cross-section. The laryngeal vestibule can also be identified. This view also shows the accessory nerve medial to the sternocleidomastoid muscle.

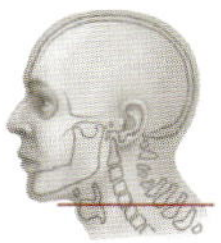

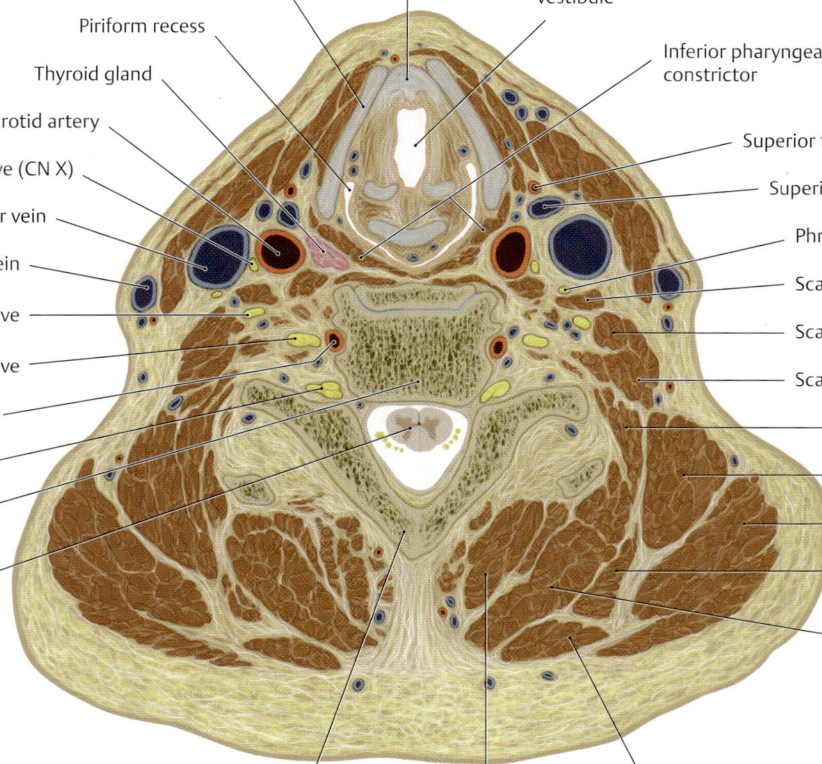

B Transverse cross-section at the level of the laryngeal vestibule, demonstrating the epiglottis (C6 vertebral body)

Caudal view. The piriform recess can be identified at this level, and the vertebral artery is visible in its course along the vertebral body. The vagus nerve lies in a posterior angle between the common carotid artery and internal jugular vein. This view shows the profile of the phrenic nerve on the scalenus anterior muscle on the left side.

7.7 Transverse Sections: Anatomy of the Neck from the T 1/T 2 to C 6/C 7 Levels

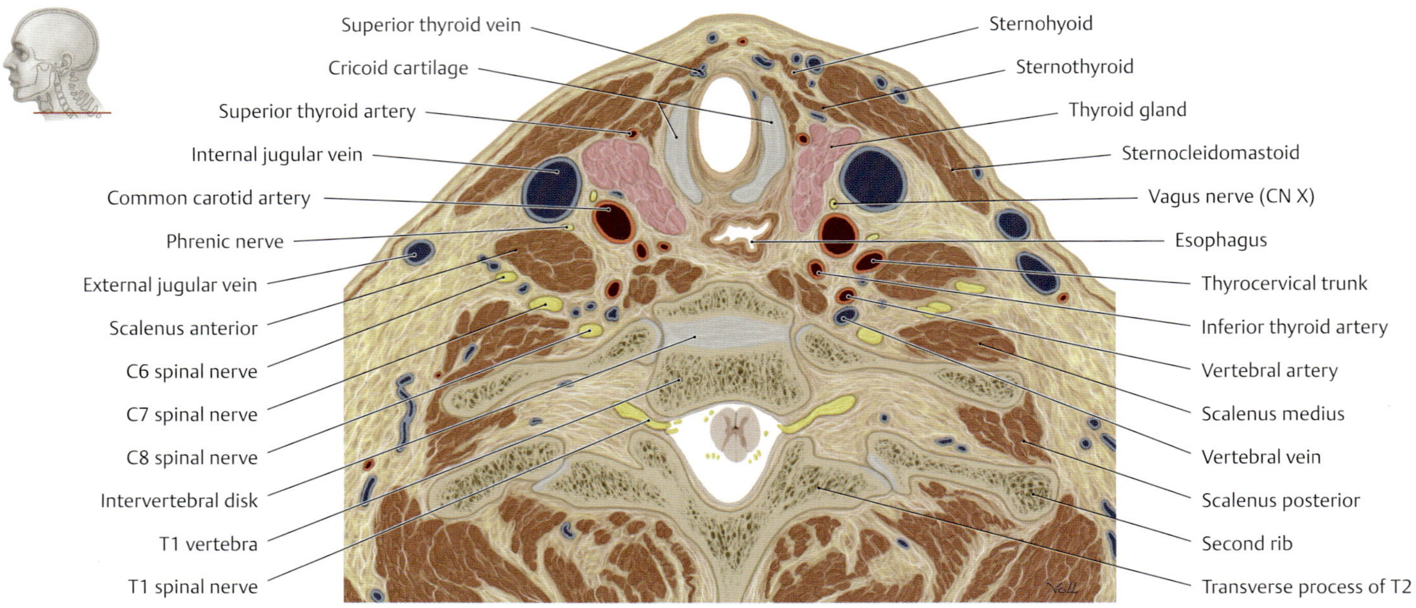

A Transverse cross-section through the lower third of the thyroid cartilage (junction of the T1/C7 vertebral bodies)
This cross-section clearly displays the scalenus anterior and medius muscles and the interval between them, which is traversed by the C6–C8 roots of the brachial plexus. Note the neurovascular structures in the carotid sheath (common carotid artery, internal jugular vein, vagus nerve).

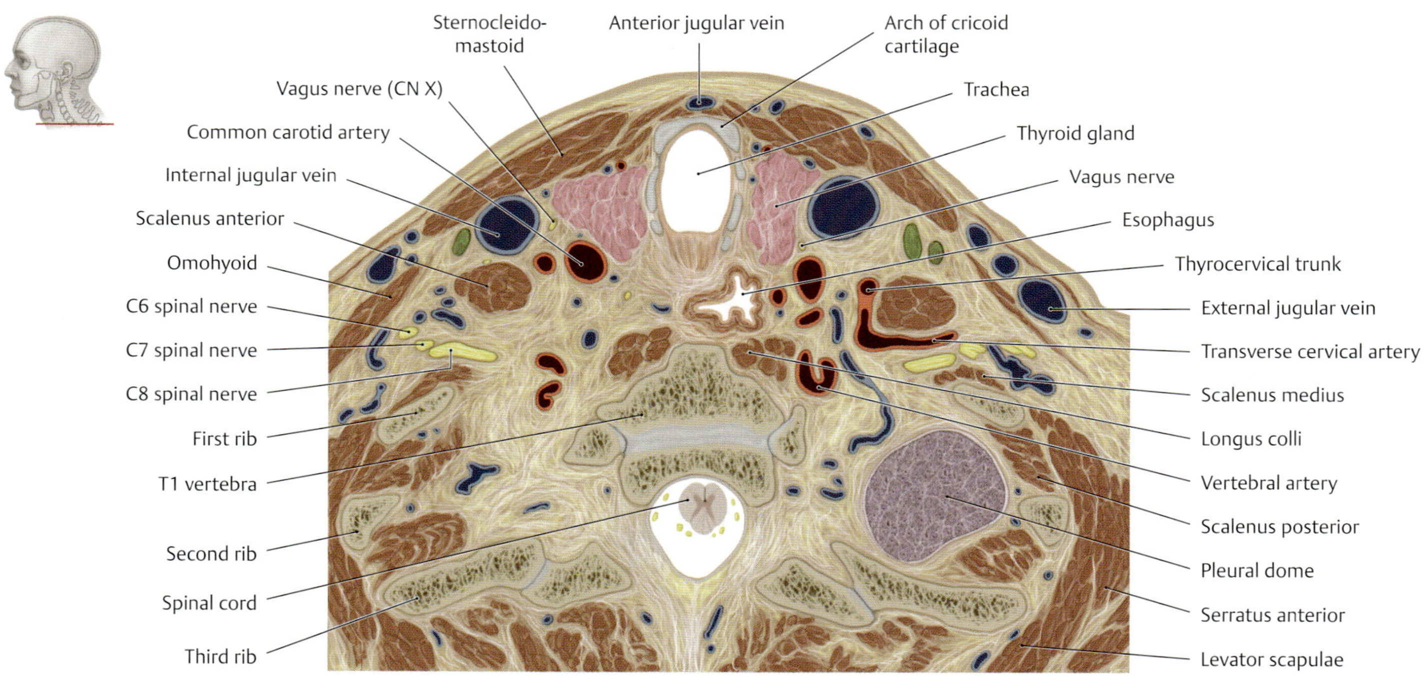

B Transverse cross-section of the neck at a level that just cuts the left pleural dome (level of the T1/T2 vertebral bodies)
Inferior view. Due to the curvature of the neck in this specimen, the section also cuts the intervertebral disk between T1 and T2.
Note that the cross-section is viewed from below like a CT scan or MRI slice. The illustrations that follow are transverse cross-sections through the neck at progressively higher (more cranial) levels (Tiedemann series).

The section in **A** includes cross-sections of the C6–C8 nerve roots of the brachial plexus and a small section of the left pleural dome. The proximity of the pulmonary apex to the brachial plexus shows why the growth of an apical lung tumor may damage the brachial plexus roots.
Note also the thyroid gland and its proximity to the trachea and neurovascular bundle in the carotid sheath (a thin fibrous sheet which is not clearly discernible in these views).

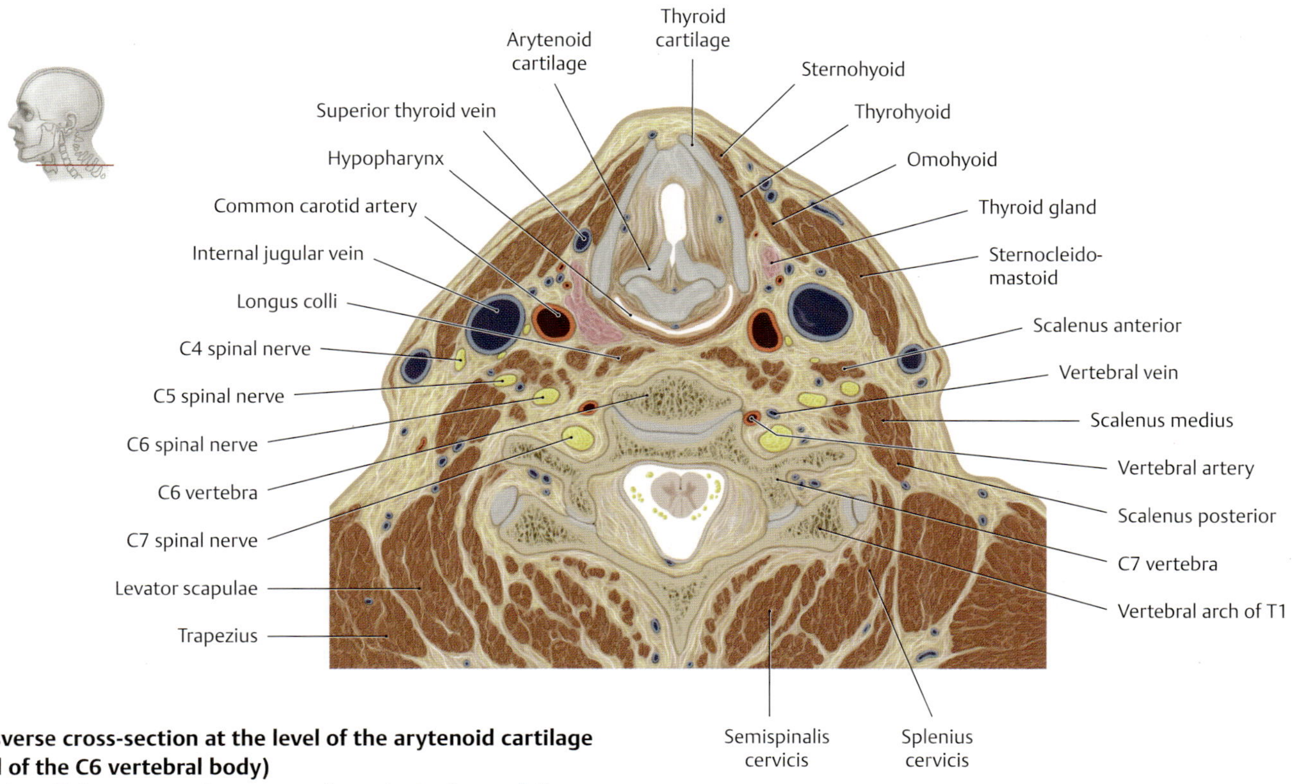

C Transverse cross-section at the level of the arytenoid cartilage (level of the C6 vertebral body)

Caudal view. This cross-section passes through the base of the arytenoid cartilage in the larynx. The hypopharynx appears as a narrow transverse cleft behind the larynx.

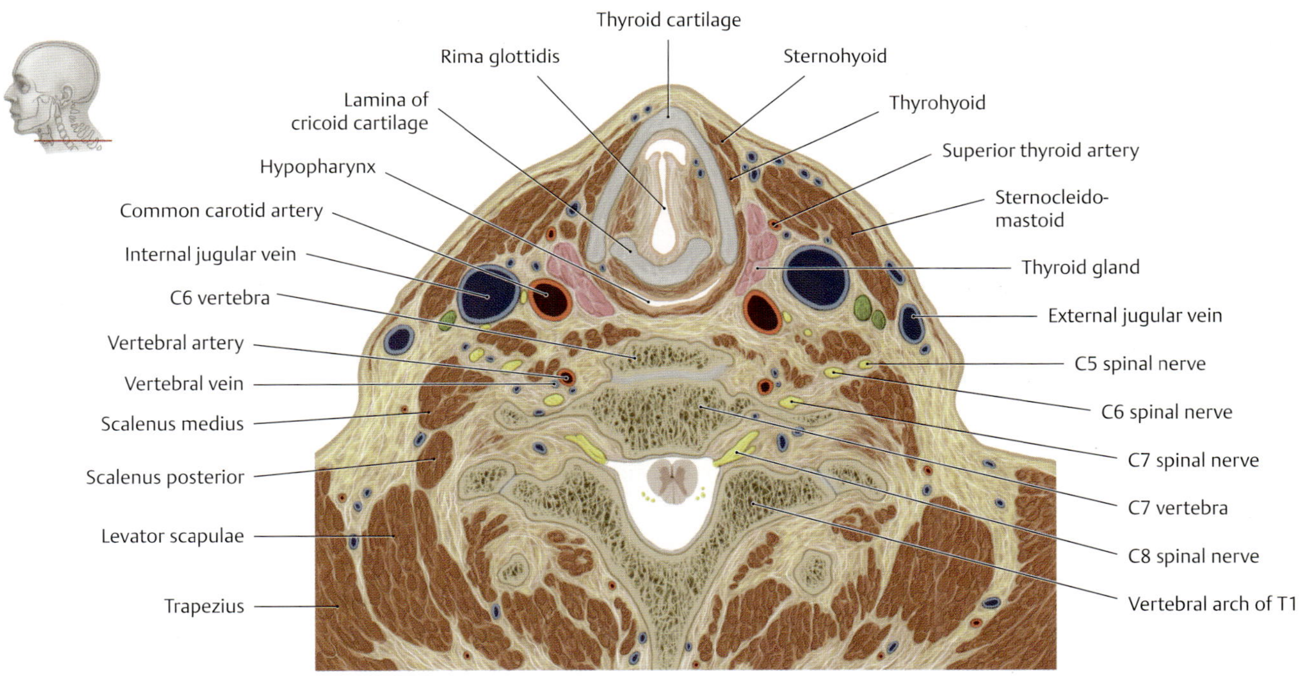

D Transverse cross-section at the level of the vocalis muscle in the larynx (junction of the C6/C7 vertebral bodies)

Caudal view. This cross-section passes through the larynx at the level of the vocal folds. The thyroid gland appears considerably smaller at this level than in views **A** and **B**.

7.8 Sagittal Sections: Nasal Septum and Medial Orbital Wall

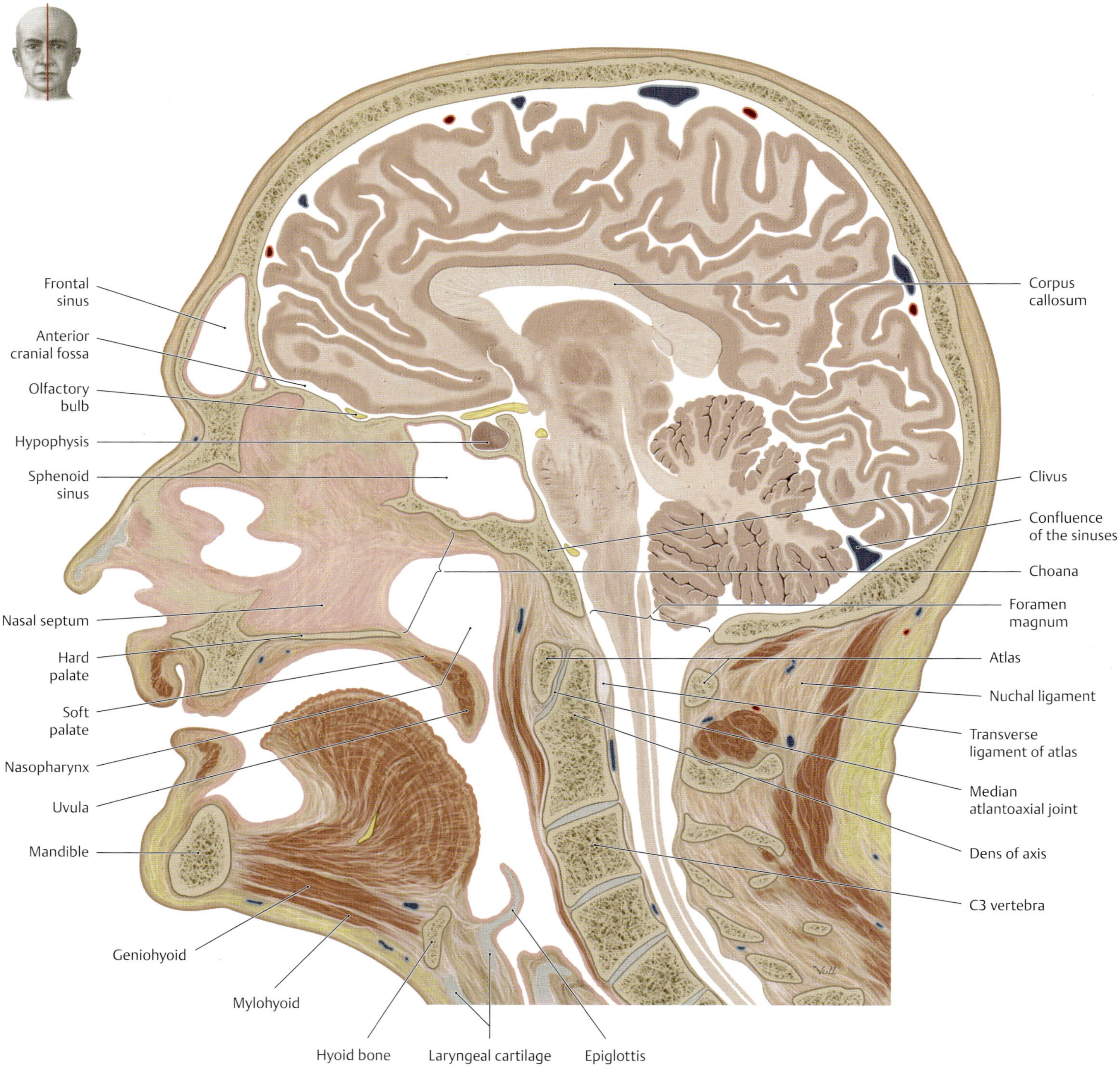

A Midsagittal section through the nasal septum
Left lateral view. The midline structures are particularly well displayed in this plane of section, and the anatomical structures at this level can be roughly assigned to the **facial skeleton** or neurocranium (cranial vault). The lowest level of the facial skeleton is formed by the oral floor muscles between the hyoid bone and mandible and the overlying skin. This section also passes through the epiglottis and the larynx below it, which are considered part of the cervical viscera. The hard and soft palate with the uvula define the boundary between the oral and nasal cavities. Posterior to the uvula is the oropharynx. The section includes the nasal septum, which divides the nasal cavity into two cavities (sectioned above and in front of the septum) that communicate with the nasopharynx through the choanae. Posterior to the frontal sinus is the anterior cranial fossa, which is part of the **neurocranium**. This section passes through the medial surface of the brain (the falx cerebri has been removed). The cut edge of the corpus callosum, the olfactory bulb, and the pituitary are also shown.
Note the median atlantoaxial joint (whose stability must be evaluated after trauma to the cervical spine).

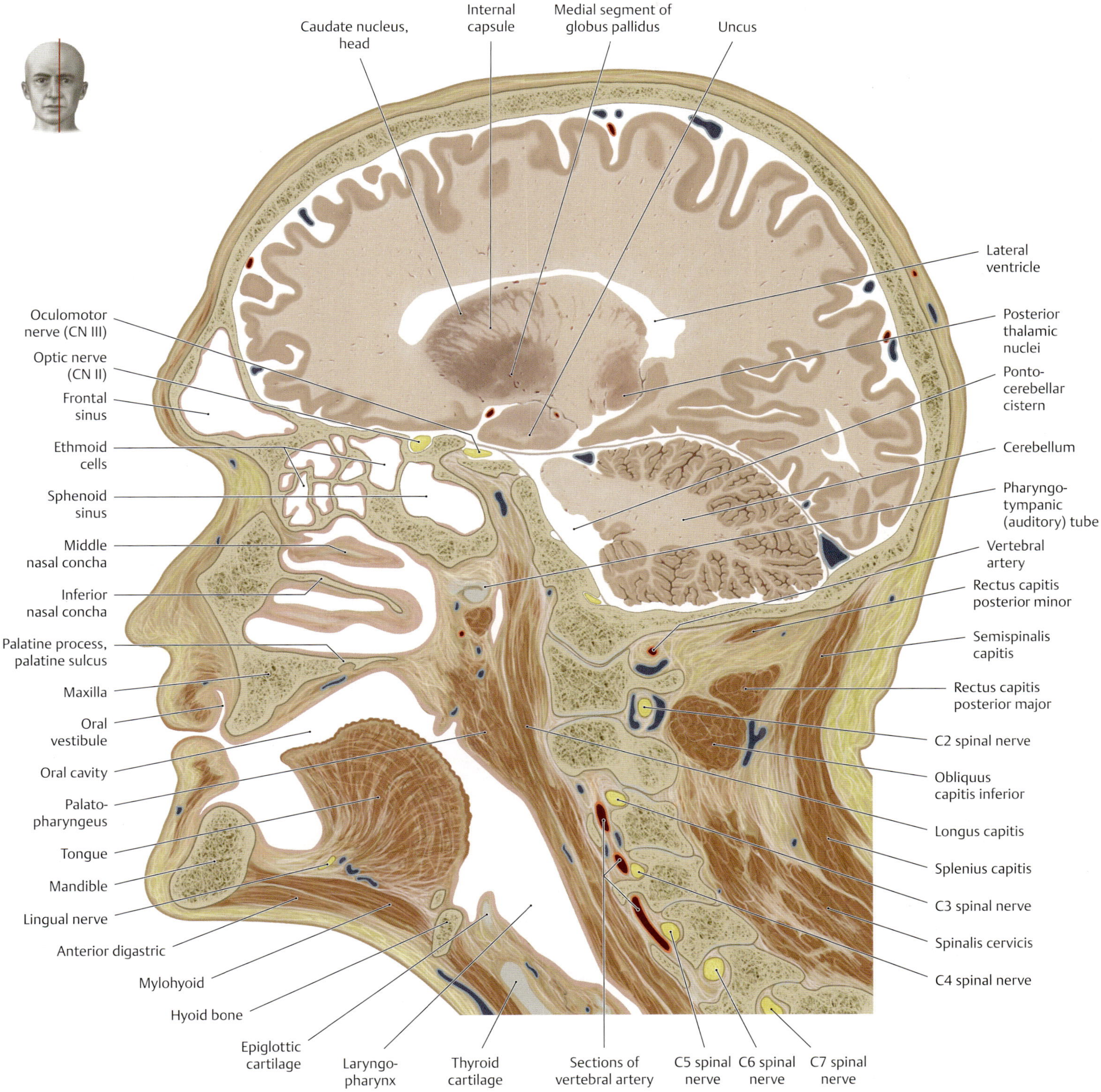

B Parasagittal section through the medial orbital wall

Left lateral view. This section passes through the inferior and middle nasal conchae within the nasal cavity. Above the middle nasal concha are the ethmoid cells. The only parts of the nasopharynx visible in this section are a small luminal area and the lateral wall, which bears a section of the cartilaginous portion of the pharyngotympanic tube. The sphenoid sinus is also displayed. In the region of the cervical spine, the section cuts the vertebral artery at multiple levels. The lateral sites where the spinal nerves emerge from the intervertebral foramina are clearly displayed.

7.9 Sagittal Sections: Inner Third and Center of the Orbit

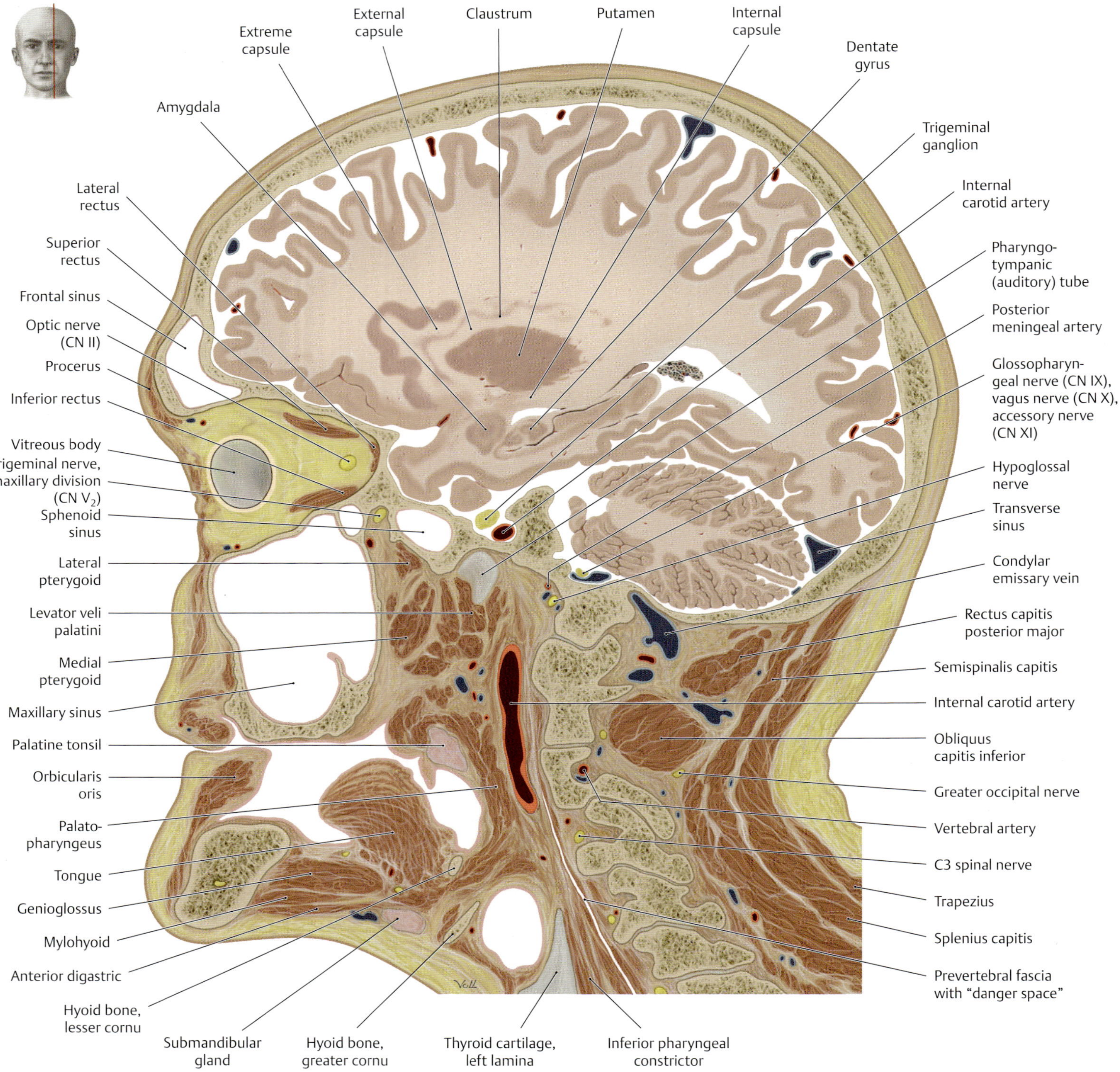

A Parasagittal section through the inner third of the orbit
Left lateral view. This section passes through the maxillary and frontal sinuses while displaying one ethmoid cell and the peripheral part of the sphenoid sinus. It passes through the medial portion of the internal carotid artery and submandibular gland. The pharyngeal and masticatory muscles are grouped about the cartilaginous part of the pharyngotympanic tube. The eyeball and optic nerve are cut peripherally by the section, which displays relatively long segments of the superior and inferior rectus muscles. Sectioned brain structures include the external and internal capsules and the intervening putamen. The amygdala and hippocampus can be identified near the base of the brain. A section of the trigeminal ganglion appears below the cerebrum.

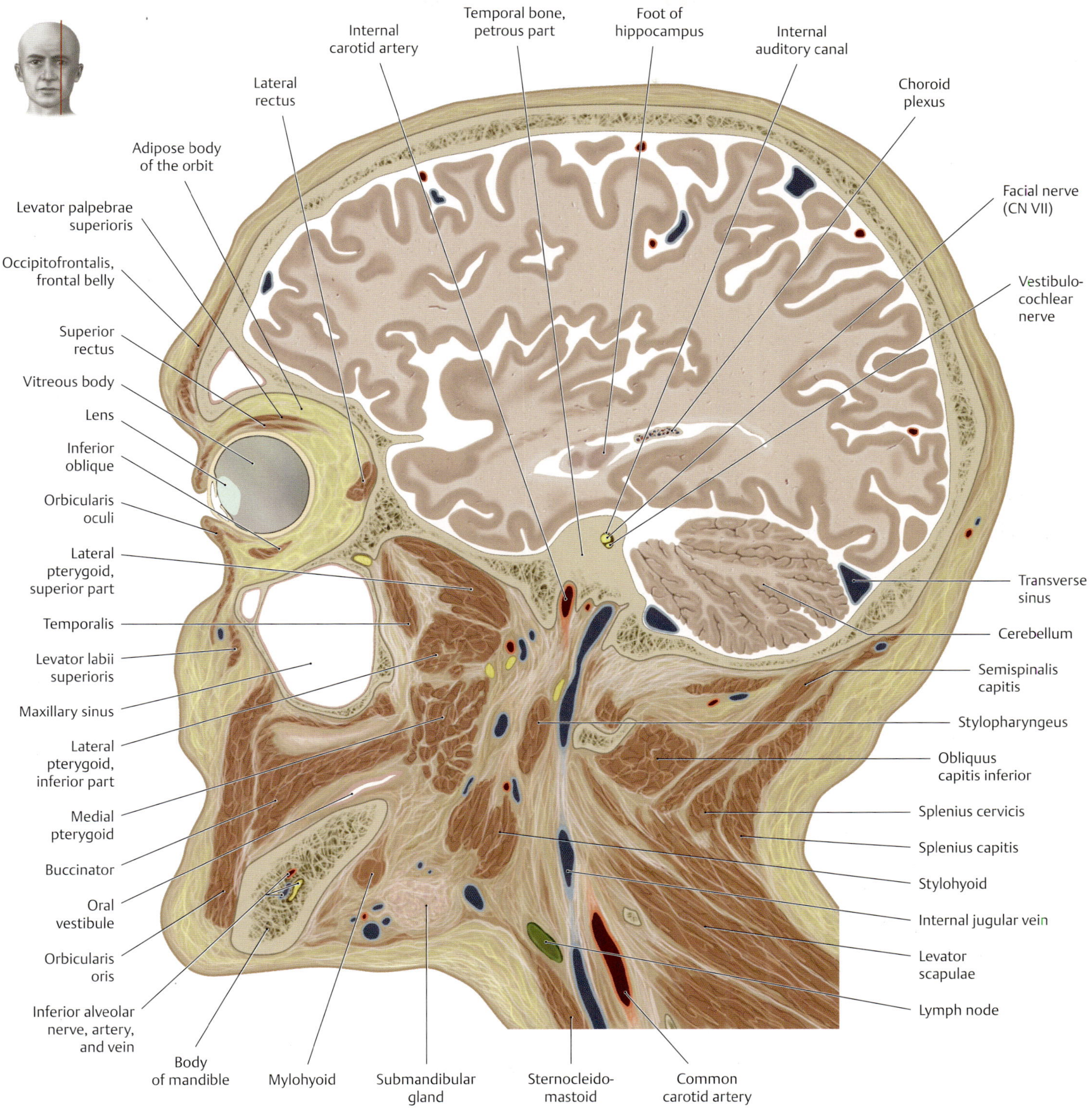

B Parasagittal section through the approximate center of the orbit
Left lateral view. Due to the obliquity of this section, the dominant structure in the oral floor region is the mandible while the oral vestibule appears as a narrow slit. The buccal and masticatory muscles are prominently displayed in this plane. Much of the orbit is occupied by the eyeball, which appears in longitudinal section. Aside from a few sections of the extraocular muscles, the orbit in this plane is filled with fatty tissue. Both the internal carotid artery and the internal jugular vein are demonstrated. Except for the foot of the hippocampus, the only visible cerebral structures are the white matter and cortex. The facial nerve and vestibulocochlear nerve can be identified in the internal auditory canal.

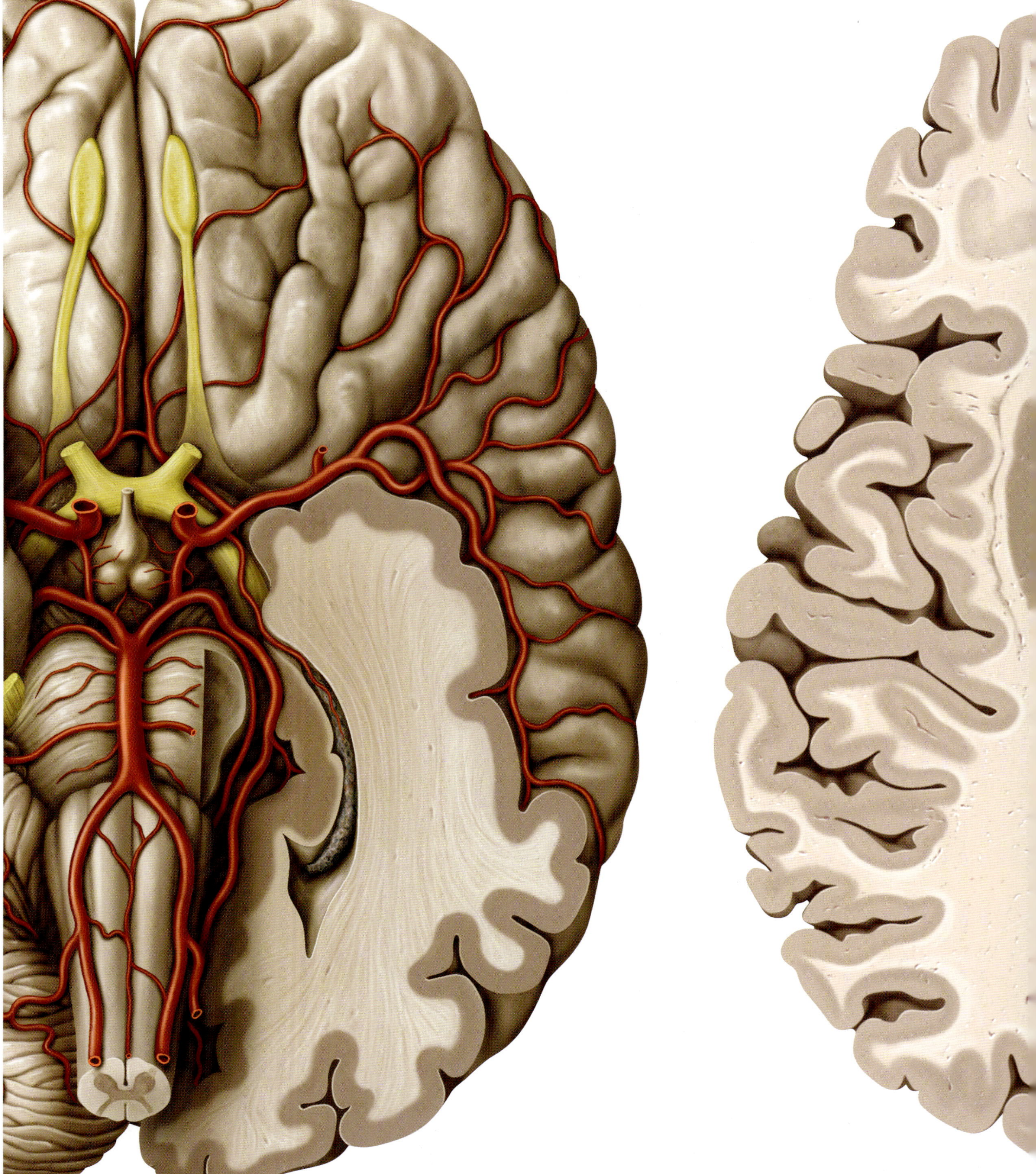

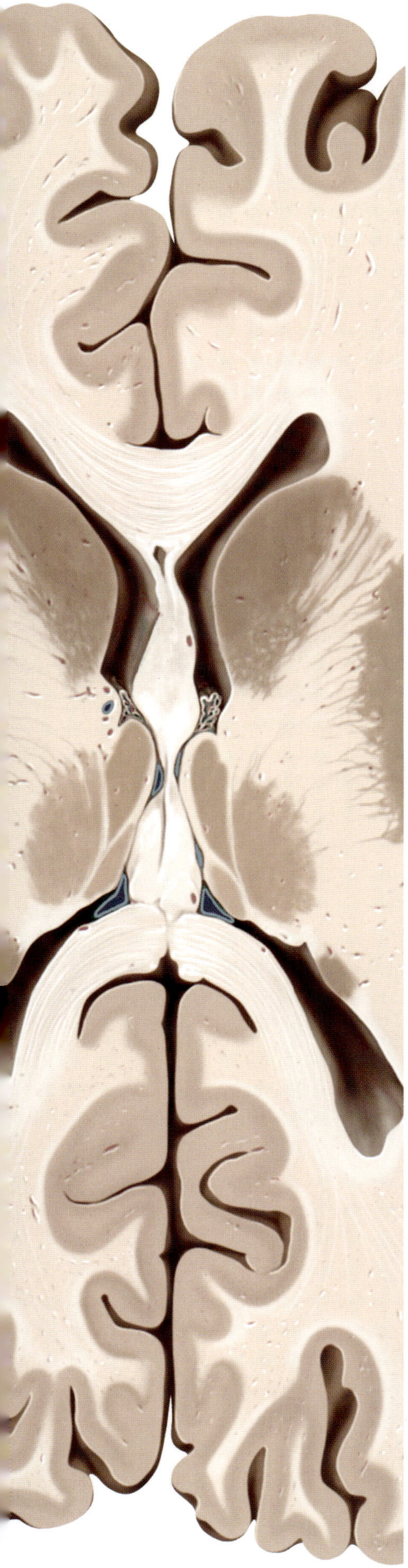

B Neuroanatomy

1.1 Organization and Basic Functions of the Nervous System

Introduction

The human nervous system is the most complex organ system to have developed in the evolution of life. Its function involves the perception of its surroundings and the detection of changes as they occur. It is responsible for responding to those changes with the help of other organ systems. At the same time, the nervous system is the only organ system with the ability to reflect upon itself and to consciously communicate with that of another human. It is this complexity and the aspect of self-awareness which makes the nervous system such an especially difficult subject of observation yet also explains our fascination with it.

Unlike the nervous system of animals, the human nervous system to a particularly large degree has the ability to learn, remember, conceptualize and show self-awareness as well as communicate with the nervous system of another individual through complex language. Disorders of the nervous system can significantly compromise the quality of life in affected patients. Thus, profound knowledge of the structure and the functions of the nervous system form the basis for prevention or treatment of diseases and are thus the foundation on which medical studies are based.

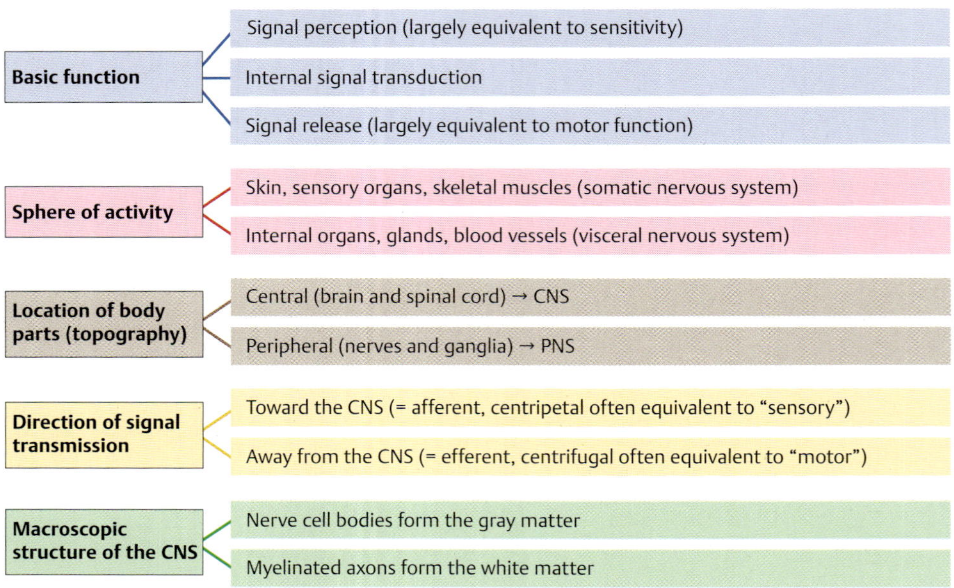

A Classification of the nervous system: Overview

The nervous system can be divided in various ways. It is this variety of criteria that makes an overall understanding of the nervous system seem initially difficult. In addition, every classification is artificial and always takes into account only specific aspects. Yet, knowledge of the structural classification makes for a much better understanding of the numerous interconnections of the nervous system without the need to memorize them all. The nervous system will be classified according to five different criteria. Each individual criterion will be explained diagramatically.

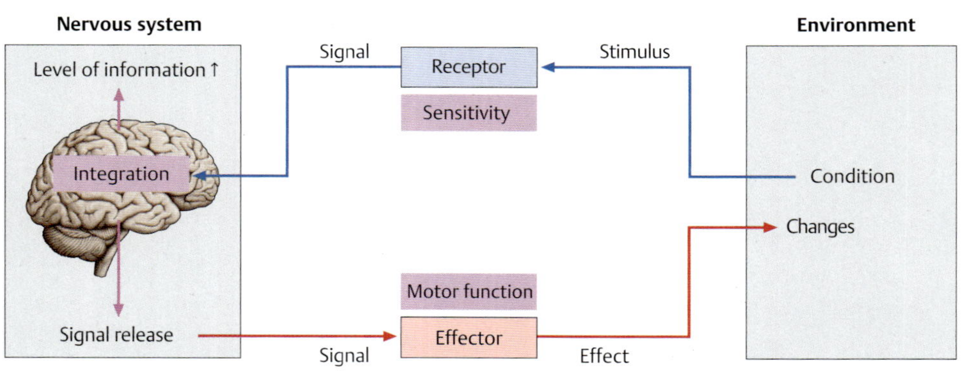

B Basic functions of the nervous system

The nervous system functions in processing information. It constantly communicates with the environment around us, both internal and external. The major functions of the nervous system are as follows:

- **Sensation** (sensory perception): The nervous system continuously receives information from the surrounding and inner environment, concerning physical and chemical stimuli. This information is
  - received by specialized receptors,
  - converted to a (mostly electrical) signal which is
  - transmitted through the nervous system.
- **Integration:** The nervous system
  - processes the information, which is coded as an electrical signal, within specialized, extremely complex structures in a very differentiated way, using electrical processing and
  - transmits it to effectors.
- **Motor function:** The effectors can now produce a response or an *effect*.

Note: The terms sensation, integration, and motor function are suitable to describe the basic functions of the CNS. That does not mean that every response initiated within the CNS can necessarily be attributed to motor function or that integration is always equivalent to signal transmission to an effector. Elevating the state of information within the nervous system (e.g., internal recognition memory, the formation of thoughts) is an integrative process, and the release of hormones is also an effect, which can be triggered by the CNS.

As a result of the diversity and complexity of particular stimuli in the environment, and receptors which are specialized in the reception of certain stimuli, comprise functional units—the *sensory organs*.

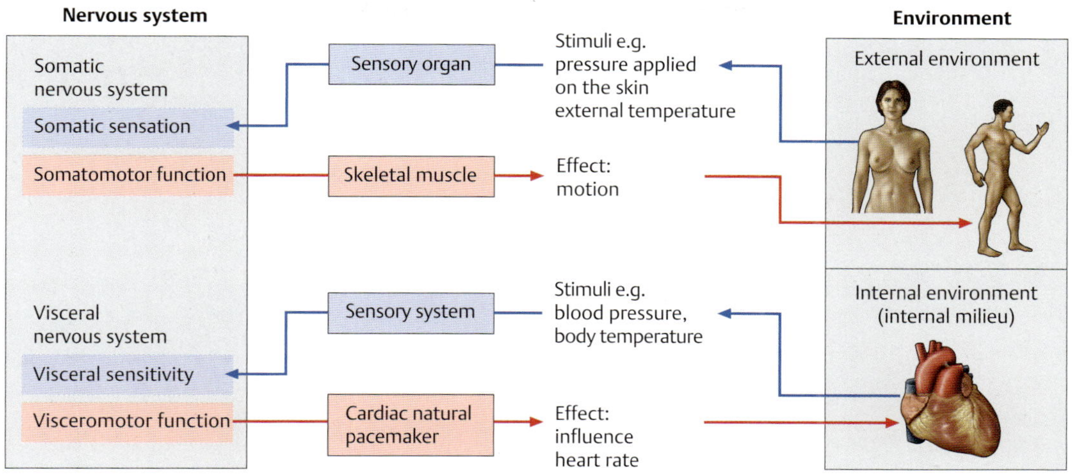

C Functional classification of the nervous system

Classifying the nervous system according to either the function (*functional classification*) or location (*topographical classification*, see **D**) of particular structures of the nervous system has proven successful, but take into consideration only certain aspects. The result is a certain degree of overlap in classifications. To a certain extent, the classification is somewhat artificial. Referring to the terms, sensation and motor function (as mentioned under **B**), requires a more precise definition of "environment":

- the "external environment" referring to the surrounding environment in which an organism lives
- the "internal environment," inside the body, with which the nervous system communicates, to maintain a state of homeostasis

Sensory perception (sensation), information about the external environment, is received through the skin or the sensory organs and the musculoskeletal system responds to those stimuli. The functional aspect of nervous system classification is represented through the *somatic* nervous system. The regulation of the internal environment occurs with the help of the viscera, with which the nervous system exchanges information. The part of the nervous system that communicates directly with the viscera is called the *visceral* nervous system. The combination of function (sensory, motor function) and location (somatic, visceral) can be subdivided:

- Interaction with the external environment is **somatomotor function** (see p. 286) or **somatic sensation** (see p. 284).
- Internal interaction is **visceromotor function** or **visceral sensation**.

Note: For visceral sensation, there are natural receptors, though they are usually not collected in their own group of sensory organs. The visceral nervous system is also commonly known as the autonomic nervous system (see p. 296).

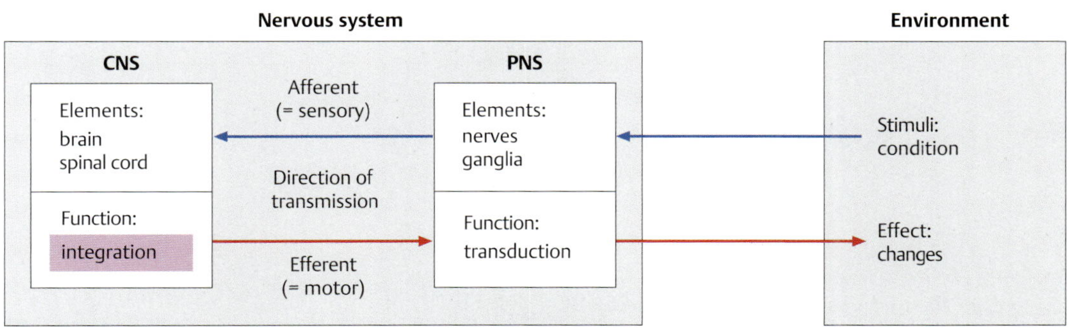

D Topographical classification and signal transmission

The nervous system can also be classified based on the *location* inside the body into

- the central nervous system (CNS) and
- the peripheral nervous system (PNS).

Note: Both the CNS and PNS contain portions of the somatic and visceral nervous system. The CNS consists of the brain and spinal cord, both of which are protected by being housed in bony enclosures (skull and vertebral column respectively). The PNS consists of nerves and ganglia (see p. 269) located outside the CNS and enclosed in a connective tissue sheath. With a few exceptions, it can be said that the function of the PNS is to carry signals and act as a "mediator" between CNS and the external environment or between CNS and effector. The direction of signal transmission in the PNS is of particular importance: carrying sensory information to the CNS is referred to as *afferent* transmission; signal transmission away from the CNS carrying motor impulses, is referred to as *efferent* transmission.

1.2 Cells, Signal Transmission, and Morphological Structure of the Nervous System

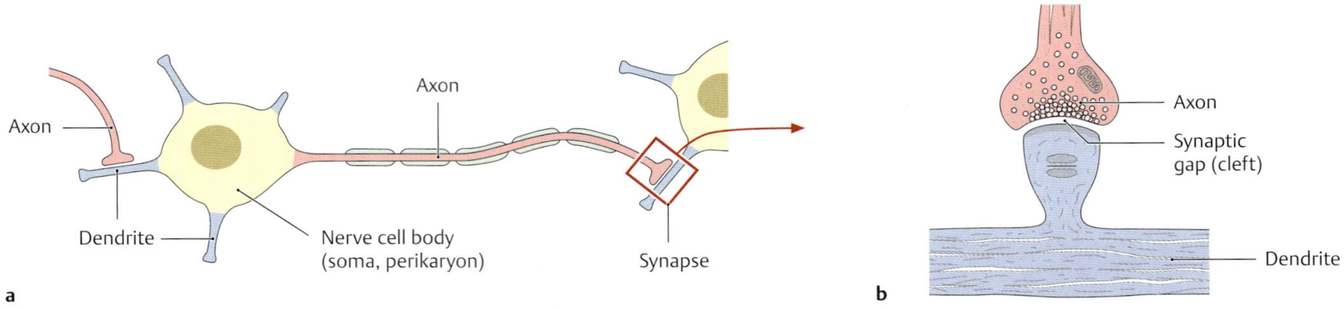

A Nerve cell and synapse

a Nerve cell: Both morphologically and functionally, the nerve cell (or neuron) is the basic structural element of the nervous system. Since nerve cells are found in both the CNS and PNS a distinction is drawn between *central* and *peripheral* neurons. Nerve cells generate electric signals, the *action potential*, and pass them on to other nerve or muscle cells. A number of types of nerve cells are classified based on their form and function. Their structure however, is largely similar. Attached to the cell body, are at least two projections of different length:

- the dendrite (dendron = tree), is typically short and highly branched (arborized); a nerve cell can possess one or more dendrites;
- the axon (neurite), which is typically longer than the dendrites and does not taper in diameter or exhibit tree-like branching; a nerve cell possesses a single axon. Axons can branch and give collaterals, which occur at roughly 90°.

In cases where there is a single dendrite, it is typically located at the opposite end of the cell body from the axon, resulting in a structural polarization, which corresponds to the functional *polarization of the neuron* (see **A**, p. 292): In dendrites, the electric signal always flows toward the cell body while in the axon it flows away from it. This flow pattern remains constant even if a nerve cell possesses numerous dendrites, some of which are not located opposite the axon.

b Synapse: Functionally speaking, nerve cells never work alone but are grouped together and transmit electric signals that are passed from cell-to-cell via junctions called *synapses*. At synapses, the axon of one nerve cell comes into very close contact with other cells. The unusual feature of this conduction is that in most cases it is discontinuous: There is a gap (synaptic gap/cleft) between the axon and the receptor cell where the electric signal is converted into a chemical signal (or transmitter). Usually, this transmitter generates another electric signal in the downstream nerve cell. The order in which signals are transmitted are electric → chemical → electric.
Note: In terms of their functions, one differentiates between *excitatory* synapses, which enhance the transmission of signals and *inhibitory* synapses, which slow down signal transmission. The nervous system is capable of producing excitatory and inhibitory signals (see **A**, p. 292).

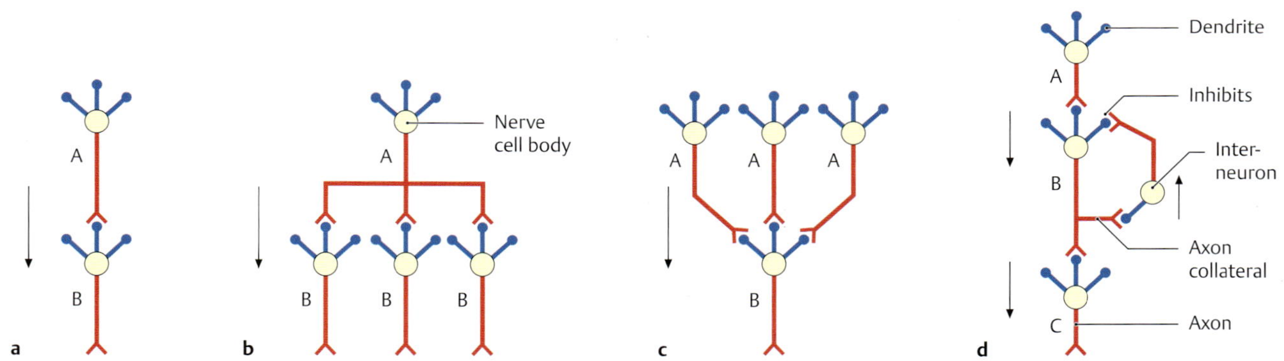

B Signal transmission within the nervous system: neural wiring
There are different ways in which neurons connect to each other to form neural networks:

a Neuron A sends its signal (projects to) neuron B: the transmission is 1:1.
b Neuron A sends its signal (via the axon‘s collateral branching) to multiple neurons B (here 3); the transmission is 1:3. There is a divergence as a result of the signal being passed to additional cells (the *megaphone effect*).
c Multiple neurons A (here 3) project to a neuron B, the transmission is 3:1. There is a convergence effect which can be used to filter information. For instance, neuron B will only pass on information if at least two A neurons send their signals simultaneously to neuron B (a *threshold* level or *filtering effect*).
d A nerve cell can be connected to other nerve cells via an interneuron. An example of this occurs in a phenomenon known as “recurrent” inhibition. A signal from neuron A stimulates neuron B which passes it on to neuron C. However, through axon collaterals, neuron B can inhibit the A → B synapse. Neuron B is temporarily numb for additional signals sent by neuron A. A time filter has been integrated: Only after a certain amount of time has expired will neuron B pass on the signals it receives from neuron A. This prevents the nervous system from being overwhelmed by continuous stimulation.

Synapse and wiring, excitation and inhibition, are important functional terms used to describe the nervous system.

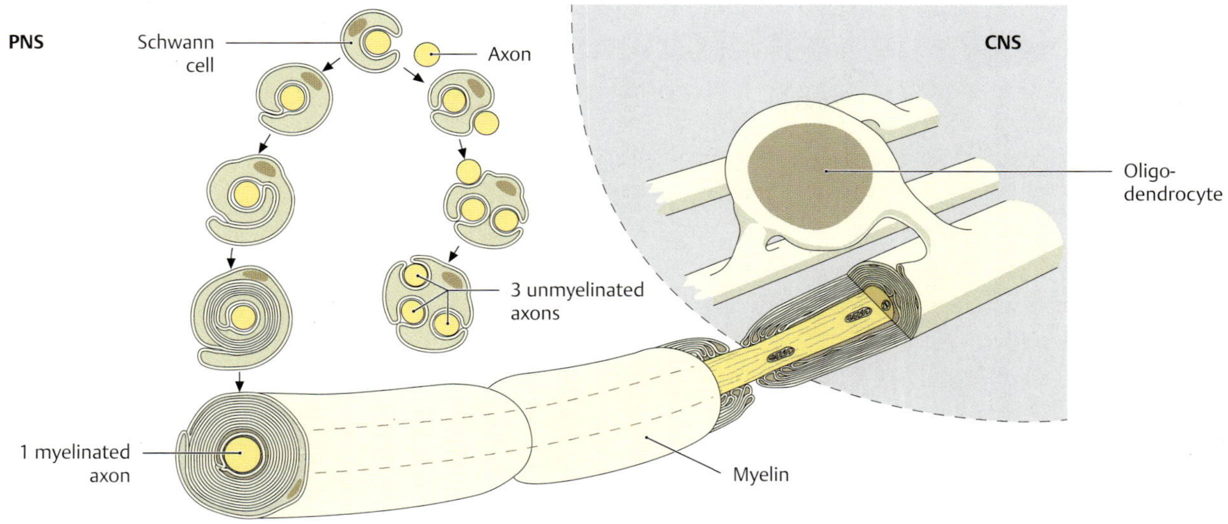

C Glial cells (neuroglia)

The other distinctive cell type of the nervous system is the glial cell (neuroglia). Some glial cells are found in the CNS (astrocytes, oligodendrocytes, ependymal cells, and microglia), while others (Schwann cells and satelite cells) are found in the PNS. Oligodendrocytes and Schwann cells don't carry nerve impulses but they are a crucial factor in determining the speed with which impulses travel through the nervous system. They accomplish this by forming sheaths around the axons of nerve cells, giving the axons different names based on shape and size of the sheath:

- **Myelinated axons:** multiple lamellar layers of glial cell membrane surround a single axon forming a distinct myelin sheath.
- **Unmyelinated axon:** a glial cell surrounds/supports multiple axons without forming a myelin sheath.

Different glial cells are responsible for myelination in each division of the nervous system. In the CNS, myelination is accomplished by oligodendrocytes; in the PNS that function is carried out by Schwann cells. Myelinated axons constitute the vast majority, outnumbering the unmyelinated ones. Since the sheath formation influences conduction velocity (myelinated axons conduct faster), this sheath is of utmost importance to the neuron's function. Other types of glial cells also support neuron function. They play an important role in regulating the environment of the nervous system (e.g., blood-brain barrier) and in providing protection against harmful agents.

Note: The axon/process + its glial sheath (myelinated or unmyelinated) = a nerve fiber. This term is very important for the following microscopic observation of the nervous system.

D Structural classification of the nervous system

Neuron cell bodies and axons are surrounded by neuroglial cells of differing types. Observed individually, they are visible only under a microscope. However, since they tend to group together, or form clusters, they are also macroscopically visible. Groups of nerve cell bodies appear gray and as such these areas are referred to as *gray* matter. The clusters of myelinated fibers appear white and are referred to as *white* matter. Dendrites, which are usually very short, and the few unmyelinated fibers get lost in the mass of cell bodies and are not observable via macroscopic observation. Depending on whether you are describing the CNS or PNS these groups of neuron cell bodies and myelinated axons/processes are described as follows (glossary, p. 502ff):

- In the **PNS**, nerve fiber-rich regions/structures are referred to as a nerve. Regions containing neuron cell bodies are referred to as *ganglia*.
- In the **CNS**, white matter is divided into tracts while the gray matter is divided into the *cortex* and *nuclei*.

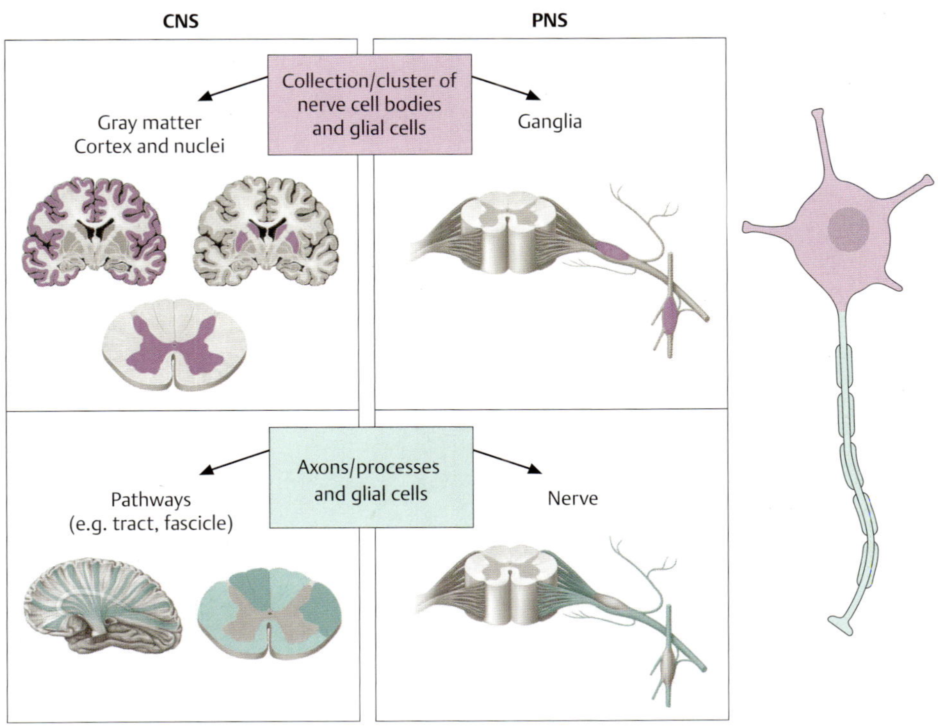

1.3 Overview of the Entire Nervous System: Morphology and Spatial Orientation

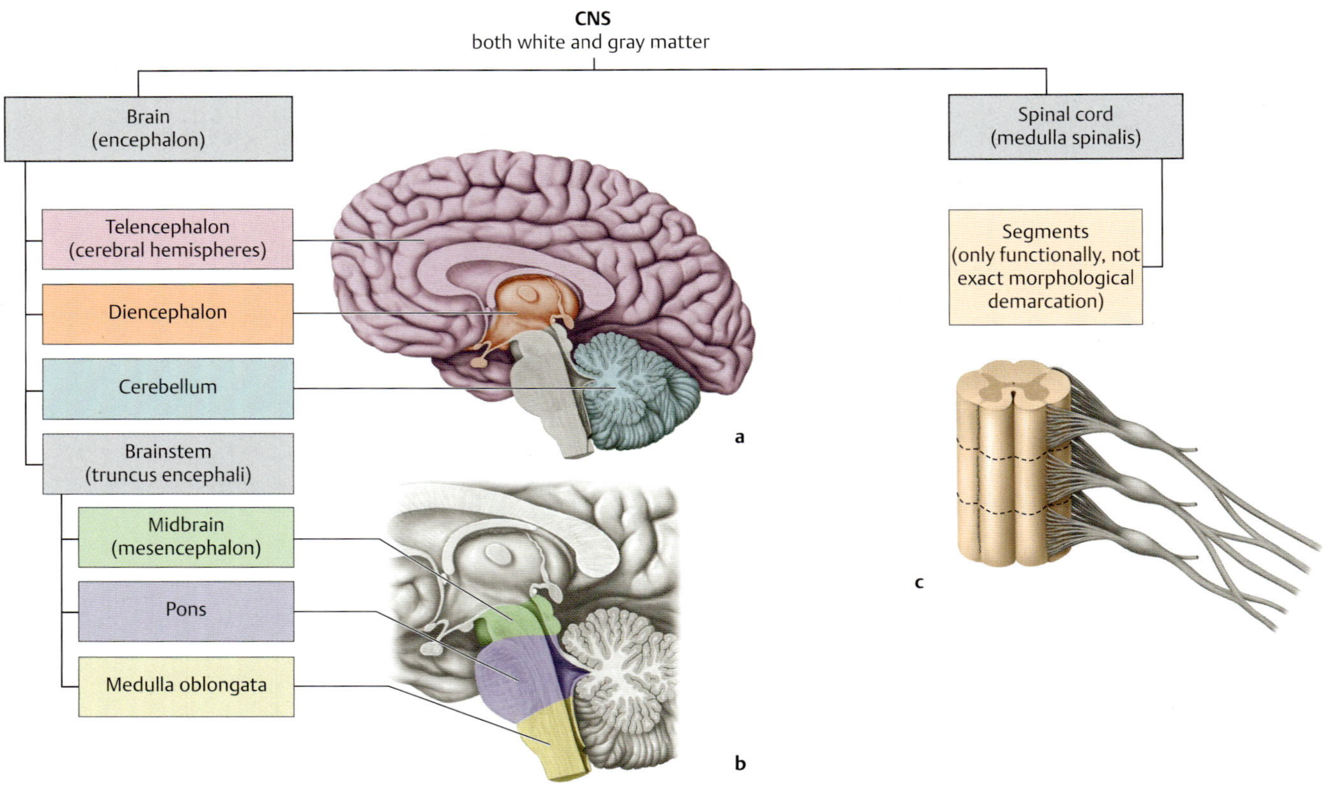

A Morphology of the central nervous system (CNS)
a and **b** Right side of the brain, medial view; **c** ventral view of a section of the spinal cord. A general morphological overview of the entire nervous system is necessary to help with understanding the material that follows. The CNS is divided into the brain and the spinal cord with the **brain** (**encephalon**) subdivided into the following regions:

- Cerebral hemispheres (telencephalon)
- Diencephalon
- Cerebellum
- Brainstem composed of the midbrain (mesencephalon), pons and medulla oblongata

In contrast, the other part of the CNS, the **spinal cord** (**medulla spinalis**) appears morphologically rather as one homogeneous structure. In terms of its functions, however, the spinal cord, can also be divided into segments. The division of gray and white matter is clearly visible:

- gray matter: centrally located, butterfly-shaped structure
- white matter: substance that surrounds the “butterfly”

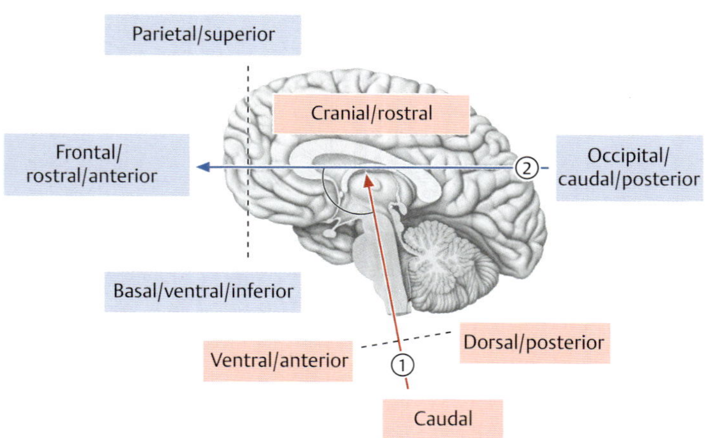

B Axes of the nervous system and directional terms
The same planes, axes and directional terms apply for both the entire body and the PNS. However, with the CNS, one differentiates between two axes:

- Axis No. 1 = Meynert axis: It corresponds to the axes of the body and is used to designate locations in the spinal cord, brainstem (truncus encephali) and cerebellum.
- Axis No. 2: Forel axis. It runs horizontally through the diencephalon and telencephalon and forms an a 80° angle to axis 1. As a result, the diencephalon and telencephalon lie “face down.”

Note: In order to avoid topographical misunderstandings, the following directional terms for axis No. 2 (Forel axis) are used:

- inferior or basal instead of ventral
- superior instead of dorsal
- frontal/rostral respectively instead of cranial
- occipital instead of caudal

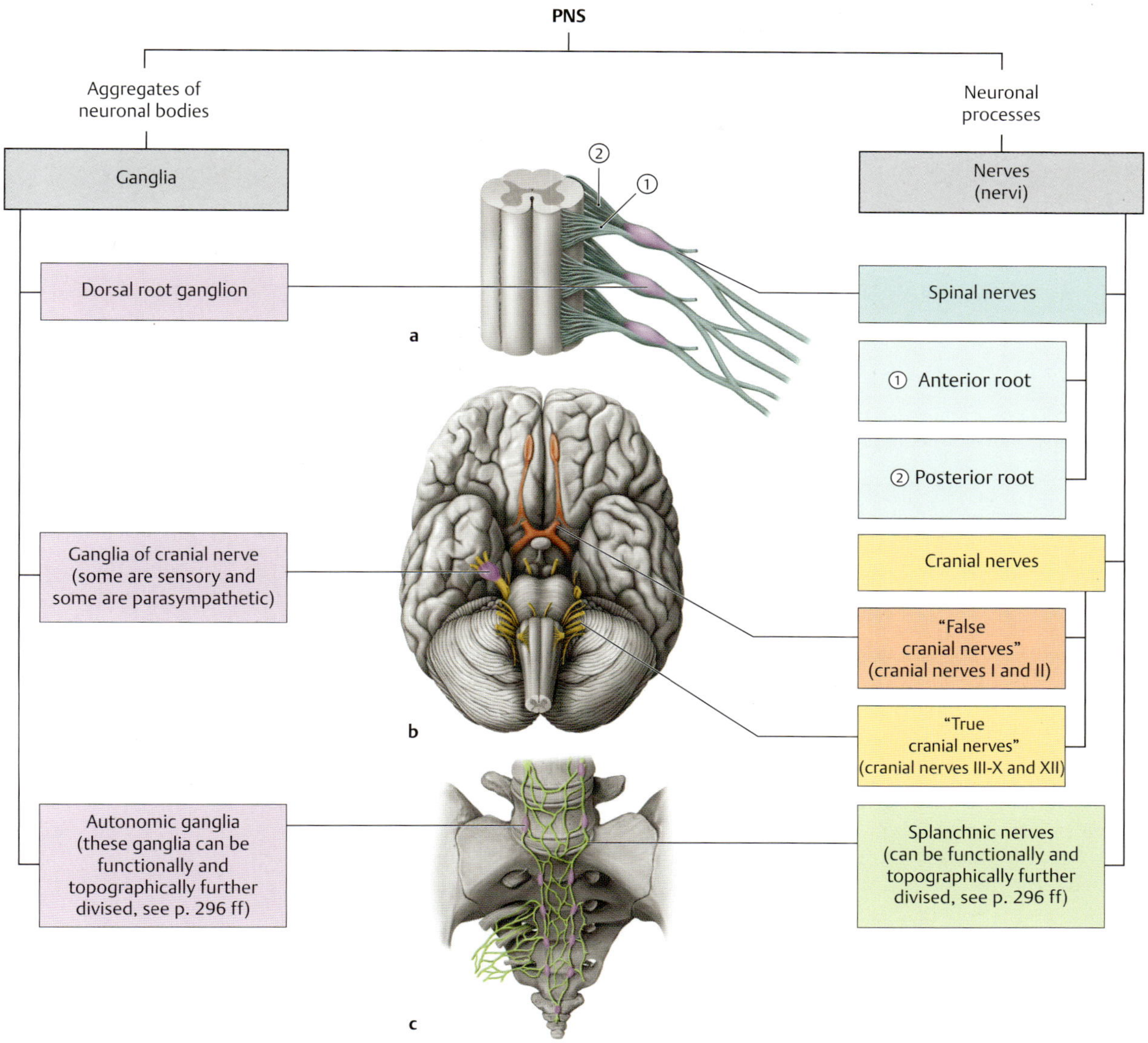

C Morphology of the peripheral nervous system

a ventral view of a segment of the spinal cord; **b** view of base of the brain; **c** view of sympathetic ganglia and nerves located anteriorly to the sacrum.

The nerves and ganglia form the peripheral nervous system and are generally named for the part of the CNS with which they are attached:

- Spinal nerves (connect the periphery of the body with the spinal cord). Usually 31 or 32 pairs. Spinal nerves (except those related to vertebral levels T2 to T11 or T12) generally have their ventral rami form plexuses for reasons of functionality (see **A**, p. 398).
- Cranial nerves (connect the periphery of the body to the brain, see p. 112 ff). 12 pairs.

Nerve cells found within ganglia (in the PNS) can be classified based on their affiliation with a particular functional division of the nervous system:

- Sensory neurons can be found within either division of nervous system. For the spinal nerves, the bodies of sensory neurons are found within the sensory (dorsal root) ganglia on the posterior (dorsal) root of the spinal nerve. For the cranial nerves, the bodies of the sensory neurons are found (with one exception) within the sensory ganglia associated with the appropriate cranial nerves that contain sensory fibers.
- Ganglia of the autonomic nervous system contain postganglionic sympathetic or parasympathetic neurons that control the organs of the body (see **C**, p. 297). Some autonomic ganglia are associated with splanchnic nerves. The autonomic nervous system also demonstrates characteristic plexus formation.

Note: The distinction discussed here applies except for a few special cases. These include the following:

- The optic nerve, which is not a true nerve but a part of the diencephalon.

For historical reasons, it has been called a "nerve," which is systematically false.

- The olfactory system: The olfactory bulb and tract are components of the CNS (not the PNS) because they have a meningeal covering. The olfactory nerve is composed of the aggregated filia olfactoria, which represent the fibers of olfactory cells. Their embryologic origin from the ectodermal olfactory placode gives this structure a special status as well.

Because of these peculiarities, the optic and olfactory nerves are often referred to as "false" cranial nerves (shown here in red) and contrasted with the "true" cranial nerves (III–X and XII, shown here in yellow), which are clearly part of the PNS. Cranial nerve XI is currently considered a spinal nerve with an atypical trajectory. In the interest of clarity, further details are omitted at this point (see p. 116).

1.4 Embryological Development of the Nervous System

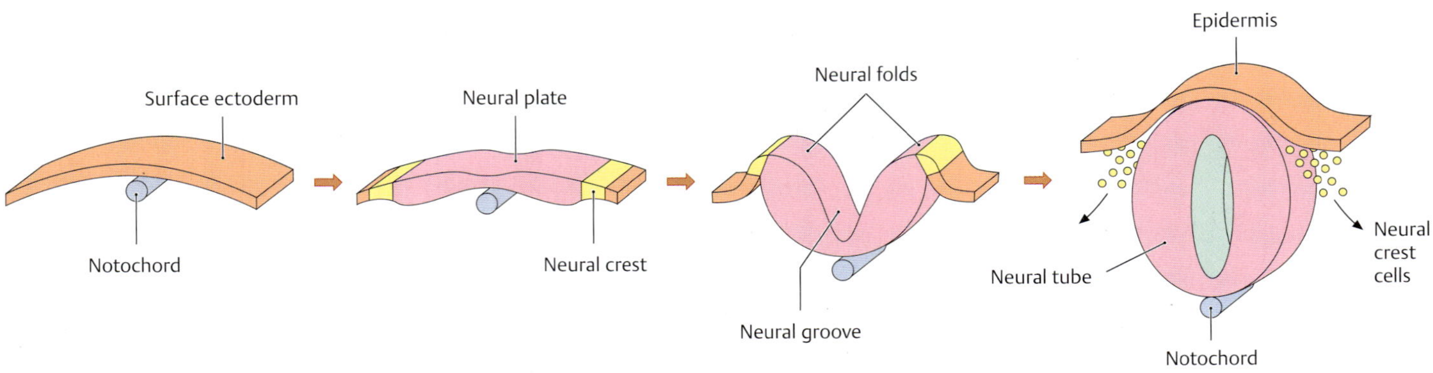

A Development of the neural tube, neural crest and their derivatives

The entire nervous system develops from the *ectoderm*, which in the third week of gestation differentiates into the *neural plate* and located laterally to it, the two neural crests. The neural plate develops a central *neural groove* between two peripheral *neural folds*. The now heavily invaginated neural plate detaches from the remaining ectoderm and closes over to form the *neural tube*. The cells of both neural crests exit the ectoderm and migrate to areas lateral to the neural tube. The **neural tube** gives rise to the following:

- In the central nervous system (CNS)
  - the brain
  - the spinal cord
  - glial cells of the CNS
- In the peripheral nervous system (PNS)
  - the somatic motor component of the spinal nerve and the preganglionic neurons of the autonomic nervous system (see **C**)

The **neural crest cells** give rise only to parts of the PNS:

- the sensory component of the spinal nerves and the sensory ganglia
- the postganglionic neurons of the autonomic nervous system
- the medullary part of the adrenal (suprarenal) gland
- glial cells of the PNS.

The cells of the neural crest give also rise to additional components such as melanoblasts (pigment cell precursors), which are not part of the nervous system.

Note: The neural *tube* provides material for the *CNS and PNS*; the neural *crest* provides material *only* for the PNS. The suprarenal (adrenal) medulla (not the cortex) is phylogenetically considered to be a part of the peripheral nervous system.

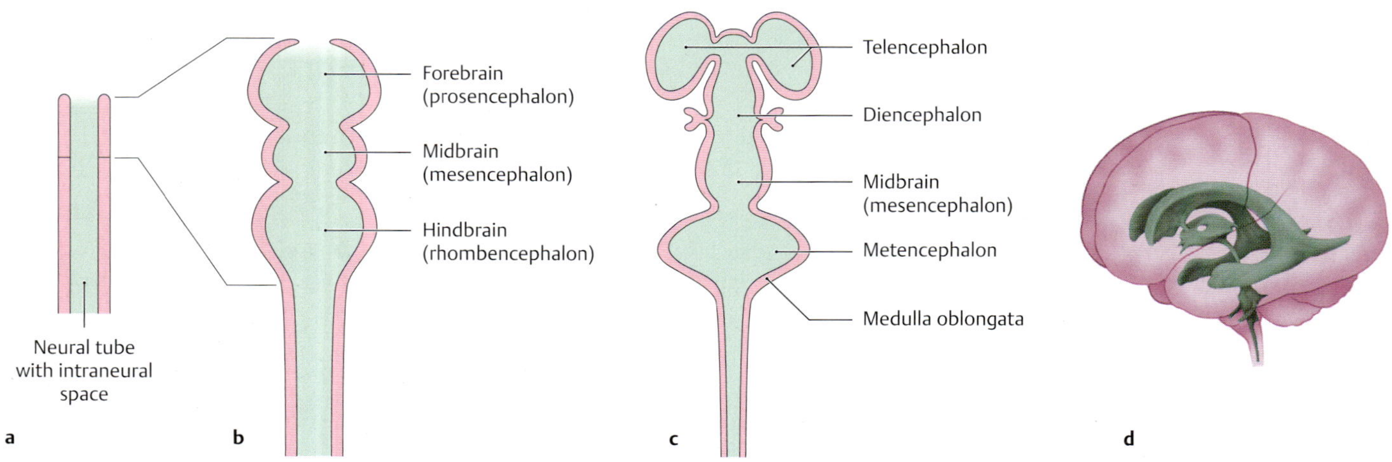

B Development of brain and subarachnoid spaces from the neural tube

Neural tube and its derivatives; dorsal view; in **a–c** the neural tube is cut open; **d** mature brain with subarachnoid spaces in situ.

From the initially undifferentiated neural tube (initially still open on both ends) (**a**), three *primary brain vesicles* develop (**b**). From these three primary vesicles the five *secondary brain vesicles* arise (**c**) from which the final components of the brain will differentiate. The lower part of the neural tube which is not involved in the development of the brain vesicles gives rise to the spinal cord. In the regions of the spinal cord, the shape of the neural tube is still visible (see **a**); in the regions of the brain, the shape of the tube is no longer discernible due to prominent vesicle formation.

Note: The cavity of the neural tube also differentiates at the same time as the brain vesicles and the spinal cord. It develops into the intraneural space, which is composed of the *four ventricles* (I–IV), the connecting *cerebral aqueduct*, and the *central canal* of the spinal cord, and will be filled with *CSF*; see p. 312.

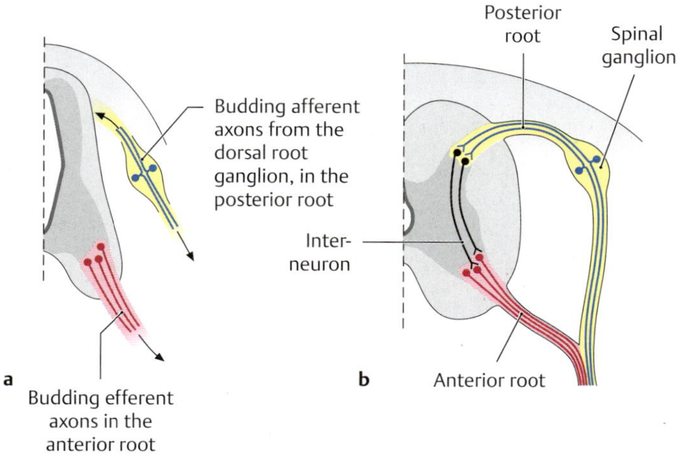

C Development of a spinal nerve
Afferent (blue) and efferent (red) axons sprout separately from the cell bodies of neurons during the early developmental stage.

- **a** The primary afferent (sensory) neurons develop in the spinal (sensory) ganglion. The α-motor neurons (anterior horn motor cells) develop in the basal plate of the spinal cord.
- **b** The interneurons (black), which form a functional connection between the two neuron types, develop at a later stage.

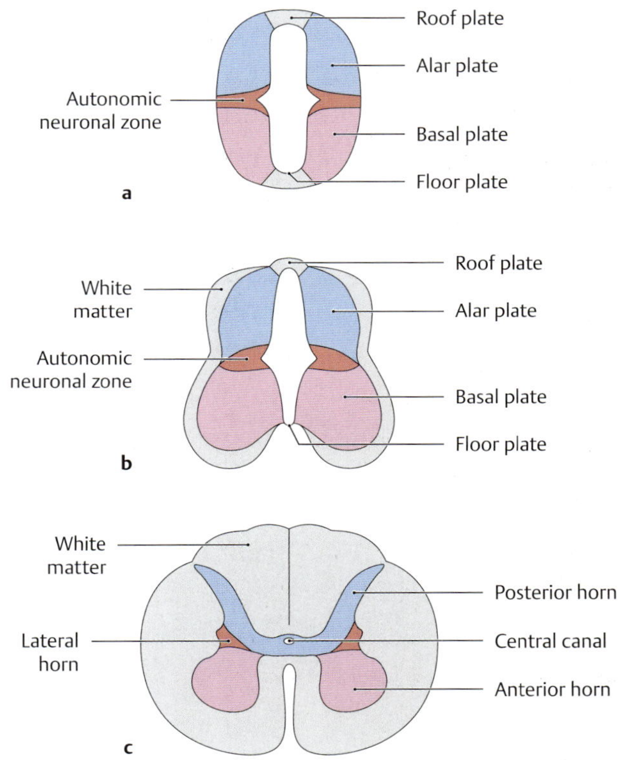

D Differentiation of the neural tube in the spinal cord region during embryonic development
Cross section, cranial view.
a early neural tube development; **b** intermediate stage; **c** final stage spinal cord.
Neurons, which originate in the basal plate of the spinal cord are efferent (*motor*) neurons; neurons, which originate in the alar plate, are afferent (*sensory*) neurons. In between—in the eventual thoracic, lumbar and sacral regions—lies an additional zone, from which the autonomic neurons originate. Roof and floor plates do not form neurons.

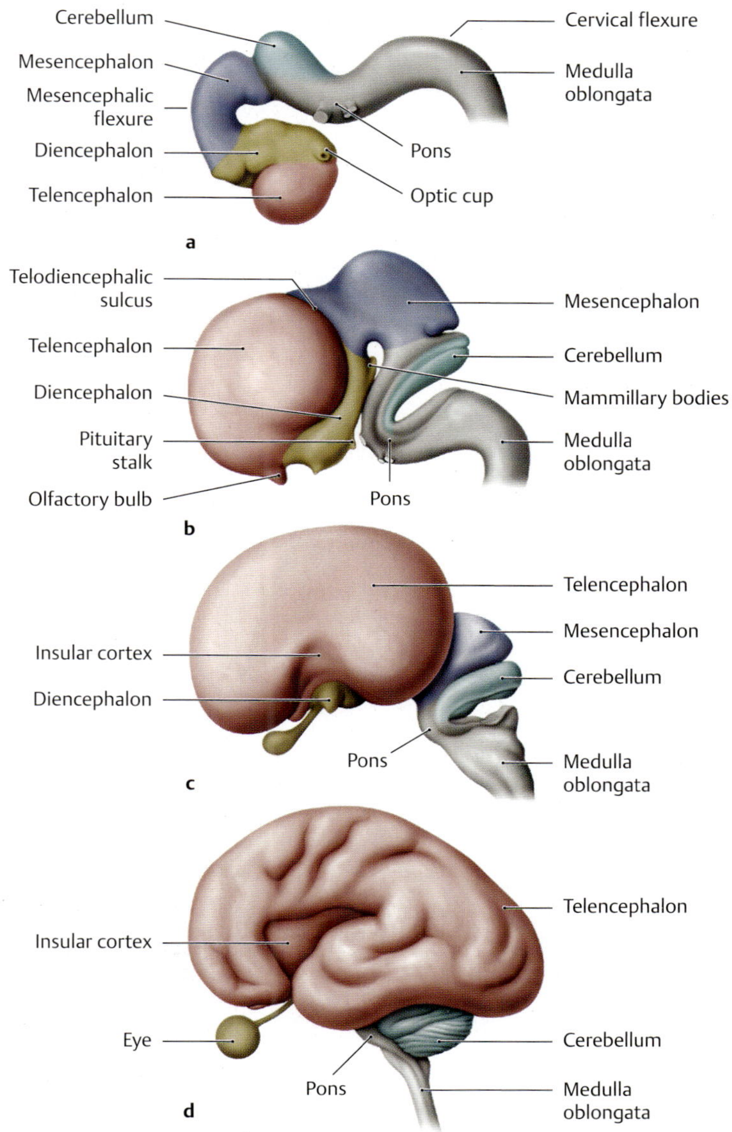

E Development of the brain from the neural tube

- **a** Embryo at a length of 10 cm, approx. second month of pregnancy. The eventual division of the brain (in its final form) is already visible:
  - Red: telencephalon
  - Dark yellow: (partially seen) diencephalon
  - Dark blue: midbrain (mesencephalon)
  - Light blue: cerebellum
  - Gray: pons and medulla oblongata

  Note: Over the course of development, the telencephalon enlarges substantially compared with the other regions of the brain.
- **b** Fetus at a length of 27mm, approx. third month of pregnancy. Telencephalon and diencephalon enlarge, the olfactory bulb develops from the telencephalon, the hypophysis (pituitary) stalk appears in the diencephalon.
- **c** Fetus at a length of 53 mm, approx. fourth month of pregnancy. The telencephalon begins to overgrow the other brain sections. The insula, which later will be covered by the other parts of the cerebral hemisphere is still visible on the brain's surface (cf. **d**).
- **d** Fetus at a length of 33mm, approx. sixth month of pregnancy. Fissures and gyri begin to form in the cerebral hemisphere.

1.5 Nervous System in situ

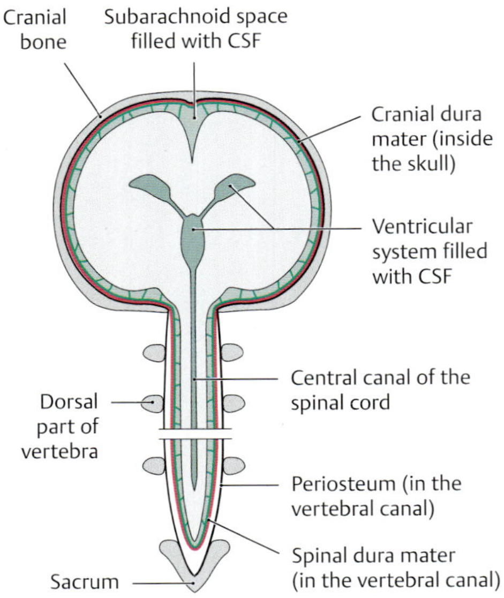

A Nervous system in situ

simplified schematic diagram of the CNS and its surroundings, coronal (frontal) section. Like any other tissue or organ, the nervous system is built into the overall structure of the human body. This integration is achieved through specific types of connective tissue, which help to provide mechanical protection against strain on the nervous system:

- **CNS:** The brain and spinal cord are surrounded by bone structures that form the cranial cavity and the vertebral canal, respectively. The connective tissue covering them are called *meninges*. These membranes completely cover the brain and spinal cord and can be divided into 3 different layers (see **B**). Meninges of the brain and spinal cord define a space which is filled with cerebrospinal fluid. The subarachnoid space can be topographically distinguished from the ventricular system (located within the CNS). Bony cavities, meninges, and the subarachnoid space accommodate the CNS into the body (for details see **B** and **C**).
- **PNS:** (not shown here, see **D**) has its nerves and ganglia surrounded by connective tissue, and as such is directly built into the body. The outer layer of connective tissue (*epineurium*) continues with the structures of the body also enveloped by connective tissue.

B The CNS and surrounding structures: The meninges

The calvarium has been removed. Superior view of the meninges; **a** and **b** brain in situ; **c** view of the dural folds after brain has been removed; **d** layers of meninges. The meninges of the brain and spinal cord—from outer to inner layer—are divided into

- **Dura mater** (pachymeninx), outermost layer surrounding the brain and spinal cord consists of tough, collagenous connective tissue. At the nerves' attachment to the CNS, dura mater merges with the epineurium covering them. Dura mater consists of an endosteal/periosteal layer and a meningeal layer. An epidural space normally exists only around the spinal cord, not around the brain. In the intracranial cavity, the meningeal layer of dura matter forms inward-directed folds that form the *falx cerebri, tentorium cerebelli*, and *falx cerebelli* that continue with each other and incompletely divide the cranial cavity into compartments (see illustration **B**, p. 298). Venous dural sinuses exist in certain locations (see illustration **C**, p. 283).
- **Leptomeninges**, which in addition to collagen fibers are composed of epithelioid cells (meningeal cells). No equivalent exists in the peripheral nerve. The leptomeninges consist of two layers:
  - *arachnoid mater:* Located directly underneath dura mater and the
  - *pia mater:* It is the innermost layer, intimately attached to the surface of the brain or spinal cord and is separated from the arachnoid mater by the subarachnoid space.

Note: Generally, the meningeal sheaths covering the brain and spinal cord are analogous.

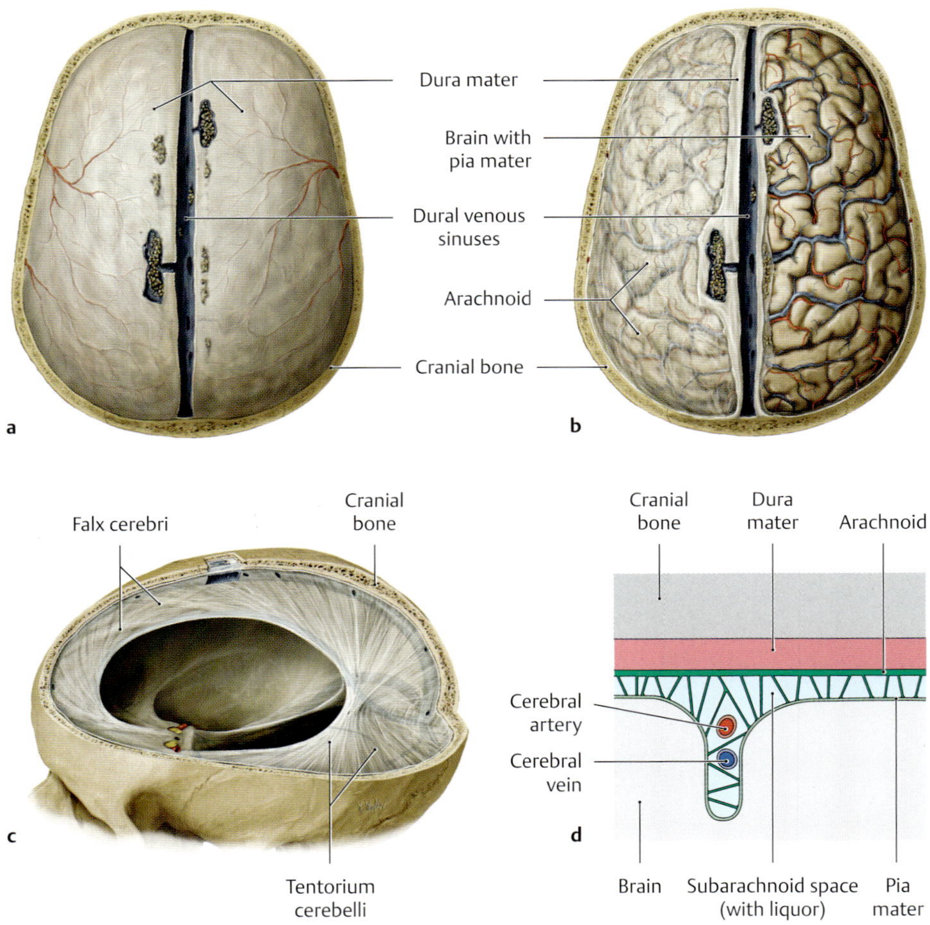

However, the relation between the dura mater (the outermost meningeal layer) and the surrounding structures in the cranial cavity vs. the vertebral canal presents differences that are clinically significant. In the *cranial cavity*, there is no epidural space under normal circumstances, whereas in the *vertebral canal*, a real space—the epidural space—separates the dura mater from the vertebral periosteum (for more details, see **D**, p. 311).

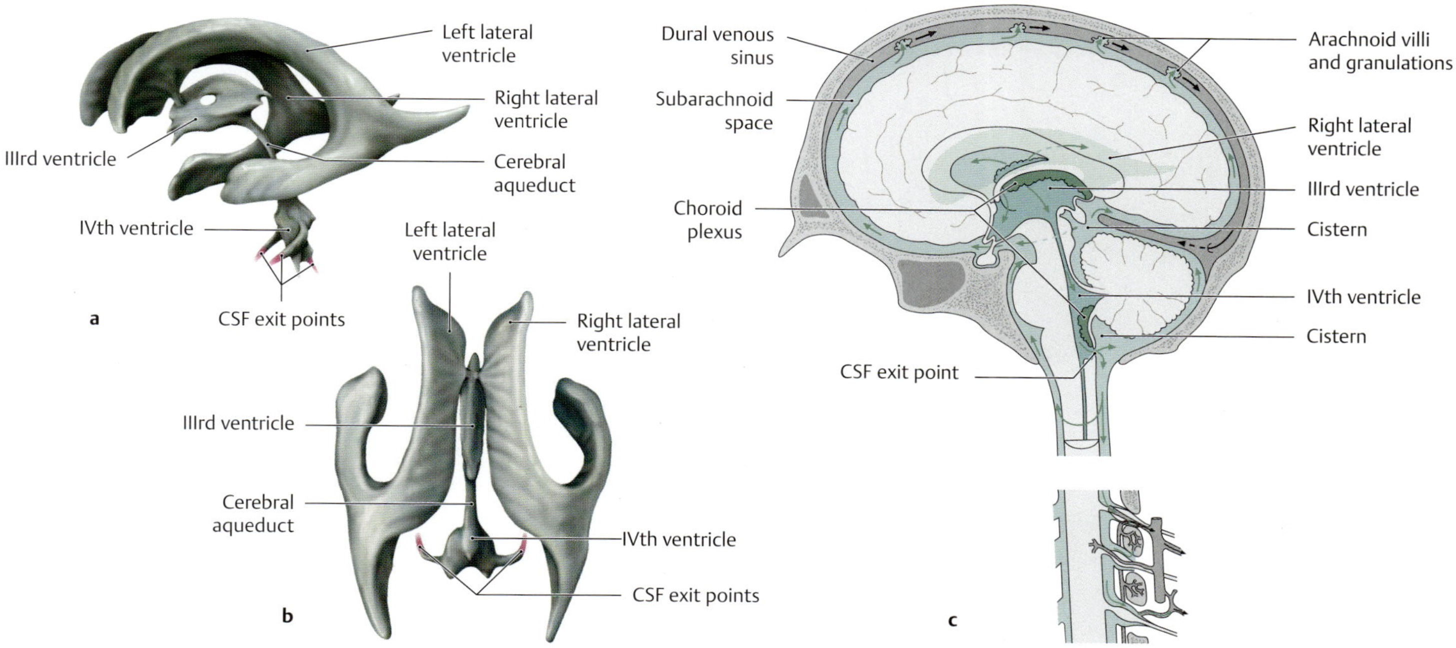

C The CNS and surrounding structures

Ventricular system, left antero-lateral view (**a**) and superior view (**b**); schematic sagittal section through the brain with the subarachnoid space and ventricular system (**c**).

The *subarachnoid space* surrounds both the brain and the spinal cord and is located between the arachnoid and pia mater. Topographically, it represents the *extraneural* CSF space that is connected with the *intraneural* CSF space—the ventricular system which is composed of four ventricles and the cerebral aqueduct (in the brain) and the central canal (in the spinal cord).

- In the four ventricles of the **ventricular system**, the cerebrospinal fluid is continuously produced by functionally specialized structures known as the choroid plexus. Due to the pressure gradient, the cerebrospinal fluid exits the fourth ventricle, located in the brain stem, through specific openings and flows into the subarachnoid space. The red-colored areas in (**b**) mark the junction/continuity of the ventricular system with the subarachnoid space.
- In the **subarachnoid space**, the cerebrospinal fluid is constantly reabsorbed into the dural venous system through functionally specialized structures—the arachnoid villi/granulations. The CSF is produced constantly, without a feedback mechanism.

The cavity of the neural tube and its folding forms the ventricular system that has a distinct shape (see **A**, p. 272). The subarachnoid space is a result of the CNS being surrounded by the meningeal layers. Its distinct shape is derived from the shape of the brain and spinal cord and how they are surrounded by the meninges. The convex surface of the brain does not conform everywhere to the internal concave surface of the cranium which leads to the creation of topographically characteristic "enlargements" of the subarachnoid spaces, known as the cisterns. They do not serve a particular function but are the inevitable result of two shapes that are not wholly congruent.

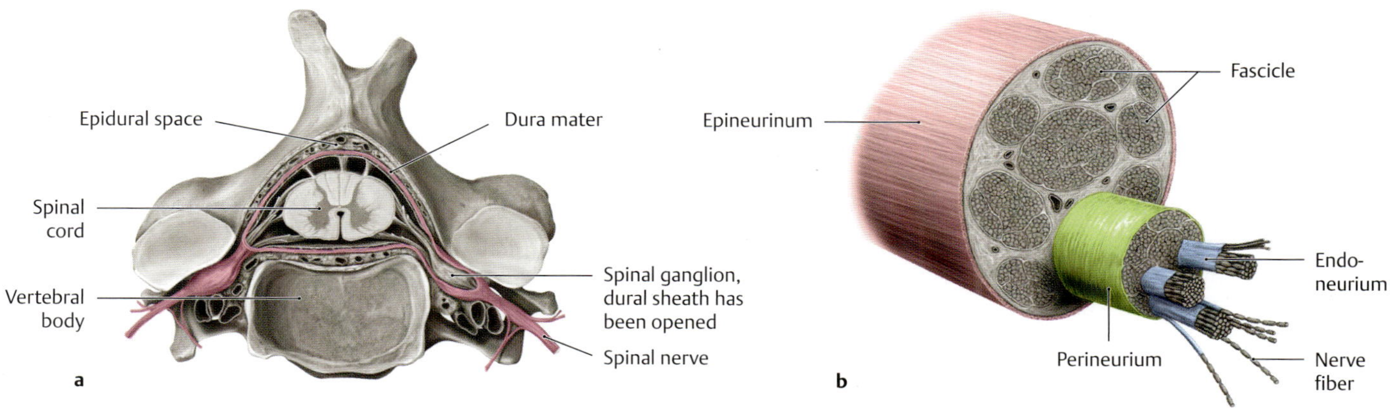

D The peripheral nerve and surrounding structures: The epineurium

a Section through the vertebral canal with spinal cord; **b** peripheral nerve, "pulled out in a telescopic fashion." The spinal cord (**a**) is surrounded by meninges in a similar way as the brain (see **B**). It is clearly visible that

- the dura mater (red in **a**) merges with the epineurium of the peripheral nerve,
- the dura mater around the spinal cord (unlike the cranial dura mater) is not firmly attached to the bone or the inner periosteum. There is a distinct epidural space filled with fat and a venous plexus.

The peripheral nerve has a cable-like structure. Its outer surface is completely covered by connective tissue, the *epineurium*. The nerve is composed of fascicles (nerve fiber bundles) which are covered by their own connective tissue sheath—the *perineurium*. In the fascicles, individual nerve fibers are covered by *endoneurium*. In cranial and spinal nerves, the epineurium is the continuation of dura mater. The connective tissue sheath that surrounds the peripheral ganglion corresponds to the epineurium.

1.6 Overview of the Brain: Telencephalon and Diencephalon

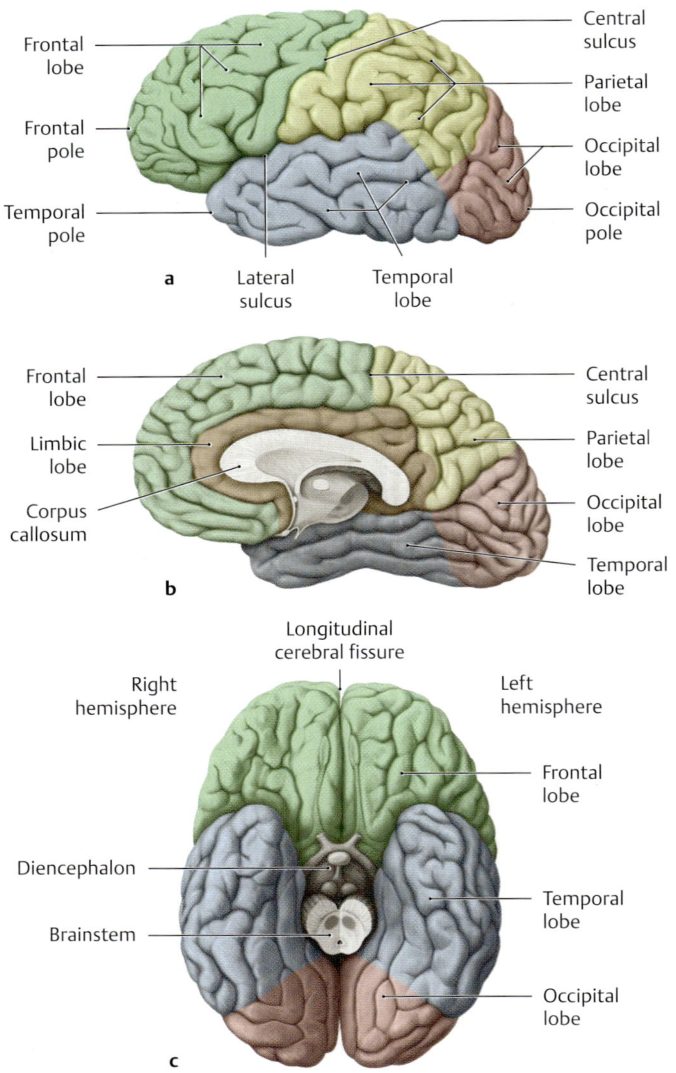

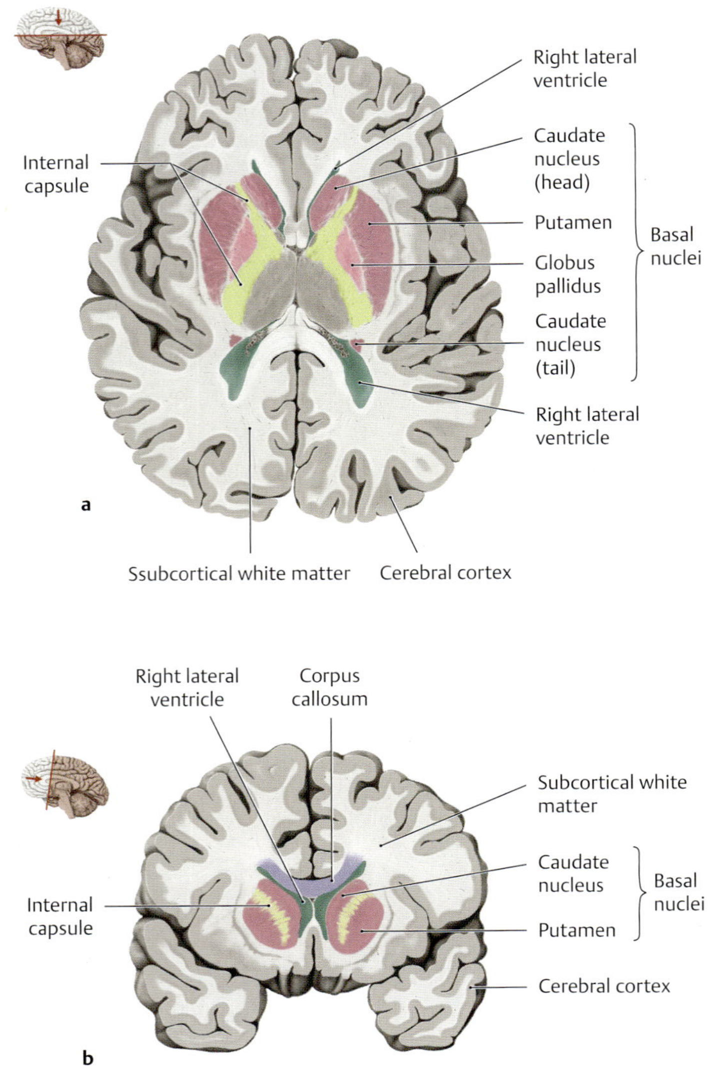

A Telencephalon: Overview and external structure

a Telencephalon, left hemisphere, lateral view; **b** right hemisphere, medial view; **c** telencephalon, basal view.

The telencephalon is the largest and most complex part of the CNS where the highest level of integration occurs in information processing. All complex motor functions, all perceptions as well as the emergence of consciousness, are tied to the functional integrity of the brain. With regard to morphology, the telencephalon is divided into two almost symmetric hemispheres which are incompletely separated by a *longitudinal fissure*. Each of the two hemispheres consists of six *lobes*: the frontal, temporal, occipital, parietal, limbic, and insular lobes. Each of the first three lobes terminate in a pole. Characteristic deep furrows, or *sulci*, define most of the borders between lobes. The surface of each lobe is made up of folds, or *gyri*, which in part are named for the lobe in which they are located. The *insula* (insular lobe) is located deep on the lateral surface of the hemisphere as it is covered by other lobes. It can only be viewed from the lateral aspect once the surrounding structures have been pushed aside (see p. 321). A medial view of the hemisphere includes gyri which are collectively referred to as the *limbic lobe*. Within the temporal lobe lies a part of the cortex called the *hippocampus* which is only visible after resection of surrounding parts of the brain (see **D**, p. 331).

B Telencephalon: internal structure

a Horizontal (axial) section, superior view; **b** coronal section, anterior view.

Like the entire CNS, the telencephalon consists of gray and white matter:

- Gray matter forms the entire outer layer or *cortex*.
- Beneath the cortex lies the *white matter*.
- Embedded in the white matter are additional isolated aggregates of gray matter or nuclei. A nucleus is typically an aggregation of bodies of neurons in the CNS that serve a similar function. An example would be the *basal nuclei* (*caudate nucleus, putamen, globus pallidus*).

Portions of the ventricular system—the *lateral ventricles*—are also visible in a horizontal section. The *white matter*, the macroscopic appearance of which is largely homogeneous, can be functionally divided into tracts that can be further differentiated depending on their course. The *internal capsule* is a white matter structure in which numerous tracts concerned with carrying sensory and motor information are closely grouped together. Phylogenetically, the cerebral cortex can be divided into *archicortex* (the oldest part of the cerebral cortex), *paleocortex*, and *neocortex* (the most recent part of the cerebral cortex). The neocortex forms the largest part of the cortex. All parts of the cerebral cortex consist of multiple layers of neurons but there are microscopic differences between paleocortex, archicortex and neocortex.

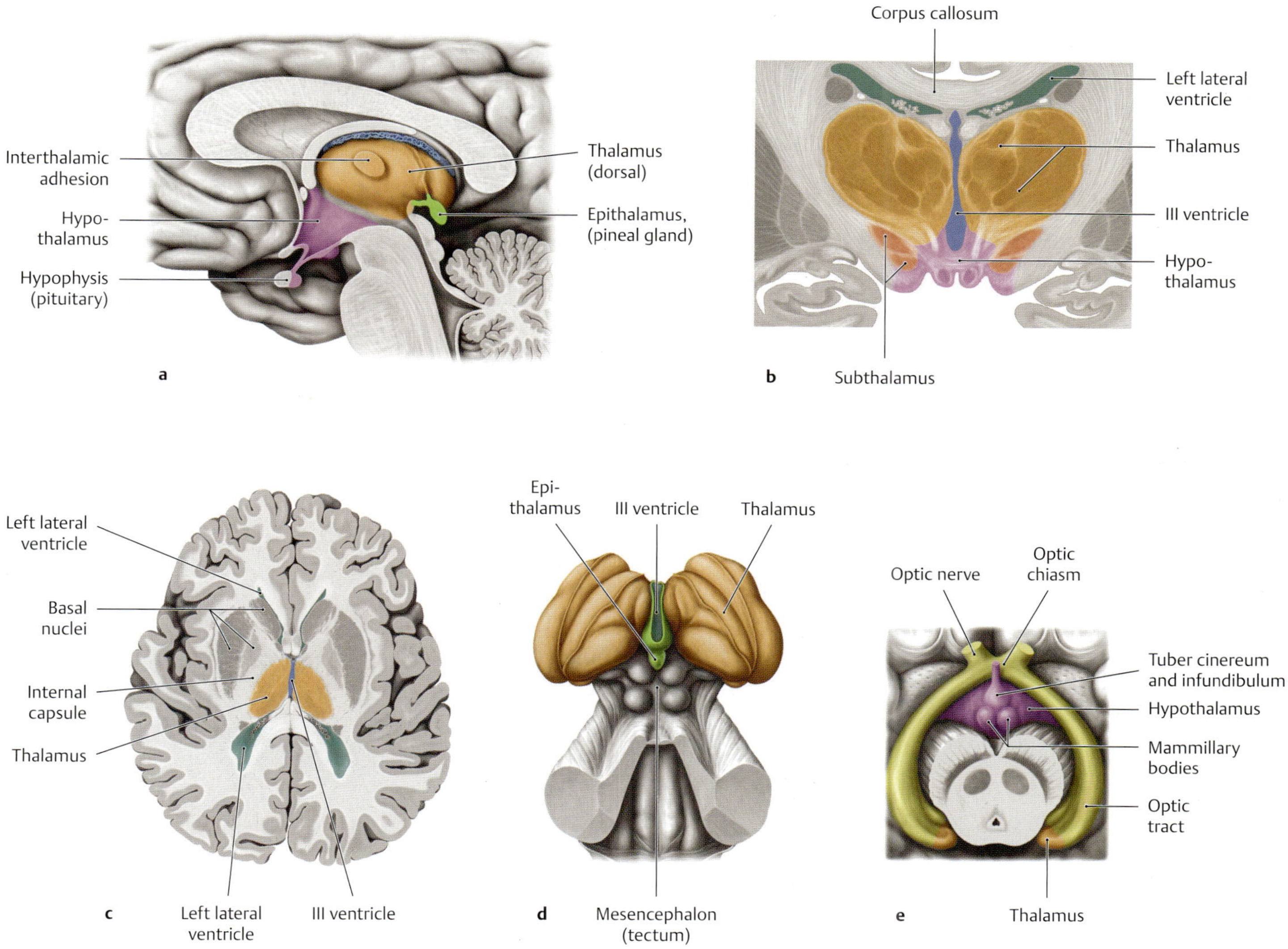

C Diencephalon: Location and classification

a Midsagittal section through the brain, medial view of the right hemisphere; **b** coronal section through the brain, anterior view; **c** horizontal section through the brain, superior view; **d** superior and posterior view of the diencephalon; e view of the base of the diencephalon.

Topographically, the diencephalon consists of structures surrounding the *third ventricle* that is located on the midline. During embryonic development, the diencephalon is located rostral to the brainstem and is largely covered by the fast growing cerebral hemispheres. In an intact brain, only the very basal aspect of the diencephalon is visible. Midsagittal, coronal, or horizontal sections through the brain could provide a good overview of the diencephalon using the third ventricle as a reference point. Due to the location of the different parts of the diencephalon related to the third ventricle, not all of the structures listed below could be seen on any single section:

- On a section through its upper part, the lateral wall of the third ventricle is formed by a large paired structure, the **thalamus** (**a–d**).Both halves of the thalamus lie very closely together and occasionally touch in the region of the *interthalamic adhesion* (**a**). The thalamus relays sensory and motor signals to the cerebral cortex.
- On a section through its lower part, the lateral wall of the third ventricle is formed by the **hypothalamus** (which, just like the thalamus, is composed of multiple nuclei). The hypothalamus can be considered the primary autonomic control center for a number of body functions (e.g., blood pressure, water balance, temperature, food intake, hormone secretion).
- Lateral to the posterior part of hypothalamus, beneath the thalamus but not involved in forming the ventricle, lies the **subthalamus** (**b**) a group of nuclei concerned with motor function.
- A small nuclear group—the **epithalamus**—is located superior and posterior to the thalamus (**d**). One of its components is the *pineal gland*. These structures are involved in photoperiodic regulation.
- Looking at the intact diencephalon from below, at the base of the hypothalamus the hypophysis as well as a group of nuclei, the **mammillary bodies** are visible. Also visible from below are the optic nerves, optic chiasm and optic tracts—all of them belong to the diencephalon and are components of the visual pathway.
- The roof of the third ventricle is formed by the body of the *fornix* that results from the union of the crura of the fornix forming a pathway that extends on each side from the hippocampus (a part of the temporal lobe) to the hypothalamus.

Note: The posterior limb of the *internal capsule* delineates the topographical border between the diencephalon and telencephalon.

1.7 Overview of the Brain: Brainstem and Cerebellum

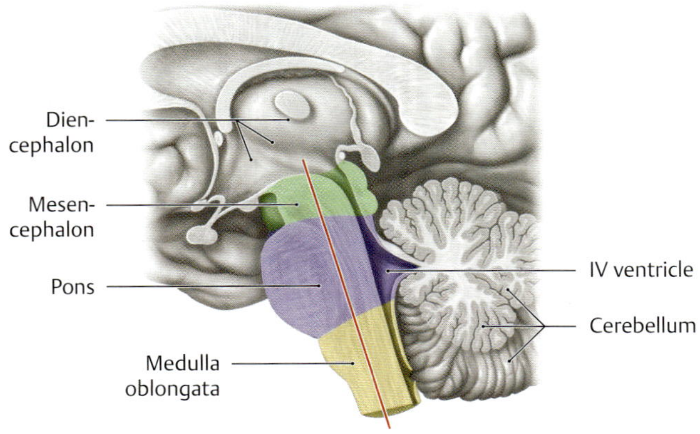

A Brainstem: Location and structure
Midsagittal section through the brain, medial view of left side of the brain.
In an intact brain, the brainstem is visible only from the basal inferior or anterior aspect since it is surrounded laterally and posteriorly by the cerebellum and the temporal lobes. It has an elongated shape which in situ has a rostral-caudal orientation that is ventrally slanted. The axis of the brainstem is described using the same terms of location and direction used for the longitudinal body axis. The brainstem consists of three parts that are (from rostral to caudal) the *mesencephalon*, *pons*, and *medulla oblongata*. The cerebellum is not part of the brainstem and is located dorsal to the brainstem to which it is attached by the cerebellar peduncles. Inside the skull, the brainstem lies close to the *clivus*, a region of the occipital bone.

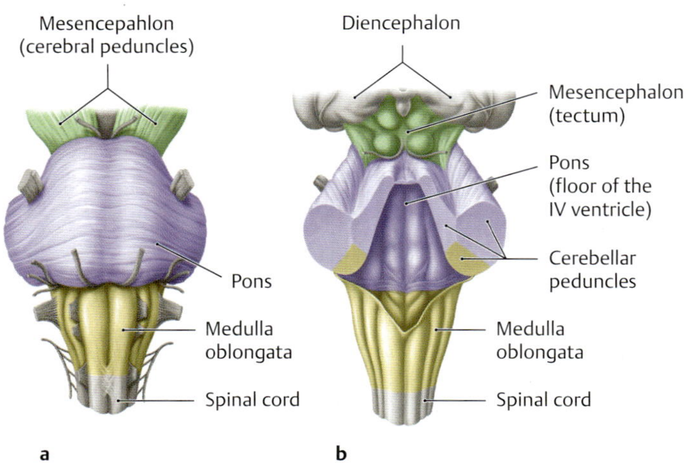

B Brainstem: external structure
The external structure of the brainstem is shaped by nuclei or pathways located within the brainstem. Visible from the outside in a **ventral** (**anterior**) **view** (**a**) are

- the cerebral peduncles (crura cerebri), composed of tracts descending to the pons, medulla oblongata and spinal cord,
- the basilar pons, containing a large tract that enters the cerebellum,
- the pyramid (formed by the pyramidal tract), and
- the olive (a group of nuclei).

In **dorsal** (**posterior**) **view** (**b**, visible only after the cerebellum has been removed):

- the quadrigeminal plate (tectum), with two paired nuclear groups for auditory and visual function, forming the roof plate of the mesencephalon,
- the medulla oblongata with two paired tubercula formed by the nuclei related to the posterior column,
- intersection of the three paired cerebellar peduncles that connect the brainstem with the cerebellum and between which lies the diamond-shaped base of the fourth ventricle (rhomboid fossa). The rhomboid fossa is formed partially by the pons and partially by the the medulla oblongata.

Note: The brainstem is the point of entry and emergence for all true cranial nerves (III–X and XII; for classification see p. 112 ff). Of the twelve pairs of cranial nerves, two cranial nerves (I: olfactory n. and II: optic n.) are not structurally nerves but tracts of the CNS (not shown here, because they don't emerge from the brainstem). In addition, cranial nerve XI is considered a spinal nerve with an unusual course.

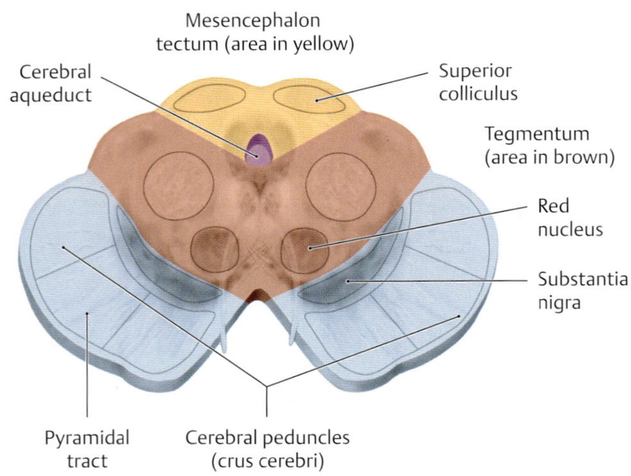

C Brainstem: compartmental organization and internal structure
Cross section of midbrain, superior view.
In anteroposterior direction, the brainstem can be divided into four segments. Although they can be found in all parts of the brainstem to a greater or lesser degree, they are most prominent in the mesencephalon. The terms for describing these segments in pons and medulla oblongata differ.

- The base, which at the mesencephalon appears as the pair of cerebral peduncles (crura), is located ventrally. The base of the brainstem usually contains large descending tracts to the brainstem, cerebellum, and spinal cord (e.g., the pyramidal tract). A continuous band of gray matter, the substantia nigra, is located directly dorsal to the cerebral peduncles.
- The midbrain tegmentum is located dorsal to the base and substantia nigra. Large groups of nuclei are found here and serve different functions (the red nucleus is particularly prominent). Multiple ascending (sensory) tracts to the telencephalon (over the thalamus in the diencephalon) and the cerebellum and a few descending tracts to the spinal also occupy the tegmentum.
- The tectum is located dorsal to the tegmentum. Depending on its location in the mesencephalon it is either called roof plate or due to its distinct shape (see **Bb**) the quadrigeminal plate. This roof region contains two superior collicular and two inferior collicular nuclei which play an important role in the visual and auditory pathways.
- Each section of the brainstem contains part of the ventricular system. In the mesencephalon this is the cerebral aqueduct.

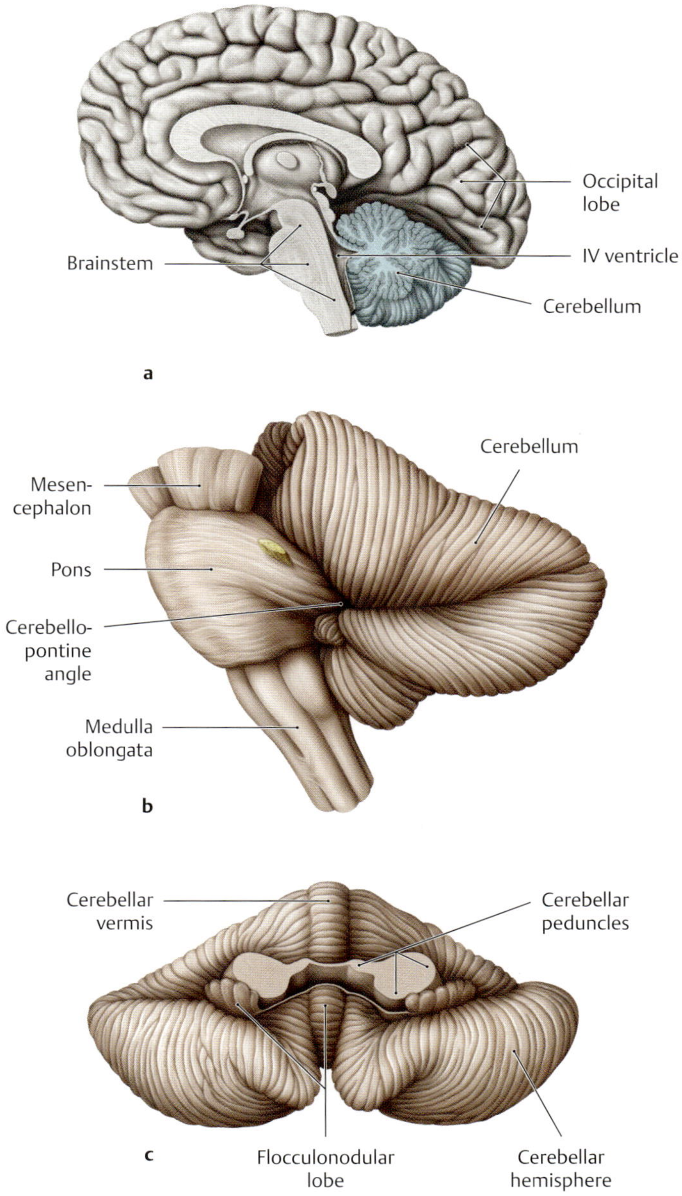

D Cerebellum: Positional relationship and external structure
a Midsagittal section through brainstem and cerebellum, medial view of the right hemisphere; **b** left lateral view of brainstem and cerebellum; **c** cerebellum, anterior view after detachment from brainstem.
The cerebellum is located dorsal to the brainstem and forms the roof of the fourth ventricle (**a**). It lies beneath the occipital lobe of the telencephalon from which it is separated by a dural fold—the tentorium cerebelli (not shown here, see p.274). Inside the skull, the cerebellum is situated in the posterior cranial fossa. Between the brainstem and cerebellum on both sides is a recess—the cerebellopontine angle (**b**) which is of clinical significance.
Like the telencephalon, the cerebellum consists of two hemispheres. They are separated by an unpaired vermis (**c**).The surface of hemispheres and vermis shows furrow-like depressions, the fissures, and separate the very thin folia. Fissures and folia of the cerebellum correspond somehow to the sulci and gyri of the telencephalon. Fissures divide the cerebellum into lobes. The flocculonodular lobe (**b**) one of the main subdivisions of the cerebellum, is located inferiorly and consists of the paired flocculi, their peduncles, and the nodule of the vermis. All tracts to and from the cerebellum pass through the three paired cerebellar peduncles.

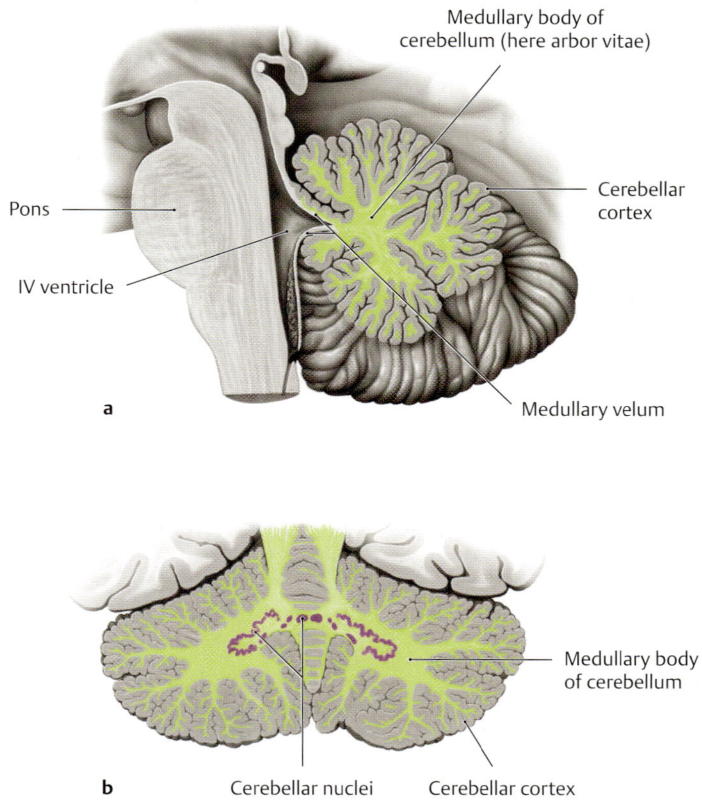

E Cerebellum: internal structure
a Midsagittal section through the cerebellum; medial view of the right cerebellar hemisphere; **b** oblique section through the cerebellum; superior view.
Similar to the telencephalon, the cerebellar vermis and hemispheres contain centrally located white matter (or medulla), surrounded by gray matter in the form of the cerebellar cortex. The morphological appearance of medulla and cortex in a midsagittal section is called the *arbor vitae* (tree of life). Embedded within the white matter are four paired deep cerebellar nuclei, composed of gray matter. The cerebellum is concerned with multiple functions including the unconscious control of balance and fine motor skills.

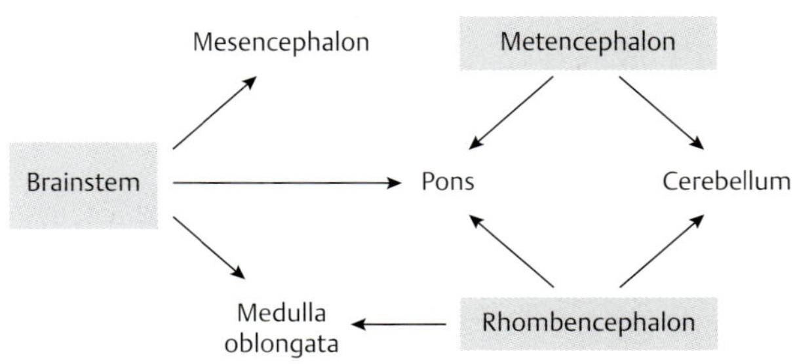

F Cerebellum and brainstem: Terminological peculiarities
Topographically, the cerebellum is not part of the brainstem, yet phylogenetically is derived from it. The pons and cerebellum are collectively known as the metencephalon. The combination of pons, cerebellum and medulla oblongata, the structures which surround the diamond-shaped fourth ventricle, is called the hindbrain or rhombencephalon.

1.8 Overview of the Spinal Cord

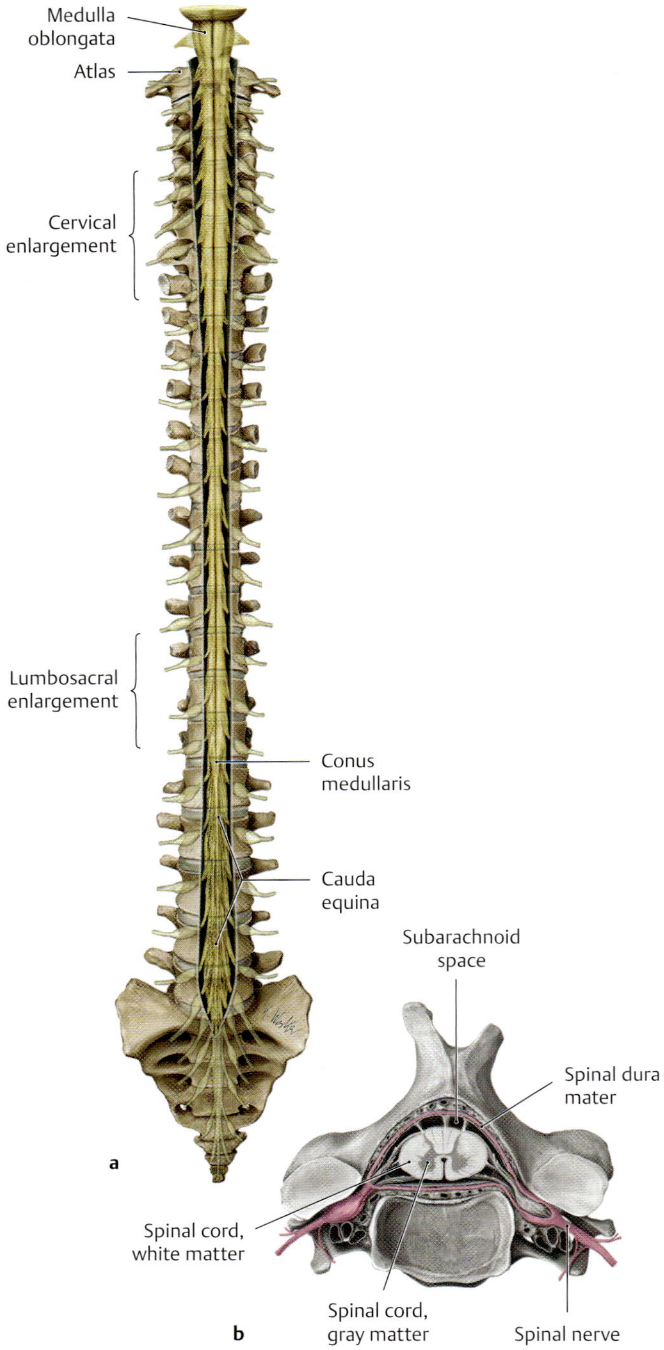

A Spinal cord: Positional relationship in the vertebral column
a Ventral (anterior) view of the opened spinal cord; **b** cross section of a vertebra and the spinal cord.
The spinal cord lies within the vertebral canal, which is formed by the vertebral foramen of all the vertebrae stacked on top of one another and the ligaments of the vertebral column traversing the vertebrae. The spinal cord which is the most caudal part of the CNS, extends caudally from the first cervical vertebra, called the atlas, to the second lumbar vertebra. From there, only certain parts of the spinal cord, the roots, extend further caudally. They are equivalent to the spinal nerves (see **D**) and are part of the PNS. Within the vertebral canal the spinal cord, as part of the CNS, is also surrounded by meninges and the subarachnoid space (see p. 311).

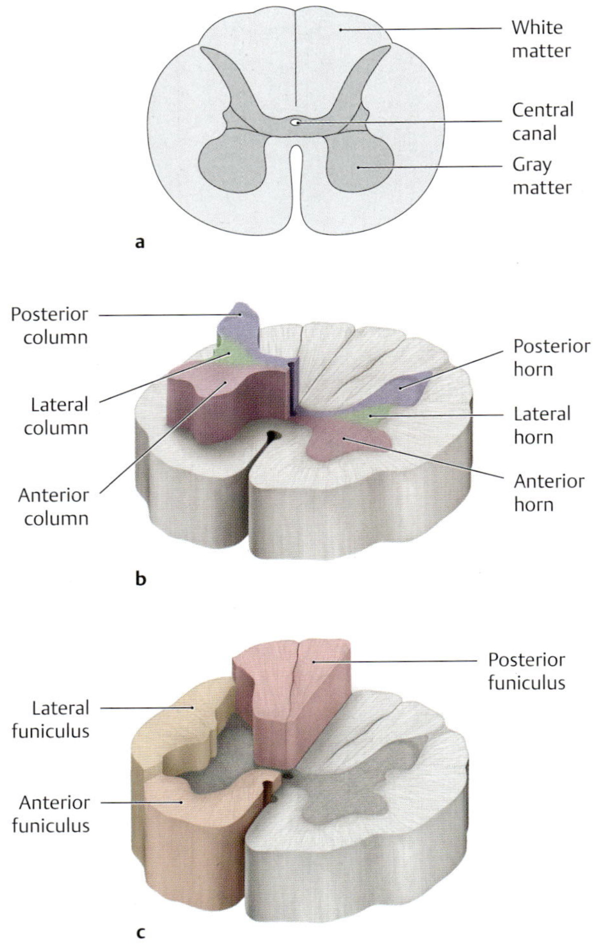

B Spinal cord: Internal structure
a Cross section of the spinal cord, superior view; **b** schematic, three-dimensional representation of the spinal cord with gray matter (**b**) and white matter (**c**) being highlighted; left anterior oblique and superior view. The spinal cord shows all characteristic structures of the CNS:

- **Gray matter**, which in cross-section appears butterfly-shaped and typically is divided into an
  - anterior horn,
  - posterior horn, and
  - lateral horn (visible only in the thoracic region).

  All gray matter horns are paired, making the spinal cord symmetrical. The gray matter contains bodies of neurons. The three-dimensional representation (**b**) shows that the term "horn" is used to describe the three-dimensional nature of the anterior, posterior, and lateral columns of gray matter. At the central core of gray matter lies part of the ventricular system, the central canal of the spinal cord. The gray matter of the spinal cord is surrounded by
- **White matter** (which is composed of tracts), forms funiculi clearly visible in the three-dimensional representation (**c**) which are analogous to the columns of gray matter and are called the anterior, posterior, and lateral funiculi. Occasionally, parts of the anterior and lateral funiculi are collectively called the anterolateral funiculus.

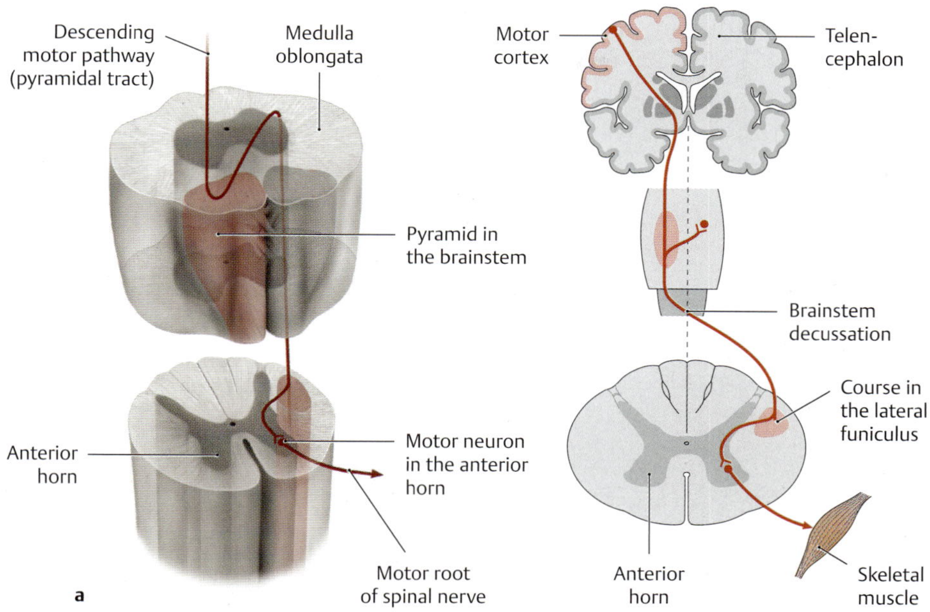

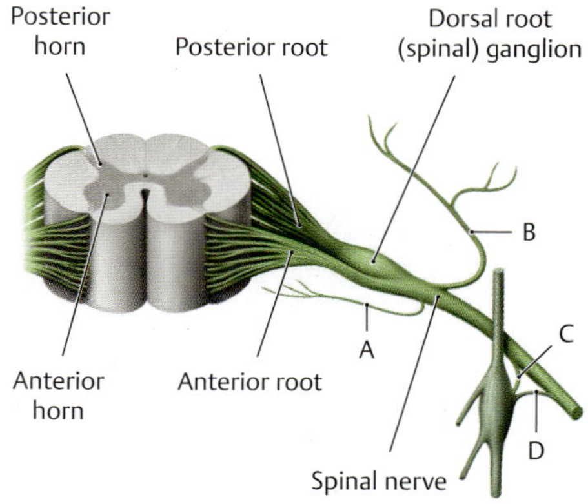

D Relationship between CNS and PNS at the spinal cord

Cross section of spinal cord, anterior oblique and superior view. All parts of the PNS are in green.

- The axons of motor neurons, located in the anterior horn, exit the anterior portion of the spinal cord via the anterior root.
- the axons of the sensory neurons, located in the spinal ganglion, enter the spinal cord via the posterior root.

Anterior and posterior roots merge to form the spinal nerve which is mixed, containing both motor and sensory modalities. **A–D** refer to: ventral primary ramus (**A**), dorsal primary ramus (**B**), gray ramus communicans (**C**), and white ramus communicans (**D**).

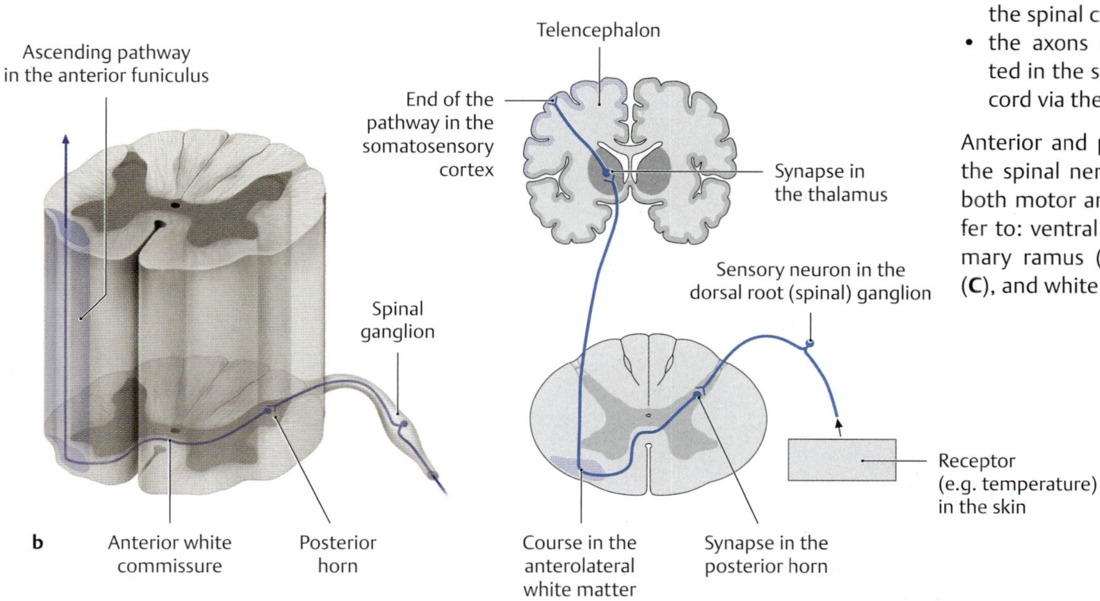

C Tracts of the spinal cord

The tracts of the spinal cord run within the white matter (funiculi) (see **Bc**). Depending on their course, they are either descending (**a**) or ascending (**b**). Descending tracts mainly affect motor function and usually originate in the higher centers of the CNS, such as the motor cortex of the cerebral cortex. Ascending tracts typically serve sensory functions and transmit the information of a sensory receptor to higher centers in the CNS.

a One example of a motor tract is the lateral corticospinal tract located in the lateral funiculus. As shown here, it is responsible for control of the voluntary motor function. It originates in the cerebral cortex and runs within the lateral funiculi of the spinal cord and reaches the anterior horn where it terminates on alpha (lower) motor neurons of the spinal cord. The lower motor neurons send their axons via the ventral root of a spinal nerve, and innervate the skeletal muscle;

b shows a sensory pathway, which runs within the anterolateral system of the spinal cord. The information comes from the skin and extends to the (somatosensory) cerebral cortex passing through intermediate stations (mainly the thalamus in the diencephalon). The body of the first-order neuron of this tract lies in the spinal ganglion and is therefore a neuron of the peripheral nervous system.

The course of both pathways helps illustrate the particular role of the **spinal cord as a “conductor for information”** between the CNS and PNS:

- The axon of the first-order sensory neuron (with the body in the spinal ganglion) enters the CNS
- The alpha (lower) motor neuron with the cell body in the anterior horn of the CNS sends the axon in the PNS

However, the spinal cord as part of the CNS can exercise its **own integrative functions**, playing an important role in reflexes. For this purpose, the spinal cord contains intersegmental fibers (lateral proper fasciculi, not shown here) located in the white matter, which are responsible for relaying information within the spinal cord without exiting it. These are intersegmental fibers that arise from cells in the gray matter, and, after a longer or shorter course, reenter the gray matter and ramify in it. In terms of their function, the tracts running through the spinal cord are called extrinsic connections and the intersegmental fibers intrinsic connections. Knowledge of location, course and function of tracts of the spinal cord is essential for understanding clinical symptoms in case of injuries to, or diseases of, the spinal cord.

1.9 Blood Supply of the Brain and Spinal Cord

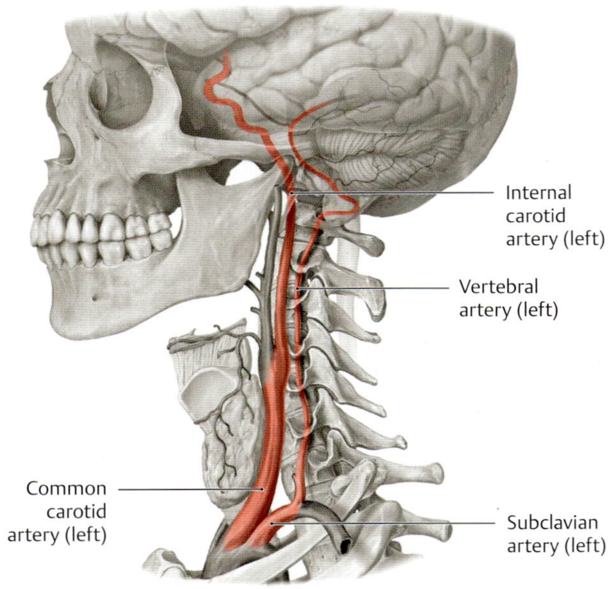

a

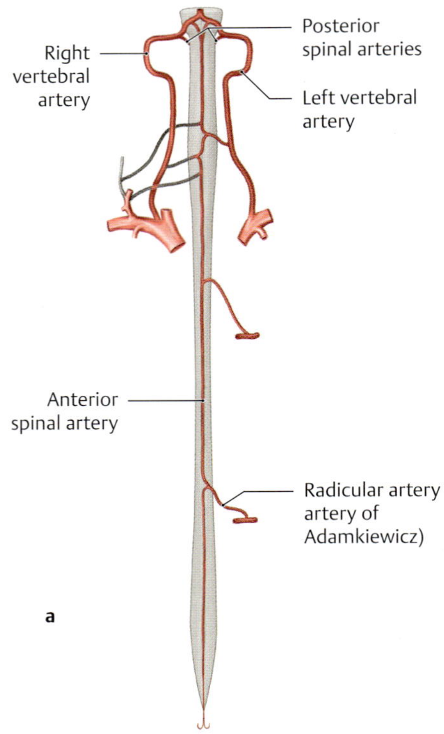

a

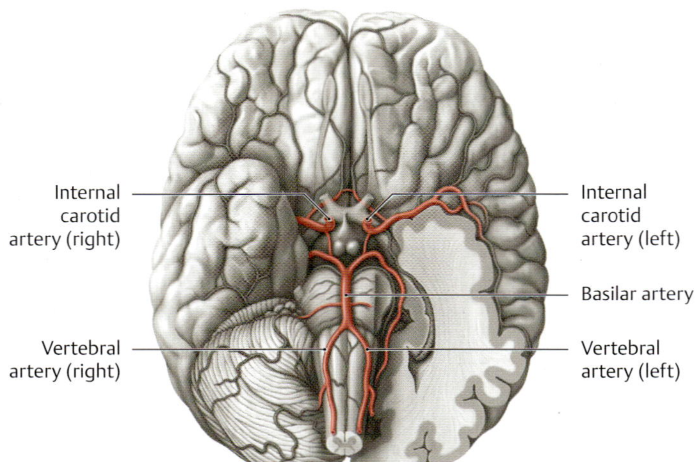

b

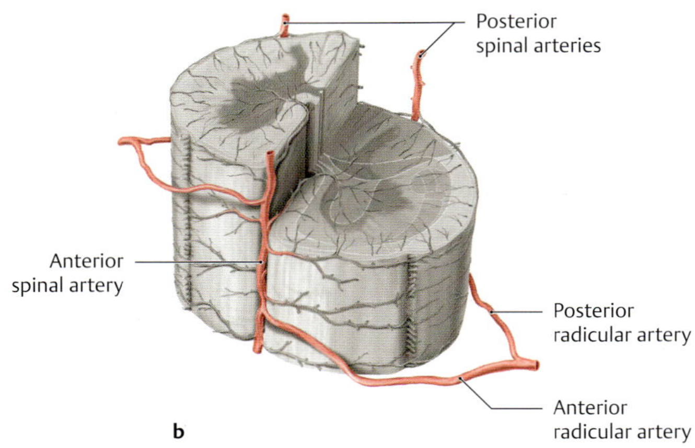

b

A Arterial supply to the brain

a Transparent skull viewed from the left; **b** basal view of brain.

The brain has a very high demand for oxygen. While it represents only 2 % of the body's weight it receives 15 % of the cardiac output. The necessary blood supply is ensured by two paired arteries (**a**): The larger internal carotid a. and the smaller caliber vertebral a., which reach the cranial cavity by passing through the carotid canal and the foramen magnum respectively. At the base of the brain—within the subarachnoid space—the branches of these four arteries merge to form a vascular ring, the arterial circle (of Willis) (**b**): The arterial circle gives off branches that supply the brain (e.g., cerebral or cerebellar aa.). Note that the arterial circle is essentially fed by three main vessels—the lt/rt internal carotid aa. and the basilar a. formed by the fusion of the lt/rt vertebral aa. The blood supply from these three sources is connected by posterior and anterior communicating aa. that result in the formation of the arterial circle. In case of impaired circulation, the merging of these arteries in a vascular ring, to a certain extent allows for compensation of decreased blood flow in one vessel with increased blood flow through another vessel.

B Arterial supply to the spinal cord

a Schematic representation of blood supply to the spinal cord; **b** cross section of spinal cord, left lateral and superior view.

The great length of the spinal cord, which lies within the narrow vertebral canal, poses significant logistical problems with regard to blood supply. The spinal cord is supplied by various branches of the vertebral a. on both sides (**a**). The anterior spinal a. and lt/rt posterior spinal aa. extend from cranial to caudal. However, the ventricular filling pressure through the vertebral a. is not sufficient to supply the entire spinal cord caudally. Segmentally derived smaller arteries, the anterior and posterior radicular aa., derived from the intercostal arteries, reach the spinal cord and constantly supply the spinal aa. From cranial to caudal direction (due to the decreasing filling pressure in this direction by the vertebral a.), these small segmental arteries become increasingly important. The goal is to guarantee a sufficient supply to the spinal aa. which extend the length of the spinal cord and send their branches into the spinal cord (**b**).

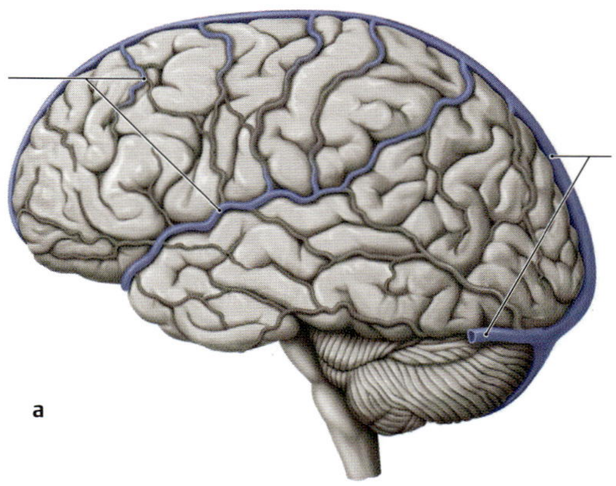

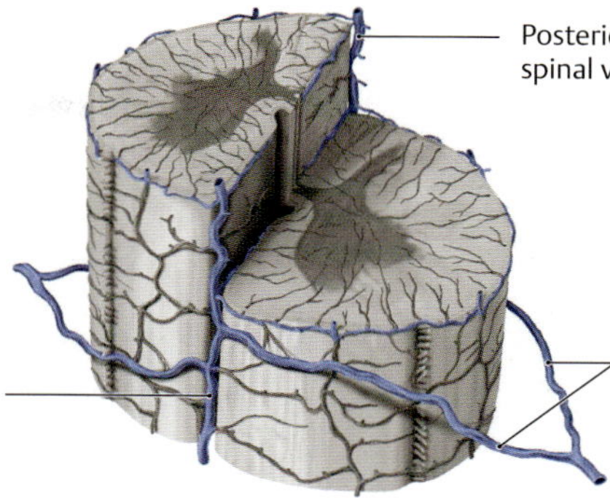

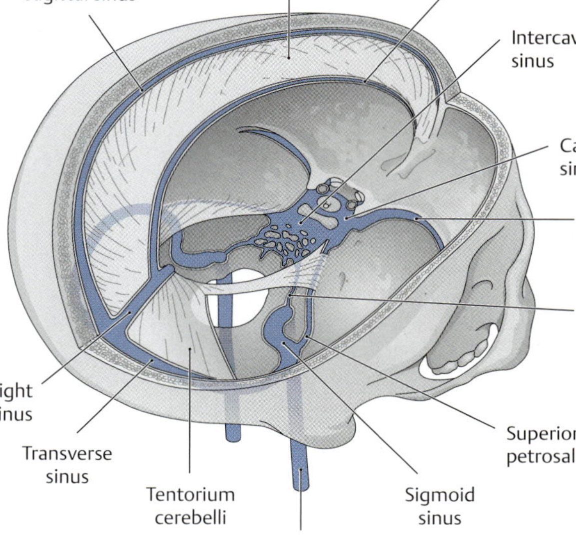

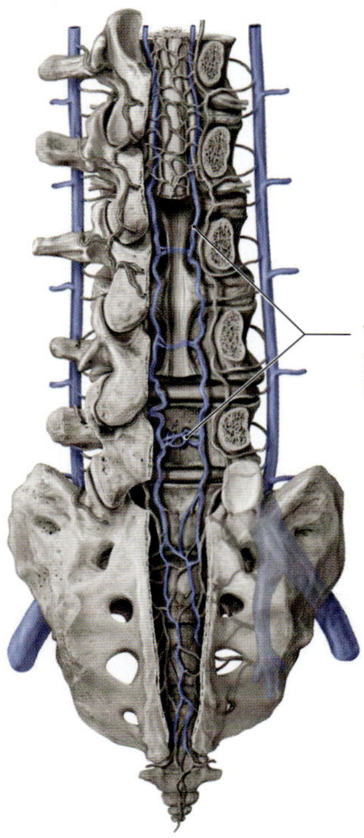

C Venous drainage of the brain

a schematic representation of superficial veins of the brain, lateral view; **b** view of the dural venous sinus system, right, posterosuperior view of the skull after the calvarium has been removed.

Superficial cerebral vv. collect and direct the blood to a series of venous sinuses generally, but not always, formed in the attached edges of dural folds in the cranial cavity. These dural venous sinuses are formed by separation of the two layers of dura generally inseparable except in these regions. Unlike true veins, there is no muscle tissue found in the walls of these venous sinuses. The dura is lined internally by only a layer of endothelium. Deep cerebral veins (not visible here) collect the blood from deeper brain regions and take it to the dural venous sinus system. The dural venous sinus system delivers the collected blood mainly to the internal jugular v. that forms at the jugular foramen of the cranial cavity. In a similar fashion to the the true veins of the head, the dural sinuses do not have valves. Blood can flow in either direction exclusively controlled by the existing pressure gradient.

Note: Dural venous sinuses are found only around the brain and not in the spinal cord, even though dura also exists in the spinal cord. The connection between the dural venous sinus system and true veins outside the skull allow bacteria to enter the cranial cavity from outside even without injury to the bone or the meninges (see p. 385).

D Venous drainage of the spinal cord

a Cross section of the spinal cord, left, anterior and superior view; **b** anterior view of the vertebral canal which has been opened and the spinal cord.

The venous blood of the spinal cord is collected by the anterior and posterior spinal vv. and delivered to large venous plexuses located in the the epidural space of the vertebral canal or directly to the intercostal vv. Unlike the brain in the skull, there is no dural venous sinus system surrounding the spinal cord within the vertebral canal.

Note: The complex venous system of the vertebral venous plexus contains many more veins than what would be required for routine blood drainage supporting spinal cord metabolism. This plexus system serves an additional function acting as a pressure equalizer in the vertebral canal. By moving large amounts of blood between internal and external vertebral venous plexuses (both of which have no valves), fluctuations in blood pressure in the vertebral canal can be accommodated (see **B** and **C**, p. 417).

1.10 Somatic Sensation

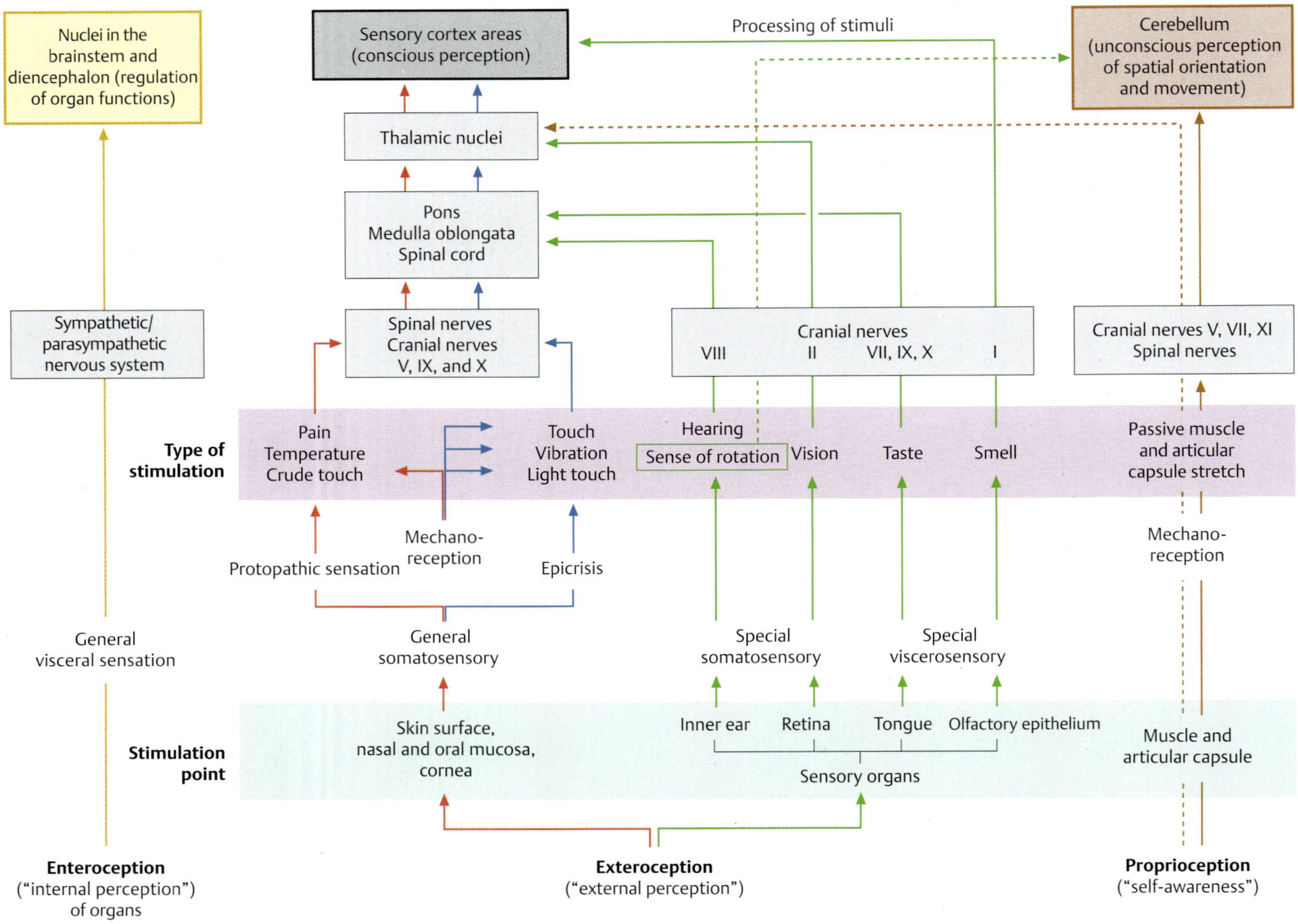

A Somatic Sensation: Classification and Overview

There are two kinds of sensation: *somatic* and *visceral*. The common *visceral sensation*—the processing of stimuli from viscera inside the body (*interoception*)—is explained on p. 297 along with visceral motor function and is only mentioned here for the sake of completeness. Somatic sensation can be distinguished based on location and type of stimulus. This distinction is important because the location and type determines the **pathway** via which the somatic signals are transmitted.

- Sensory signals originating on the skin, the nasal or oral mucosa, or the ocular surface (not vision) are referred to as external perception (exteroception, superficial/cutaneous sensation).
- If the stimulus location is a stretch receptor (strain measurement) within a muscle, a tendon or an articular capsule, it is referred to as proprioception—deep sensation of the musculoskeletal system important for controlling the body position sense.

Classification based on **type** of stimulus: Only the external perception, meaning *exteroception*, is further divided into

- epicritic sensation (sense of touch, vibration, light touch, light pressure or subtle mechanoreception) is contrasted with
- protopathic sensation (pain, temperature, crude mechanical stimuli or crude mechanoreception).

Although proprioception is a form of mechanoreception, it is not further differentiated.

Both exteroception and proprioception are conveyed via spinal nerves (information from torso, neck, limbs) or cranial nerves. Cranial nerves V_1–V_3, IX, and X convey exteroception; cranial nerves V_3, VII, and XI convey proprioception.

Perception through the sensory organs is ultimately a form of *exteroception*. It is transmitted exclusively via cranial nerves. Regarding the sensory organs, *chemical* stimuli (taste, smell) and *electromagnetic* waves (optics) in addition to *mechanical* stimuli (acoustics) play a role. However, for phylogenic and terminological reasons, the perception of *physical stimuli* (optics and acoustics) is referred to as "*specific somatosensation*" and the perception of chemical stimuli is referred to as "*specific visceral sensation*."

Note: The specific visceral sensitivity in the case of chemical stimuli to two sensory organs should not be confused with the "general visceral sensation" of the internal organs (yellow arrow on far left).

The different ways of **processing stimuli in the CNS**—conscious or subconscious—is a factor in distinguishing various types of sensation. For a sensory stimulus to reach consciousness (*conscious* sensation), it has to reach the sensory cortex of the telencephalon. Usually, the stimuli are conveyed via the thalamus. Sensory stimuli, which are not transmitted to the cerebral cortex, but only reach other, secondary regions of the CNS are not perceived consciously (*unconscious* sensation). In addition to location and type of stimulus, the final destination of the signal transmission can be distinguished in sensory stimuli. Analogous to somatomotor function, specific terms for specific sensory perceptions are used to describe somatic sensation.

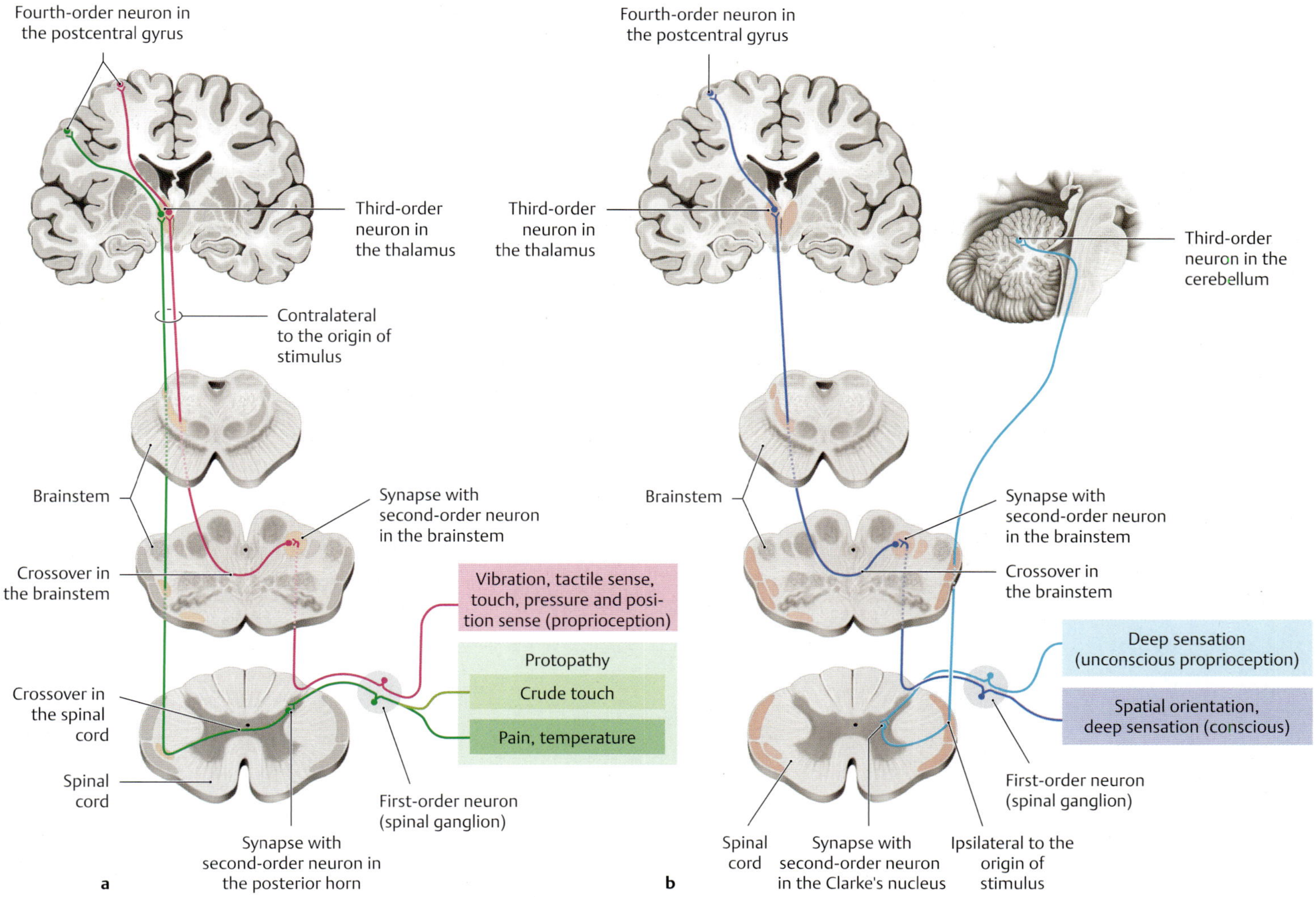

B Somatic sensation: Interconnections and the anatomical structures involved

The CNS, PNS and a receptor are involved in somatic sensation.

a Transmission of a sensory stimulus from the skin to the telencephalon (epicritic and protopathic, conscious perception)

b Transmission of a signal from skeletal muscle (stretch in muscle), which is perceived via specialized stretch receptors (proprioception) to the cerebellum (unconscious) and to the telencephalon (conscious)

A cranial or spinal nerve transmits the signal from the respective sensory receptor. The impulse is conveyed to the CNS, via afferent transmission. Like the motor neurons, the somatic neurons, are numbered and defined using a signal chronology:

- *Four* neurons carry information to the *telencephalon* (conscious).
- *Three* neurons carry information to the *cerebellum* (unconscious).

In each instance, the *first-order neuron in the PNS* lies in a spinal ganglion or a cranial nerve ganglion (not shown here), the *second-order neuron* is located *in the CNS* (spinal cord or the brainstem nuclei). From this point, the number of neurons differ. The reason for an additional neuron carrying information to the telencephalon is that all impulses conducted by neurons to the telencephalon first pass through a particular group of nuclei located in the diencephalon—the *thalamus*. This is the central relay station for conscious sensation, and also plays an important role in filtering information ("what has the highest priority?"). The *third-order neuron* is found In the thalamus (the "filter neuron"). The *fourth-order neuron* is the sensory endpoint. It is located in the *postcentral gyrus* of the telencephalon. For signals that are relayed to the cerebellum, by only three neurons, the third-order neuron lies in the cerebellar cortex.

Note: Signals to the cerebellum don't pass through the thalamus and are therefore relayed by only three neurons.

Pain, temperature, and crude touch mechanoreception of the skin and mucosae are transmitted in the spinal cord via the sensory spinothalamic tract. Subtle mechanoreception (vibration, precise touch, pressure, and position sense [proprioception]) is transmitted in the spinal cord via the dorsal column (fasciculus gracilis and/or cuneatus).

Note:

- All tracts that carry *exteroceptive* impulses, cross over to the opposite side in the CNS. It is always the axon of the second-order neuron that crosses over. Thus, a stimulus in the left arm will pass through the thalamus and be relayed to, and received by, the right cerebral cortex.
- In the spinal cord, *proprioceptive* impulses are mainly transmitted via the spinocerebellar tract. The cell body of the first-order neuron lies in the spinal ganglion. For the posterior spinocerebellar tract, the cell body of the second-order neuron is located in the Clarke's nucleus. This information processing is not conscious.

Within the head, all parts of somatic sensation pass via the trigeminal n. (CN V) and the central trigeminal tract.

Note: To a lesser extent, proprioceptive impulses can also be relayed to the cerebral cortex to perceive positional sense via the dorsal column: Epicrisis (as part of exteroception) and proprioception run parallel in the same tract, but terminate at different nuclei. For more details see p. 402 ff.

1.11 Somatomotor Function

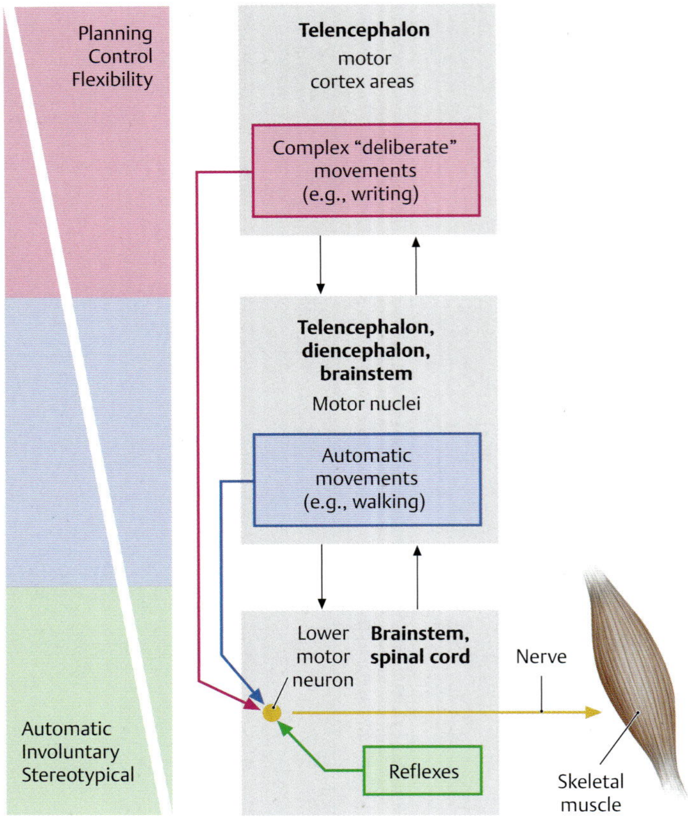

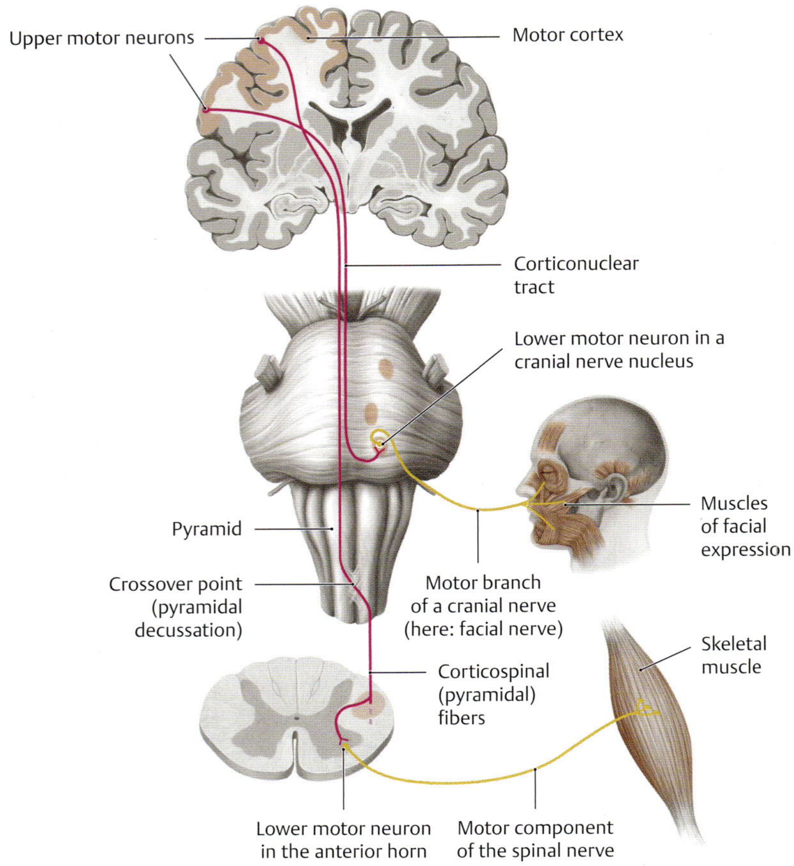

A Somatomotor function: An overview

The classification of somatomotor function is less complex than that of somatic sensation. *Somatomotor function* is the activation of skeletal muscle fibers. This process is mainly associated with the musculoskeletal system. However, muscles used for facial expression, mastication, or movement of the eyeball, are also skeletal muscle, but are in a stricter sense not part of the musculoskeletal system even if they move something such as the mandible. Occasionally specific terms (see p. 112) are used to describe those specific somatomotor movements. Only the somatomotor function is described here; for visceromotor function, also referred to as organ motility, see p. 296.

Somatomotor function can be characterized based on whether the movement happens entirely *automatically* or is *deliberately* controlled, both of which are linked to a high degree of flexibility in movement pattern. Typically, movements are combinations of automatic movements and deliberate, controlled actions. All necessary interconnections in the CNS for such somatomotor functions share a common final segment/pathway: They terminate at a motor neuron which lies in the spinal cord (for spinal nerves) and in brainstem motor nuclei (for cranial nerves). This motor neuron sends signals to the muscle. Physiologically a distinction is drawn between α- and γ-motor neurons. To put it simply, the α-motor neuron causes muscle contractions that generate movement whereas the γ-motor neuron, independent of concrete movement, regulates normal muscle tone. The differing complexity of movements corresponds with the unequal participation of different complex parts of the nervous system concerned with interconnections. Simple reflexes occur only at the spinal cord level, the more complex voluntary motor functions involve participation of the cerebral cortex and cerebellum.

B Somatomotor function: Neuronal wiring

The CNS and the PNS are involved in somatomotor function. Shown here is the deliberate activation of a muscle—the effector—by the telencephalon.

A neuron in the CNS sends a signal via its axon to another neuron in a different part of the CNS. This neuron receives the signal and transmits it via its own axon through the PNS to the effector organ. Due to the direction of signal transmission (away from the CNS), it is considered to be an *efferent* transmission (see p. 266) and the participating neurons can be named in hierarchical order: upper and lower motor neurons. In the white matter of the CNS, the axons of many first-order neurons form a tract (e.g., corticospinal tract). The axons of many lower motor neurons, since they exit the CNS, form a nerve in the PNS (see **C**, p. 295). The axon of the lower motor neuron terminates at the muscle in a specific structure at the *motor endplate*, where the signal transfer from nerve to muscle takes place.

The upper motor neuron lies in a motor area of the telencephalon in the motor cortex. A lower motor neuron found in the gray matter of the spinal cord has its axon reaching the muscle of the musculoskeletal system via a spinal nerve. If the lower motor neuron lies in a specific brainstem nucleus, its axon reaches the muscles of the head and neck, used for facial expression, mastication or movement of the eyeball and tongue, via a cranial nerve.

Note: The somatomotor system has only centrally located cell bodies of neurons. Only the axon of the lower motor neuron extends in the PNS.

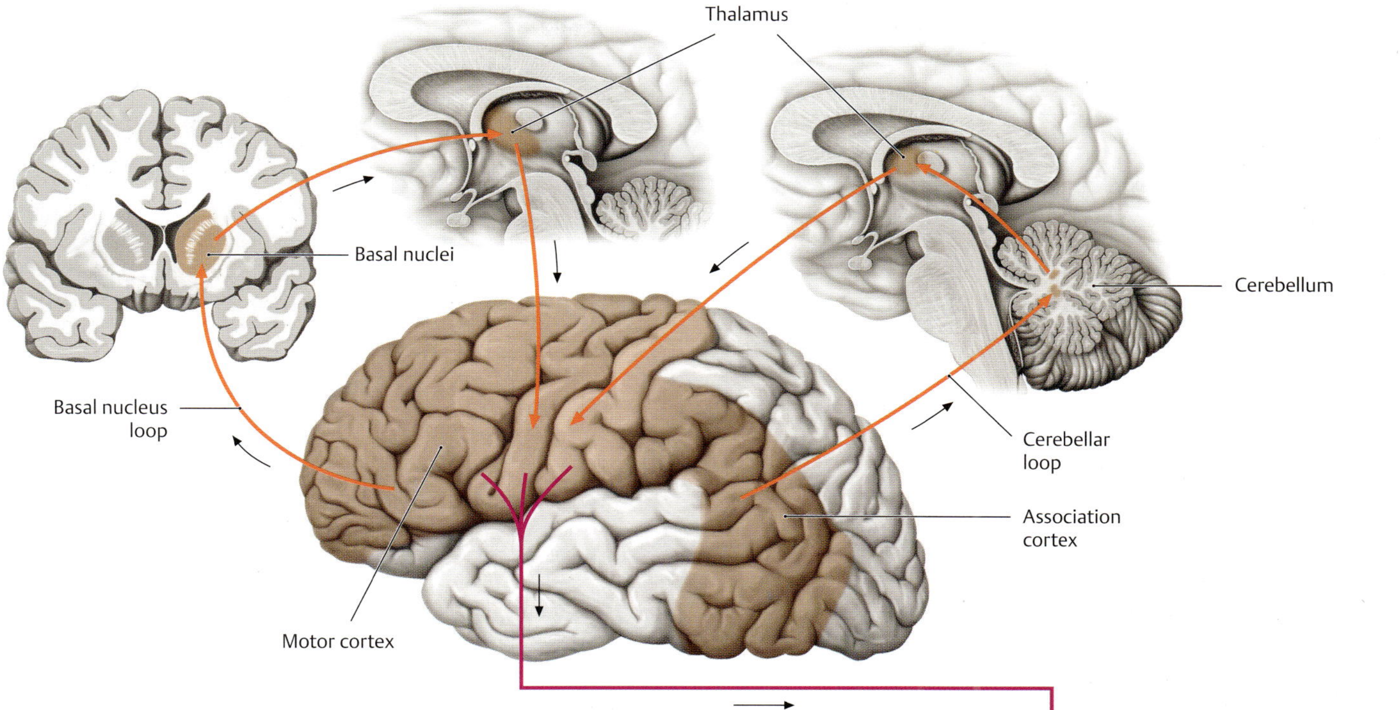

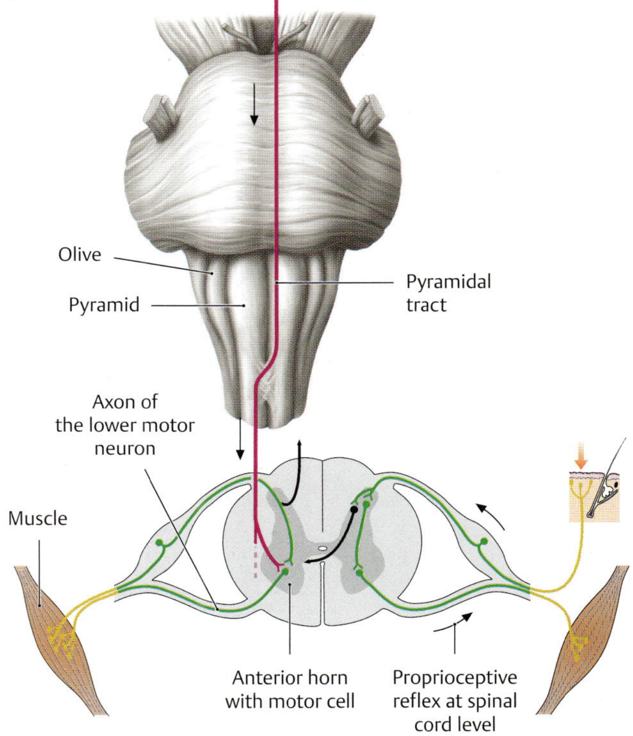

C Somatomotor function: the anatomical structures involved

The general planning and initiation of movement takes place in different areas of the cerebral cortex, e.g. in the motor cortex and the association cortex. To eventually carry out the movement, however, the participation of additional neuronal centers, such as the cerebellum (for balance control) and nuclei in other different brain regions, is required. The latter are referred to as *subcortical motor centers*, since topographically, they are all located beneath the motor cortex. They include

- the *basal nuclei* in the telencephalon,
- motor areas of the *thalamus* in the diencephalon,
- the *red nucleus*, the *substantia nigra* (not shown here), the *subthalamic nucleus*, and the *inferior olive* in the brainstem.

The subcortical motor centers are responsible for muscular coordination and fine motor control. Feedback loops link the cerebral cortex with the cerebellum and the basal nuclei. The tract of the motor cortex to the spinal cord, shown in fig. **B**, passes in the brainstem through a structure which, due to its shape, is called the pyramid, the tract is referred to as the pyramidal tract. Tracts of the subcortical centers of the brainstem do not travel through the pyramid and are therefore called extrapyramidal tracts. Both types of tracts reach the spinal cord by descending and eventually terminating in the anterior horn of the spinal cord at the lower motor neuron, the axon of which extends to the muscle. The pyramidal tract (corticospinal tract) is the tract which in the end generates movement. Extrapyramidal tracts of the subcortical centers in the brainstem play a role in planning and fine-tuning the movement.

Note: The cortico*nuclear* tract, which like the cortico*spinal* tract comes from the motor cortex, terminates at motor nuclei of the brainstem, which functionally corresponds to the anterior horns of the spinal cord. It conveys the same type of motor function as the corticospinal tract. However, it does not travel through the pyramid but terminates above it (the pyramid is located in the lowest part of the brainstem). Due to its analogous motor function, the corticonuclear tract is usually referred to as part of the pyramidal tract. Most axons of the upper motor neuron cross. Motor impulses of the right hemisphere travel to the left side of the spinal cord and reach via the left spinal nerve, an effector skeletal muscle located on the left side of the spinal cord. Very simple motor processes such as reflexes can be carried out directly at the spinal cord level (spinal cord reflexes) or the brainstem (brainstem reflexes) without including higher centers of the CNS.

1.12 Sensory Organs

Overview

Sensory organs are specialized for detecting stimuli. Specific receptors are grouped together forming the organ—a morphologically definable unit—and are not scattered across the skin. Typically, sensory organs are able to perceive very complex stimulus patterns, referred to as higher senses, contrasted to the more simple sensory functions performed by the skin. Detection of the stimulus, however, exhibits no difference between the sensory organs and sensory functions of the skin. However, detecting particularly complex stimuli, an ability that only sensory organs have, in most cases requires complex central nervous system processing. The level of sensory integration (see p. 256) for such stimuli is usually very high. The five classic senses include olfaction (smell), vision, gustation (taste), auditory sense (hearing), and vestibular sense (balance and sense of acceleration).

Note: The order in which the senses have been outlined above, which also matches the following descriptions, is based on the sequence of participating neuronal structures—in this case the cranial nerves involved. Smell and taste, which are often mentioned together, are separated here as they are processed by completely different parts of the nervous system.

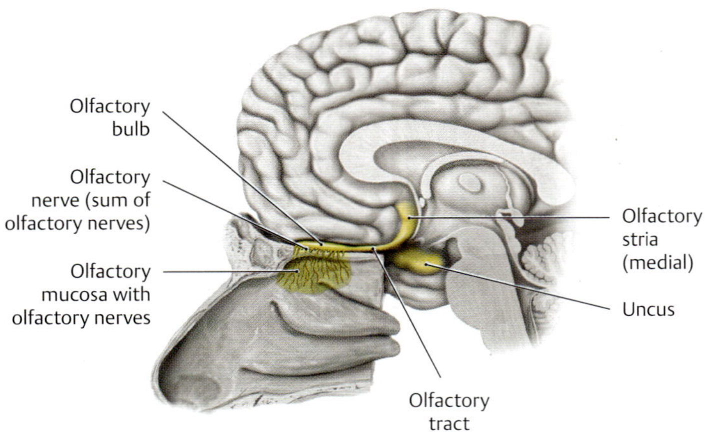

A Olfaction

Olfactory stimuli are detected by specific receptors in olfactory cells in the nasal mucosa. The axons of these olfactory cells combine to form olfactory fila. The receptor cells transmit their information directly to the CNS without involvement of a ganglion. The two other readily visible components of the olfactory system, the *olfactory bulb* and *olfactory tract*, are extensions of the brain and thus integral components of the CNS (not the PNS).

From the olfactory n., the olfactory information is carried via different relay stations (olfactory bulb, olfactory tract) to very old cortex portions (the *paleocortex*, mainly located in the temporal lobe close to the uncus) in both cerebral hemispheres where it is consciously processed. In perception of odors the olfactory sense is triggered by a chemical stimulus, the odorant—that attaches to a receptor in the nasal mucosa.

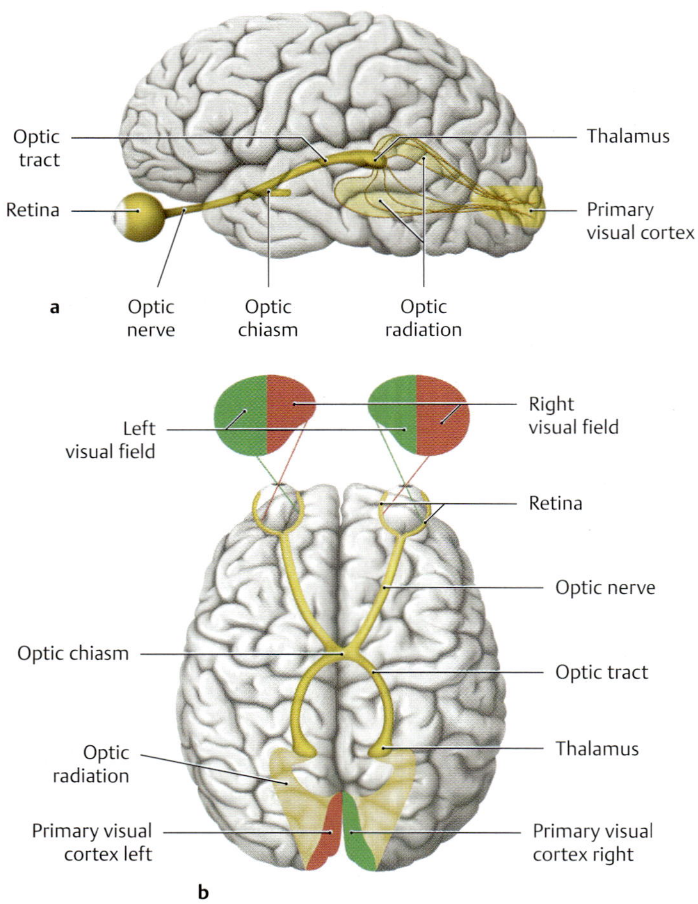

B Vision

Light stimuli (in the form of *photons*) are also exclusively received by the CNS: the light sensitive *retina* of the eye is an evaginated part of the diencephalon and again, the *optic n.* (CN II) is considered not to be a true nerve but structurally a tract. There is also no ganglion. From the retina (first-order to third-order neuron) where a neuronal processing of the light stimulus has already taken place, the axons (of the third-order neuron) extend via the optic n. and the optic tract to the thalamus (fourth-order neuron) in the cerebellum and from there as optic radiation to the so-called primary visual cortex (fifth-order neuron) at the occipital pole (**a**). The visual information crosses over to the opposite side at the optic chiasm. Visual impressions from the left visual field reach, and are interpreted in, the right hemisphere, and vice versa (**b**).

Note: The retina has a concave surface resembling the structure of a concave mirror. This means the images formed on the retina are upside down—up and down is reversed. Through a neuronal process up and down are placed in the correct position again. In terms of perception, the visual sense is triggered by a physical stimulus, electromagnetic waves, in a certain frequency range.

The perception of warmth on the skin is a physical stimulus, also triggered by electromagnetic waves. Light in the infrared region (which receptors in the eye can't detect) stimulates temperature receptors. Some animals (e.g., some types of snakes) possess infrared receptors and are able to see the warmth radiating off their prey.

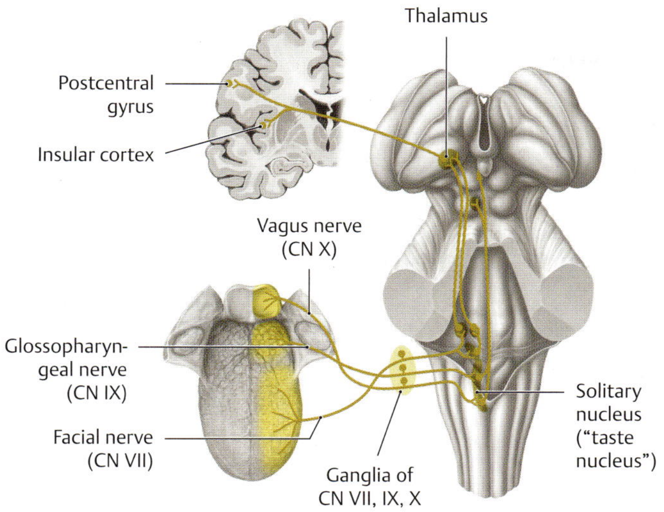

C Gustatory sense (of taste)
Taste perception takes place in the taste buds of the tongue. Three cranial nerves are responsible for the sense of taste: CN VII (facial n.) covers the anterior two thirds of the dorsum of the tongue; CN IX (glossopharyngeal n.) covers the posterior one third of the tongue, and CN X (vagus n.) covers the epiglottic region. From this distribution, it is evident that the facial n. (CN VII) plays the largest role in taste perception. All three nerves are true cranial nn. and as such, the first-order neuron lies in a sensory ganglion, and the second-order neuron is located in a brainstem nucleus shared by the three nerves, the nucleus solitarius. The third-order neuron of the gustatory tract uses the thalamus to reach the cerebral cortex of both hemispheres where the fourth-order neuron is located. The interesting point to note is that they terminate on both sides of two cortical regions—the postcentral gyrus and the insular lobe. In terms of perception, the gustatory sense is triggered by a chemical stimulus, a chemical compound or flavor, that attaches to a receptor in a taste bud on the surface of the tongue. Among the five senses, the gustatory sense is the simplest.

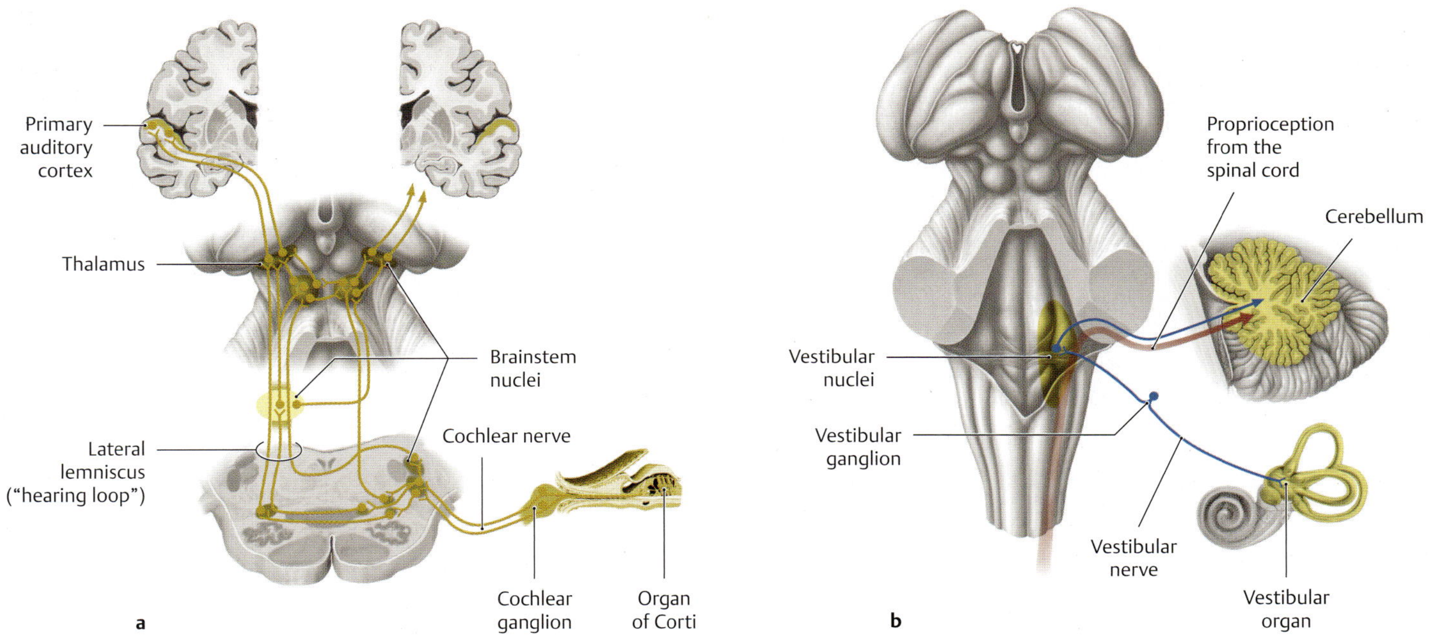

D Auditory and vestibular senses
In each case, information comes from an organ in the inner ear and is transmitted via the vestibulocochlear n., which is why they are discussed together here.

a Auditory sense: the auditory sense is a specific form of *mechanoreception:* air pressure fluctuations are perceived and analyzed. Loud music in the bass range can even be felt as vibration in visceral organs. The auditory sense is usually not considered part of mechanoreception. The perception of acoustic stimuli, which are transmitted to the inner ear through the middle ear in the form of pressure fluctuation, is achieved through sensory cells in the inner ear—*auditory hair cells* in the *organ of Corti*—and is carried to the CNS via the *cochlear n*. The cochlear n. is a peripheral nerve, the first-order neuron lies in the *cochlear ganglion*. The axon of this first-order neuron enters the CNS at the brainstem. Via neuronal pathways in the brainstem nuclei (primarily pons and mesencephalon), the information reaches the *primary auditory cortex* in the temporal lobes of both hemispheres after passing through the thalamus. This is where conscious auditory perception takes place. The entire auditory pathway in the brainstem is referred to as the *lateral lemniscus*. There are multiple crossing points of fibers in the auditory pathway. The fact that auditory information from the ear reaches both hemispheres is a precondition for directional hearing.

b Vestibular sense: The term "vestibular sense" is not precise, as balance is not a sensory perception triggered by each single stimulus, but the inner representation of a state of motion or rest of the body. It is based on the processing of different sensory impressions. The most vital region for maintenance of balance is the *cerebellum*. From the inner ear, the *vestibular organ* provides information about angular acceleration (circular motion) or transverse acceleration (e.g., through gravitational force) via the *vestibular n*. The first-order neuron is located in the vestibular ganglion where it synapses with neurons that reach then the cerebellum. Some axons travel directly from the vestibular ganglion to the cerebellum. Through proprioception, the cerebellum receives information about the position of head and limbs and their alignment to the trunk from receptors in skeletal muscle. Based on body posture and its spatial orientation, the cerebellum calculates the desired movement to control balance. Together the cochlear n. (hearing) and vestibular n. (acceleration) form the *vestibulocochlear n*. Auditory and vestibular sense in the vestibular apparatus are referred to as *specific somatic sensation*.

1.13 Principles of the Neurological Examination

In order to conduct a neurological examination and interpret its findings, the examiner has to be knowledgeable about basic neuroanatomy. This learning unit describes selected aspects of the neuroanatomical examination and explains why a neuroanatomical background is essential and indispensable for detecting and analyzing symptoms. The neurological examination as described below is a part of the general examination of a patient.

A Testing sensation

Sensation is the perception of different stimuli on the skin, mucosae, muscles, joints and internal organs. When assessing sensation, different qualities of sensory are being tested. Different receptors are responsible for different stimuli, which are transmitted to the brain via different pathways. The receptors and their pathways will be discussed in greater detail later on. *For* now, knowledge about the different sensory qualities and how to test them is sufficient. During all tests described here, the patient should keep the eyes closed in order to prevent a correction of the results by being able to see them. In addition, all tests should be conducted on both sides to detect damage affecting only one side of the body.

Note: All tests described here require the cooperation of the patient. They can only be conducted on a patient who is alert.

- **a Touch sensation** is assessed using a paintbrush, a cotton ball, or the fingertips. The examiner strokes the skin and the patient has to say whether they can feel the touch. A reduced sensation is referred to as *hypesthesia*; a total loss of sensation is referred to as *anesthesia*.
- **b Sensation of pain** is assessed using the pointed tip of an injection needle. A reduced sensation is referred to as *hypalgesia*, a loss of sensation is referred to as *analgesia*.
- **c Temperature sensation** is assessed using a warm or cold metallic object or a test tube filled with either cold or warm water. It is important that the water is not so hot that it generates temperature and in addition, pain sensation. Impaired temperature sensation is referred to as *thermohypesthesia*; a total loss of sensation is referred to as *thermoanesthesia*.
  Pain and temperature sensitivity are referred to as *protopathic sensitivity* (see p. 284).
- **d** The **vibratory sensation** is assessed using a tuning fork (64 or 128 Hz). A vibrating tuning fork is placed near the patient's ankle or held above the tibia. The patient is asked if they feel a vibration in their bones. A reduced sensation is referred to as *pallhypesthesia*; a total loss of sensation is referred to as *pallesthesia*.

Another sensory quality not described here is the **sense of position** (proprioception). It provides information about the spatial position of the limbs. The examiner moves one limb and asks the patient about the its position (e.g., bent or extended). The decisive stimulus is the elongation (tension) of muscles and articular capsules. The stimulus does not come from the body's surface but from deep within (deep sensation).

The sensory qualities listed here are found all over the body. In classical neuroanatomy, they are referred to as "sensitivity." The senses perceived by specific sensory organs (the five "classical" senses: olfactory, visual, gustatory, auditory and vestibular; see p. 288) were initially referred to as "sensation." However, since perception and transmission of impulses are in principle the same for sensibility and sensation, they are both referred to now as sensation.

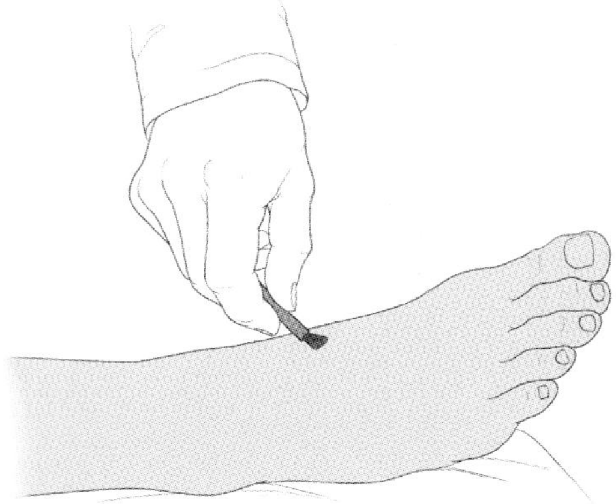

a

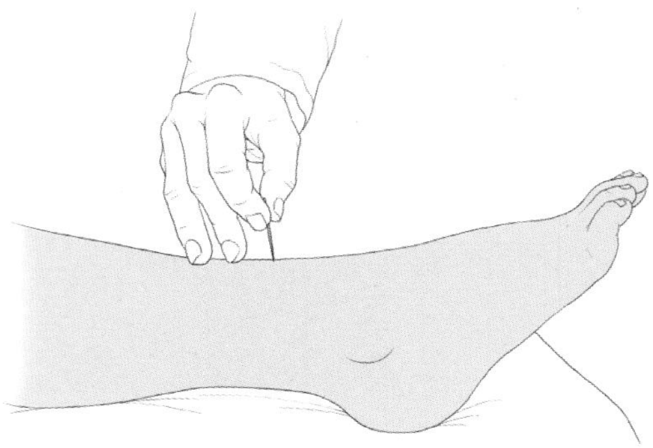

b

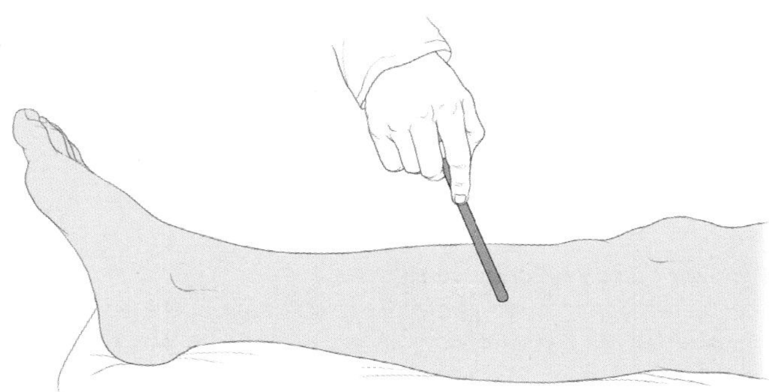

c

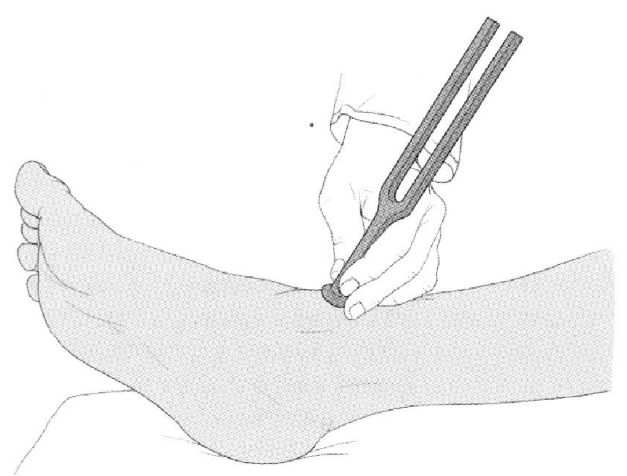

d

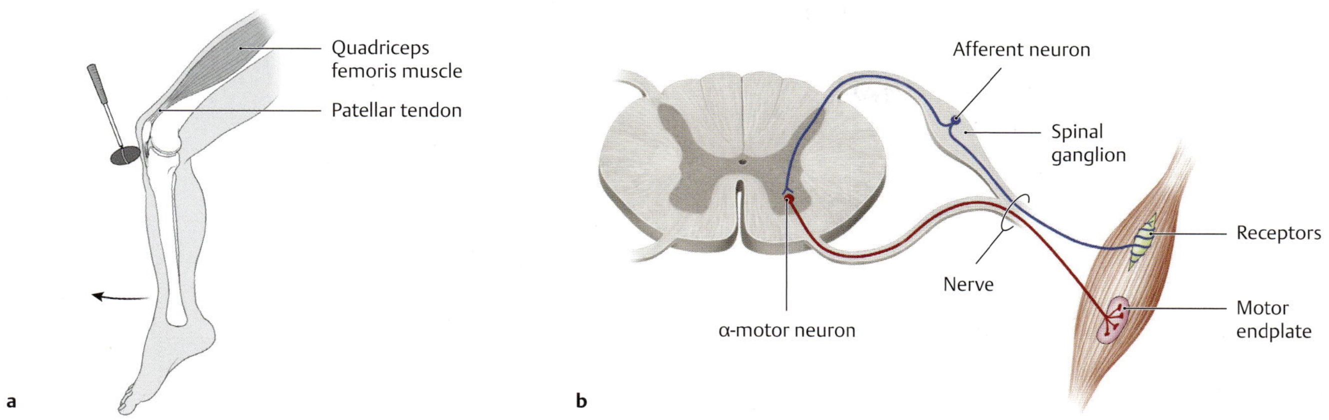

B Testing motor function

The efferent systems, which generate movements of the skeletal muscles, are referred to as "motor systems" or "motor function." They are assessed by examining the reflexes. One example listed here is the patellar tendon reflex (**a**). When tapping the patellar tendon with a reflex hammer, the quadriceps m. contracts. As a result, it shortens to such an extent that it causes the knee to extend. If that happens, the reflex arc is intact (**b**). By tapping the tendon, the muscle is pulled and elongates. This muscle elongation is perceived by muscle receptors and relayed to the spinal cord. The cell body of the stimulated afferent neuron lies in the spinal ganglion. Its axon releases a transmitter at the α-motoneuron in the spinal cord. This transmitter stimulates the α-motoneuron, which itself releases transmitters at the motor endplate. This transmitter stimulates the muscle which will then contract and the knee extends. The leg kicks forward.

Note: For the α-motoneuron to be stimulated, sensory input pathways must be intact. With regard to reflexes, sensation and motor function are closely related, which is why in physiology the term sensorimotor function is often used. Intact sensation is a precondition for intact motor function, and has been described in a previous chapter in this book.

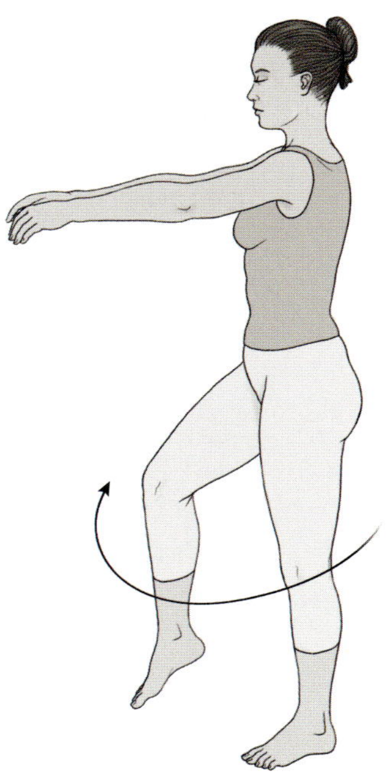

C Coordination assessment

In addition to tests for assessing sensation and reflexes, the neurological exam also includes the assessment of more complex pathways of information processing. One example is Unterberger's stepping test. With eyes closed and arms extended forward, the patient is asked to walk on the spot. Performing this task requires the coordination of several sensory systems. It is especially challenging to provide information about the position of the head for which the inner ear is responsible (see p. 289). A malfunctioning of the vestibular parts of the inner ear (the semicircular canals) leads to increased spinning of the affected side. In the example shown here, a turn to the right (illustrated by the arrow) is caused by right inner ear malfunction.

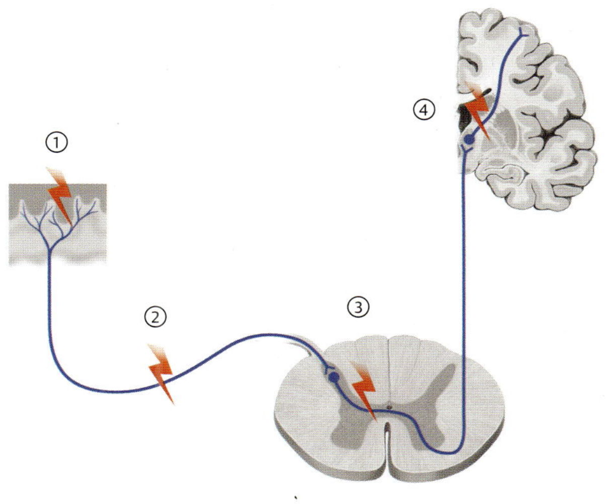

D Problems in neurological-topical diagnostics

The figure illustrates a pain pathway extending from the body surface to the sensory cortex. If the pathway is disrupted, the pain information does not reach the sensory cortex. Location of the disruption can be in either the receptive field (1), in the peripheral nerve (2), in the spinal cord (3), or the brain itself (4). Disruption in any of these locations prevents the sensory cortex from perceiving the pain. This explains why the brain always localizes disruption in the receptive field (1) even though the disruption can be located in the spinal cord (3). The physician is confronted with the problem of "tricking" the brain and to identify the location of the disruption, since the therapy differs depending on where the pathway has been damaged. The process of identifying the damaged location is referred to as neurological-topical diagnostics. This is why intimate knowledge of important pathways is essential when examining a patient.

2.1 Neurons

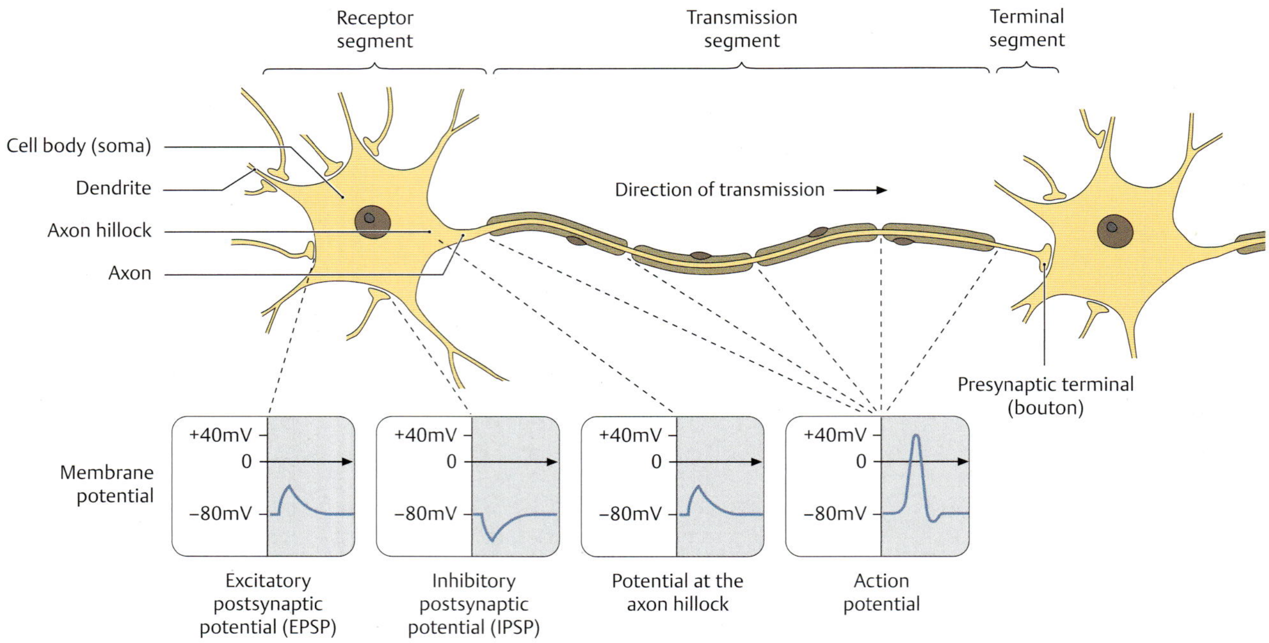

A The nerve cell (neuron)
The basic structure of a nerve cell (neuron) has already been explained on p. 268, fig. **A**. The terms "signal input," "signal output" and "signal exchange" as mentioned in the previous chapter can also be used to describe the "functional classification" of neurons. The **three segments** are as follows:

- The *receptor segment*; corresponds to the cell body and the dentrites.
- The *transmission segment*; carries the information to the target cell. Physiologically and morphologically, this segment is called the axon. Where a rapid transfer of information is required, the axon has a myelin sheath (for structure see **C**, p. 295). Fast reaction speed is usually needed in the CNS.
- The *terminal segment* is responsible for relaying the information to the target cell. It is identical to the structures that form a synapse.

The axons of other neurons, which also form synapses with the target neuron, (cf. **D**) terminate at the receptor segment of the target cell. It is in these synapses that the release of either excitatory or inhibitory neurotransmitters occurs. These transmitters released at the end of the axon bind to receptors at the cell membrane of the target cell, creating either a local increase in membrane potential (excitatory postsynaptic potential EPSP) or a decrease (inhibitory postsynaptic potential IPSP).

A neuron constantly receives inhibitory and excitatory signals. The integration of these local potentials takes place at the axon hillock. A preponderance of excitatory over inhibitory signals leads to action potential generation at the axon hillock. The action potential arrives at the axon terminal (bouton) and triggers the release of transmitters at this axonal site. Receptors at the target cell recognize the released transmitters and the local membrane potential is either decreased (IPSP) or increased (EPSP) depending on the transmitter and its receptor. This last portion represents the terminal segment, the synapse.
Note: The transfer of information between nerve cells is made possible through neurotransmitters. The presynaptic neuron releases the transmitter, which is detected by a receptor on a postsynaptic membrane. As a result, the local membrane potential of a nerve cell increases (EPSP) or decreases (IPSP). These local potential changes occur only in dendrites and the neuron cell body.
In the axon, during the transfer of information, potential changes occur according to the all-or-none principle. In a myelinated axon, the potential change can be measured only at specific myelin-free sections (the nodes of Ranvier, see **B**, p. 294).

B Electron microscopy of the neuron
The organelles of neurons can be resolved with an electron microscope. Neurons are rich in rough endoplasmic reticulum (protein synthesis, active metabolism). This endoplasmic reticulum (called *Nissl substance* under a light microscope) is easily demonstrated by light microscopy when it is stained with cationic dyes (which bind to the anionic mRNA and nRNA of the ribosomes). The distribution pattern of the Nissl substance is used in neuropathology to evaluate the functional integrity of neurons. The neurotubules and neurofilaments that are visible by electron microscopy are referred to collectively in *light microscopy* as neurofibrils, as they are too fine to be resolved as separate structures under the light microscope. Neurofibrils can be demonstrated in light microscopy by impregnating the nerve tissue with silver salts. This is important in neuropathology, for example, because the clumping of neurofibrils is an important histological feature of Alzheimer's disease.

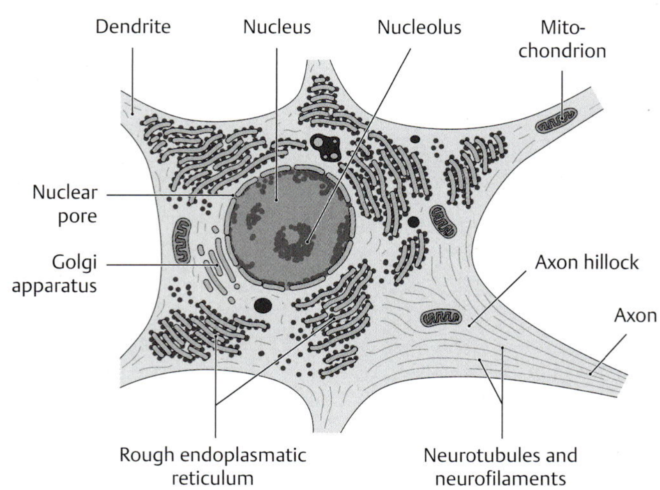

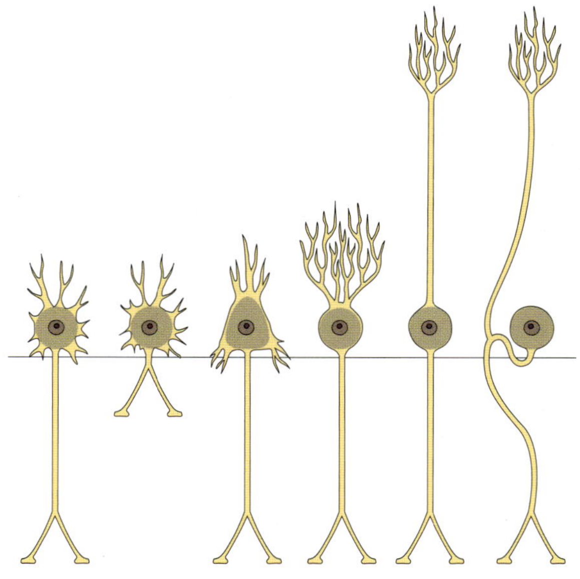

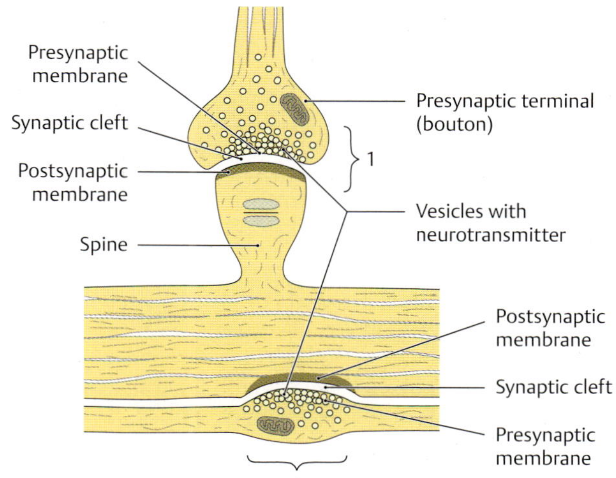

C Basic forms of the neuron and its functionally adapted variants
The horizontal line marks the region of the axon hillock, which represents the initial segment of the axon. (The structure of a peripheral nerve, which consists only of axons and sheath tissue, is shown on p. 275, see **D**.)

a Multipolar neuron (multiple dendrites) with a long axon (= long transmission path). Examples are projection neurons such as alpha motor neurons in the spinal cord.
b Multipolar neuron with a short axon (= short transmission path). Examples are interneurons like those in the gray matter of the brain and spinal cord.
c Pyramidal cell: Dendrites are present only at the apex and base of the triangular cell body, and the axon is long. Examples are efferent neurons of the cerebral motor cortex (see pp. 327 and 457).
d Purkinje cell: An elaborately branched dendritic tree arises from one circumscribed site on the cell body. The Purkinje cell of the cerebellum has many synaptic contacts with other neurons (see p. 369).
e Bipolar neuron: The dendrite arborizes in the periphery. The bipolar cells of the retina are an example (see **Ab**, p. 476).
f Pseudounipolar neuron: The dendrite and axon are not separated by the cell body. An example is the primary afferent (sensory) neuron in the spinal (dorsal root) ganglion (see p. 444 and **C**, p. 273).
Note: In pseudounipolar cells, the single dendrite also has a myelin sheath for fast signal transduction, and unlike the usually short dendrite of multipolar neurons, the dendrite of a unipolar neuron is generally long (e.g., from a receptor at the sole of the foot to the neuron in the spinal ganglion is about 1 meter in length). In these cells the axon and dendrite can not be distinguished from each other based on their structure but their stimulus conduction can be used. The dendrite moves stimuli to the nerve cell body; the axon takes it away from the nerve cell body.

D Electron microscopic appearance of the two most common types of synapse in the CNS
Synapses—in terms of their structure correlate to the terminal segment (see **A**)—display a structure visible under the electron microscope. They consist of a presynaptic membrane, a synaptic gap and a postsynaptic membrane. In case of a synapse with a dendritic spine (1), the terminal bouton of the axon contacts a specialized protrusion (or spine) found on a dendrite of the target cell. The side-by-side synapse of an axon with the flat surface of a target neuron is called a parallel contact or *bouton en passage* (2). The vesicles in the presynaptic expansions contain the neurotransmitters that are released into the synaptic cleft by exocytosis when the axon fires. From there the neurotransmitters diffuse to the postsynaptic membrane, where their receptors are located. A variety of drugs and toxins act upon synaptic transmission (antidepressants, muscle relaxants, nerve gases, botulinum toxin).

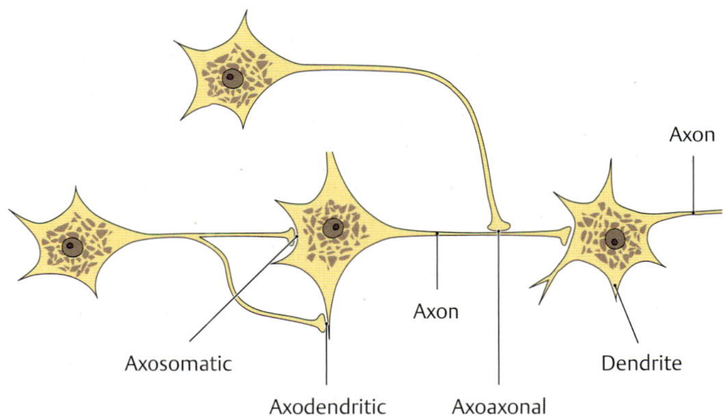

E Synaptic patterns in a small group of neurons
Axons may terminate at various sites on the target neuron and form synapses there. The synaptic patterns are described as axodendritic, axosomatic, or axoaxonal. Axodendritic synapses are the most common (see also **A**). The cerebral cortex consists of many small groups of neurons that are collected into functional units called columns (see p. 327).

2.2 Neuroglia and Myelination

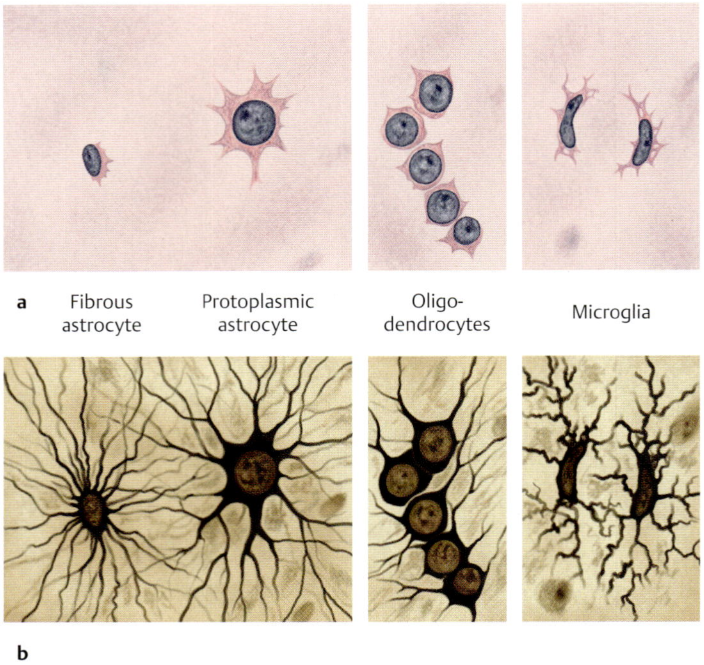

A Cells of the neuroglia in the CNS
Neuroglial cells surround the neurons, providing them with structural and functional support (see **D**). Various staining methods are used in light microscopy to define specific portions of the neuroglial cells:

a Cell nuclei demonstrated with a basic stain
b Cell body demonstrated by silver impregnation

Recent studies have found that in the CNS neurons and neuroglia exist at a ratio ranging from 1:1 up to 1.6. Neuroglial cells provide critical support functions for neurons. For example, astrocytes absorb excess neurotransmitters from the extracellular milieu, helping to maintain a constant internal environment. While neurons are, almost without exception, permanently post-mitotic, some neuroglial cells continue to divide throughout life. For this reason, most primary brain tumors originate from neuroglial cells and are named for their morphological similarity to normal neuroglial cells: astrocytoma, oligodendroglioma, and glioblastoma. Developmentally, most neuroglial cells arise from the same progenitor cells as neurons. This may not apply to microglial cells, which develop from precursor cells in the blood from the monocyte lineage.

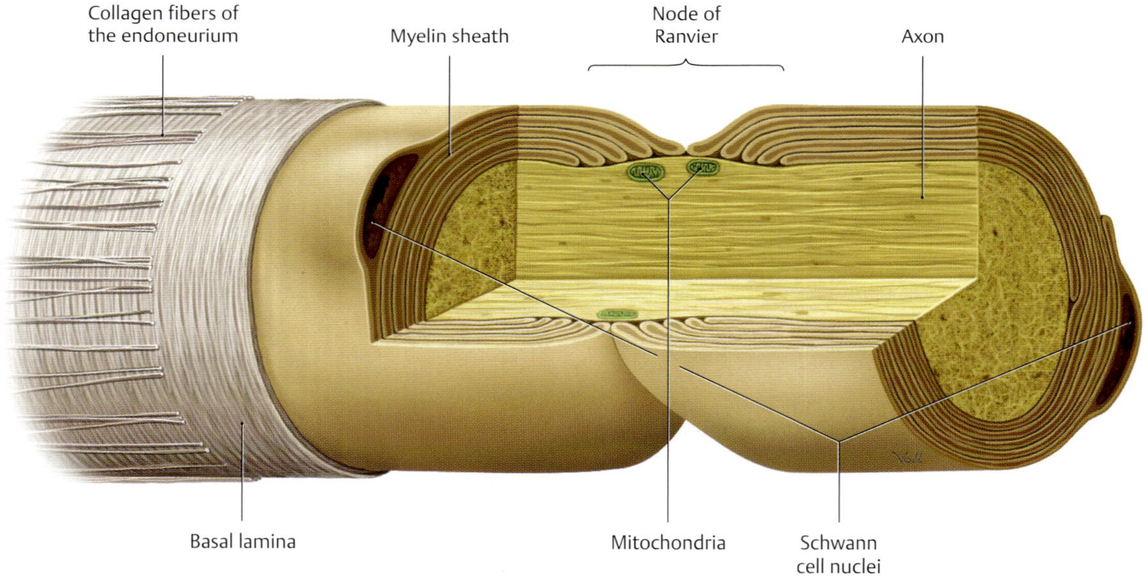

B Myelinated axon in the PNS
Most axons in the peripheral nervous system are insulated by a myelin sheath, although unmyelinated axons are also found in the PNS (see **C**). The myelin sheath enables impulses to travel faster along the axon as they "jump" from one *node of Ranvier* to the next (saltatory nerve conduction), rather than travel continuously as in an unmyelinated axon. Mitochondria concentrate in the nodes of Ranvier to ensure the energy supply of Na/K ATPase.

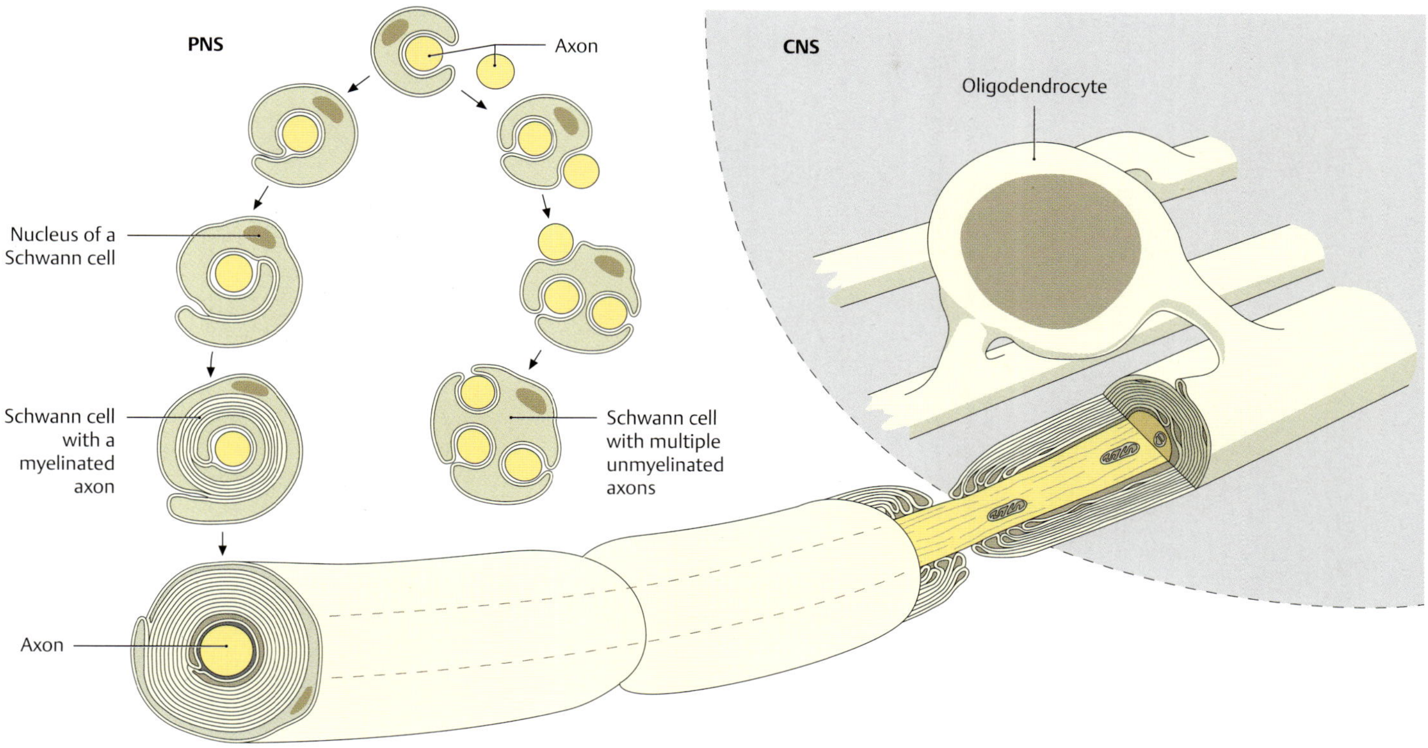

C Myelination differences in the PNS and CNS
The purpose of myelination is to insulate the axons electrically. This significantly boosts the nerve conduction velocity as a result of saltatory conduction (i.e., potentials jumping from one node of Ranvier to the next). While almost all axons in the CNS are myelinated, this is not the case in the PNS. The axons of the PNS are myelinated in regions where fast reaction speeds are needed (e.g., skeletal muscle contraction) and unmyelinated in regions that do not require rapid information transfer (e.g., the transmission of muscle spindle and tendon tension sensation). The very lipid-rich membranes of myelinating cells are wrapped around the axons to insulate them. There are differences between the myelinating cells of the central and peripheral nervous systems. Schwann cells (left) myelinate the axons in the PNS, whereas oligodendrocytes (right) form the myelin sheaths in the CNS.

Note: In the CNS, one oligodendrocyte always wraps around multiple axons; however, Schwann cells ensheathe either one myelinated axon or multiple unmyelinated axons.

This difference in myelination has important clinical implications. In multiple sclerosis, the oligodendrocytes are damaged but the Schwann cells are not. As a result, the peripheral myelin sheaths remain intact in MS while the central myelin sheaths degenerate.

D Summary: Cells of the central nervous system (CNS) and peripheral nervous system (PNS) and their functional importance

Cell type	Function
Neurons (CNS and PNS)	1. Impulse formation 2. Impulse conduction 3. Information processing
Glial cells	
Astrocytes (CNS only) (also called *macroglia*)	1. Maintain a constant internal milieu in the CNS 2. Help to form the blood–brain barrier 3. Phagocytosis of nonfunctioning synapses 4. Scar formation in the CNS (e.g., after cerebral infarction or in multiple sclerosis) 5. Absorb excess neurotransmitters and K^+
Microglial cells (CNS only)	Cells specialized for phagocytosis and antigen processing (brain macrophages, part of the mononuclear phagocyte system); secrete cytokines and growth factors
Oligodendrocytes (CNS only)	Form the myelin sheaths in the CNS
Ependymal cells (CNS only)	Line ventricular system cavities in the CNS
Cells of the choroid plexus (CNS only)	Secrete cerebrospinal fluid
Schwann cells (PNS only)	Form the myelin sheaths in the PNS
Satellite cells (PNS only) (also called *mantle cells*)	Modified Schwann cells; surround the cell body of neurons in PNS ganglia

3.1 Sympathetic and Parasympathetic Nervous Systems, Organization

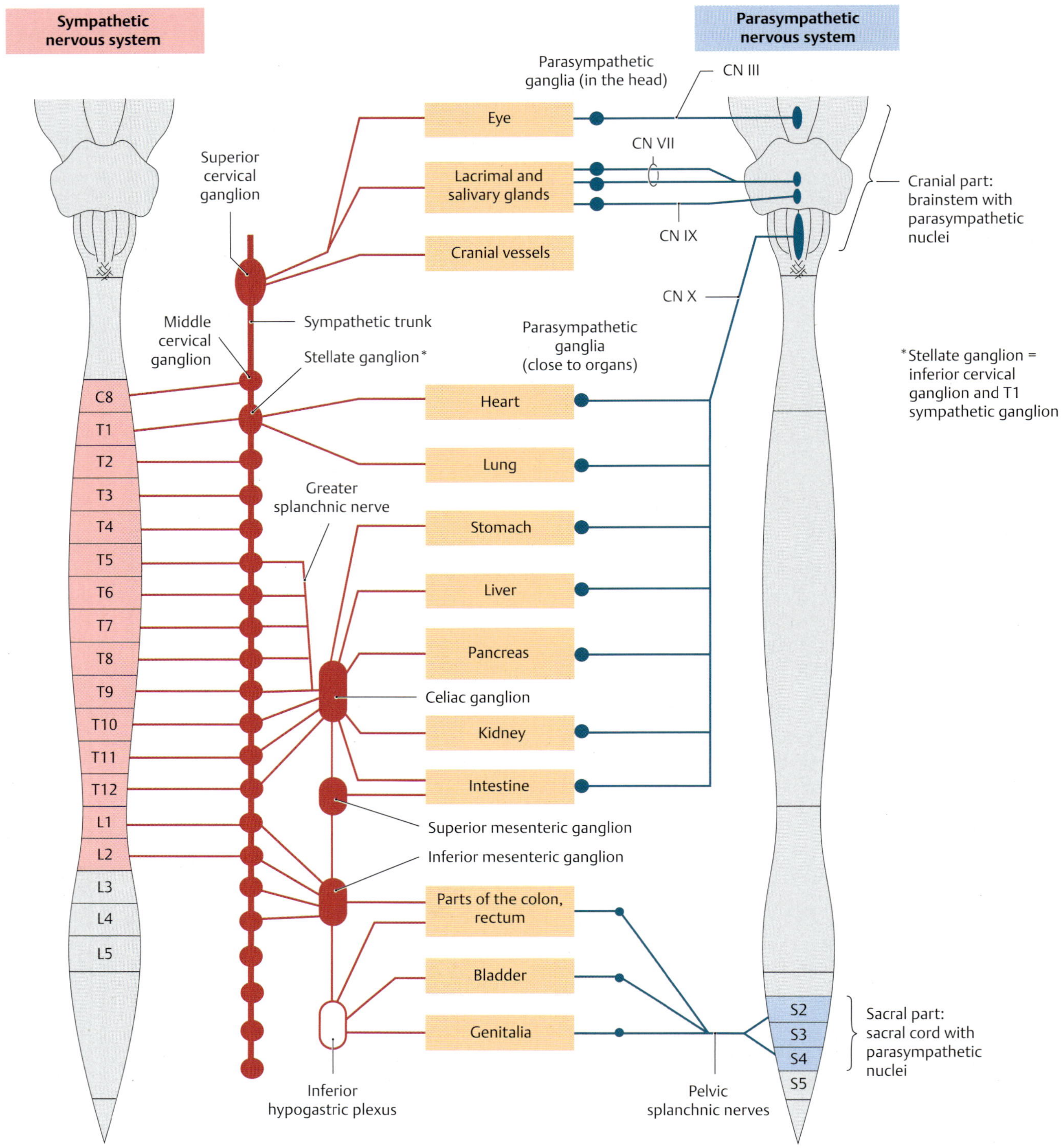

A Structure of the autonomic nervous system

The somatic nervous system, which innervates skeletal muscles, is contrasted with the autonomic nervous system. This is further subdivided into the *sympathetic* (red) and *parasympathetic* (blue) nervous systems (for their function see **C**). The preganglionic neurons of the sympathetic system have their bodies located in the lateral horns of thoracic and lumbar spinal cord (T1–L2). The preganglionic neurons of the parasympathetic system have their bodies located in parts of the brainstem and in the sacral spinal cord. In the sympathetic system, the preganglionic neurons synapse with the postganglionic neurons in sympathetic ganglia (either paravertebral ganglia or prevertebral ganglia). Axons of the preganglionic sympathetic neurons that will synapse in the prevertebral ganglia form the splanchnic nerves (visceral nerves). In the parasympathetic system the preganglionic neurons synapse with the postganglionic neurons in parasympathetic ganglia associated with cranial nerves or in the wall of target structures. Langley (1905) restricted the terms sympathetic and parasympathetic systems to the efferent neurons and their axons (visceral efferent fibers; only those are shown here). Meanwhile, it has been proven that the sympathetic and parasympathetic systems contain also afferent fibers (visceral afferents, pain and stretch receptors; not shown here, see p. 302). The *enteric nervous* system is now regarded as an independent part of the autonomic nervous system (see p. 304).

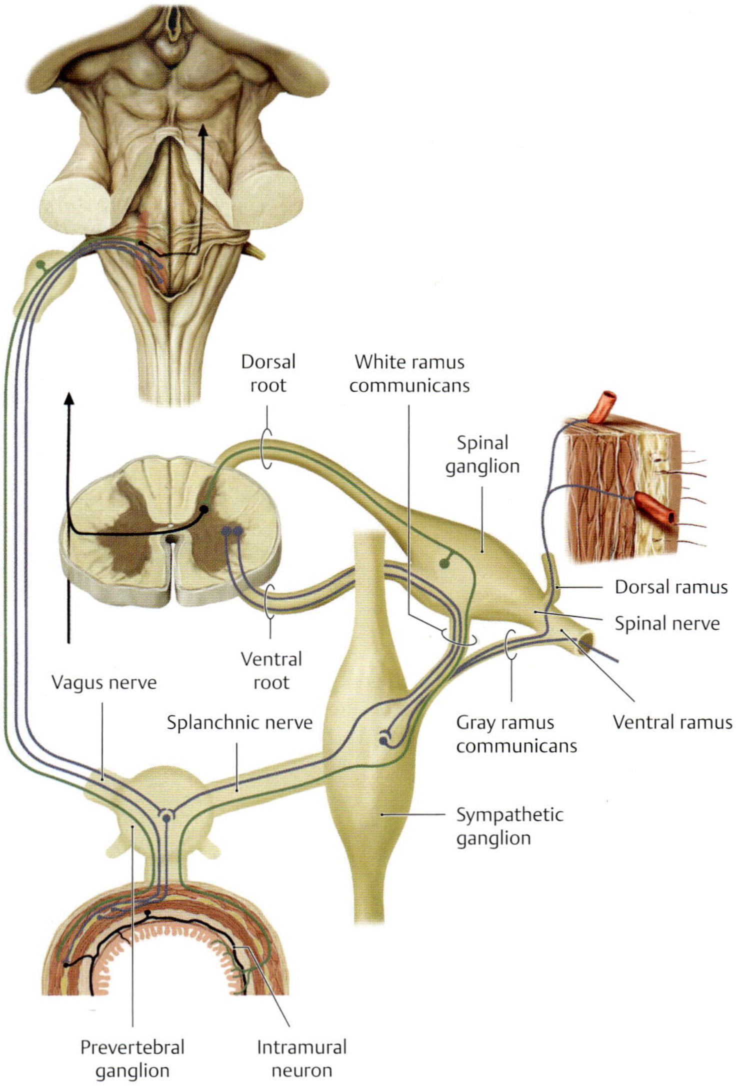

B Synaptic organization of the autonomic nervous system

The sympathetic and parasympathetic portions of the nervous systems innervate many of the same targets, but use different transmitters, often with antagonistic effects (see **C**). These antagonistic systems also have differing patterns of organization, including unique paths to their targets and connections to the CNS. The cell bodies of the preganglionic motor neurons of the **sympathetic system** are located in the lateral horn of spinal cord segments T1 to L2. Their axons leave the spinal cord through thoracolumbar ventral roots, briefly travel in spinal nerves, and enter the paravertebral sympathetic trunk via white rami communicantes (white = myelinated). These axons terminate in synapses with postganglionic neurons at three different levels:

1. Sympathetic ganglia along the paravertebral chain: The postganglionic neurons send their axons back into the spinal nerves via gray rami communicantes (gray = unmyelinated). These axons travel in the ventral or dorsal rami to innervate local blood vessels, sweat glands, etc.
2. Prevertebral sympathetic ganglia: The postganglionic neurons send their axons along arterial plexuses to the bowel, kidneys, etc., providing innervation to both the organs and their vasculature (see p. 304).
3. Adrenal medulla (not shown): Adrenal medullary (endocrine) cells are developmentally sympathetic ganglion cells, and receive direct innervation from presynaptic sympathetic axons.

In contrast, the preganglionic neurons of the **parasympathetic system** are located in the CNS in the brainstem (nuclei related to cranial nerves III, VII, IX, and X) and sacral spinal cord (S2–S4). The preganglionic axons leave the CNS via the cranial nerves noted above (the vagus nerve [CN X] is the example shown here), and pelvic splanchnic nerves. These presynaptic axons synapse with postganglionic neurons in discrete cranial ganglia (ciliary, pterygopalatine, submandibular, and otic), which in turn send their axons via other cranial nerves to the target organ. Preganglionic neurons in the vagus nerve and the pelvic splanchnic nerves synapse with the postganglionic neurons in small ganglia within the wall of the target organs. Afferent fibers (shown in green), originating from pseudounipolar neurons in spinal (dorsal root) and cranial sensory ganglia, travel with autonomic motor axons. These sensory fibers carry information from visceral nociceptors (pain) and stretch receptors into the CNS. Efferent fibers are shown in purple, the ascending pain pathway in gray. For detailed description of the autonomic innervation of the viscera, see *Volume 2, Internal Organs.*

C Synopsis of the sympathetic and parasympathetic nervous systems

This table summarizes the effects of the sympathetic and parasympathetic nervous systems on specific organs.

1. The *sympathetic* nervous system is the excitatory part of the autonomic nervous system (fight or flight).
2. The *parasympathetic* nervous system coordinates rest and digestive processes (rest and digest).
3. Although the two systems have separate nuclei, they establish close anatomical and functional connections in the periphery.
4. The transmitter at the target organ is *acetylcholine* in the parasympathetic and *norepinephrine* in the sympathetic nervous system (except for the adrenal medulla).
5. Stimulation of the sympathetic or parasympathetic nervous system produces the following effects in specific organs (see table):

Organ	Sympathetic nervous system	Parasympathetic nervous system
Eye	Pupillary dilation	Pupillary constriction and increased curvature of the lens
Salivary glands	Decreased salivation (scant, viscous)	Increased salivation (copious, watery)
Heart	Increased heart rate	Decreased heart rate
Lungs	Decreased bronchial secretions and bronchodilation	Increased bronchial secretions and bronchoconstriction
Gastrointestinal tract	Decrease in secretions and motility	Increase in secretions and motility
Pancreas	Decreased exocrine secretions	Increased exocrine secretions
Male sex organs	Ejaculation	Erection
Skin	Vasoconstriction, sweating, piloerection	No effect

3.2 Autonomic Nervous System, Actions and Regulation

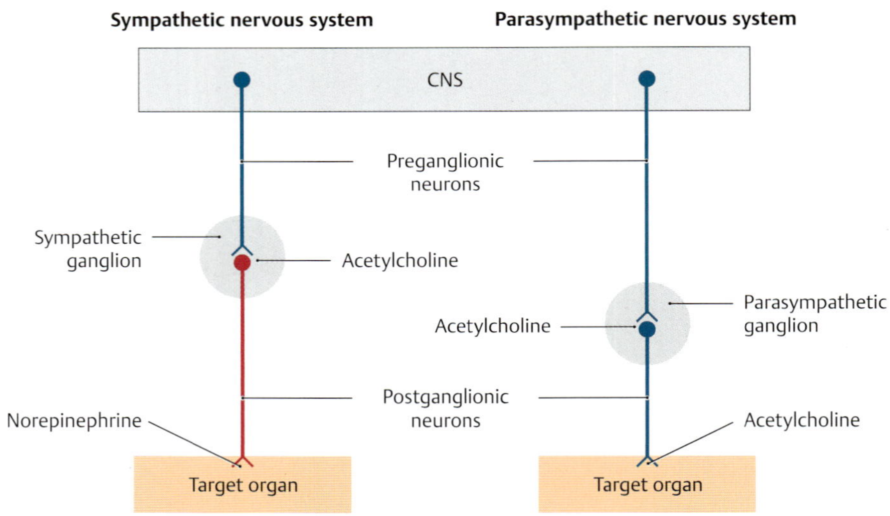

A Circuit diagram of the autonomic nervous system
The preganglionic neuron is located in the central nervous system and uses acetylcholine as a neurotransmitter in both the sympathetic and parasympathetic nervous systems (cholinergic neuron, shown in blue). Acetylcholine is also used as a neurotransmitter by the postganglionic neuron in the parasympathetic nervous system. In the sympathetic nervous system, norepinephrine is used by the noradrenergic neuron (shown in red).
Note: The target cell membrane contains different types of receptors for acetylcholine and norepinephrine. Each neurotransmitter can produce entirely different effects, depending on the type of receptor.

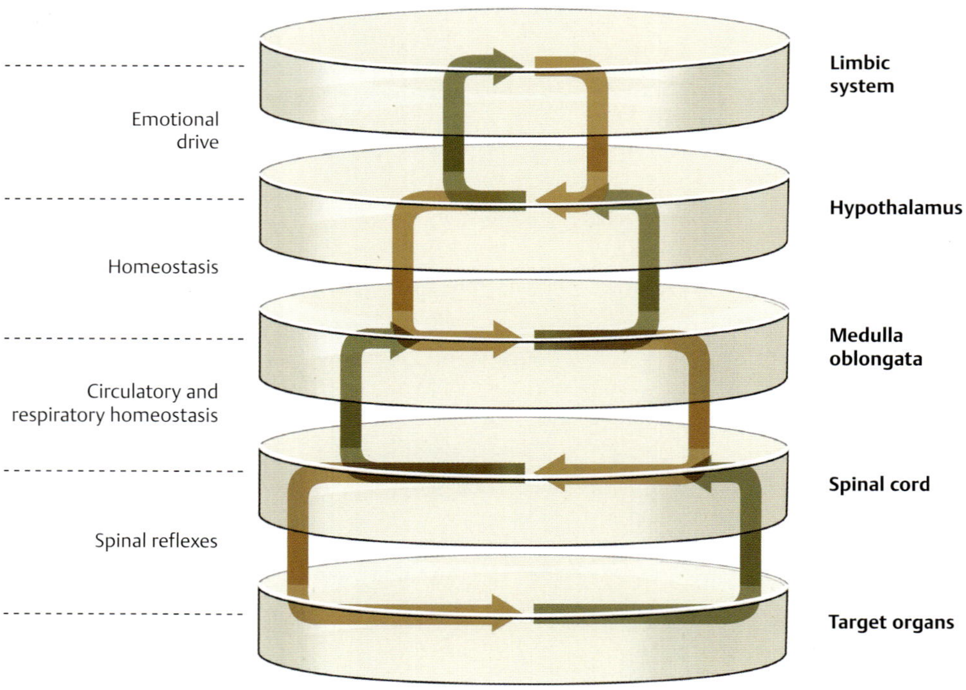

B Control of the peripheral autonomic nervous system
(after Klinke and Silbernagl)
The peripheral actions of the autonomic nervous system are subject to control at various levels, the highest being the limbic system. The efferent fibers act on the peripheral target organs (e.g., heart, lung, bowel). The sympathetic tone and cutaneous blood flow are also affected through centers in the hypothalamus, medulla oblongata, and spinal cord. The higher the control center, the more subtle and complex its effect on the target organ. The limbic system receives signals from its target organs via afferent feedback mechanisms.

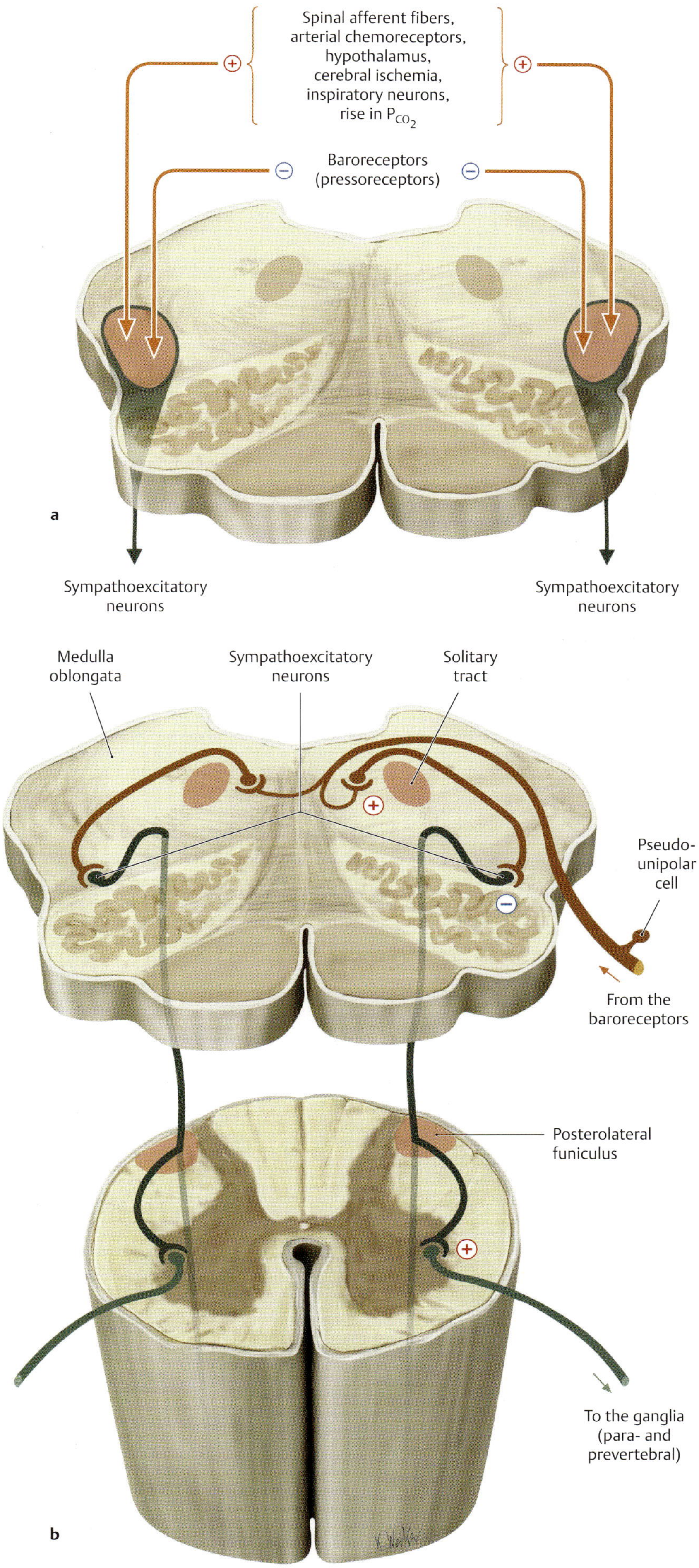

C Excitatory and inhibitory effects on sympathoexcitatory neurons in the medulla oblongata

a Cross-section through the brainstem at the level of the medulla oblongata. To generate a baseline level of sympathetic outflow, the presynaptic visceral efferent sympathetic neurons in the spinal cord (intermediolateral nuclei) must be stimulated by sympathoexcitatory neurons in the hypothalamus and anterolateral part of the medulla oblongata. Numerous factors can inhibit or enhance the activity of these neurons which play a critical role in the regulation of blood pressure. If the blood pressure is too high, for example, afferent impulses from the baroreceptors (pressoreceptors) will inhibit sympathetic outflow.

b Afferent impulses from the factors listed in **a** are relayed in the medial nuclei of the solitary tract nucleus to secondary neurons, whose axons project back to the sympathoexcitatory neurons. When these neurons are inhibited, the peripheral resistance vessels relax and the blood pressure falls. The axons from these sympathoexcitatory neurons pass ipsilaterally through the posterolateral funiculus to presynaptic sympathetic neurons in the lateral horn of the spinal cord. Sensory neurons are shown in orange, motor neurons in green.

3.3 Parasympathetic Nervous System, Overview and Connections

A Overview: parasympathetic nervous system (cranial part)

There are four parasympathetic nuclei in the brainstem. The visceral efferent fibers of these nuclei travel along particular cranial nerves, listed below.

- Visceral oculomotor (Edinger–Westphal) nucleus: oculomotor nerve (CN III)
- Superior salivatory nucleus: facial nerve (CN VII)
- Inferior salivatory nucleus: glossopharyngeal nerve (CN IX)
- Dorsal vagal nucleus: vagus nerve (CN X)

The presynaptic parasympathetic fibers often travel with multiple cranial nerves to reach their target organs (for details see p. 528 and **E**, p. 130). The vagus nerve supplies all of the thoracic and abdominal organs as far as a point near the left colic flexure.

Note: The sympathetic fibers to the head travel along the arteries to their target organs.

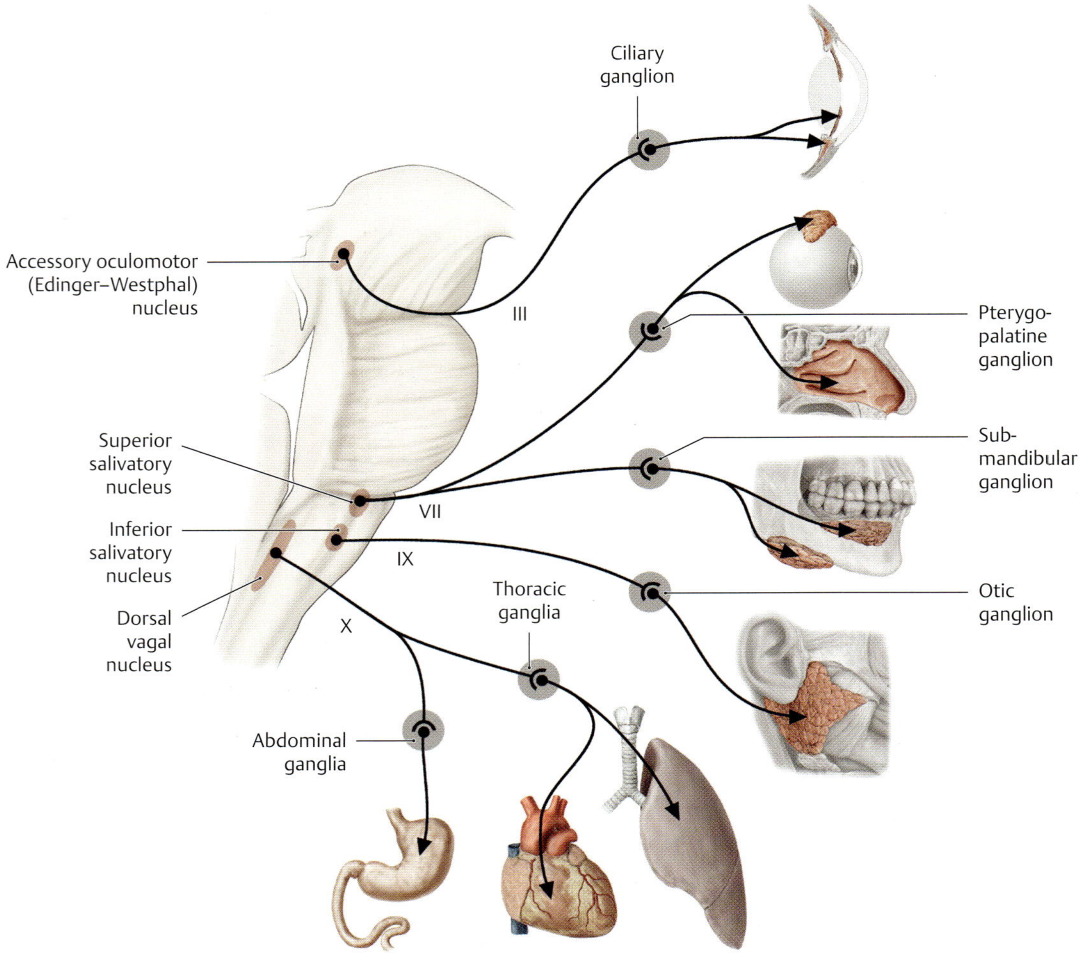

B Parasympathetic ganglia in the head

Nucleus	Path of presynaptic fibers	Ganglion	Postsynaptic fibers	Target organs
• Accessory oculomotor (Edinger–Westphal) nucleus	• Oculomotor nerve	• Ciliary ganglion	• Short ciliary nerves	• Ciliary muscle (accommodation) • Pupillary sphincter (miosis)
• Superior salivatory nucleus	• Nervus intermedius (facial nerve root) divides into:		• Maxillary nerve → zygomatic nerve → anastomosis → lacrimal nerve	• Lacrimal gland
	1. Greater petrosal nerve → nerve of pterygoid canal	• Pterygopalatine ganglion	• Orbital branches • Lateral posterior nasal branches • Nasopalatine nerve • Palatine nerves	• Glands on: – posterior ethmoid cells – nasal conchae – anterior palate – hard and soft palate
	2. Chorda tympani → lingual nerve	• Submandibular ganglion	• Glandular branches	• Submandibular gland • Sublingual gland
• Inferior salivatory nucleus	• Glossopharyngeal nerve → tympanic nerve → lesser petrosal nerve	• Otic ganglion	• Auriculotemporal nerve (CN V_3)	• Parotid gland
• Dorsal vagal nucleus	• Vagus nerve	• Ganglia near organs	• Fine fibers in organs, not individually named	• Thoracic and abdominal viscera

→ = is continuous with

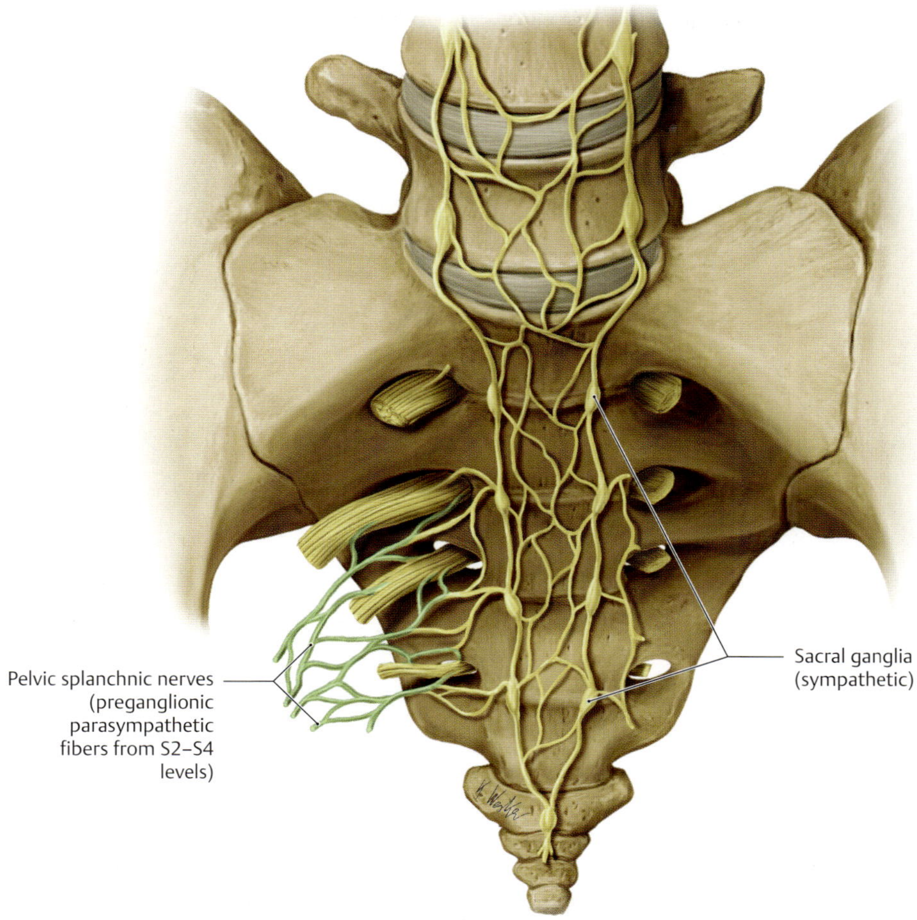

C Overview: parasympathetic nervous system (lumbrosacral part)
The portions of the bowel past the left colic flexure and the pelvic viscera are supplied by the sacral part of the parasympathetic nervous system. Efferent fibers emerge from the anterior sacral foramina in the anterior (ventral) roots of segments S2–S4. The fibers are collected into bundles to form the pelvic splanchnic nerves. They blend with the sympathetic fibers and synapse in the ganglia in or near the organs.

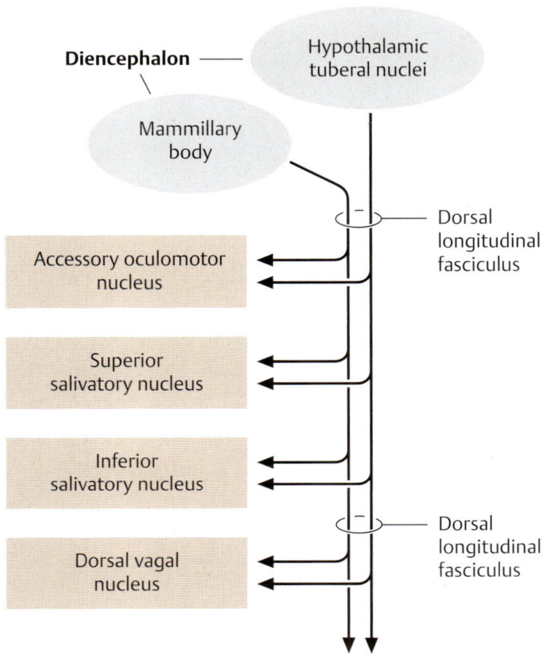

D Connections of the dorsal longitudinal fasciculus
Increased salivation during eating results from stimulation of the salivary glands by the parasympathetic nervous system. To produce the coordinated stimulation of various glands, the cranial parasympathetic nuclei require excitatory impulses from higher centers (tuberal nuclei, mammillary bodies). The parasympathetic nuclei are then stimulated to increase the flow of saliva. The dorsal longitudinal fasciculus establishes the necessary connections with the higher centers. Besides the fibers that coordinate the parasympathetic nuclei, the fasciculus contains other fiber systems that are not shown in the diagram.

3.4 Autonomic Nervous System: Pain Conduction

A Pain afferents conducted from the viscera by the sympathetic and parasympathetic nervous systems

a Sympathetic pain fibers, **b** parasympathetic pain fibers.

It was originally thought that the sympathetic and parasympathetic nervous systems conveyed only efferent fibers to the viscera. More recent research has shown, however, that both systems also carry afferent nociceptive (pain) fibers (shown in green), many running parallel to visceral efferent fibers (shown in purple). It is likely that many of these fibers (which make up only 5 % of all the afferent pain fibers in the body) are inactive during normal processes and may become active in response to organ lesions, for example.

a The pain-conducting (nociceptive) axons from the viscera course in the splanchnic nerves to the sympathetic ganglia and reach the spinal nerve by way of the white ramus communicans. The cell bodies of these neurons are located in the spinal ganglion. From the spinal nerve, the neurons pass through the dorsal roots to the posterior horn of the spinal cord. There they are relayed to establish a connection with the ascending pain pathway. Alternatively, a reflex arc may be established through interneurons (see **B**).
Note: Unlike the efferent system, the afferent nociceptive fibers of the sympathetic and parasympathetic systems are not relayed in the peripheral ganglia.

b The cell bodies of the pain-conducting pseudounipolar neurons in the *cranial* parasympathetic system are located in the inferior or superior ganglion of the vagus nerve (CN X). Those of the *sacral* parasympathetic system are located in the sacral spinal ganglia of S2–S4. Their fibers run parallel to the efferent vagal fibers and establish a central connection with the pain-processing systems.

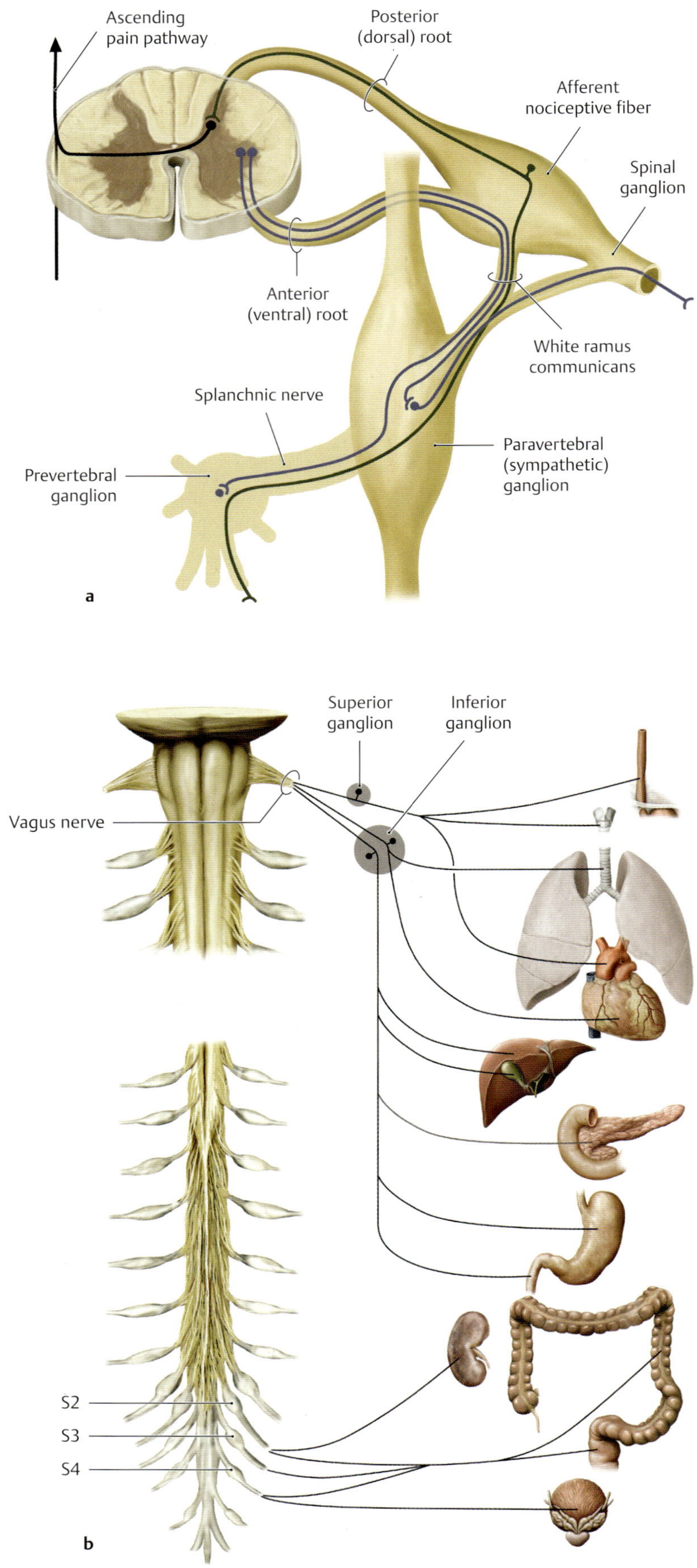

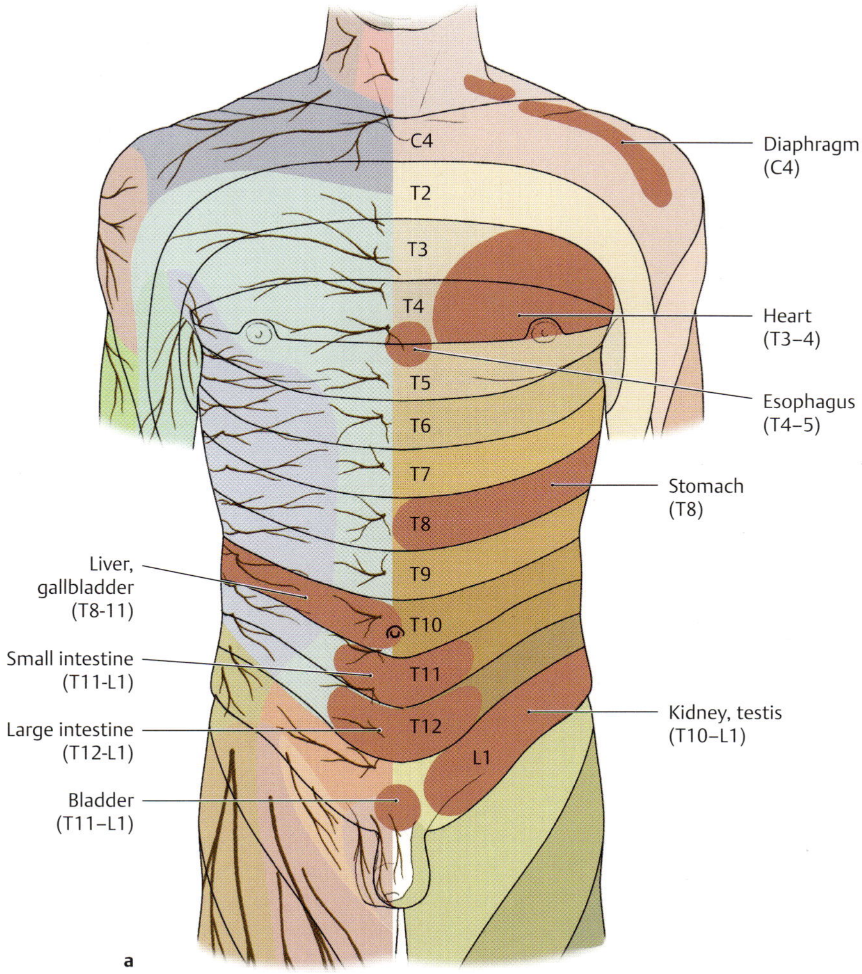

a

B Referred pain

It is believed that nociceptive afferent fibers from dermatomes (somatic pain) and internal organs (visceral pain) terminate on the same relay neurons in the posterior horn of the spinal cord. The convergence of somatic and visceral afferent fibers (see **b**) confuses the relationship between the perceived and actual sites of pain, a phenomenon known as referred pain. The pain is typically perceived at the somatic site given that somatic pain is well-localized while visceral pain is not. Pain impulses from a particular internal organ are consistently projected to the same well-defined skin area (**a**); the pattern of pain projection is very helpful in determining the affected organ. The skin regions on which certain organs project their pain impulses are referred to as *Head zones* after *Sir Henry Head*, the English neurologist who first described them. In this figure the main areas of the Head zones are marked. Due to the diffuse nature of pain, it can occasionally extend to adjacent dermatomes (see numbers). This explanatory model considers only the peripheral processing of impulses that are perceived in the cortex as pain. It remains unclear why, in the opposite case, somatic pain is not perceived as visceral pain. On the whole the problem of pain is complex and requires central processing in addition to peripheral processing (see **A**, p. 450).

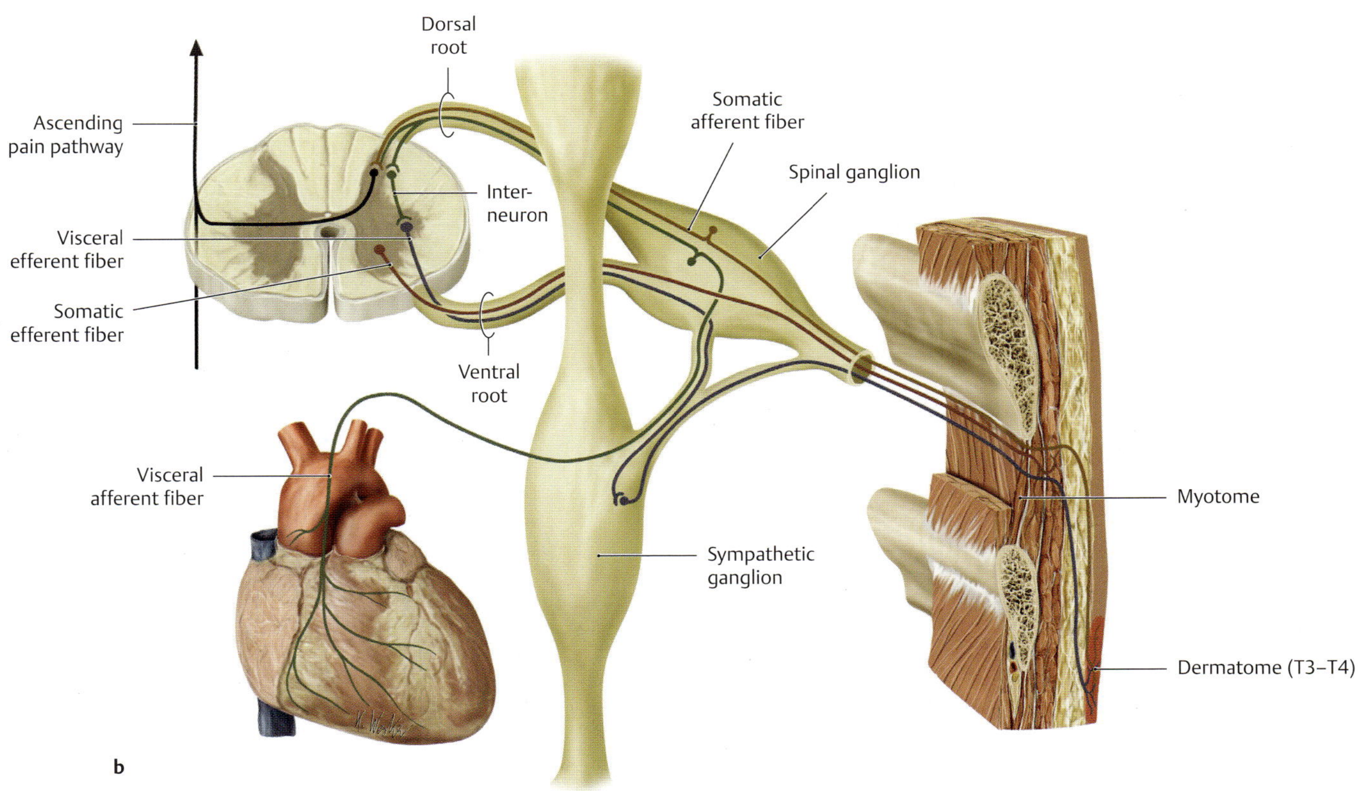

b

3.5 Enteric Nervous System

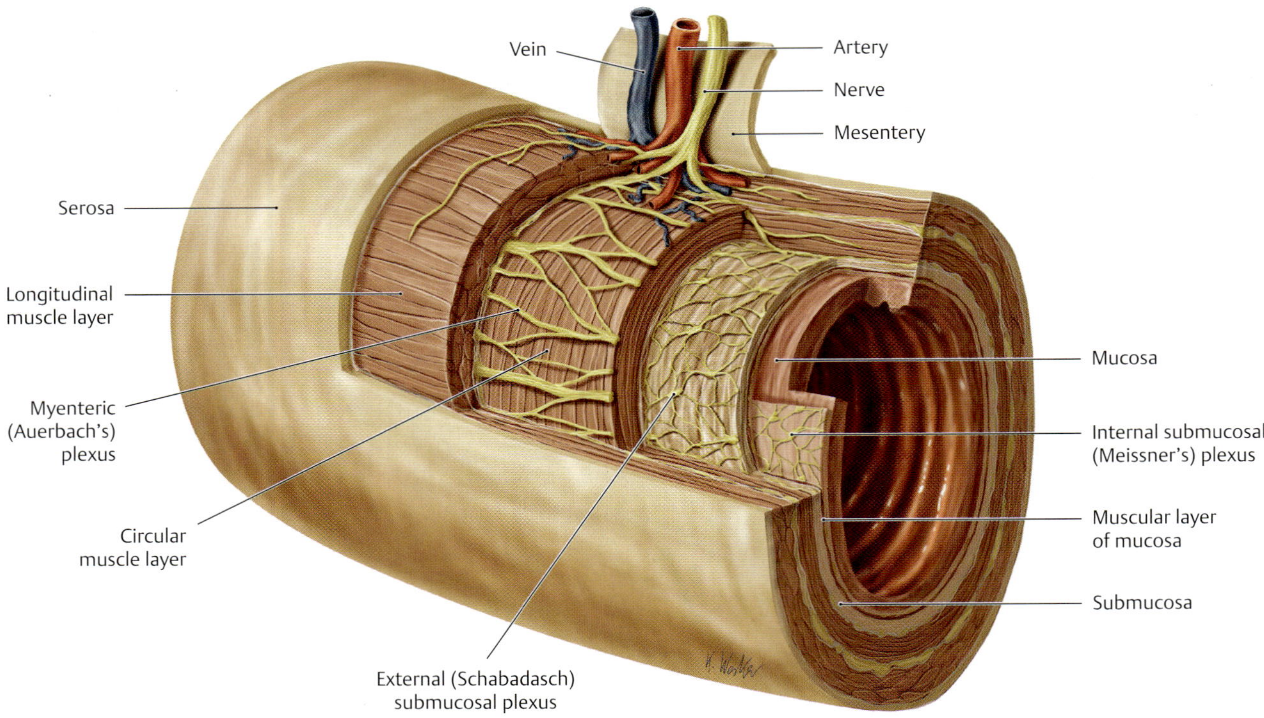

A Enteric nervous system in the small intestine
The enteric nervous system is the intrinsic nervous system of the bowel, consisting of small groups of neurons that form interconnected, microscopically visible ganglia in the wall of the digestive tube. Its two main divisions are the *myenteric* (Auerbach) *plexus* (located between the longitudinal and circular muscle fibers) and the *submucosal plexus* (located in the submucosa), which is subdivided into external (Schabadasch) and *internal* (Meissner) *submucosal plexuses*. (Details on the fine lamination of the enteric nervous system can be found in textbooks of histology.) These networks of neurons are the foundation for autonomic reflex pathways. In principle they can function without external innervation, but their activity is intensely modulated by the sympathetic and parasympathetic nervous systems. Activities influenced by the enteric nervous system include enteric motility, secretion into the digestive tube, and local intestinal blood flow.

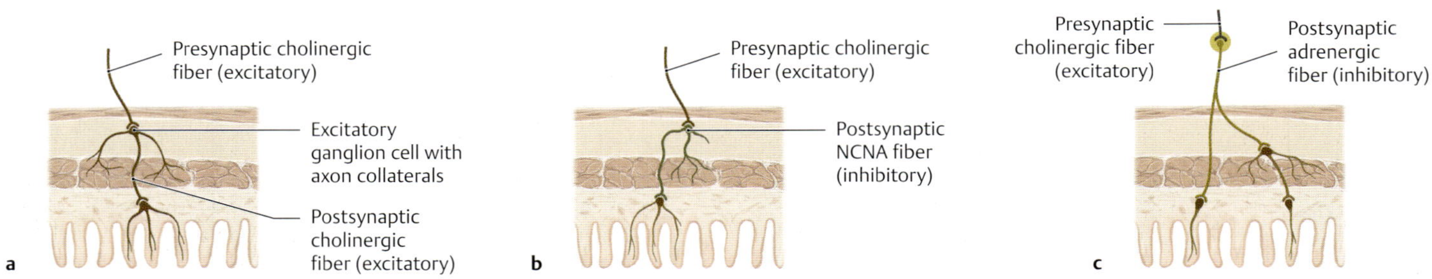

B Modulation of intestinal innervation by the autonomic nervous system
Although the parasympathetic nervous system ("rest and digest") generally promotes the activities of the digestive tube (secretion, motility), it may also produce inhibitory effects.

- **a** Excitatory presynaptic cholinergic parasympathetic fibers terminate on excitatory cholinergic neurons that promote intestinal motility (mixing of the bowel contents to facilitate absorption).
- **b** An inhibitory parasympathetic fiber synapses with an inhibitory ganglion cell that uses noncholinergic, nonadrenergic (NCNA) transmitters. These NCNA transmitters are usually neuropeptides that inhibit intestinal motility.
- **c** Sympathetic fibers are not abundant in the muscular layers of the bowel wall. Postsynaptic adrenergic fibers inhibit the motor and secretory neurons in the plexuses.

The clinical importance of autonomic bowel innervation is illustrated below:

- During shock, the vessels in the bowel are constricted and the intestinal mucosa is accordingly deprived of oxygen. This results in disruption of the epithelial barrier, which may then be penetrated by microorganisms from the bowel lumen. This is an important mechanism contributing to multisystem failure in shock.
- There may be a cessation of intestinal motility (atonic bowel) after intestinal operations involving surgical manipulation of the digestive tube.
- Medications (especially opiates) may suppress the motility of the enteric nervous system, causing constipation.

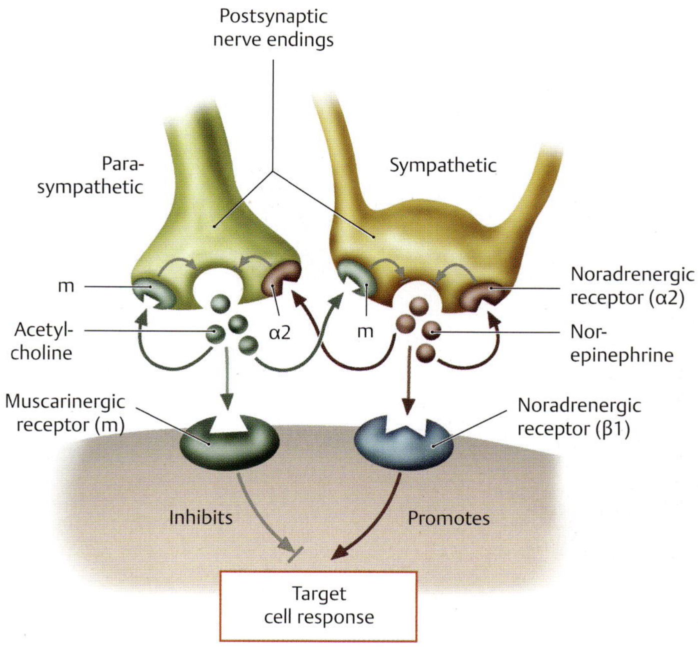

C Functional interactions of the sympathetic and parasympathetic nervous systems at the target organ

The transmitters of the sympathetic and parasympathetic nervous systems (norepinephrine and acetylcholine, respectively) act upon both the target organ and the (para)sympathetic nerve endings at the synapse. Noradrenergic receptors on the target tissue (β_1, shown in blue) and nerve endings themselves (α_2, shown in pink) modulate target cell responses on two levels: norepinephrine binding to the β_1 receptor directly promotes a cellular response in heart tissue, while similar binding to the α_2 receptors on the postsynaptic nerve endings allows for regulation of subsequent neurotransmitter release, through positive and negative feedback loops. The muscarinergic receptors (m, shown in green) mediate a similar process upon binding of acetylcholine. The neurotransmitters of the autonomic nervous system can therefore self- and cross-regulate in a multifaceted control mechanism.

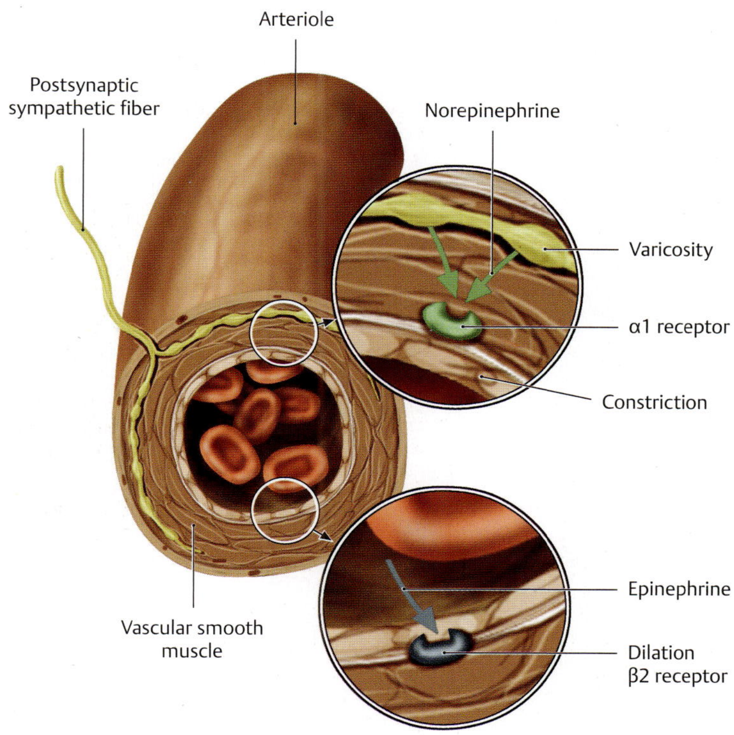

D Sympathetic effects on arteries

An important function of the sympathetic nervous system is to regulate the caliber of the arterioles (blood pressure regulation). When sympathetic fibers release norepinephrine into the media of the arterioles, the α1 receptor mediates contraction of the vascular smooth muscle, and the blood pressure rises. Meanwhile, epinephrine from the blood acts on the β_2 receptors in the sarcolemma of the same vascular smooth muscle cells, inducing vasodilation and a corresponding drop in blood pressure.

Note: Parasympathetic fibers do not terminate on blood vessels.

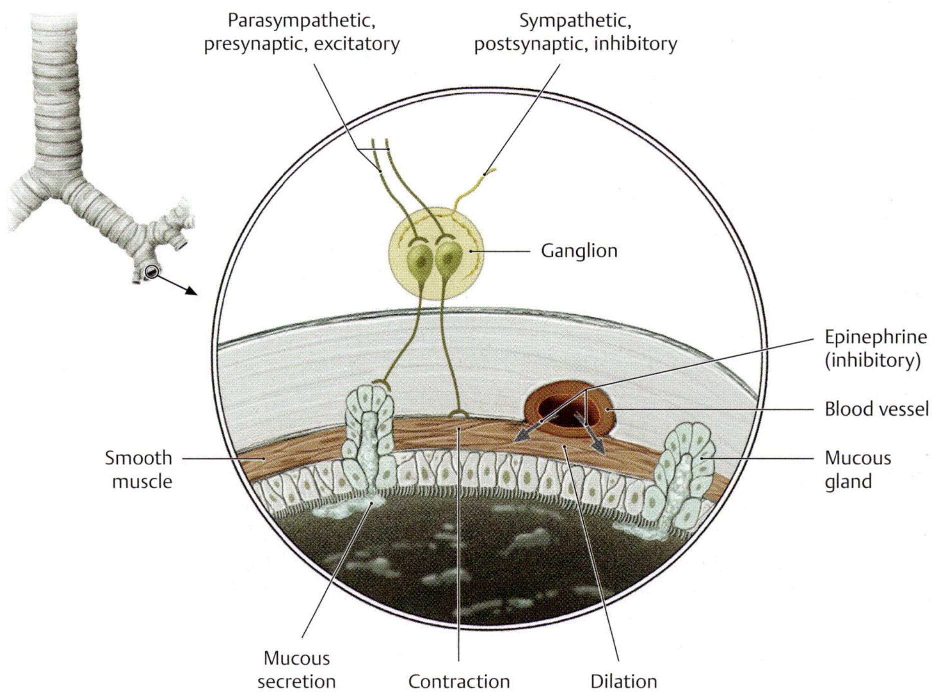

E Autonomic innervation of the trachea and bronchi

Parasympathetic stimulation of the local ganglia promotes secretion by the bronchial glands and narrowing of the bronchial passages. For this reason, the preparations for bronchoscopy include the administration of a drug (atropine) which blocks parasympathetic innervation, ensuring that mucous secretions will not obscure the bronchial mucosa. A similar reduction in bronchial secretions can be achieved through *sympathetic* stimulation. Epinephrine from the bloodstream acts on adrenergic β_2 receptors to induce bronchodilation. This effect is used to treat severe asthma attacks.

4.1 Brain and Meninges in situ

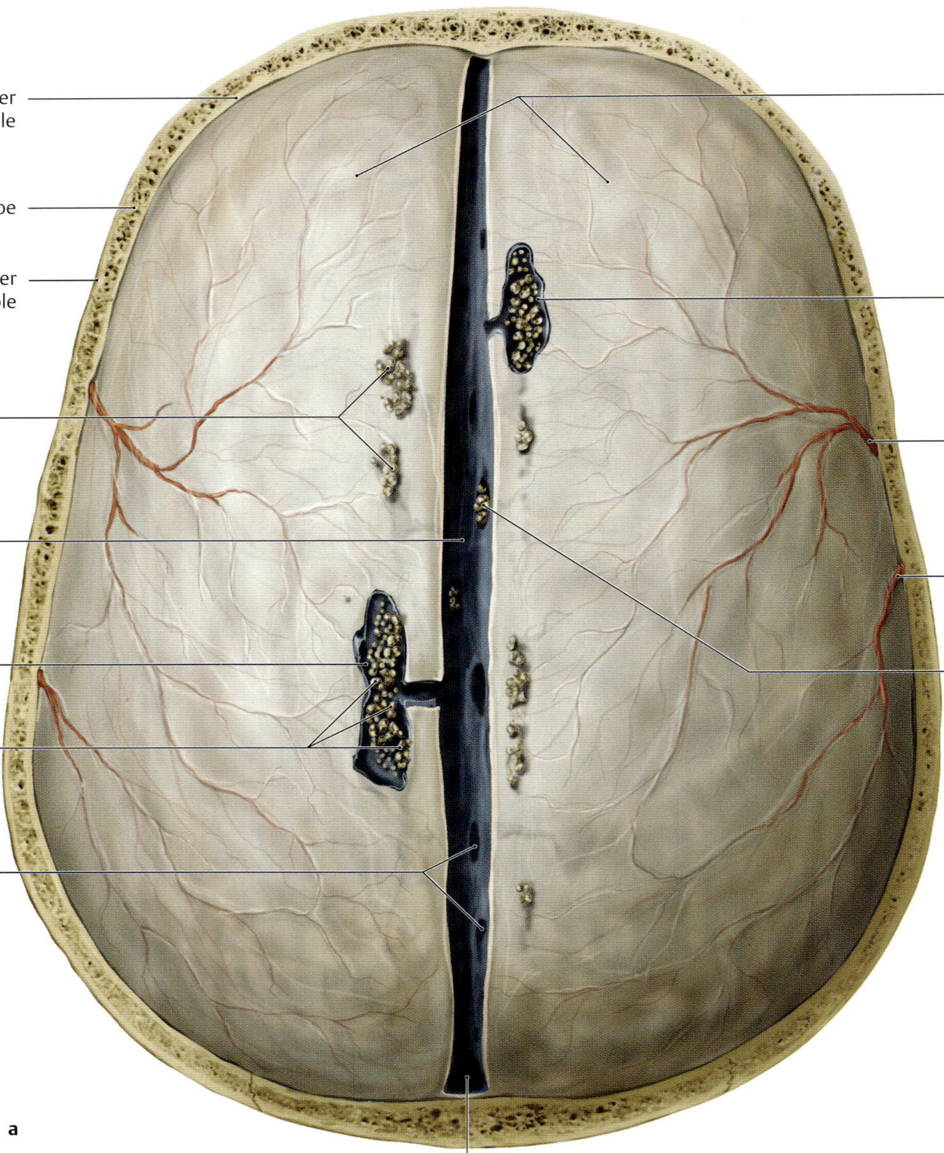

A Brain and meninges in situ
Superior view of the cranial cavity with the calvarium removed. **a** The calvarium has been removed, and the superior sagittal sinus and its lateral lacunae have been opened; **b** after removal of dura mater (left hemisphere) and dura mater and arachnoid (right hemisphere).

a The first structure encountered when the calvarium has been removed is the outer layer of the meninges, the endosteal (periosteal) layer of the dura mater. It contains a very dense network of collagen fibers that lend mechanical strength and make it impossible to tear without scissors or a scalpel. Hair-like collagen fibers can be seen torn out of the calvarium—Sharpey's fibers of the outermost endosteal layer of dura. On its surface, branches of the epidurally located meningeal aa. are visible. They run in grooves—arterial sulci (see fig. **A**, p. 18)—on the internal surface of the calvarial bones. They are located directly between dura and bone, which is significant with regard to the localization and spreading of epidural hematoma (see **Aa**, p. 390) which are caused by ruptured or injured meningeal arteries. The dura mater of the cranial cavity is formed of two inseparable layers—the outer endosteal (periosteal) layer (seen here) and the inner meningeal layer. (not visible here, see **C**, p. 311). In certain regions the layers separate to form a dural venous sinus—the superior sagittal sinus, one

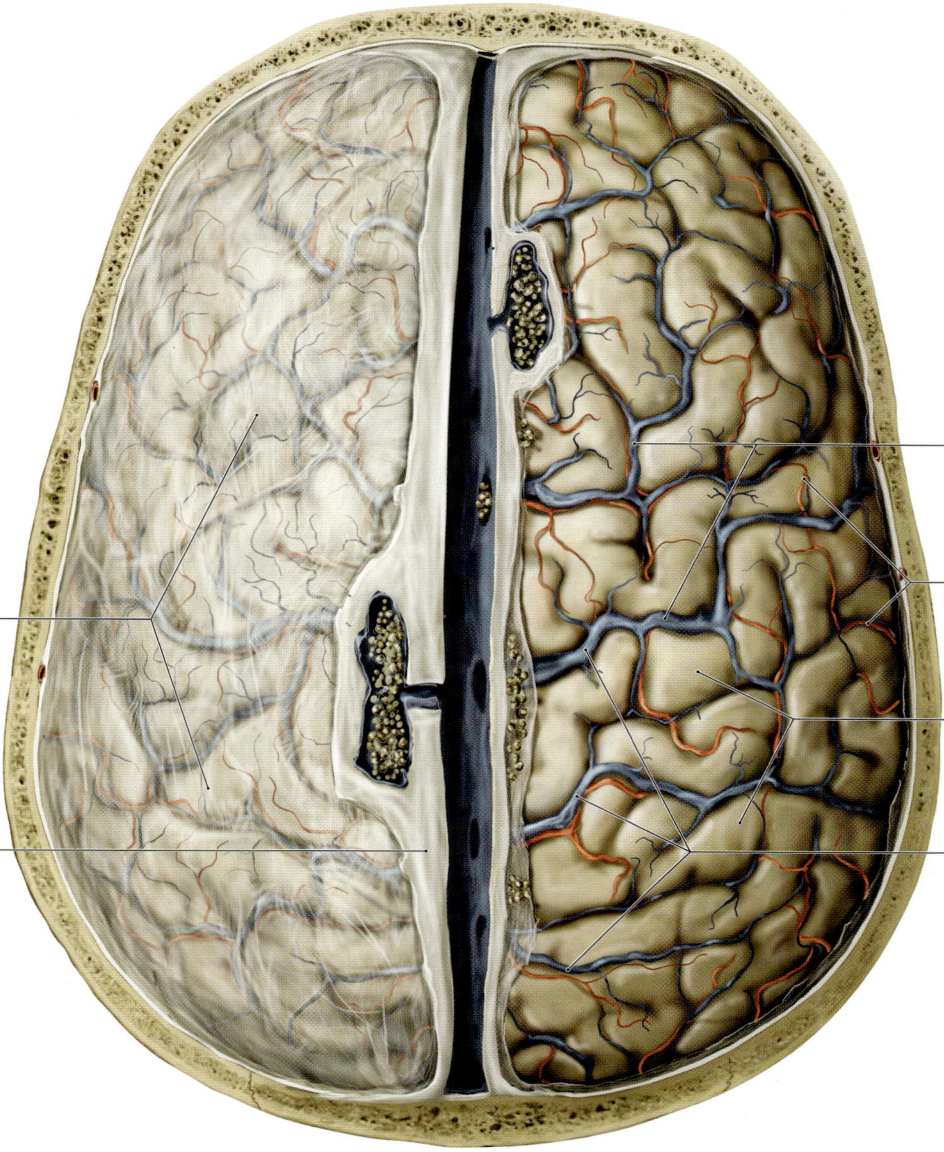

of the largest venous sinuses (see p. 382 ff) is seen here opened along its entire length. In figure **b** the arachnoid is now visible after removal of the dura mater from the left cerebral hemisphere. On the right side, the arachnoid has also been removed so that the brain enclosed by pia mater (the innermost layer) is visible. Unlike the arachnoid, the pia mater extends into the sulci. The subarachnoid space, which is filled with cerebrospinal fluid, lies between the arachnoid and the pia mater (see fig. **C**, p. 311). The space remains covered on the left side but opened on the right. In addition to the cerebral arteries, the superficial cerebral veins pass through the subarachnoid space. The veins open into the superior sagittal sinus via bridging veins. Some open into pools or lateral lacunae that then drain into the superior sagittal sinus. Protruding into the sinus and the lacunae are arachnoid granulations—overgrown arachnoid villi. These structures are important for the reabsorption of CSF (for further details see **A**, p. 314).

Note: Unlike the CNS which develops from the neural tube, the meninges originate from embryonic connective tissue (mesenchyme) which surrounds the neural tube. Therefore, the meninges are not brain tissue derivatives. In the CNS the pia mater is separated from the surface of the brain by a layer of glial cells (astrocytes) which are derived from the neural tube in the form of a superficial glial membrane. This membrane is only visible under the microscope. The pia mater appears intimately applied to the surface of the brain and cannot be separated from it.

4.2 Meninges and Dural Septa

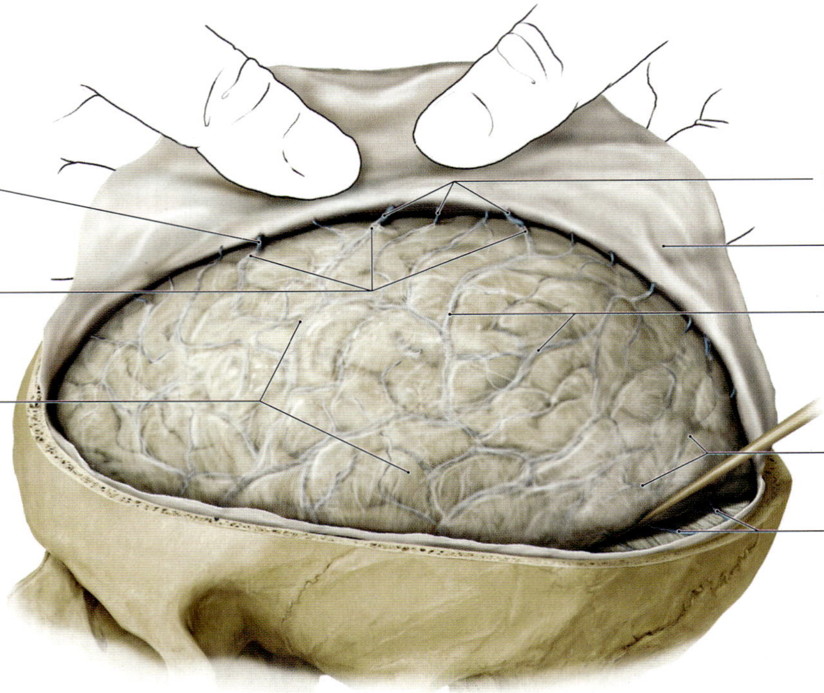

A Brain in situ with the dura partially dissected from the arachnoid

Viewed from upper left. The dura has been opened and reflected upward, leaving the underlying arachnoid and pia mater on the brain. Because the arachnoid is so thin, we can see the underlying subarachnoid space and the vessels that lie within it (see **C**). The subarachnoid space no longer contains cerebrospinal fluid at this stage of the dissection and is therefore collapsed. Before the superficial cerebral veins terminate in the sinus, they leave the subarachnoid space for a short distance and course between the neurothelium of the arachnoid and the meningeal layer of the dura to the superior sagittal sinus. These segments of the cerebral veins are called *bridging veins* (see **C**). Some of the bridging veins, especially the inferior cerebral veins, open into the transverse sinus. Injury to the bridging veins leads to subdural hemorrhage (see p. 311 and **A**, p. 390).

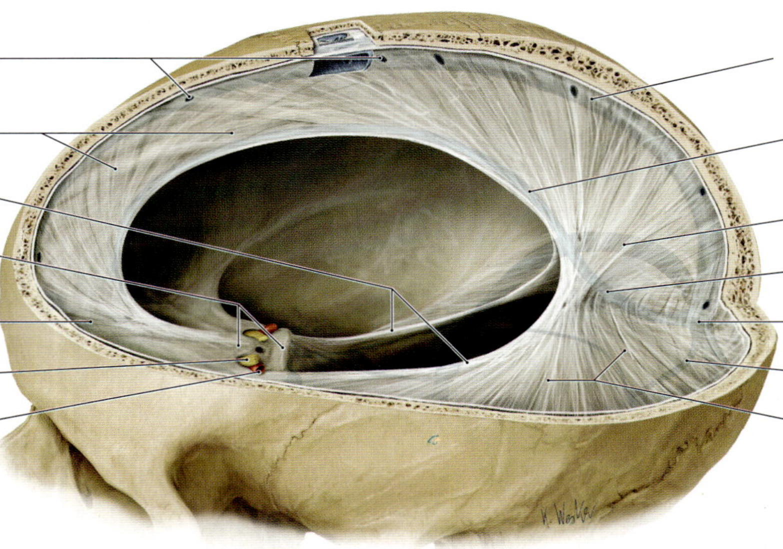

B Dural (folds) septa

Left anterior oblique view. The brain has been removed to demonstrate the dural folds or septa. The falx cerebri appears as a fibrous sheet that arises from the crista galli of the ethmoid bone and separates the two cerebral hemispheres. At its site of attachment to the calvaria, the falx cerebri separates to form the superior sagittal sinus. Additional septa are the tentorium cerebelli and falx cerebelli (not shown here). The tentorium cerebelli fans out into the groove between the cerebrum and cerebellum and houses the transverse sinus in its attached margin. The falx cerebelli separates the two hemispheres of the cerebellum and has the occipital sinus in its attached margin. Because the dural septa are rigid structures, portions of the brain may herniate beneath their free edges (see **D**). The midbrain passes through an opening in the tentorium cerebelli called the tentorial notch.

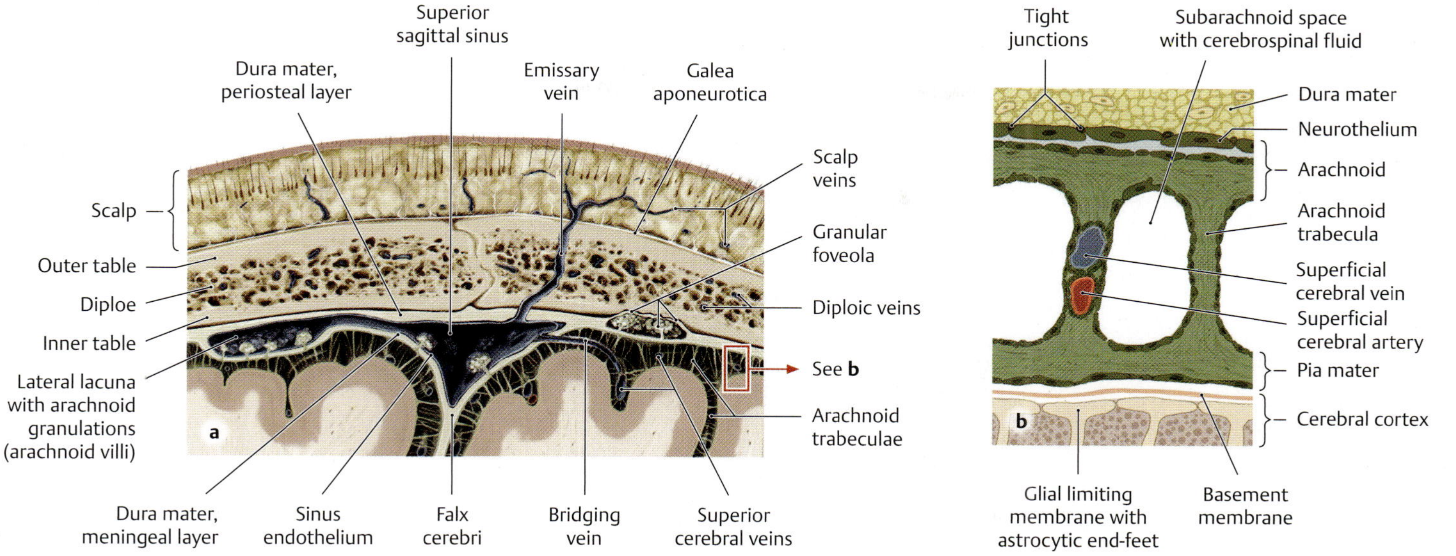

C Relationship of the meninges to the calvarium

a Coronal section through the vertex of the skull, anterior view. The dura mater and internal periosteum of the skull form an inseparable structural unit. They are composed of a tough meshwork of collagen fibers. The part of the dura facing the bone takes on the task of the periosteum (periosteal/endosteal layer). The meningeal layer of dura, facing the brain, forms septae that extend between cerebral areas—dural folds. A dural fold is said to be composed of two layers of meningeal dura. In the vertex region pictured here, the septum shown is the falx cerebri (other septa are shown in **B**). Located within the dura, between its endosteal and meningeal layers, are the principal venous channels of the brain, the dural venous sinuses (e.g., the superior sagittal sinus). Their walls are composed of dura and endothelium. Arachnoid villi, which protrude into the dural venous sinus, provide drainage of cerebrospinal fluid from the subarachnoid space into the blood stream (details see p. 314 ff). With age, the arachnoid villi grow across the sinus and produce pits in the inner table of the skull (granular foveolae, see p. 18). A schematic close-up (**b**) shows the relationship of the pia-arachnoid, which contains the slit-like subarachnoid space. This space is subdivided by arachnoid trabeculae that extend from the outer layer (arachnoid) to the inner layer (pia mater). At its boundary with the dura, the arachnoid is covered by flat cells which, unlike other meningeal cells, are joined together by "tight junctions" (neurothelium) to create a diffusion barrier between the blood and cerebrospinal fluid (see p. 317).

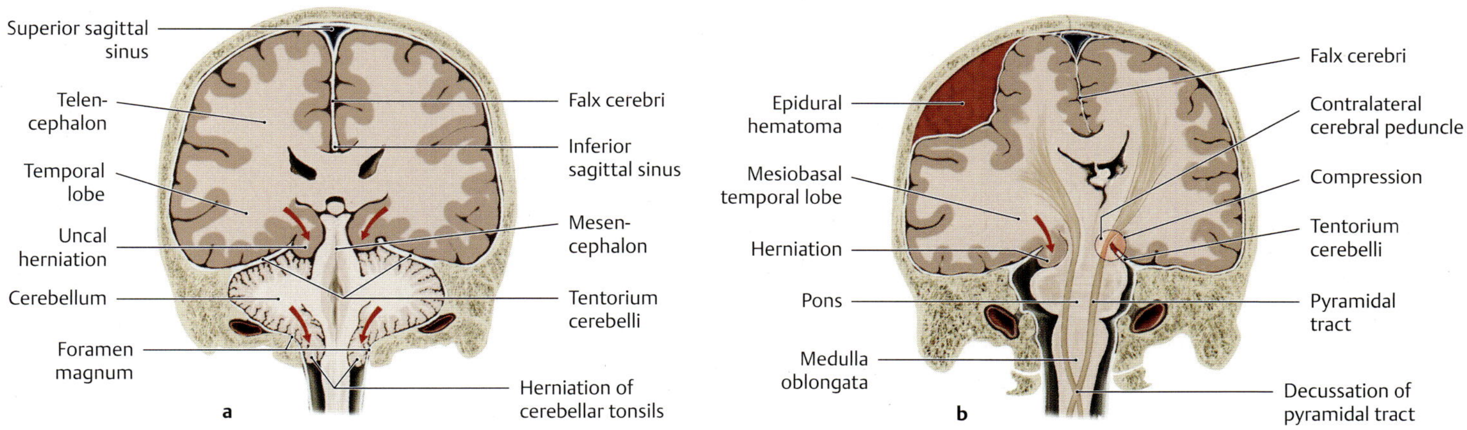

D Potential sites of brain herniation beneath the free edges of the meninges

Coronal section, anterior view. The tentorium cerebelli divides the cranial cavity into a supratentorial and an infratentorial space. The telencephalon is supratentorial, and the cerebellum is infratentorial (**a**). Because the dura is composed of tough, collagenous connective tissue, it creates a rigid intracranial framework. As a result, a mass lesion within the cranium may displace the cerebral tissue and cause portions of the cerebrum to become entrapped (herniate) beneath the rigid dural septa (duplication of the meningeal layer of the dura).

a Axial herniation. This type of herniation is usually caused by generalized brain edema. It is a symmetrical herniation in which the middle and lower portions of both temporal lobes of the cerebrum herniate down through the tentorial notch, exerting pressure on the upper portion of the midbrain (bilateral uncal herniation). If the pressure persists, it will force the cerebellar tonsils through the foramen magnum and also compress the lower part of the brainstem (tonsillar herniation). Because respiratory and circulatory centers are located in the brainstem, this type of herniation is life-threatening. Concomitant vascular compression may cause brainstem infarction.

b Lateral herniation. This type is caused by a unilateral mass effect (e.g., from a brain tumor or intracranial hematoma), as illustrated here on the right side. Compression of the ipsilateral cerebral peduncle usually produces contralateral hemiparesis. Sometimes, the herniating mesiobasal portions of the temporal lobe press the opposite cerebral peduncle against the sharp edge of the tentorium. This damages the pyramidal tract above the level of its decussation, causing hemiparesis to develop on the side opposite the injury (compression).

4.3 Meninges of the Brain and Spinal Cord

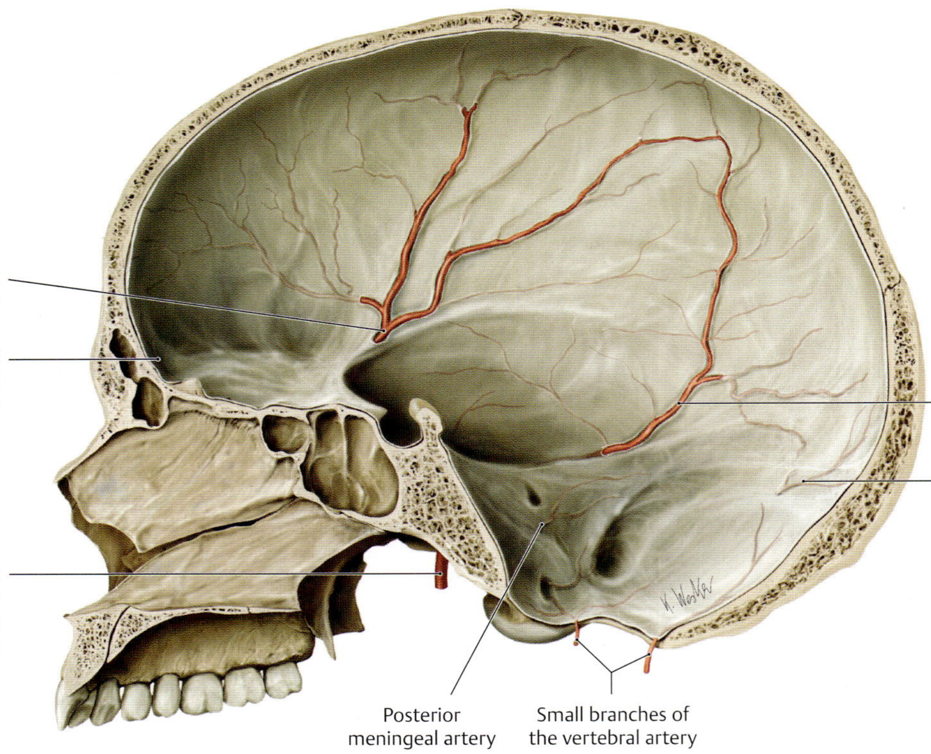

A Blood supply of the dura mater
Midsagittal section, left lateral view with branches of the middle meningeal artery exposed at several sites. Most of the dura mater in the cranial cavity receives its blood supply from the middle meningeal artery, a branch of the maxillary artery within the infratemporal fossa. The other vessels shown here are of minor clinical importance. The essential function of the middle meningeal artery is to supply the calvarium. Head injuries may cause the middle meningeal artery to rupture, leading to life-threatening complications (epidural hematoma; see **C**, and pp. 309 and 390).

B Innervation of the dura mater in the cranial cavity
Superior view with the tentorium cerebelli removed on the right side. The intracranial meninges are supplied by meningeal branches from all three divisions of the trigeminal nerve and also by branches of the vagus nerve and the first two cervical nerves. Irritation of these sensory fibers due to meningitis is manifested clinically by headache and reflex nuchal stiffness (the neck is hyperextended in an attempt to relieve tension on the inflamed meninges). The brain itself is insensitive to pain.

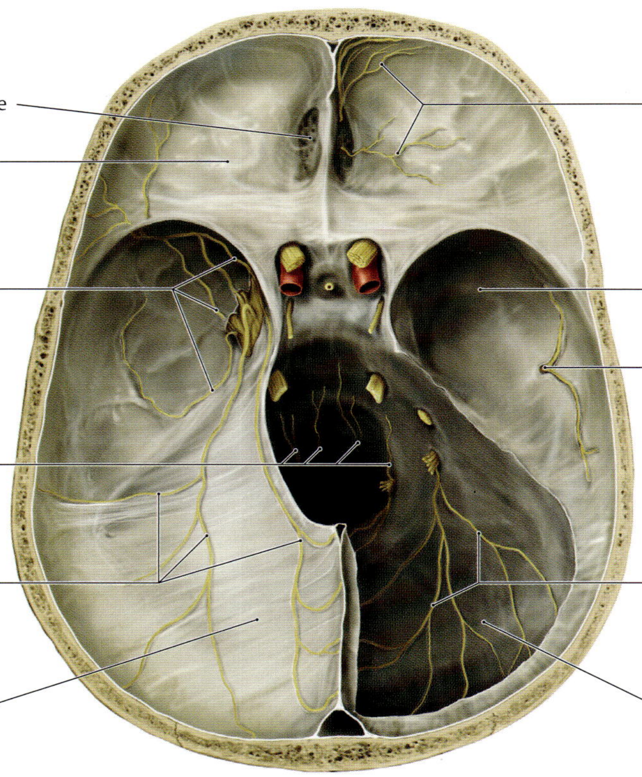

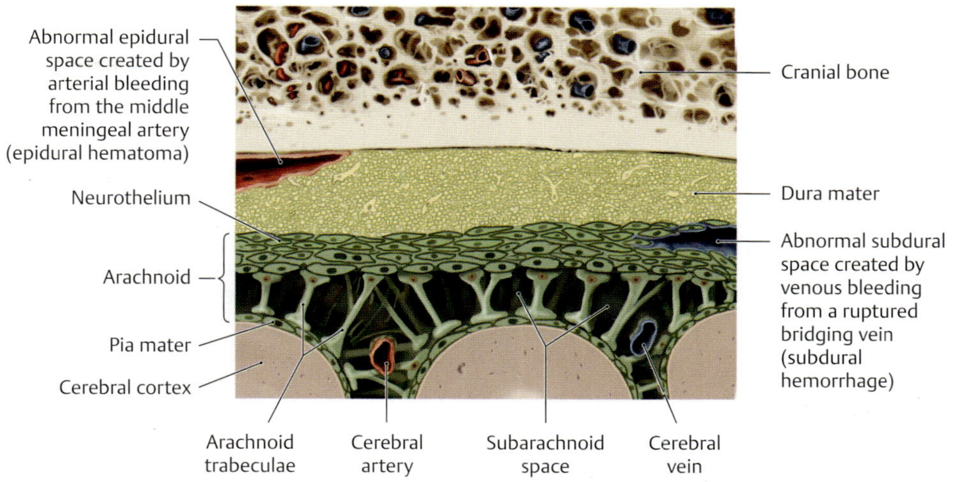

C Meninges and their spaces

Transverse section through the calvaria (schematic). The meninges have two spaces that do not exist under normal conditions, as well as one physiological space:

- Epidural space: This space is not normally present around the brain (contrast with **E**, which shows the physiological epidural space in the spinal canal). It develops in response to bleeding from the middle meningeal artery or one of its branches (arterial bleeding). The extravasated blood separates the dura mater from the bone, dissecting an epidural space between the inner table of the calvaria and the dura (epidural hematoma, see p. 390).
- Subdural space: Bleeding from the bridging veins artificially opens the subdural space between the meningeal layer of the dura mater and upper layer of the arachnoid membrane (subdural hematoma, see p. 390). The cells of the uppermost layer of the arachnoid (neurothelium) are interconnected by a dense network of tight junctions, creating a tissue barrier (blood-cerebrospinal fluid barrier).
- Subarachnoid space: This physiologically normal space lies just beneath the arachnoid. It is filled with cerebrospinal fluid and is traversed by blood vessels. Bleeding into this space (subarachnoid hemorrhage) is usually arterial bleeding from an aneurysm (abnormal circumscribed dilation) of the basal cerebral arteries (see p. 390).

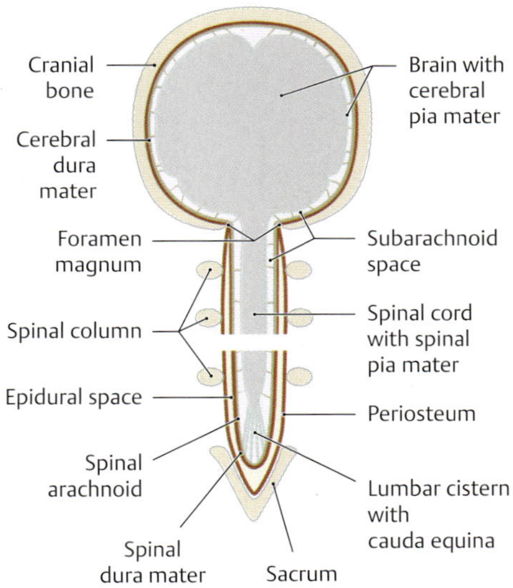

D Meninges in the cranial cavity and spinal canal

The two layers of the dura mater (meningeal and endosteal) form one inseparable structural unit in the cranial cavity. The dura mater of the spinal canal is separated from the periosteum beginning at the foramen magnum. Due to the mobility of the spinal column, the periosteum of the vertebrae must be free to move relative to the dural sac. This is accomplished by the presence of the epidural space, which exists physiologically only within the spinal canal. It contains fat and venous plexuses (see **E**). This space has major clinical importance because it is the compartment into which epidural anesthetics are injected.

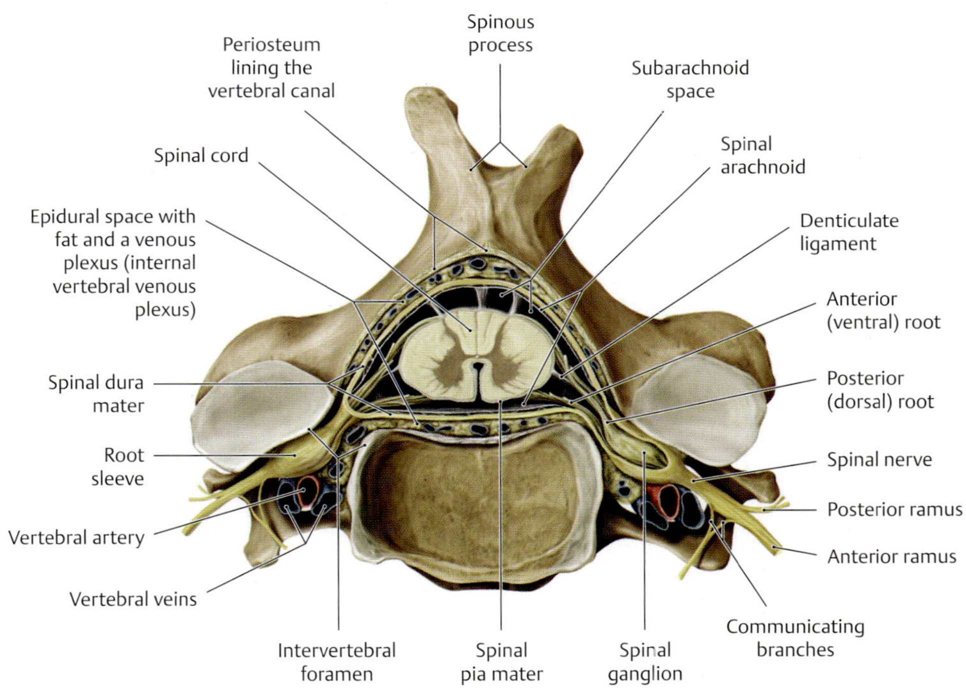

E Spinal cord in cross section

Cross-section of a cervical vertebra, cranial view. The dura mater and periosteum in the vertebral canal separate from each other to define the epidural space. This space is occupied by fatty tissue and venous plexuses functioning to cushion the spinal cord when it moves within the vertebral canal as a result of movements of the vertebral column. The dorsal and ventral roots of the spinal nerves course within the dural sac of the spinal cord and collectively form the cauda equina in the lower part of the sac (not shown here). The posterior and anterior roots unite within a dural sleeve at the intervertebral foramina to form the spinal nerves. After the two roots have fused lateral to the spinal ganglion, the spinal nerve emerges from the dural sac. The pia mater invests the surfaces of the brain and spinal cord in the same fashion. The denticulate ligaments are sheets of pial connective tissue that pass from the spinal cord to the dura and are oriented in the coronal plane.

5.1 Ventricular System, Overview

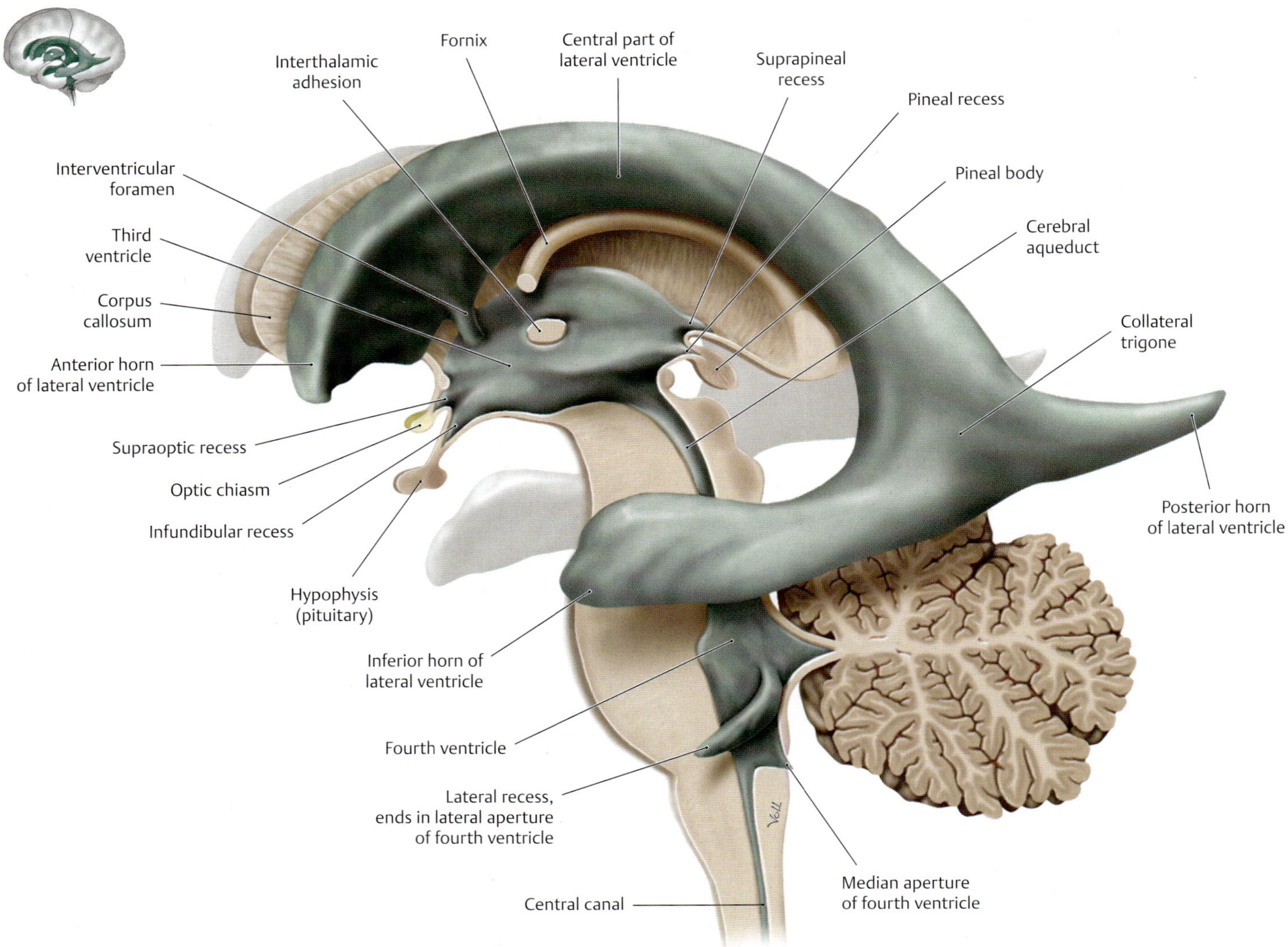

A Overview of the ventricular system and neighboring structures
Left lateral view. The ventricular system in the brain and the central canal in the spinal cord develops from the cavity of the neural tube. Topographically, they form what is referred to as the ventricular system. The complex form of the ventricles results from the development of brain vesicles. Ventricles and central canal are lined with a specialized type of epithelium, the ependyma (see fig. **D**, p. 317), which prevents direct contact between the cerebrospinal fluid and the surrounding brain tissue. The four ventricles are as follows:

- The *two* lateral ventricles, each of which communicates through an interventricular foramen with the
- third ventricle, which in turn communicates through the cerebral aqueduct with the
- fourth ventricle. This ventricle communicates with the subarachnoid space via median and lateral apertures (cf. **B**).

The largest ventricles are the lateral ventricles, each of which consists of an anterior, inferior, and posterior horn and a central part. Certain portions of the ventricular system can be assigned to specific parts of the brain: the anterior (frontal) horn to the frontal lobe of the cerebrum, the inferior (temporal) horn to the temporal lobe, the posterior (occipital) horn to the occipital lobe, the third ventricle to the diencephalon, the aqueduct to the midbrain (mesencephalon), and the fourth ventricle to the hindbrain (rhombencephalon). The anatomical relationships of the ventricular system can also be appreciated in coronal and transverse sections (see pp. 420 ff and 432 ff).
Cerebrospinal fluid is formed mainly by the choroid plexus, a network of vessels that is present to some degree in each of the four ventricles (see p. 315). Another site of cerebrospinal fluid production is the ependyma. Certain diseases (e.g., atrophy of brain tissue in Alzheimer's disease and internal hydrocephalus) are characterized by abnormal enlargement of the ventricular system and are diagnosed from the size of the ventricles in sectional images of the brain.

This unit deals with the ventricular system and neighboring structures. The next unit will trace the path of the cerebrospinal fluid from its production to its reabsorption. The last unit on the cerebrospinal fluid spaces will deal with the specialized functions of the ependyma, the circumventricular organs, and the physiological tissue barriers in the brain.

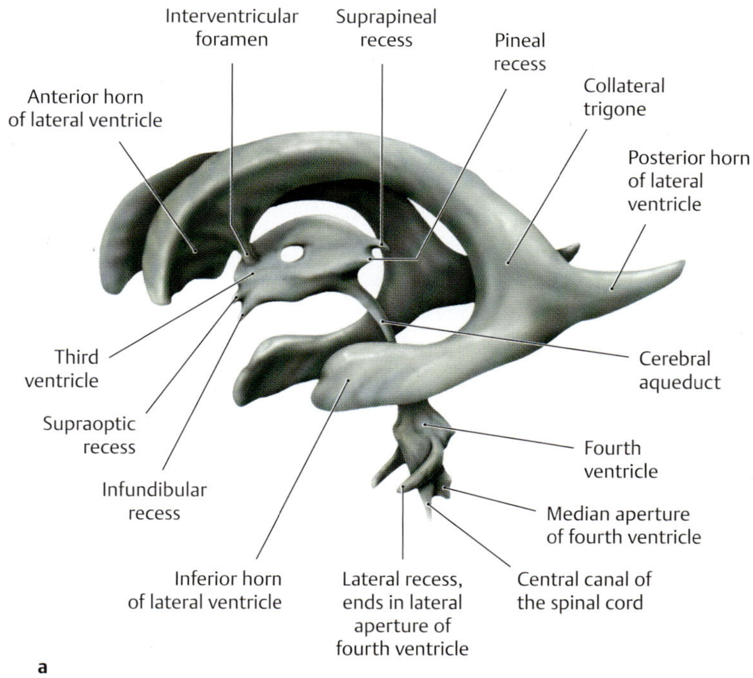

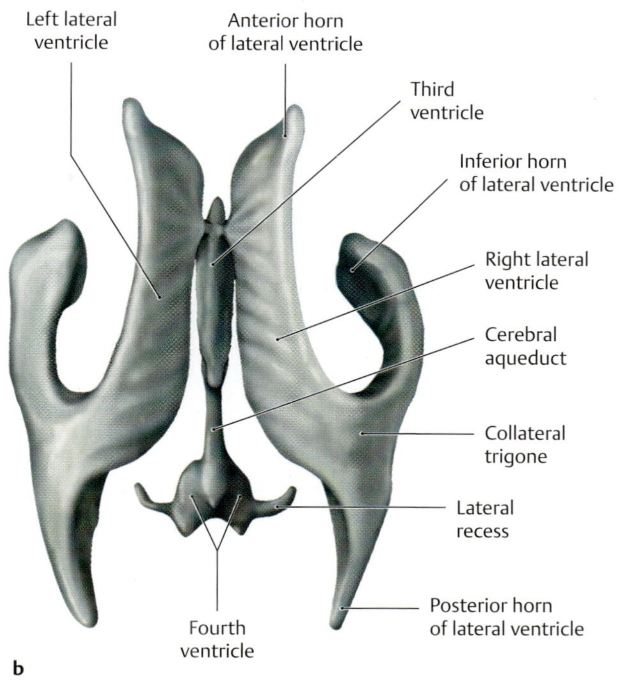

B Cast of the ventricular system
Left lateral view (**a**) and superior view (**b**). Cast specimens are used to demonstrate the connections between the ventricular cavities. Each lateral ventricle communicates with the third ventricle through an interventricular foramen. The third ventricle communicates through the cerebral aqueduct with the fourth ventricle in the rhombencephalon.

The ventricular system has a fluid capacity of approximately 30 ml, while the subarachnoid space has a capacity of approximately 120 ml. *Note* the three apertures (paired lateral apertures [foramina of Luschka] and an unpaired median aperture [foramen of Magendie]), through which cerebrospinal fluid flows from the deeper ventricular system into the more superficial subarachnoid space.

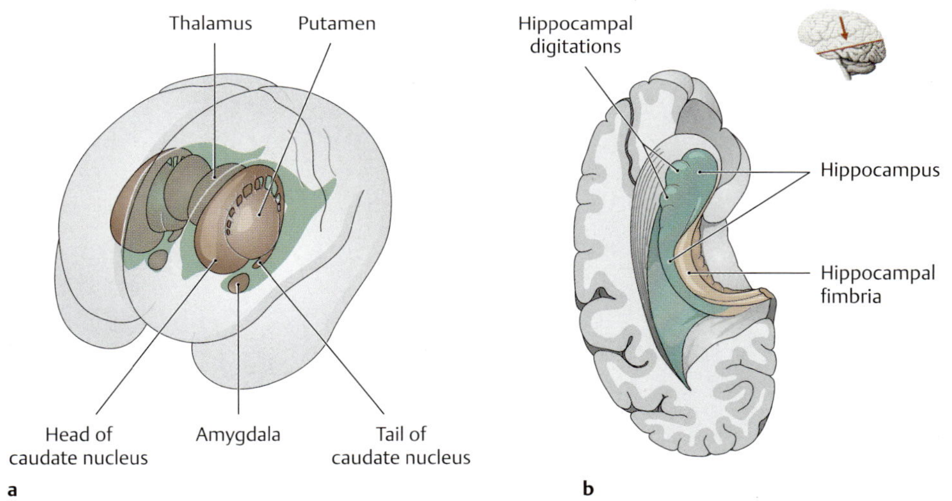

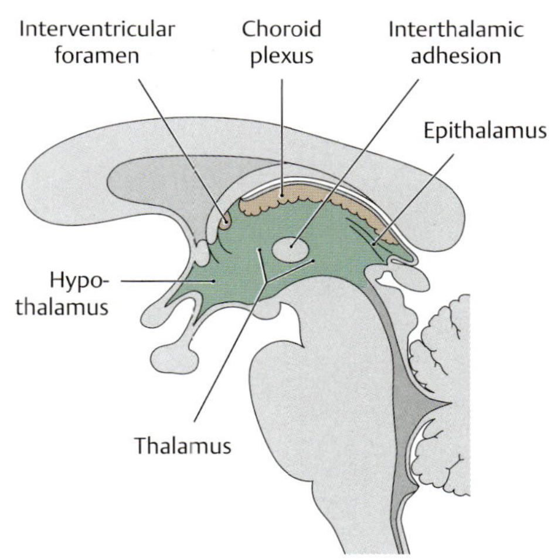

C Important structures neighboring the lateral ventricles

a View of the brain from upper left.
b View of the inferior horn of the left lateral ventricle in the opened temporal lobe.

a The following brain structures border on the lateral ventricles:
- The caudate nucleus (anterolateral wall of the anterior horn)
- The thalamus (posterolateral wall of the anterior horn)
- The putamen, which is lateral to the lateral ventricle and does not border it directly

b The hippocampus (see p. 333) is visible in the anterior part of the floor of the inferior horn. Its anterior portions with the hippocampal digitations protrude into the ventricular cavity.

D Lateral wall of the third ventricle
Midsagittal section, left lateral view. The lateral wall of the third ventricle is formed by structures of the diencephalon (epithalamus, thalamus, hypothalamus). Protrusions of the thalami on both sides may touch each other (interthalamic adhesion) but are not functionally or anatomically connected and thus do not constitute a commissural tract.

5.2 Cerebrospinal Fluid, Circulation, and Cisterns

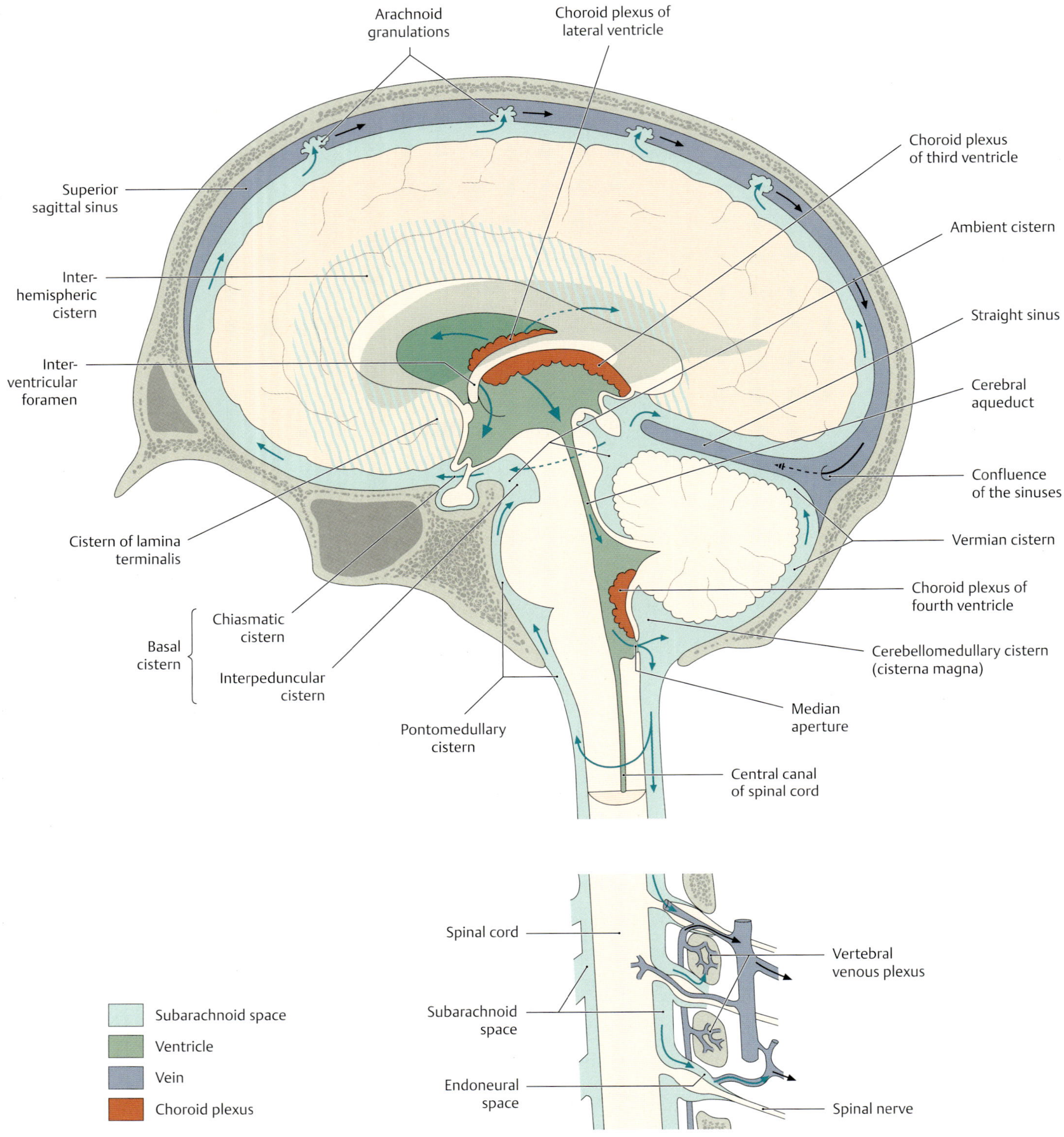

A Cerebrospinal fluid circulation and the cisterns

Cerebrospinal fluid (CSF) is produced in the choroid plexus, which is present to some extent in each of the four cerebral ventricles. It flows through the median aperture and paired lateral apertures (not shown; see p. 312 for location) into the subarachnoid space, which contains expansions called cisterns. The cerebrospinal fluid drains from the subarachnoid space through the arachnoid villi (and/or granulations) in the cranial cavity or along the spinal nerve root sleeves into the venous plexuses or lymphatic pathways of the epidural space in the spinal cord. Recent studies have initiated a discussion about additional drainage of the CSF in the cranial cavity through capillaries and superficial cerebral veins (not shown here). The cerebral ventricles and subarachnoid space have a combined capacity of approximately 150 ml of CSF (20% in the ventricles and 80% in the subarachnoid space). This volume is completely replaced two to four times daily, so that approximately 500 ml of CSF are produced each day. Obstruction of CSF drainage will therefore cause a rise in intracranial pressure (see **E**, p. 317).

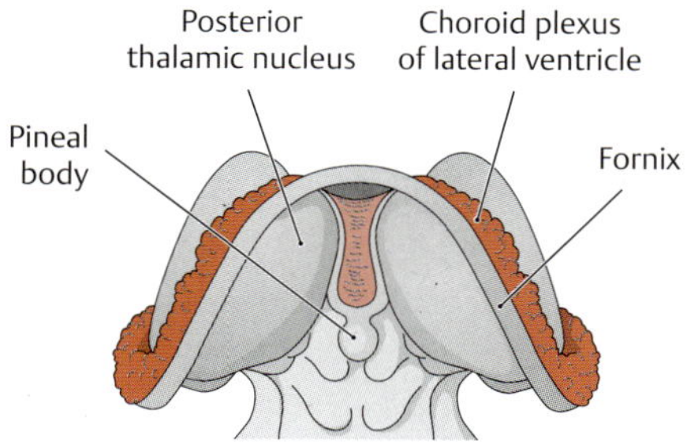

B Choroid plexus in the lateral ventricles
Rear view of the thalamus. Surrounding brain tissue has been removed down to the floor of the lateral ventricles, where the choroid plexus originates. The plexus is adherent to the ventricular wall at only one site (see **D**) and can thus float freely in the ventricular system.

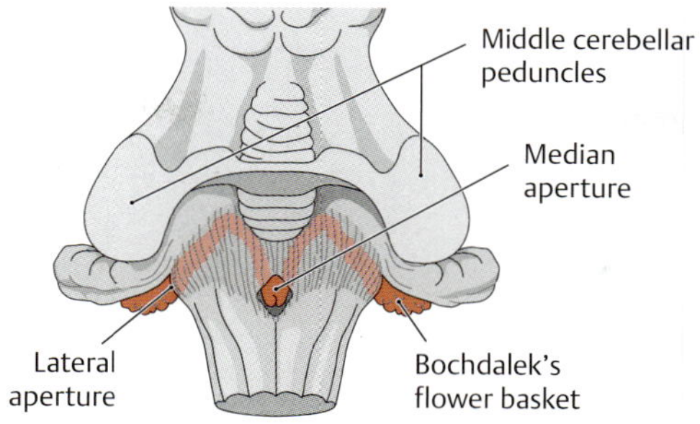

C Choroid plexus in the fourth ventricle
Posterior view of the partially opened rhomboid fossa (with the cerebellum removed). Portions of the choroid plexus are attached to the roof of the fourth ventricle and run along the lateral aperture. Free ends of the choroid plexus may extend through the lateral apertures into the subarachnoid space on both sides ("Bochdalek's flower basket").

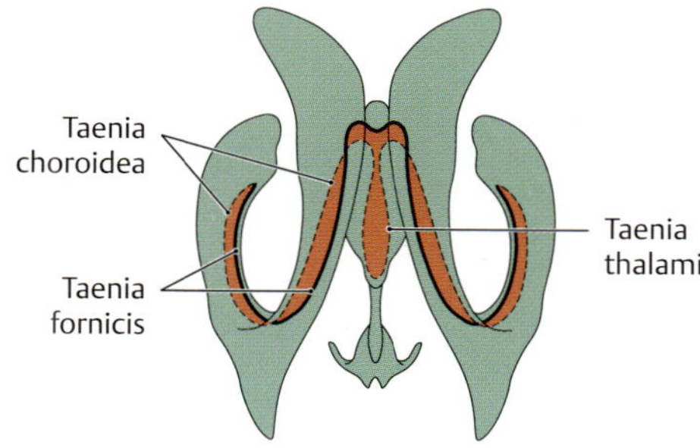

D Taeniae of the choroid plexus
Superior view of the ventricular system. The choroid plexus is formed by the ingrowth of vascular loops into the ependyma, which firmly attach it to the wall of the associated ventricle (see **F**). When the plexus tissue is removed with a forceps, its lines of attachment, called taeniae, can be seen.

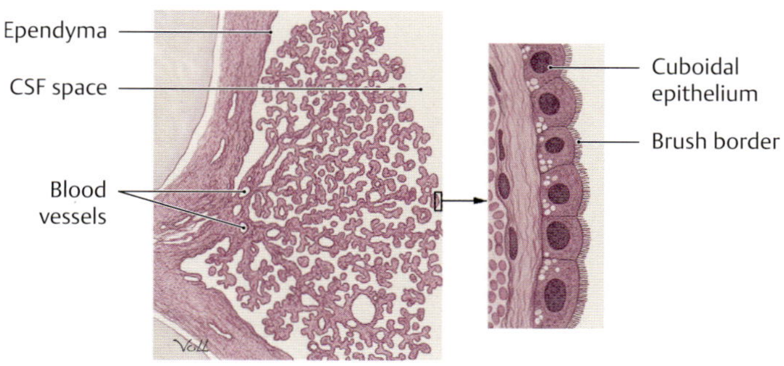

E Histological section of the choroid plexus, with a detail showing the structure of the plexus epithelium (after Kahle)
The choroid plexus is a protrusion of the ventricular wall. It is often likened to a cauliflower because of its extensive surface folds. The epithelium of the choroid plexus consists of a single layer of cuboidal cells and has a brush border on its apical surface (to increase the surface area).

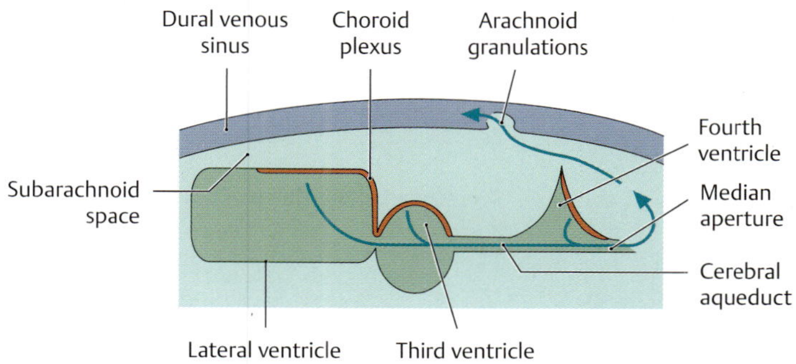

F Schematic diagram of cerebrospinal fluid circulation
As noted earlier, the choroid plexus is present to some extent in each of the four cerebral ventricles. It produces CSF, which flows through the two lateral apertures (not shown) and median aperture into the subarachnoid space. At this point, the largest amount of CSF enters the systemic circulation (lymphatic vessels, venous blood) by escaping at the dural sleeve of each spinal nerve exiting the intervertebral foramen.

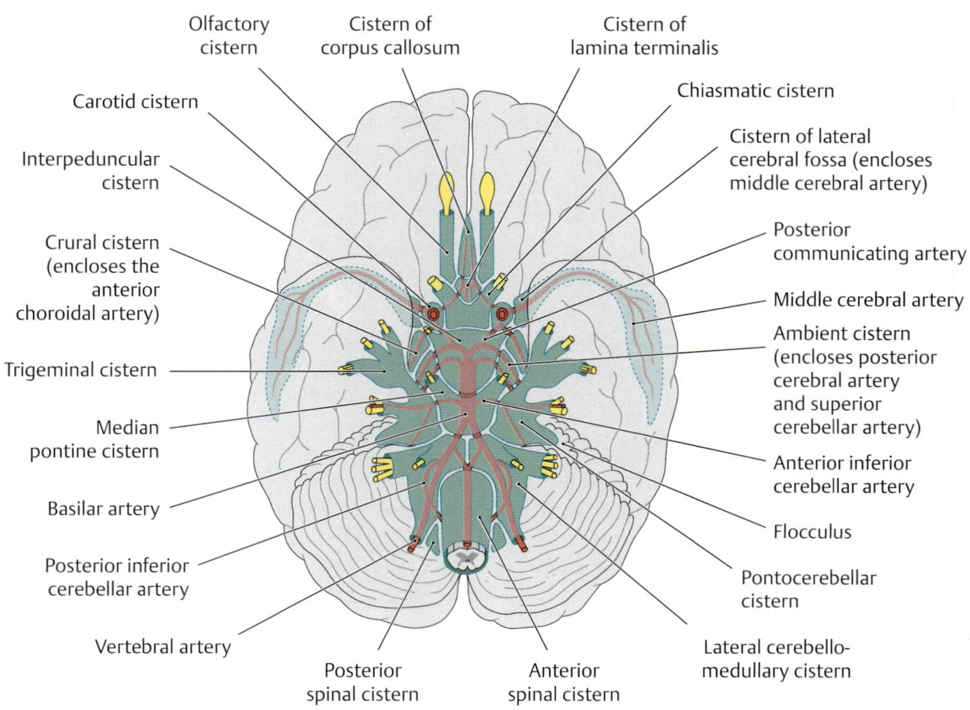

G Subarachnoid cisterns
Basal view. The cisterns are CSF-filled expansions of the subarachnoid space. They contain the proximal portions of some cranial nerves and basal cerebral arteries (veins are not shown). When arterial bleeding occurs (as from a ruptured aneurysm), blood will leak into the subarachnoid space and enter the CSF. A ruptured intracranial aneurysm is a frequent cause of blood in the CSF (methods of sampling the CSF are described on p. 317).

5.3 Circumventricular Organs and Tissue Barriers in the Brain

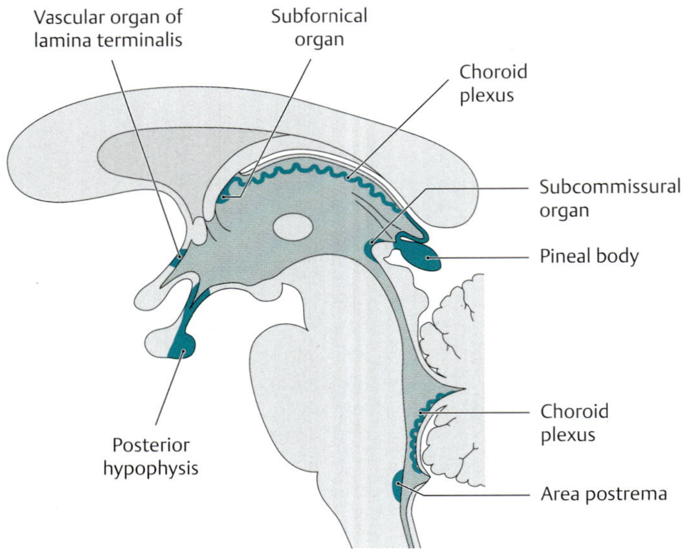

A Location of the circumventricular organs
Midsagittal section, left lateral view. The circumventricular organs include the following:

- Posterior hypophysis with the neurohemal region (see p. 350)
- Choroid plexus (see p. 315)
- Pineal body (see **D** on p. 353)
- Vascular organ of the lamina terminalis, subfornical organ, subcommissural organ, and area postrema (see **B**)

The circumventricular or ependymal organs all have several features in common. They are composed of modified ependyma, they usually border on the ventricular and subarachnoid CSF spaces, and they are located in the median plane (except the choroid plexus, though it does develop from an unpaired primordium in the median plane). The blood–brain barrier is usually absent in these organs (see **C** and **D**; except the subcommissural organ).

B Summary of the smaller circumventricular organs
In addition to the four regions listed below, the circumventricular organs include the posterior hypophysis, choroid plexus, and pineal body. The functional descriptions are based largely on experimental studies in animals.

Organ	Location	Function
Vascular organ of the lamina terminalis (VOLT)	Vascular loops in the rostral wall of the third ventricle (lamina terminalis); rudimentary in humans	Secretes the regulatory hormones somatostatin, luliberin, and motilin; contains cells sensitive to angiotensin II; is a neuroendocrine mediator
Subfornical organ (SFO)	Fenestrated capillaries between the interventricular foramina and below the fornices	Secretes somatostatin and luliberin from nerve endings; contains cells sensitive to angiotensin II; plays a central role in the regulation of fluid balance ("organ of thirst")
Sub-commissural organ (SCO)	Borders on the pineal body; overlies the epithalamic commissure at the junction of the third ventricle and cerebral aqueduct	Secretes glycoproteins into the aqueduct that condense to form the Reissner fiber, which may extend into the central canal of the spinal cord; blood–brain barrier is intact; function is not completely understood
Area postrema (AP)	Paired organs in the floor of the caudal end of the rhomboid fossa, richly vascularized	Trigger zone for the emetic reflex (absence of the blood–brain barrier); atrophies in humans after middle age

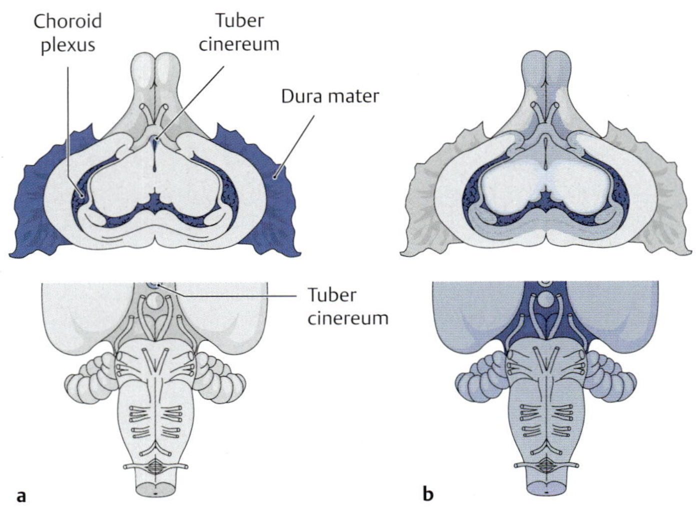

C Demonstration of tissue barriers in the brain (after Kahle)
a Blood–brain barrier, **b** blood–CSF barrier. The upper drawings show an inferior view of a transverse section through a rabbit brain, and the lower drawings show the brainstem from the basal aspect. The function of these barriers is to protect the brain from harmful substances in the bloodstream. These include macromolecular as well as small molecular pharmaceutical compounds.

a Demonstration of the blood–brain barrier: The *intravenous injection* of trypan blue dye (first Goldmann test) stains almost all organs blue except the brain and spinal cord. Even the dura and choroid plexus show heavy blue staining. Faint blue staining is noted in the tuber cinereum (neurohemal region of the posterior hypophysis), area postrema, and spinal ganglia (absence of the blood–brain barrier in these regions). The same pattern of color distribution occurs naturally in *jaundice*, where bile pigment stains all organs but the brain and spinal cord, analogous to trypan blue in the first Goldmann test.

b Demonstration of the blood–CSF barrier: When the dye is injected *into the* CSF (second Goldmann test), the brain and spinal cord (CNS) show diffuse superficial staining while the rest of the body remains unstained. This shows that a barrier exists between the CSF and blood, but not between the CSF and the CNS.

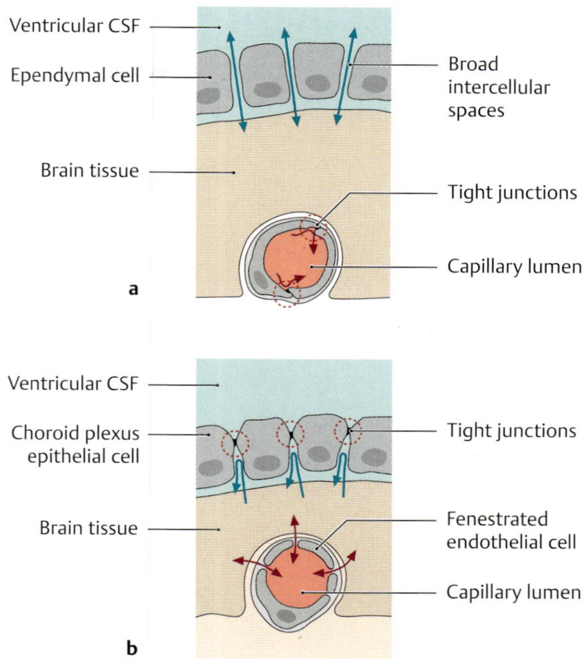

D D Blood–brain barrier and blood–CSF barrier

a Normal brain tissue with an intact blood–brain barrier; **b** Blood–CSF barrier in the choroid plexus.

a The blood–brain barrier in normal brain tissue consists mainly of the tight junctions between capillary endothelial cells. It prevents the paracellular diffusion of hydrophilic substances from CNS capillaries into surrounding tissues and in the opposite direction as well. Essential hydrophilic substances that are needed by CNS must be channeled through the barrier with the aid of specific transport mechanisms (e.g., glucose through the insulin-independent transporter GLUT 1).

b The blood–brain barrier is absent at fenestrated capillary endothelial cells in the choroid plexus and other circumventricular organs (see **A**), which allow substances to pass freely from the bloodstream into the brain tissue and vice versa. Tight junctions in the overlying ependyma (choroid plexus epithelium) create a two-way barrier between the brain tissue and ventricular CSF in these regions. The diffusion barrier shifts from the vascular endothelium to the cells of the ependyma and choroid plexus.

a

b

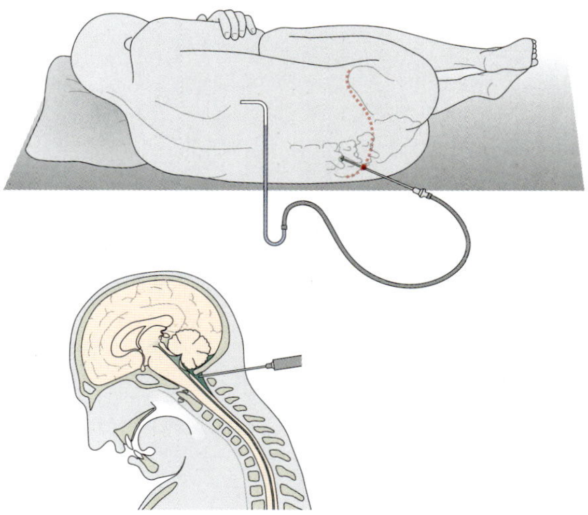

E Obtaining cerebrospinal fluid samples

a **Lumbar puncture:** This is the *method of choice* for sampling the CSF. A needle is inserted precisely in the midline between the spinous processes of L3 and L4 and is advanced into the dural sac (lumbar cistern). At this time a fluid sample can be drawn and the CSF pressure can be measured for diagnostic purposes by connecting a manometer to the needle. Lumbar puncture is contraindicated if the intracranial pressure is markedly increased because it may cause a precipitous cranial to spinal pressure gradient, causing the brainstem and/or cerebellar tonsils to herniate through the foramen magnum. This would exert pressure on vitally important centers in the medulla oblongata, with a potentially fatal outcome. Thus, the physician should always check for signs of increased intracranial pressure (e.g., papilledema, see p. 171) before performing a lumbar puncture.

b **Suboccipital puncture:** This technique should be used only in *exceptional cases* where a lumbar puncture is contraindicated (e.g., by a spinal cord tumor), because it may, in rare cases, produce a fatal complication. The mortality risk results from the need to pass a needle through the cerebellomedullary cistern (cisterna magna), which may endanger vital centers in the medulla oblongata.

F Comparison of cerebrospinal fluid and blood serum

Infection of the brain and its coverings (meningitis), subarachnoid hemorrhage, and tumor metastases can all be diagnosed by CSF examination. As the table indicates, CSF is more than a simple ultrafiltrate of blood serum. Its primary function is to impart buoyancy of the brain (the brain has an effective weight of only about 50 g despite a mass of 1300 g). Decreased CSF production therefore increases pressure on the spine and also renders the brain more susceptible to injury (less cushioning).

	CSF	**Serum**
Pressure	50–180 mm H_2O	
Volume	100–160 mL	
Osmolarity	292–297 mOsm/l	285–295 mOsm/l
Electrolytes		
Sodium	137–145 mM	136–145 mM
Potassium	2.7–3.9 mM	3.5–5.0 mM
Calcium	1–1.5 mM	2.2–2.6 mM
Chloride	116–122 mM	98–106 mM
pH	7.31–7.34	7.38–7.44
Glucose	2.2–3.9 mM	4.2–6.4 mM
CSF/serum glucose ratio	> 0.5–0.6	
Lactate	1–2 mM	0.6–1.7 mM
Total protein	0.2–0.5 g/l	55–80 g/l
Albumin	56–75 %	50–60 %
IgG	0.01–0.014 g/l	8–15 g/l
Leukocytes	< 4 cells/μL	
Lymphocytes	60–70 %	

5.4 In Situ Projection of the Ventricular and Dural Venous Sinus Systems in the Cranial Cavity

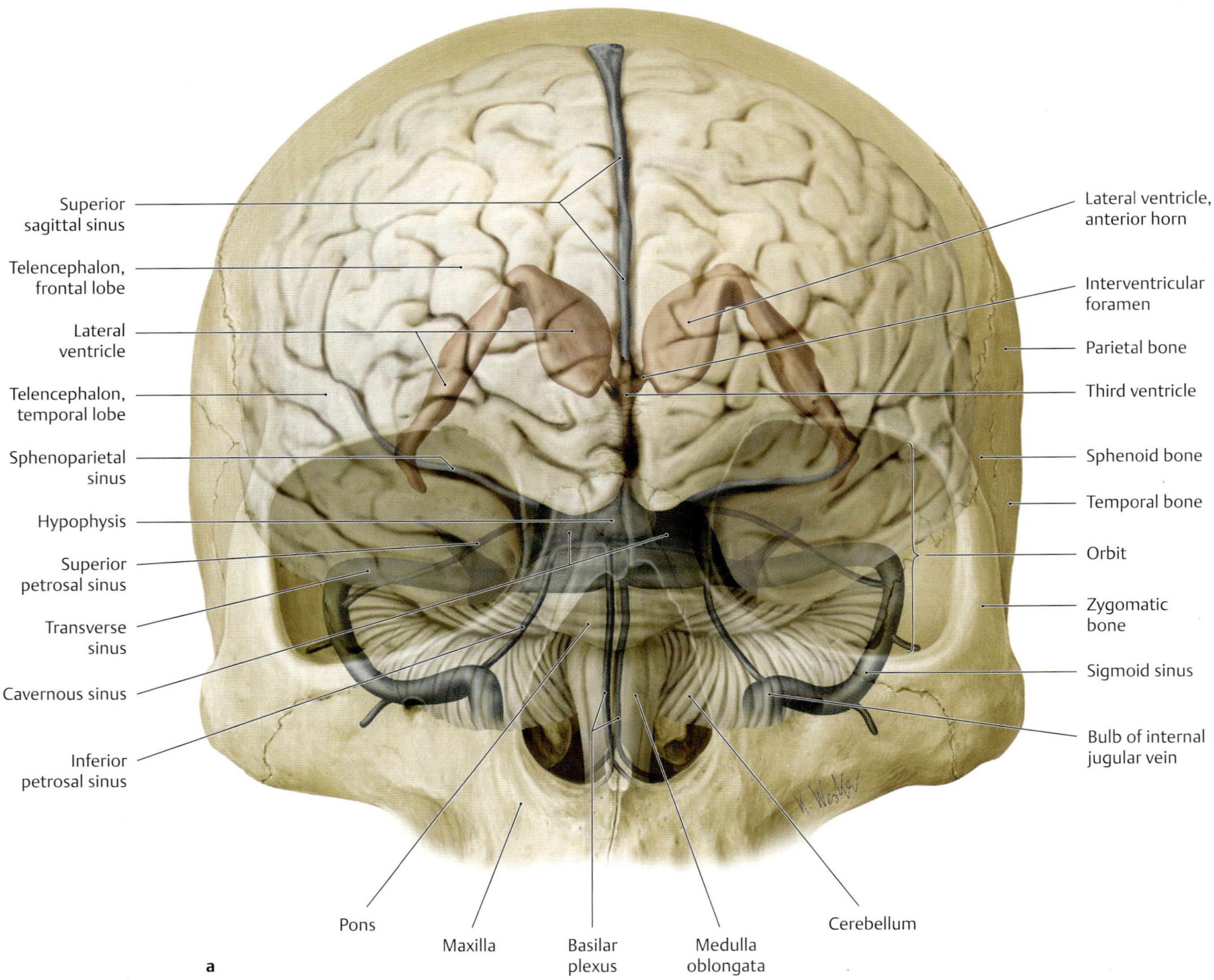

A Projection of important brain structures onto the skull
a Anterior view; **b** left lateral view.
The largest structures of the cerebrum (telencephalon) are the frontal and temporal lobes. The falx cerebri separates the two cerebral hemispheres in the midline (not visible here). In the brainstem, we can identify the pons and medulla oblongata on both sides of the midline below the telencephalon. The superior sagittal sinus and the paired sigmoid sinuses can also be seen. The anterior horns of the two lateral ventricles are projected onto the forehead.

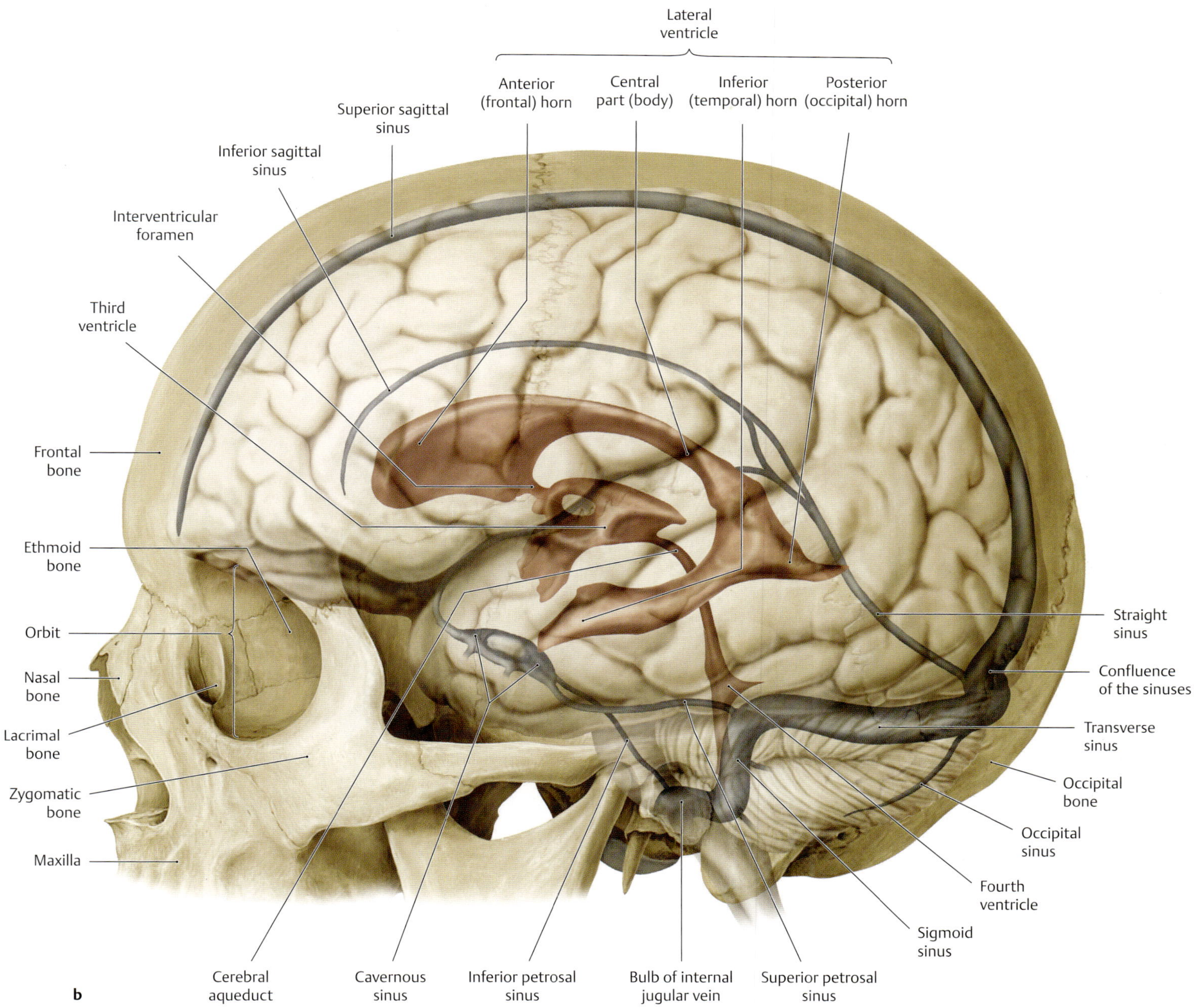

b

Viewed from left (**b**), the additional relationship between individual brain lobes and the cranial fossae becomes visible. The frontal lobe lies in the anterior cranial fossa, the temporal lobe in the middle cranial fossa, and the cerebellum in the posterior cranial fossa. The following dural venous sinuses can be identified: the superior and inferior sagittal sinus, straight sinus, transverse sinus, sigmoid sinus, cavernous sinus, superior and inferior petrosal sinus, and occipital sinus.

6.1 Telencephalon, Development and External Structure

A Division of the cerebral hemispheres into lobes

a Lateral view of the left hemisphere; **b** Medial view of the right hemisphere; **c** Basal view of the intact telencephalon; optic n. cut off on both sides, brainstem removed showing the cut surface of the mesencephalon.

Although *morphologically* both hemispheres are roughly symmetrical, textbooks more commonly depict the left hemisphere because of the *functional* asymmetry of the brain: some functions—for instance speech production and speech comprehension—are localized in only one hemisphere and more often in the left than in the right. The left hemisphere is considered to be dominant since in most people it contains the person's language centers. The sulci and gyri which are visible on the hemispheres increase the cortical surface area to roughly 2200 cm^2. Some anatomic landmarks are well suited to serve as reference points:

- Precentral and postcentral gyri are separated by the central sulcus.
- Above the superior temporal gyrus lies the lateral sulcus which terminates blindly at the supramarginal gyrus (see p. 322).
- Close to the posterior end of each cerebral hemisphere—visible on the medial surface—lies the parieto-occpital sulcus.
- The medial surface of the hemisphere shows the corpus callosum and the cingulate gyrus that is located above it.

With the help of these structures, the telencephalon can be divided into 6 lobes. This distinction is based in part on phylogenetic grounds but is also arbitrary in a topographical sense

- Topographically: the central sulcus separates the *frontal and parietal lobes* (**a**); the lateral sulcus defines the superior border of the *temporal lobe* (**a**); the *insular lobe* (Insula, **Ba**) is located deep within the lateral sulcus; the parietooccipitalis sulcus separates the *occipital* and *parietal lobes* (**b**).
- Phylogenetically: the *limbic lobe*—mainly visible on the medial surface through the cingulate gyrus (**b**)—is older than the previously mentioned lobes.

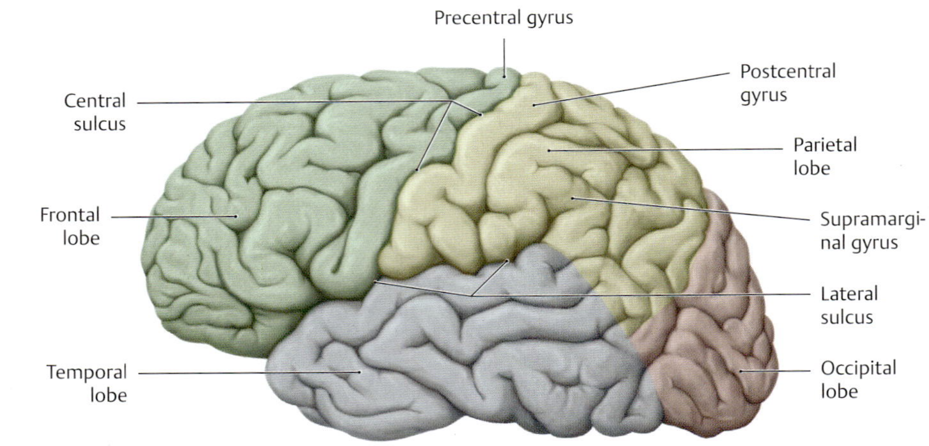

a

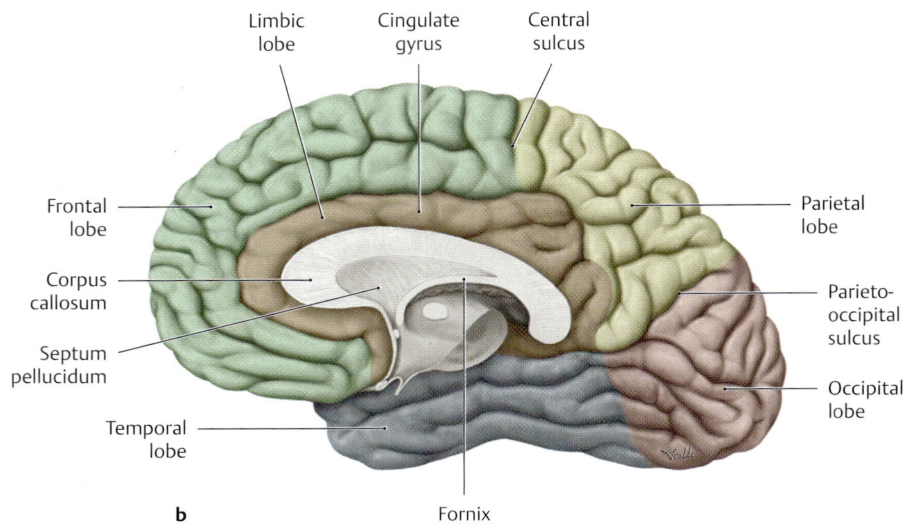

b

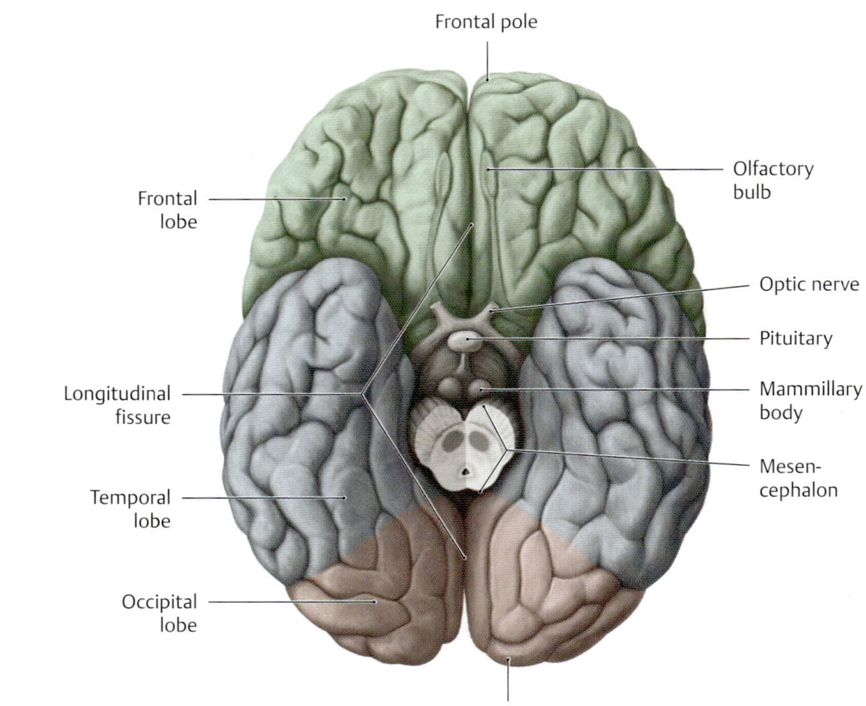

c

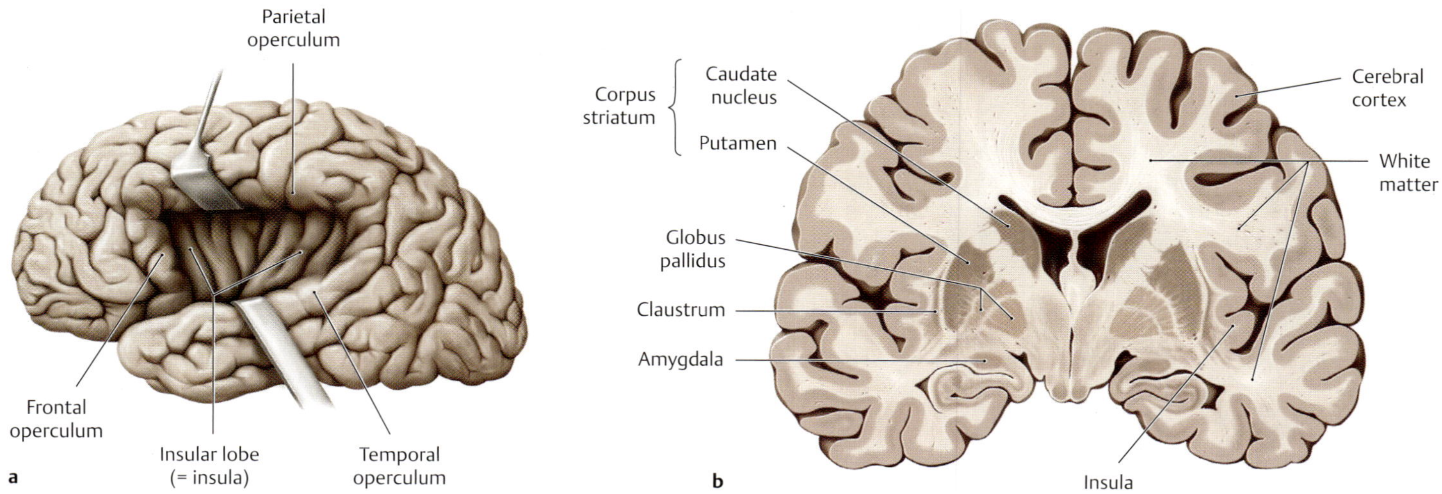

B Gray and white matter in the telencephalon

a Left cerebral hemisphere, lateral view, lateral sulcus spread open; **b** Coronal section of the brain.

a The insula located in the depth of the cerebral hemisphere becomes visible only after the lateral sulcus has been spread open. In an intact brain it is covered by neighboring lobes. These parts are referred to as little lids (opercula).

b The coronal section shows the distribution of gray and white matter. Based on the division of the pallium, the cortex is divided into neo-, archi-, and paleocortex. The modern neocortex (also called isocortex) is composed of six layers. The archi- and paleocortex (collectively called allocortex) consist of fewer layers. For further detail see p. 326 and 330. Embedded subcortically in the white matter are the neuron groups or nuclei. Due to their location at the base of the telencephalon, the caudate nucleus (tail), putamen (or shell, owing to the striation collectively called corpus striatum [or striped body]) and globus pallidus (pale globe) are also referred to as basal nuclei and are often misnamed basal ganglia. Additional nuclei, which anatomically are part of the basal nuclei, are the amygdala (an almond-shaped structure) in the temporal lobe and the claustrum (front wall) a subcortical structure found deep to the insular lobe. Thus the insula, the previously mentioned nuclei, and the exposed lateral ventricles dominate the cross section.

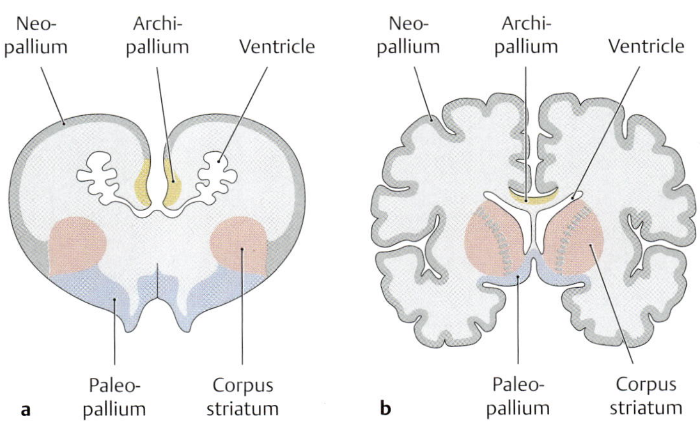

C Development of cerebral cortex and basal nuclei

a Embryonic brain; **b** Adult brain; frontal sections.

Phylogenetically, the entire telencephalon can be roughly divided into 3 parts of varying age. For this purpose, white matter and the overlying gray matter (cortex) are collectively referred to as mantle or pallium. In chronological order, a distinction is drawn between *paleopallium*, *archipallium* and *neopallium* (for further detail see **D**). The newer the part of the pallium, the larger its share of the telencephalon. During embryonic development, a large part of the neopallium is invaginated to form the insula (see **Ba**). Additionally, neurons from the neopallium migrate into the deeper regions where they form a portion of the basal nuclei (the striatum, see p. 336). Insula and basal nuclei are thus anatomical reference structures on a frontal section.

D Phylogenetic origins of major components of the telencephalon

Phylogenetic term	Structure in the embryonic brain	Structure(s) in the adult brain	Cortical structure
Paleopallium (oldest part)	Floor of the hemispheres	• Rhinencephalon (olfactory bulb plus surrounding region)	Allocortex (see p. 330)
Archipallium (old part)	Medial portion of hemispheric wall	• Ammon's horn (largest part, not shown here) • Indusium griseum • Fornix (see p. 332 f)	Allocortex
Neopallium (newest part)	Most of the brain surface plus the deeper corpus striatum	• Neocortex (cortex), largest part of the cerebral cortex • Insula • Corpus striatum	Isocortex (see p. 326)

6.2 Gyri and Sulci of the Telencephalon: Convex Surface of the Cerebral Hemispheres and Base of the Brain

Introduction

Morphologically, the surface of the telencephalon is defined by numerous ridges or *gyri* which are separated from one another by furrows or *sulci*. This form follows a basic pattern in humans which can vary significantly from one individual to another. Some brains even show differences between the left and right hemisphere. This explains why the surface morphology of the brain is not the same in every textbook. A textbook can only present an average anatomical image of the brain. The following illustrations show the gyri and sulci, that are officially recognized by the Terminologia Anatomica.

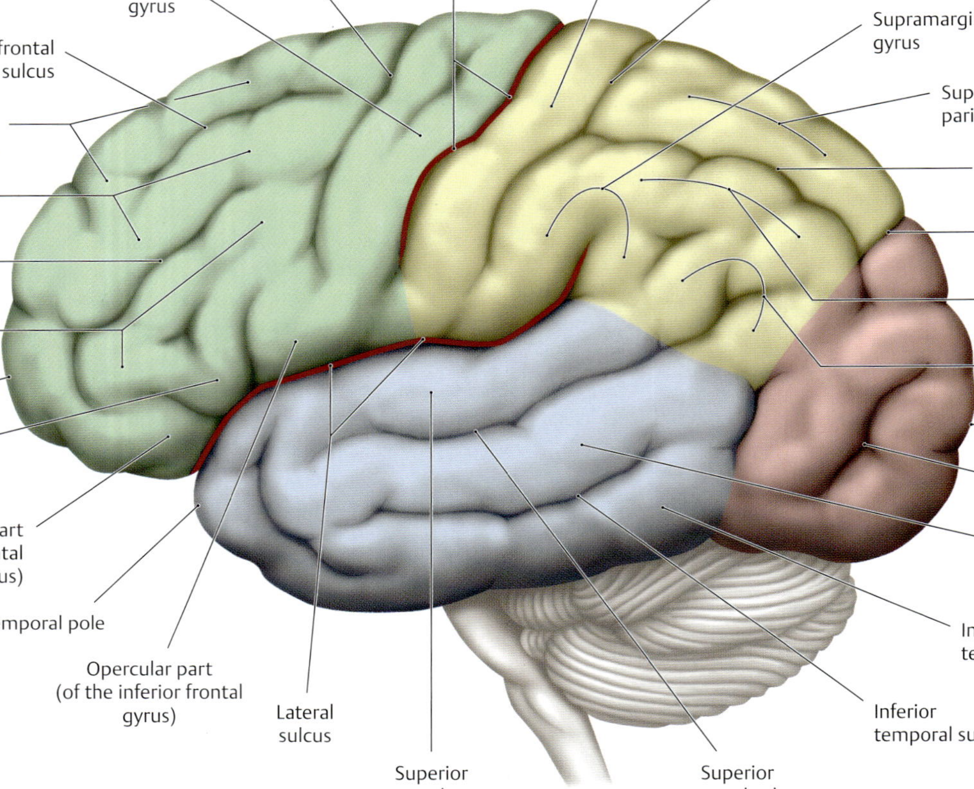

A Gyri and sulci of the convex surface

Left hemisphere, lateral view. The important reference point of the brain is the *central sulcus*, which is clearly visible here. It should not be confused with the neighboring *pre-* and *postcentral sulci*. Often three morphological characteristics are ascribed to the central sulcus:

- it is the longest sulcus of the brain,
- it extends across the superior margin of the brain to the medial surface of the brain (see **A**, p. 324),
- it is joined by the lateral suclus, which is also clearly visible here.

In actuality, the central sulcus rarely exhibits all these three characteristics. In this case, it helps to use the "two finger rule" to locate the central sulcus on the surface of the brain. With the index and middle finger of one hand held close together, they are placed above the hemisphere so that the fingers are above the convolutions which most closely correspond to the longitudinal direction of the fingers and as such run more or less parallel. The index finger is located on the precentral gyrus and the middle finger lies on the postcentral gyrus. The gap between the fingers corresponds to the central sulcus.

Note: Many gyri are named for their location in a specific lobe (e.g., the superior frontal gyrus is located on the superior portion of the frontal lobe).

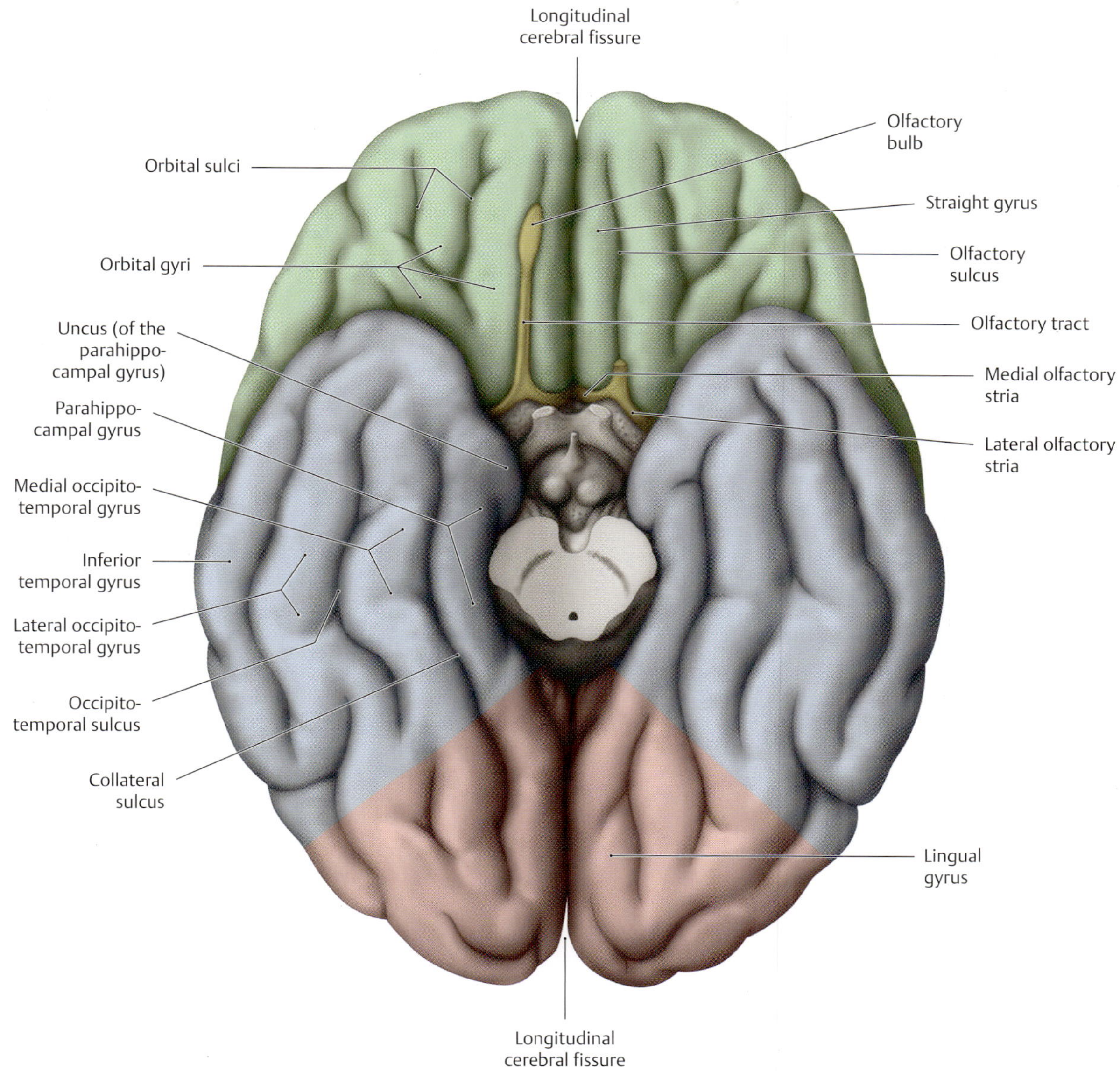

B Gyri and sulci at the base of the brain

Basal view of the telencephalon (from below).

The gyri at the base of the temporal lobe are sometimes topographically barely distinguishable. This is the case with both the *occipitotemporal gyri*. For this reason the anatomical illustrations in textbooks may differ. In contrast, the *straight gyri* are located in the frontal lobe and the *orbital gyri*, are situated in the cranium directly above the roof of the orbit. The comparison with **Aa** shows the "edge position" of the *inferior temporal gyrus*: it is visible in both the lateral view (as the lower border of the temporal lobe) and the basal view (as lateral border of the temporal lobe). What is apparent at the base of the brain, is a paleocortical part of the telencephalon, which morphologically resembles a nerve rather than a part of the cortex since it does not have any gyri: the olfactory bulb and *tract*. Histologically, this part of the paleocortex does not exhibit a cortical structure.

Note: In the occipital lobe very close to the longitudinal cerebral fissure lies the lingual gyrus. Its shape, which resembles the tongue, is only visible when viewed from medial aspect (see **A**, p. 324). Although morphologically, it seems to be the posterior extension of the parahippocampal gyrus (which is the most medial of the gyri) functionally these gyri have nothing to do with each other: The *parahippocampal gyrus* is part of the limbic system, while the *lingual gyrus* is part of visual cortex. The separation between the two gyri is visible in fig. **A**, p. 324.

6.3 Gyri and Sulci of the Telencephalon: Medial Surface and Insula

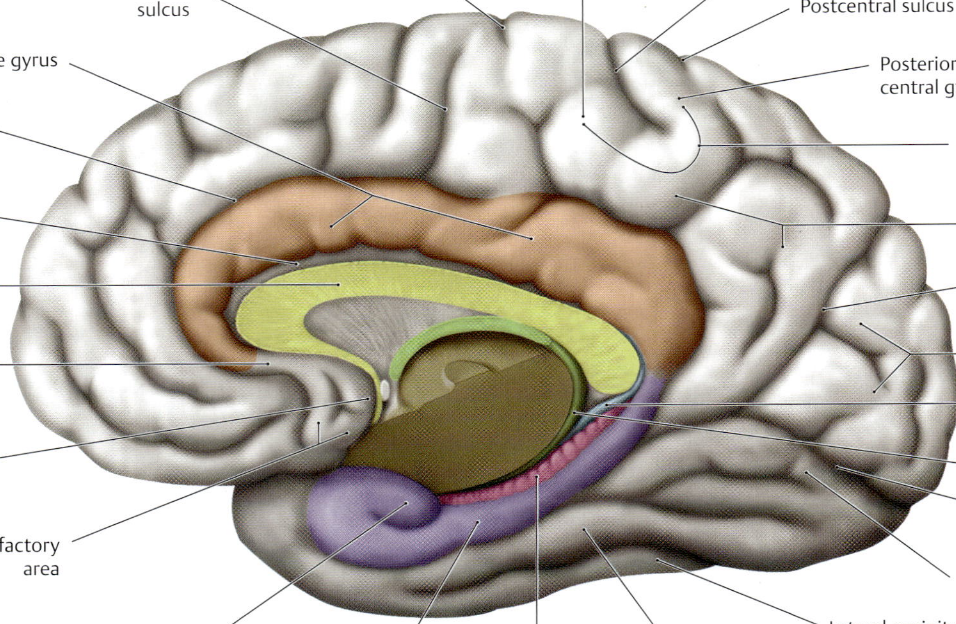

A Gyri and sulci of the medial surface

Right hemisphere, medial view; brainstem and basal parts of the diencephalon have been removed.

This midsagittal section provides a view of the medial surface of the brain. The corpus callosum serves as an anatomical reference point. Clearly visible are the following structures:

- Located directly above the corpus callosum and surrounding it like a belt (Latin cingulum: belt, girdle) is the *cingulate gyrus*, which is part of the limbic system.
- Located ventral to the corpus callosum are structures which are often referred to as the "hippocampal formation." The sections of the hippocampal formation are not easily visible from the outside. They are the *hippocampus proper* and the *dentate gyrus* with its tooth-like surface. To provide an unobstructed view of the dentate gyrus, in this specimen the neighboring gyri would either have to be removed or pushed out of the way. The dentate gyrus lies above and somewhat medial to the hippocampus proper, which is why the latter is still not visible here. The dentate gyrus and in particular the hippocampus proper are almost rolled up in the temporal lobe of the brain; both structures are part of the limbic system and process information related to learning, memory, and emotions (for a description of the hippocampus proper see pp. 330–333). The fornix, which is also clearly visible, is a tract of the limbic system which extends from the hippocampus to the diencephalon.

The midsagittal section also shows additional morphological characteristics, which are less clearly visible when looking at the convex or basal cerebral surfaces:

- The cingulate gyrus has a C shape. Its superior border is marked by the cingulate sulcus.
- Adjacent to it is a wedge-shaped region of the brain known by the Latin name cuneus which in turn is demarcated by the parieto-occipital sulcus. Adjacent to the cuneus is the precuneus. The calcarine sulcus separates the cuneus from the lingula. The primary visual cortex is found on each side of the calcarine sulcus (see p. 329).
- The separation between the lingual and parahippocampal gyri is visible.
- The parahippocampal gyrus continues posteriorly and superiorly with the cingulate gyrus. Both gyri are connected through a long association tract—the cingulum—which is located in the white matter of the gyri and therefore not visible here.
- The anterior end of the parahippocampal gyrus is uncinated or bent like a hook.

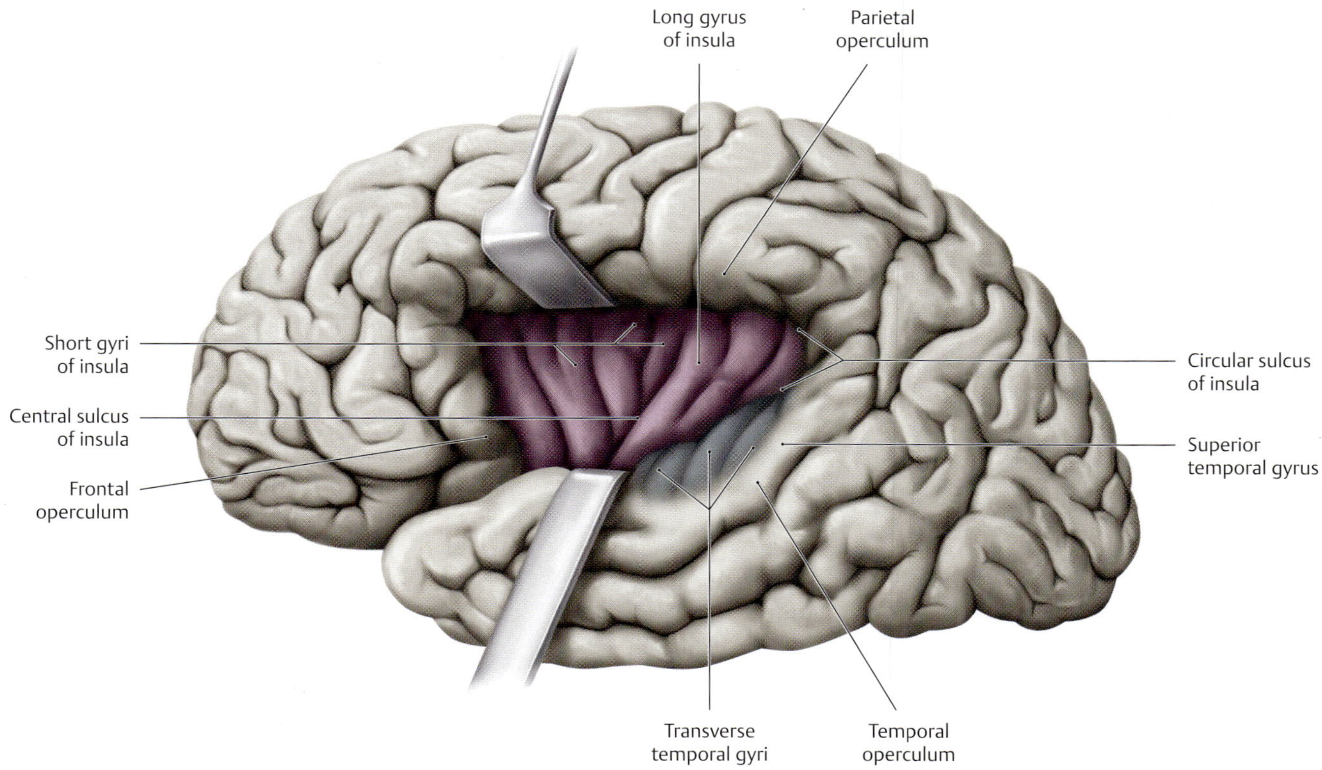

B Gyri and sulci of the insula

Left hemisphere, lateral view; lateral sulcus spread open by retractors. As a result, the following structures become visible:

- the insula (not visible in an intact brain) along with the *insular gyri* as well as
- the *transverse temporal gyri* (transverse gyri of Heschl—the primary auditory cortex) on the surface of the superior temporal gyrus at its posterior end.

Transverse temporal gyri and insular gyri do not touch but are separated by the circular insular sulcus. The insula is not isolated as its cortex connects it to the cortices of the neighboring lobes. The portions of those lobes which cover the insula in an intact brain from above and below like "little lids" (opercula) have been pulled aside with retractors:

- The *parietal operculum* (part of the parietal lobe, which covers the superior part of the insula)
- The *temporal operculum* (part of the temporal lobe which covers the inferior part of the insula)
- A small part of the frontal lobe, which covers the anterior part of the insula, the *frontal operculum*, has been left in its place. It is significant in that in the frontal operculum—found in most people on the left side—is where the motor speech center of *Broca* is located.

C Gyri and sulci: variants

The previous illustrations depicting gyri and sulci (cf. p. 322 f) show a quasi-standardized basic arrangement pattern. However, there are significant individual variants regarding both the form of the gyri and the shape of the sulci located between them. In particular, the sulci can show enormous differences in depth but neighboring gyri are always connected at the bottom of the sulci. At points where sulci are typically much less dense, the range of variation can make them difficult to identify. Thus, gyri which are seemingly separated by such a sulcus are no longer recognizable as two separate units. The connection between these gyri is visible at the surface. In such a brain, it can be impossible to identify individual gyri due to a lack of demarcations between them. This is most often the case at the base of the brain where a demarcation between the occipitotemporal gyri does not exist. Assigning names to individual gyri here might not be possible.

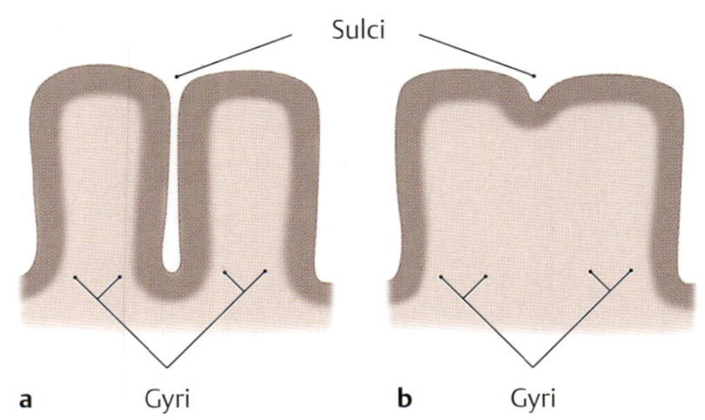

The diagram shows a cross-section of two neighboring gyri with the sulcus located between them: In **a**, the sulcus is very deep and both gyri are clearly separated; in **b**, the sulcus is so shallow that it might not even be recognizable when viewed from the surface; in such a case, the morphological distinction of the two gyri would be impossible.

6.4 Cerebral Cortex, Histological Structure and Functional Organization

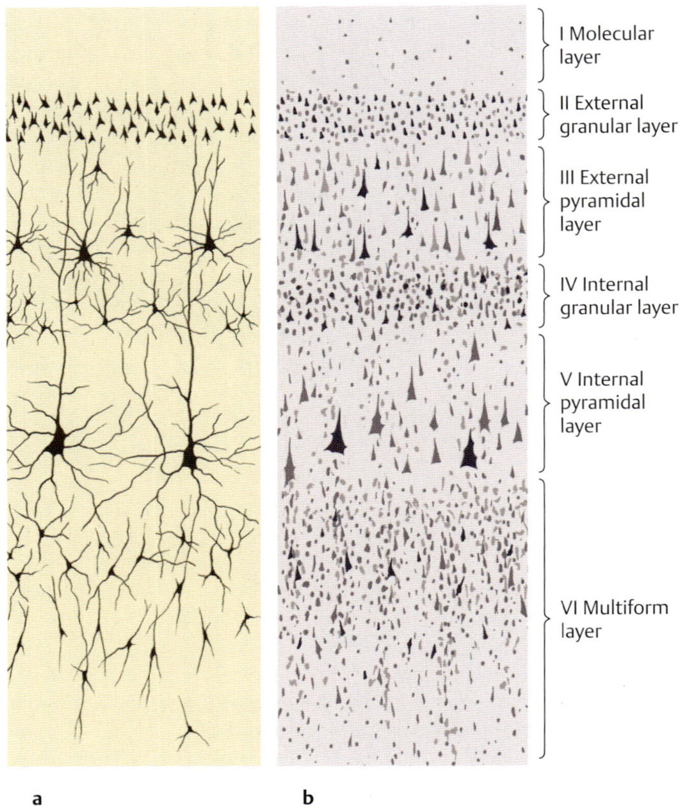

A Histological structure of the cerebral cortex
six-layered (laminar) structure is found throughout most of the neocortex. The silver impregnation (**a**) or Nissl staining of the cell bodies (**b**) allows for histological division of the neocortex according to the dominant structure of each layer:

- I Molecular layer: (outermost layer); relatively few neurons
- II External granular layer: mostly stellate and scattered small pyramidal neurons
- III External pyramidal layer: small pyramidal neurons
- IV Internal granular layer: stellate and small pyramidal neurons
- V Internal pyramidal layer: large pyramidal neurons
- VI Multiform layer: (innermost layer); neurons of varied shape and size

Cortical areas that are concerned primarily with information processing (e.g., primary somatosensory cortex) are rich in granule cells; the granular layers of these regions (*granular cortex*, see **Ba**) are also exceptionally thick. Areas in which information is transmitted out of the cortex (e.g., the primary motor cortex) are distinguished by prominent layers of pyramidal cells and known as the *agranular cortex* (see **Bb**). Analysis of the distribution of nerve cells in the cerebral cortex allows for identification of functionally distinct areas (*cytoarchitectonics*, see **A**, p. 328).

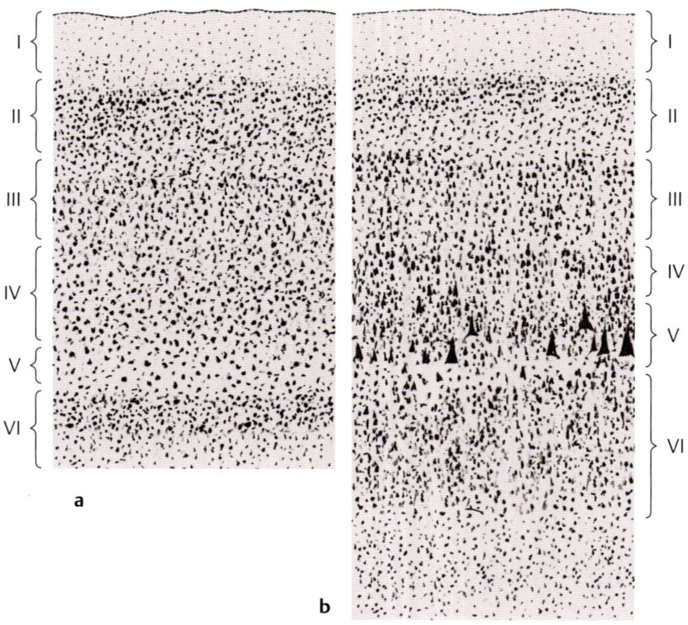

B Examples of granular and agranular cortex

a Granular cortex (koniocortex from the Greek konis = sand): The primary somato*sensory* cortex, in which the afferents from the thalamus terminate (at layer IV), is located in the *post*central gyrus. It is thinner overall than the primary somato*motor* cortex (see **b**). A striking feature in the primary somatosensory cortex is that the external and internal granular layers (II and IV) where the large sensory tracts terminate are markedly widened. By contrast, the pyramidal cell layers (III and V) are thinned.

b Agranular cortex: The efferents fibers that project to the motor nuclei of the cranial nerves and motor columns of the spinal cord originate in the primary somato*motor* cortex, located in the *precentral* gyrus. Its pyramidal layers (III and V) are greatly enlarged. Exceptionally large pyramidal neurons (Betz cells after the author who first described them) are found in the some areas of layer V. Their long axons extend as far as the sacral spinal cord.

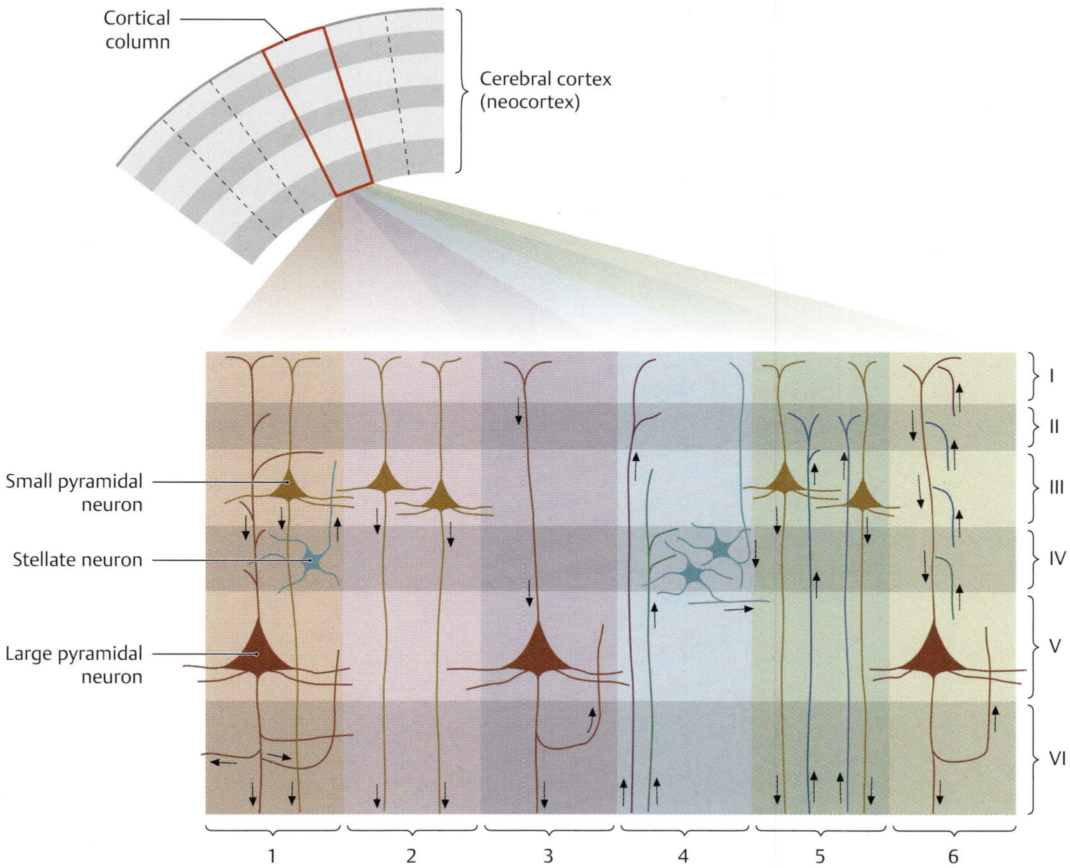

C Columnar organization of the cortex (after Klinke and Silbernagl)
While morphological considerations divide the cerebral cortex into horizontal layers (see **A**), functional considerations lead to its division into distinct units or modules (see **C**). Encompassing all six layers, these modules consist of vertically arranged *cortical columns* of neurons that are interconnected to serve a common function, despite showing no distinct histological boundaries. In total, there are several million of such modules in the cerebral cortex, with a variable width between 50 and 500 µm each. One cortical column has been magnified here to display its constituent neurons and connections in separate panels. Panels **1–3** show the principal types of cells participating in a cortical column: several thousand *stellate neurons* of various subtypes and one hundred or so large and small pyramidal neurons (panel **1**). Panel **2** isolates the small pyramidal cells whose axons tend to terminate within the cortex itself. In contrast, the deeper, large pyramidal neurons (panel **3**) have axons that generally project to subcortical structures. Large pyramidal cells are responsible for tracts of corticobulbar and corticospinal motor axons, which project to the brainstem and spinal cord, respectively. They may also send recurrent collateral fibers which end in the local cortex. Panels **4–6** contain axons projecting *into* the cerebral cortex. Panel **4** isolates thalamocortical projections that enter from the thalamus and synapse mostly on the stellate neurons of layer IV. Incoming association fibers of the nearby cortex and commissural fibers of the contralateral hemisphere frequently terminate on the dendrites of the small pyramidal neurons (panel **5**). Panel **6** shows the large pyramidal neurons whose apical dendrites reach from layer V to layer I. These large pyramidal neurons integrate inputs from various other local neurons and incoming fibers.

D Types of neuron in the cerebral cortex (simplified)

Neuron	Definition	Properties
Stellate neuron (layers II and IV)	Cell with short axon for local information processing; various types: basket, candelabra, double-bouquet cells	Inhibitory interneuron in most cortical areas; primary information-processing neuron (in layer II), especially in primary sensory areas
Small pyramidal neuron (layer III)	Cell with long axon that often ends within the cortex, either as • Association fiber: axon ends in same hemisphere but different cortical area, or as • Commissural fiber: axon ends in opposite hemisphere but cortical area of similar function	Projection neuron whose axons end within the cortex
Large pyramidal neuron (layer V)	Cell with very long axon that projects outside the cortex, sometimes reaching distant structures	Excitatory projection neuron whose axons end outside the cortex
Granule cell (layers II and IV)	Generic term for small neuron, most often with stellate morphology	Depends on the cell type (see entries for stellate and small pyramidal neurons)

6.5 Neocortex, Cortical Areas

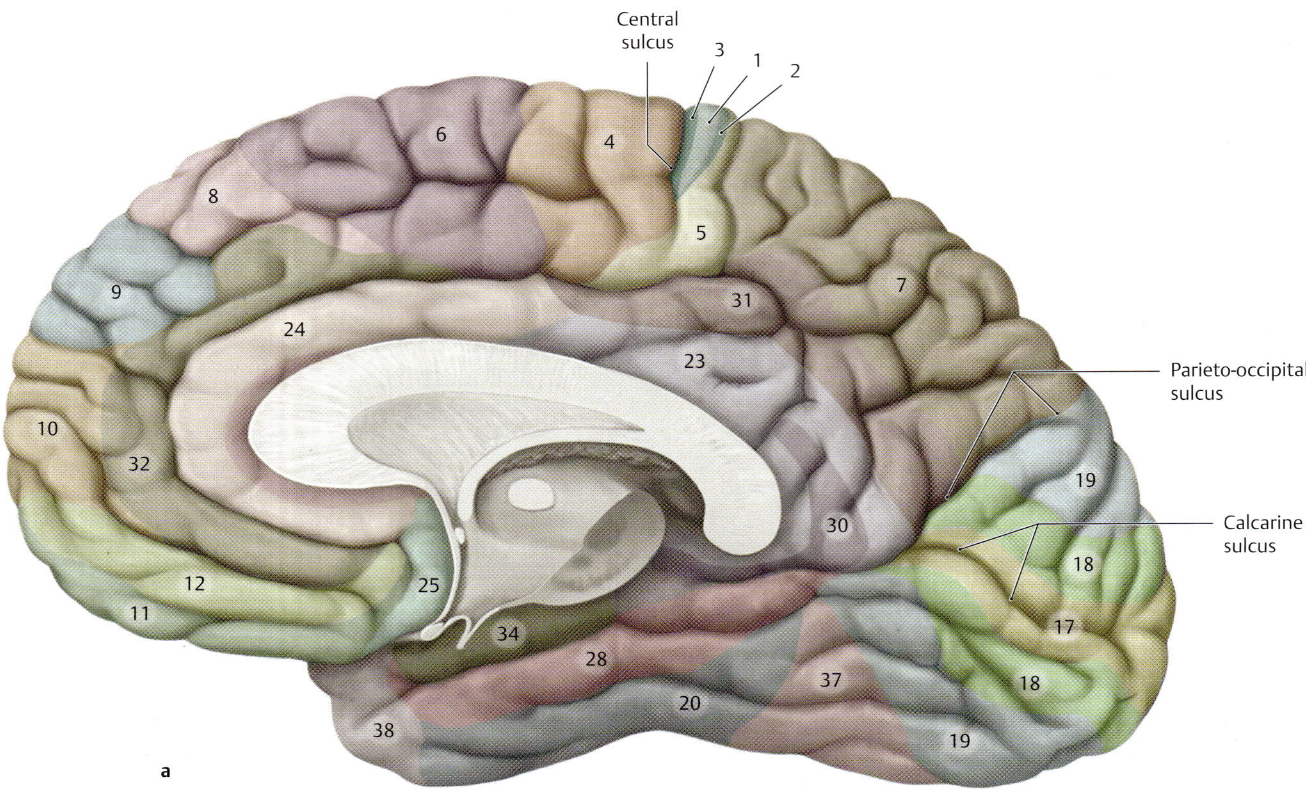

a

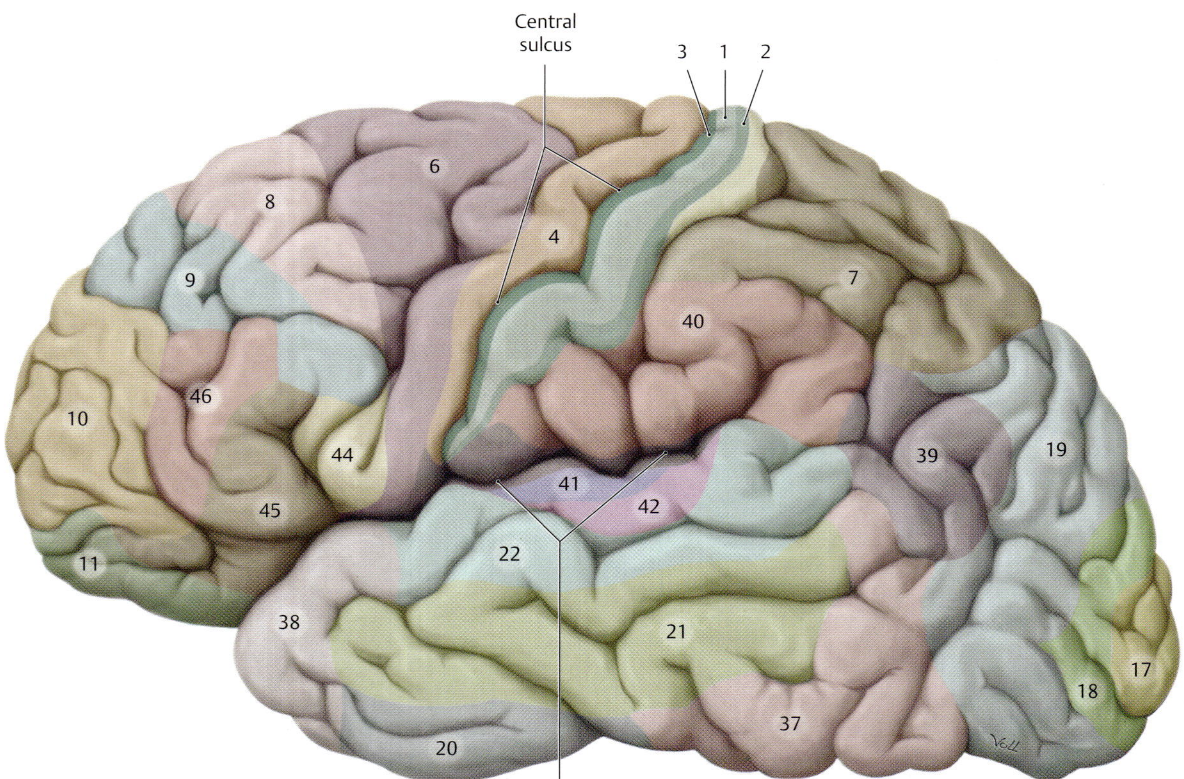

b

A Brodmann areas in the neocortex

a Midsagittal section of the right cerebral hemisphere, viewed from the left side; **b** Lateral view of the left cerebral hemisphere.

As noted earlier, the surface of the brain consists macroscopically of lobes, gyri, and sulci. Microscopically, however, subtle differences can be found in the distribution of the cortical neurons, and some of these differences do not conform to the gross surface anatomy of the brain. Portions of the cerebral cortex that have the same basic microscopic features are called *cortical areas* or *cortical fields*. This organization into cortical areas is based on the distribution of neurons in the different layers of the cortex (*cytoarchitectonics*, see **A**, p. 326). In the brain map shown at left, these areas are indicated by different colors. Although the size of the cortical areas may vary between individuals, the brain map pictured here is still used today as a standard reference chart. It was developed in the early 20th century by the anatomist Korbinian Brodmann (1868–1918), who spent years painstakingly examining the cellular architecture of the cortex in a single brain. It has long been thought that the map created by Brodmann accurately reflects the functional organization of the cortex, and indeed, modern imaging techniques have shown that many of the cytologically defined areas are associated with specific functions. There is no need, of course, to memorize the location of all the cortical areas, but the following areas are of special interest:

- Areas 1, 2, and 3: primary somatosensory cortex
- Area 4 primary motor cortex
- Area 17: primary visual cortex (striate area, the extent of which is best appreciated in the midsagittal section)
- Areas 41 and 42: auditory cortex

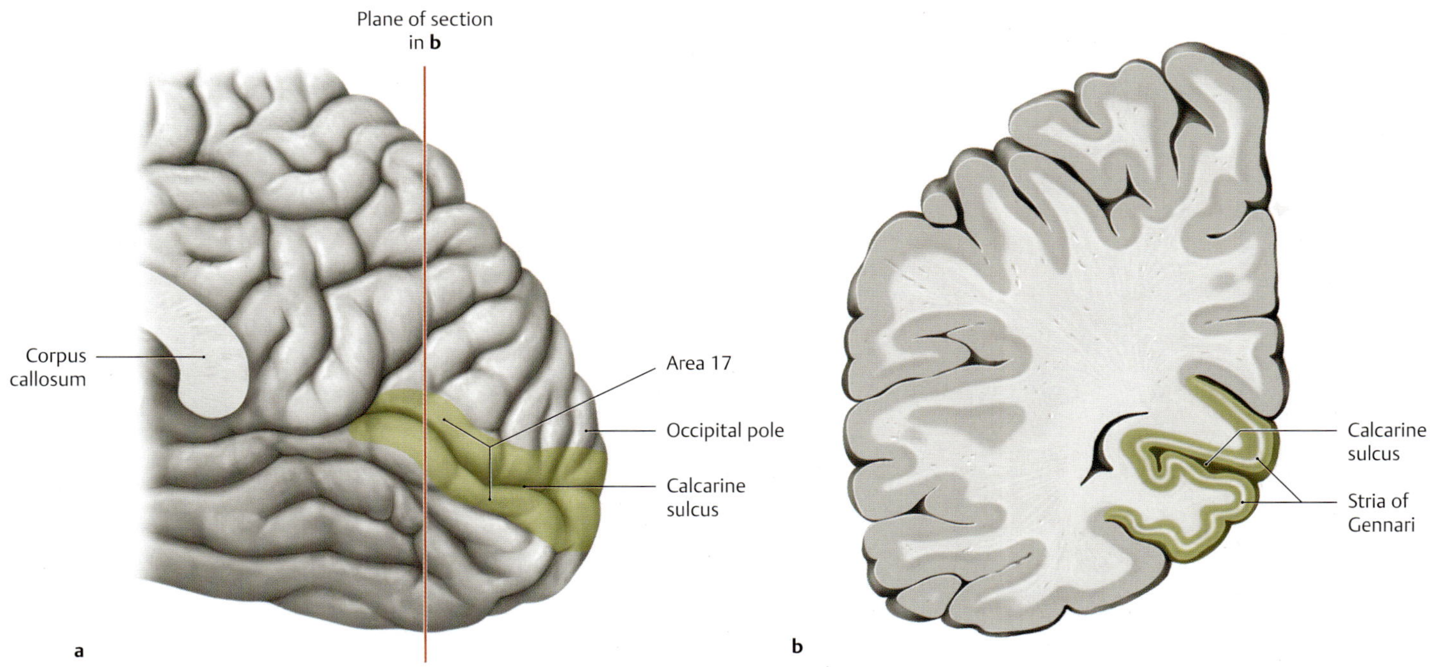

B Visual cortex (striate area)

a Medial aspect of the right hemisphere viewed from the left side; **b** Coronal section (plane of section shown in **a**), anterior view.

The primary visual cortex (striate area, shaded yellow) is the only cortical area that can be clearly recognized by its macroscopic appearance. It extends along both sides of the calcarine sulcus at the occipital pole. In an unstained coronal section (**b**), the *stria of Gennari* can be identified as a prominent white stripe within the gray cortical area. This stripe contains cortical association fibers that synapse with the neurons of the internal granular layer (IV). The pyramidal cell layers (efferent fibers) are attenuated in the visual cortex, while the granular cell layers where the afferent fibers from the lateral geniculate nucleus terminate are markedly enlarged.

6.6 Allocortex, Overview

A Overview of the allocortex

View of the base of the brain (**a**) and the medial surface of the right hemisphere (**b**). Structures belonging to the allocortex are indicated by colored shading.

The allocortex consists of the phylogenetically old part of the cerebral cortex. It is very small in relation to the cortex as a whole. Unlike the isocortex, which has a six-layered structure, the allocortex (*allo* = "other") usually consists of *three* layers that encompass the paleo- and archicortexes. Additionally, there exist *four*-layered transitional areas between the allocortex and isocortex: the *peri*paleocortex (not indicated separately in the drawing) and the *peri*archicortex (indicated by pink shading). An important part of the allocortex is the *rhinencephalon* ("olfactory brain"). Olfactory impulses that are perceived by the olfactory bulb are the only sensory afferent impulses that do not reach the cerebral cortex by way of the dorsal thalamus. Another important part of the allocortex is the hippocampus and its associated nuclei (see p. 332). As in the isocortex, the gyral patterns of the allocortex do not always conform to its histological organization.

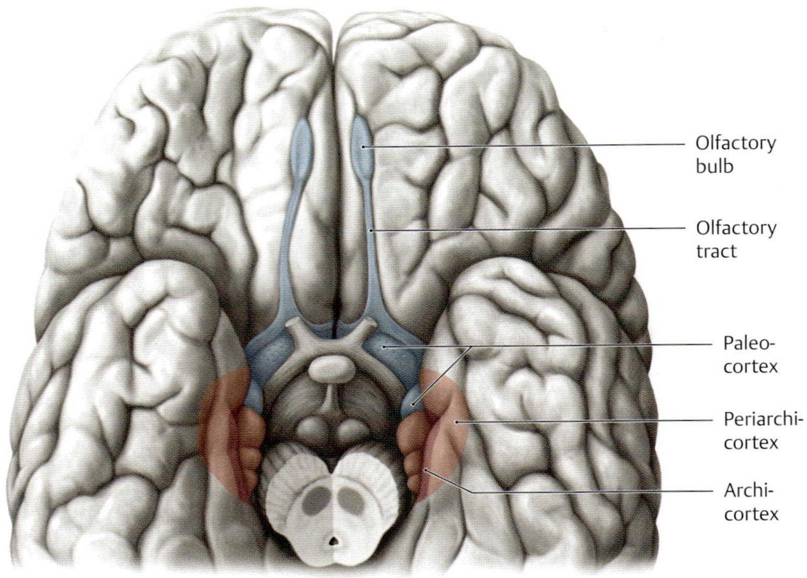

a

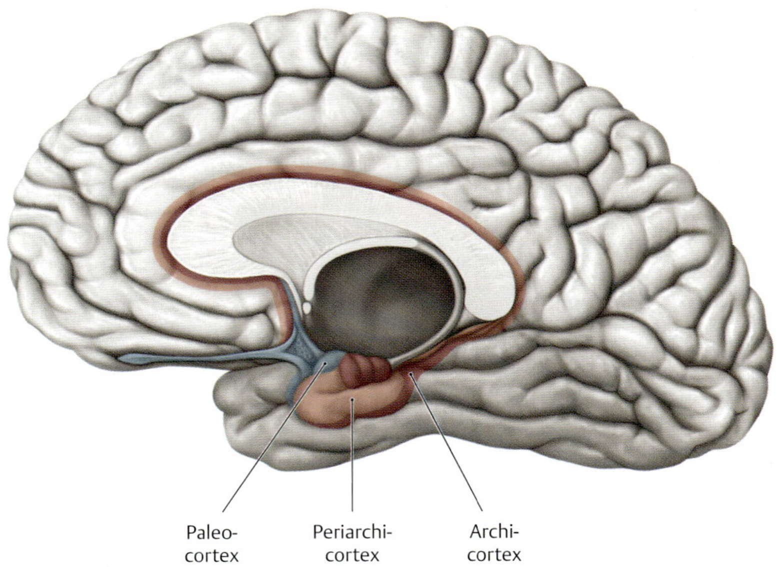

b

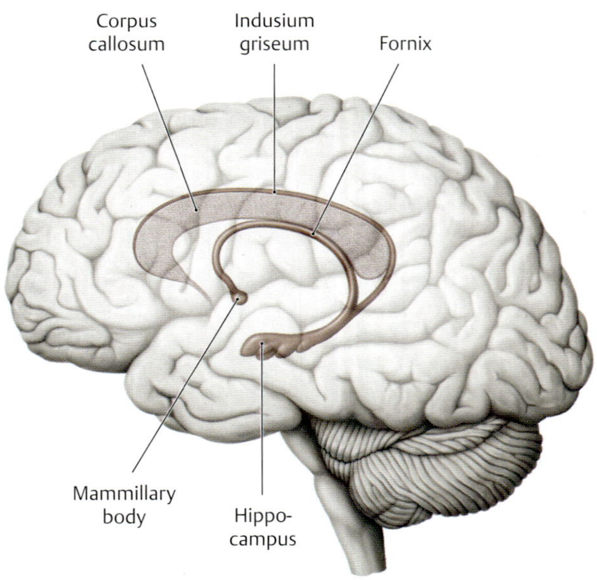

B Organization of the archipallium: deeper parts

Lateral view of the left hemisphere. The archicortex described in **A** is the *only* part of the archipallium that is located on the brain surface. The deeper parts of the archipallium, which lie within the white matter, are the hippocampus ("sea horse"), indusium griseum ("gray covering"), and fornix ("arch"). All three structures are part of the *limbic system* (see p. 492), and together form a border ("limbus") around the corpus callosum as a result of their arrangement during development.

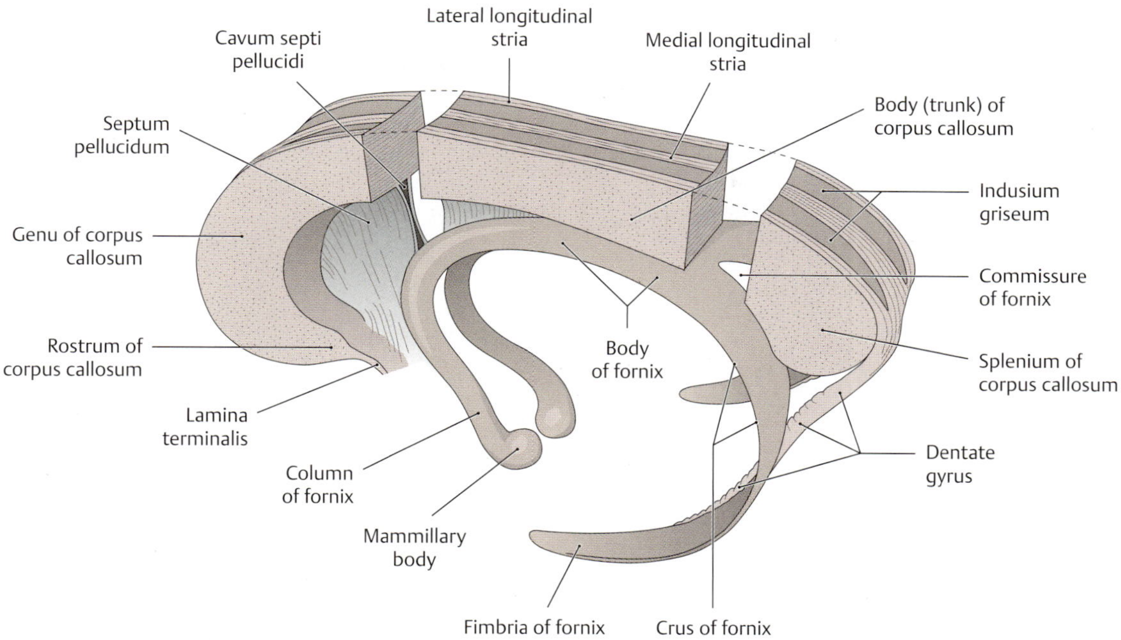

C Topography of the fornix, corpus callosum, and septum pellucidum (after Feneis)
Occipital view from upper left. The fornix is a tract of the archicortex that is closely apposed but functionally unrelated to the corpus callosum. The corpus callosum is the largest neocortical commissural tract between the hemispheres, serving to interconnect cortical areas of similar function in the two hemispheres (see **D**, p. 335). The septum pellucidum is a thin plate that stretches between the corpus callosum and fornix, forming the medial boundary of the lateral ventricles. Between the two septa is a cavity of variable size, the *cavum septi pellucidi*. The cholinergic nuclei in the septa, which are involved in the organization of memory, are connected to the hippocampus by the fornix (see p. 332).

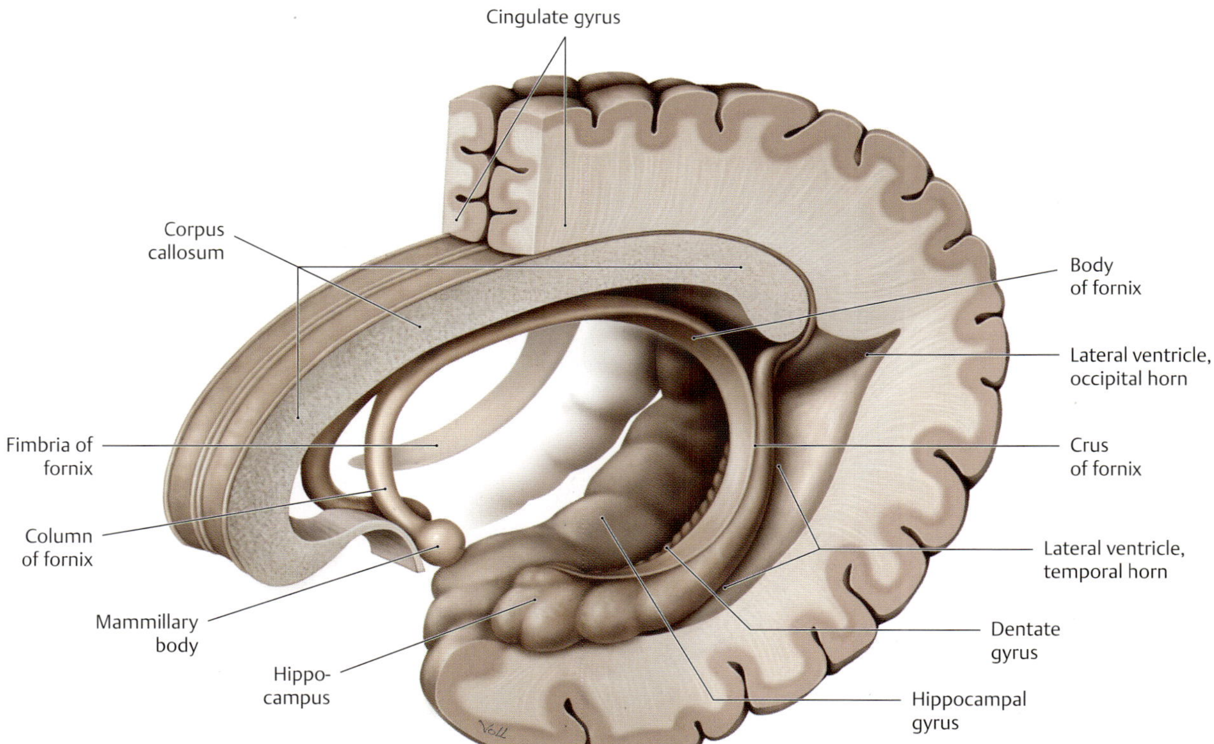

D Topography of the hippocampus, fornix, and corpus callosum
Viewed from the upper left and anterior aspect. This drawing shows the hippocampus on the floor of the inferior horn of the lateral ventricle. The left and right *crura of the fornix* unite to form the *commissure of the fornix* (see **C**) and the *body of the fornix*, which divides anteriorly into left and right bundles, the *columns of the fornix*. The fornix is a white matter tract connecting the hippocampus to the mammillary bodies in the diencephalon. Fimbria is a band of white matter along the hippocampus. Neurons project their axons to the septum, mammillary bodies, contralateral hippocampus, and other structures. In it run efferent pathways between hippocampus and hypothalamus. This important pathway is part of the limbic system.

6.7 Allocortex: Hippocampus and Amygdala

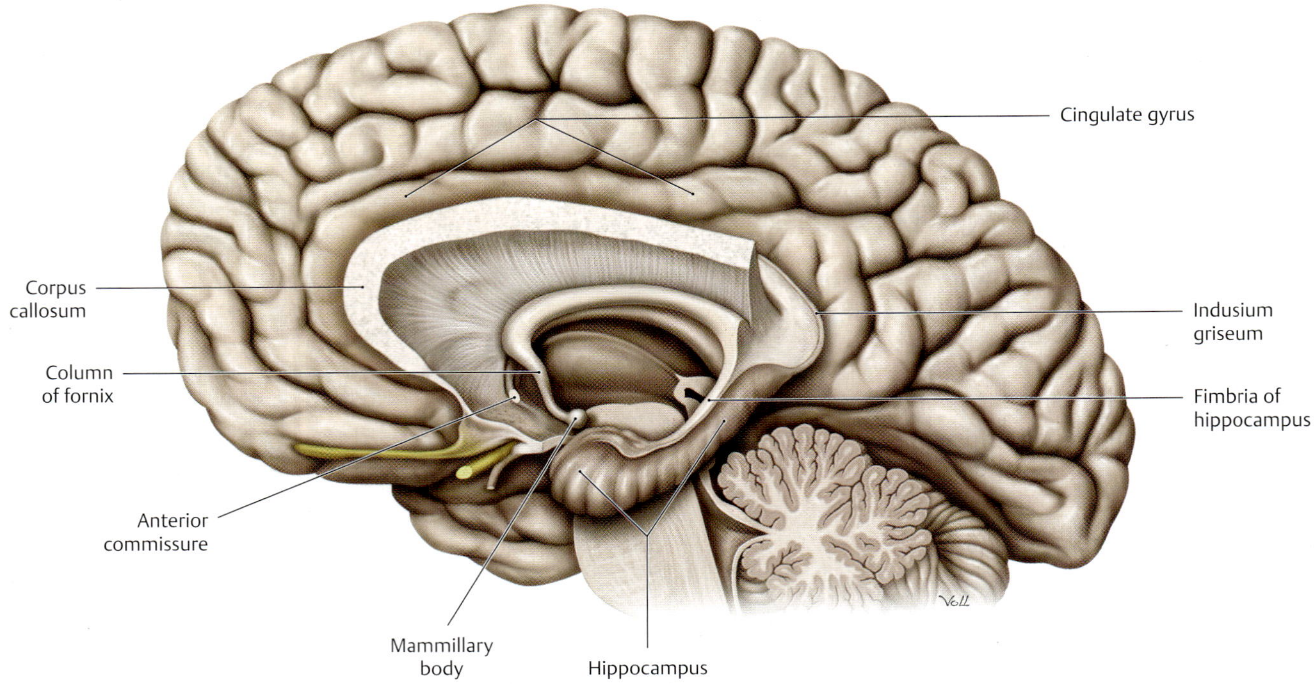

A Left hippocampal formation
Medial view of hippocampus and fornix. Most of the left hemisphere has been dissected and removed, leaving only the corpus callosum, fornix, and hippocampus. The intact right hemisphere is visible in the background.
The hippocampal formation is an important component of the limbic system (see p. 492). It consists of three parts:

- Subiculum (see **Cb**)
- Hippocampus proper (Ammon's horn)
- Dentate gyrus (fascia dentata)

The fiber tract of the fornix connects the hippocampus to the mammillary body. The hippocampus integrates information from various brain areas and influences endocrime, visceral, and emotional processes via its efferent output. It is particulary associated with the establishment of short-term memory. Lesions of the hippocampus can therefore cause specific defects in memory formation (see **B**, p. 498).
Besides the hippocampus, which is the largest part of the archicortex, we can recognize another component of the archicortex, the indusium griseum.

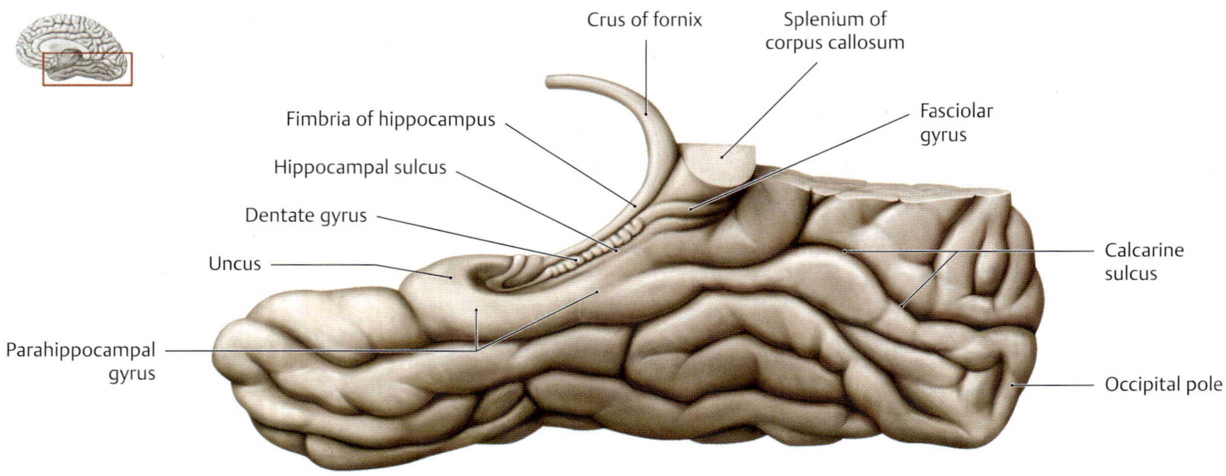

B Right hippocampal formation and the caudal part of the fornix
Medial view. Compare this medial view of the right hippocampal formation with the lateral view in **A** above. A useful landmark is the calcarine sulcus, which leads to the occipital pole. The cortical areas that border the hippocampus (e.g., the parahippocampal gyrus) are particularly visible in this view.

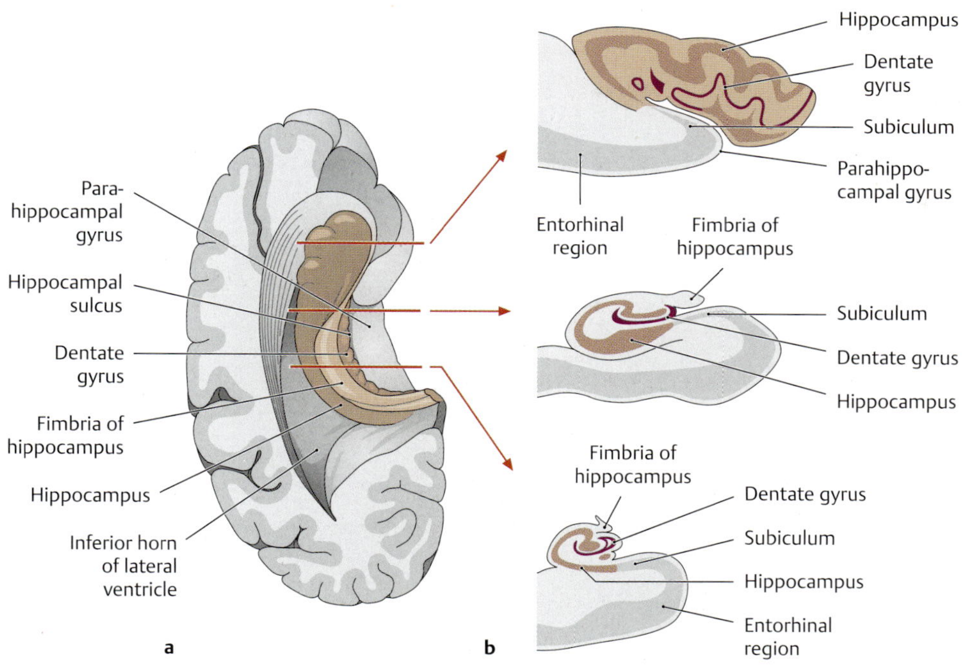

C Left temporal lobe with the inferior horn of the lateral ventricle exposed

a Transverse section, posterior view of the hippocampus on the floor of the inferior (temporal) horn. The following structures can be identified from lateral to medial: hippocampus, fimbria, dentate gyrus, hippocampal sulcus, and parahippocampal gyrus.

b Coronal sections of the left hippocampus. The hippocampus appears here as a curled band (Ammon's horn = the hippocampus proper), which shows considerable structural diversity in its different portions. The junction between the entorhinal cortex (entorhinal region) in the parahippocampal gyrus and Ammon's horn is formed by a transitional area, the subiculum. The entorhinal region is the "gateway" to the hippocampus, through which the hippocampus receives most of its afferent fibers.

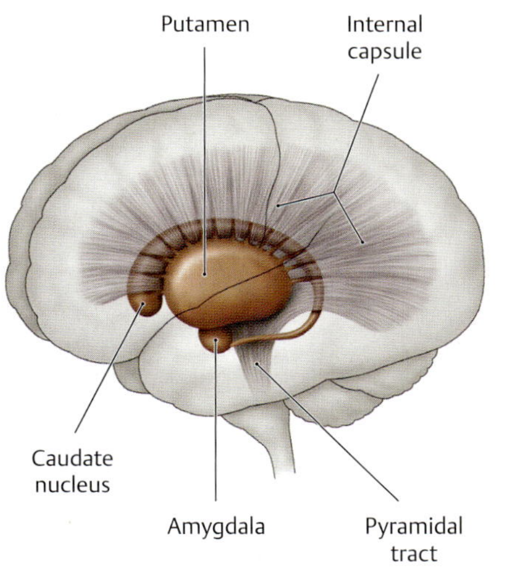

D Relationship of the amygdala to internal brain structures

Lateral view of the left hemisphere. The amygdala (amygdaloid body) is located below the putamen and anterior to the tail of the caudate nucleus. The fibers of the pyramidal tract run posterior and medial to the amygdala.

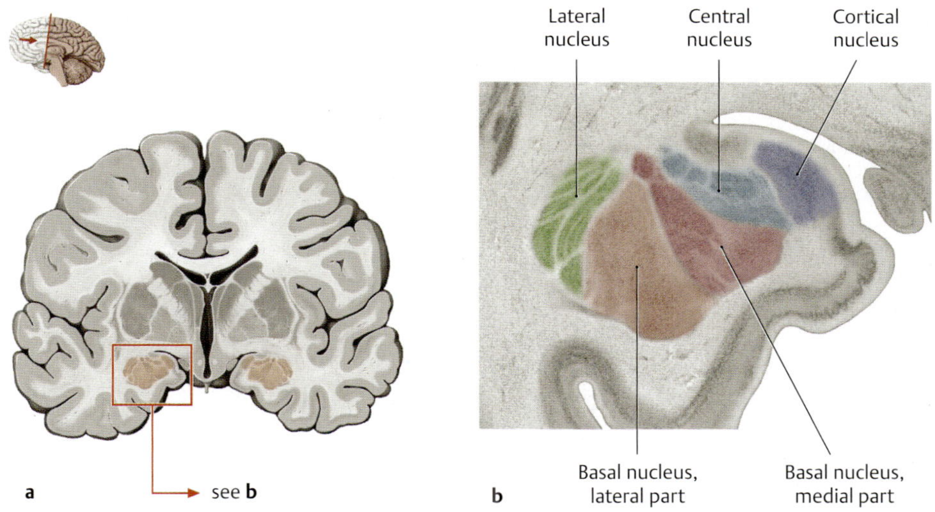

E Amygdala

a Coronal section at the level of the interventricular foramen. The amygdala extends medially to the inferior surface of the cortex of the temporal lobe. For this reason, it is considered to be part of the cortex as well as a nuclear complex that has migrated into the white matter. Stimulation of the amygdala in humans leads to changes in mood, ranging from rage and fear to rest and relaxation depending on the emotional state of the patient immediately prior to stimulation. Since the amygdala functions as an "emotional amplifier," lesions affect the patient's evaluation of events' emotional significance. The surrounding periamygdaline cortex and the corticomedial half of the amygdala are part of the primary olfactory cortex. Hence these portions of the amygdala are considered part of the paleocortex, while the deeper portion is characterized as "nuclear."

b Detail from **a** showing the two main groups of nuclei in the amygdala:

- Phylogenetically old corticomedial group:
  - Cortical nucleus
  - Central nucleus
- Phylogenetically new basolateral group:
  - Basal nucleus
  - Lateral nucleus

The basal nucleus can be subdivided into a parvocellular medial part and a macrocellular lateral part.

6.8 The White Matter

A White matter in the telencephalon
a Midsagittal view of the right hemisphere viewed from the left; **b** Parasagittal view of left hemisphere viewed from the left, a *fiber dissection specimen*. The fan-shaped pattern of the inner capsule with ascending and descending fibers is referred to as the corona radiata.
In the intact central nervous system, the white matter appears structurally homogeneous. With the help of special preparation techniques that utilize the different water content of various structures of the CNS, it can be shown that the white matter is composed of tracts (see **D**, p. 269), of myelinated axons. Axons are responsible for signal transduction. Tracts are therefore "data highways" for the rapid signal transmission in the CNS. Although all of the white matter in the CNS consists of tracts, they can be most easily shown in the white matter of the telencephalon. The tracts are distinguished based on the direction of information flow and the localization of the tract connecting parts of the CNS:

- projection tracts
- commissural tracts (see **D**)
- association tracts (see **C**)

If tracts are destroyed (e.g., in the case of multiple sclerosis) the functions assigned to one tract are no longer executed. Due to the functional variety of tracts, the disruption can lead to a range of symptoms including paralysis, impaired somatosensation, visual disturbances, and/or memory loss. Since tracts always connect two structures in the CNS, is is very important when studying those tracts, to learn the involved structures, signal sender and signal receiver. For more detail see **B**.

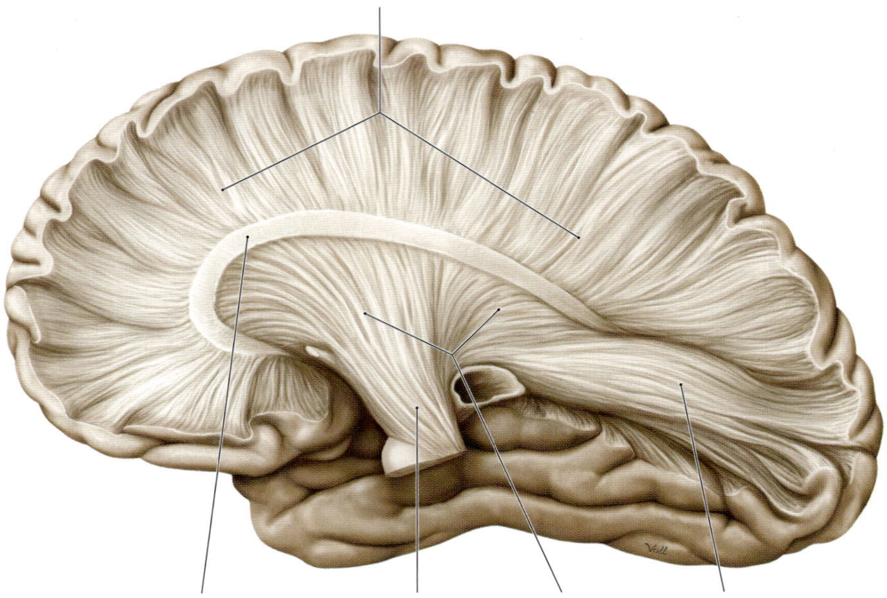

a

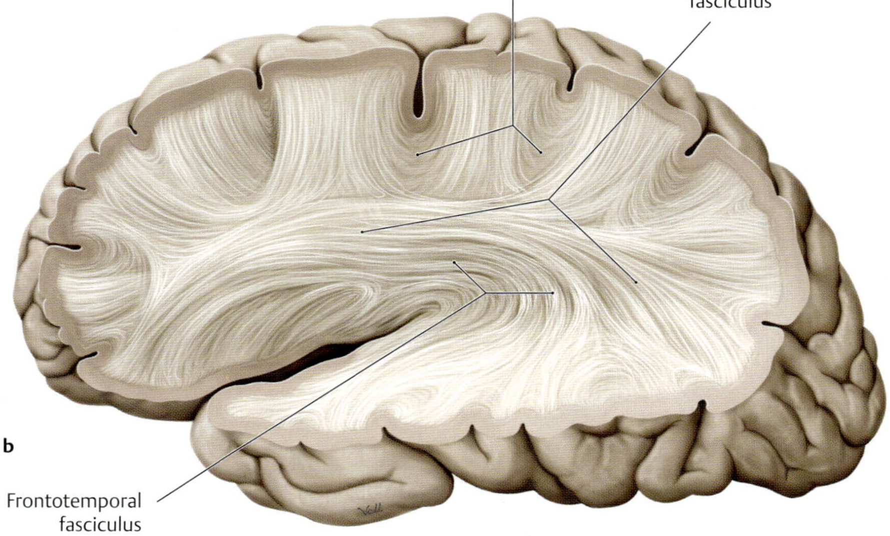

b

B Pathways of the CNS
Classification of pathways. Two pathways are usually macroscopically visible in a brain even if it has not been specifically prepared: fornix (vault) and corpus callosum.

Projection fibers	Connect different levels of organization within the CNS, either ascending or descending (Fornix = special projection tract of the limbic system)
• **Corticopetal fibers**	Ascending fibers, especially to the cerebral cortex
• **Corticofugal fibers**	Descending fibers, especially from the cerebral cortex
Association fibers	Connect different cortical areas within one hemisphere (see **C**)
Commissural fibers	Connect similar cortical areas in both hemispheres (see **D**) (= interhemispheric association fibers); Corpus callosum = largest commissural tract in the brain

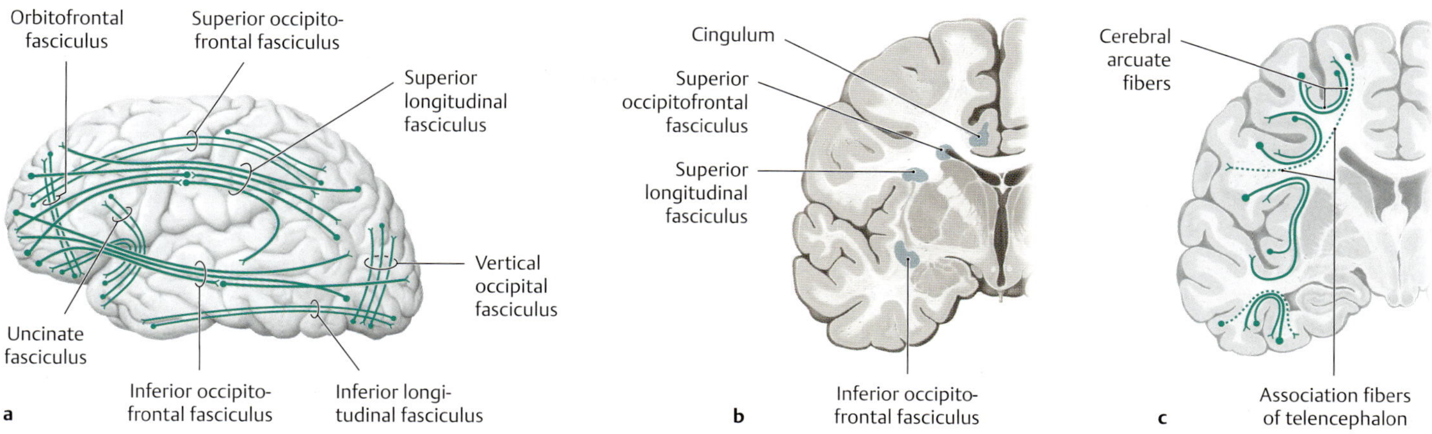

C Association fibers

a Lateral view of the left hemisphere. **b** Anterior view of coronal section of the right hemisphere. **c** Anterior view of short association fibers.

Long association fibers interconnect different brain areas that are located in different lobes, whereas short association fibers interconnect cortical areas within the same lobe. Adjacent cortical areas are interconnected by short, U-shaped arcuate fibers, which run just below the cortex.

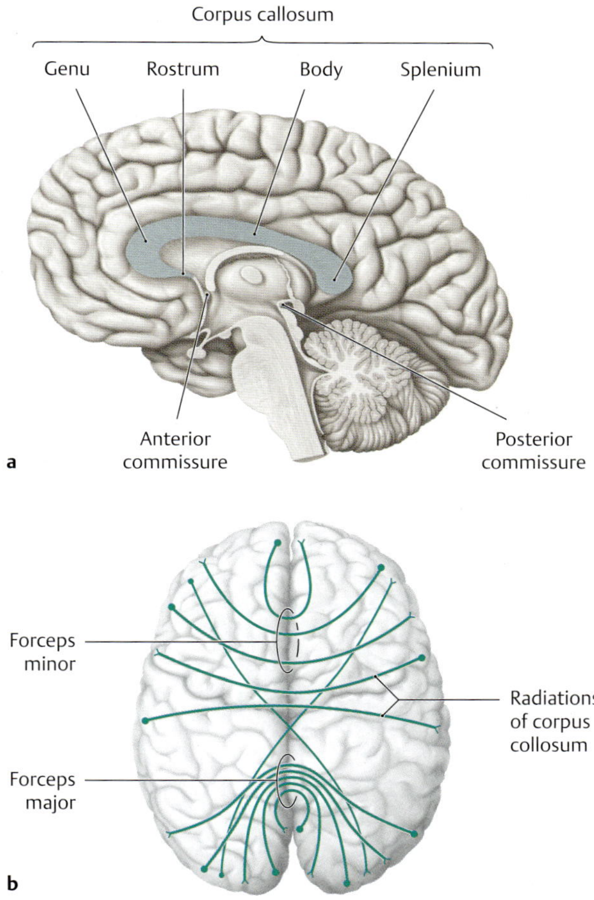

D Commissural fibers

a Medial view of the right hemisphere. **b** Superior view of the transparent brain.

Commissural fibers interconnect the two hemispheres of the brain. The most important connecting structure between the hemispheres is the corpus callosum. If the corpus callosum is intentionally divided, as in a neurosurgical procedure, the two halves of the brain can no longer communicate with each other ("split-brain" patient, see p. 496). There are other, smaller commissural tracts besides the corpus callosum (anterior commissure, fornical commissure).

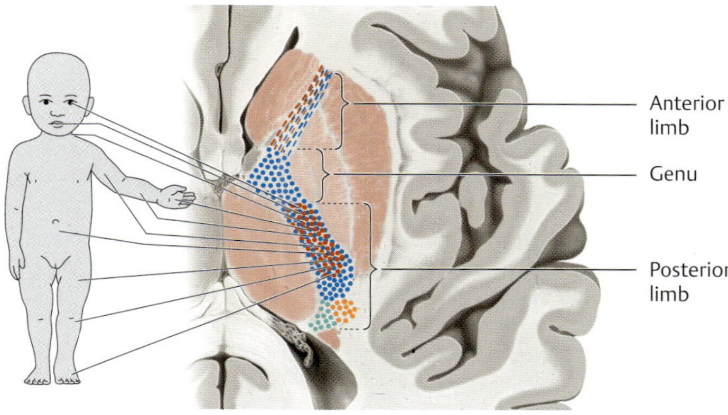

E Projection tracts

Horizontal section through the right hemisphere, superior view of the internal capsule. Both ascending and descending projection fibers pass through the internal capsule. If blood flow to the internal capsule is interrupted, as by a stroke, these ascending and descending tracts undergo irreversible damage. The figure of the child shows how the sites where the pyramidal tract fibers pass through the internal capsule can be assigned to peripheral areas of the human body. Thus, we see that smaller lesions of the internal capsule may cause a loss of upper motor neuron control (= spastic paralysis) of certain areas of the body. This accounts for the great clinical importance of this structure. The internal capsule is bounded medially by the thalamus and the head of the caudate nucleus, and laterally by the globus pallidus and putamen. The internal capsule consists of an anterior limb, a genu, and a posterior limb, which are traversed by specific tracts (cf. Holodny et al. 2005 and Kim et al. 2008):

Anterior limb	• Frontopontine tracts (red dashes) • Anterior thalamic peduncle (blue dashes)
Genu of internal capsule	• Dorsal thalamic peduncle (blue dots)
Posterior limb	• Corticobulbar tracts (red dots) • Corticospinal fibers (red dots) • Posterior thalamic peduncle (blue dots) • Temporopontine tract (orange dots) • Occipitopontine tract (green dots)

6.9 Basal Nuclei

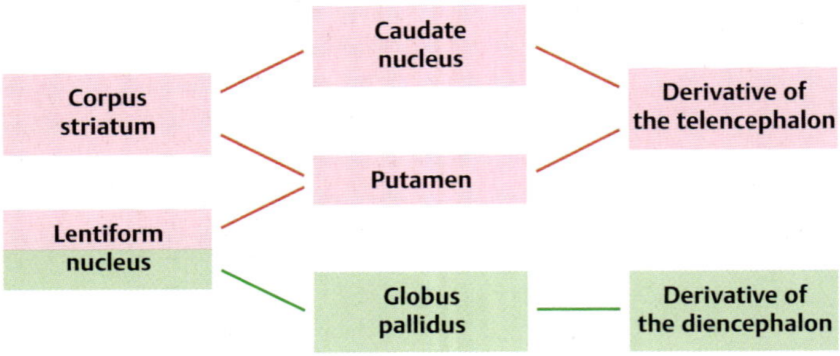

A Definition and classification of basal nuclei
The term "basal nuclei" includes three paired large nuclear regions, which are topographically located at the base of the telencephalon at its border with the diencephalon. The "official" term is telencephalic basal nuclei to explicitly distinguish them from the thalamic basal nuclei located in the diencephalon. *Anatomically*, the basal nuclei include the caudate nucleus (tail), the putamen (dish), and the globus pallidus (pale globe). Based purely on morphological grounds, two basal nuclei are grouped together under one name: Putamen and caudate nucleus are collectively called corpus striatum (striated body). Developmentally, they derive from telencephalon. Putamen and globus pallidus are referred to as lentiform nucleus (lentil-shaped nucleus). It is not uncommon, especially in the clinical literature, to find the term "basal ganglia" used. From a strictly anatomic point of view, this is incorrect because "ganglia" are only found in the PNS. Here in the CNS, true nuclei exist.
Note: The basal nuclei are involved in motor control. They share these functions with other central areas: subthalamic nucleus (part of the diencephalon) and substantia nigra (part of the mesencephalon). Physiologically, these two structures are considered components of basal nuclei/ganglia. This is functionally justified. In the following chapters, the term "basal nuclei" exclusively refers to the nuclear complex as that anatomically defined above.

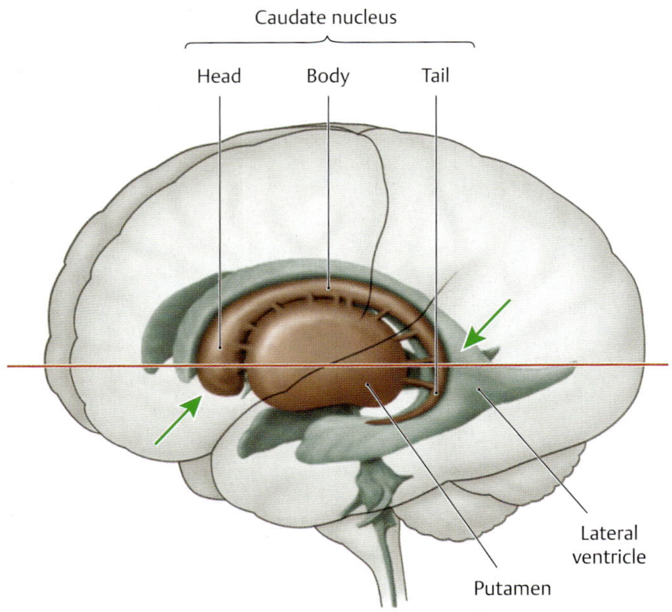

a

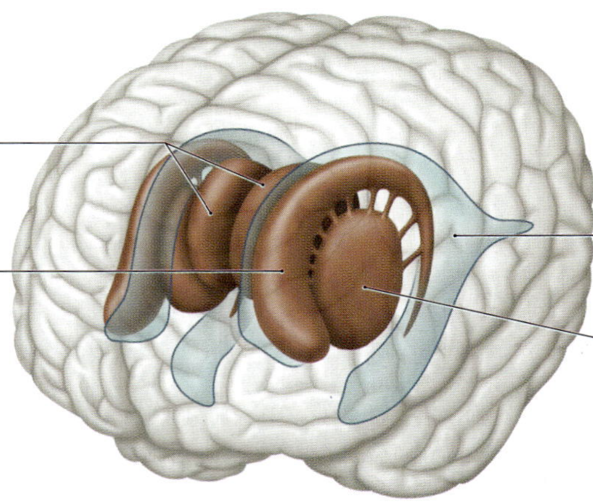

b

B Location and projection of basal nuclei
Telencephalon. **a** Left lateral view of the brain: basal nuclei located anteriorly; **b** Left anterior oblique view.
The location of the basal nuclei leads to complex topographical relationships, which can be best understood with the help of a conceptual combination of three-dimensional representations and parts (see **C**). The caudate nucleus with its sections head, body, and tail virtually "nestles" into the concave wall of the lateral ventricle and follows it along its entire length down to the temporal lobe (**a**). Located on the concave side of the caudate nucleus is the putamen. The comparatively small globus pallidus lies hidden medially to the putamen and is not visible here. The oblique view (**b**) additionally shows the thalamus which is part of the diencephalon. In the lateral view (**a**) the thalamus is also hidden by the putamen. The thalamus is *not a basal nucleus*, yet it is located adjacent to the basal nuclei, since they lie at the base of the telencephalon at the border with the diencephalon. The thalamus is mentioned here because it is a significant anatomical landmark for the demarcation of the internal capsule (see **D**, p. 339).
Note: In both horizontal and coronal sections, with a suitable sectional plane, the caudate nucleus can be cut twice (green arrows in **a**) due to its curved nature.

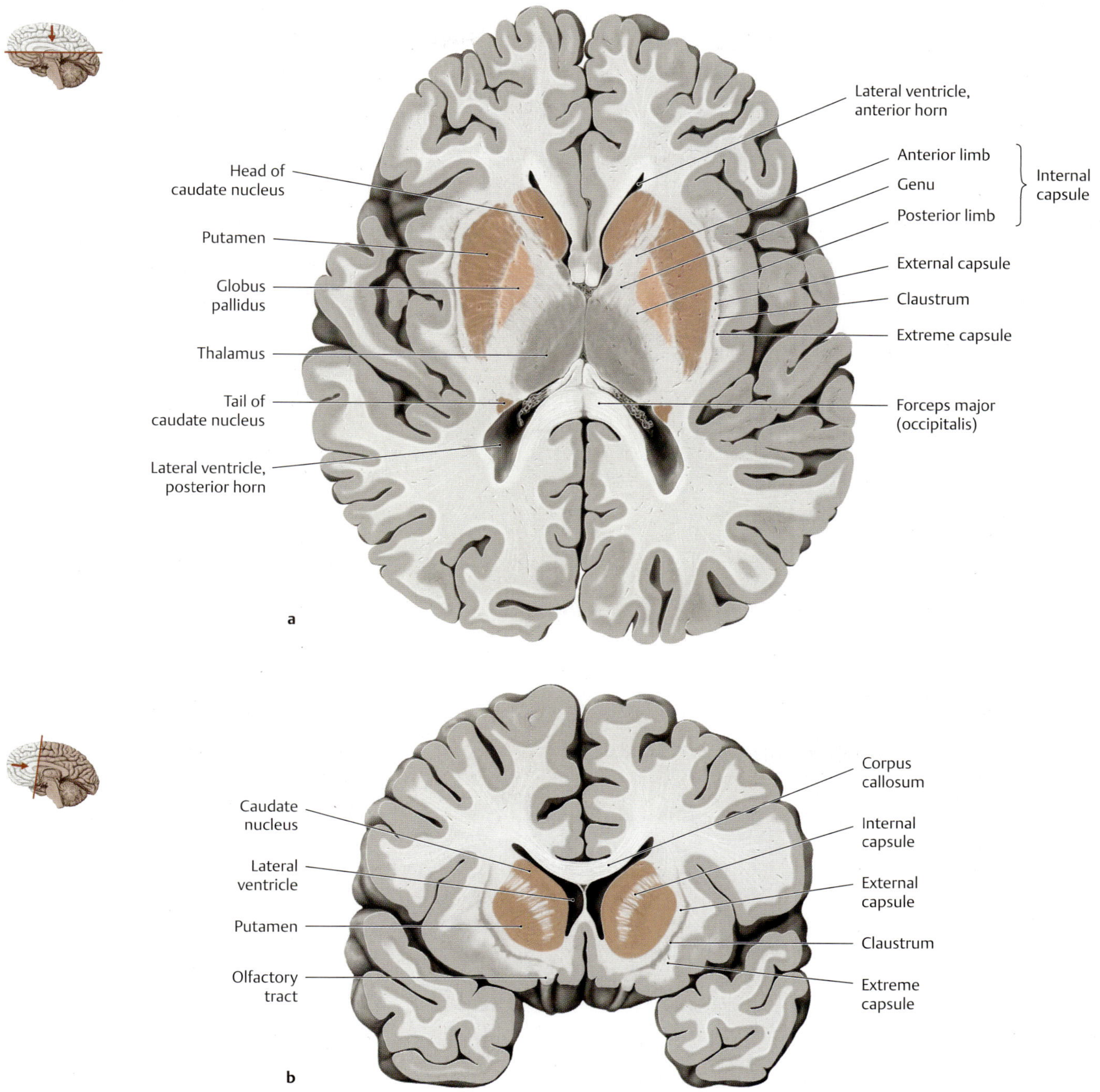

C Basal nuclei on the brain section: neighborhood relationships
a Horizontal section through the brain at the telencephalon–diencephalon border, superior view; **b** Coronal section through the telencephalon, anterior view.

If the brain is cut horizontally at the border between telencephalon and diencephalon, all basal nuclei are visible. The caudate nucleus is cut twice (head and tail and topographically closely associated with the lateral ventricle's anterior and posterior horns). The small globus pallidus is located medially to the putamen (thus not visible in the lateral view, see **B**). The thalamus lies on both sides of the very narrow third ventricle. The internal capsule, a boomerang-shaped area of white matter, which contains ascending and descending projection tracts, is surrounded by basal nuclei and the thalamus (see **A**, p. 334). The anterior limb of the internal capsule, runs between the head of the caudate nucleus and lentiform nucleus; the genu, and the posterior limb are located between the thalamus and the lentiform nucleus, thus at the border between telencephalon and diencephalon.

Note: Lateral to the putamen, directly medial to the insular cortex, lies a nucleus that is referred to as claustrum (front wall). It is surrounded by white matter of the external and extreme capsules. The claustrum is not a basal nucleus (though it once was referred to as one); its function is largely unknown; it is believed to be involved in regulating sexual behavior.

The coronal section that was chosen here, cuts though the head of the caudate nucleus, which protrudes into the anterior horn of the lateral ventricle. In this section, no parts of the diencephalon are visible. Third ventricle, thalamus and globus pallidus are not present in this section. The anterior limb of the internal capsule passes between the basal nuclei, which are located close to one another, and due to the alternating arrangement of gray and white matter gives the gray matter of the nuclei a striated appearance (corpus striatum). The coronal section (**b**) illustrates the close topographical relationship between the caudate nucleus and the corpus callosum, which in this image is located superomedial to the caudate nucleus and forms the roof of the lateral ventricle.

7.1 Diencephalon, Overview and Development

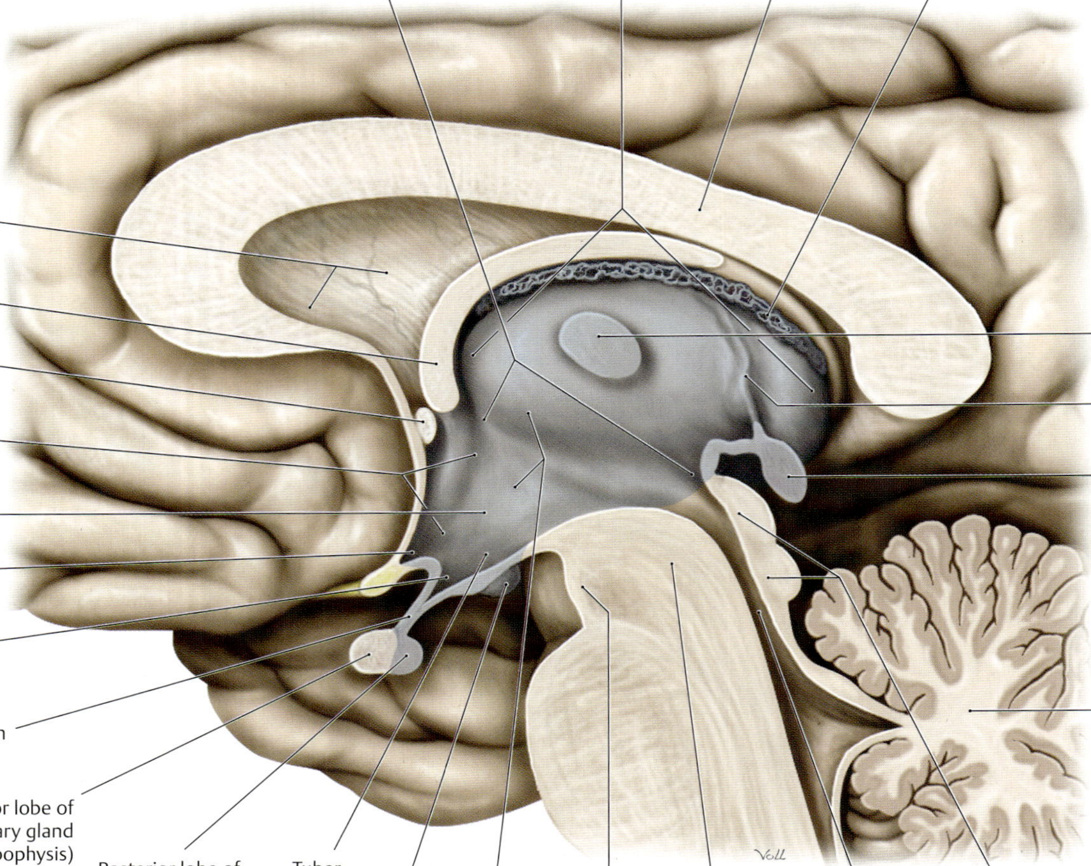

A The diencephalon in situ

Midsagittal section; left lateral view of right hemisphere. The diencephalon is located beneath the two cerebral hemispheres and above the brainstem. The anterior, superior, and lateral parts of the diencephalon directly adjoint the telencephalon. Posteriorly a small section in the area around the pineal gland (see also fig. **B**, p. 352) lies exposed. The base of the diencephalon is composed of two parts. The posterior part of the base is located at the poorly defined border with the mesencephalon, the anterior part—defined by the hypothalamus—has been exposed. The third ventricle located in the median plane divides the diencephalon into symmetrical halves which either contain paired structures (in the lateral wall of the third ventricle, e.g., the thalamus, which are not cut in midsagittal sections), or unpaired structures (located in the midline; therefore they always appear cut on a midsagittal section). As a result of the position of the individual parts of the diencephalon, the third ventricle has several extensions, or recesses. The corpus callosum and the septum pellucidum (the partition between the lateral ventricles) are clearly visible and therefore helpful anatomical reference points.

Located beneath the corpus callosum, the thalamus occupies the largest area of the lateral wall of the third ventricle. Due to its projection into the ventricular lumen, the third ventricle is separated from the smooth wall of the hypothalamus by a furrow: the hypothalamic sulcus. The fornix (arch) is an arch-shaped structure that passes above the thalamus and surrounds it. It extends between the (hippocampus which is part of the telencephalon) and the mammillary bodies. As a projection tract, it is, topographically and functionally, part of both the telencephalon and the diencephalon. Topographically, the fornix is occasionally referred to as the roof of the third ventricle. Functionally, the diencephalon is extremely multifaceted: It acts as a relay station for most sensorial modalities, represents a station for the control of motor functions, regulates the circadian rhythm and endocrine activity and is the supreme authority for important autonomic functions of the body. *Note:* One part of the diencephalon, which is particularly important for motor functions, the subthalamus, due to its far lateral location, can never be seen on the midsagittal section but only on coronal (see **B**, p. 343; **E**, p. 353, and p. 420 ff and p. 433 f) or horizontal sections.

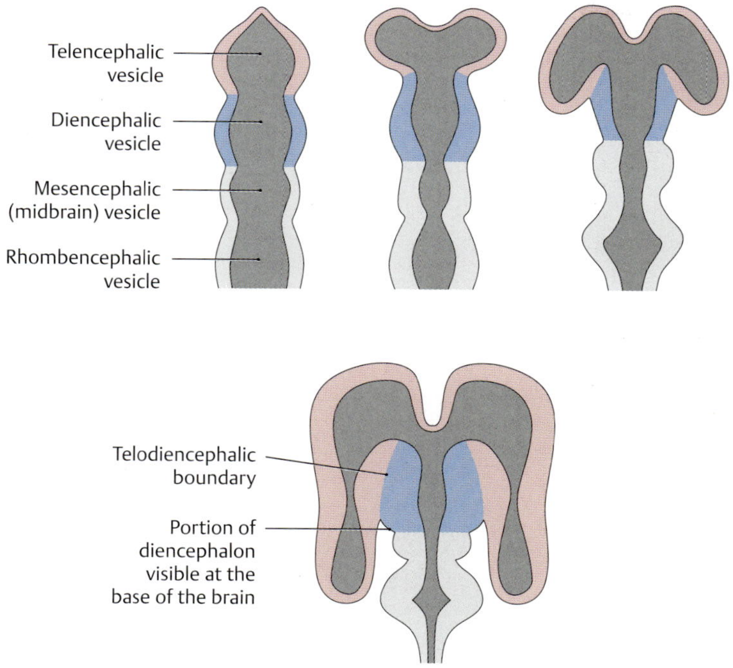

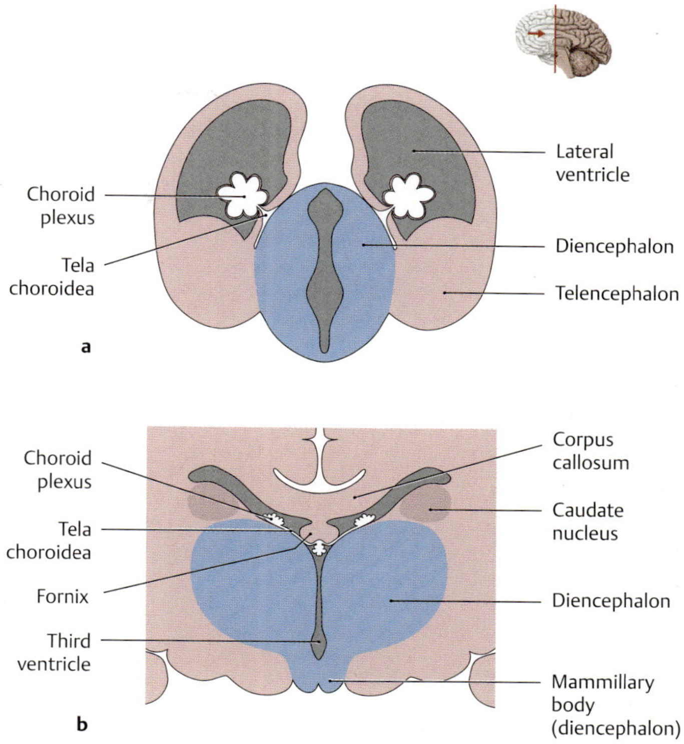

B Development of the diencephalon from the cranial neural tube
Anterior view. To understand the location and extent of the diencephalon in the adult brain, it is necessary to know how it develops from the neural tube. The diencephalon and telencephalon both develop from the prosencephalon, or forebrain (see p. 273). As development proceeds, the two hemispheres of the telencephalic vesicle (red) expand, overgrowing the diencephalic vesicle (blue). This process shifts the boundary between the telencephalon and diencephalon until only a small area of the diencephalon can be seen at the base of the developed brain (see **A**).

C Posterior telodiencephalic boundary
Coronal sections.

a Embryonic brain. The development of the telencephalon (red) has progressed considerably in relation to **B**. The lateral ventricles containing the choroid plexus have already completely overgrown the diencephalon (blue) from behind. The medial wall of the lateral ventricles is very thin and has not yet fused to the diencephalon. Between the telencephalon and diencephalon is a vascularized sheet of connective tissue, the *tela choroidea*.

b Adult brain. By the adult stage, the tela choroidea and the medial wall of the lateral ventricle have become fused to the diencephalon. Removing the choroid plexus and the thin tela choroidea affords a direct view of the posteromedial boundary of the diencephalon (see **B**, p. 340).

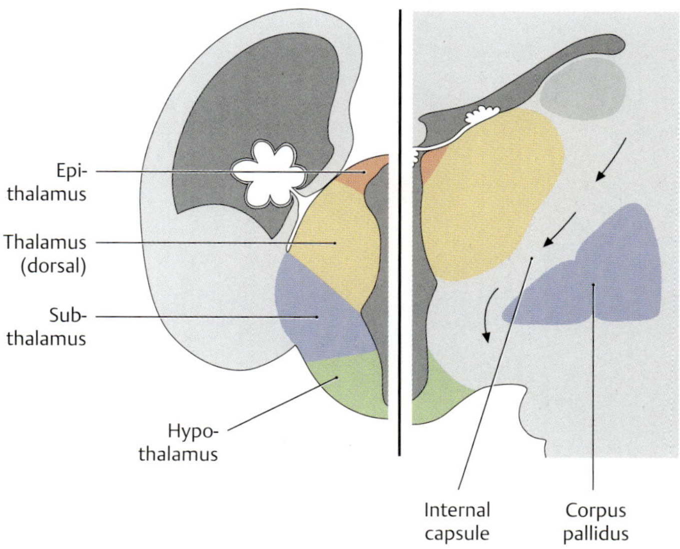

D Organization of the diencephalon during embryonic development
Coronal section of an embryonic brain (left) and an adult brain (right) demonstrating the parts of the diencephalon.
Because the diencephalon of the adult brain lies between the telencephalon and mesencephalon, the ascending and descending axons must penetrate this part of the brain during development, forming the internal capsule. As development proceeds, the axon bundles that form the internal capsule pass through the subthalamus (black arrows), displacing the greater portion of it laterally. This laterally displaced part of the subthalamus is called the *globus pallidus*. Although the globus pallidus is displaced anatomically into the telencephalon and is considered part of the telencephalon in a topographical sense, it still retains close functional ties with the subthalamus because both are part of the extrapyramidal motor system. The *medial* part of the subthalamus remains in the diencephalon as the true *subthalamus* (not visible in this plane of section). As a result, the internal capsule of the telencephalon forms the lateral boundary of the diencephalon.
The different parts of the diencephalon grow to reach different definitive sizes. The thalamus grows disproportionately and eventually occupies four-fifths of the mature diencephalon.

7.2 Diencephalon, External Structure

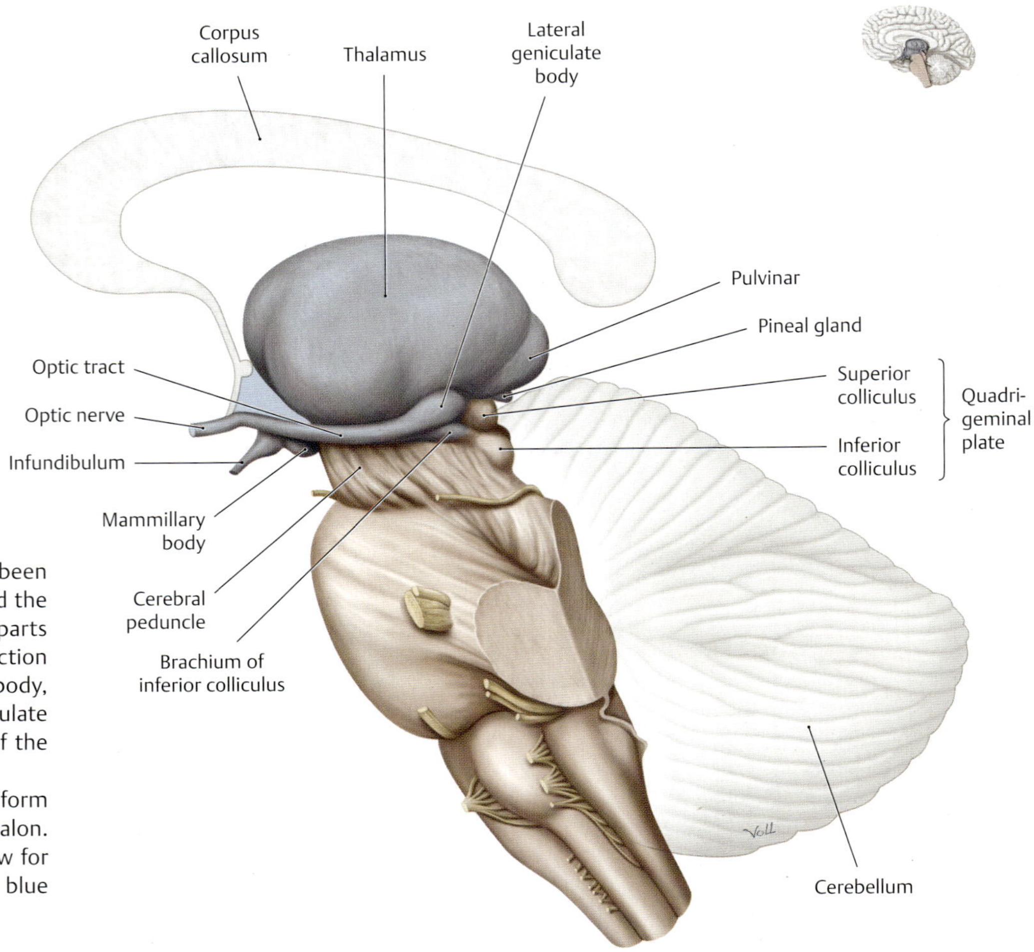

A The diencephalon and brainstem
Left lateral view. The telencephalon has been removed from around the thalamus, and the cerebellum has also been removed. The parts of the diencephalon visible in this dissection are the thalamus, the lateral geniculate body, and the optic tract. The lateral geniculate body and optic tract are components of the visual pathway.
The retina and associated optic nerve form an anterior extension of the diencephalon. Departing from the convention of yellow for nerves, we have colored the optic nerve blue to emphasize this relationship.

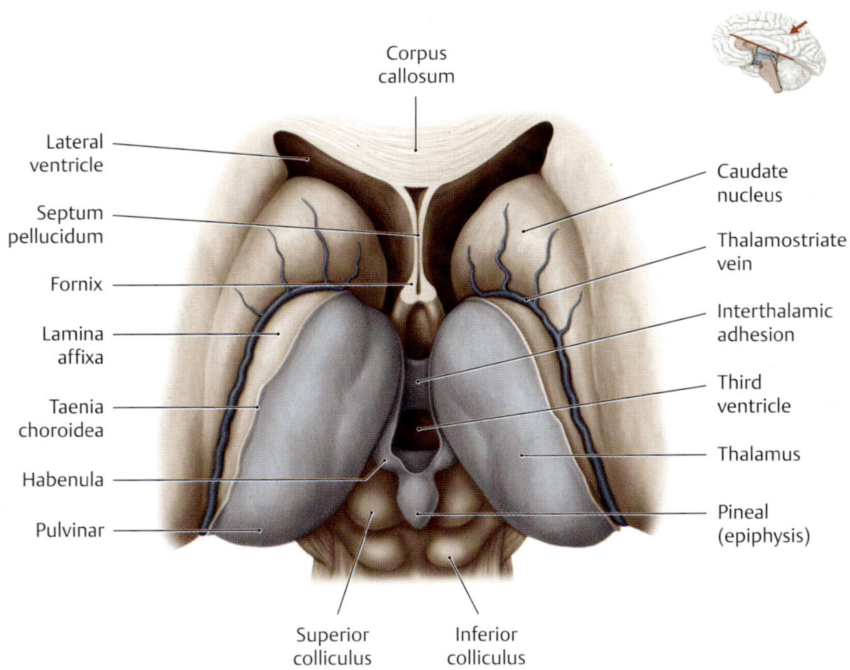

B Arrangement of the diencephalon around the third ventricle
Posterior superior view of an oblique transverse section through the telencephalon with the corpus callosum, fornix, and choroid plexus removed. Removal of the choroid plexus leaves behind its line of attachment, the *taenia choroidea*. The thin wall of the third ventricle has been removed with the choroid plexus to expose the thalamic surface medial to the boundary line of the taenia choroidea. The thin ventricular wall has been left on the thalamus lateral to the taenia choroidea. This thin layer of telencephalon, called the *lamina affixa*, is colored brown in the drawing and covers the thalamus (part of the diencephalon), shown in blue. Because the thalamostriate vein marks this boundary between the diencephalon and telencephalon, it is featured prominently in the drawing. Lateral to the vein is the caudate nucleus, which is part of the telencephalon (compare with **D**, p. 339).

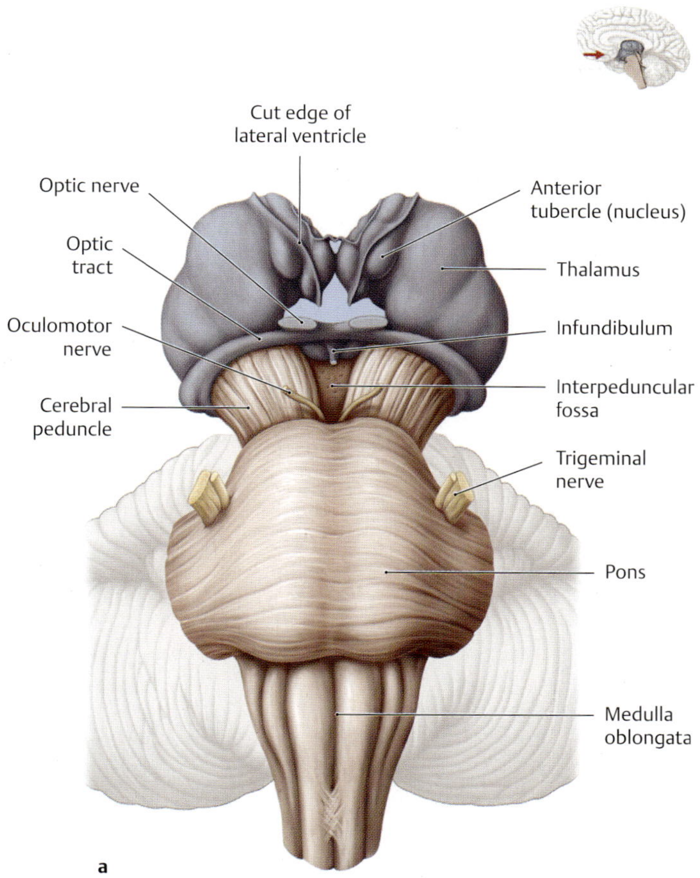

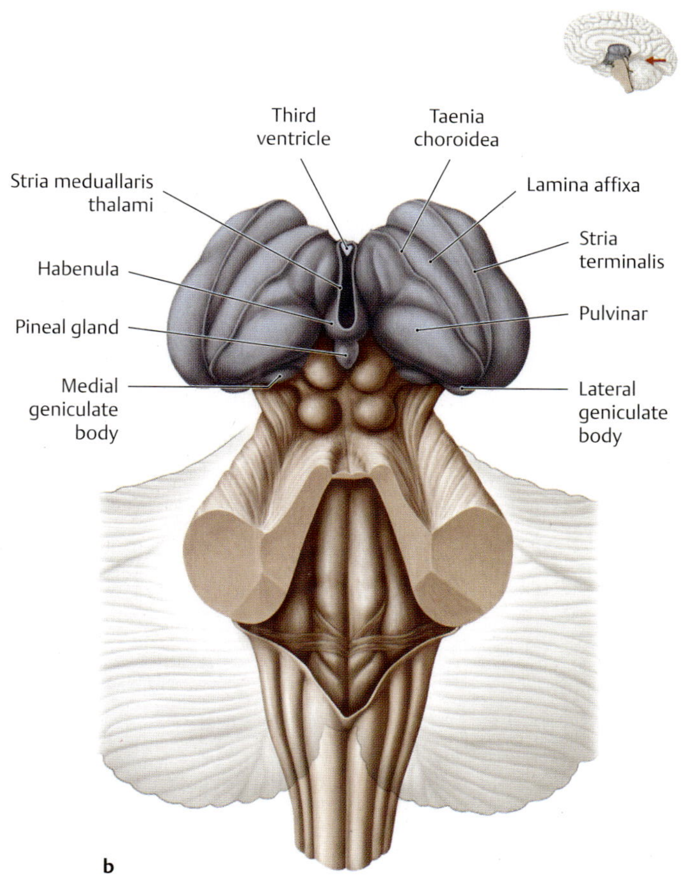

C The diencephalon and brainstem

a Anterior view, **b** posterior view with the cerebellum and telencephalon removed.

a The optic tract marks the lateral boundary of the diencephalon. It winds around the cerebral peduncles (crura cerebri), which are part of the adjacent midbrain (mesencephalon).

b The epithalamus, which is formed by the pineal and the two habenulae ("reins"), is well displayed in this posterior view. The lateral geniculate body is an important relay station in the visual pathway, just as the medial geniculate body is an important relay station in the auditory pathway. They are also collectively referred to as *metathalamus* and represent an extension of the nuclear regions of the thalamus proper. There are close functional connections with regard to the auditory pathway, particularly between the medial geniculate body and the inferior colliculus of the mesencephalon. The pulvinar ("pillow"), which encompasses the posterior thalamic nuclei, is seen particularly well in this section. It too is assigned complex functions, including relations with the visual and auditory connectivity.

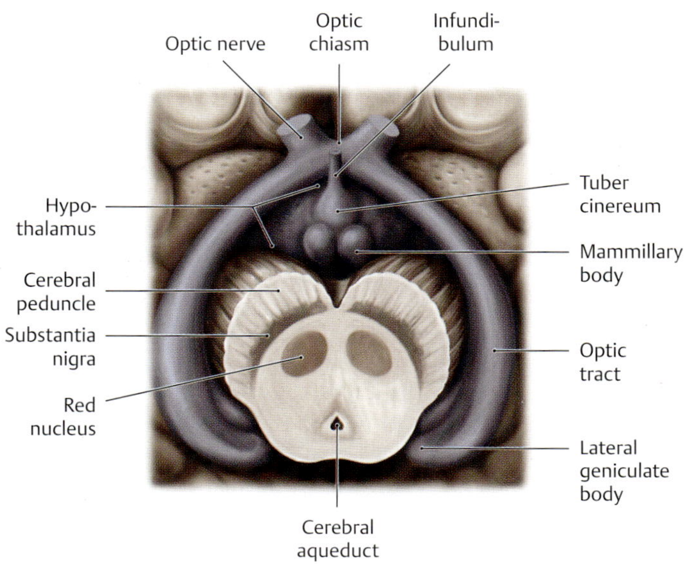

D Location of the diencephalon in the adult brain

Basal view of the brain (the brainstem has been sectioned at the level of the mesencephalon). The structures that can be identified in this view represent the parts of the diencephalon situated on the basal surface of the brain. Due to the expansion of the telencephalon, only a few structures of the diencephalon can be seen on the undersurface of the brain:

- Optic nerve
- Optic chiasm
- Optic tract
- Tuber cinereum with the infundibulum
- Mammillary bodies
- Medial geniculate body (see **Cb**)
- Lateral geniculate body
- Posterior lobe of the pituitary gland (neurohypophysis, see p. 350)

This view also demonstrates how the optic tract, which is part of the diencephalon, winds around the cerebral peduncles of the mesencephalon.

7.3 Diencephalon, Internal Structure

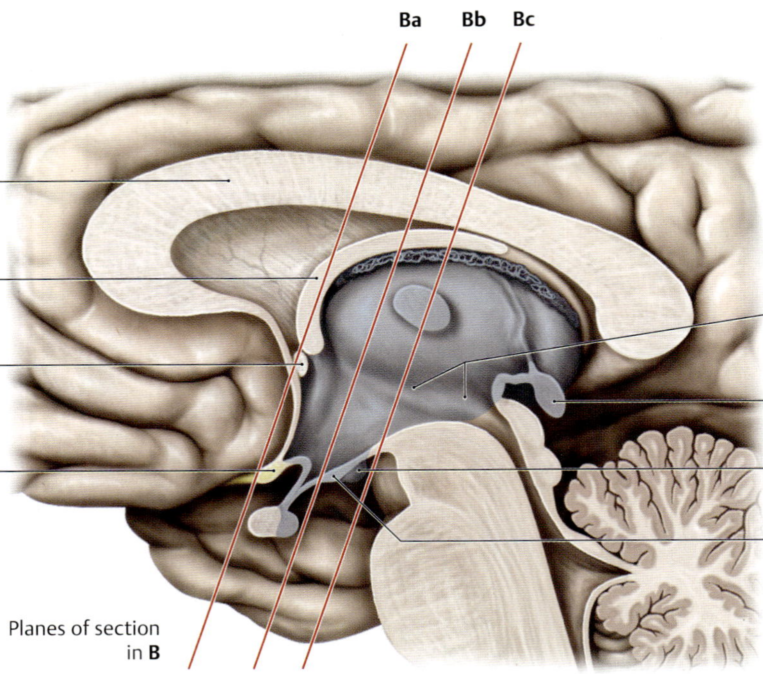

A The four parts of the diencephalon

Boundary line	Part	Structure	Function
	Epithalamus	• Pineal gland • Habenulae	• Regulation of circadian rhythms; linking of olfactory system to brainstem
Dorsal diencephalic sulcus			
	Thalamus	• Thalamus	• Relay of sensory information; assistance in regulation of motor function
Middle diencephalic sulcus			
	Subthalamus	• Subthalamic nucleus • Zona incerta • Globus pallidus (see **E**, p. 353)	• Relay of sensory information (somatomotor zone of diencephalon)
Ventral diencephalic sulcus (= hypothalamic sulcus)*			
	Hypothalamus	• Optic chiasm, optic tract • Tuber cinereum, neurohypophysis • Mammillary bodies	• Coordination of autonomic nervous system with endocrine system; participation in visual pathway

* This is the only sulcus shown in **A**

B Coronal sections through the diencephalon at three different levels

a Level of the optic chiasm: Portions of the diencephalon and telencephalon appear in this section, which clearly shows the position of the diencephalon on both sides of the third ventricle. An outpouching of the third ventricle, the preoptic recess, is located above the optic chiasm. Its connection to the third ventricle lies outside this plane of section.

b Level of the tuber cinereum, just behind the interventricular foramen: The boundary between the diencephalon and telencephalon is clearly defined only in the region about the ventricles; the underlying nuclear areas blend together with no apparent boundary. Along the lateral ventricles, the boundary between the diencephalon and telencephalon is marked by the lamina affixa, a narrow strip of telencephalon that overlies the thalamus (see **Bc**). It can be seen that layers of gray matter permeate the internal capsule in its dorsal portion.

c Level of the mammillary bodies: This section displays the thalamic nuclei. More than 120 separate nuclei may be counted, depending on the system of nomenclature used. Most of these nuclei cannot be grossly identified in anatomical specimens. Their classification is reviewed on p. 344 (after Kahle and Frotscher, quoted from Villinger and Ludwig).

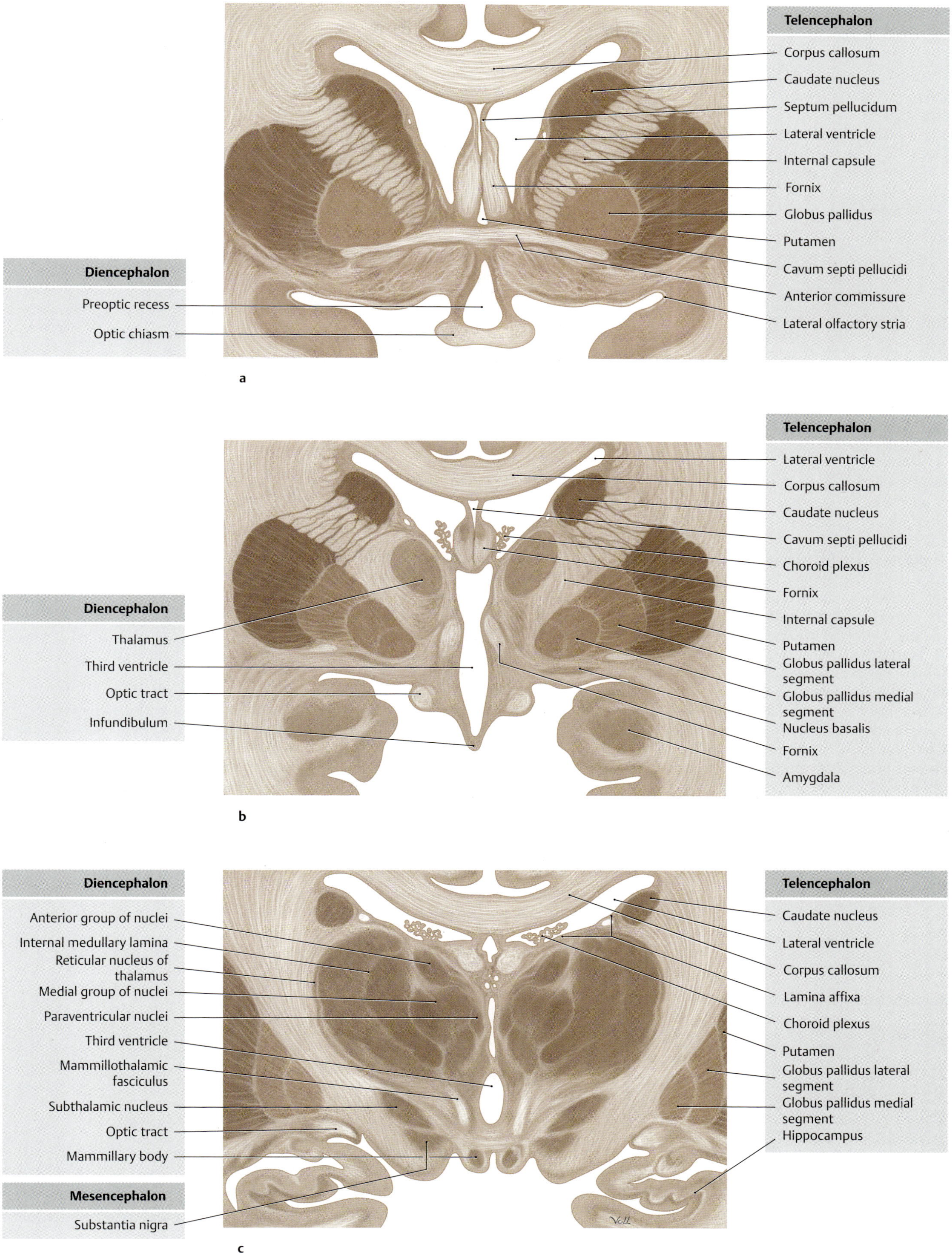
Telencephalon
Corpus callosum
Caudate nucleus
Septum pellucidum
Lateral ventricle
Internal capsule
Fornix
Globus pallidus
Putamen
Cavum septi pellucidi
Anterior commissure
Lateral olfactory stria
Diencephalon
Preoptic recess
Optic chiasm
a
Telencephalon
Lateral ventricle
Corpus callosum
Caudate nucleus
Cavum septi pellucidi
Choroid plexus
Fornix
Internal capsule
Putamen
Globus pallidus lateral segment
Globus pallidus medial segment
Nucleus basalis
Fornix
Amygdala
Diencephalon
Thalamus
Third ventricle
Optic tract
Infundibulum
b
Diencephalon
Anterior group of nuclei
Internal medullary lamina
Reticular nucleus of thalamus
Medial group of nuclei
Paraventricular nuclei
Third ventricle
Mammillothalamic fasciculus
Subthalamic nucleus
Optic tract
Mammillary body
Mesencephalon
Substantia nigra
Telencephalon
Caudate nucleus
Lateral ventricle
Corpus callosum
Lamina affixa
Choroid plexus
Putamen
Globus pallidus lateral segment
Globus pallidus medial segment
Hippocampus
c

7.4 Thalamus: Thalamic Nuclei

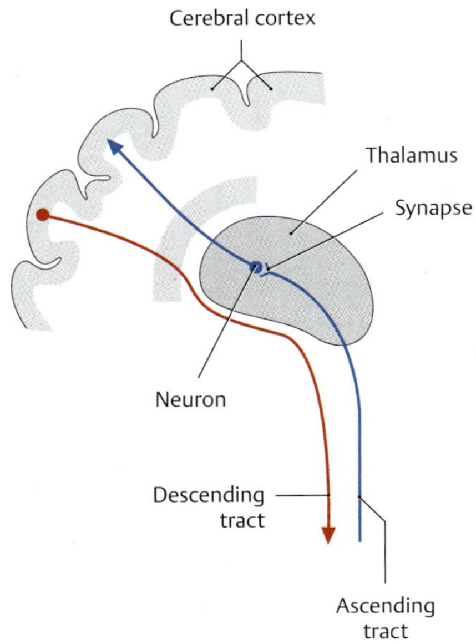

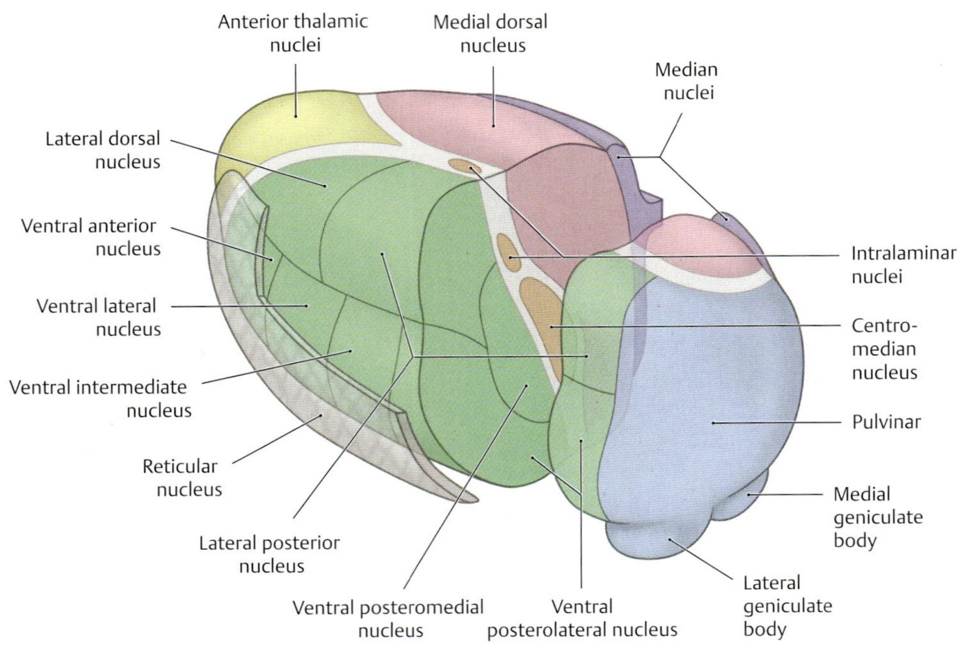

A Functional organization of the thalamus
Almost all of the sensory pathways are relayed via the thalamus and project to the cerebral cortex (see **G**, thalamic radiation). Consequently, a lesion of the thalamus or its cortical projection fibers caused by a stroke or other disease leads to sensory disturbances. Although a diffuse kind of sensory perception may take place at the thalamic level (especially pain perception), cortical processing (by the telencephalon) is necessary in order to transform unconscious perception into conscious perception. The olfactory system is an exception to this rule, although its olfactory bulb is still an extension of the telencephalon. *Note:* Major descending motor tracts from the cerebral cortex generally bypass the thalamus.

B Spatial arrangement of the thalamic nuclear groups
Left thalamus viewed from the lateral and occipital aspect, slightly rotated relative to the views on p. 340. The thalamus is a collection of approximately 120 nuclei that process extensive sensory, motor, and limbic information. They are broadly classified as specific or nonspecific:

- *Specific* nuclei and the fibers arising from them (thalamic radiation, see **G**) have direct connections with specific areas of the *cerebral cortex.*
- *Nonspecific* nuclei have no direct connections with the cerebral cortex. Part of a general arousal system, they are connected directly to the brainstem. The only nonspecific nuclei shown in this diagram (orange, see **F** for further details) are the centromedian nucleus and the intralaminar nuclei.

The specific thalamic nuclei are subdivided into four groups:

- Anterior nuclei (yellow)
- Medial nuclei (red)
- Lateral nuclei (green)
- Dorsal nuclei (blue)

The dorsal nuclei are in contact with the the medial and lateral geniculate bodies. Located beneath the pulvinar, these two nuclear bodies contain the *nuclei of the medial and lateral geniculate bodies*, and are collectively called the *metathalamus*. Like the pulvinar, they belong to the category of specific thalamic nuclei.

C Nomenclature of the thalamic nuclei

Name	Alternative name	Properties
Specific thalamic nuclei (cortically dependent)	Palliothalamus	Project to the cerebral cortex (pallium)
Nonspecific thalamic nuclei (cortically independent)	Truncothalamus	Project to the brainstem, diencephalon, and corpus striatum
Integration nuclei		Project to other nuclei within the thalamus (classified as nonspecific thalamic nuclei)
Intralaminar nuclei		Nuclei in the white matter of the internal medullary lamina (classified as nonspecific thalamic nuclei)

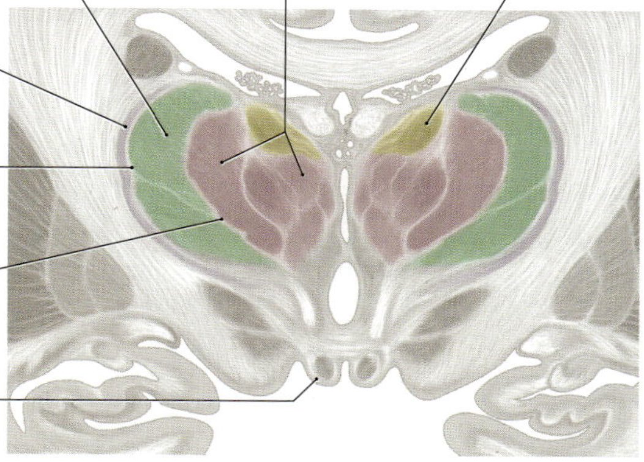

D Division of the thalamic nuclei by the medullary laminae
Coronal section at the level of the mammillary bodies. Several groups of thalamic nuclei are grossly separated into larger nuclear complexes by fibrous sheets called medullary laminae. The following laminae are shown in the diagram:

- Internal medullary lamina between the medial and ventrolateral thalamic nuclei
- External medullary lamina between the lateral nuclei and the reticular nucleus of the thalamus.

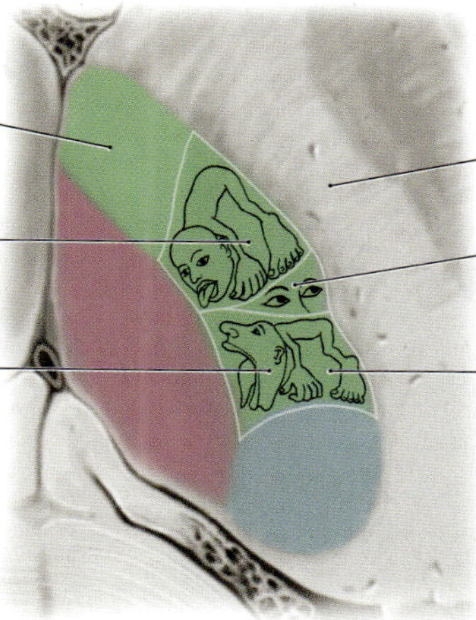

E Somatotopic organization of the specific thalamic nuclei
Transverse section. The specific thalamic nuclei (defined in **C**) are topographically arranged according to their functional relation to specific regions of the body. Afferent fibers from the spinal cord, brainstem, and cerebellum are localized to specific areas of the thalamus, where the corresponding thalamic nuclei are clustered. This pattern of somatotopic arrangement, a recurring theme in neural organization, is here illustrated for the ventrolateral thalamic nuclei (green in **B, D, E**). Axons from the crossed superior cerebellar peduncle terminate in the ventral lateral nucleus of the thalamus (**2**); information on body position, coordination and muscle tone travels by this pathway to the motor cortex, which also shows a pattern of somatotopic organization (see **B**, p. 457). The *lateral* part of the ventral lateral nucleus relays impulses from the trunk and limbs, while the *medial* part relays impulses from the head. The ventral intermediate nucleus (**3**) receives afferent input from the vestibular nuclei concerning the coordination of gaze toward the ipsilateral side. The large sensory pathways of the spinal cord (the tracts of the dorsal column) are relayed to the nuclei cuneatus and gracilus, which send their axons through the medial lemniscus to terminate in the ventral posterolateral nucleus (**4**), while the trigeminal sensory pathways from the head terminate in the ventral posteromedial nucleus (**5**, trigeminal lemniscus, see p. 545). Topographical localization according to function is a basic principle of neural organization.

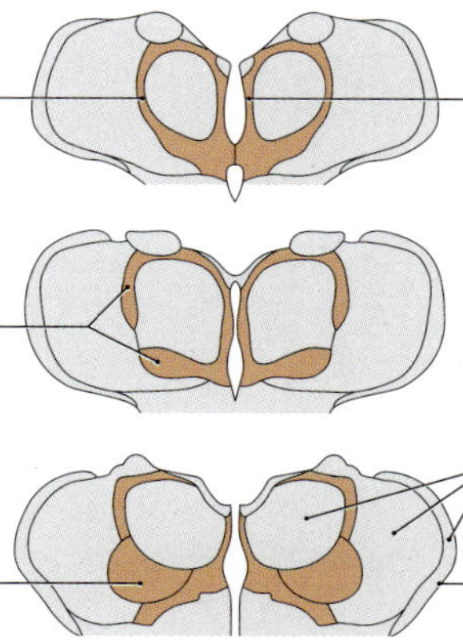

F Nonspecific thalamic nuclei
Coronal sections presented in an oral-to-caudal series. The nonspecific thalamic nuclei project to the brainstem, to other nuclei in the diencephalon (including other thalamic nuclei), and to the corpus striatum. They have no direct connections with the cerebral cortex, acting only indirectly on the cortex. The medial *nonspecific* thalamic nuclei are subdivided into two groups:

- Nuclei of the central thalamic gray matter (midline nuclei): small groups of cells distributed along the wall of the third ventricle
- Intralaminar nuclei, located in the internal medullary lamina.

The largest nucleus of this group is the centromedian nucleus.
The lateral *specific* thalamic nucleus shown in the diagram is the reticular nucleus of the thalamus, which is situated lateral to the other specific thalamic nuclei. The reticular nucleus is the source of the electrical impulses recorded in an electroencephalogram (EEG).

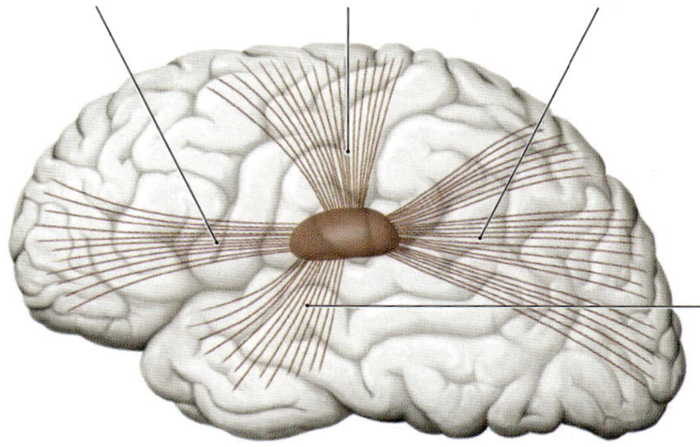

G Thalamic radiations
Lateral ventricle of the left hemisphere. The axons of the specific thalamic nuclei (so called because their fibers project to specific cortical areas) are collected into tracts that form the thalamic radiations. The arrangement of the fibers shows that the specific thalamic nuclei have connections with all areas of the cortex. The anterior thalamic radiation projects to the frontal lobe, the central thalamic radiation to the parietal lobe, the posterior thalamic radiation to the occipital lobe, and the inferior thalamic radiation to the temporal lobe.

7.5 Thalamus: Projections of the Thalamic Nuclei

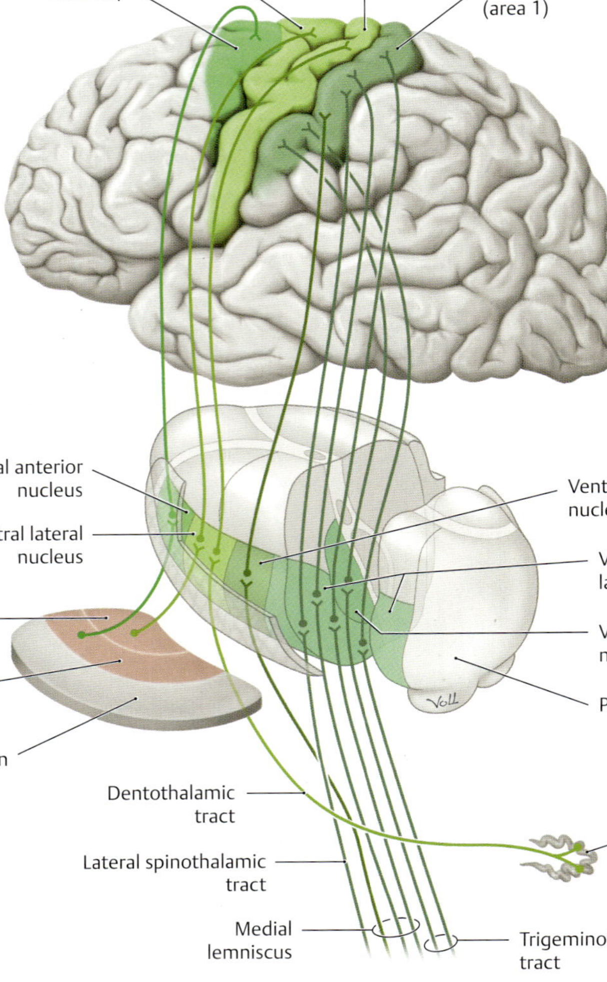

A Ventrolateral thalamic nuclei: afferent and efferent connections

The **ventral posterolateral nucleus** (VPL) and **ventral posteromedial nucleus** (VPM) are the major thalamic relay centers for somatosensory information.

- The *medial lemniscus* ends in the *VPL*. It contains sensory fibers for position sense, vibration, pressure, discrimination, and touch that are relayed from the nucleus gracilis and nucleus cuneatus.
- Pain and temperature fibers from the trunk and limbs travel through the lateral *spinothalamic tract* to lateral portions of the *VPL*. These sensations are relayed from this nucleus to the somatosensory cortex.
- Pain and temperature information from the head region is conveyed by the *trigeminal system* to the *VPM*. As in the VPL, they synapse with third order thalamic neurons that project to the postcentral gyrus (somatosensory cortex).

A *lesion of the VPL* leads to contralateral disturbances of superficial and deep sensation with dysesthesia and an abnormal feeling of heaviness in the limbs (lesion of the medial lemniscus). Because the pain fibers of the spinothalamic tract terminate in the basal portions of the VPL, lesions in that region may additionally cause severe pain ("thalamic pain"). The **ventral lateral nucleus** (VL) projects to somatomotor cortical areas (6aα and 6aβ). The VL nuclei form a feedback loop with the motor areas of the cortex, and so lesions of these nuclei are characterized by motor deficits.

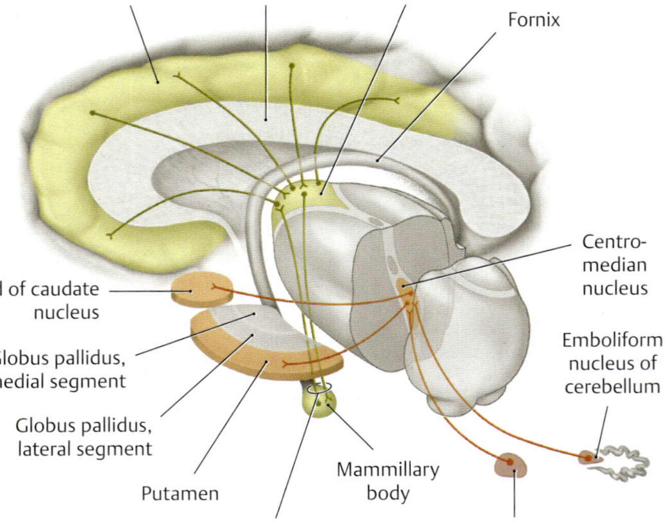

B Anterior nucleus and centromedian nucleus: afferent and efferent connections

The anterior nucleus receives *afferent fibers* from the mammillary body by way of the mammillothalamic fasciculus (bundle of Vicq-d'Azyr). The anterior nucleus establishes both afferent and efferent connections with the cingulate gyrus of the telencephalon. The largest nonspecific thalamic nucleus is the centromedian nucleus, which is one of the intralaminar nuclei. It receives *afferent fibers* from the cerebellum, reticular formation, and medial pallidus. Its *efferent fibers* project to the head of the caudate nucleus and the putamen. The centromedian nucleus is an important component of the **a**scending **r**eticular **a**ctivation **s**ystem (ARAS, arousal system). Essential for maintaining the waking state, the ARAS begins in the reticular formation of the brainstem and is relayed in the centromedian nucleus.

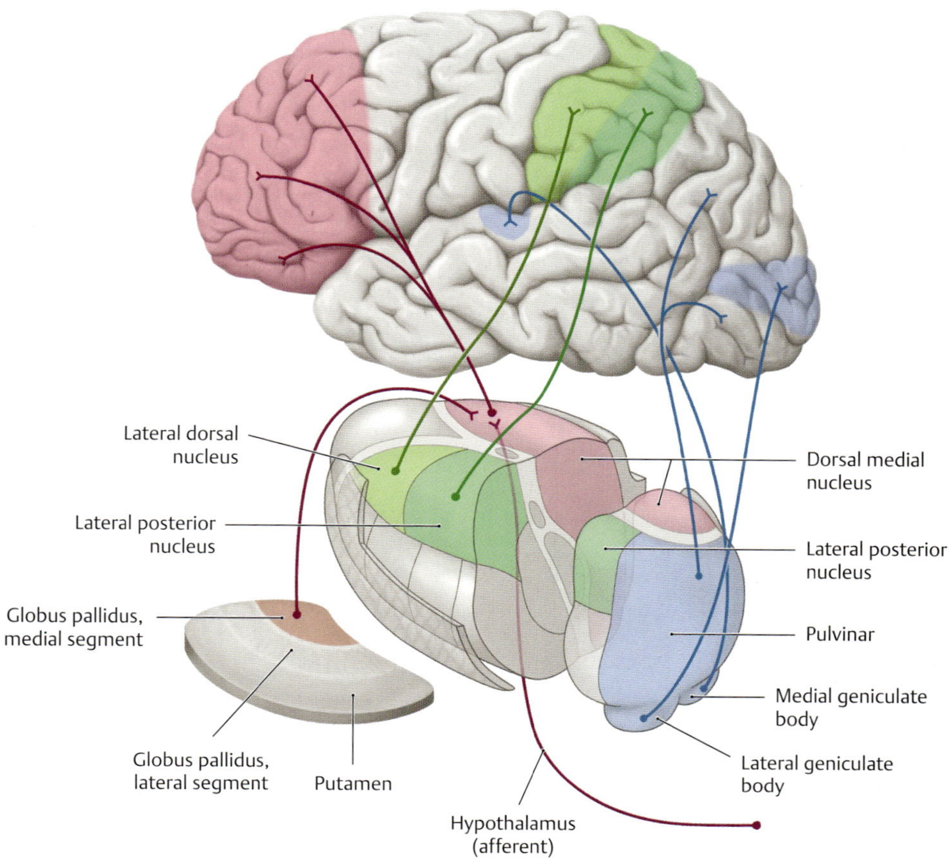

C Medial, posterior, and lateral thalamic nuclei: afferent and efferent connections

The **medial thalamic nuclei** receive their afferent input from ventral and intralaminar thalamic nuclei (not shown), the hypothalamus, the mesencephalon, and the globus pallidus. Their efferent fibers project to the frontal lobe and premotor cortex, and afferent fibers from these regions return to the nuclei. The destruction of these tracts leads to *frontal lobe syndrome*, which is characterized by a loss of self-control (episodes of childish jocularity alternating with suspicion and petulance). The **posterior nuclei** are formed by the pulvinar, which is the largest nuclear complex of the thalamus. The pulvinar receives afferent fibers from other thalamic nuclei, particularly the intralaminar nuclei (not shown). Its efferent fibers terminate in the association areas of the parietal and occipital lobes, which have reciprocal connections with the pulvinar. The lateral geniculate body (part of the visual pathway) projects to the visual cortex, while the medial geniculate body (part of the auditory pathway) projects to the auditory cortex. The **lateral nuclei** consist of the lateral dorsal nucleus and lateral posterior nucleus. They represent the dorsal portion of the ventrolateral group and receive their input from other thalamic nuclei (hence the term "integration nuclei," see p. 344). Their efferent fibers terminate in the parietal lobe of the brain.

D Synopsis of some clinically important connections of the specific thalamic nuclei

The specific thalamic nuclei project to the cerebral cortex. The table below lists the origins of the tracts that terminate in the nuclei, the nuclei themselves, and the sites to which their afferent fibers project.

Thalamic afferents (structures that project *to* the thalamus)	**Thalamic nucleus (abbreviation)**	**Thalamic efferents (structure to *which* the thalamus projects)**
Mammillary body (mammillothalamic fasciclus)	Anterior nucleus (AN)	Cingulate gyrus (limbic system)
Cerebellum, red nucleus	Ventral lateral nucleus (VL)	Premotor cortex (6a) Motor cortex (area 4)
Posterior funiculus, lateral funiculus (somatosensory input, limbs, trunk)	Ventral posterolateral nucleus (VPL)	Postcentral gyrus (= somatosensory cortex) (see **A**)
Trigeminothalamic tract (somatosensory input, head)	Ventral posteromedial nucleus (VPM)	Postcentral gyrus (= somatosensory cortex) (see **A**)
Inferior brachium (part of the auditory pathway)	Medial geniculate nucleus (body) (MGB)	Transverse temporal gyri (auditory cortex)
Optic tract (part of the visual pathway)	Lateral geniculate nucleus (body) (LGB)	Striate area (visual cortex)

7.6 Hypothalamus

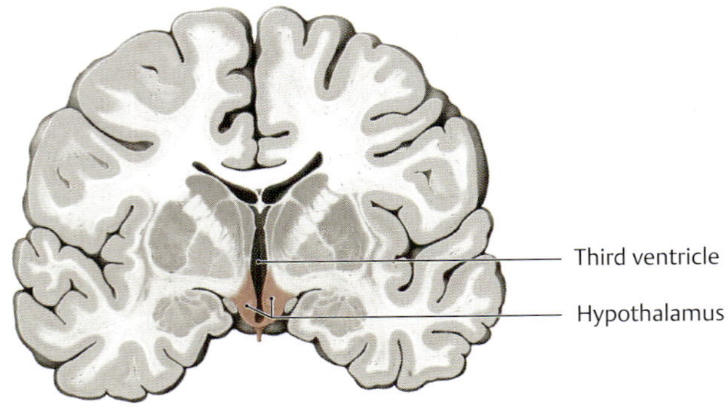

A Location of the hypothalamus
Coronal section. The hypothalamus is the lowest level of the diencephalon, situated below the thalamus. It is the only externally visible portion of the diencephalon (see **D**, p. 341). Located on either side of the third ventricle, its size is most clearly appreciated in a midsagittal section that bisects the third ventricle (see **Ba**).

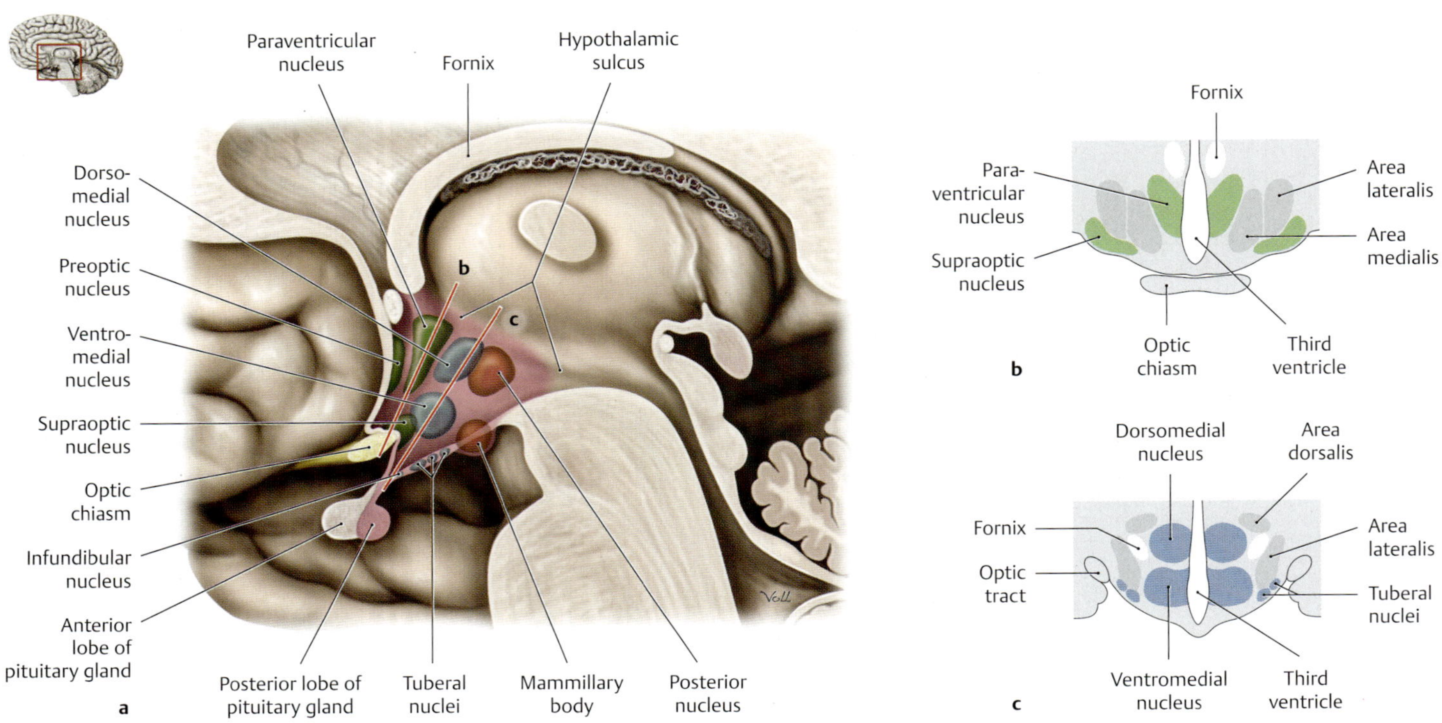

B Nuclei in the right hypothalamus
a Midsagittal section of the right hemisphere viewed from the medial side.**b**, **c** Coronal sections. The hypothalamus is a small nuclear complex located ventral to the thalamus and separated from it by the hypothalamic sulcus. Despite its small size, the hypothalamus is the command center for all autonomic functions in the body. The Terminologia Anatomica lists over 30 hypothalamic nuclei located in the lateral wall and floor of the third ventricle. Only a few of the larger, more clinically important nuclei are mentioned in this unit. Three groups of nuclei are listed below in a rostral-to-caudal sequence, and their functions are briefly described:

- The anterior (rostral) group of nuclei (green) synthesizes the hormones released from the posterior lobe of the pituitary gland, and consists of the
  - preoptic nucleus,
  - paraventricular nucleus, and
  - supraoptic nucleus.
- The middle (tuberal) group of nuclei (blue) controls hormone release from the anterior lobe of the pituitary gland, and consists of the
  - dorsomedial nucleus,
  - ventromedial nucleus, and
  - tuberal nuclei.
- The posterior (mammillary) group of nuclei (red) activates the sympathetic nervous system when stimulated. It consists of the
  - posterior nucleus and
  - mammillary nuclei located in the mammillary bodies.

The coronal section (**c**) shows the further subdivision of the hypothalamus by the fornix into lateral and medial zones. The three nuclear groups described above are part of the *medial* zone, whereas the nuclei in the *lateral* zone are not subdivided into specific groups (e.g., the area lateralis takes the place of a nucleus; the course of the fornix is described on p. 331). Bilateral lesions of the mammillary bodies and their nuclei are manifested by the *Korsakoff syndrome*, which is frequently associated with alcoholism (cause: vitamin B1 [thiamine] deficiency). The memory impairment that occurs in this syndrome mainly affects short-term memory, and the patient may fill in the memory gaps with fabricated information. A major neuropathological finding is the presence of hemorrhages in the mammillary bodies, which are sectioned at autopsy to confirm the diagnosis.

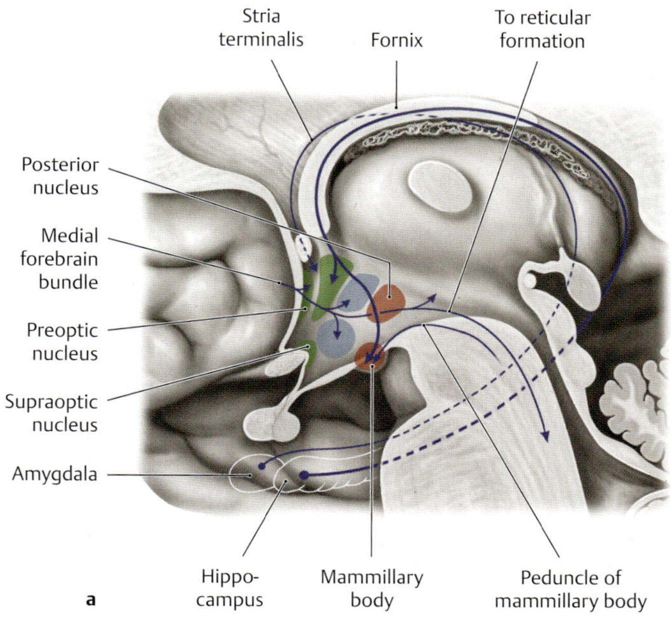

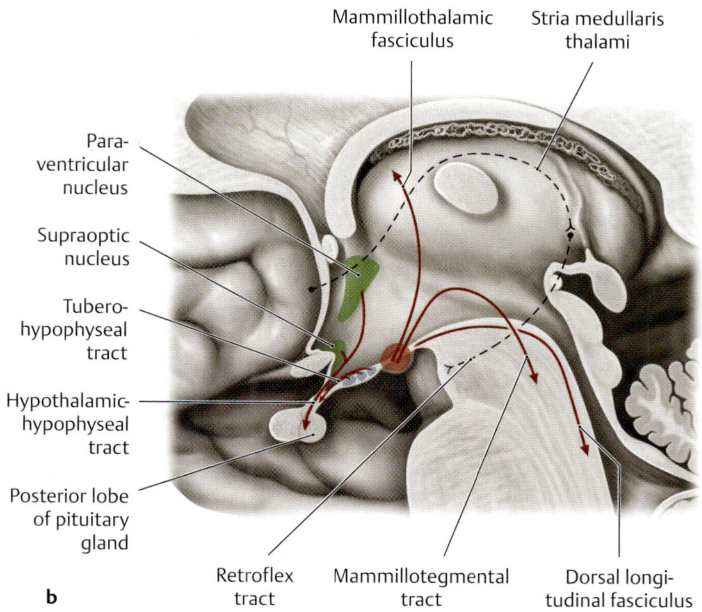

C Important afferent and efferent connections of the hypothalamus

Midsagittal section of the right hemisphere viewed from the medial side. Because the hypothalamus coordinates all the autonomic functions in the body, it establishes afferent (blue) and efferent (red) connections with many brain regions. The following are particularly important:

a Afferent connections (to the hypothalamus):

- The fornix conveys afferent fibers from the hippocampus; it is an important fiber tract of the limbic system.
- The medial forebrain bundle transmits afferent fibers from the olfactory areas to the preoptic nuclei.
- The stria terminalis conveys afferent fibers from the amygdala.
- The peduncle of the mammillary bodies transmits visceral afferent fibers and impulses from erogenous zones (nipples, genitalia).

b Efferent connections (from the hypothalamus):

- The dorsal longitudinal fasciculus passes to the brainstem where it is relayed several times before reaching the parasympathetic nuclei.
- The mammillotegmental tract distributes efferent fibers to the tegmentum of the midbrain; these are then relayed to the reticular formation. The fibers of this tract mediate the exchange of autonomic information between the hypothalamus, cranial nerve nuclei, and spinal cord.
- The mammillothalamic fasciculus (bundle of Vicq d'Azyr) conveys efferent fibers to the anterior thalamic nucleus, which is connected to the cingulated gyrus. This is part of the limbic system (see p. 492).
- The hypothalamic–hypophyseal and tuberohypophyseal tracts are efferent tracts to the pituitary gland (see p. 350 f).

D Functions of the hypothalamus

The hypothalamus is the coordinating center of the autonomic nervous system. There is no specific sympathetic or parasympathetic control center. Certain functions can be assigned to specific regions or nuclei in the hypothalamus, and these relationships are outlined in the table. Not all of the regions or nuclei listed in the table are shown in the drawings.

Region or nucleus	Function
Anterior preoptic region	Maintains constant body temperature; **Lesion:** central hypothermia
Posterior region	Responds to temperature changes, e.g., sweating; **Lesion:** hypothermia
Midanterior and posterior regions	Activate sympathetic nervous system
Paraventricular and anterior regions	Activate parasympathetic nervous system
Supraoptic and paraventricular nuclei	Regulate water balance; **Lesion:** Diabetes insipidus, also lack of thirst response resulting in hyponatremia
Anterior nuclei • Medial part • Lateral part	Regulate appetite and food intake • **Lesion:** Obesity • **Lesion:** Anorexia and emaciation

7.7 Pituitary Gland (Hypophysis)

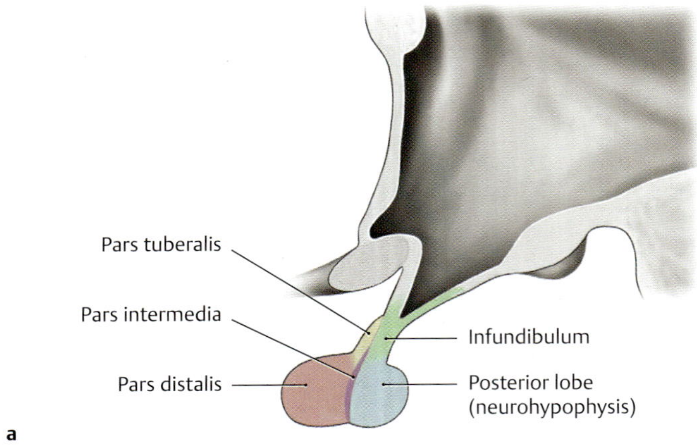

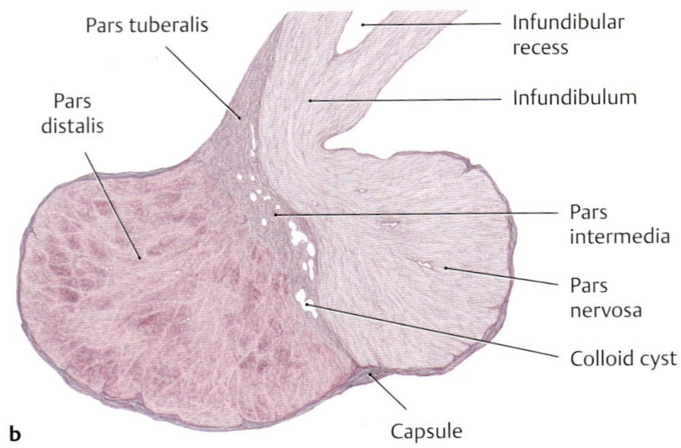

A Divisions of the pituitary gland

Midsagittal sections: **a** Schematic representation. **b** Histological appearance. The pituitary gland (hypophysis) consists of two lobes:

- Anterior lobe (adenohypophysis), which is a hormone-*producing* and releasing part (see **D** and **E**), and
- Posterior lobe (neurohypophysis), which is a hormone-*releasing* part for hormones produced in the hypothalamus.

While the posterior pituitary lobe is an extension of the diencephalon, the anterior pituitary lobe is derived from the epithelium of the roof of the pharynx. The two lobes establish contact during embryonic development. The pituitary stalk (infundibulum) attaches both lobes of the gland to the hypothalamus. The pituitary gland is surrounded by a fibrous capsule and lies in the *sella turcica* over the sphenoid sinus, which provides a route of surgical access to pituitary tumors.

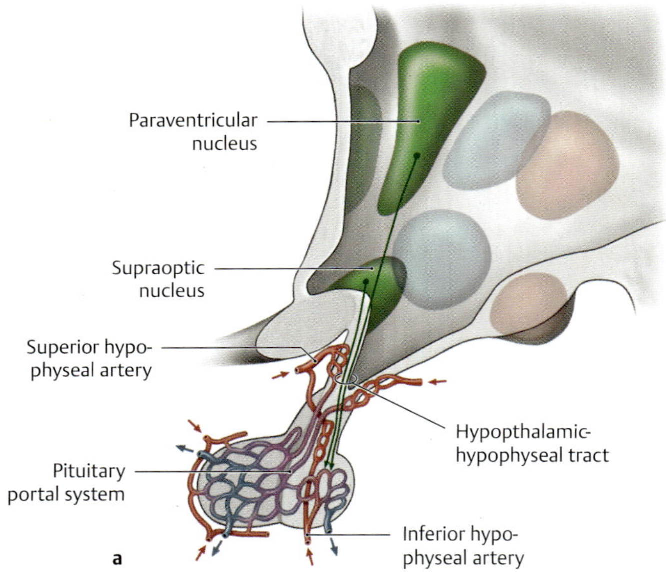

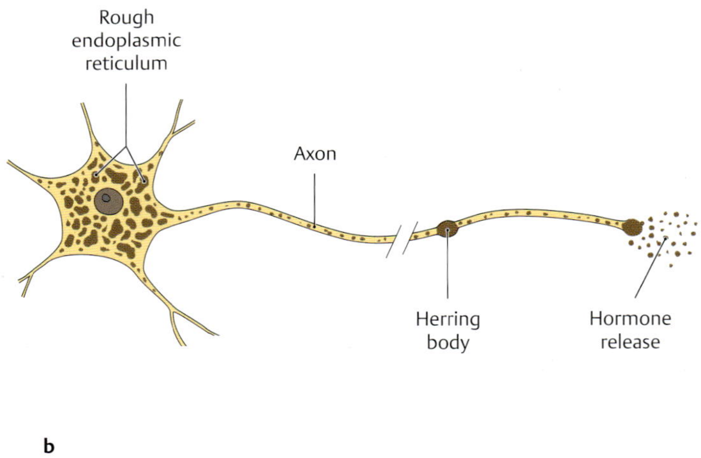

B Connections of the hypothalamic nuclei to the posterior lobe of the pituitary gland

a Hypothalamic–(neuro)pituitary axis. **b** Neurosecretory neuron in the hypothalamic nucleus.

Pituitary hormones are not synthesized in the *posterior pituitary lobe* (neurohypophysis) but in neurons located in the paraventricular nucleus and supraoptic nucleus of the hypothalamus. They are then transported by axons of the hypothalamic–hypophyseal tract to the neurohypophysis, where they are released as needed. Terminals of the paraventricular and supraoptic hypothalamic nuclei release two hormones in the posterior pituitary lobe:

- **Oxytocin** from the neurons of the paraventricular nucleus
- **Antidiuretic hormone** (ADH) or **vasopressin** from the neurons of the supraoptic nucleus

The axons from both nuclei pass through the pituitary stalk to the posterior lobe of the pituitary gland. The peptide hormones are stored in vesicles (aggregated into large "Herring bodies") in the cell bodies of the neurosecretory neurons and are carried to the posterior lobe by anterograde axoplasmic transport.

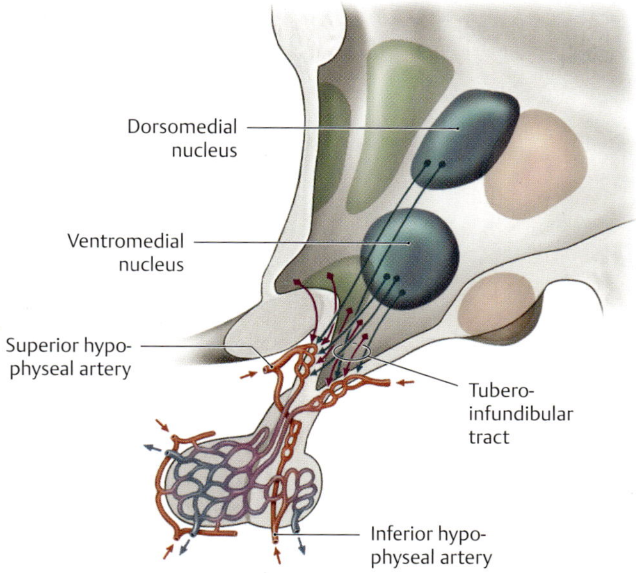

C Hypophyseal portal circulation and connections of the hypothalamic nuclei to the anterior pituitary lobe

The superior hypophyseal arteries from each side of the body form a vascular plexus around the infundibulum (pituitary stalk). The axons from neurons of the hypothalamic nuclei (dark red and dark blue arrows) terminate at this plexus and secrete hormones that have been produced in smaller (parvocellular) neurons of the hypothalamus. The secreted hypothalamic hormones are of two types:

- Releasing factors which stimulate hormone release from cells of the anterior pituitary lobe
- Inhibiting factors which inhibit the hormonal release from these cells

These hormones are carried by the hypophyseal (pituitary) portal venous system (named after the portal circulation of the liver) to capillaries in the anterior lobe, establishing communication between the hypothalamus and endocrine cells of the anterior pituitary.

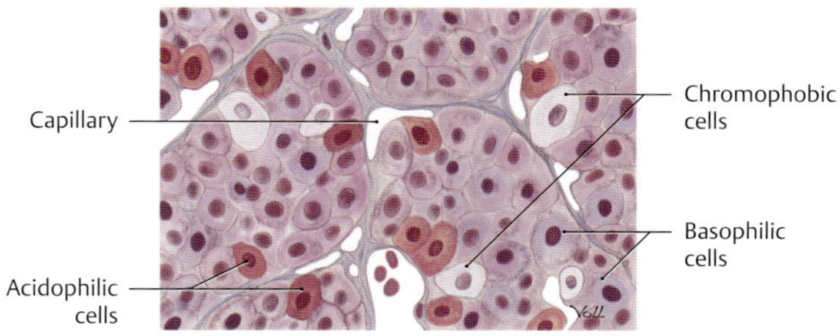

D Histology of the anterior pituitary gland

Three types of cells can be distinguished in the anterior pituitary gland using classic histologic methods: acidophilic cells, basophilic cells, and chromophobic cells. The latter have already released their hormones, and are therefore negative in immunohistochemical tests that specifically detect peptide hormones; they are not listed in **E**. The acidophilic (**a**) cells secrete hormones that act directly on target cells (non-glandotropic hormones) while the basophilic (**b**) cells stimulate subordinate endocrine cells (glandotropic hormones).

E Hormones of the anterior pituitary lobe (adenohypophysis)

Hormones and synonyms	Cell designation*	Hormone actions
Somatotropin (STH) Growth hormone (GH) Somatotropic hormone	Somatotropic (a)	Stimulates longitudinal growth; acts on carbohydrate and lipid metabolism
Prolactin (PRL or LTH) Luteotropic hormone Mammotropic hormone	Mammotropic (a)	Stimulates lactation and proliferation of glandular breast tissue
Follitropin (FSH) Follicle-stimulating hormone	Gonadotropic (b)	Acts on the gonads; stimulates follicular maturation, spermatogenesis, estrogen production, expression of lutropin receptors and proliferation of granulosa cells
Lutropin (LH) Interstitial cell stimulating hormone – ICSH Luteinizing hormone	Gonadotropic (b)	Triggers ovulation; stimulates proliferation of follicular epithelial cells, production of testosterone in interstitial Leydig cells of the testis, and synthesis of progesterone; has general anabolic activity
Thyrotropin (TSH) Thyroid stimulating hormone Thyrotropic hormone	Thyrotropic (b)	Stimulates thyroid gland activity; increases O_2 consumption and protein synthesis; influences carbohydrate and lipid metabolism
Corticotropin (ACTH) Adrenocorticotropic hormone	Adrenotropic (b)	Stimulates hormone production in adrenal cortex; influences water and electrolyte balance; acts on carbohydrate formation in liver
Alpha/beta **Melanotropin (MSH)**	Melanotropic (b)	Aids in melanin formation and skin pigmentation; protects against UV radiation**

* Cells are classified as either acidophilic (a) or basophilic (b).
** In humans, melanotropin serves as a neurotransmitter in various brain regions.

7.8 Epithalamus and Subthalamus

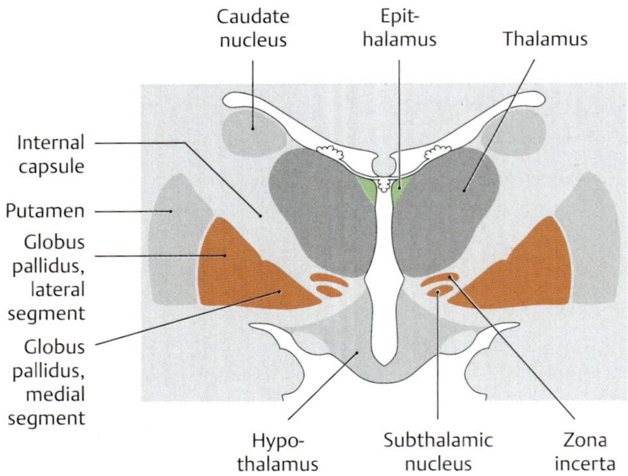

A Location of the epithalamus and subthalamus

Coronal section. The appropriateness of the term "epithalamus" can be appreciated in this plane of section, which shows the epithalamus riding upon the thalamus (epi = "upon"). The **epithalamus** (green) consists of the following structures:

- Pineal gland (epiphysis), see **B**.
- Habenulae with the habenular nuclei, see **D**.
- Habenular commissure, see **C**.
- Stria medullaris, see **D**.

The posterior commissure that lies rostral to the pineal gland, see **Ca**, contains fibers from mesencephalic nuclei and is therefore regarded as a functional part of the midbrain. The region of the **subthalamus** (orange), formerly called the ventral thalamus, initially lies directly below the thalamus, but during embryonic development is displaced laterally into the telencephalon by fibers of the internal capsule, forming the *globus pallidus* (see **D**, p. 339). The subthalamus contains nuclei of the medial motor system (motor zones of the diencephalon), and has connections with the motor nuclei of the tegmentum. In fact, the subthalamus can be considered the cranial extension of the tegmentum.

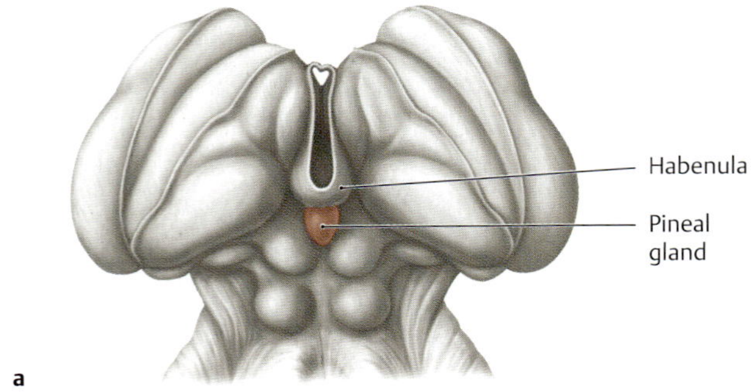

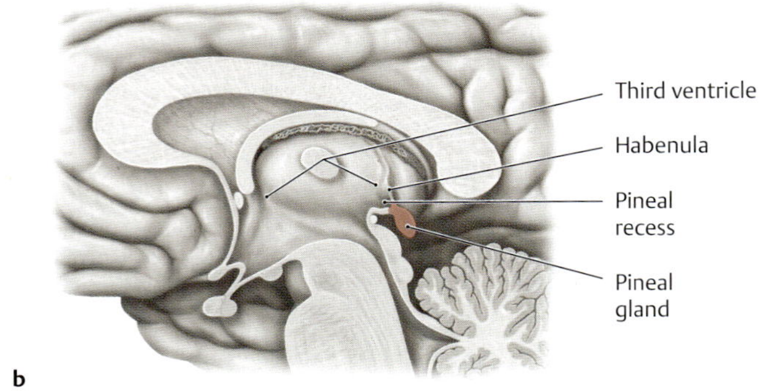

B Location of the pineal

a Posterior view. **b** Midsagittal section of the right hemisphere viewed from the medial side.

The pineal gland resembles a pine cone when viewed from behind. It is connected to the diencephalon by the habenula, which contains both afferent and efferent tracts. Its topographical relationship to the third ventricle is seen particularly well in midsagittal section (pineal recess). In reptiles, the calvaria over the pineal gland is thinned so that it is receptive to light stimuli. This is not the case in humans, although retinal afferents still communicate with the pineal through relay stations in the hypothalamus and the superior cervical (sympathetic) ganglion, helping to regulate circadian rhythms.

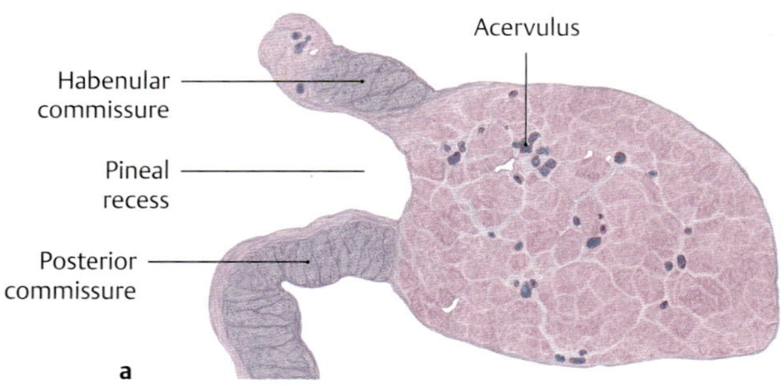

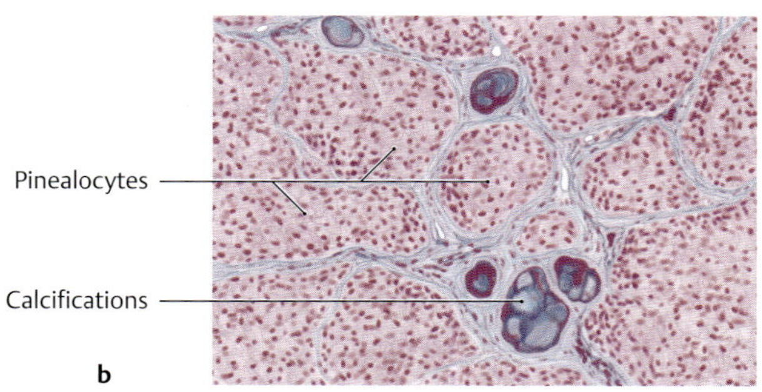

C Structure of the pineal gland

a Gross midsagittal tissue section. **b** Histological section.

a In the gross tissue section, the habenular commissure can be identified at the rostral end of the pineal gland. Below it is the posterior (epithalamic) commissure. Between the two commissures is the CSF-filled pineal recess of the third ventricle. Calcifications (corpora arenacea, "brain sand") are frequently present and may be visible on radiographs; they have no pathological significance.

b The histological section demonstrates the specific cells of the pineal, the *pinealocytes*, which are embedded in a connective-tissue stroma and are surrounded by astrocytes. The pinealocytes produce *melatonin*, which plays a role in the regulation of circadian rhythms; it may be taken prophylactically, for example, to moderate the effects of jet lag. If the pineal ceases to function during childhood, the individual may undergo precocious puberty given that the pineal has significant, mostly inhibitory, effects on endocrine systems.

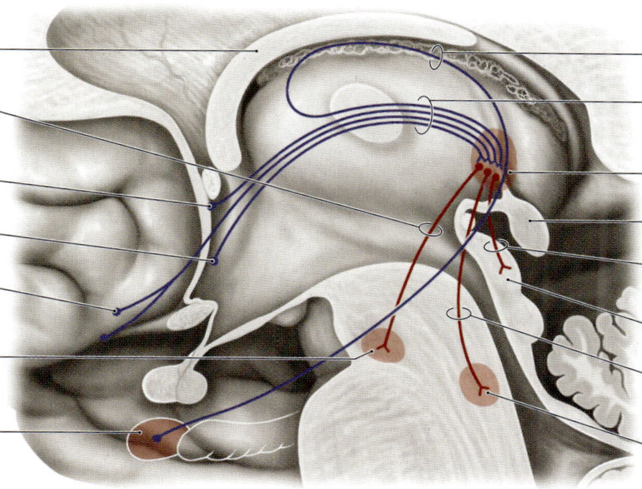

D Habenular nuclei and their fiber connections
Midsagittal section of the right hemisphere viewed from the medial side. The habenula ("reins") and their nuclei function as a relay station for afferent olfactory impulses. After their relay in the habenular nuclei, their efferent fibers are distributed to the salivatory and motor nuclei (mastication) in the brainstem.

Afferent connections (blue): Afferent impulses from the anterior perforated substance (olfactory area), septal nuclei, and preoptic region are transmitted by the stria medullaris to the habenular nuclei. These nuclei also receive impulses from the amygdala via the stria terminalis.

Efferent connections (red): Efferent fibers from the habenular nuclei are projected to the midbrain along three tracts:

- Habenulotectal tract: terminates in the roof of the mesencephalon, the quadrigeminal plate, supplying it with olfactory impulses.
- Habenulotegmental tract: terminates in the dorsal tegmental nucleus, establishing connections with the dorsal longitudinal fasciculus and with the salivatory and motor cranial nerve nuclei. (The smell of food stimulates salivation and gastric acid secretion: e.g., Pavlovian response.)
- Habenulointerpeduncular tract: terminates in the interpeduncular nucleus, which then connects with the reticular formation.

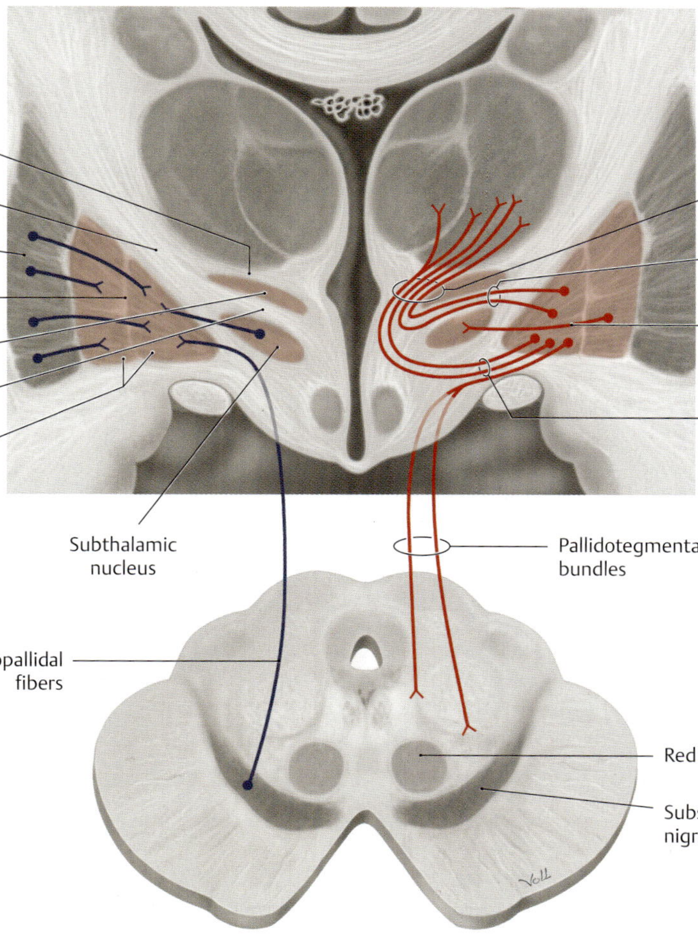

E Subthalamic nuclei with their afferent (blue) and efferent (red) connections
The principal nucleus of the subthalamus is the *globus pallidus*, which is displaced laterally during development into the telencephalon by the internal capsule. A lamina of white divides the globus pallidus into a medial (internal) and lateral (external) segment. Certain small nuclei are exempt from this migration and remain near the midline: these are the *zona incerta* and *subthalamic nucleus*. The subthalamic nucleus, substantia nigra, and putamen send afferent fibers to the globus pallidus. The globus pallidus in turn distributes efferent fibers to these regions and also to the thalamus through a tract called the lenticular fasciculus. Functionally, these nuclei are classified as portions of the basal nuclei. Lesions of these nuclei lead to a movement disorder called contralateral hemiballismus (the functional role of the subthalamus is described on p. 458 f).

8.1 Brainstem, Organization and External Structure

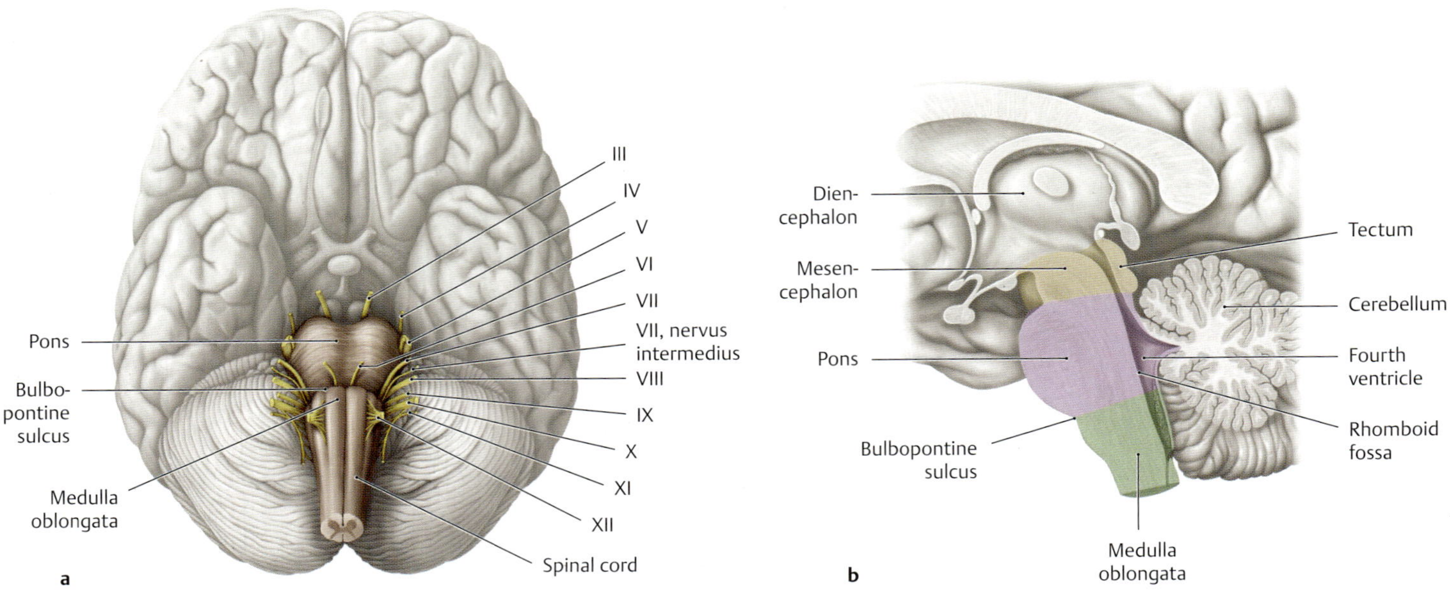

A Brainstem (truncus encephali)

a View of the intact brain from below; **b** Midsagittal section, left lateral view.

Compared to the telencephalon, the brainstem is so small that its parts become better visible in midsagittal section (**b**). Features of the brainstem:

- Part of the brain that is most connected to the PNS.
- It is only at the brainstem that the ventricular system (via the fourth ventricle) communicates with the subarachnoid space (see **A**, p. 312 and **C**, p. 315).
- The brainstem is connected to the spinal cord.
- The cerebellum is situated on the dorsal aspect of the brainstem that connects it to the other parts of the CNS (see **A** and **B**, p. 370).

The purely *topographical* demarcation of zones in the brainstem from rostral to caudal is based on its external, macroscopic structure. The mesencephalon is located between the diencephalon and the pons, which at its caudal end is separated from the medulla oblongata by the bulbopontine sulcus. The brainstem extends caudally to the point of exit of the first spinal nerve after which the spinal cord begins. The external structure of the brainstem does not match its internal structure. Here, nuclear columns of cranial nerves are located, which developmentally follow a specific arrangement pattern, which applies to the entire brainstem (see p. 114). Also purely topographical criteria are used to subdivide each brainstem section into four parts (see **B**). According to its many functions, the brainstem's internal structure can be roughly divided into the following:

- Nuclear regions (collection of neuronal cell bodies), in which the wiring takes place—roughly divided into nuclei, of cranial nerves and nuclei that are not associated with cranial nerves (e.g., red nucleus and substantia nigra, both part of the motor system, and nuclei of the reticular formation)
- Since the brainstem is located between diencephalon and spinal cord, axons, which are bundled together in tracts, pass through it. All communication between the spinal cord and the more rostral regions of the brain passes though these tracts within the brainstem. Depending on the flow of information, a distinction is drawn between ascending (afferent, to the telencephalon) and descending (efferent, away from the telencephalon) tracts.

Note: Since so many nuclei and tracts lie so closely together in the brainstem, even small lesions, for example in case of brainstem stroke, can cause severe damage.

B Overview of the brainstem

Topographical organization
- *Craniocaudal direction:*
  - Mesencephalon (midbrain)
  - Pons
  - Medulla oblongata
- *Anteroposterior direction:*
  - Base (mesencephalon: cerebral peduncles; pons: basal part; medulla oblongata: pyramids)
  - Tegmentum (present as such in all three parts)
  - Section of ventricular system (cerebral aqueduct, fourth ventricle, central canal)
  - Tectum ("roof"; present only in the mesencephalon; quadrigeminal plate)
- The cerebellum adjoins the brainstem dorsally.

Functional organization
- *Brainstem as "control center"*
  - nuclei for cranial nerves III–XII and XII (divided into four longitudinal nuclear columns)
  - coordination center for motor control (red nucleus, substantia nigra)
  - reticular formation (motor function; respiration; blood circulation; autonomic functions)
  - pontine nuclei (connected to the cerebellum)
  - nuclei of the posterior funiculus (termination point of sensory pathways)
  - interconnection of auditory and visual stimuli (lamina tecti)
- *Brainstem as "passage for tracts"*
  - toward and away from the brain: descending (motor) and ascending (sensory) tracts
  - toward and/or away from the cerebellum: cerebellar connection with spinal cord, brainstem, diencephalon and telencephalon (via pons and thalamus)
  - descending autonomic tracts

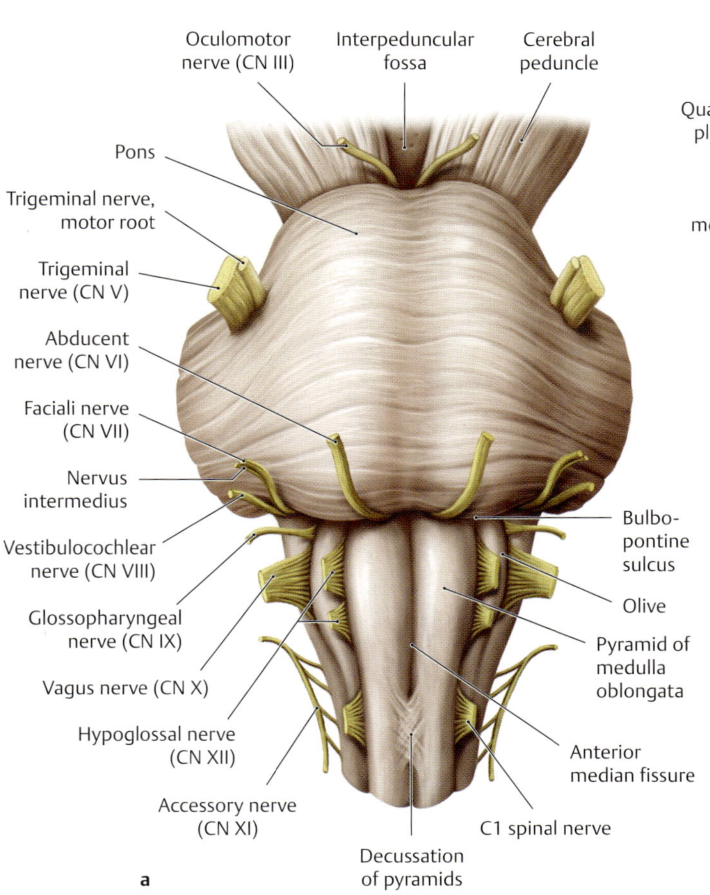

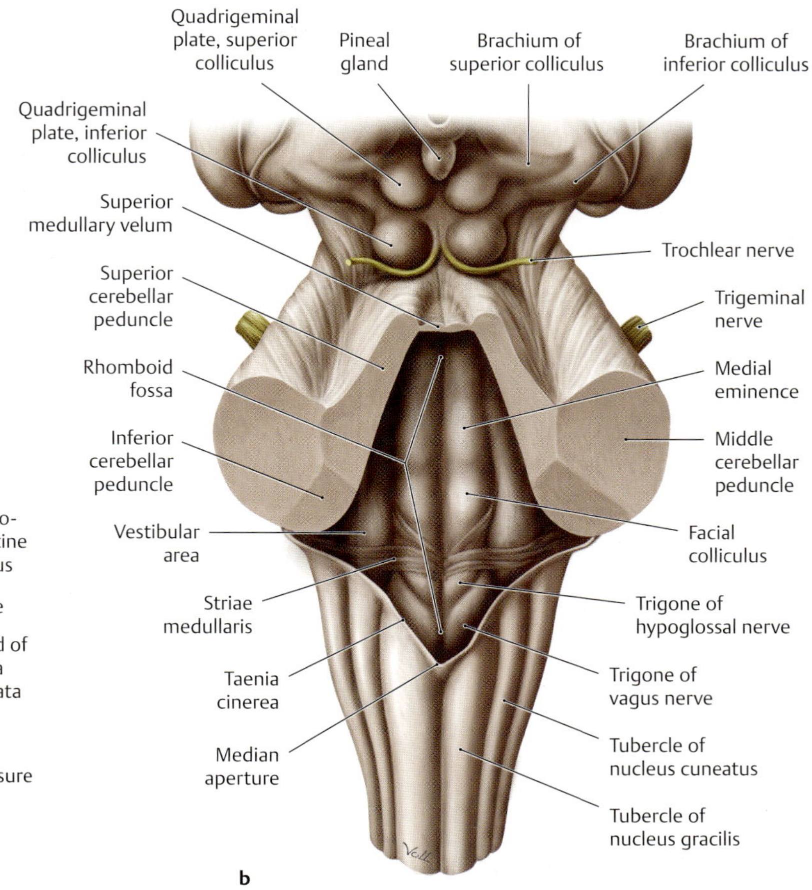

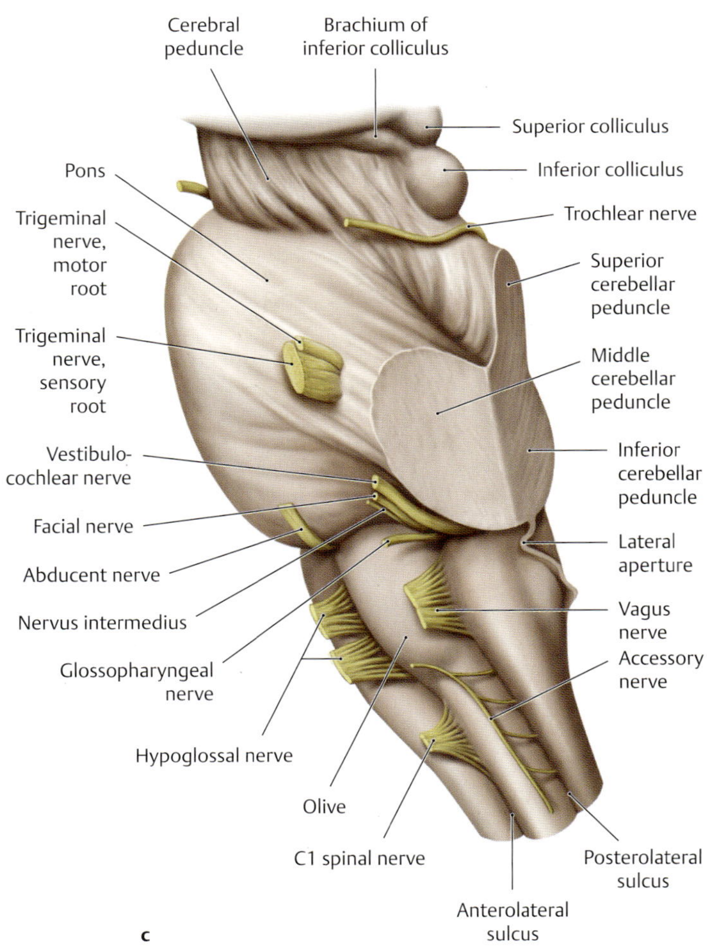

C Brainstem: external structure

a Ventral view. The ventral view is dominated by the pons (a small bridge, which appears to traverse the brainstem oriented lengthwise). The attachment points of cranial nerves III and V–XII are on this side of the brainstem (CN IV is the only cranial nerve to emerge dorsally, see **b**). Cranial to the pons lie the crus cerebri, which contain descending motor pathways. A part of these fibers travel to the pyramids of the medulla oblongata and most of them cross over in the pyramidal decussation. The olive, located lateral to the pyramid, contains a large motor nuclear group, the inferior olivary nuclei.
Note: Therefore, the pyramidal decussation lies very close to the border between medulla oblongata and spinal cord.

b Dorsal view. What is striking is the view of the diamond-shaped floor of the fourth ventricle known as the rhomboid fossa. The rhomboid fossa is outlined by several cranial nerve nuclei. Located cranially is the roof of the mesencephalon with the lamina tecti, from which CN IV emerges. The lamina tecti contains four colliculi (lamina quadrigemina). The superior colliculi are integrative centers related to visual information and the inferior colliculi are relay stations of the auditory pathway. The brachium ("arm") of the superior colliculus and the brachium of the inferior colliculus connect these colliculi with their corresponding thalamic nuclei. Lateral to the fourth ventricle, as a topographic connection between cerebellum and brainstem, are three paired cerebellar peduncles: the superior, middle, and inferior cerebellar peduncles.

c Lateral view from left. Very clearly displayed in this view is the fact that the ventral curvature of the pons extends into the middle cerebellar peduncle, which connects the pons with the cerebellum. The nuclei necessary for this cross-wiring lie within the pons (pontine nuclei). The trigeminal nerve (cranial nerve V) emerges directly from the pons. Immediately caudal to the pons the left olive is visible.

8.2 Brainstem: Cranial Nerve Nuclei, Red Nucleus, and Substantia Nigra

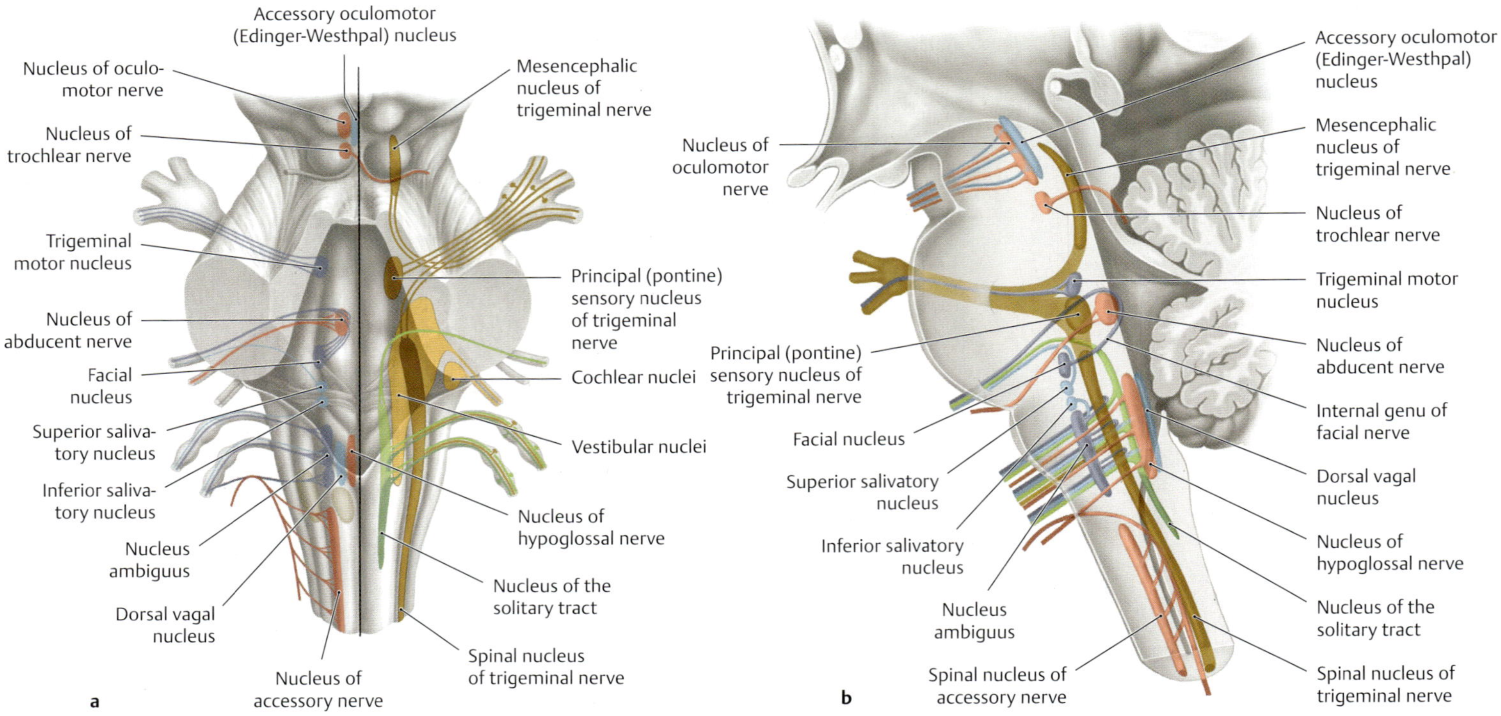

A Cranial nerve nuclei in the brainstem
a Posterior view with the cerebellum removed, exposing the rhomboid fossa; **b** Midsagittal section of the right half of the brainstem viewed from the left side.
The diagrams show the nuclei themselves and the course of the nerves (to save space, the vestibular and cochlear nuclei are not shown).
The arrangement of the cranial nerve nuclei is easier to understand when we divide them into functional nuclear columns. The *motor nuclei*, which give rise to the efferent fibers, are shown on the left side of diagram **a**, and the *sensory nuclei*, where the afferent fibers terminate, are shown in **b**. The arrangement of these nuclei can be derived from the arrangement of the nuclei in the spinal cord (see p. 114). The function and connections of some of these cranial nerves can be clinically evaluated by testing the *brainstem reflexes* (whose relay centers are located in the brainstem). These reflexes are important in the evaluation of comatose patients. A prime example is the pupillary reflexes, which are further described on p. 481.

B Overview of the nuclei of cranial nerves III–XII

Motor nuclei: give rise to efferent (motor) fibers, left in **Aa**	**Sensory nuclei:** where afferent (sensory) fibers terminate, right in **Aa**
Somatic efferent or somatic motor nuclei (red): – Nucleus of oculomotor nerve (CN III) – Nucleus of trochlear nerve (CN IV) – Nucleus of abducent nerve (CN VI) – Nucleus of accessory nerve (CN XI) – Nucleus of hypoglossal nerve (CN XII) **Visceral efferent (visceral motor) nuclei:** • *Nuclei associated with the parasympathetic nervous system (light blue):* – Accessory oculomotor (Edinger–Westphal) nucleus (CN III) – Superior salivatory nucleus (facial nerve, CN VII) – Inferior salivatory nucleus (glossopharyngeal nerve, CN IX) – Dorsal vagal nucleus (CN X) • *Nuclei associated with the innervation of muscles derived from branchial arches (dark blue):* – Trigeminal motor nucleus (CN V) – Facial nucleus (CN VII) – Nucleus ambiguus (CN IX; CN X)	**Somatic afferent (somatic or main sensory) and vestibulocochlear nuclei (yellow):** • *Sensory nuclei associated with the trigeminal nerve (CN V):* – Mesencephalic nucleus of trigeminal nerve (special feature: pseudounipolar ganglion cells ("displaced sensory ganglion"), provide direct sensory innervation for muscles of mastication) – Principal (pontine) sensory nucleus of trigeminal nerve – Spinal nucleus of trigeminal nerve *Nuclei of the vestibulocochlear nerve (CN VIII):* • Vestibular part: – Medial vestibular nucleus – Lateral vestibular nucleus – Superior vestibular nucleus – Inferior vestibular nucleus • Cochlear part: – Anterior cochlear nucleus – Posterior cochlear nucleus **Visceral afferent (visceral sensory) nuclei (green):** • Nucleus of the solitary tract (nuclear complex): • Superior part: – Special visceral afferents (taste) from CN VII, CN IX, and CN X • Inferior part: – General visceral afferents from CN IX and CN X

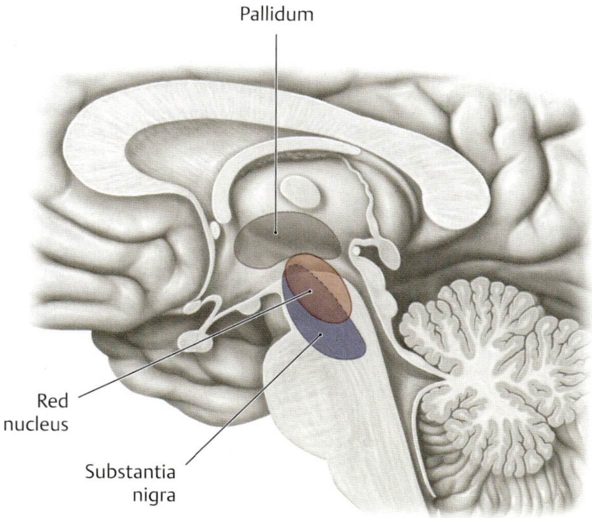

C Location of the substantia nigra and red nucleus in the mesencephalon

Both of these nuclei, like the cranial nerve nuclei, are well-defined structures that belong functionally to the *extrapyramidal motor* system. Anatomically, the substantia nigra is part of the cerebral peduncles and therefore is not located in the tegmentum of the mesencephalon (see **A**, p. 362). Owing to their high respective contents of melanin and iron, the substantia nigra and red nucleus appear brown and red, respectively, in sections of fresh brain tissue. Both nuclei extend into the diencephalon and are connected to its nuclei by fiber tracts (see **E**).

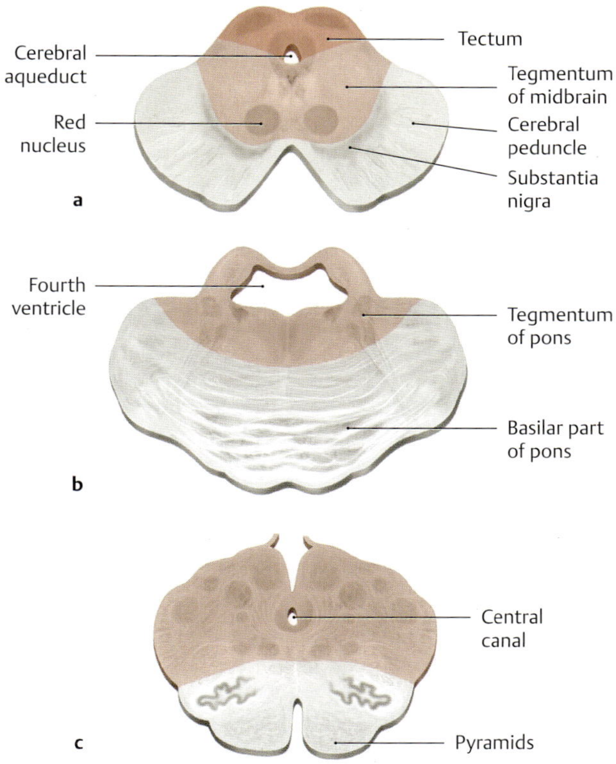

D Cross-sectional structure of the brainstem at different levels

Transverse sections through the **a** mesencephalon, **b** pons, and **c** medulla oblongata, viewed from above.

A feature common to all three sections is the dorsally situated tegmentum ("hood," medium gray), the phylogenetically old part of the brainstem. The tegmentum of the adult brain contains the brainstem nuclei. Anterior to the tegmentum are the large ascending and descending tracts that run to and from the telencephalon. This region is called the cerebral peduncle (crus cerebri) in the mesencephalon, the basilar part (base) of the pons at the pontine level, and the pyramids in the medulla oblongata. The tegmentum is covered dorsally by the tectum (= "roof") only in the region of the mesencephalon. In the mature brain pictured here, this structure forms the quadrigeminal plate containing the superior and inferior colliculi ("little hills"), shown faintly in **Da**. The brainstem is covered by the cerebellum at the level of the medulla oblongata and pons and therefore lacks a tectal covering at those levels.

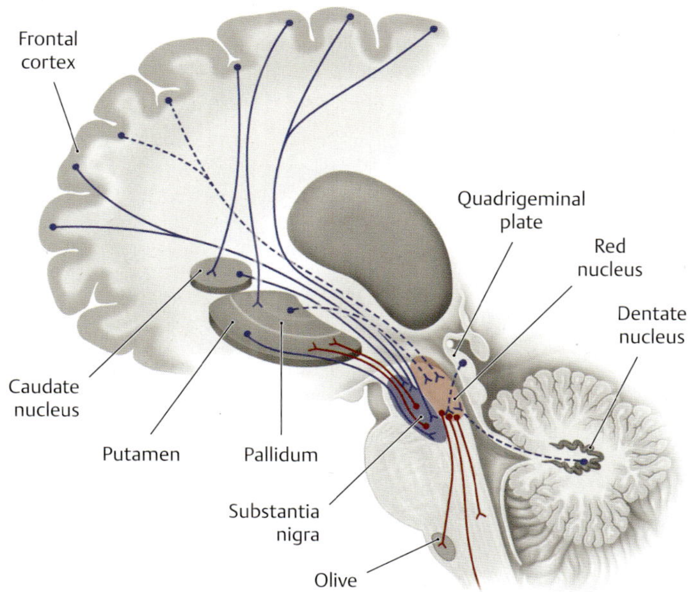

E Afferent (blue) and efferent (red) connections of the red nucleus and substantia nigra

These two nuclei are important relay stations in the motor system. The **red nucleus** consists of a larger *neorubrum* and a smaller *paleorubrum*. It receives afferent axons from the dentate nucleus (dentatorubral tract), superior colliculi (tectorubral tract), inner pallidum (pallidorubral tract), and cerebral cortex (corticorubral tract).

The red nucleus sends its axons to the olive (rubro-olivary fibers and reticulo-olivary fibers, part of the central tegmental tract) and to the spinal cord (rubrospinal tract). It coordinates muscle tone, body position, and gait. A lesion of the red nucleus produces resting tremor, abnormal muscle tone (tested as involuntary muscular resistance of the joints in the relaxed patient), and choreoathetosis (involuntary writhing movements, usually involving the distal parts of the limbs).

The **substantia nigra** consists of a *compact part* (dark, contains melanin) and a *reticular part* (reddish, contains iron; for simplicity, the entire substantia nigra appears dark in the drawing). Most of its axons project diffusely to other brain areas and are not collected into tracts. Some axons from the caudate nucleus and putamen (striatonigral fibers), and precentral cortex (corticonigral fibers) terminate in the substantia nigra.

8.3 Brainstem: Reticular Formation

A Definition, demarcation and organization

The *Reticular Formation (RF)* is a phylogenetically old, morphologically ill-defined collection of numerous small nuclei in the *tegmentum* of the brainstem. These nuclei serve entirely different functions. The morphological term "*reticular formation*" incorrectly implies a homogeneity when in fact it represents different centers. Thus, it would be better to refer to them as *reticular nuclei*, which morphologically are difficult to distinguish from one another. The reticular nuclei use different neurotransmitters to serve their different functions. Considering these facts, the reticular formation can be classified as follows:

- Cytoarchitectonics (morphological classification) takes into account the shape and architecture of the reticular nuclei (see **C**).
- Transmitter architectonics (chemical classification) takes into account the type of neurotransmitters used by the cells (see **C**).
- The classification based on functional centers (physiological classification) covers the functions associated with the nuclei (see **B**).

Note: Cranial nerve nuclei, which are mainly located in the tegmentum of the brainstem (but are usually very well defined morphologically) are not part of the RF but are functionally closely linked with it. Neither the nuclear regions of the "red nucleus" or "substantia nigra" located in the tegmentum of the mesencephalon nor the pontine nuclei are part of the RF.

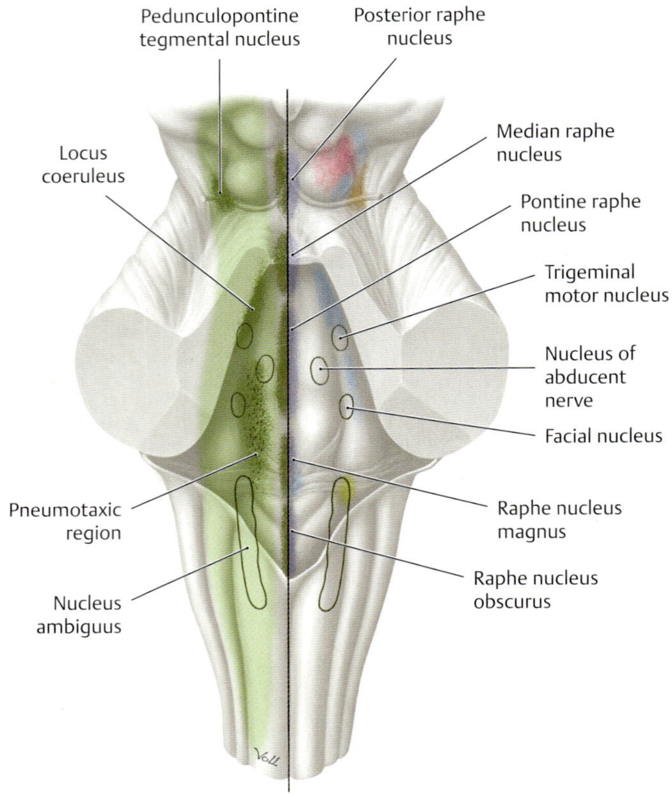

C Cyto- and transmitter architectonics

Dorsal view of the brainstem after the cerebellum has been removed; left hemisphere: cytoarchitectonics; right hemisphere: transmitter architectonics. With the help of cytoarchitectonics, the reticular nuclei can be divided already in the RF on both sides into three longitudinal zones each:

- *lateral zone* with small-cell nuclei (parvocellular zone),
- *medial zone* with large-cell nuclei (magnocellular zone)
- *median zone* (it lies on both sides of the midline = raphe of the brainstem; the large-cell nuclei located in this zone are thus also referred to as "raphe nuclei").

The axons of the medial and median zone, after a long course, reach other nuclei of the CNS either in cranial direction up to the telencephalon or in caudal direction up to the sacral spinal region. These two zones are mostly responsible for connecting the RF with other regions of the CNS. They are thus called "effectory." However, the axons of the lateral zone largely remain inside the brainstem, connecting individual portions of the RF with one another or interconnecting with cranial nerve nuclei in the brainstem. They are thus also referred to as "association areas." Some nuclei have been labeled as examples.

Note: The division into three longitudinal zones is not equally visible in all portions of the brainstem. It is best visible in the medulla oblongata. As a reference point, the cranial nerve nuclei (they are not part of the RF, see introduction), which are closely interconnected with the RF, have also been marked.

Transmitter architectonics can help identify areas in which neurons with a specific transmitter predominate. Catecholamines (adrenaline, in **C** yellow; noradrenaline, in **C** light blue; dopamine, in **C** orange) as well as serotonin (in **C** violet) and acetylcholine (in **C** red) are examples shown here.

Note: Raphe nuclei (median zone), which send their axons to the limbic system (modulation of moods and feelings) use serotonin as a transmitter. Pharmacologically, influencing the effect of serotonin is said to effectively modulate emotions.

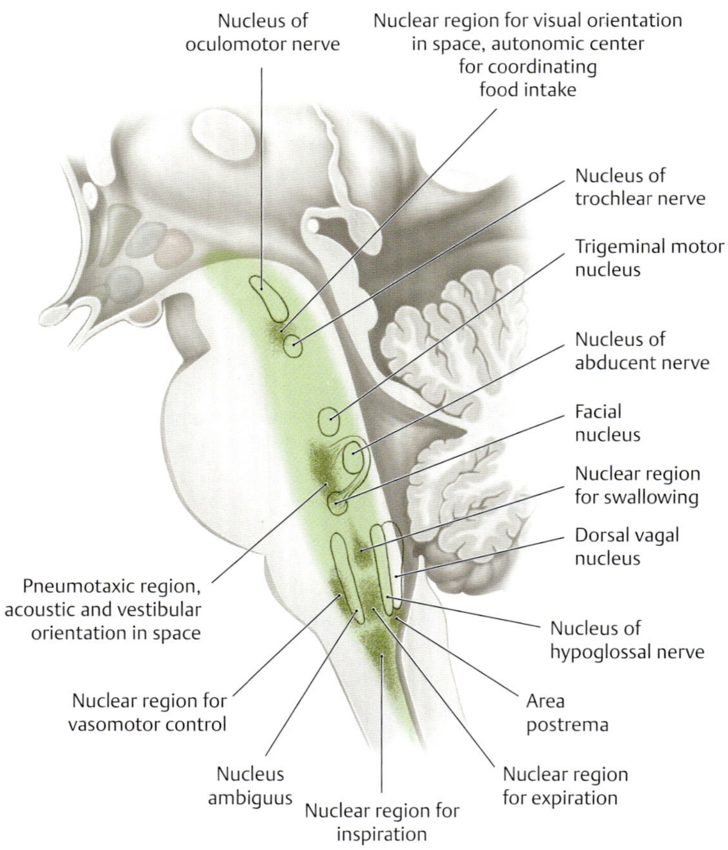

B Functional centers

Left lateral view of the brainstem bisected. Displayed is the position of functional centers as well as the position of functionally relevant cranial nerve nuclei. For further details of the functional centers see **D**.

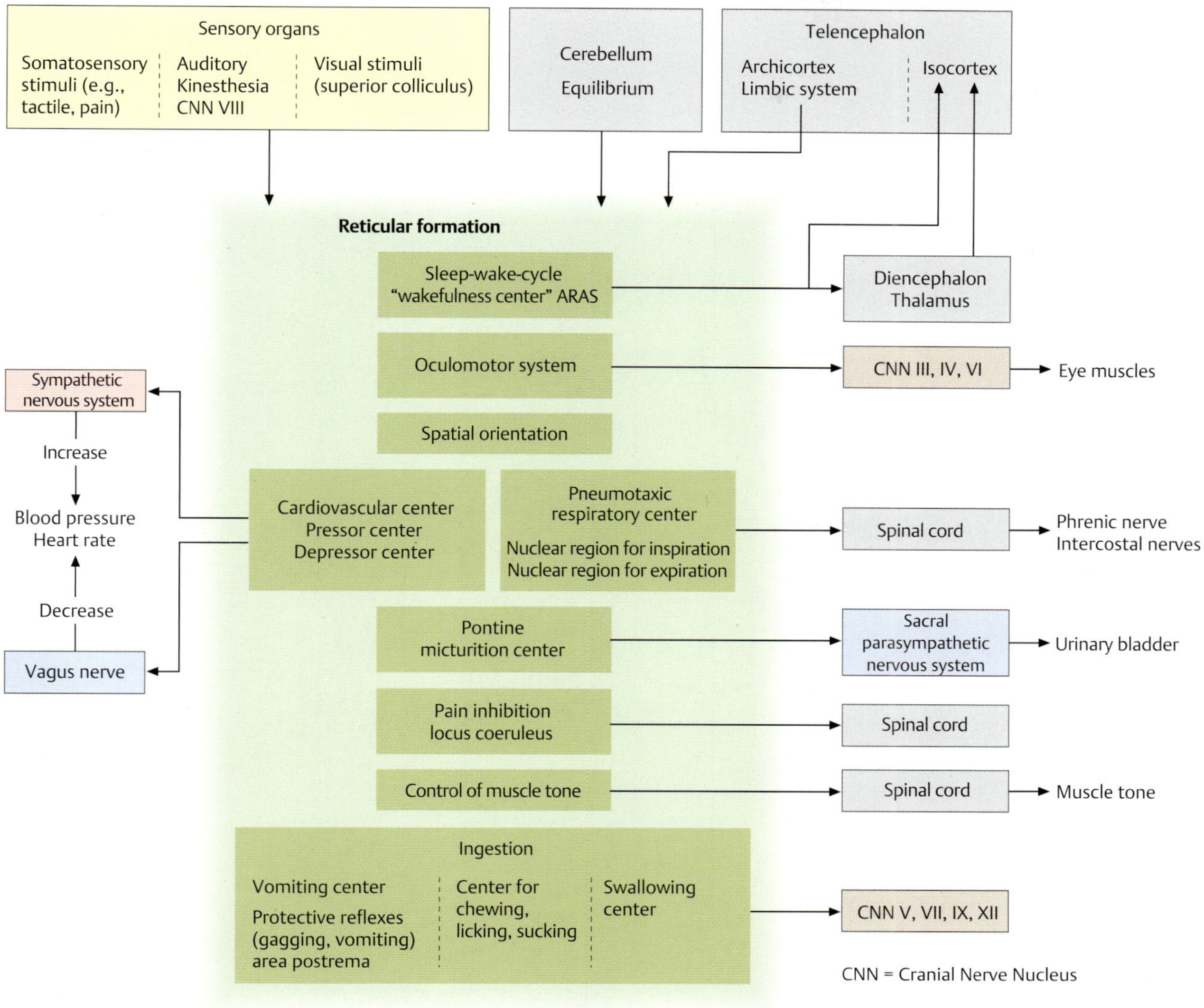

D Overview of the functions of the reticular formation

A distinction is drawn between the following functional relationships of the reticular formation with other centers in the CNS:

- **Afferents to the reticular formation:** These originate from nuclei of almost all sensory organs, the telencephalon, diencephalon as well as the cerebellum and spinal cord. They carry auditory, visual and tactile impulses and to a special degree, pain sensation, but also carry information regarding muscle relaxation, equilibrium, blood pressure, oxygen saturation and parameters of ingestion.
- **Efferents of the reticular formation:** These extend to the telencephalon and diencephalon but also to the motor nuclei of the cranial nerves and the spinal cord. These efferents have very different effects:
  - regulating sleep-wake transitions and level of alertness of the telencephalon (so-called "*ARAS*": **A**scending **R**eticular **A**ctivitating **S**ystem),
  - regulating eye movement,
  - "vital" functions such as regulating blood pressure and respiration,
  - functions of ingestion such as licking, sucking and chewing,
  - protective reflexes such as gagging and vomiting,
  - control of micturition,
  - regulating muscle tone in the spinal cord, and
  - pain inhibition in the spinal cord

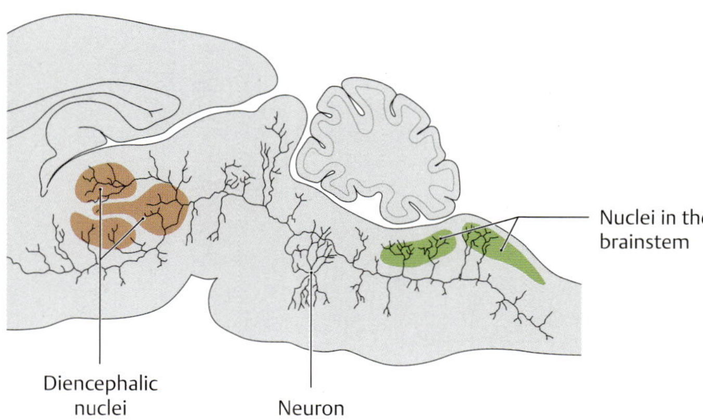

E Branching pattern of a neuron in the reticular formation of the rat brainstem

Midsagittal section viewed from the left side. Neurons can be selectively visualized with the silver-impregnation (Golgi) staining method. The axon of the neuron shown here divides into an ascending branch, which comes into contact with the diencephalic nuclei (shown in brown) and a descending branch, which establishes connections with cranial nerve nuclei (green) in the pons and medulla oblongata. This extensive arborization allows neurons of the reticular formation to have widespread effects on multiple brain regions

8.4 Brainstem: Descending and Ascending Tracts

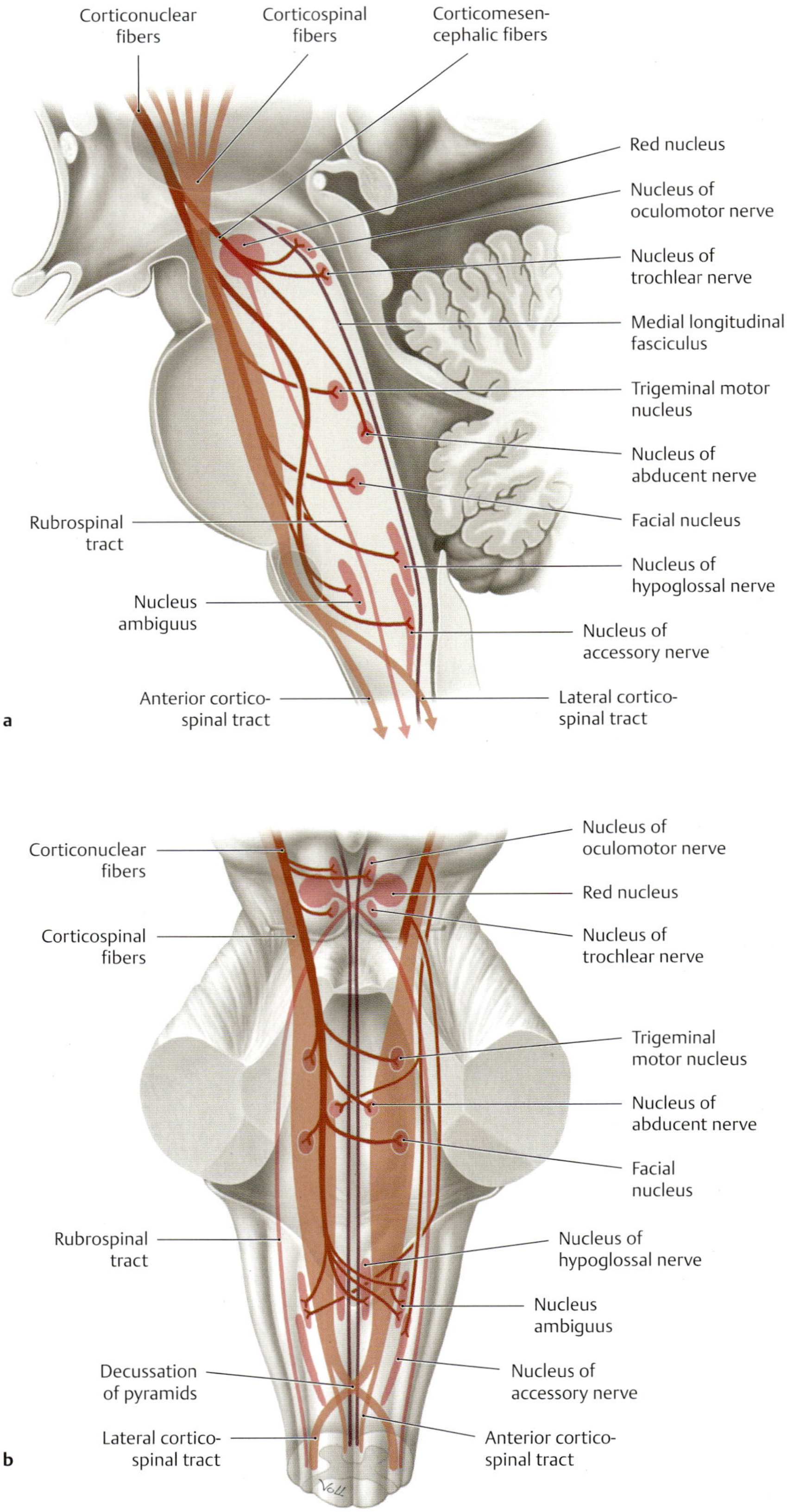

A Descending tracts in the brainstem

a Midsagittal section viewed from the left side. **b** Posterior view with the cerebellum removed.

The descending tracts shown here begin in the telencephalon and terminate partly in the brainstem but mostly in the spinal cord. The most prominent tract that descends through the brainstem, the *corticospinal tract*, terminates in the spinal cord. Its axons arise from large pyramidal neurons of the primary motor cortex and terminate on or near alpha motor neurons in the anterior horn of the spinal cord. Most of the axons cross to the opposite side (decussate) at the level of the pyramids. The fibers in this part of the pyramidal tract that descend through the brainstem are called *corticospinal fibers*. Those fibers in the pyramidal tract that terminate in the brainstem are called *corticonuclear fibers*. Corticonuclear axons connect the motor cortex to the brainstem motor nuclei of the cranial nerves.

Note: Direct cortical projections to the brainstem nuclei are predominantly

- *bilaterally supplied:*
  - III (oculomotor nucleus),
  - V (trigeminal motor nucleus),
  - part of the facial motor nucleus controlling the forehead muscles,
  - X (nucleus ambiguus);
- *others only contralaterally:*
  - VI (nucleus of the abducent nerve),
  - part of the facial motor nucleus controlling muscles of facial expression, except for the forehead,
  - XII (nucleus of the hypoglossal nerve), or
- *only ipsilaterally:*
  - IV (nucleus of the trochlear nerve).

The pattern of corticonuclear innervation is important in the diagnosis of different lesions, particularly involving the facial nerve (CN VII; see **D**, p. 124).

The *medial longitudinal fasciculus* is a brainstem tract containing both ascending and descending fibers that interconnects the nuclei of the brainstem (for its function see **C**, p. 483).

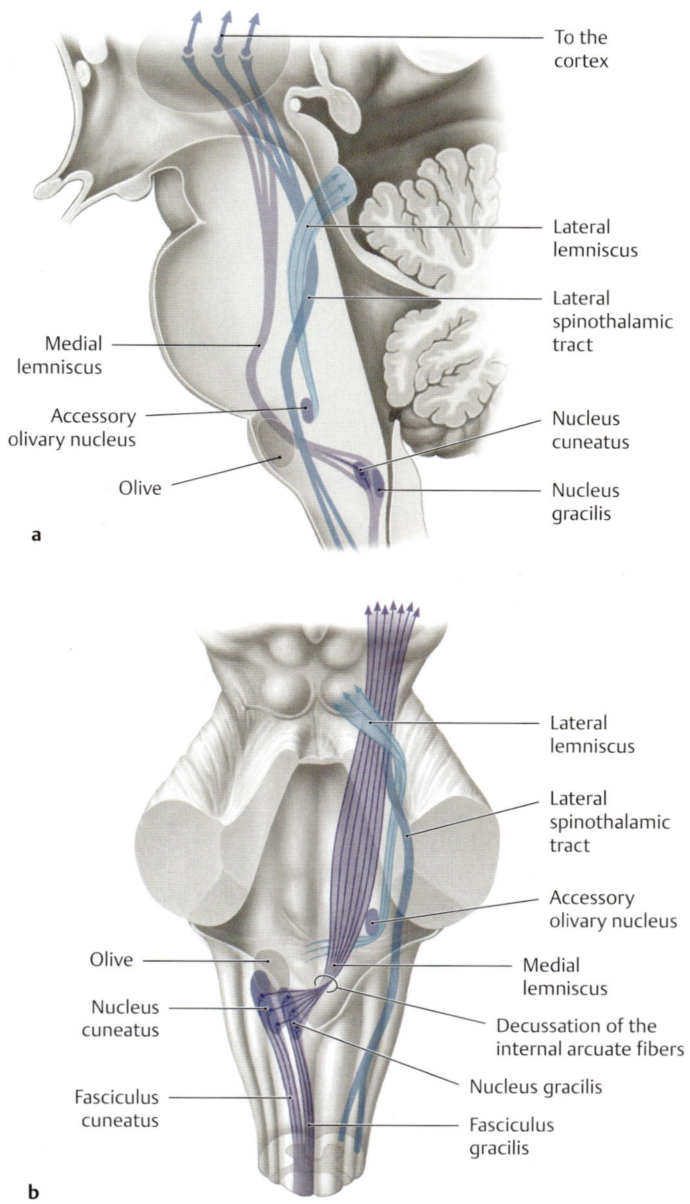

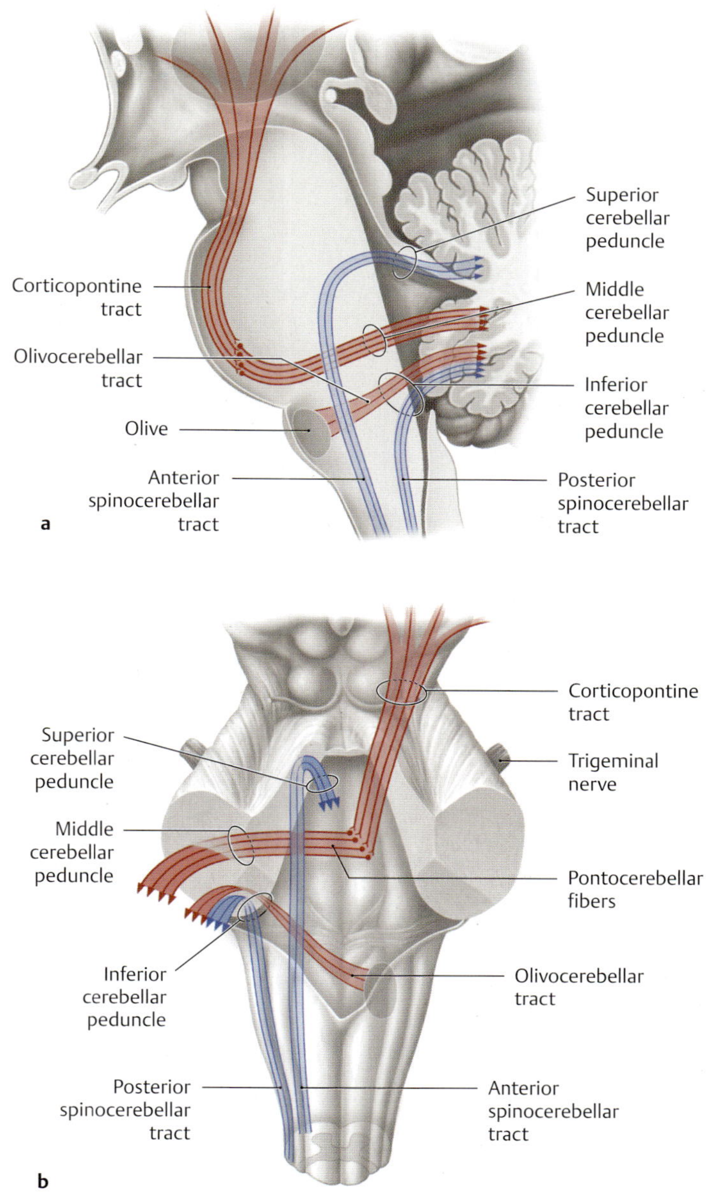

B Courses of ascending tracts through the brainstem
a Midsagittal section viewed from the left side; **b** Posterior view.
Two major ascending spinal cord tracts, the lateral spinothalamic tract and posterior funiculus carry somatosensory information from the spinal cord to the thalamus (diencephalon, see pp. 344 and 346). Two of the ribbon-like tracts are recognizable in the brainstem (see p. 545), the *medial lemniscus* and the *lateral lemniscus*:

- The **medial lemniscus** consists of axons of the second neurons with the cell bodies in the gracilis and cuneatus nuclei. Afferents to these nuclei come from the fasciculus gracilis or fasciculus cuneatus (e.g., pressure, vibration). Spinothalamic tract axons (pain, temperature) join the medial lemniscus before approaching the thalamus.
- The **lateral lemniscus** contains axons from the cochlear nuclei and other stations on the auditory pathway that ascend to the inferior colliculus of the quadrigeminal plate.

The anterior spinothalamic tract is not shown because its location in the brainstem is disputed. The anterior spinothalamic tract together with the lateral spinothalamic tract is sometimes referred to as the spinal lemniscus.

C Courses of the major cerebellar tracts through the brainstem
a Midsagittal section viewed from the left side; **b** Posterior view (cerebellum has been removed).
The cerebellum is involved in the coordination of fine motor movements and the regulation of muscle tone. Its tracts are composed of ascending (blue) and descending (red) pathways. They enter the cerebellum through the three cerebellar peduncles (superior, middle, and inferior).

- **Superior cerebellar peduncle:** Most of the efferent tracts from the cerebellar nuclei run through the superior cerebellar peduncle (see p. 370). The only afferent tract entering the cerebellum through the superior peduncle is the anterior spinocerebellar tract.
- **Middle cerebellar peduncle:** Contains only afferent fibers to the cerebellum. They belong to a pathway that originates in the different lobes (corticopontine tract). The axons of the corticopontine tract synapse with neurons in the pontine nuclei and the axons of these neurons form the pontocerebellar fibers that cross over and run within the opposite middle cerebellar peduncle to the contralateral cerebellum.
- **Inferior cerebellar peduncle:** It is mainly afferent to the cerebellum. The posterior spinocerebellar tract, the cuneocerebellar tract and the olivocerebellar tract enter the cerebellum through the inferior peduncle.

The diagram shows the course and location of the distinct cerebellar tracts.

8.5 Mesencephalon and Pons, Transverse Section

A Transverse section through the mesencephalon (midbrain)

Superior view.

Nuclei: The most rostral cranial nerve nucleus is the relatively small *nucleus of the oculomotor nerve* (see **B**, p. 356 and p. 114). In the same transverse section plan the *mesencephalic nucleus of the trigeminal nerve* is also present; other trigeminal nuclei can be identified in sections at caudal levels (see **C**). Unique in the CNS, the mesencephalic nucleus of the trigeminal nerve contains displaced pseudounipolar sensory neurons, closely related to the PNS neurons of the trigeminal ganglion (both populations are derived embryologically from the neural crest). The peripheral processes of these mesencephalic neurons are proprioceptors in the muscles of mastication. The *nucleus of the superior colliculus* is part of the visual system. The *red nucleus* and *substantia nigra* are involved in coordination of motor activity. The red nucleus and all of the cranial nerve nuclei are located in the tegmentum of the mesencephalon, the superior colliculus is in the tectum (roof) of the mesencephalon, and the substantia nigra is in the cerebral peduncle (see **C**, p. 357). Different parts of the reticular formation, a diffuse aggregation of nuclear groups, are visible here and in sections below.

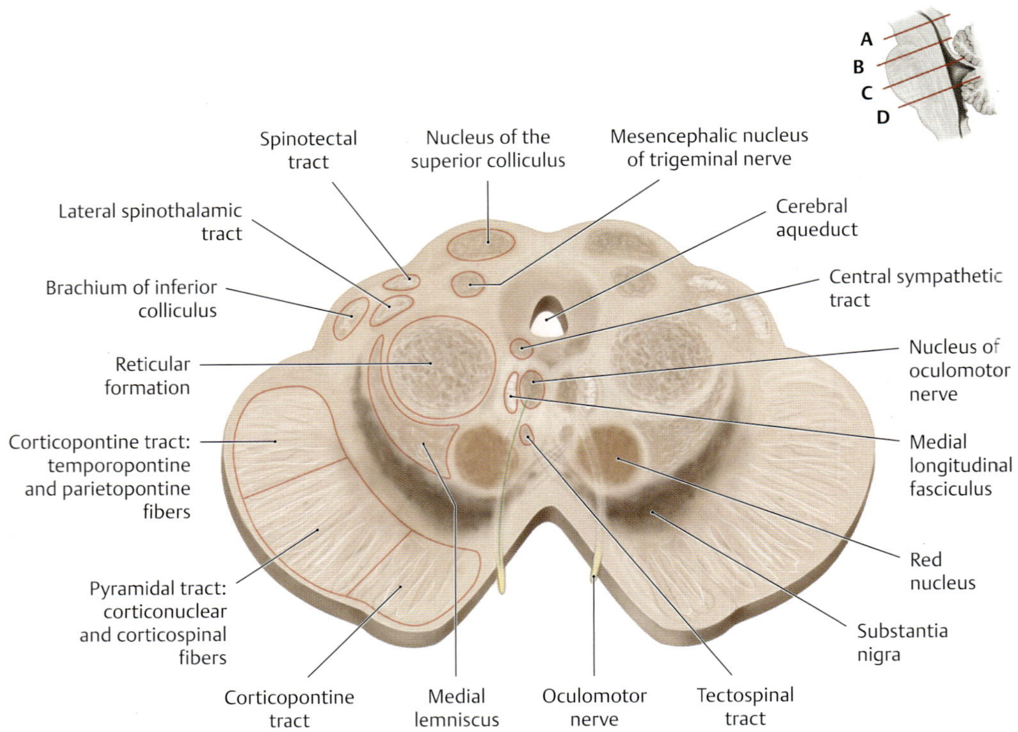

Tracts: The tracts at this level run anterior to the nuclear regions. Prominent descending tracts seen at this level include the pyramidal tract and the corticonuclear fibers. Ascending tracts visible at this level include the lateral spinothalamic tract and the medial lemniscus, both of which terminate in the thalamus.

B Transverse section through the upper pons

Nuclei: The only cranial nerve nucleus appearing in this plane of section is the mesencephalic trigeminal nucleus. It can be seen that the fibers from the nucleus of the trochlear nerve (CN IV) cross to the opposite side (decussate) while still within the brainstem.

Tracts: The ascending and descending tract systems are the same as in **A** and **C**. The pyramidal tract appears less compact at this level compared with the previous section due to the presence of intermingled pontine nuclei. This section cuts the tracts (mostly efferent) that exit the cerebellum through the superior cerebellar peduncle. The lateral lemniscus at the dorsal surface of the section is part of the auditory pathway. The relatively large *medial* longitudinal fasciculus extends from the mesencephalon (see **A**) into the spinal cord. It interconnects the brainstem nuclei and contains a variety of fibers that enter and emerge at various levels (“*highway of the brainstem nuclei*”). The smaller *dorsal* longitudinal fasciculus connects hypothalamic nuclei with the parasympathetic cranial nerve nuclei. The size and location of the nuclei of the reticular formation, which here are shown graphically within a compact area, vary with the plane of the section. This diagram indicates only the approximate location of the reticular formation, and other smaller nuclei and fibers may be found within these regions.

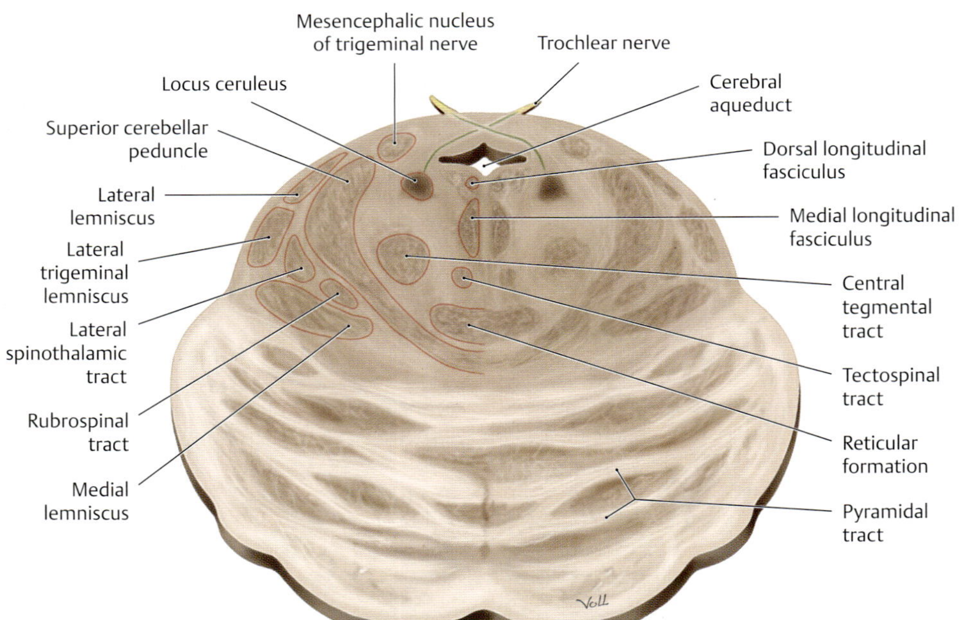

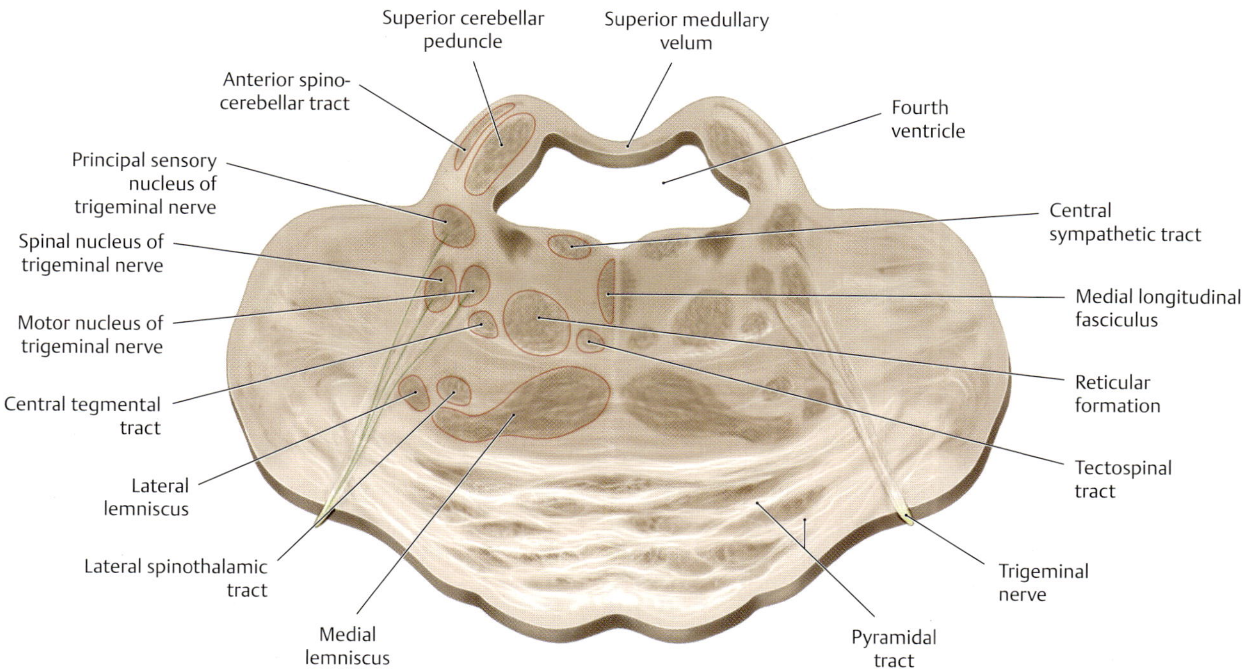

C Transverse section through the midportion of the pons

Nuclei: The trigeminal nerve leaves the brainstem at the midlevel of the pons, its various nuclei dominating the pontine tegmentum. The *principal sensory nucleus* of the trigeminal nerve relays afferents for touch and discrimination, while its *spinal nucleus* relays pain and temperature fibers. The trigeminal motor nucleus contains the motor neurons for the muscles of mastication.

Tracts: This section cuts the anterior spinocerebellar tract, which passes to the cerebellum, immediately dorsal to the pons.

CSF space: At this level the cerebral aqueduct has given way to the fourth ventricle, which appears in cross-section. It is covered dorsally by the medullary velum.

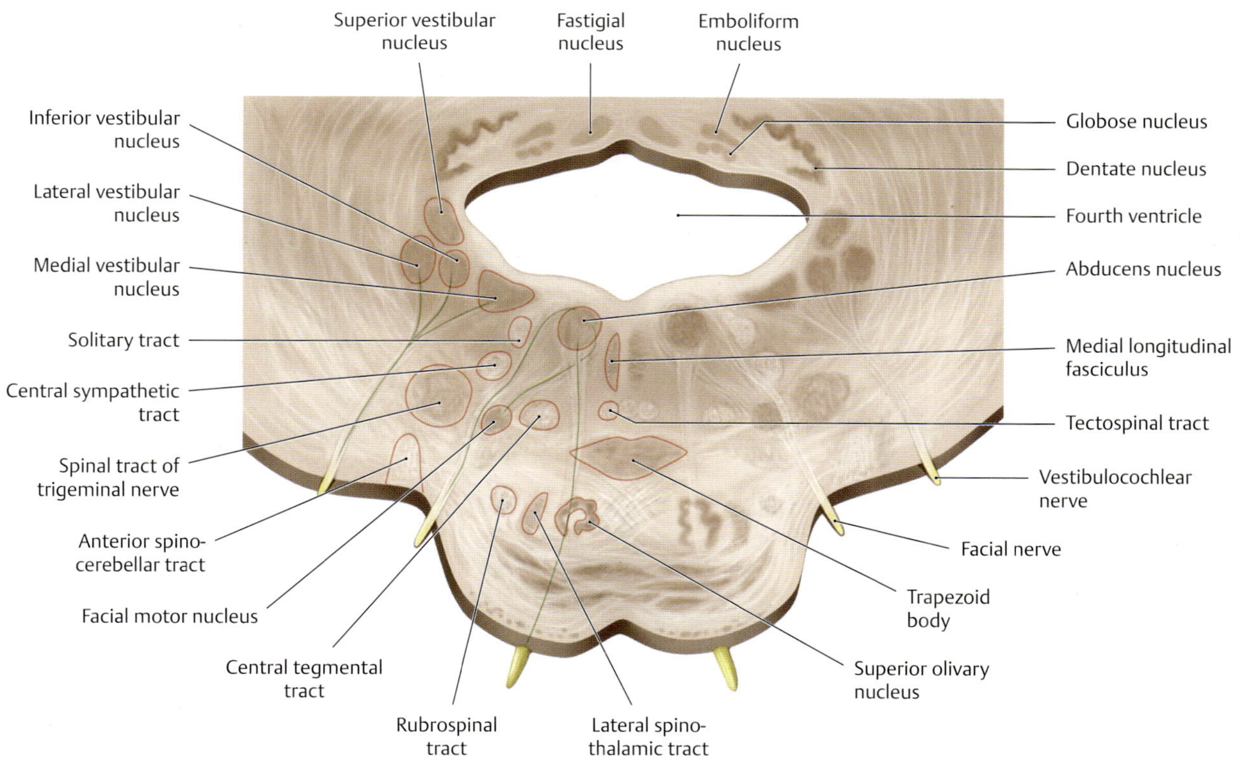

D Transverse section through the lower pons

Nuclei: The lower pons contains a number of cranial nerve nuclei including the nuclei of the vestibulocochlear and abducens nerves, and the facial (motor) nucleus. The rhomboid fossa is covered dorsally by the cerebellum, whose nuclei also appear in this section—the fastigial, emboliform, globose, and dentate nuclei.

Tracts: The trapezoid body with its subnuclei is an important relay station and crossing point in the auditory pathway (see p. 484). The *central tegmental tract* is an important pathway in the motor system.

8.6 Medulla Oblongata, Transverse Section

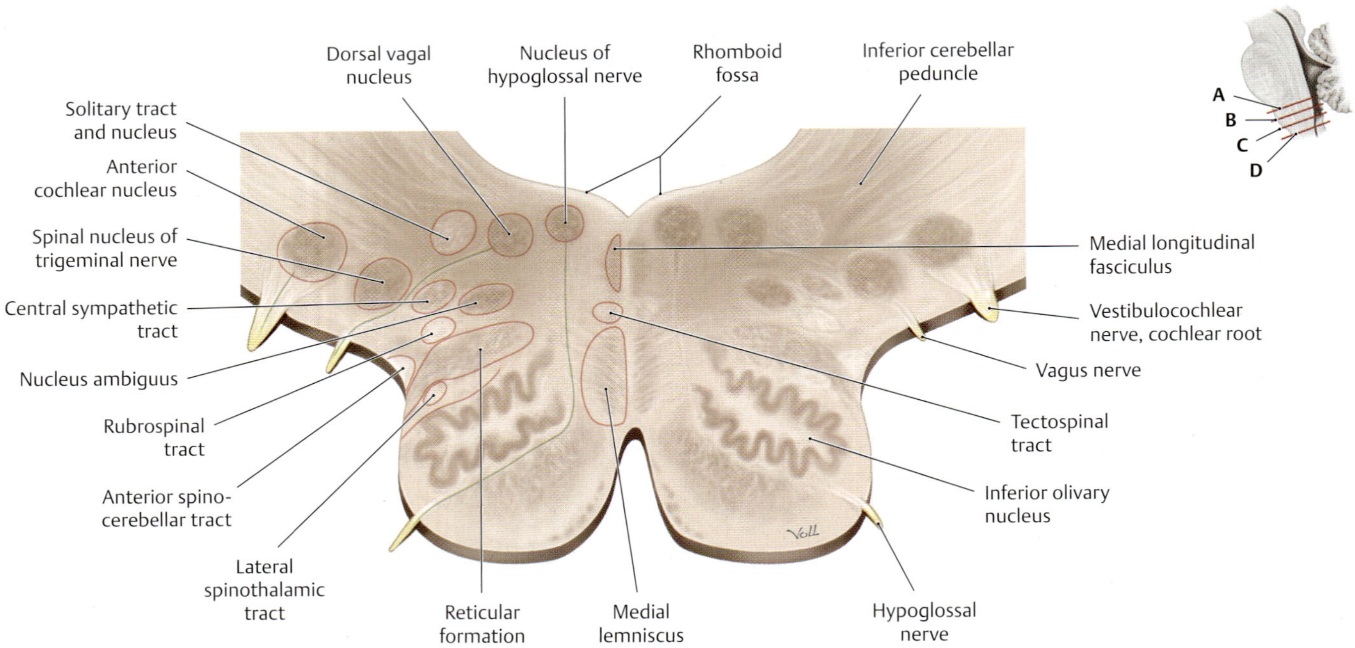

A Transverse section through the upper medulla oblongata

Nuclei: The nuclei of the hypoglossal nerve, vagus nerve, vestibulocochlear nerve, and the spinal nucleus of the trigeminal nerve appear in the *dorsal* part of the medulla oblongata. The inferior olivary nucleus, which belongs to the motor system, is located in the *ventral* part of the medulla oblongata. The reticular formation is interposed between the cranial nerve nuclei and the inferior olivary nucleus. It appears in all the transverse sections of this unit.

Tracts: Most of the ascending and descending tracts are the same as in the previous unit. A new structure appearing at this level is the *inferior cerebellar peduncle*, through which afferent tracts pass to the cerebellum (see p. 361).

CSF space: The floor of the fourth ventricle is the rhomboid fossa, which marks the dorsal boundary of this section.

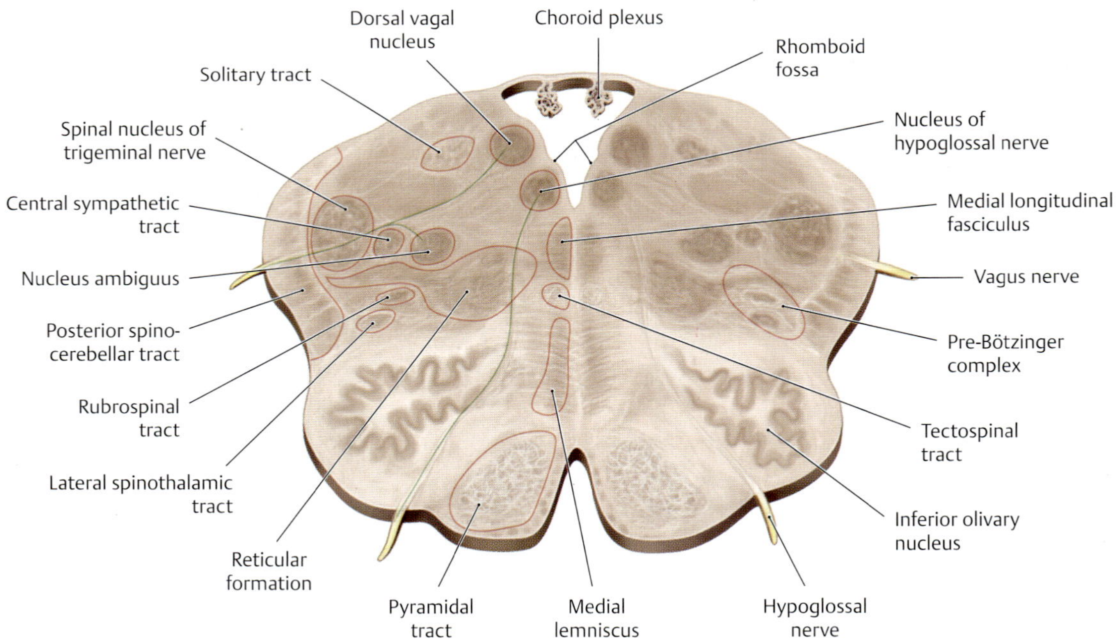

B Transverse section just above the middle of the medulla oblongata

Nuclei: Of the cranial nerve nuclei, only those of the hypoglossal, vagus, and trigeminal nerves remain in the posterior part of the tegmentum. The section passes through the anterior inferior olivary nucleus as well as the pre-Bötzinger complex. It consists of a sparse array of small, lipofuscin-rich neurons that form an integral part of the respiratory network and thus of the mammalian respiratory impulse in the medulla oblongata.

Tracts: The ascending and descending tracts are the same as in the previous unit. The *medial lemniscus* is formed by decussated axons originating in the nuclei gracilis and cuneatus (see p. 404). The solitary tract carries the gustatory fibers of cranial nerves VII, IX, and X. Dorsolateral to it is the *nucleus of the solitary* tract (not shown). The *pyramidal tract* again appears as a compact structure at this level due to the absence of interspersed nuclei and decussating fibers.

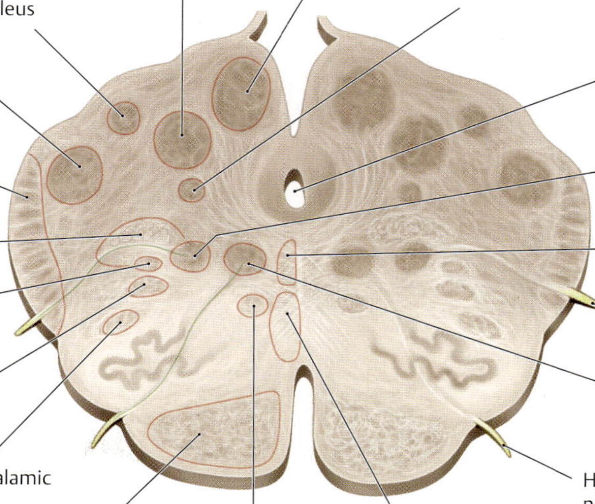

C Transverse section just below the middle of the medulla oblongata

Nuclei: The nuclei of the hypoglossal, and vagus as well as the spinal trigeminal nucleus appear at this level. The irregular outline of the inferior olivary nucleus is still just visible in the ventral medulla. The nuclei that relay signals from the posterior funiculus—the nucleus cuneatus and nucleus gracilis—appear prominently in the dorsal part of the section. The axons that arise from these nuclei decussate and form the medial lemniscus (see above).

Tracts: The ascending and descending tracts correspond to those in the previous diagrams. The rhomboid fossa, which is the floor of the fourth ventricle, has narrowed substantially at this level to become the central canal.

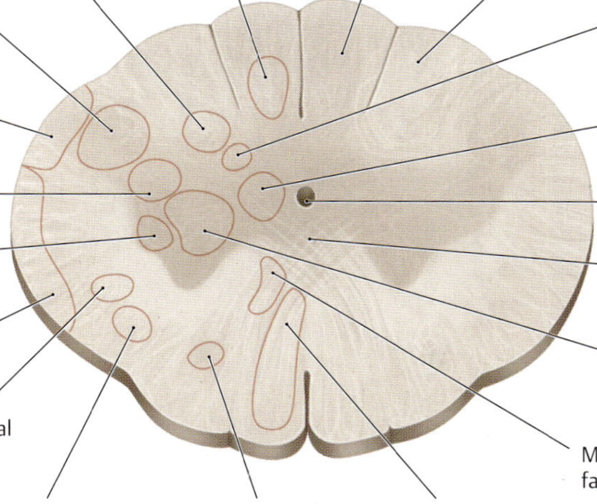

D Transverse section through the lower medulla oblongata

The medulla oblongata is continuous with the spinal cord at this level, showing no distinct transition.

Nuclei: The cranial nerve nuclei visible at this level are the spinal part of the spinal trigeminal nucleus and the nucleus of the accessory nerve. This section passes through the caudal end of the nuclei in the nucleus cuneatus and nucleus gracilis, which are a relay station for the posterior funiculus.

Tracts: The ascending and descending tracts correspond to those in the previous diagrams of this unit. The section passes through the decussation of the pyramids, and we can now distinguish the anterior pyramidal tract (uncrossed) from the lateral pyramidal tract (crossed; see pp. 409 and 461).

CSF space: This section passes through a portion of the central canal, which is markedly smaller at this level than in **C**. It may even be obliterated at some sites, but this has no clinical significance.

9.1 Cerebellum, External Structure

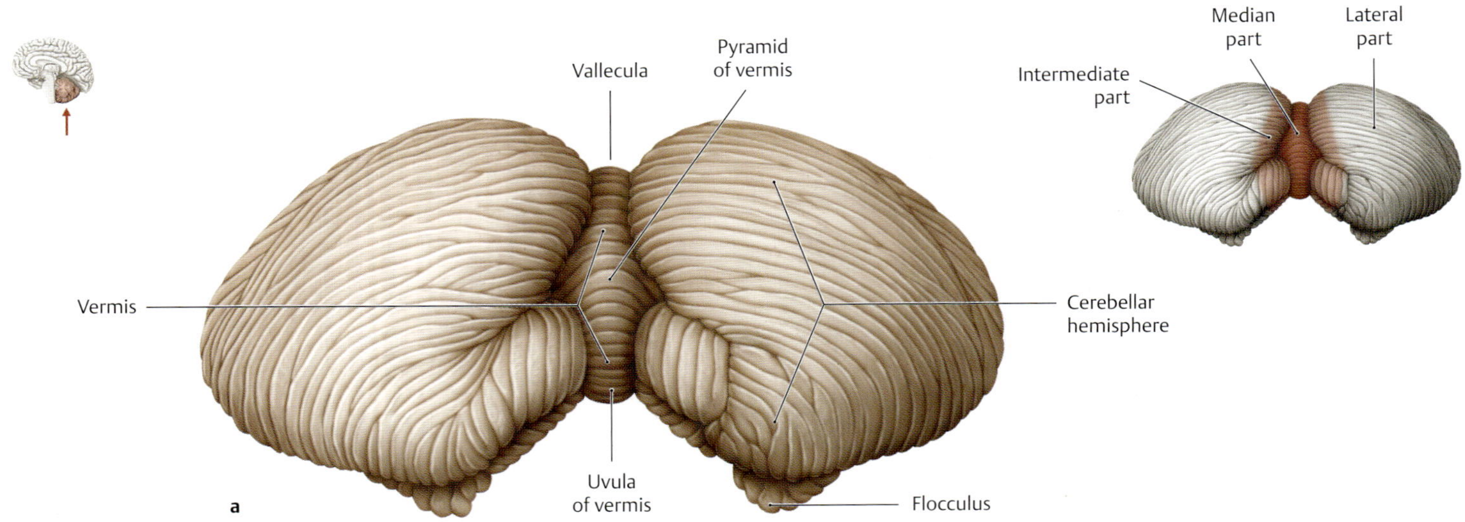

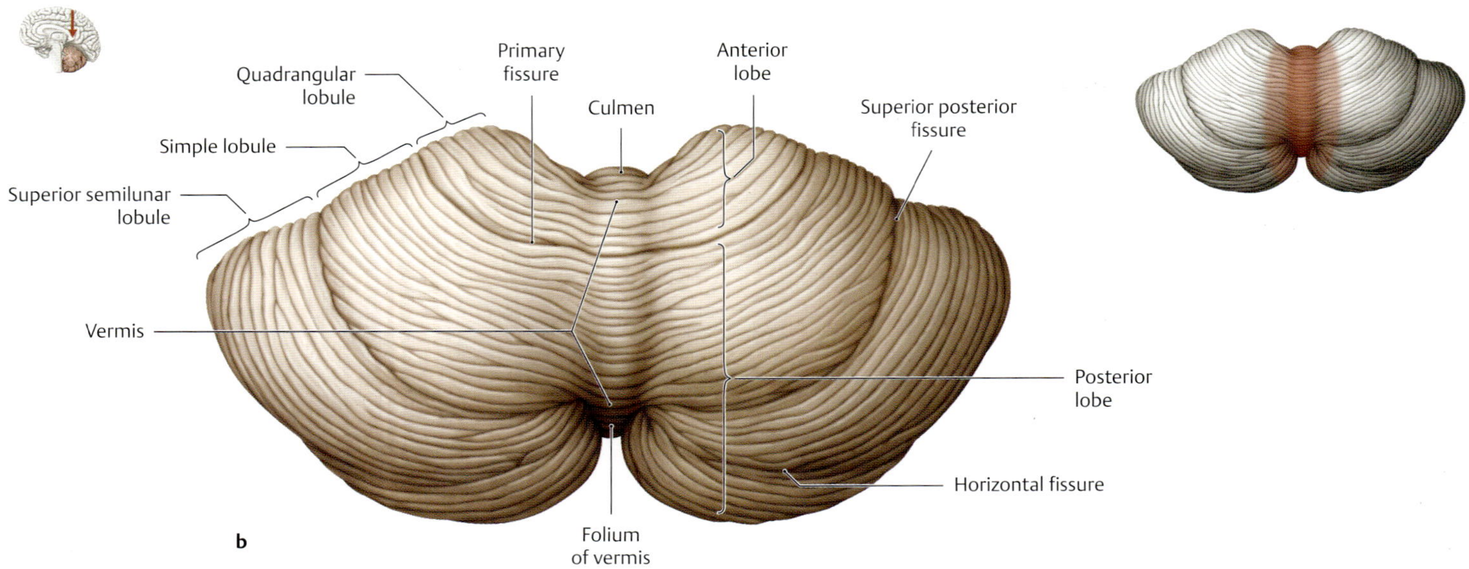

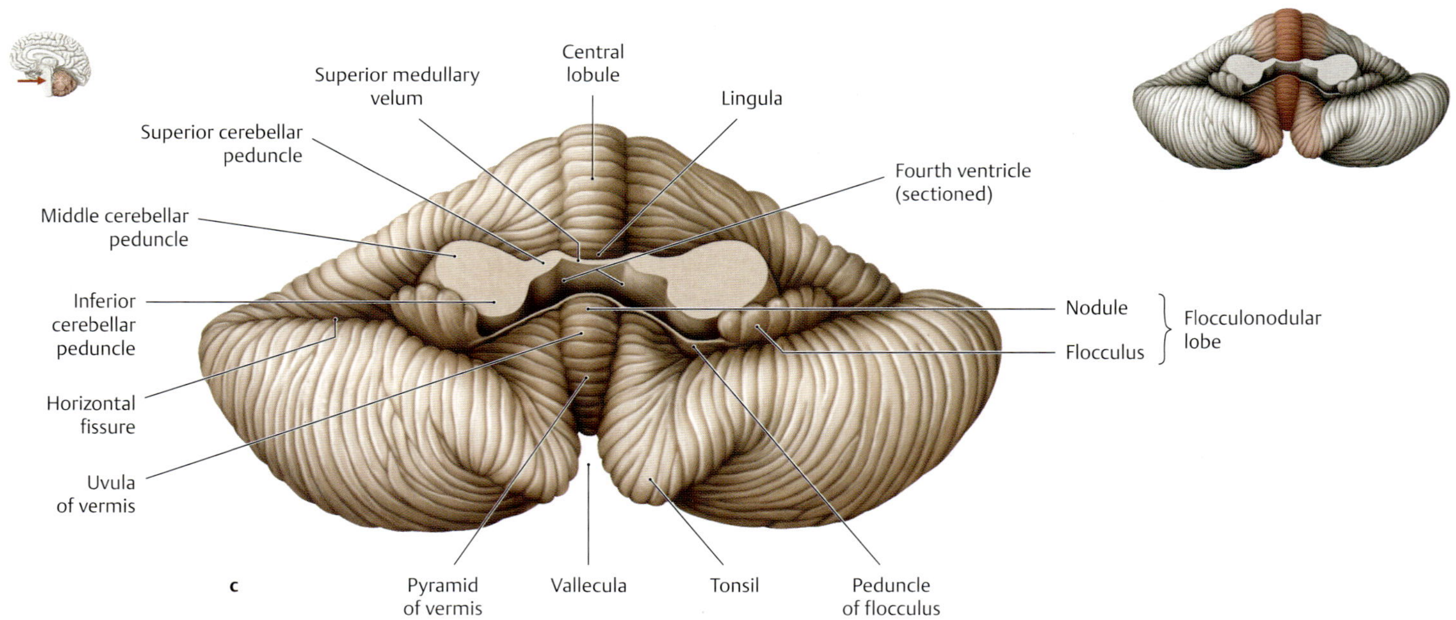

A Isolated cerebellum
a Inferior view, **b** superior view, c anterior view. Cerebellum with the cerebellar peduncles detached from the brainstem.
Functionally, the cerebellum is largely part of the motor system. However, it does not trigger any conscious movements but is responsible for planning and execution of ongoing movements (unconscious coordination and fine-tuning of movements) (see **B**, p. 372). Just like the telencephalon, the cerebellum consists of two hemispheres. The two cerebral hemispheres, are largely separated from one another but connected by commissural tracts of axons. Between cerebellar hemispheres lies an unpaired, worm-shaped structure—the cerebellar vermis. It is a portion of the cerebellum which exhibits the same structure as the hemispheres. Unlike the telencephalon, where all gyri and sulci are individually named, the cerebellar folia and fissures are not. However, similar to the gyri and sulci, their role is also to increase the surface area of the cortex. Cerebellar fissures further subdivide the cerebellum into lobes. In particular:

- The primary fissure separates the anterior lobe of the cerebellum from the posterior lobe (see **b**).
- The posterolateral fissure separates the posterior lobe of the cerebellum from the flocculonodular lobe (see **B**).

Other, less important fissures have no clinical or functional significance and are not described here. Besides these anatomical divisions, the parts of the cerebellum can also be distinguished according to *phylogenetic* and *functional* criteria (see **B**, p. 372). The cerebellum is connected to the brainstem via the three pairs of cerebellar peduncles (superior, middle, and inferior cerebellar peduncles [see **c**]). The cerebral peduncles are not equal in size. They contain the afferent and efferent tracts that connect the cerebellum with other parts of the CNS. The brainstem shows the analogous sections of the cerebellar peduncles (see **C**, **b** and **c**, p. 355). The superior medullary velum stretches between the two superior cerebellar peduncles and forms part of the roof of the fourth ventricle (see **c**). The cerebellar tonsils protrude downward near the midline on each side, almost to the foramen magnum at the base of the skull (not shown). Increased intracranial pressure may cause the cerebellar tonsils to herniate into the foramen magnum, impinging upon vital centers in the brainstem and posing a threat to life (see **D**, p. 309). Functionally, the medial part of the *cerebellum* (red) is distinguished from the *intermediate part* (pale red) and *lateral part* (gray). This functional classification does not conform to the anatomically defined lobar boundaries. Each of these parts projects to a specific cerebellar nucleus (see p. 368).

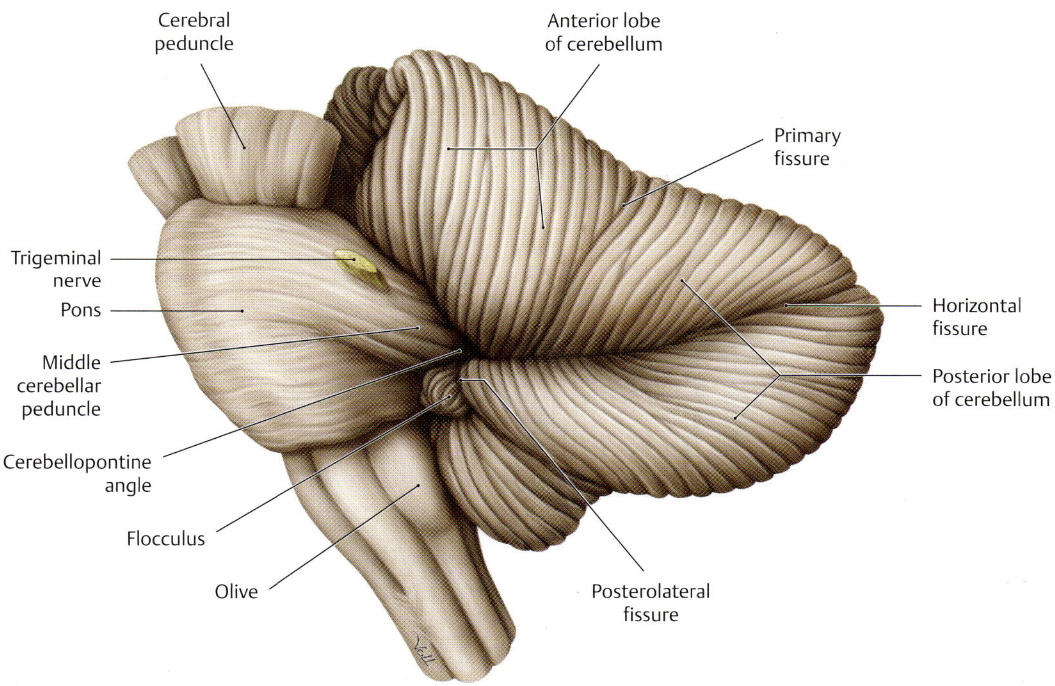

B Cerebellum on the brainstem
Left lateral view. For the brainstem and cerebellum, which overlies the dorsal aspect of the brainstem, the same terms of location and direction are used. In the lateral view, only the cerebellar hemispheres and the flocculus are visible as well as, the middle cerebellar peduncle along with its origin in the pons. At the angle formed at the junction of the pons and cerebellum (the cerebellopontine angle), cranial nerves VII and VIII are attached to the brainstem (not shown here, see **Ca**, p. 355). Occasionally, the vestibulocochlear nerve (cranial nerve VIII) develops an acoustic neuroma. Based on their localization, these tumors are referred to as cerebellopontine angle tumors (see **D**, p. 151). Due to the damage to cranial nerve VIII, affected patients mainly suffer from impaired hearing or balance.

C Synopsis of cerebellar classifications

Phylogenetic classification	Anatomical classification	Functional classification based on the origin of afferents
• Archicerebellum	• Flocculonodular lobe	• Vestibulocerebellum: maintenance of equilibrium and eye movement control
• Paleocerebellum	• Anterior lobe of cerebellum • Portions of the vermis • Medial portions of the posterior lobe	• Spinocerebellum: regulation of muscle tone
• Neocerebellum	• Lateral portions of the posterior lobe	• Pontocerebellum (= cerebrocerebellum): skilled movements, especially of distal part of the limbs

9.2 Cerebellum, Internal Structure

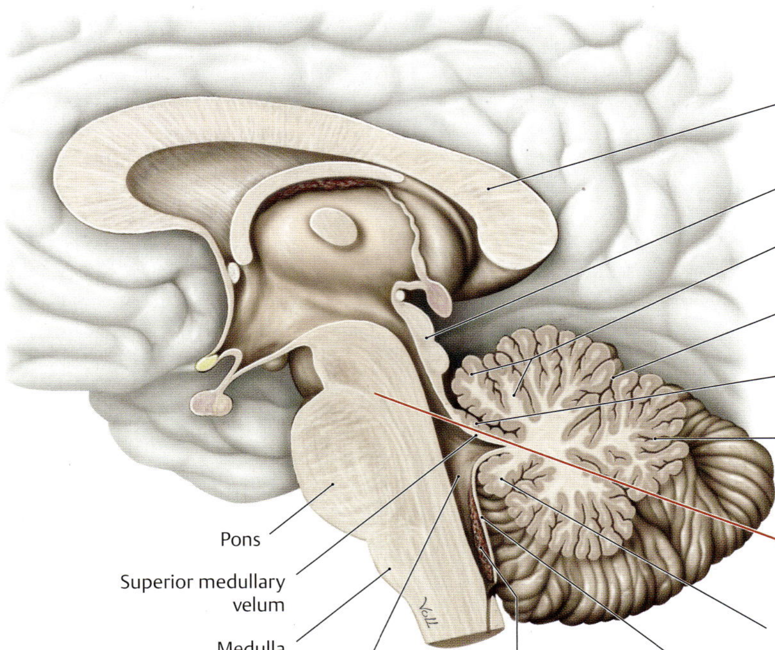

A Cerebellum: Positional relationship and cut surface
Midsagittal section, left lateral view. The cerebellum extends along almost the entire dorsal surface of the brainstem and abuts the tectum of the mesencephalon in the rostral direction and the medulla oblongata in the caudal direction. Its superior and inferior medullary vela form the roof of the fourth ventricle. The cerebellar lingula overlies the superior medullary velum and the inferior medullary velum lies below the nodulus. Such a midsagittal section shows only the part of the medially located unpaired vermis. The laterally located hemispheres remain intact. The primary fissure (that slants superiorly and dorsally) separates the anterior and posterior lobes, which, due to their lateral position, are not visible here (see **C**, p. 368). The (deep) cerebellar nuclei, which are located in the white matter of the cerebellum are barely visible on midsagittal sections. A slightly dorsocaudal-oblique view displays all the cerebellar nuclei (see **B**).

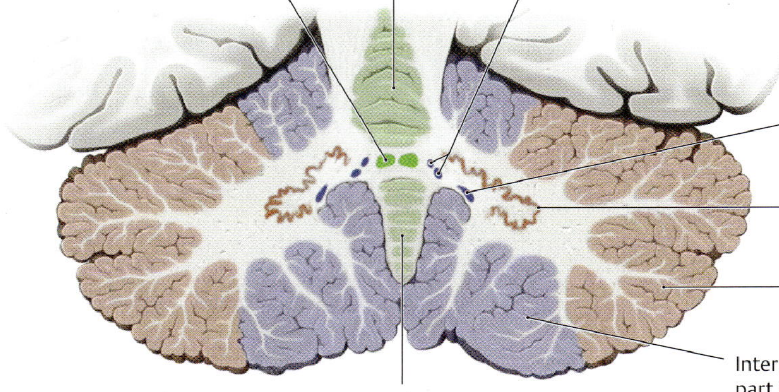

B Nuclei of the cerebellum
Section through the superior cerebellar peduncles (plane of section shown in **A**), viewed from behind. Deep within the cerebellar white matter are four pairs of nuclei that contain most of the *efferent* neurons of the cerebellum:

- Fastigial nucleus (green)
- Emboliform nucleus (blue)
- Globose nuclei (blue)
- Dentate nucleus (pink).

The cortical regions have been color-coded to match their corresponding nuclei. The dentate nucleus is the largest of the cerebellar nuclei and extends into the cerebellar hemispheres. The cerebellar nuclei receive projections from Purkinje cells in the cerebellar cortex (cf. p. 366). While the *efferent fibers* of the cerebellum can be assigned rather easily to anatomical structures, this is not true of the afferent fibers. Their sources are examined on p. 372.

C Cerebellar nuclei and the regions of the cortex from which they receive projections (cf. p. 371)

Cerebellar nucleus	Synonyms	Regions of the cerebellar cortex that send axons to the nucleus
Dentate nucleus	Lateral cerebellar nucleus	Lateral part (lateral portions of the cerebellar hemispheres)
Emboliform nucleus	Anterior interpositus nucleus	Intermediate part (medial portions of the cerebellar hemispheres)
Globose nuclei	Posterior interpositus nucleus	Intermediate part (medial portions of the cerebellar hemispheres)
Fastigial nucleus	Medial cerebellar nucleus	Median part (cerebellar vermis) and flocculonodulus

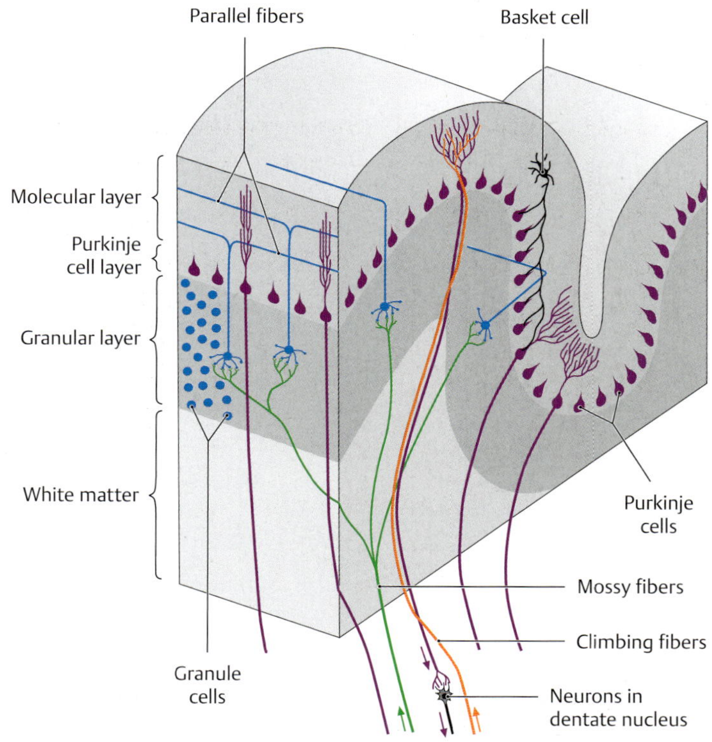

D Diagram of synaptic circuitry within the cerebellar cortex

The cerebellar cortex consists of three layers:

- Molecular layer: outer layer; contains *parallel fibers*, which are the axons of granule cells (blue) from the granular layer. They run parallel to the cerebellar folia and terminate in the molecular layer, where they synapse on the dendrites of the Purkinje cells. This layer also contains also contains *climbing fibers* (which are axons from the inferior olive and its accessory nuclei), as well as inhibitory interneurons (*basket and stellate cells*).
- Purkinje layer: contains the cell bodies of *Purkinje cells* (purple).
- Granular layer: contains mostly *granule cells* (blue), as well as *mossy* and *climbing fibers* (green and orange, respectively), and *Golgi cells* (not shown; the cell types are viewed in **F**).

The white matter of the cerebellum is located under the granular layer.

Note: The Purkinje cells are the only efferent cells of the cerebellar cortex and project to the cerebellar and vestibular nuclei.

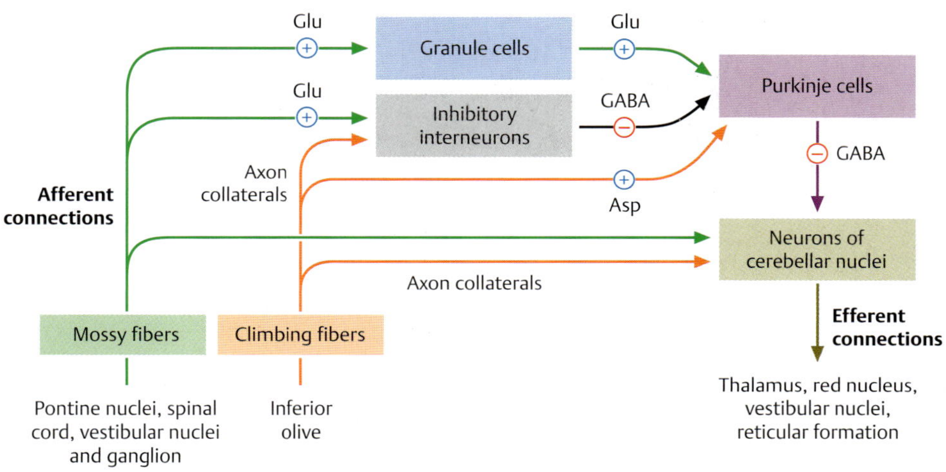

E Synaptic circuitry of the cerebellum
(after Bähr and Frotscher)

Afferents on the left, efferents on the right. The cerebellum comprises 10% of the mass of the brain, but slightly more than 50% of its neurons. This is in indication of the complexity of the motor circuitry in the cerebellum. The **afferents** reach the cerebellum via climbing fibers and mossy fibers: The *climbing fibers* end in the dendritic tree of Purkinje cells, where they release their excitatory transmitter aspartic acid (ASP; see **D**). Their axon collaterals extend to inhibitory intermediate neurons and especially to the neurons of the cerebellar nuclei. The *mossy fibers* branch out and give off numerous axon collaterals. Some of the mossy fibers form synapses on the dendrites of the granule cells whose neurotransmitter glutamate has an excitatory effect on Purkinje cells. Another part of the mossy fibers ends at inhibitory intermediate neurons, which inhibit Purkinje cells by means of their inhibitory neurotransmitter GABA. The mossy fibers also send axon collaterals to the cerebellum which are important for function. As mentioned above, the **efferents** of the cerebellum are localized in the cerebellum. Their neurons send basically efferent, excitatory impulses to the periphery. Impulses from the cerebellum are specifically inhibited by the Purkinje cells, which also contain the inhibitory neurotransmitter GABA, as well as by the adjacent vestibular nuclei. This ensures a coordinated sequence of movements. When the Purkinje cells themselves are inhibited by inhibitory intermediate neurons (see black arrow), the impulses from the cerebellum are transmitted without inhibition so that the motion sequences are impaired (see p. 373).

F Principal neurons and fiber types in the cerebellar cortex

Name	Definition
Climbing fibers	Axons of neurons in the inferior olive and its associated nuclei
Mossy fibers	Axons of neurons in the pontine nuclei, the spinal cord, and vestibular nuclei (pontocerebellar, spinocerebellar, and vestibular tracts)
Parallel fibers (see **D**)	Axons of granule cells
Granule cells	Interneurons of the cerebellar cortex
Purkinje cells	The only efferent cells of the cerebellar cortex; exert an inhibitory effect

9.3 Cerebellar Peduncles and Tracts

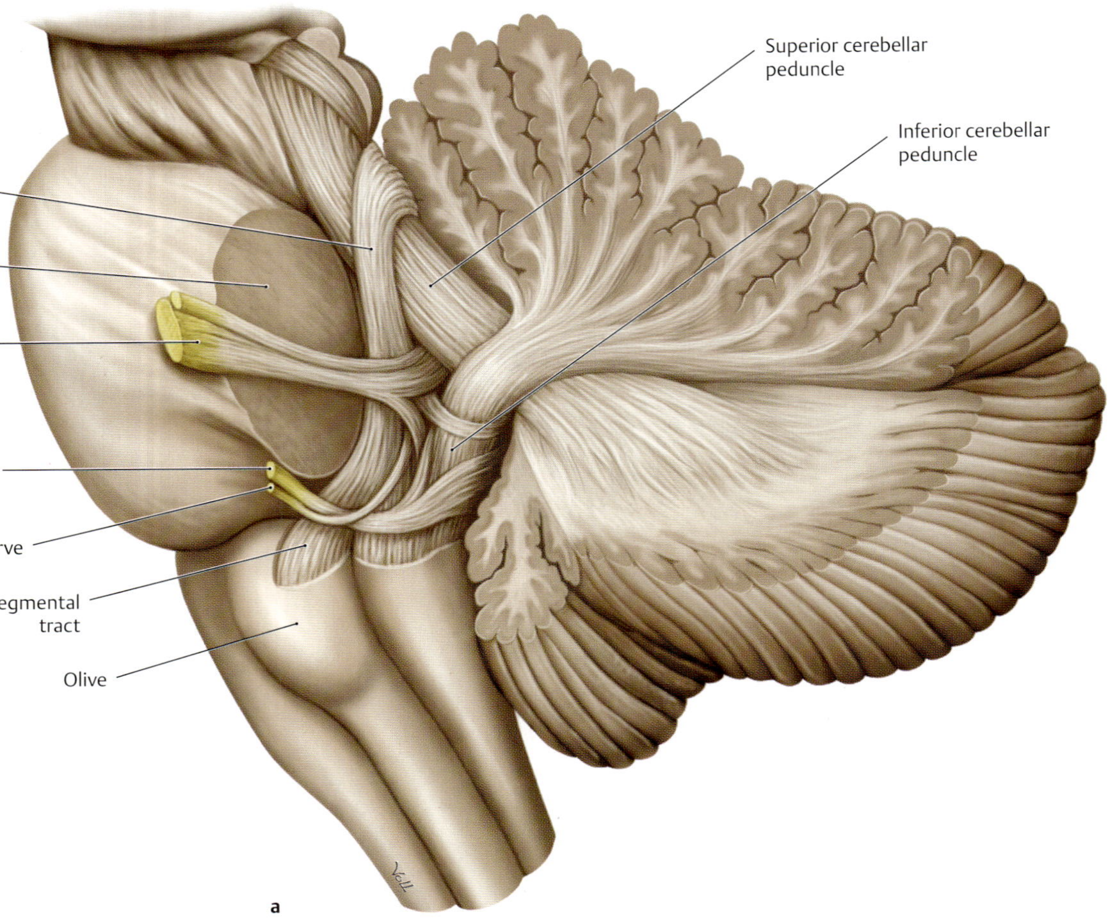

a

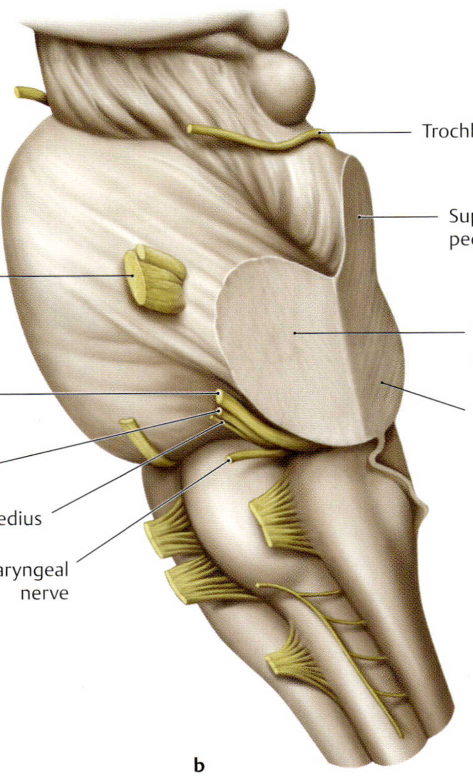

b

A Cerebellar peduncles

a Left lateral view with the upper portion of the cerebellum and lateral portions of the pons removed. This dissection, which has been prepared to show fiber structure, clearly shows the course of the cerebellar tracts. The size of the cerebellar peduncles, and thus the mass of entering and emerging axons, is substantial and reflects the extensive neural connections in the cerebellum (see p. 369). The cerebellum requires these numerous connections because it is an integrating center for the coordination of fine movements. In particular, it contains and processes vestibular and proprioceptive afferents and it modulates motor nuclei in other brain regions and in the spinal cord. The principal afferent and efferent connections of the cerebellum are reviewed in **B**.

b Left lateral view. Here the cerebellum has been sharply detached from its peduncles to demonstrate the complementary cut surface of the peduncles on the brainstem (compare with **Ac**, p. 366).

B Synopsis of the cerebellar peduncles and their tracts

Tracts made up of afferent and efferent axons enter or leave the cerebellum through the cerebellar peduncles. The afferent axons originate in the spinal cord, vestibular organs, inferior olive and pons, while the efferent axons originate in the cerebellar nuclei (see p. 368). The representation of the body in the cerebellum, unlike in the cerebrum, is ipsilateral. Ascending cerebellar pathways thus are either uncrossed or cross (decussate) twice in order to reach the same side. Compare the synopsis of the distinct tract systems (p. 445).

Cerebellar peduncle and constituent parts*	Origin**	Site of termination
Superior cerebellar peduncle: contains mostly efferent tracts from the cerebellar nuclei. Some tracts cross in the decussation of the superior cerebellar peduncles, then divide into a *descending* part (to the pons) and an *ascending* part (to the midbrain and thalamus).		
Descending parts (**e**)	Fastigial and globose nuclei	Reticular formation and vestibular nuclei (projection is mostly *contralateral*)
Ascending parts (**e**)	Dentate nucleus	Red nucleus and thalamus (both *contralateral*)
Anterior spinocerebellar tract (**a**)	Secondary neurons in intermediate gray matter, lumbosacral spinal cord. Relay proprioception stimuli related to lower limbs and trunk (muscle spindles, tendon receptors, etc.) received from the dorsal root ganglion. Fibers cross locally and then re-cross in the pons to return to the ipsilateral side.	Vermis and intermediate part of anterior lobe of cerebellum (they bring information from the ipsilateral side of the body since this pathway crosses twice on its way from the spinal cord to the cerebellum). Terminate as mossy fibers.
Middle cerebellar peduncle: contains only afferent tracts to the cerebellum		
Pontocerebellar fibers (**a**)	Basal pontine nuclei. Relay cerebropontine to pontocerebellar projections (source of 90% of the axons in middle peduncle)	Lateral regions of posterior and anterior lobes of cerebellum (*contralateral* to the origin of these fibers in pons; terminate as mossy fibers; branches to dentate nucleus, also contralateral to the origin in pons)
Inferior cerebellar peduncle: contains both afferent and efferent tracts		
Posterior spinocerebellar tract (**a**)	Clarke's nucleus/column. Relays proprioception and cutaneous sensation from the lower limb. Contains large axons with high conduction velocity.	Vermis and nearby anterior lobe of cerebellum, pyramid, and nearby posterior lobe of cerebellum. (*ipsilateral*; terminates as mossy fibers)
Cuneocerebellar tract (**a**)	Nucleus cuneatus and external cuneate nucleus. Relays proprioception (external cuneate nucleus) and cutaneous sensation (nucleus cuneatus) from the upper limb, with fast transmission, functionally corresponding to the posterior spinocerebellar tract.	Posterior part of anterior lobe of cerebellum (*ipsilateral*; terminates as mossy fibers).
Olivocerebellar tract (**a**)	Inferior olivary nuclear complex. Inferior olive receives numerous inputs from sensory and motor systems, including a large contralateral projection from the cerebellum itself (dentate nucleus, see below).	Molecular layer of cerebellar cortex (*contralateral*, terminates as climbing fibers)
Vestibulocerebellar tract (**a**)	Semicircular canals (vestibular ganglion) and vestibular nuclei. Transmits balance and body position/motion information either directly (vestibular axons via vestibulocochlear nerve [CN VIII], *ipsilateral*) or via synaptic relay in vestibular nuclei (*bilateral*).	Nodule, flocculus, anterior lobe, and vermis of cerebellum (*bilateral*, see left; terminates as mossy fibers)
Trigeminocerebellar fibers (**a**)	Trigeminal sensory nuclei in the brainstem. Relay proprioception and cutaneous sensation from the head.	Rostral part of posterior lobe of cerebellum (*ipsilateral*; terminate as mossy fibers)
Cerebello-olivary fibers (**e**)	Dentate nucleus	Inferior olive (*contralateral*)

* Subentries for constituent parts are classified as efferent (**e**) or afferent (**a**).

** In the case of afferents, the type of afferent is listed along with the site of origin.

9.4 Cerebellum, Simplified Functional Anatomy and Lesions

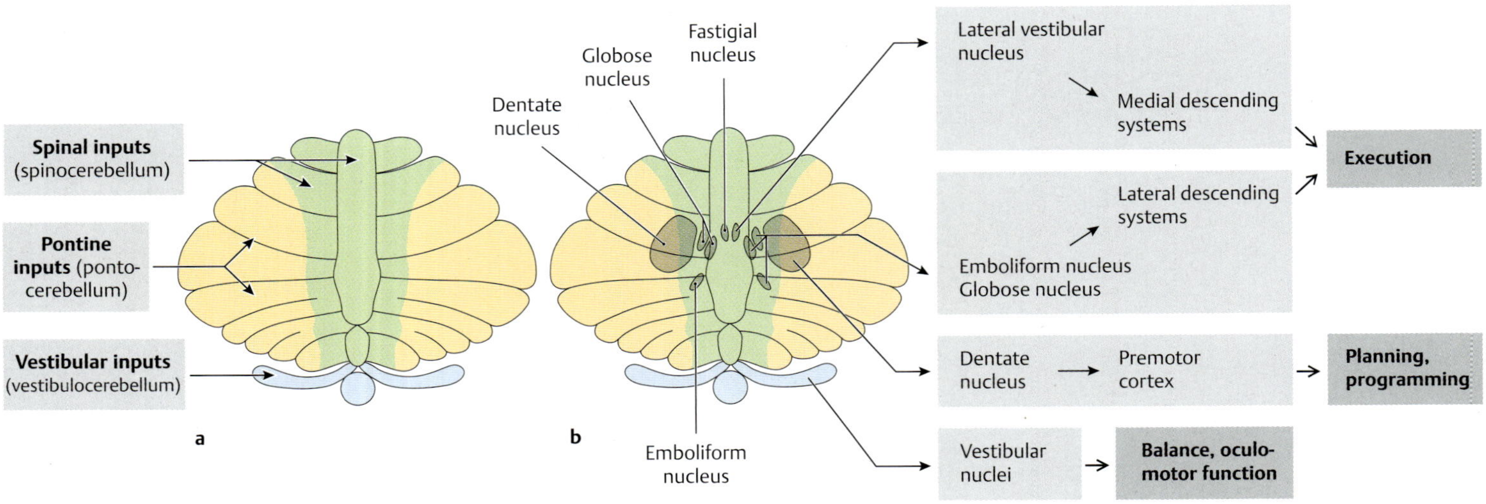

A Simplified functional anatomy of the cerebellum

Two-dimensional representation of the cerebellum. From a functional standpoint, the cerebellum can be divided into three sections. They are named according to the CNS structures from which they receive information via afferent tracts:

- The *spino*cerebellum (green) receives information from the *spinal cord* about the posture and position of the trunk and extremities.
- The *ponto*cerebellum (yellow) receives information from the telencephalon that was previously relayed by nuclei in the *pons*. This is primarily information about fine motor function.
- The *vestibulo*cerebellum (blue) receives information about the position and motion of the skull in space from the *vestibular* nuclei in the brainstem.

After the afferent information has been processed, the cerebellar cortex sends *efferent* impulses to the *cerebellar nuclei*, the eventual cerebellar efferents (shown on the right side).

- The fastigial nucleus and lateral vestibular nucleus coordinate the activity of skeletal muscles and thus movement via the *medial* descending systems; emboliform and globose nuclei via the *lateral* descending systems (see p. 410).
- The dentate nucleus projects to the cerebral cortex and thus exerts influences on the planning and programming of movements.
- Efferents from the vestibulocerebellum control balance and oculomotor functions.

Visual inputs have not been considered here.

B Synopsis of cerebellar classifications and their relationships to motor deficits

Some cerebellar lesions cause subtle cognitive deficits that cannot be explained simply as a loss of muscle coordination.

Phylogenetic classification	Anatomical classification	Functional classification	Deficit symptoms (see **C**)
• Archicerebellum	• Flocculonodular lobe	• Vestibulocerebellum	• Truncal, stance, and gait ataxia • Oculomotor dysfunction • Vertigo • Nystagmus • Vomiting
• Paleocerebellum	• Anterior lobe, parts of vermis • Posterior lobe, medial parts	• Spinocerebellum	• Ataxia, chiefly affecting the lower limb • Speech disorder (asynergy of speech muscles)
• Neocerebellum	• Posterior lobe, hemispheres	• Pontocerebellum (= cerebrocerebellum)	• Dysmetria/hypermetria (positive rebound) • Dysdiadochokinesia • Intention tremor • Nystagmus • Decreased muscle tone

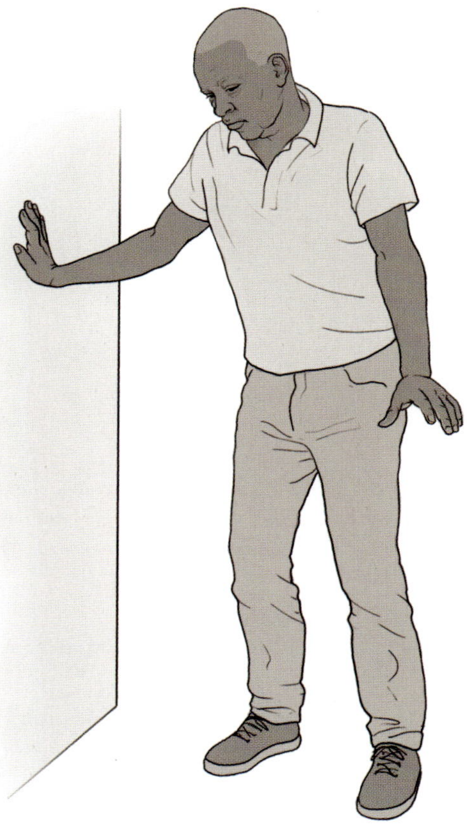

a

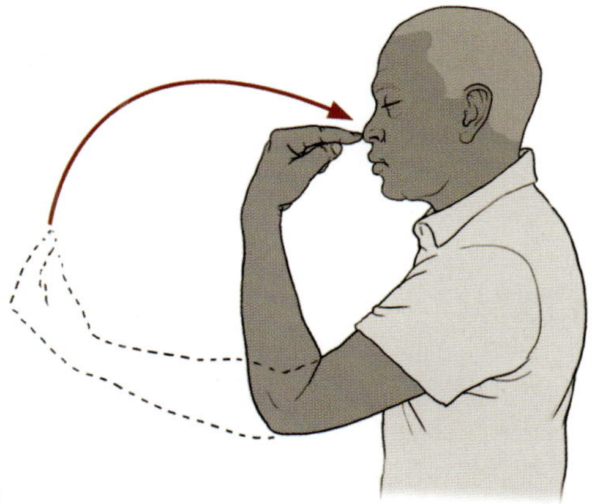

b

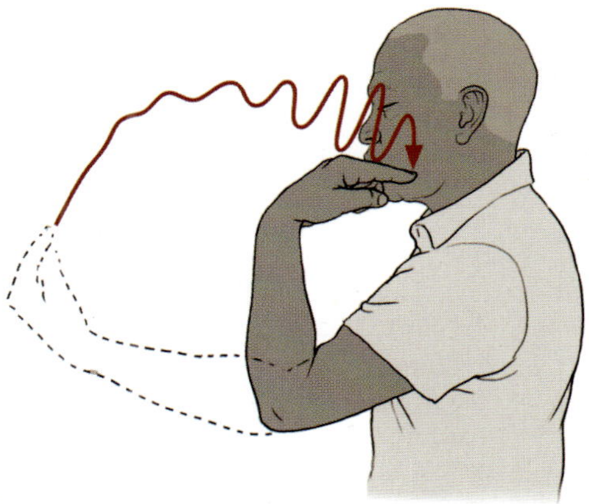

c

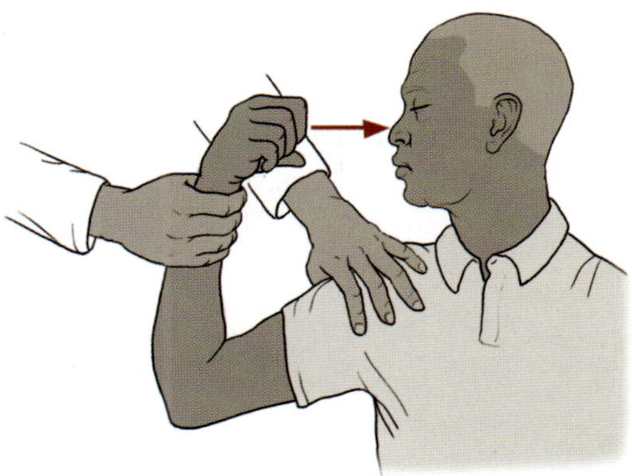

d

C Cerebellar lesions

Cerebellar lesions may remain clinically silent for some time because other brain regions can functionally compensate for them with reasonable effectiveness. Exceptions are direct lesions of the efferent cerebellar nuclei, which cannot be clinically compensated.

Cerebellar symptoms:

Asynergy	Lack of coordination among different muscle groups, especially in the performance of fine movements.
Ataxia	Uncoordinated sequence of movements. Truncal ataxia (patient cannot sit quietly upright) is distinguished from stance and gait ataxia (impaired limb movements, such as an unsteady gait in inebriation). The patient stands with the legs spread apart and places his hand on the wall for stability (**a**).
Decreased muscle tone	Ipsilateral muscle weakness and rapid fatigability (asthenia).
Intention tremor	Involuntary, rhythmical wavering movement of the hand when a purposeful movement is attempted, as in the finger-nose test: normal test (**b**), test indicating a cerebellar lesion (**c**).
Rebound phenomenon	The patient, with eyes closed, is told to move the arm against a resistance from the examiner (**d**). When the examiner suddenly releases the arm, it forcefully "rebounds" toward the patient (hypermetria).

10.1 Arteries of the Brain: Blood Supply and the Circle of Willis

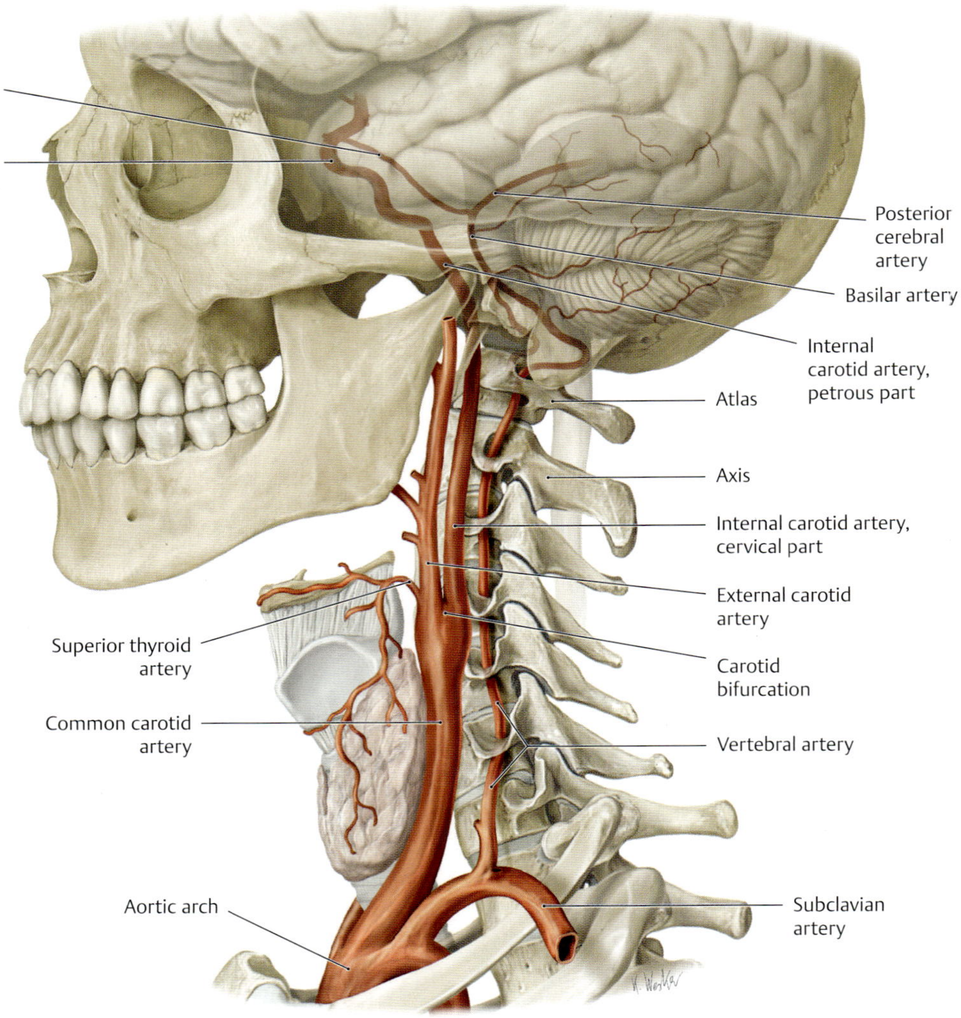

A Overview of the arterial supply to the brain

Left lateral view. The internal carotid a. primarily supplies parts of the brain in the anterior and middle cranial fossae (carotid territory), whereas parts in the posterior cranial fossa (including cerebellum and brainstem) receive their blood supply from the vertebral aa. or basilar a. (vertebrobasilar territory). The carotid and vertebrobasilar territories are connected by the arterial circle (of Willis) at the base of the brain, which in many cases ensures compensation of decreased blood flow in one vessel with increased blood flow through another vessel. That can lead to the shifting of blood from one side to the other or from posterior to anterior and vice versa. The pulse of the large internal carotid a. is so strong that its wave makes the brain vibrate. *Note:* The vertebral a. runs through the transverse foramen of the cervical vertebrae from C6 to C1. If narrowing of the foramina due to pathological processes occurs, the compression of the vertebral a. can lead to impaired blood supply of occipital areas of the cerebrum and the cerebellum. The primary symptom for this would be vertigo.

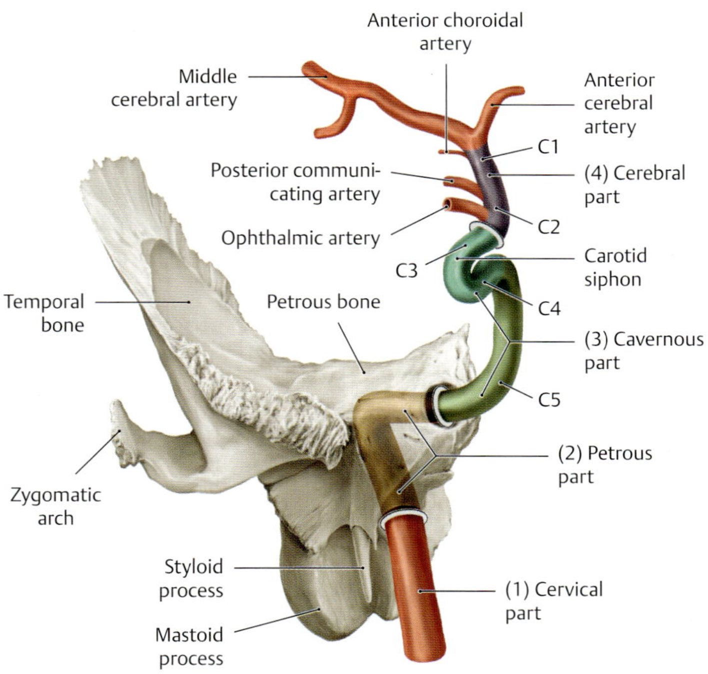

B The four anatomical divisions of the internal carotid artery

Anterior view of the left internal carotid artery. The internal carotid artery consists of four topographically distinct parts between the carotid bifurcation (see **A**) and the point where it divides into the anterior and middle cerebral arteries. The parts (separated in the figure by white disks) are as follows:

(1) Cervical part (red): located in the lateral pharyngeal space.
(2) Petrous part (yellow): located in the carotid canal of the petrous bone.
(3) Cavernous part (green): follows an S-shaped curve in the cavernous sinus.
(4) Cerebral part (purple): located in the chiasmatic cistern of the subarachnoid space

Except for the cervical part which generally does not give off branches, all the other parts of the internal carotid artery give off numerous branches (see p. 102). The *intracranial* parts of the internal carotid artery are subdivided into five segments (C1–C5) based on clinical criteria:

- C1–C2: the supraclinoid segments, located within the cerebral part. C1 and C2 lie above the anterior clinoid process of the lesser wing of the sphenoid bone.
- C3–C5: the infraclinoid segments, located within the cavernous sinus

The segments C2–C4 form the carotid siphon.

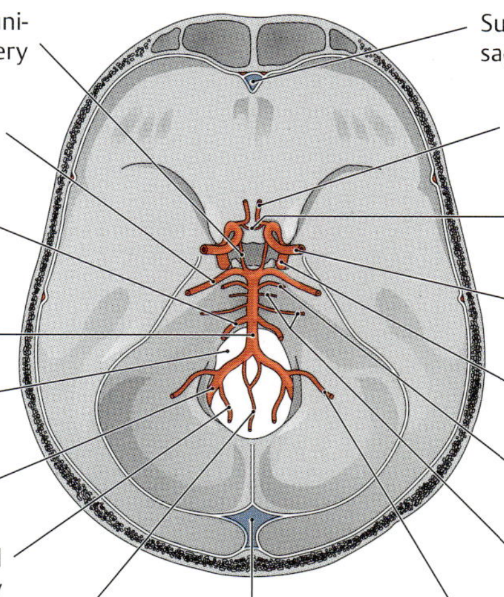

C Projection of the circle of Willis onto the base of the skull

Superior view. The two vertebral arteries enter the skull through the foramen magnum and unite behind the clivus to form the unpaired basilar artery. This vessel then divides into the two posterior cerebral arteries (additional vessels that normally contribute to the circle of Willis are shown in **D**).

Note: Each middle cerebral artery (MCA) is the direct continuation of the internal carotid artery on that side. Clots ejected by the left heart will frequently embolize to the MCA territory.

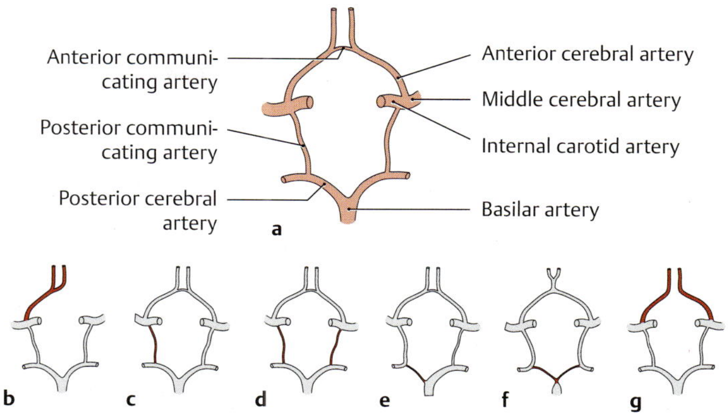

D Variants of the circle of Willis
(after Lippert and Pabst)

The vascular connections within the circle of Willis are subject to considerable variation. As a rule, the segmental hypoplasias shown here do not significantly alter the normal functions of the arterial ring.

- **a** In most cases, the circle of Willis is formed by the following arteries: the anterior, middle, and posterior cerebral arteries; the anterior and posterior communicating arteries; the internal carotid arteries; and the basilar artery.
- **b** Both anterior cerebral arteries may arise from one internal carotid artery (10% of cases).
- **c** The posterior communicating artery may be absent or hypoplastic on one side (10% of cases).
- **d** The posterior communicating artery may be absent or hypoplastic on both sides (10% of cases).
- **e** The posterior cerebral artery may arise from the internal carotid artery on one side (10% of cases).
- **f** The posterior cerebral artery may arise from the internal carotid artery both sides (5% of cases).
- **g** The anterior communicating artery may be absent (1% of cases).

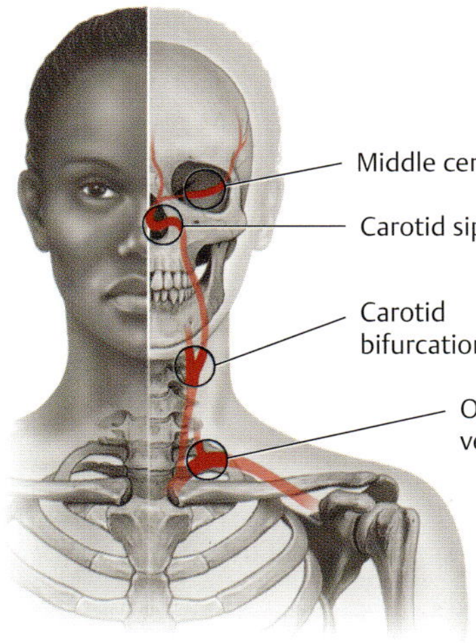

E Stenoses and occlusions of arteries supplying the brain

Atherosclerotic lesions in older patients may cause the narrowing (stenosis) or complete obstruction (occlusion) of arteries that supply the brain. Stenoses most commonly occur at arterial bifurcations, and the sites of predilection are shown. Isolated stenoses that develop gradually may be compensated for by collateral vessels. When stenoses occur simultaneously at multiple sites, the circle of Willis cannot compensate for the diminished blood supply, and cerebral blood flow becomes impaired (varying degrees of cerebral ischemia, see p. 392).

Note: The damage is manifested clinically in the brain, but the cause is located in the vessels that supply the brain. Because stenoses are treatable, their diagnosis has major therapeutic implications.

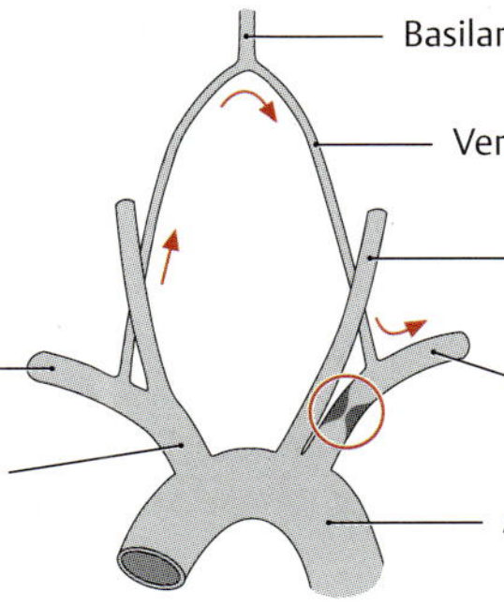

F Anatomical basis of subclavian steal syndrome

"Subclavian steal" usually results from stenosis of the left subclavian artery (red circle) located proximal to the origin of the vertebral artery. This syndrome involves a stealing of blood from the *vertebral artery* by the subclavian artery. When the left arm is exercised, as during yard work, insufficient blood may be supplied to the arm to accommodate the increased muscular effort (the patient complains of muscle weakness). As a result, blood is "stolen" from the vertebral artery circulation and there is a reversal of blood flow in the vertebral artery on the *affected* side (arrows). This leads to deficient blood flow in the basilar artery and may deprive the brain of blood, producing a feeling of lightheadedness.

10.2 Arteries of the Cerebrum

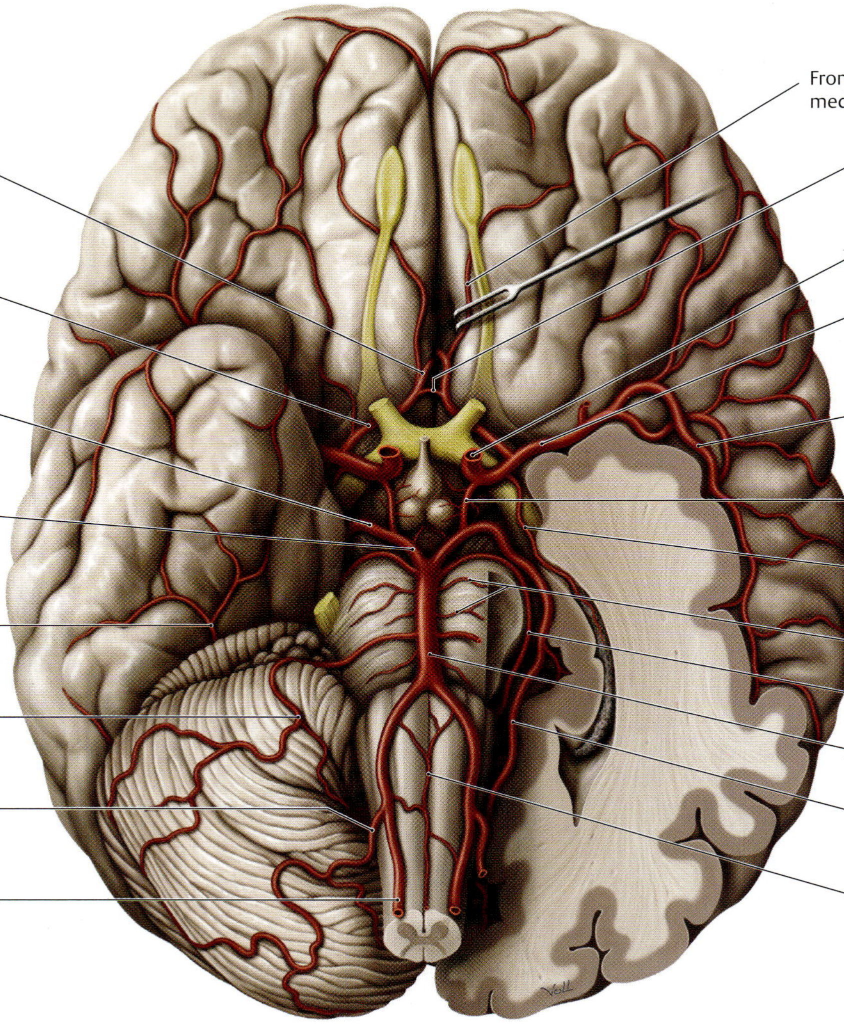

A Arteries at the base of the brain

As this view shows, most of the arteries that supply the brain enter the cerebrum from its basal aspect. The cerebellum and temporal lobe have been removed on the left side to display the course of the posterior cerebral artery. Note the three principal arteries of the cerebrum, the anterior, middle, and posterior cerebral arteries. The first two arteries are branches of the internal carotid artery; the latter artery arises from the flow tract of the vertebral arteries (see p. 374 f).

The vertebral arteries also distribute branches to the spinal cord, brainstem, and cerebellum (anterior spinal artery, posterior spinal arteries, superior cerebellar artery, and anterior and posterior inferior cerebellar arteries). Immediately after its origin, the anterior cerebral artery courses around the corpus callosum to supply the medial aspect of the brain with blood. As a result, practically the only visible portion of the postcommunicating part of the anterior cerebral artery in this view of the underside of the brain is its branch, the medial frontobasal artery.

Note: If one of the main vessels of the arterial circle rupture due to a defect in the vascular wall (aneurysm, see **B**, p. 391), blood flows directly into the subarachnoid space resulting in subarachnoid hemorrhage.

B Segments of the anterior, middle, and posterior cerebral arteries

Artery	Parts	Segments
Anterior cerebral artery	• Precommunicating part • Postcommunicating part	• A1 = segment proximal to the anterior communicating artery • A2 = segment distal to the anterior communicating artery
Middle cerebral artery (MCA)	• Sphenoidal part • Insular part	• M1 = first horizontal segment of the artery (horizontal part) • M2 = segment on the insula
Posterior cerebral artery	• Precommunicating part • Postcommunicating part	• P1 = segment between the basilar artery bifurcation and posterior communicating artery • P2 = segment between the posterior communicating artery and anterior temporal branches • P3 = lateral occipital artery • P4 = medial occipital artery

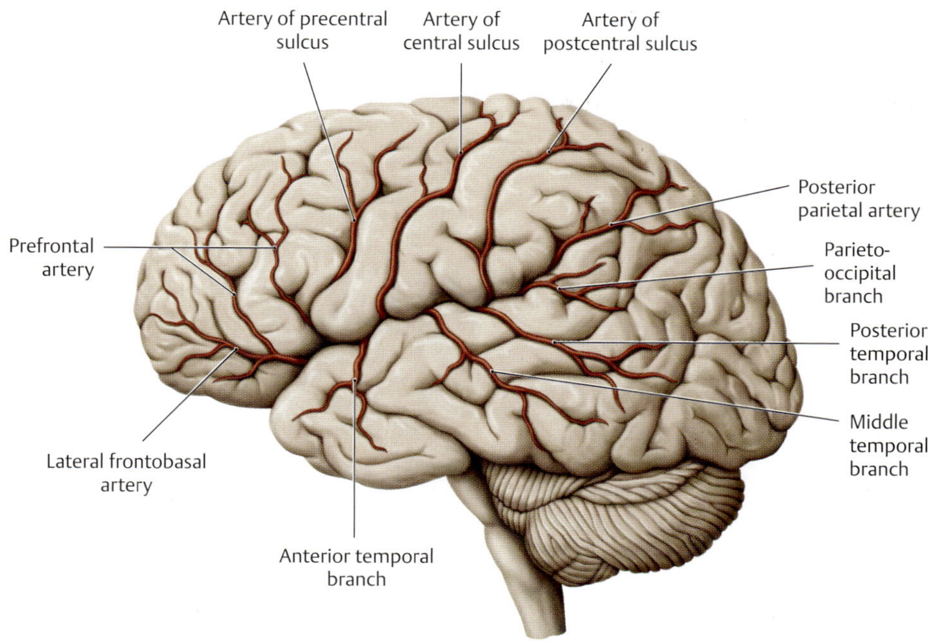

C Terminal branches of the middle cerebral artery on the lateral cerebral hemisphere

Left lateral view. Most of the blood vessels on the lateral surface of the brain are terminal branches of the middle cerebral artery (MCA). They can be subdivided into two main groups:

- Inferior terminal (cortical) branches: supply the temporal lobe cortex
- Superior terminal (cortical) branches: supply the frontal and parietal lobe cortex.

Deeper structures supplied by these branches are not shown in the diagram (see p. 378).

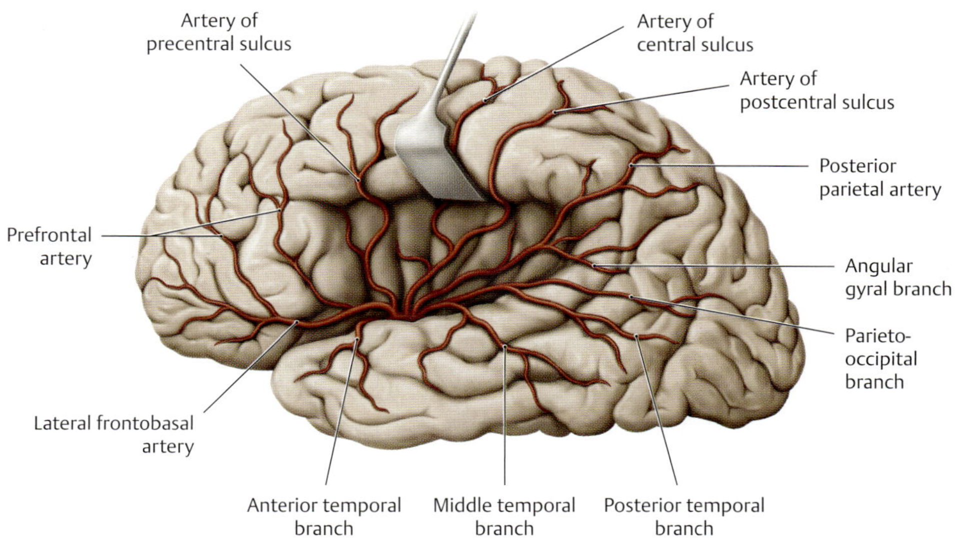

D Course of the middle cerebral artery in the interior of the lateral sulcus

Left lateral view. On its way to the lateral surface of the cerebral hemisphere, the middle cerebral artery first courses on the base of the brain; this is the sphenoidal part of the MCA. It then continues through the lateral sulcus along the insula, which is the sunken portion of the cerebral cortex. When the temporal and parietal lobes are spread apart with a retractor, as shown here, we can see the arteries of the insula (which receive their blood from the insular part of the middle cerebral artery; see **A**). When viewed in an angiogram, the branches of the insular part of the MCA resemble the arms of a candelabrum, giving rise to the term "candelabrum artery" for that arterial segment.

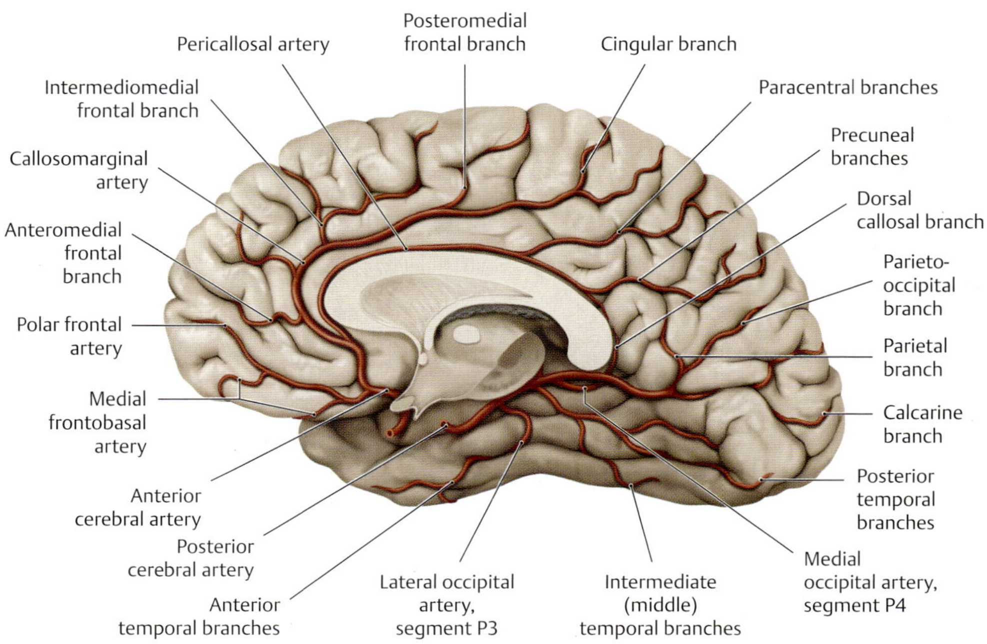

E Branches of the anterior and posterior cerebral arteries on the medial surface of the cerebrum

Right cerebral hemisphere viewed from the medial side, with the left cerebral hemisphere and brainstem removed. The medial surface of the brain is supplied by branches of the anterior and posterior cerebral arteries. While the *anterior cerebral artery* arises from the internal carotid artery, the *posterior cerebral artery* arises from the basilar artery (which is formed by the junction of the left and right vertebral arteries).

10.3 Arteries of the Cerebrum, Distribution

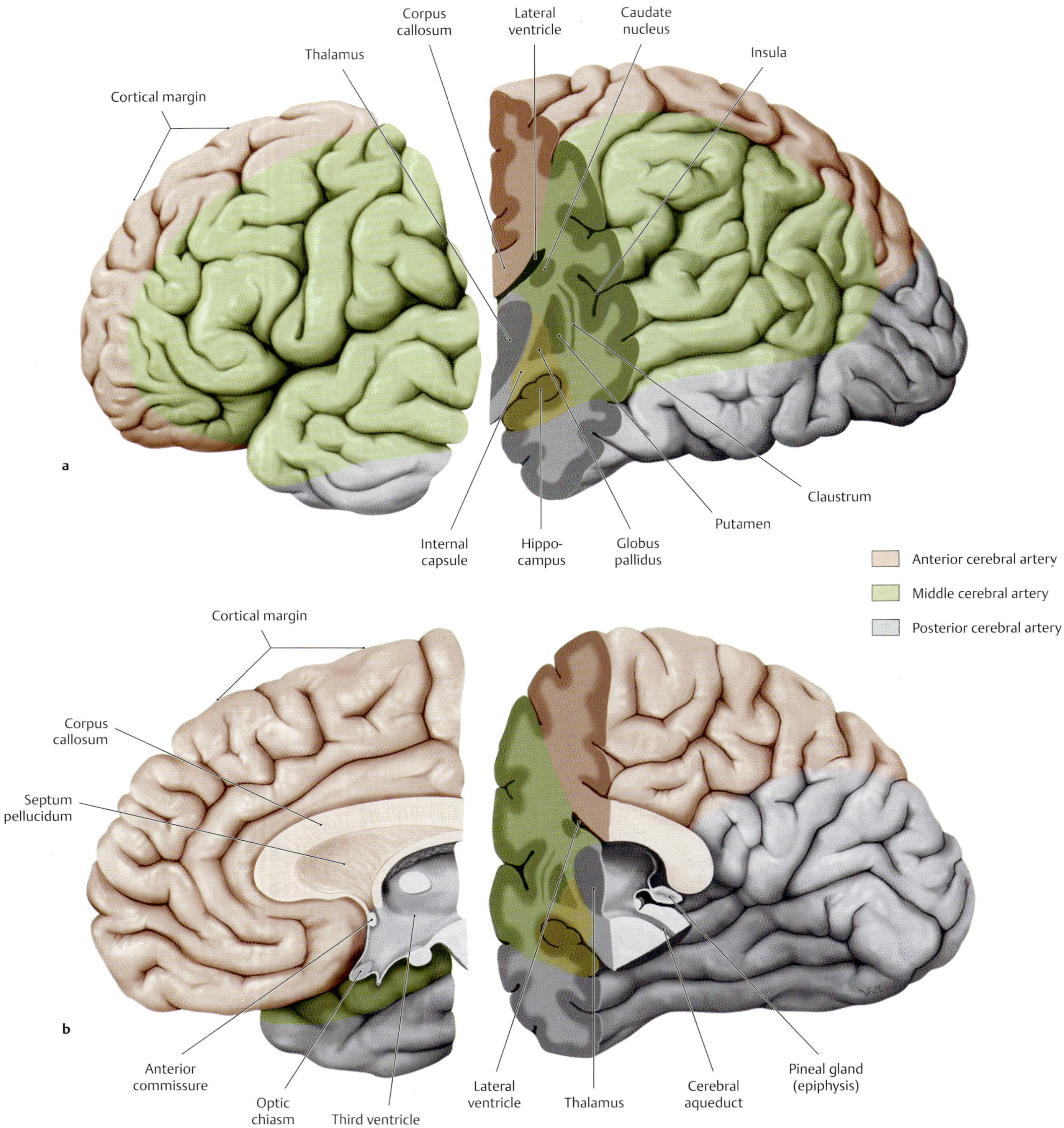

A Distribution areas of the main cerebral arteries

a Lateral view of the left cerebral hemisphere; **b** Medial view of the right cerebral hemisphere. Most of the lateral surface of the brain is supplied by the *middle* cerebral artery (green), whose branches ascend to the cortex from the depths of the insula. The branches of the *anterior* cerebral artery supply the frontal pole of the brain and the cortical areas near the cortical margin (red and pink). The *posterior* cerebral artery supplies the occipital pole and lower portions of the temporal lobe (blue). The central gray and white matter have a complex blood supply (yellow) that includes the anterior choroidal artery. The anterior and posterior cerebral arteries supply most of the medial surface of the brain.

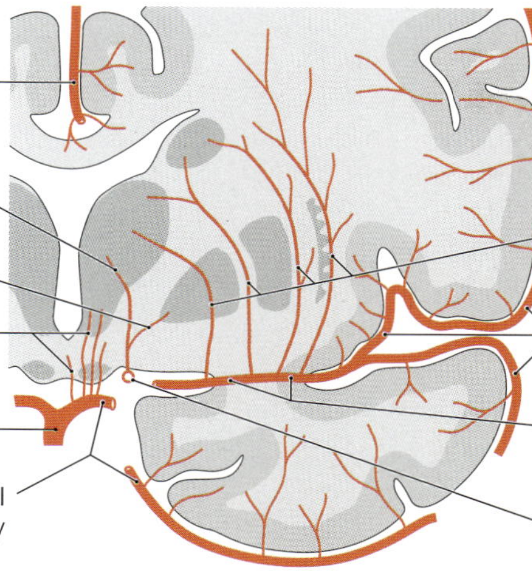

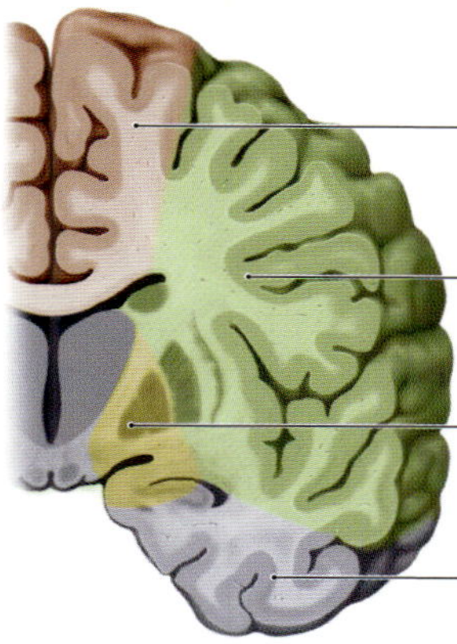

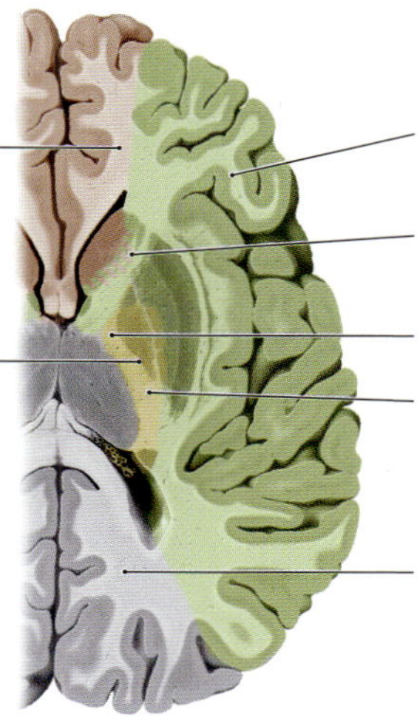

B Distribution of the three main cerebral arteries in transverse and coronal sections

a, b Coronal sections at the level of the mammillary bodies. **c** Transverse section at the level of the internal capsule. The internal capsule, basal nuclei, and thalamus derive most of their blood supply from perforating branches of the following vessels at the base of the brain:

- Anterior choroidal artery (direct branch from the internal carotid artery, see **Ab**, p. 102)
- Anterolateral central arteries (lenticulostriate arteries and striate branches) with their terminal branches (from the middle cerebral artery)
- Posteromedial central arteries (from the posterior cerebral artery)
- Perforating branches (from the posterior communicating artery)

The internal capsule, which is traversed by the pyramidal tract and other structures, receives most of its blood supply from the middle cerebral artery (anterior limb and genu) and from the anterior choroidal artery (posterior limb). If these vessels become occluded, the pyramidal tract and other structures will be interrupted, causing paralysis on the contralateral side of the body (stroke: central paralysis, see **C** on p. 393).

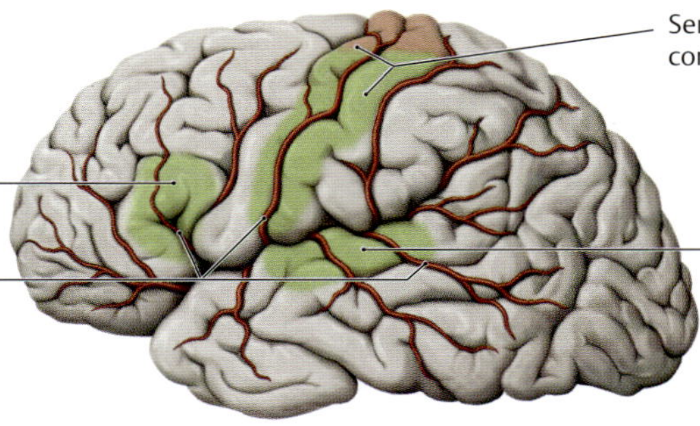

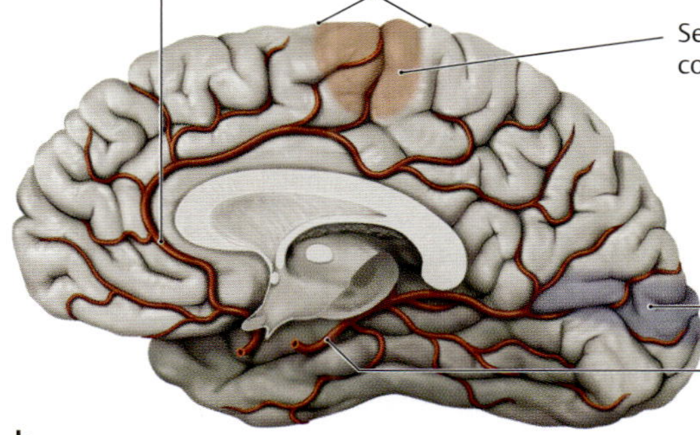

C Functional centers on the surface of the cerebrum

a Left lateral view of the telencephalon; regions supplied by branches of the middle cerebral a. are shaded green; **b** Medial view of the right cerebral hemisphere; regions supplied by the anterior cerebral a. are shaded red; regions supplied by the branches of the posterior cerebral a. are shaded blue.

Specific functions can be assigned to well-defined areas of the telencephalon. These areas are supplied by branches of the three main cerebral arteries:

- The sensorimotor cortex e.g. of branches of *middle* cerebral a. (precentral and postcentral gyri, see **a**) *and* of branches of the *anterior* cerebral a. (the superior margin of the cerebral hemisphere, see **b**);
- Broca's area and Wernicke's areas (motor and sensory speech centers) e.g., by branches of the *middle* cerebral a. (see **a**);
- Visual cortex by branches of the *posterior* cerebral a. (see **b**).

Certain disorders or deficits are indicative of arterial occlusion in a certain territory. A failure, deficit, or outage of the speech center suggests an occlusion of the middle cerebral a., hemianopsia suggests an occlusion of the posterior cerebral a., and paralysis and sensory disturbances in the lower limbs suggest an occlusion of the anterior cerebral a. (cf. p. 393).

10.4 Arteries of the Brainstem and Cerebellum

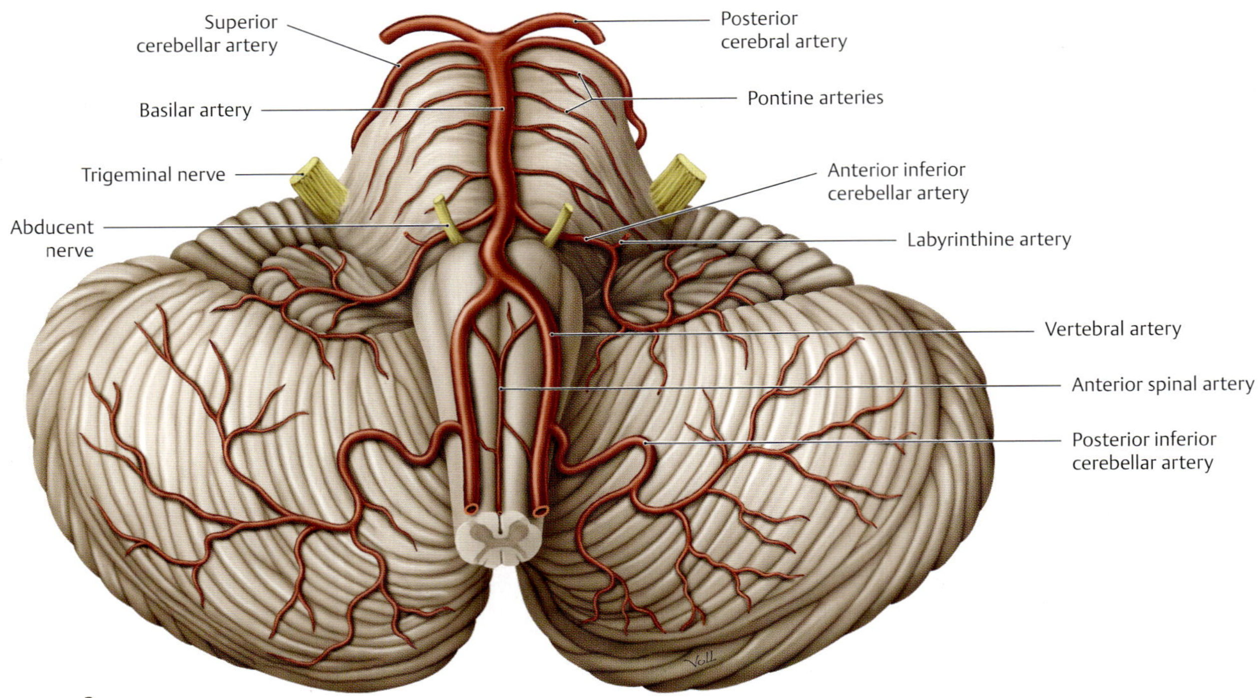

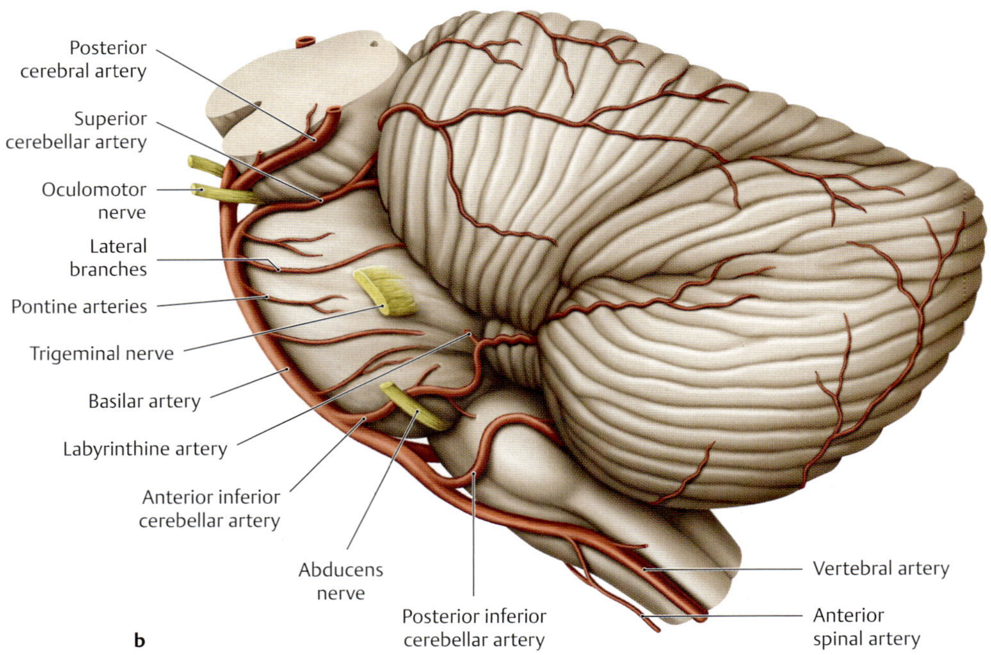

A Arteries of the brainstem and cerebellum

a Basal view; **b** Left lateral view.

The brainstem and cerebellum are supplied by the basilar and cerebellar arteries (see below). Because the basilar artery is formed by the union of the two vertebral arteries, blood supplied by the basilar artery is said to come from the *vertebrobasilar complex* (or *system*). The vessels that supply the **brainstem** (mesencephalon, pons, and medulla oblongata) arise either directly from the basilar artery (e.g., the pontine arteries) and vertebral arteries or from their branches. The branches are classified by their sites of entry and distribution as medial, mediolateral, or lateral (paramedian branches; short and long circumferential branches). Decreased perfusion in or occlusion of these vessels leads to transient or permanent impairment of blood flow (brainstem syndrome) and may produce a great variety of clinical symptoms, given the many nuclei and tract systems that exist in the brainstem. The **spinal cord** receives a portion of its blood supply from the anterior spinal artery (see **b**), which arises from the vertebral artery (see p. 414). The **cerebellum** is supplied by three large arteries:

- Posterior inferior cerebellar artery (PICA), the largest branch of the vertebral artery. This vessel is usually referred to by its acronym, PICA.
- Anterior inferior cerebellar artery (AICA), the first major branch of the basilar artery
- Superior cerebellar artery (SCA), the last major branch of the basilar artery before it divides into the posterior cerebral arteries

Note the labyrinthine artery which supplies the inner ear (see also **D**, p. 157) *usually* arises from the anterior inferior cerebellar artery, as pictured here, although it may also spring directly from the basilar artery. Impaired blood flow in the labyrinthine artery leads to an acute loss of hearing (sudden sensorineural hearing loss), frequently accompanied by tinnitus (see **D**, p. 151).

B Distribution of the arteries of the brainstem and cerebellum in midsagittal section

All of the brain sections shown here and below are supplied by the vertebrobasilar complex. The transverse sections are presented in a caudal-to-cranial series corresponding to the direction of the vertebrobasilar blood supply.

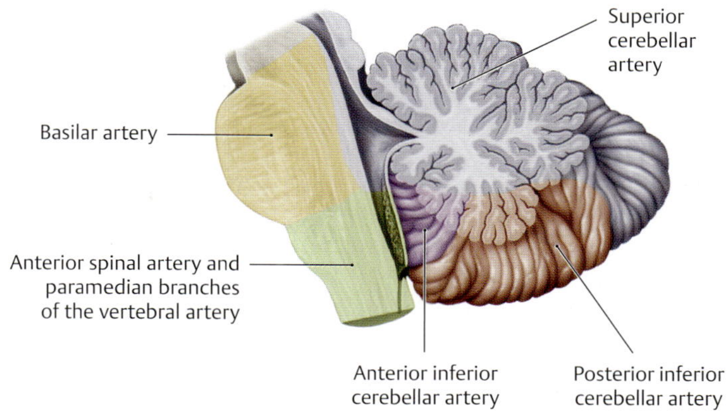

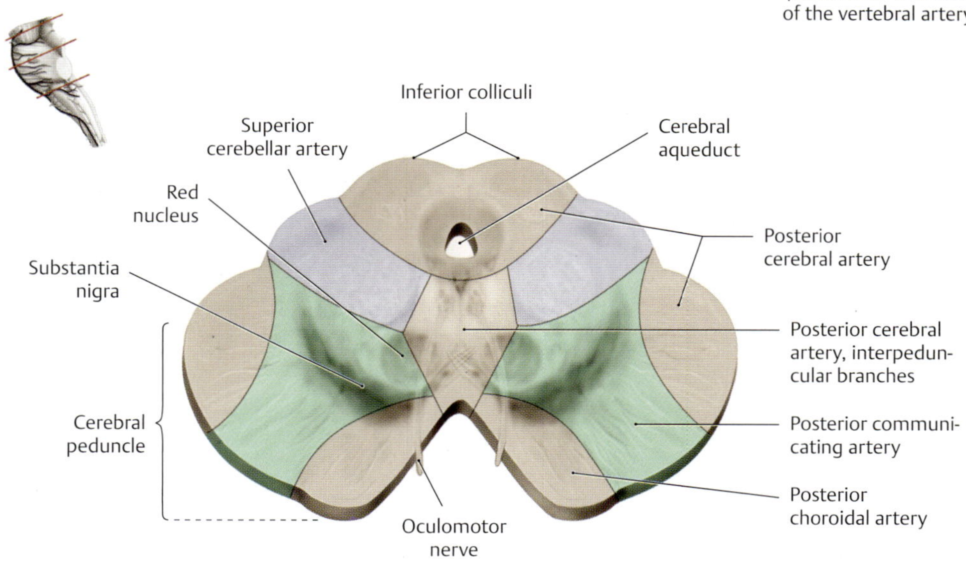

C Distribution of the arteries of the mesencephalon in transverse section

Besides branches from the superior cerebellar artery, the mesencephalon is supplied chiefly by branches of the posterior cerebral artery and posterior communicating artery.

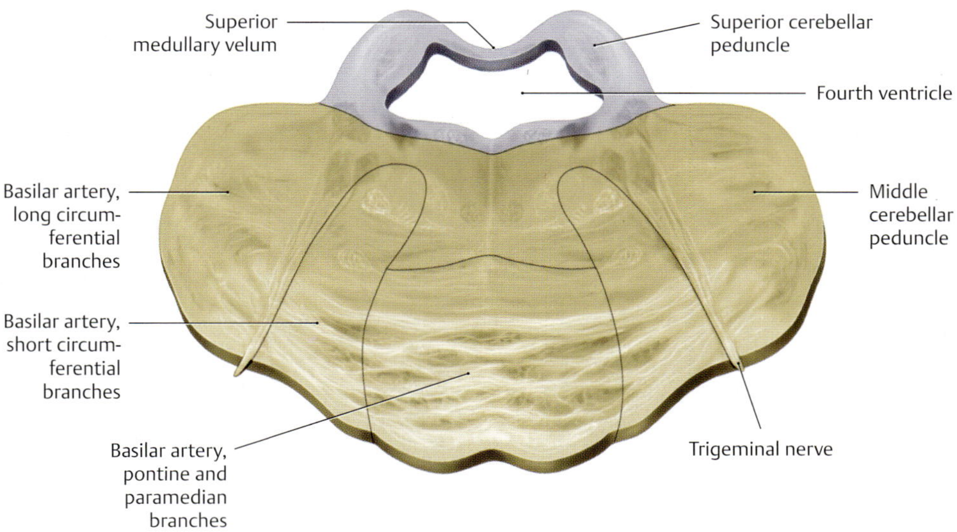

D Distribution of the arteries of the pons in transverse section

The pons derives its blood supply from short and long branches of the basilar artery.

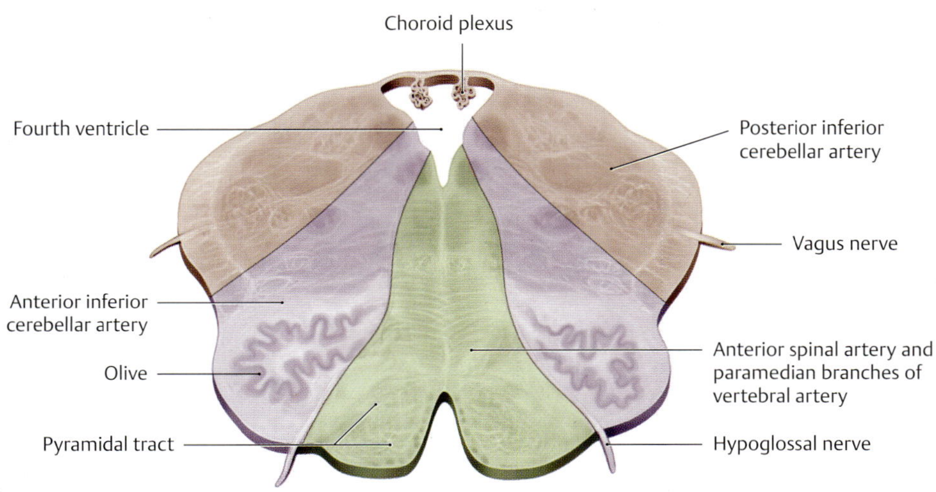

E Distribution of the arteries of the medulla oblongata in transverse section

The medulla oblongata is supplied by branches of the anterior spinal artery, posterior inferior cerebellar artery (both arising from the vertebral artery), as well as the anterior inferior cerebellar artery (first large branch of the basilar artery).

10.5 Dural Sinuses, Overview

A Relationship of the principal dural sinuses to the skull

Oblique posterior view from the right side (brain removed and tentorium windowed on the right side). Dural venous sinuses are located either in the attached or free margins of the dural folds. The falx cerebri has a dural venous sinus on both edges. The larger venous sinuses are those attached to the inside to the cranial bone (e.g., superior sagittal, transverse, sigmoid sinuses). The wall of the venous sinus is stiff, consisting only of dura and an endothelial lining. The absence of muscle in the sinus wall prevents sinuses from contracting if injured and, unlike veins, don't contribute to the control of bleeding. Bleeding from a venous sinus caused by cranial injury can be life-threatening. Venous sinuses collect blood from the brain, orbital cavity, and calvaria. Since sinuses do not have valves, the direction of blood flow depends on the position of the head. When lying down or holding the head upright, the sinuses convey blood to the internal jugular vv. which are located on both sides at the deepest point of the posterior cranial fossa. The system of dural sinuses is divided into an upper group and a lower group:

- **Upper group:** superior and inferior sagittal sinuses, straight sinus, occipital sinus, transverse sinus, sigmoid sinus, and the confluence of the sinuses
- **Lower group:** cavernous sinus with anterior and posterior intercavernous sinuses, sphenoparietal sinus, superior and inferior petrosal sinuses

The upper and lower groups of dural sinuses communicate with the venous plexuses of the vertebral canal through the marginal sinus at the inlet to the foramen magnum and through the basilar plexus on the clivus (see **C**).

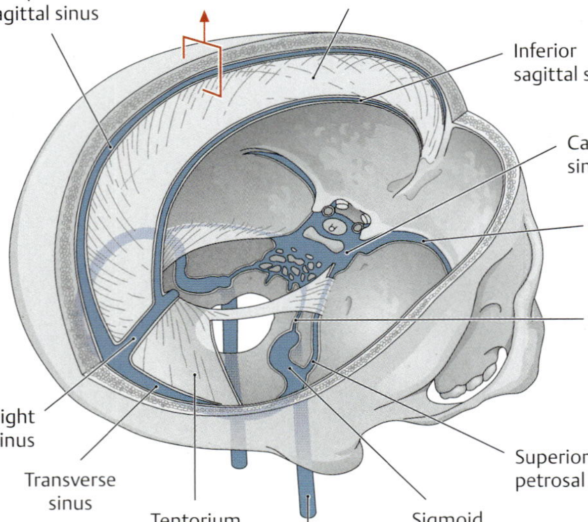

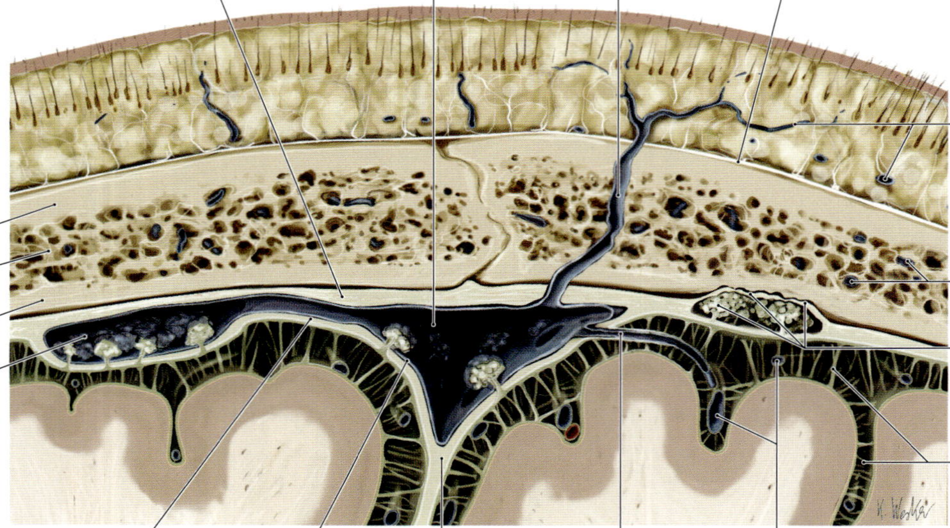

B Structure of a dural sinus, shown here for the superior sagittal sinus

Transverse section, occipital view (detail from **A**). The sinus wall is composed of endothelium and tough, collagenous dural connective tissue with a periosteal and meningeal layer. Between the two layers is the sinus lumen.

Note the lateral lacunae, where the arachnoid villi open into the venous system. Superficial cerebral veins (superior cerebral veins, bridging veins, see pp. 306 and 308) open into the sinus itself along with diploic veins from the adjacent cranial bone. The sinus also receives emissary veins—valveless veins that establish connections among the sinuses, the diploic veins, and the extracranial veins of the scalp.

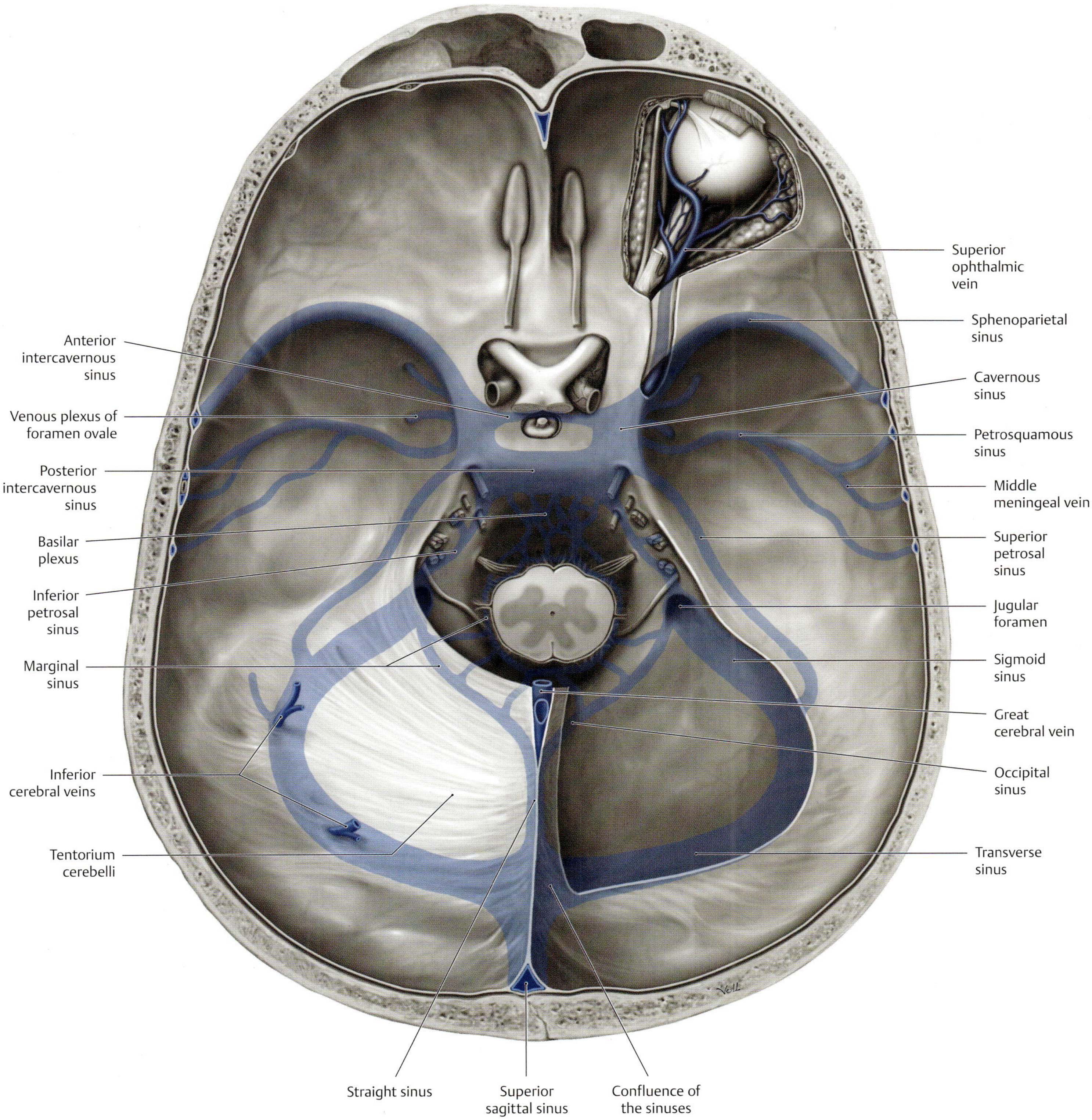

C Dural sinuses at the skull base
Transverse section at the level of the tentorium cerebelli, viewed from above (brain removed, orbital roof and tentorium windowed on the right side). The cavernous sinus forms a ring around the sella turcica, its left and right parts being interconnected at the front and behind by an anterior and a posterior intercavernous sinus. Behind the posterior intercavernous sinus, on the clivus, is the basilar plexus. This plexus also contributes to the drainage of the cavernous sinus.

10.6 Dural Sinuses: Tributaries and Accessory Draining Vessels

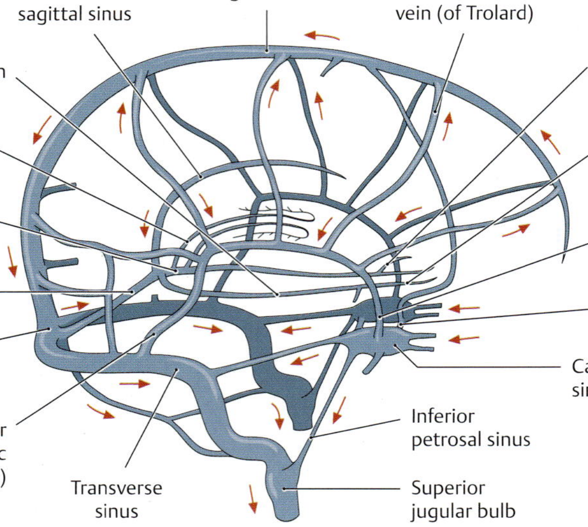

A Dural sinus tributaries from the cerebral veins

Right lateral view. Venous blood collected deep within the brain drains to the dural sinuses through *superficial* and deep cerebral veins (see p. 386). The red arrows in the diagram show the principal directions of venous blood flow in the major sinuses. Because of the numerous anastomoses, the isolated occlusion of even a complete sinus segment may produce no clinical symptoms.

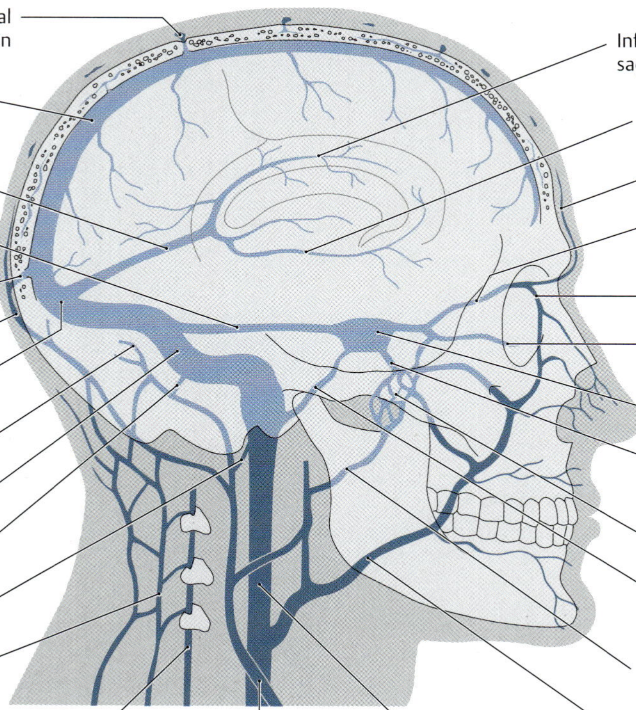

B Accessory drainage pathways of the dural sinuses

Right lateral view. The dural sinuses have many accessory drainage pathways besides their principal drainage into the two internal jugular veins. The connections between the dural sinuses and extracranial veins mainly serve to equalize pressure and regulate temperature. These anastomoses are of clinical interest because their normal direction of blood flow may reverse (no venous valves), allowing blood from extracranial veins to reflux into the dural sinuses. Bacteria can spread via the superficial veins to the sinus which can lead to life-threatening bacterial venous sinus thrombosis. The most important accessory drainage vessels include the following:

- Emissary veins (diploic and superior scalp veins), see **C**
- Superior ophthalmic vein (angular and facial veins)
- Venous plexus of foramen ovale (pterygoid plexus, retromandibular vein)
- Marginal sinus and basilar plexus (internal and external vertebral venous plexus), see **C**

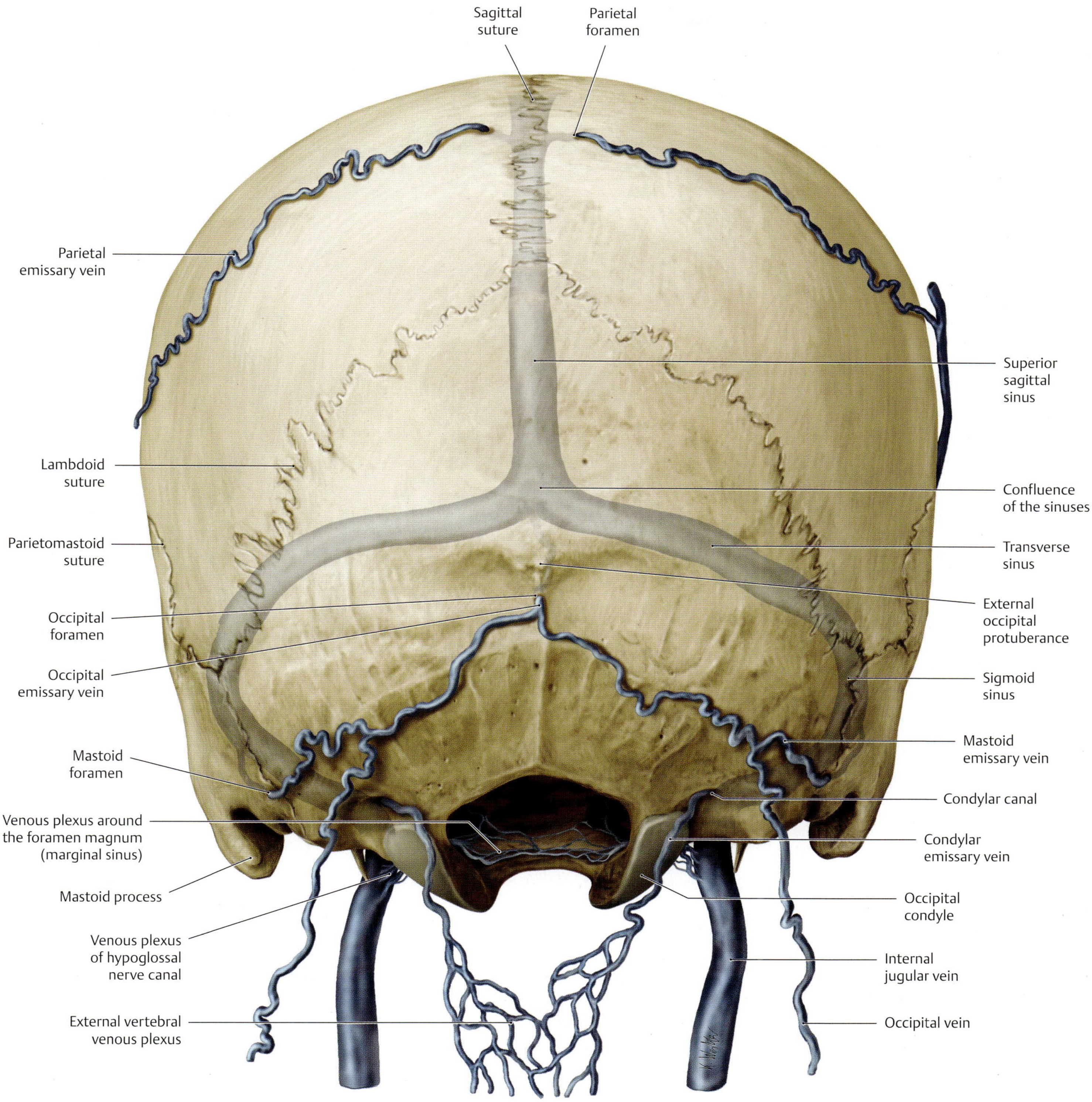

C Occipital emissary veins

Emissary veins establish a direct connection between the intracranial dural sinuses and extracranial veins. They run through small cranial openings such as the parietal and mastoid foramina. Emissary veins are of clinical interest because they create a potential route by which bacteria from the scalp may spread to the dura mater and dural venous sinuses.

10.7 Veins of the Brain: Superficial and Deep Veins

Because the veins of the brain do not run parallel to the arteries, marked differences are noted between the regions of arterial supply and venous drainage. While all of the cerebral arteries enter the brain at its base, venous blood is drained from the entire surface of the brain, including the base, and also from the interior of the brain by two groups of veins: the *superficial cerebral veins* and the *deep cerebral veins*. The superficial veins drain blood from the cerebral cortex (via cortical veins) and white matter (via medullary veins) directly into the dural sinuses. The deep veins drain blood from the deeper portions of the white matter, basal nuclei, corpus callosum, and diencephalon into the great cerebral vein, which enters the straight sinus. The two venous regions (those of the superficial and deep veins) are interconnected by numerous intracerebral anastomoses (see **D**).

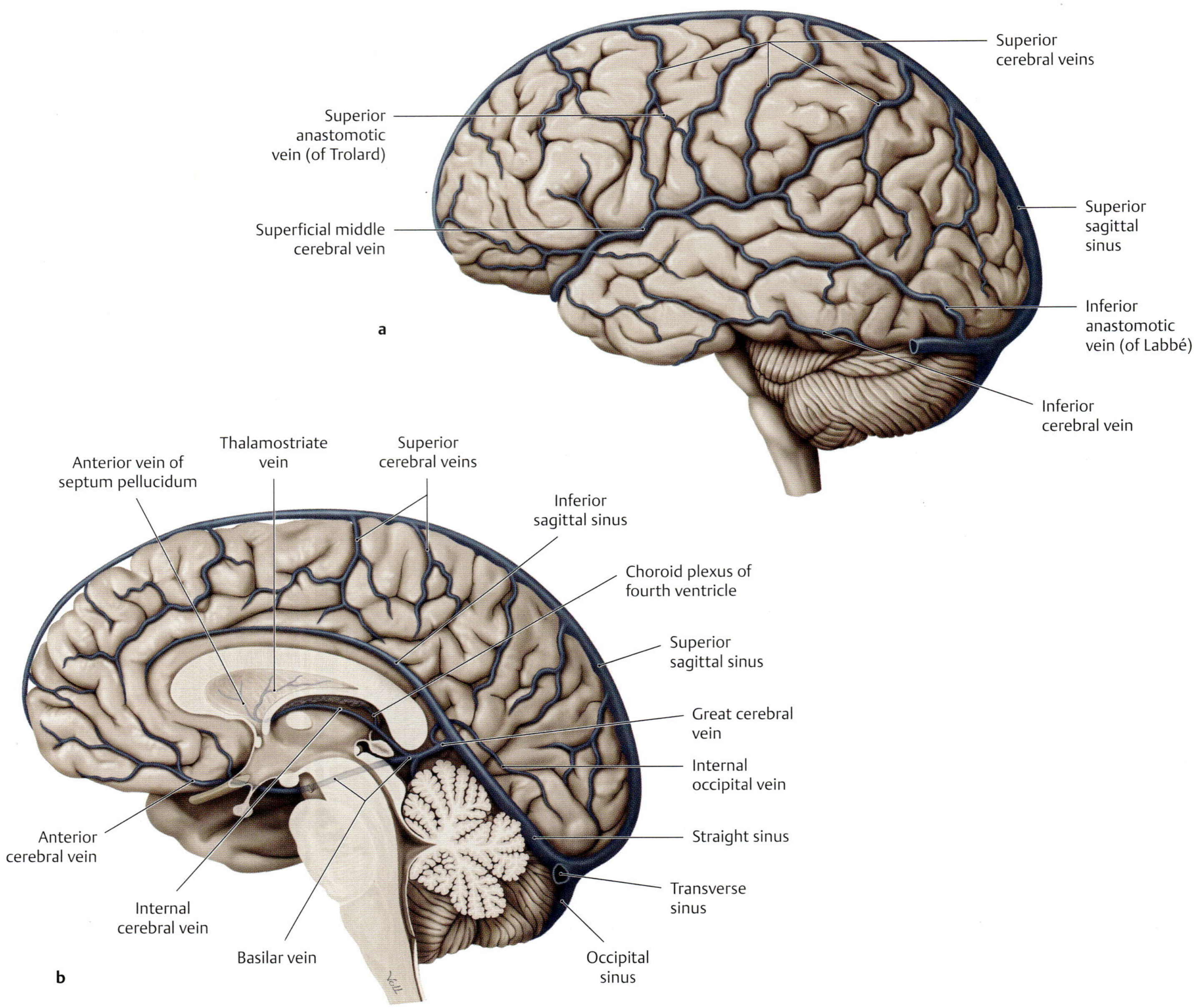

A Superficial veins of the brain (superficial cerebral veins)
Left lateral view (**a**) and medial view (**b**).
a, b The superficial cerebral veins drain blood from the short cortical veins and long medullary veins in the white matter (see **D**) into the dural sinuses. (The deep cerebral veins are described in **C**, p. 389.) Their course is extremely variable, and veins in the subarachnoid space do not follow arteries, gyri, or sulci. Consequently, only the most important of these vessels are named here. Just before terminating in the dural sinuses, the veins leave the subarachnoid space and run a short subdural course between the dura mater and arachnoid. These short subdural venous segments are called bridging veins. The bridging veins have great clinical importance because they may be ruptured by head trauma, resulting in a subdural hematoma (see p. 390).

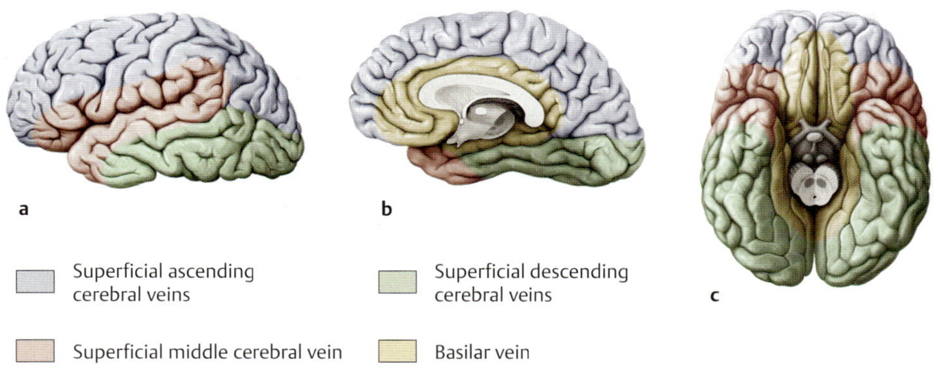

B Regions drained by the superficial cerebral veins

a Left lateral view, **b** view of the medial surface of the right hemisphere, **c** basal view.
The veins on the lateral surface of the brain are classified by their direction of drainage as ascending (draining into the superior sagittal sinus) or descending (draining into the transverse sinus). The superficial middle cerebral vein drains into both the cavernous and transverse sinuses (see **A**, p. 384).

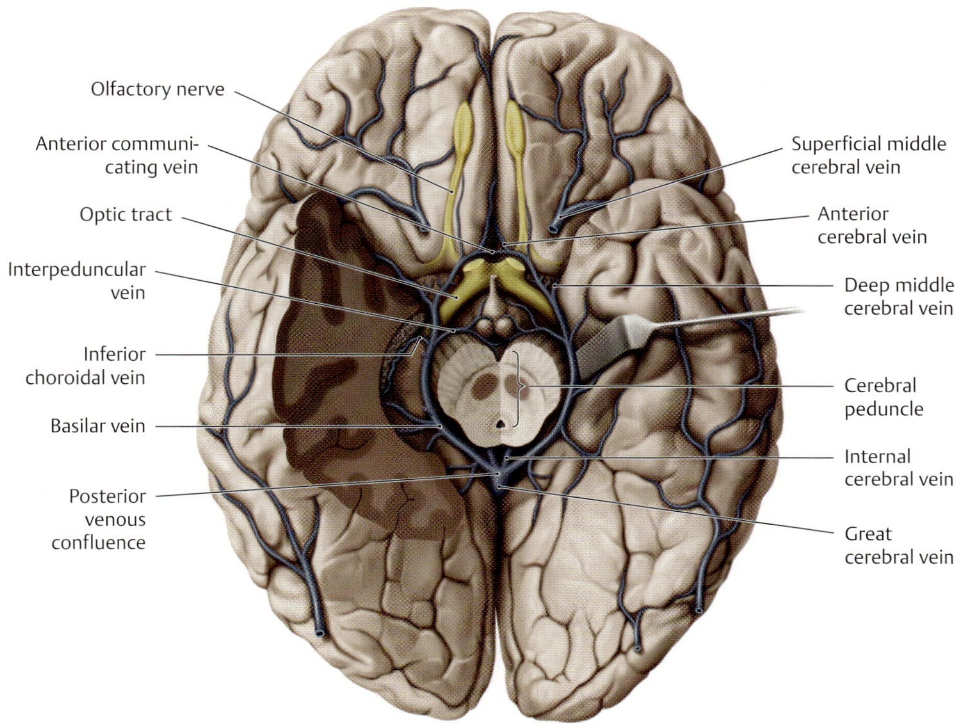

C Basal cerebral venous system

The basal cerebral venous system drains blood from both superficial and deep cerebral veins. A venous circle formed by the basilar veins (of Rosenthal, see below) exists at the base of the brain, analogous to the arterial circle of Willis. The basilar vein is formed in the anterior perforate substance by the union of the anterior cerebral and deep middle cerebral veins. Following the course of the optic tract, the basilar vein runs posteriorly around the cerebral peduncle and unites with the basilar vein from the opposite side on the dorsal aspect of the mesencephalon. The two internal cerebral veins also terminate at this venous junction, the posterior venous confluence. This junction gives rise to the midline great cerebral vein, which enters the straight sinus. The basilar vein receives tributaries from deep brain regions in its course (e.g., veins from the thalamus and hypothalamus, choroid plexus of the inferior horn, etc.). The two anterior cerebral veins are interconnected by the anterior communicating vein, creating a closed, ring-shaped drainage system.

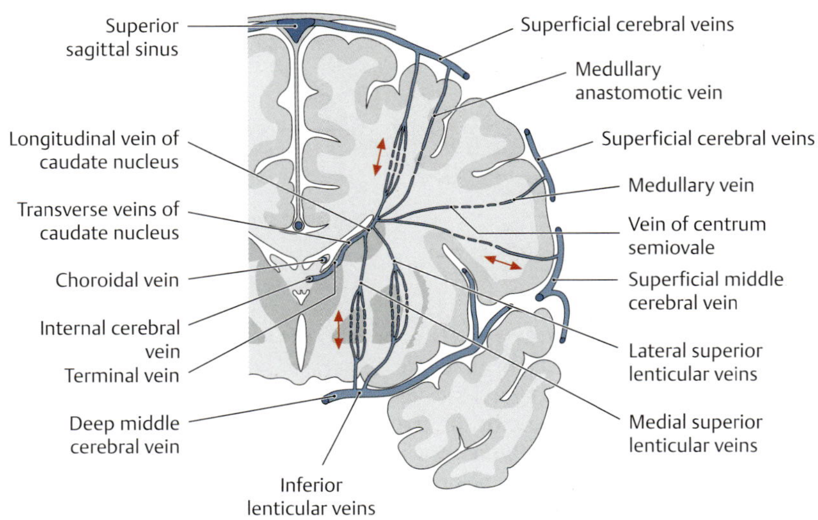

D Anastomoses between the superficial and deep cerebral veins

Transverse section through the left hemisphere, anterior view. The superficial cerebral veins communicate with the deep cerebral veins through the anastomoses shown here (see p. 388). Flow reversal (double arrows) may occur in the boundary zones between two territories.

10.8 Veins of the Brainstem and Cerebellum: Deep Veins

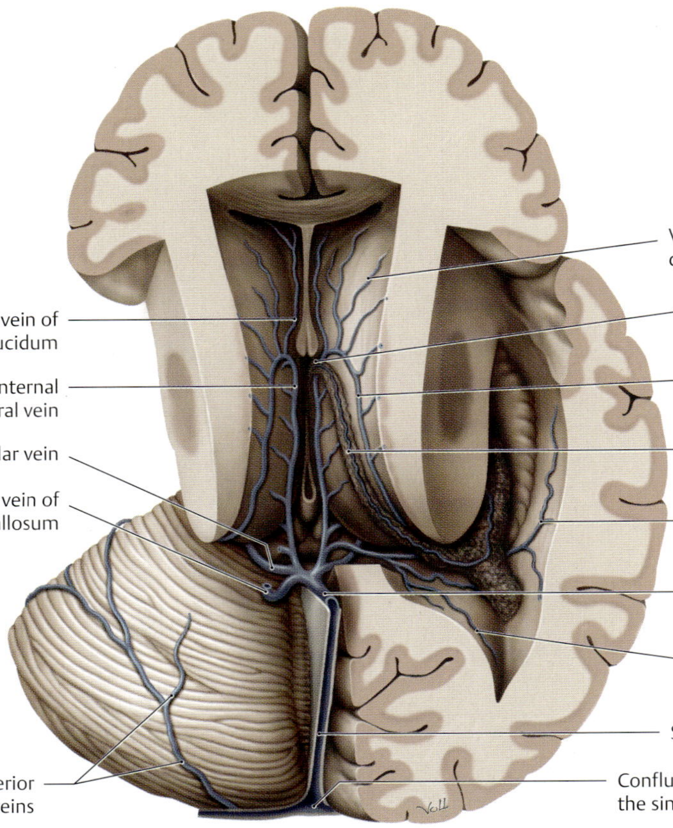

A Deep cerebral veins
Multiplanar transverse section (combining multiple transverse planes) with a superior view of the opened lateral ventricles. The temporal and occipital lobes and tentorium cerebelli have been removed on the left side to demonstrate the upper surface of the cerebellum and the superior cerebellar veins. On the lateral walls of the anterior horns of both lateral ventricles, the superior thalamostriate vein runs toward the interventricular foramen in the groove between the thalamus and caudate nucleus. After receiving the anterior vein of the septum pellucidum and the superior choroidal vein, it forms the internal cerebral vein and passes through the interventricular foramen along the roof of the diencephalon toward the quadrigeminal plate, which contains the superior and inferior colliculi. There it unites with the internal cerebral vein of the opposite side, and the basal veins to form the posterior venous confluence, which gives rise to the great cerebral vein.

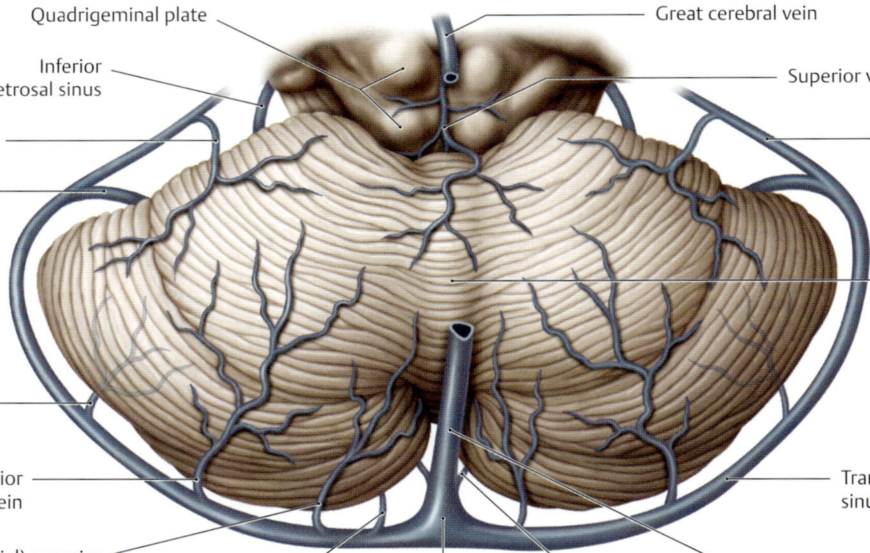

B Cerebellar veins
Posterior view. Like the other veins of the brain, the cerebellar veins are distributed independently of the cerebellar arteries. Larger trunks cross over gyri and sulci, running mainly in the sagittal direction. A *medial* and a *lateral* group can be distinguished based on their gross topographical anatomy. The medial group of cerebellar veins drains the vermis and adjacent portions of the cerebellar hemispheres (precentral vein, superior and inferior veins of the vermis) and the medial portions of the superior and inferior cerebellar veins. The *lateral group* (petrosal vein and lateral portions of the superior and inferior cerebellar veins) drains most of the two cerebellar hemispheres. All of the cerebellar veins anastomose with one another; their outflow is exclusively infratentorial (i.e., below the tentorium cerebelli).

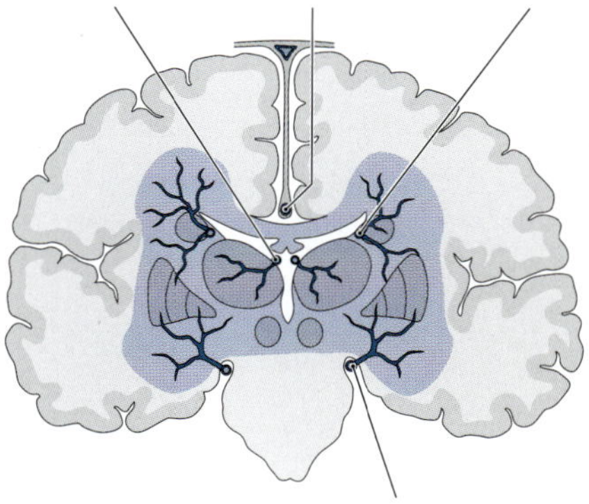

C Region drained by the deep cerebral veins

Coronal section. Three principal venous segments can be identified in each hemisphere:

- Thalamostriate vein
- Internal cerebral vein
- Basal vein

The region drained by the deep cerebral veins encompasses large portions of the base of the cerebrum, the basal nuclei, the internal capsule, the choroid plexuses of the lateral and third ventricles, the corpus callosum, and portions of the diencephalon and mesencephalon.

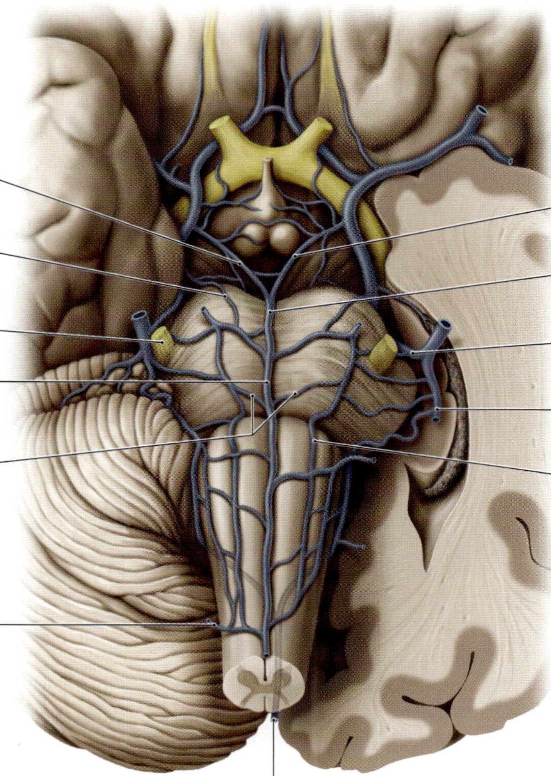

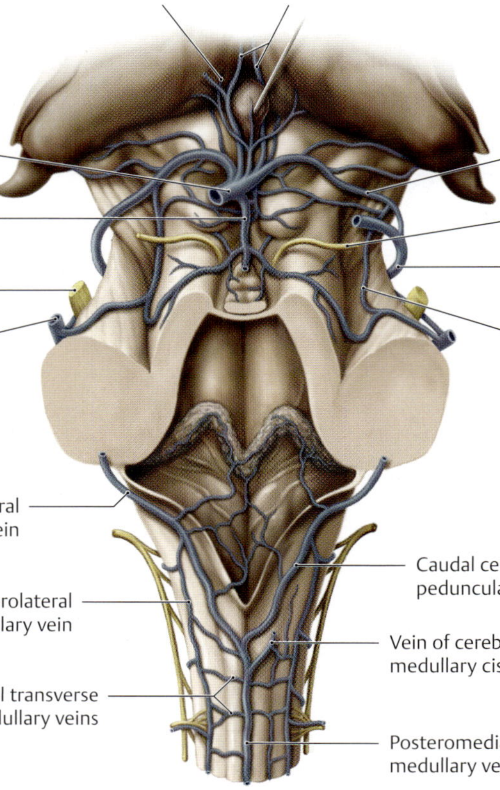

D Veins of the brainstem

a Anterior view of the brainstem in situ (the cerebellum and part of the occipital lobe have been removed on the left side). **b** Posterior view of the isolated brainstem with the cerebellum removed.

The veins of the brainstem are a continuation of the veins of the spinal cord and connect them with the basal veins of the brain. As on the spinal cord, the veins on the lower part of the brainstem form a venous plexus consisting of a powerfully developed *longitudinal* system and a more branched *transverse* system. The veins of the medulla oblongata, pons, and cerebellum make up the infratentorial venous system. Various anastomoses (e.g., anteromedial and lateral) exist at the boundary between the infra- and supratentorial systems.

10.9 Blood Vessels of the Brain: Intracranial Hemorrhage

Intracranial hemorrhages may be extracerebral (see **A**) or intracerebral (see **C**).

A Extracerebral hemorrhages

Extracerebral hemorrhages are defined as bleeding between the calvaria and brain. Because the bony calvaria is immobile, the developing hematoma exerts pressure on the soft brain. Depending on the source of the hemorrhage (arterial or venous), this may produce a rapidly or slowly developing incompressible mass with a rise of intracranial pressure that may damage not only the brain tissue at the bleeding site but also in more remote brain areas. Three types of intracranial hemorrhage can be distinguished based on their relationship to the dura mater:

- **a** **Epidural hematoma** (epidural = above the dura). This type generally develops after a head injury involving a skull fracture. The bleeding most commonly occurs from a ruptured middle meningeal artery (due to the close proximity of the middle meningeal artery to the calvaria, a sharp bone fragment may lacerate the artery). The hematoma forms between the calvaria and the periosteal layer of the dura mater. Pressure from the hematoma separates the dura from the calvaria and displaces the brain. Typically there is an initial transient loss of consciousness caused by the impact, followed 1–5 hours later by a second decline in the level of consciousness, this time due to compression of the brain by the arterial hemorrhage. The interval between the first and second loss of consciousness is called the *lucid interval* (occurs in approximately 30–40% of all epidural hematomas). Detection of the hemorrhage (CT scanning of the head) and prompt evacuation of the hematoma are life-saving.
- **b** **Subdural hematoma** (subdural = below the dura). Trauma to the head causes the rupture of a *bridging vein* (see p. 308) that bleeds between the dura mater and arachnoid. The bleeding occurs into a potential "subdural space," which exists only when extravasated blood has dissected the arachnoid membrane from the dura (the spaces are described in **C**, p. 311). Because the bleeding source is venous, the increased intracranial pressure and mass effect develop more slowly than with an arterial epidural hemorrhage. Consequently, a subdural hematoma may develop *chronically* over a period of weeks, even after a relatively mild head injury.
- **c** **Subarachnoid hemorrhage** is an arterial bleed caused by the rupture of an aneurysm (abnormal outpouching) of an artery at the base of the brain (see **B**). It is typically caused by a brief, sudden rise in blood pressure, like that produced by a sudden rise of intra-abdominal pressure (straining at stool or urine, lifting a heavy object, etc.). Because the hemorrhage is into the CSF-filled subarachnoid space, blood can be detected in the cerebrospinal fluid by means of lumbar puncture. The cardinal symptom of a subarachnoid hemorrhage is a sudden, excruciating headache accompanied by a stiff neck caused by meningeal irritation.

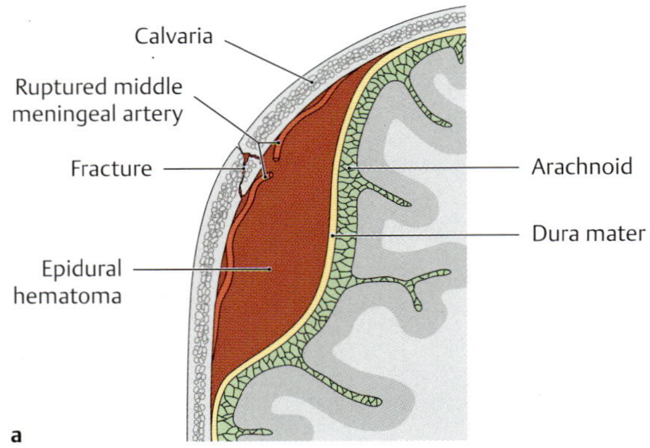

a

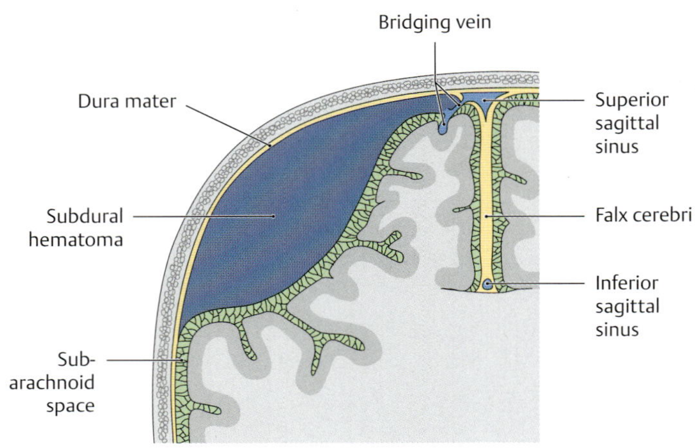

b

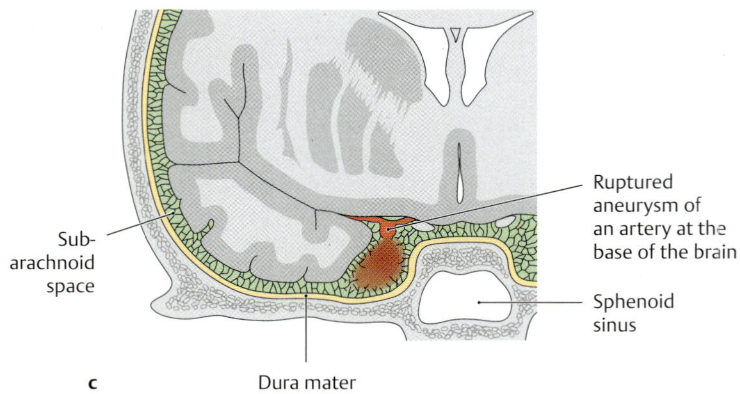

c

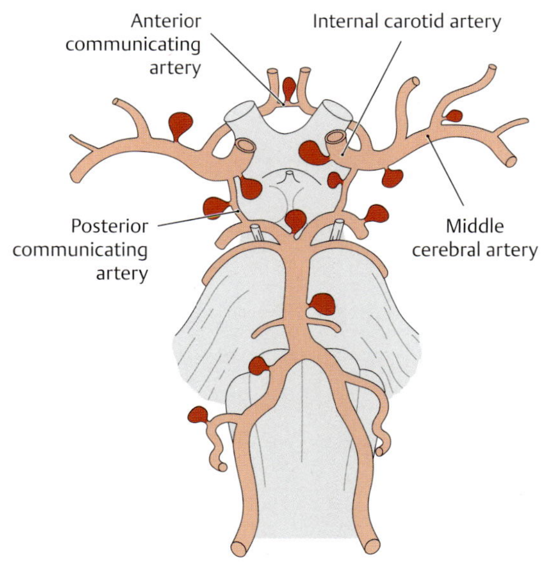

B Sites of berry aneurysms at the base of the brain
(after Bähr and Frotscher)
The rupture of congenital or acquired arterial aneurysms at the base of the brain is the most frequent cause of subarachnoid hemorrhage and accounts for approximately 5% of all strokes. These are abnormal saccular dilations of the circle of Willis and are especially common at the site of branching. When one of these thin-walled aneurysms ruptures, arterial blood escapes into the subarachnoid space. The most common site is the junction between the anterior cerebral and anterior communicating arteries; the second most likely site is the branching of the posterior communicating artery from the internal carotid artery.

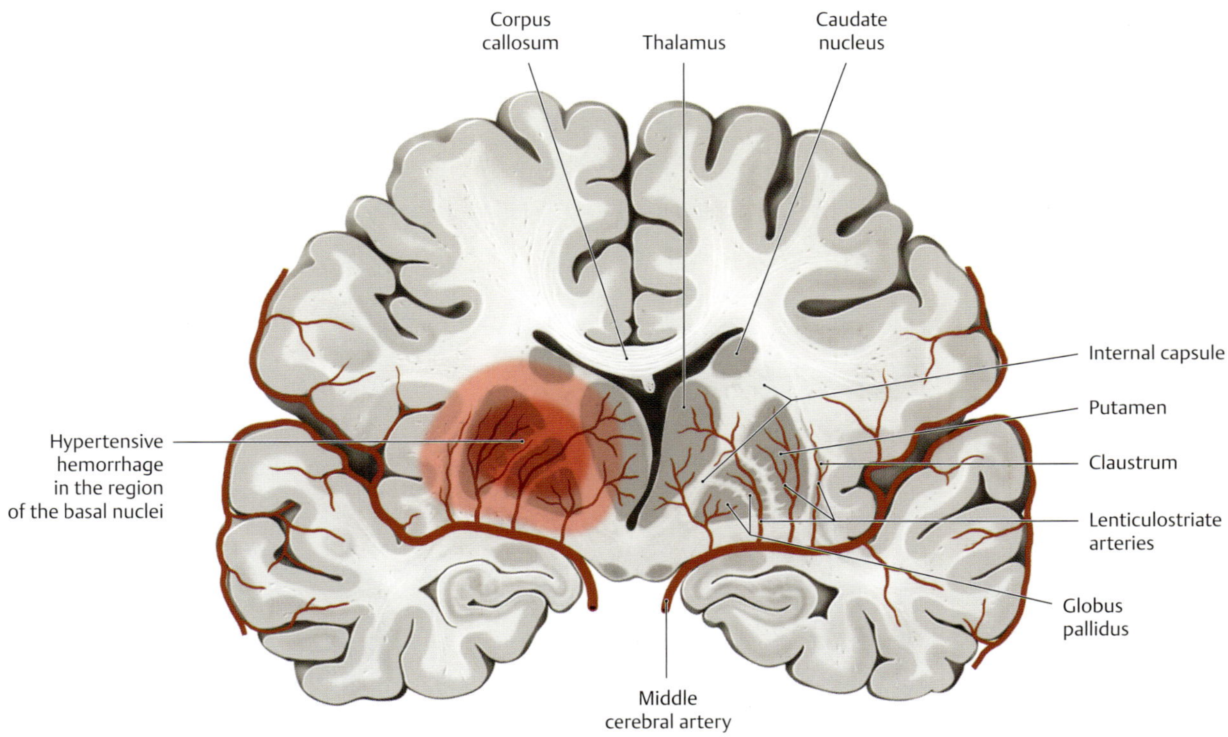

C Intracerebral hemorrhage
Coronal section through the mamillary bodies. Unlike the intracranial extracerebral hemorrhages (see **A**), intracerebral hemorrhage involves bleeding directly into the substance of the brain. Because the soft brain tissue offers very little resistance, a massive hemorrhage can develop which, in contrast to extracerebral bleeding, cannot be controlled by surgical hemostasis. The most frequent cause of intracerebral hemorrhage (hemorrhagic stroke) is high blood pressure. The hemorrhage produces a stroke with a central (dark red) area of necrosis surrounded by a lighter halo. This halo is known as a penumbra (Latin *paene* "almost" and *umbra* "shadow") and is readily distinguishable from the central necrotic area on MRI. The penumbra is an area of relative oxygen deficiency. As a result, there is an initial total loss of function in the affected area of the brain. In contrast to the irreversibly destroyed brain tissue in the area of necrosis, the ischemic tissue in the penumbra can recover in certain cases. The most common sites of vascular rupture are what are known as the "stroke arteries," the lenticulostriate arteries in the region of the internal capsule. Because the pyramidal tract passes through the internal capsule (see **E**, p. 335), there is a loss of pyramidal tract function below the lesion. This is manifested clinically by spastic paralysis of the limbs on the opposite side to the injury (as the pyramidal tracts cross below the level of the lesion). Aside from massive hemorrhages, smaller bleeds may occur in the territories of the three main cerebral arteries, producing a typical clinical presentation.

10.10 Blood Vessels of the Brain: Cerebrovascular Disease

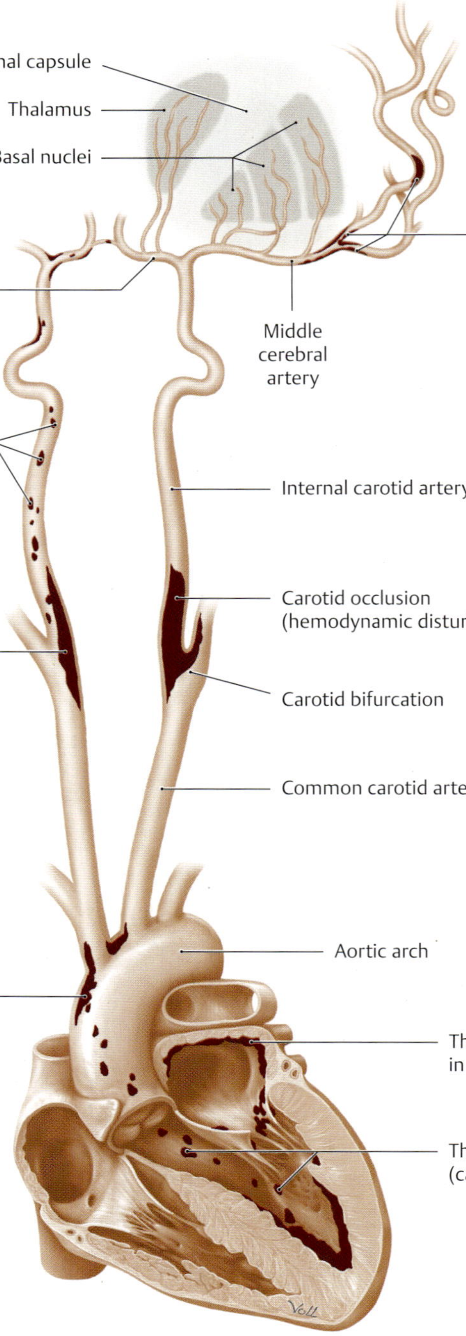

A Frequent causes of cerebrovascular disease

Disturbances of cerebral blood flow that deprive the brain of oxygen (cerebral ischemia) are the most frequent cause of central neurological deficits. The most serious complication is stroke: the vast majority of all strokes are caused by cerebral *ischemic* disease. Stroke has become the third leading cause of death in western industrialized countries (approximately 700,000 strokes occur in the United States each year). Cerebral ischemia is caused by a prolonged diminution or interruption of blood flow and involves *the distribution area of the internal carotid artery* in up to 90% of cases. Much less commonly, cerebral ischemia is caused by an obstruction of venous outflow due to cerebral venous thrombosis (see **B**). A decrease of arterial blood flow in the carotid system most commonly results from an embolic or local thrombotic occlusion. Most emboli originate from atheromatous lesions at the carotid bifurcation (arterioarterial emboli) or from the expulsion of thrombotic material from the left ventricle (cardiac emboli). Blood clots (thrombi) may be dislodged from the heart as a result of valvular disease or atrial fibrillation. This produces emboli that may be carried by the bloodstream to the brain, where they may cause the functional occlusion of an artery supplying the brain. The most common example of this involves all of the distribution region of the middle cerebral artery, which is a direct continuation of the internal carotid artery.

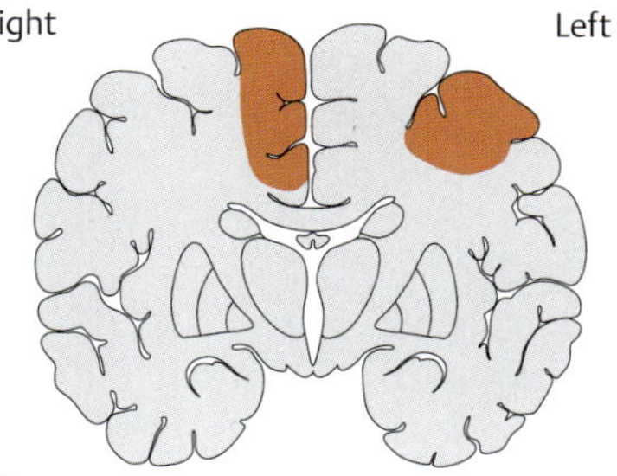

B Cerebral venous thrombosis

Coronal section, anterior view. The cerebral veins, like the cerebral arteries, serve specific territories (see pp. 386 and 388). Though much less common than decreased arterial flow, the obstruction of venous outflow is an important potential cause of ischemia and infarction. With a thrombotic occlusion, for example, the quantity of blood and thus the venous pressure are increased in the tributary region of the occluded vein. This causes a drop in the capillary pressure gradient, with an increased extravasation of fluid from the capillary bed into the brain tissue (edema). There is a concomitant reduction of arterial inflow into the affected region, depriving it of oxygen. The occlusion of specific cerebral veins (e.g., due to cerebral venous thrombosis) leads to brain infarctions at characteristic locations:

a Superior cerebral veins: Thrombosis and infarction in the areas drained by the
- Medial superior cerebral veins (right, *symptoms*: contralateral lower limb weakness)
- Posterior superior cerebral veins (left, *symptoms*: contralateral hemiparesis) Motor aphasia occurs if the infarction involves the motor speech center in the dominant hemisphere.

b Inferior cerebral veins: Thrombosis of the right inferior cerebral veins leads to infarction of the right temporal lobe (*symptoms*: sensory aphasia, contralateral hemianopia).

c Internal cerebral veins: Bilateral thrombosis leads to a symmetrical infarction affecting the thalamus and basal nuclei. This is characterized by a rapid deterioration of consciousness ranging to coma.

Because the dural sinuses have extensive anastomoses, a limited occlusion affecting part of a sinus often does not cause pronounced clinical symptoms, unlike the venous thromboses described here (see p. 384).

Vascular territory	Main neurological symptoms	
Anterior cerebral artery	Paralysis of lower limb (with or without hemisensory deficit) 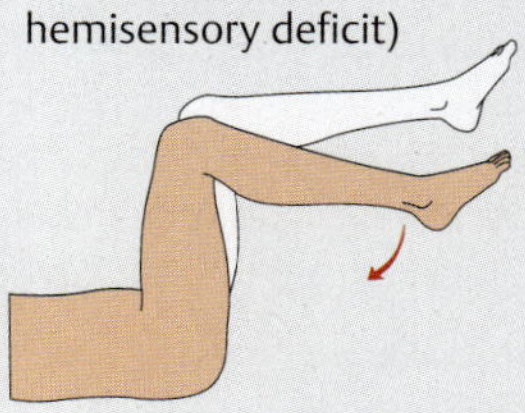	Bladder dysfunction 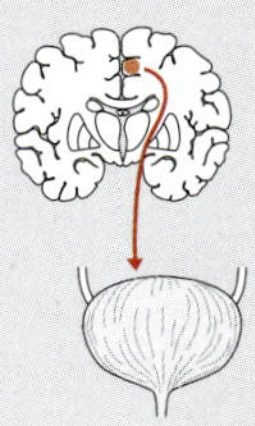
Middle cerebral artery	Hemiparesis (with or without hemisensory deficit) mainly affecting the upper limb and face 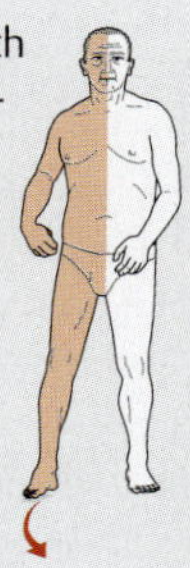	Aphasia 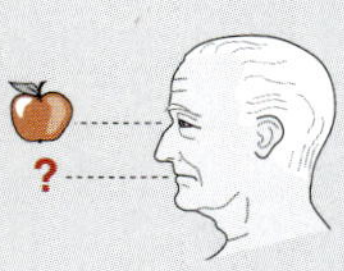
Posterior cerebral artery	Hemisensory losses 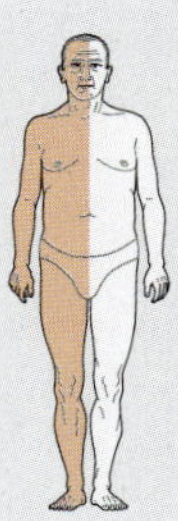	Hemianopia 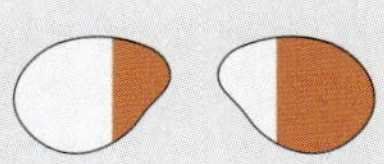

C Cardinal symptoms of occlusion of the three main cerebral arteries (after Masuhr and Neumann)

When the *anterior*, *middle*, or *posterior cerebral artery* becomes occluded, characteristic functional deficits occur in the oxygen-deprived brain areas supplied by the occluded vessel (see p. 378). In many cases the affected artery can be identified based on the associated neurological deficit:

- Bladder weakness (cortical bladder center) and paralysis of the lower limb (with or without hemisensory deficit, predominantly affecting the leg) on the side opposite the occlusion (see motor and sensory homunculi, pp. 447 and 457) indicate an infarction in the territory of the **anterior cerebral artery**.
- Contralateral hemiplegia affecting the arm and face more than the leg indicates an infarction in the territory of the **middle cerebral artery**. If the dominant hemisphere is affected, aphasia also occurs (the patient cannot name objects, for example).
- Visual disturbances affecting the contralateral visual field (contralateral homonymous hemianopsia) may signify an infarction in the territory of the **posterior cerebral artery**, because the structures supplied by this artery include the visual cortex in the calcarine sulcus of the occipital lobe. If branches to the thalamus are also affected, the patient may also exhibit a contralateral hemisensory deficit because the afferent sensory fibers have already crossed below the thalamus.

The extent of the infarction depends partly on whether the occlusion is proximal or distal. Generally a proximal occlusion will cause a much more extensive infarction than a distal occlusion. MCA infarctions are the most common because the middle cerebral artery is essentially a direct continuation of the internal carotid artery.

11.1 Spinal Cord: Segmental Organization

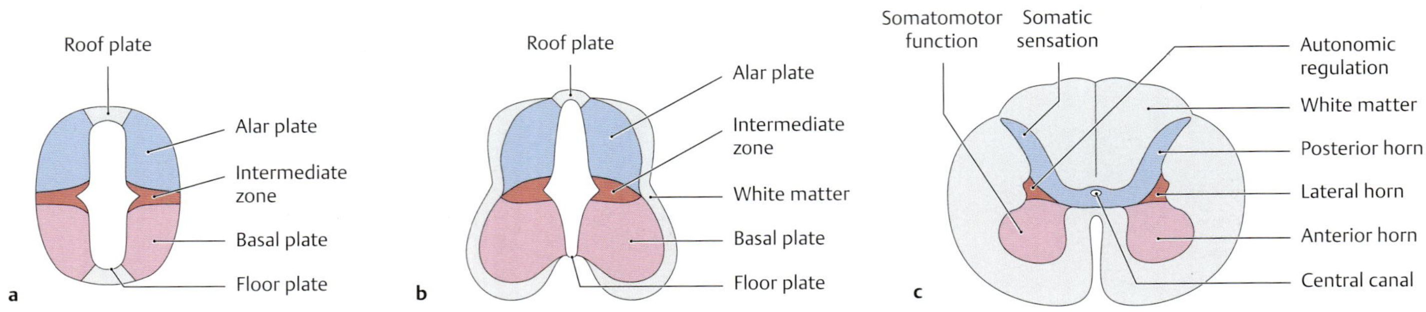

A Embryological development of the spinal cord

Cross-section through the neural tube at the level where the spinal cord eventually develops; cranial view.

a Early neural tube; **b** Intermediate stage; **c** Adult spinal cord.

The development of the spinal cord has already been explained on p. 273. More than any other part of the CNS, knowledge of the embryological development of the spinal cord facilitates the understanding of its structure and function after birth. This is why its development will be briefly reviewed and highlighted.

- The spinal cord as a part of the CNS derives from the neural tube. A cross-section through the early neural tube (**a**) shows a central fluid filled (cerebrospinal fluid) lumen, which is surrounded by so-called "plates":
  - the unpaired floor and roof plate as well as
  - the paired basal and alar plates.

  Between basal and alar plates lies an *intermediate* zone (zona intermedia). Numerous neurons develop In the basal and alar plate as well as in the intermediate zone. They form the **gray matter** as a result of which these areas enlarge and increasingly constrict the lumen leading to the formation of the central canal of the spinal cord (**c**), which may become even obstructed in some regions. In the adult spinal cord, the three gray columns are referred to as anterior, lateral, and posterior horns.
- The processes (axons) emerging from neurons or the axons arriving from other neurons form the **white matter**, which topographically can be divided into three columns (funiculi) and functionally into numerous tracts (see p. 396). The white matter surrounds the gray matter.

Morphologically, the gray matter which is surrounded by white matter on all sides, is considered a nucleus or nuclear group. Each of the three horns can be assigned one main function according to their neurons: anterior horn: somatomotor function; posterior horn: somatic sensation; lateral horn: control of the autonomic functions of organs.

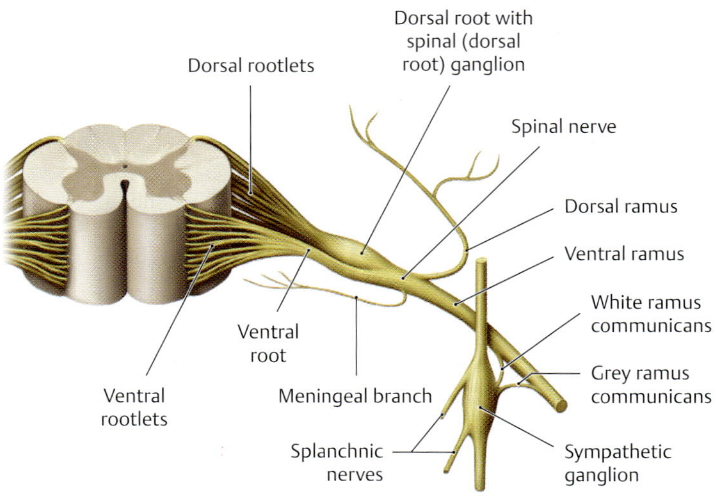

B Structure of a spinal cord segment

Anteriosuperior view of a spinal cord segment as well as a spinal nerve. The spinal cord is a continuous structure located in the vertebral canal. A segmental functional or morphological distinction is not precisely identifiable. The spinal cord as part of the CNS is continuously connected with the PNS via **nerve rootlets**. These nerve rootlets are groups of axons, which

- exit the spinal cord on its anterior aspect (typically axons of motor neurons, which terminate in an target organ or autonomic ganglion) or
- enter the spinal cord on its posterior aspect (typically axons of sensory neurons, which carry information from a receptor).

The spinal columns consist of segments—corresponding to the individual vertebrae—which means that the vertebral canal itself is divided (see **C**). It virtually determines a segmental arrangement of the continuous spinal cord. It is only at the openings *between* individual vertebrae—at the *inter*vertebral foramina—that the rootlets that form the spinal nerves can either enter or exit the vertebral canal. They don't do that individually but in bundles in form of a **root (radix)**:

- The anterior rootlets form an anterior root.
- The posterior rootlets form a posterior root.

Both roots merge to form the **spinal nerve (n. spinalis)**. The rootlets, roots, and spinal nerve are parts of the PNS. Functionally, a spinal cord segment is based a longitudinal division of the spinal cord, which contains the cell bodies of motor neurons that form precisely one anterior root. Each spinal segment (which is a *continuous* part of the CNS) is therefore connected with a spinal nerve (which is a *discontinuous* part of the PNS).

Note: The posterior root is not "involved" in the functional definition because the fibers entering the spinal cord through the posterior root don't always end on neurons located at the same level of the spinal cord (i.e., in certain cases they will end in the medulla oblongata). Since the spinal nerve consists of (motor) anterior root and (sensory) posterior root, it has mixed functions. The only exception among the spinal nerves: the spinal nerve from the C1 segment does not have a posterior root (thus there are no posterior rootlets): it is exclusively motor. For all other spinal nerves, it could be said that in morphological terms, a segment of the spinal cord is the part where *the rootlets, which merge to form a spinal nerve*, enter or exit the spinal cord.

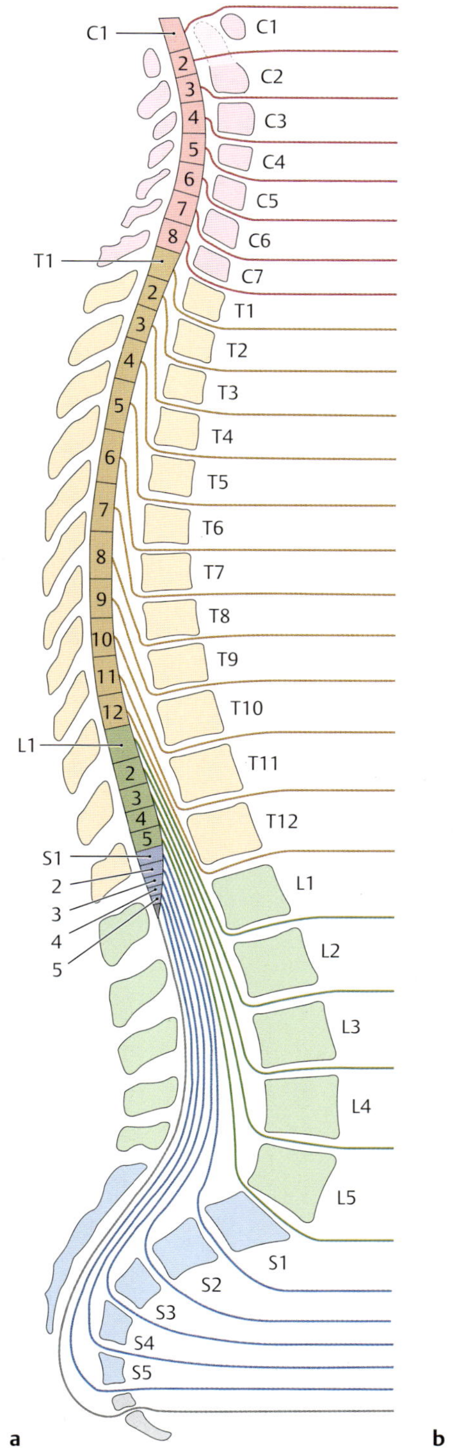

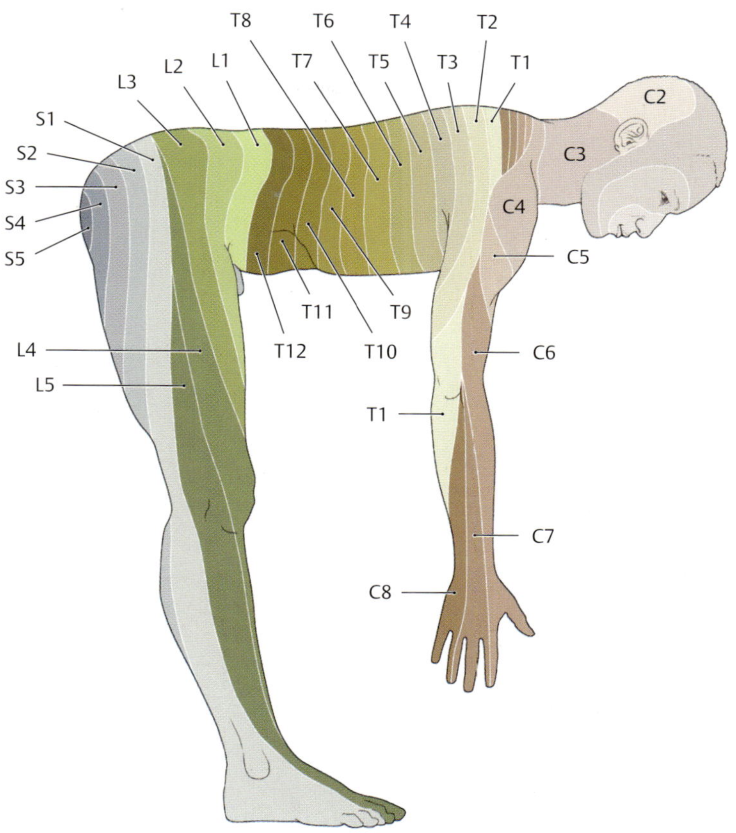

D Simplified schematic representation of the segmental innervation of the skin

Distribution of the dermatomes on the body. Sensory innervation of the skin correlates with the sensory roots of the spinal nerves. Every spinal cord segment (except for C1, see below) innervates a particular skin area (dermatome). From a clinical standpoint, it is important to know the precise correlation of dermatomes with spinal cord segments so that the level of a spinal cord lesion can be deter-mined based on the location of the affected dermatome. For example, a lesion of the C8 spinal nerve root is characterized by a loss of sensation on the ulnar (small-finger) side of the hand.

Note: There is no C1 dermatome because there is no posterior root. Proprioceptive fibers from the short neck muscles in the suboccipital nerve course via the posterior cervical plexus into the posterior root of C2.

Spinal cord segment	Vertebral body	Spinous process
C8	Inferior margin of C 6, superior margin of C 7	C 6
T 6	T 5	T 4
T 12	T 10	T 9
L 5	T 11	T 10
S 1	T 12	T 12

C Relation between spinal cord segments and spinal column in adults

a Midsagittal section of the spinal column, viewed from the right side; **b** Spinal cord segments (selected).

A spinal cord segment is named according to the vertebra related to which "its" spinal nerve emerges.

- The first spinal nerve, which emerges above the first cervical vertebra (C1), is referred to as C1.
- The spinal nerve which emerges above the second cervical vertebra (C2) is referred to as C2, and so on.

Note: As the first spinal nerve emerges from the spinal column between the occipital bone and the first cervical vertebra, that is superior to the first cervical vertebra, there are eight cervical spinal nerves (C1–C8) whereas there are only seven cervical vertebrae.

As a result of this counting convention, the first thoracic vertebra (T1) is unique in that the eighth cervical spinal nerve (C8) emerges superior to it whereas the first thoracic spinal nerve (T1) emerges *inferior* to it. From T1 to the distal end of the spinal column, all spinal nerves emerge *inferior* to their respective vertebrae. Spinal nerve S5 courses through the sacral canal as there are only four available sacral intervertebral foramina through which spinal nerves S1–S4 emerge. It is apparent that the spinal column is significantly longer than the spinal cord. Therefore, as one moves distally, the spinal cord segments and their respective vertebrae are increasingly found to be at different levels (in contrast to their location in the embryo). The most distal spinal cord segment, with coccygeal segment 1/2, lies at the level of the first lumbar vertebra (L1) and not at the level of the corresponding coccygeal vertebra 1 or 2. This gives rise to what is known as the cauda equina (horse tail); the roots of the spinal nerves which must follow an ever longer course from their spinal cord segment to "their" vertebra. Spinal injuries distal to L1 thus do not damage the spinal cord itself but the anterior or posterior root of the respective spinal nerve (*cauda equina syndrome*). Knowledge of these topographical relationships is important when performing a lumbar puncture (see **C** and **E**, p. 419).

11.2 Spinal Cord: Organization of Spinal Cord Segments

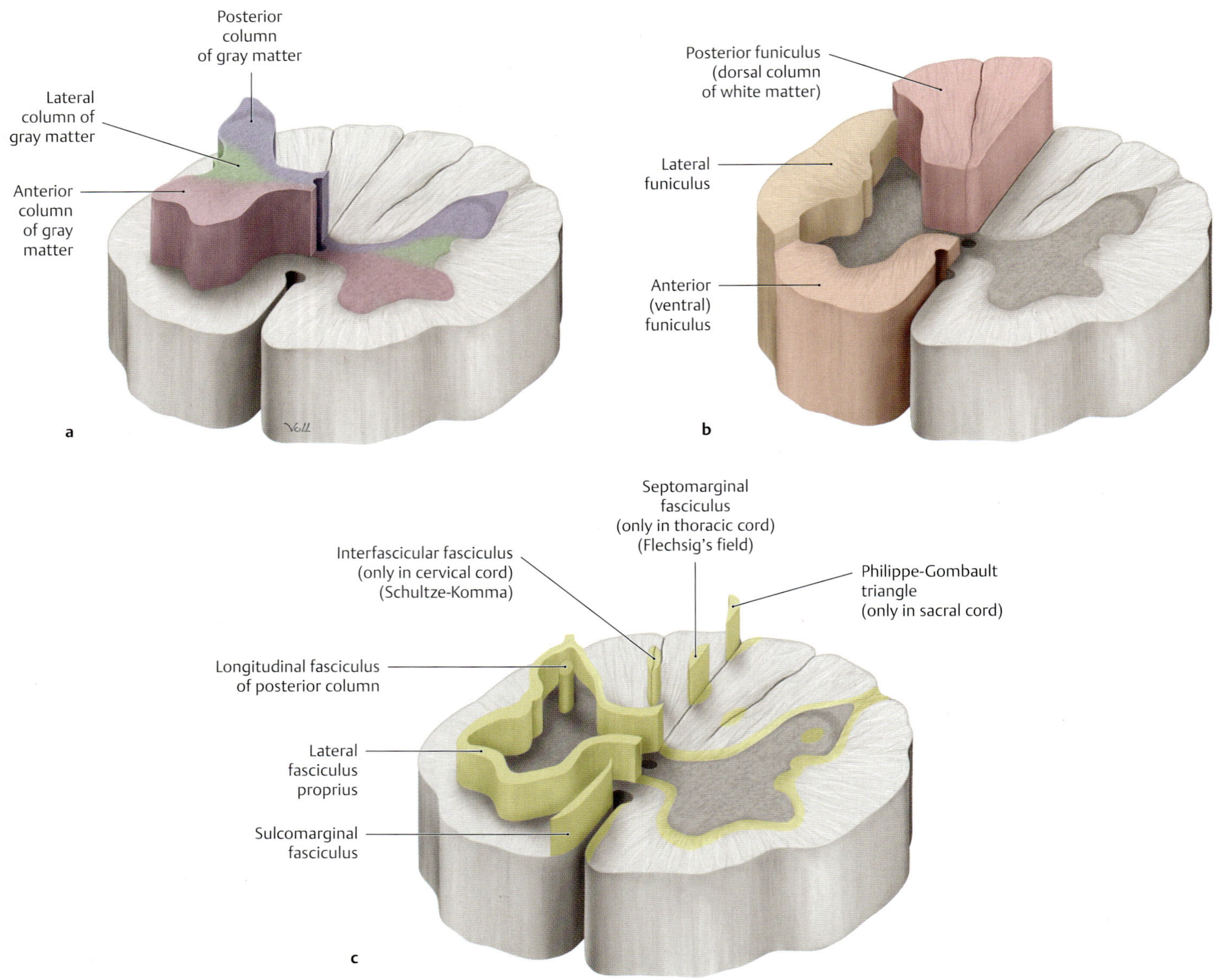

A Gray and white matter of the spinal cord

Three dimensional representation of the spinal cord, oblique anterior view from upper left.

a Gray matter; **b** White matter: the funiculi; **c** White matter: propriospinal fasciculi.

The typical cross-sectional view of the spinal cord simplifies the fact that the functional arrangement of neurons occurs in columns (called nuclear columns) (see **A**, p. 398). Thus, the representation of the gray matter in three columns (**a**), anterior, lateral, and posterior, the cross-section of which shows the respective horn, is more than a topographic aspect. For the functional understanding of muscles through nuclear columns on one hand (see p. 398) and for knowledge about the function of propriospinal fasciculi (see **c**) on the other hand, the concept of the columns is essential. With reference to the definition of a segment (see **B**, p. 394), the anterior *column* is the place where all motor neurons that form the anterior *root* are located. The lateral or posterior column contain autonomic or sensory neurons as it has already been mentioned in **A**, p. 394, in connection with the respective horns. The white matter consists of tracts. They can generally be distinguished based on their *destination*:

- **b** Tracts, which run through the spinal cord—p.r.n after interconnecting inside the spinal cord—and permit communication with other parts of the CNS. With respect to the spinal cord's extrinsic circuits, the white matter is divided into three funiculi or white matter columns: anterior, lateral, and posterior.
- **c** Tracts that interconnect neurons in the columns inside the spinal cord and are responsible for the "intrinsic circuits" of the spinal cord. The axons of these tracts belong to interneurons that are arranged around the gray matter. The intrinsic circuit is organized as propriospinal fasciculi, typically located adjacent to the gray matter. These fibers can also run horizontally and interconnect neurons of one level (not shown here).

In both circuits, the tracts can be ascending or descending. In the extrinsic circuits, ascending tracts are sensory while descending tracts are motor.

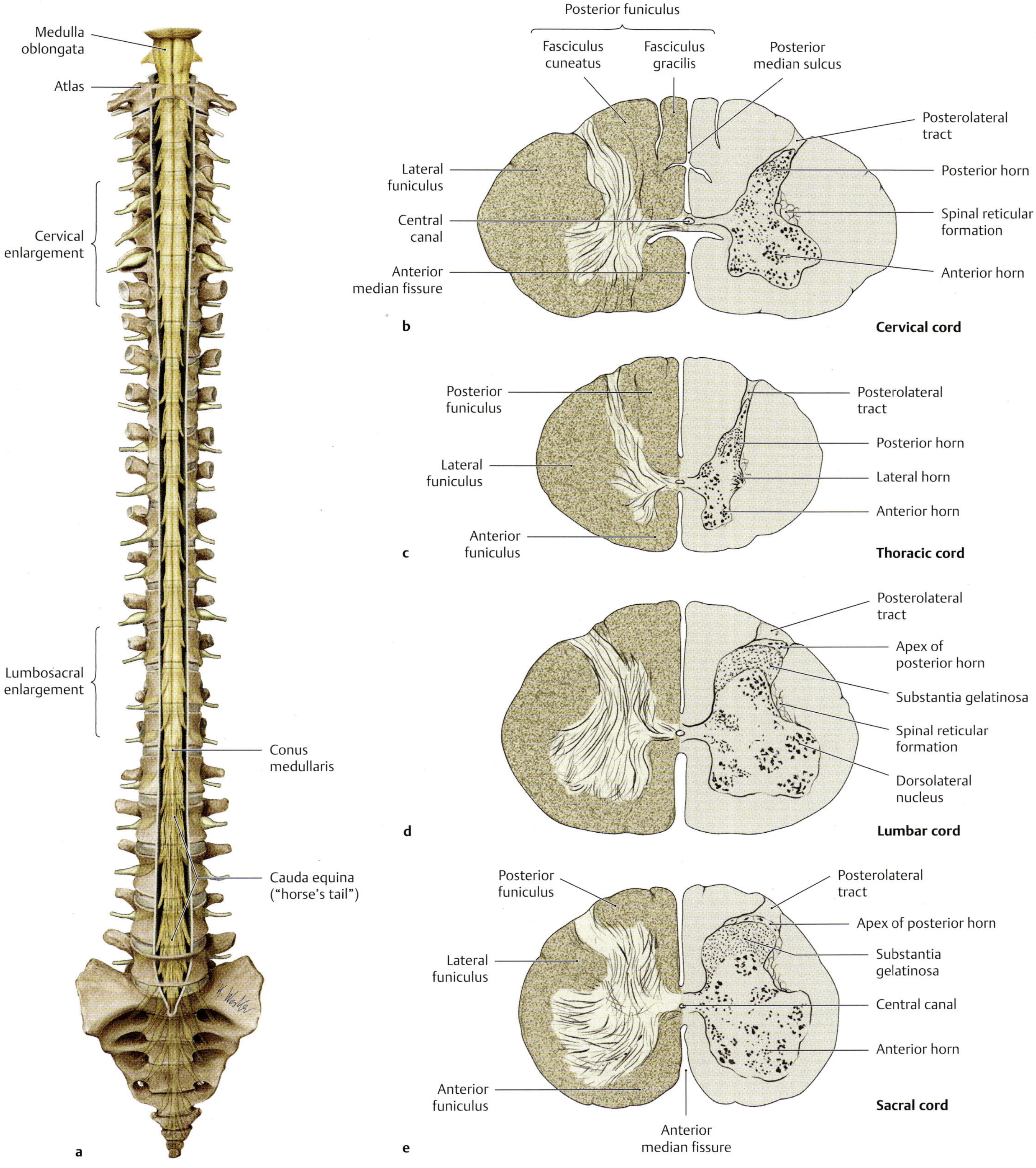

B Position of the spinal cord in the dural sac
a Anterior view with the vertebral bodies partially removed to display the anterior aspect of the spinal cord. The transverse sections (**b–e**) depict fiber tracts (left side, myelin stain) and neuron cell bodies (right side, Nissl stain) at different levels of the spinal cord. The areas of the cervical and lumbosacral enlargements have been demarcated (**a**). In these areas, which provide innervation to the limbs, the gray matter is significantly expanded.

11.3 Spinal Cord: Internal Divisions of the Gray Matter

A Organizational principles of the anterior column of the spinal cord

Motor neurons that innervate specific muscles are arranged into vertical columns in the anterior (ventral) horn of the gray matter of the spinal cord. Analogous to the brainstem motor nuclei, these columns can themselves be called nuclei, and are arranged in a somatotopic fashion (see **B** for a mapping of these nuclei to their target muscles). The motor columns innervating the trunk have a relatively simple arrangement that follows the linear segmental organization of spinal nerves and dermatomes. The cervical and lumbrosacral enlargements, which innervate the limbs, have a more complex pattern of innervation than the trunk muscles: during the migratory processes of embryonic development, muscle precursors "carry" their original innervation with them, generating a motor column that sends its axons through multiple nerve roots from multiple spinal cord levels. The muscles innervated by such a column are accordingly called *multisegmental muscles* (see **B**, p. 400). Muscles whose motor neurons are situated entirely within one segment are referred to as *indicator muscles*; testing the function of indicator muscles is valuable in clinical assessment.
Note: Although one muscle may be innervated by axons from multiple spinal segments, those axons arise from a *single* motor column.

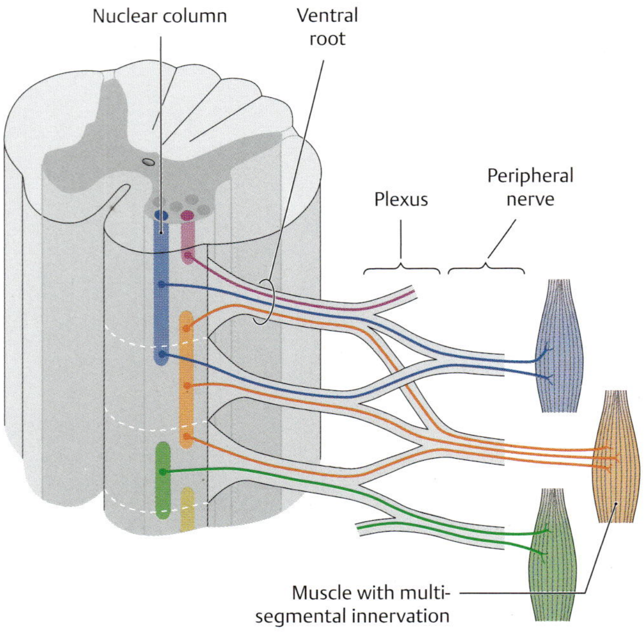

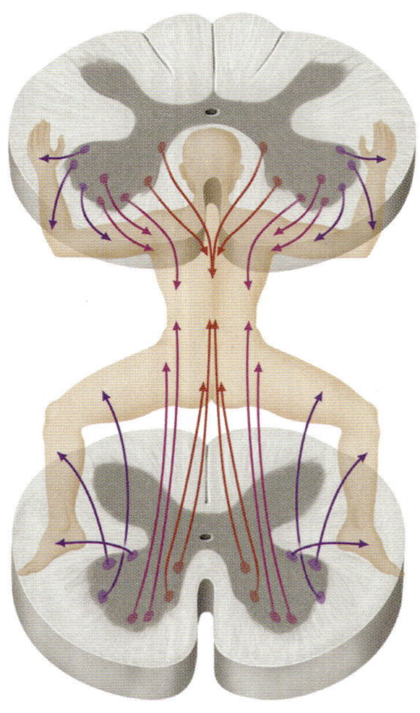

a

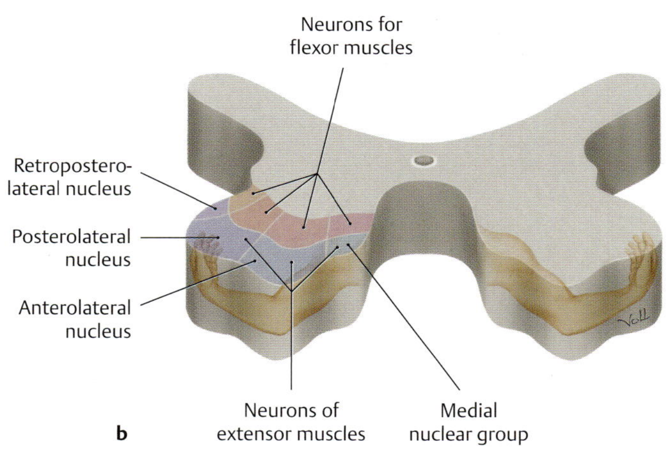

b

B Somatotopic organization of nuclear columns of the anterior horn

a Common pattern of organization in the spinal cord. More medial nuclear columns of the anterior horn innervate muscles close to the midline, while more lateral nuclear columns tend to innervate muscles outside the trunk.

b Enlargement of cervical cord. The same pattern of medial-to-lateral organization exists (see **a**) with medial nuclei innervating axial muscles and lateral nuclei innervating muscles at the extremities. However, there is also an anterior-to-posterior segregation of motor columns. Neurons serving extensor muscles (shades of blue) are found in the most anterior parts of the anterior horn, while those serving flexor muscles (shades of pink) are found in the more posterior regions. These nuclei are further divided into the following:

- Medial nuclei: innervate nuchal, back, intercostal, and abdominal muscles
- Anterolateral nucleus: innervates shoulder girdle and upper arm muscles
- Posterolateral nucleus: innervates forearm muscles
- Retroposterolateral nucleus: innervates small muscles of the fingers.

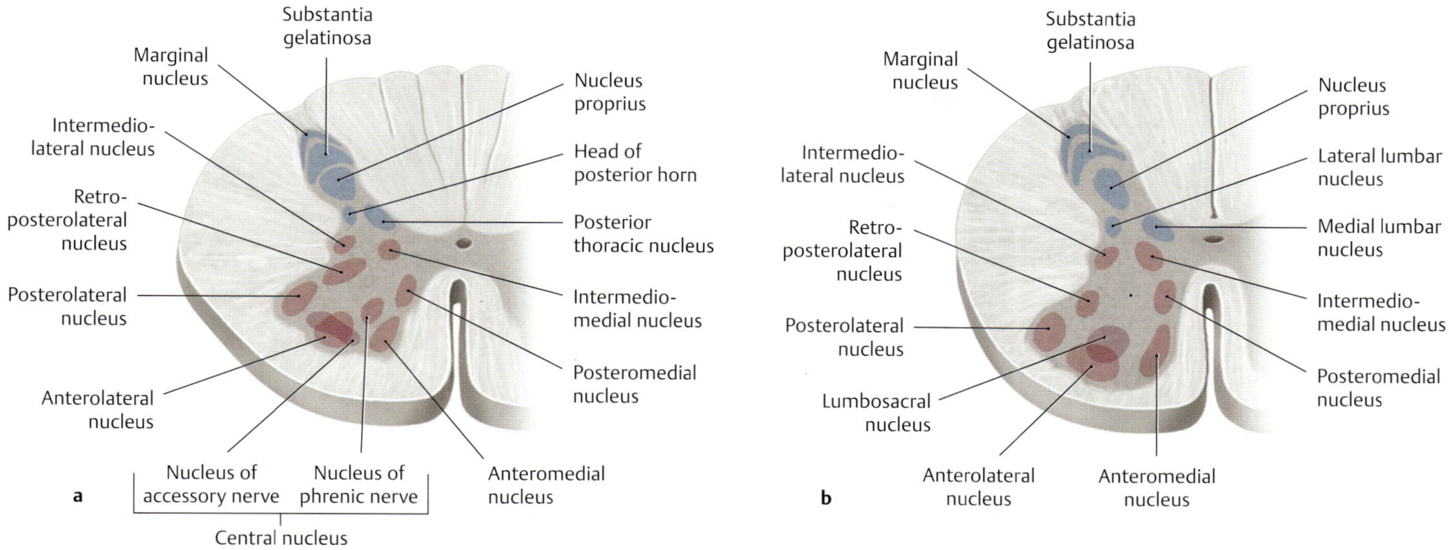

C Cell groups in the gray matter of the spinal cord

a Cervical cord; **b** Lumbar cord. The neurons in the gray matter of the spinal cord are classified in cell groups (nuclei) according to their shape and position. When one excludes the neurons not involved in local information processing, the anterior horn essentially contains the somatoefferent motor neurons. As a result, the anterior horn is significantly larger than the posterior horn, which essentially contains the projection neurons of the ascending pathways. As the positions of the nuclear groups can vary in the different sections, the illustration shows the cervical and lumbar cord. A few cell columns are specific to the respective segment of the spinal cord. For example, the nucleus for the phrenic nerve is found only in the cervical cord. The **sacral cord** (not shown here) contains a small nucleus (on average 625 neurons), nucleus X after Onuf, on the anterior aspect of lamina IX (see **D**) at the level of (S1)–S2–S3. This nucleus contains the motor neurons of the pudendal nerve, which are responsible for urinary and fecal continence (external sphincters for the anus and urethra) and for orgasm (ischiocavernosus and bulbocavernosus).

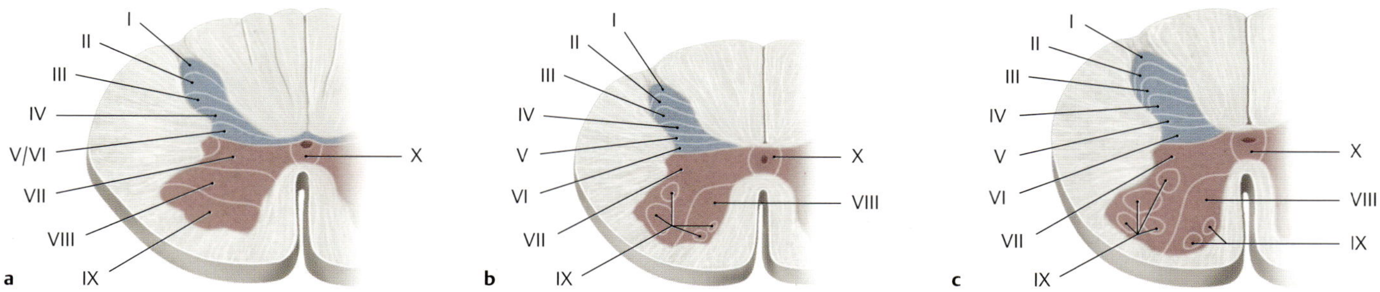

D Classification of the nuclei in layers after Rexed

a Cervical cord; **b** Thoracic cord; **c** Lumbar cord. The complex organization of the CNS means that there are different ways to classify the gray matter. Aside from the division described above, the gray matter can also be divided into cytoarchitectural layers (laminae I–X) after Rexed. This laminar architecture is especially well defined in the posterior (dorsal) horn; in the anterior horn, the arrangement of the laminae resembles that of the nuclei (see **C**). The site at which the sensory axons of the spinal ganglia end is often specified as the lamina after Rexed. This figure can serve as a reference.

E Gray matter neurons of the spinal cord

Root cells

Neurons whose axons exit from the anterior root. These are further differentiated as follows:

- Somatomotor root cells (extend to the skeletal muscles; α and γ motor neurons)
- Visceral motor root cells (extending to the viscera)

Intrinsic neurons

Neurons whose axons do not leave the CNS. These are further differentiated as follows:

- *Projection neurons:* Intrinsic neurons in the posterior column whose axons leave the gray matter and extend in the white matter as ascending pathways to higher centers. They represent the second sensory neuron; the first lies in the spinal ganglion (see p. 403). Because their axons terminate in higher centers, they are referred to collectively as projection neurons (analogously to the descending projection neurons).
- *Interneurons:* Neurons distributed throughout the gray matter whose axons do not leave the gray matter. These are further differentiated as follows:
  - Relay cells: Neurons whose axons terminate within one side on a single segment level (see **C**, S. 401)
  - Commissural cells: Neurons whose axons extend in the white commissure to the opposite side (see **C**, S. 401)
  - Associative cells: Neurons whose axons interconnect various segments on one side; intersegmental correlation system (see **C**, S. 401)
  - Renshaw cells: Neurons which are stimulated by axon collaterals of the excitatory alpha motor neuron. They then release and inhibitory neurotransmitter that acts in a retrograde manner on the stimulating alpha motor neuron (retrograde inhibition; see **D**, p. 401).

11.4 Spinal Cord: Reflex Arcs and Intrinsic Circuits

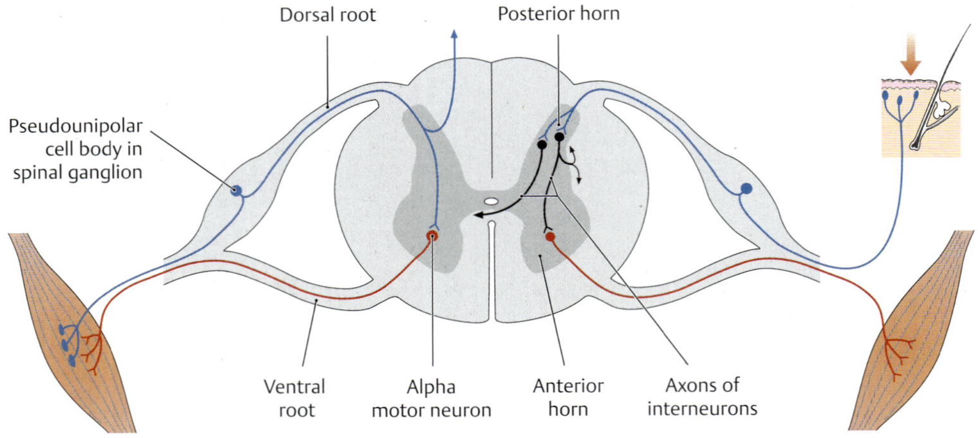

A Integrative function of the gray matter of the spinal cord: reflexes

Afferent nerves are shown in blue, efferent nerves in red. Black indicates neurons of the spinal reflex circuit.

The gray matter of the spinal cord supports muscular function at the unconscious (reflex) level, holding the body upright during stance and enabling us to walk and run without conscious control. To perform this coordinating function, the neurons of the gray matter must receive information from the muscles and their surroundings; this information enters the posterior horn of the spinal cord via the axons of neurons in the spinal ganglia (see p. 446). Two types of reflex exist:

- **Monosynaptic reflex** (left): intrinsic reflex in which information from the periphery (e.g., on muscle length and stretch) comes from the muscle itself. Receptors in the muscle transmit signals to alpha motor neurons via neurons whose cell bodies are in the dorsal root ganglia. These afferent neurons release excitatory neurotransmitters which cause the alpha motor neurons to stimulate muscle contraction (see **D**).
- **Polysynaptic reflex** (right): reflex mediated by receptors in the skin or other sites *outside* the muscle. These receptors act via *interneurons* (see **C**) to stimulate muscular contraction.

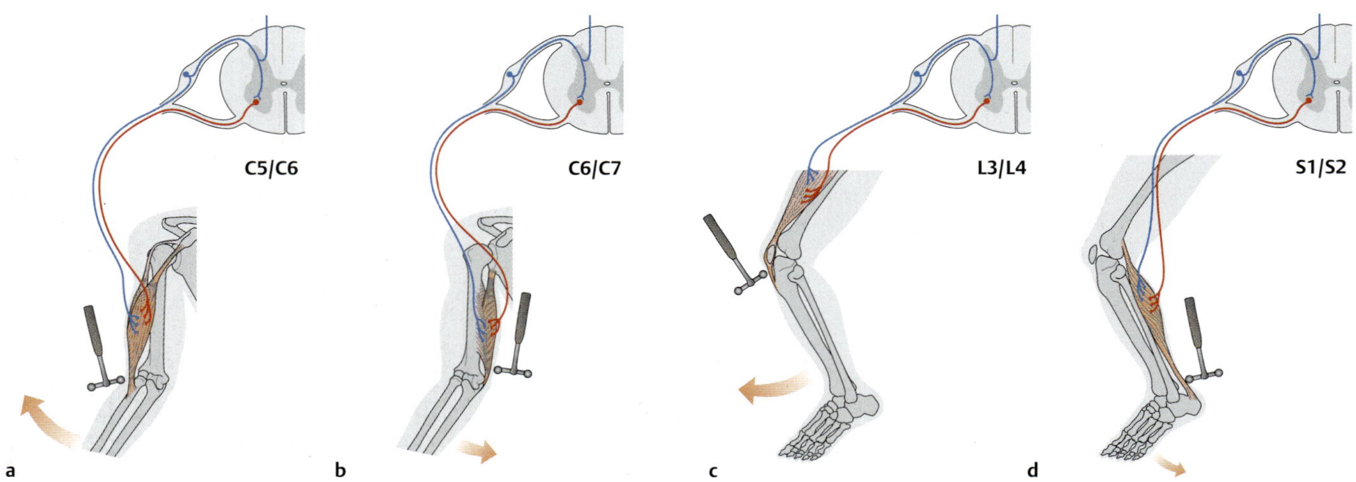

B Clinically important monosynaptic reflexes

a Biceps reflex; **b** Triceps reflex; **c** Patellar reflex (quadriceps reflex); **d** Achilles tendon reflex.

The drawings show the muscles, the trigger points for eliciting the reflexes, the nerves involved in the reflexes (afferent nerves in blue, efferent nerves in red), and the corresponding spinal cord segments.

The principal monosynaptic reflexes should be tested in every physical examination. Each reflex is elicited by briskly tapping the appropriate tendon with a reflex hammer to stretch the muscle. If the muscle contracts in response to this stretch, the reflex arc is intact. Although each test involves just one muscle and one peripheral nerve supplying the muscle, the innervation involves several spinal cord segments (multisegmental muscles, see **A**, p. 398). The right and left sides should always be compared in clinical reflex testing because this is the only way to recognize a *unilateral* increase, decrease, or other abnormality.

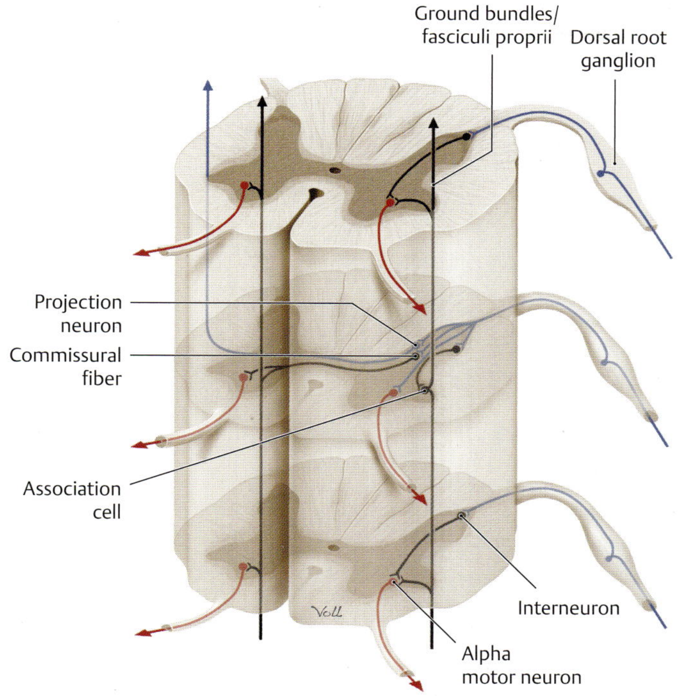

C Components of the intrinsic circuits of the spinal cord
Afferent neurons are shown in blue, efferent neurons in red. The neurons of the spinal reflex circuits are shown in black. Polysynaptic reflexes often must be coordinated at the spinal cord level by multiple segments. Interneurons, some of whose axons show a T-shaped branching pattern, convey the afferent signals to higher and lower segments along crossed and uncrossed pathways (types of interneurons are described in **E**, p. 399). These chains of interneurons, which are entirely contained within the spinal cord, make up the *intrinsic circuits* of the cord. The axons of the neurons in the intrinsic circuits pass to adjacent segments in intrinsic fascicles (fasciculi proprii) located as the edge of the gray matter (see **A**, p. 396). These fascicles are the conduction apparatus of the intrinsic circuits.

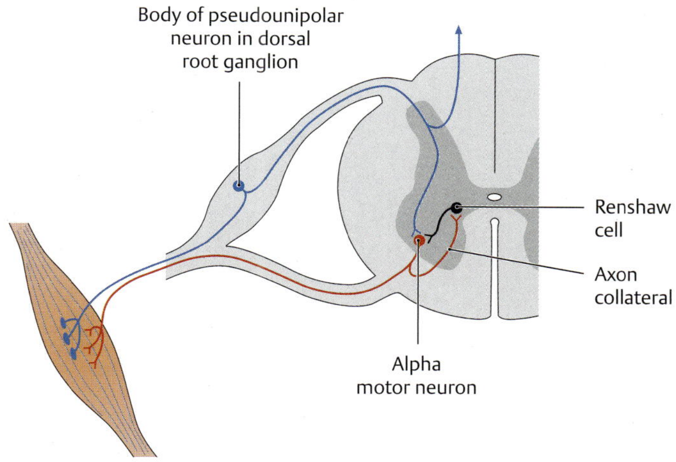

D Effects of the Renshaw cell on the alpha motor neuron
The afferent fibers in a monosynaptic reflex originate in neurons of the dorsal root ganglia. They terminate on the alpha motor neurons, where they release the excitatory transmitter acetylcholine. In response to this transmitter release, the alpha motor neuron transmits excitatory impulses to the neuromuscular junction (the transmitter is also acetylcholine). The excitatory alpha motor neuron has axon collaterals that enable it to exert a stimulatory effect on an inhibitory interneuron called a Renshaw cell. In response to this stimulation, the Renshaw cell releases the *inhibitory* transmitter glycine. This self-inhibiting mechanism serves to prevent overexcitation of the alpha motor neurons (recurrent inhibition). The clinical importance of the Renshaw cells is dramatically illustrated in patients with tetanus. The tetanus toxin inhibits the release of glycine from the Renshaw cells. Inhibition of the alpha motor neurons fails to occur, and so the patient experiences sustained (tetanic) muscle contractions.

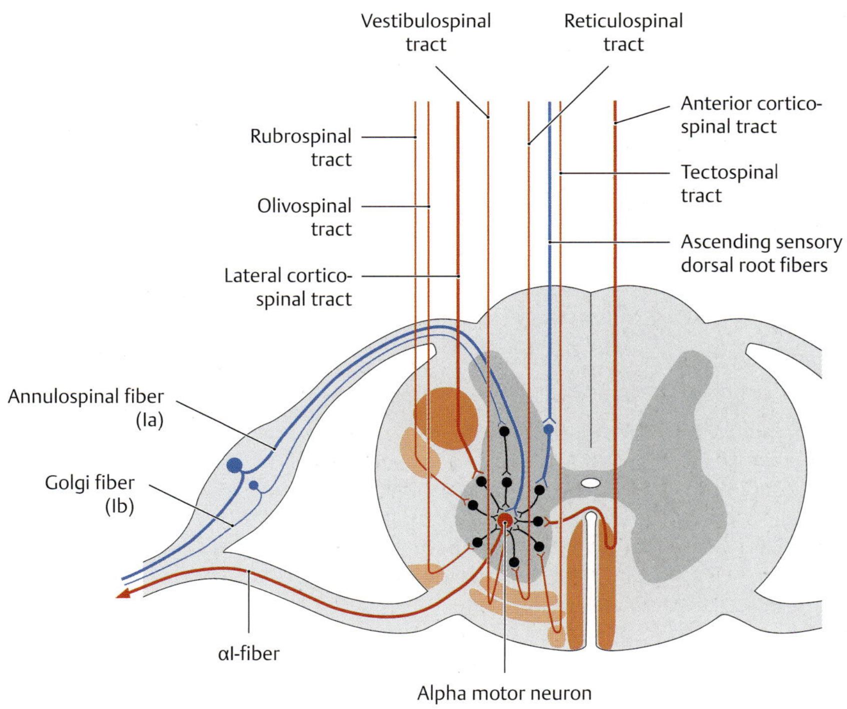

E Effects of long tracts on the alpha motor neuron
The alpha motor neuron not only receives afferent fibers from the spinal cord itself, but is also strongly modulated by fibers from long tracts that originate in the brain. Most of these fibers have an inhibitory effect on the alpha motor neuron. If these effects are abolished due to a complete cord lesion above the alpha motor neuron, for example, the disproportionately strong influence of the spinal intrinsic circuits will lead to spastic paralysis (see p. 461).

11.5 Ascending Tracts of the Spinal Cord: Spinothalamic Tracts

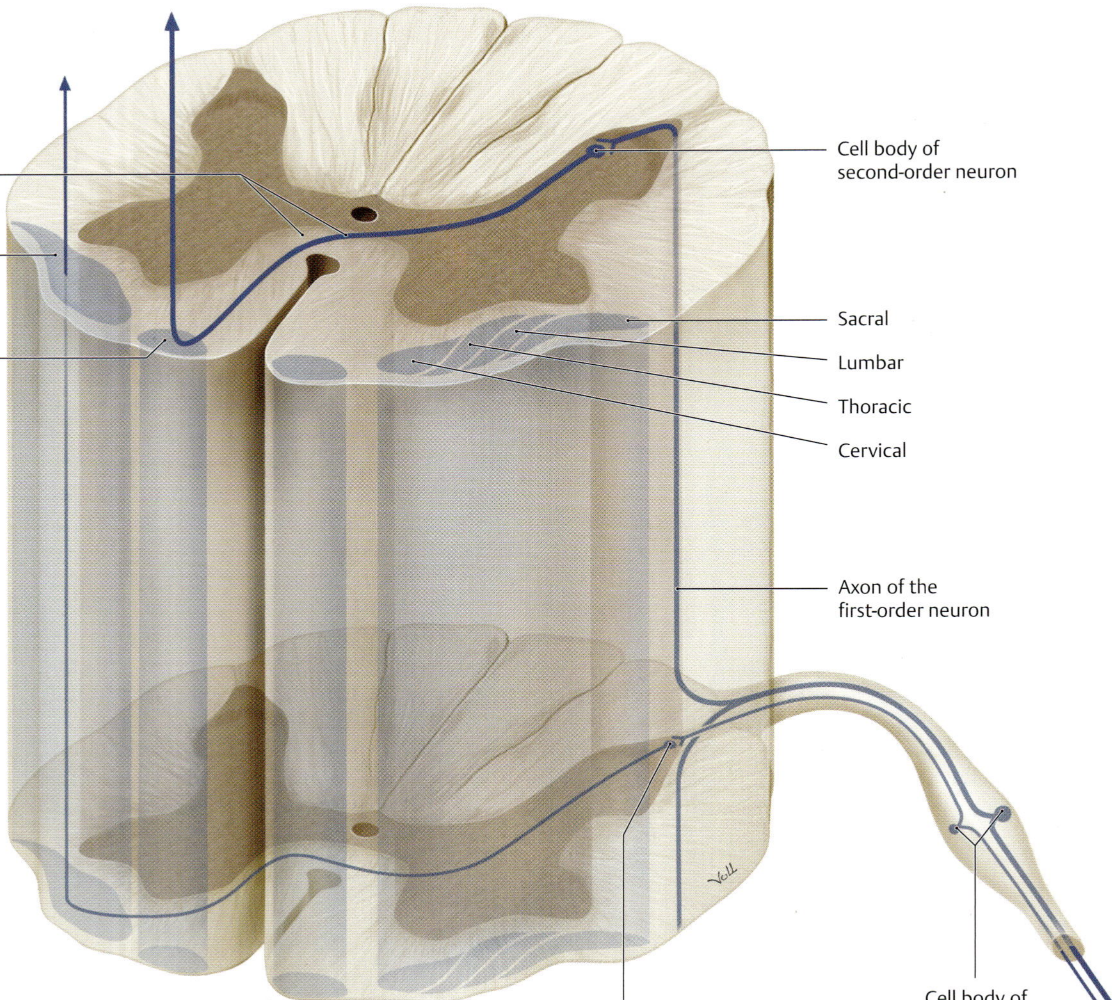

A Course of the anterior and lateral spinothalamic tracts in a transverse section of the spinal cord

The axons of the anterior spinothalamic tract run in the anterior funiculus of the spinal cord, while those of the lateral spinothalamic tract run in both the anterior and lateral funiculi. (These two tracts are sometimes referred to collectively as the *anterolateral system*.) The anterior spinothalamic tract is the pathway for crude touch and pressure sensation, while the lateral spinothalamic tract conveys pain, temperature, tickle, itch, and sexual sensation. The cell bodies of the primary afferent neurons for both tracts are located in the dorsal root ganglia. Both tracts contain second neurons that crossed in the anterior commissure. The somatotopic organization of the lateral spinothalamic tract is shown on the left side of the diagram. Starting dorsally and moving clockwise, we successively encounter the sacral, lumbar, thoracic, and cervical fibers. In older terminology a distinction is sometimes drawn between *epicritic* and *protopathic* sensation. According to this terminology, the anterior and lateral spinothalamic tracts are classified as *protopathic pathways* while the tracts of the posterior funiculus are classified as an *epicritic sensory pathway*. Today the original classification has been dropped because it does not correspond well to the assignment of sensory modalities of anatomically defined tracts.

Note: The spinothalamic tract is formed by fibers that cross (decussate) in the anterior white commissure but is not part of the anterior white commissure. The anterior white commissure, just like the posterior white commissure (not represented here), is a true commissure, in which fibers cross between the right and left halves of the spinal cord. The anterior white commissure is not to be confused with the anterior commissure, which is also a true commissure. However, it is not located in the spinal cord but in the telencephalon where it connects the left and right temporal lobes as well as the left and right olfactory nuclei. The posterior white commissure is not to be confused with the posterior commissure, which is a true commissure located in the diencephalon.

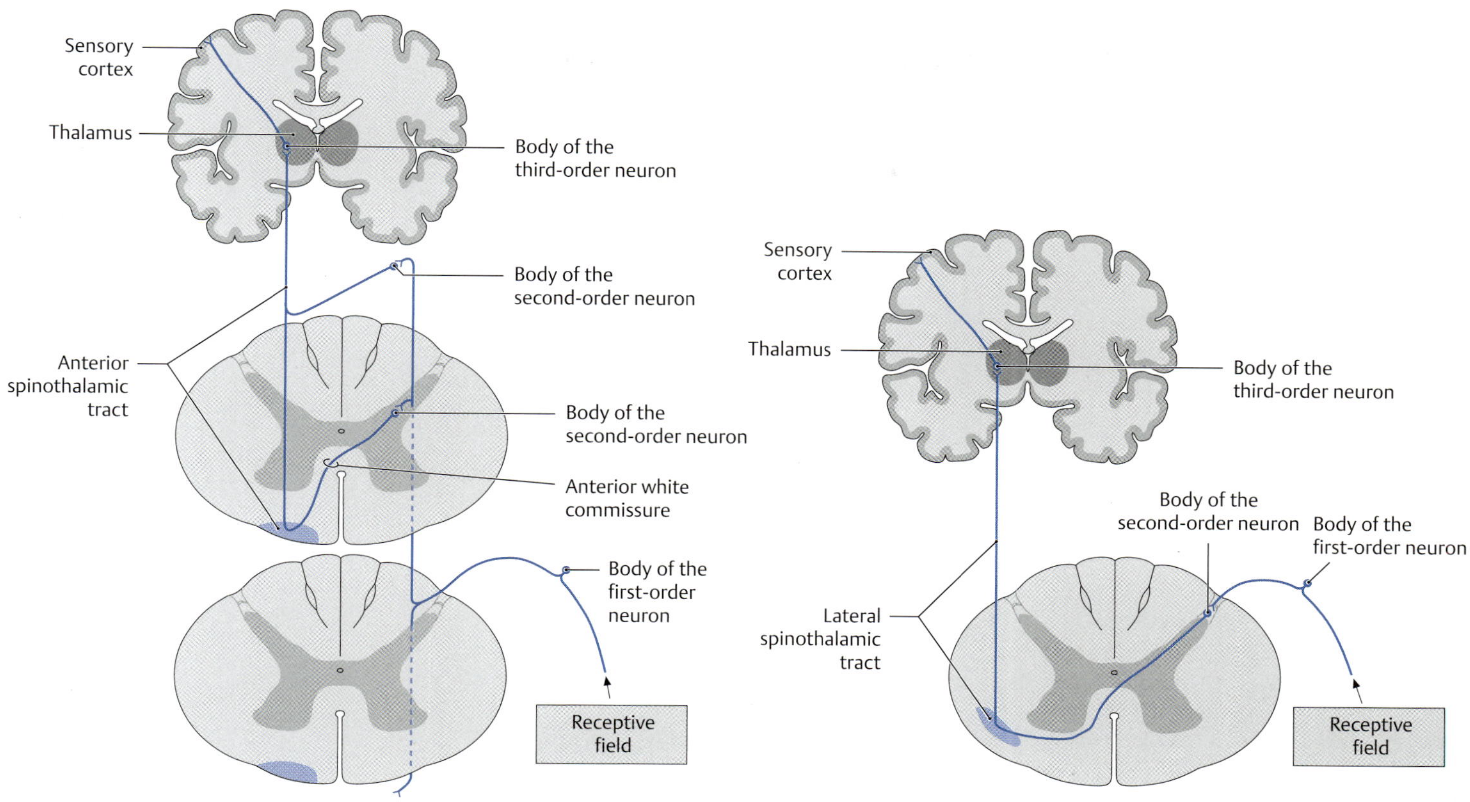

B The spinothalamic tracts and their central connections

a Anterior spinothalamic tract; **b** Lateral spinothalamic tract. Both spinothalamic tracts deal with stimuli received from cutaneous receptors but each of them relays information related to different **types of sensation:**

- The *anterior* spinothalamic tract carries impulses via tactile corpuscles found in the skin as well as hair follicle receptors mechanoreceptors through moderately myelinated peripheral neuronal processes (dendritic axons).
- The *lateral* spinothalamic tract carries information about pain and temperature from the free nerve endings in the skin.

In both tracts, the cell bodies of the first-order neurons (primary neurons) are located in the dorsal root ganglia. There are other similarities regarding the further course of the spinothalamic tracts. Both tracts transmit information toward the sensory cortex in the postcentral gyrus. Thus, the impulses they carry are consciously processed in the brain. However, there is one, also clinically significant, difference between the two tracts regarding their pathway:

- In the case of the *anterior* spinothalamic tract:
  (**a**) The axons of the first-order neuron initially branch in a T-shaped pattern. After entering the spinal cord, they descend 1–2 segments and ascend 2–15 segments. Only then, and not at the level where they enter the spinal cord segment, do they synapse with neurons in the posterior horn (second neurons). Axons of these second-order neurons than cross in the anterior white commissure and ascend in the opposite anterior funiculus.
- In the case of the *lateral* spinothalamic tract:
  (**b**) The axons of the first-order neurons synapse with the second-order neurons as soon as they enter the gray matter of the spinal cord, thus on the same level where they enter it! The axons of the second-order neurons, also, cross the midline in the anterior white commissure and ascend in the opposite lateral funiculus. Knowledge about these differences can be significant when evaluating a patient with *Brown–Séquard Syndrome* (see **E**, p. 473).

Both spinothalamic tracts (which in the brainstem are also referred to as spinothalamic fibers) ascend in the brainstem in a composite bundle of tracts, called the spinal lemniscus, to the ventral posterolateral nucleus of the thalamus where they synapse with the third-order neurons. The axons of the third-order neurons pass through the internal capsule and reach the fourth-order neurons in the postcentral gyrus.

Note: A lesion to the spinothalamic tracts leads to reduced or complete loss of sensation to different sensory stimuli such as pain, temperature and crude touch. Since both tracts are hardly separable, an isolated lesion to only one of them is practically never encountered. A lesion affecting the spinothalamic tracts will always result in clinical deficit that is contralateral to the side of the lesion; therefore on the same side with the dorsal root ganglion that contains the bodies of the first-order neurons of the pathway. Moreover, based on the crossing of the second-order neurons of these tracts, a lesion of the left first-order neuron of the same pathway (part of the PNS) or the left second-order neuron (part of the CNS) before it crosses the midline will result in a deficit on the left side of the patient. A lesion of the right third and fourth-order neurons (both of them in the CNS) will result in a deficit on the left side of the patient.

11.6 Ascending Tracts of the Spinal Cord: Fasciculus gracilis and Fasciculus cuneatus

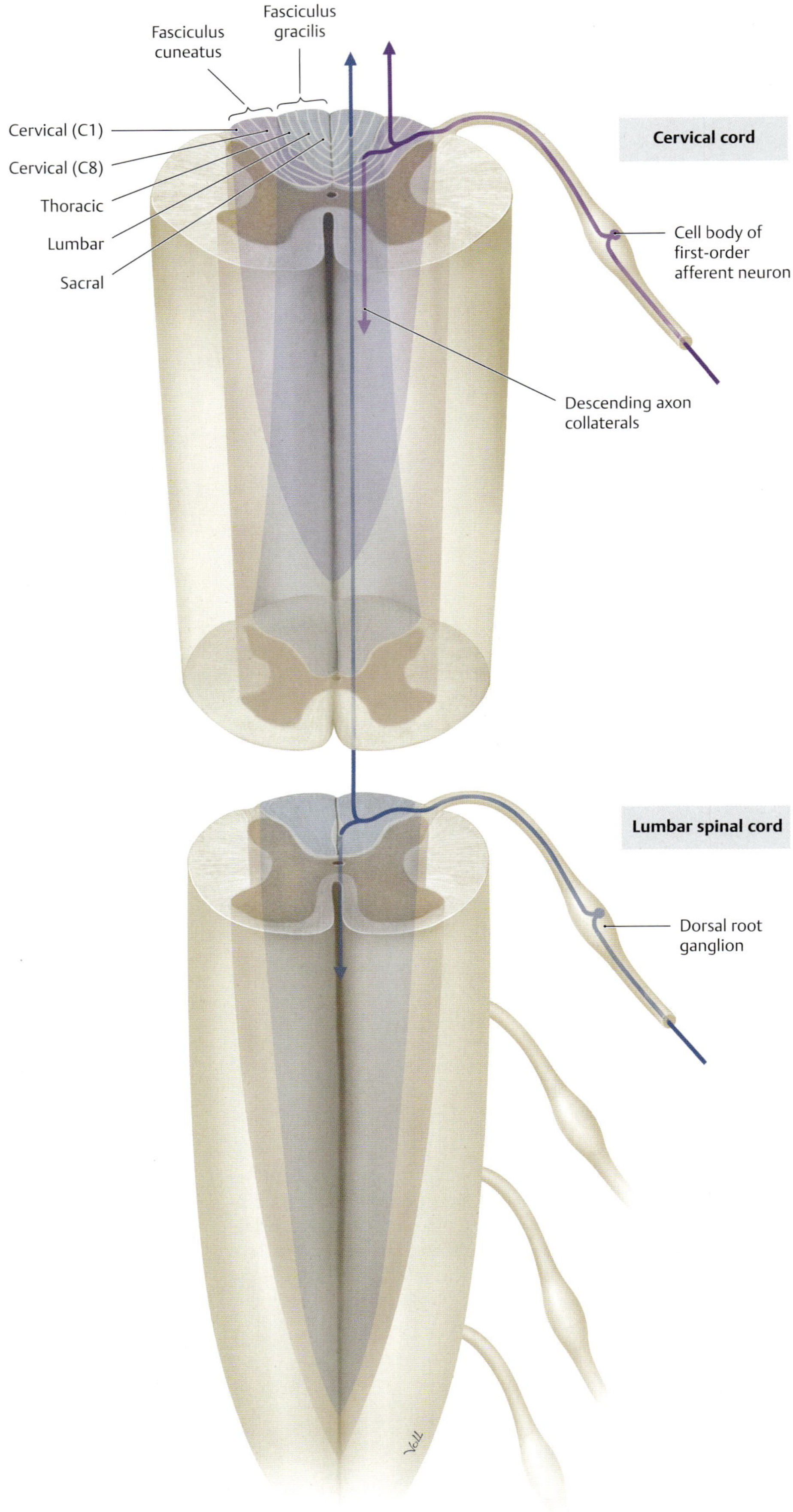

A Ascending axons in the fasciculus gracilis and fasciculus cuneatus

The fasciculus gracilis ("slender fasciculus") and fasciculus cuneatus ("wedge-shaped fasciculus") are the two large ascending tracts in the posterior funiculus. Since these tracts largely run analogous to the spinothalamic tract and also carry information about conscious perception to the telencephalon, they are depicted immediately hereafter. Both tracts convey fibers for position sense (conscious proprioception) and fine cutaneous sensation (touch, vibration, fine pressure sense, two-point discrimination). The fasciculus gracilis carries fibers from the lower limbs, while the fasciculus cuneatus carries fibers only from the upper limbs and is therefore not present in the spinal cord below the T 6 level. The cell bodies of the first-order neuron are located in the dorsal root ganglion. Their fibers are heavily myelinated and therefore conduct impulses rapidly. They pass uncrossed (the level of the decussation is shown in **C**) to the dorsal column nuclei (nucleus gracilis and cuneatus, see **C**). Both nuclei are located in the caudal portion of the medulla oblongata. The fasciculi are somatotopically organized.

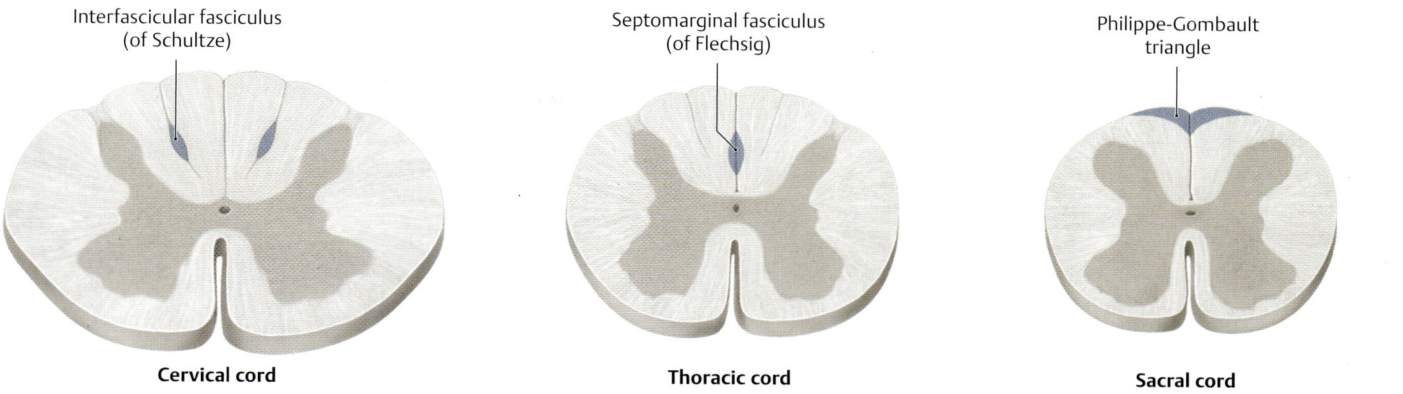

B Descending axons
Besides the ascending axons contained in the fasciculus gracilis and fasciculus cuneatus (both shown in **A**), there are also descending axon collaterals that are distributed to lower segments. This pathway takes different shapes at different levels, appearing as the comma tract of Schultze (interfascicular fasciculus) in the cervical cord, the oval area of Flechsig (septomarginal fasciculus) in the thoracic cord, and the Philippe–Gombault triangle in the sacral cord. These tracts are concerned with sensorimotor innervation at the spinal cord level and are thus considered part of the intrinsic circuits of the spinal cord (see pp. 396 and 400).

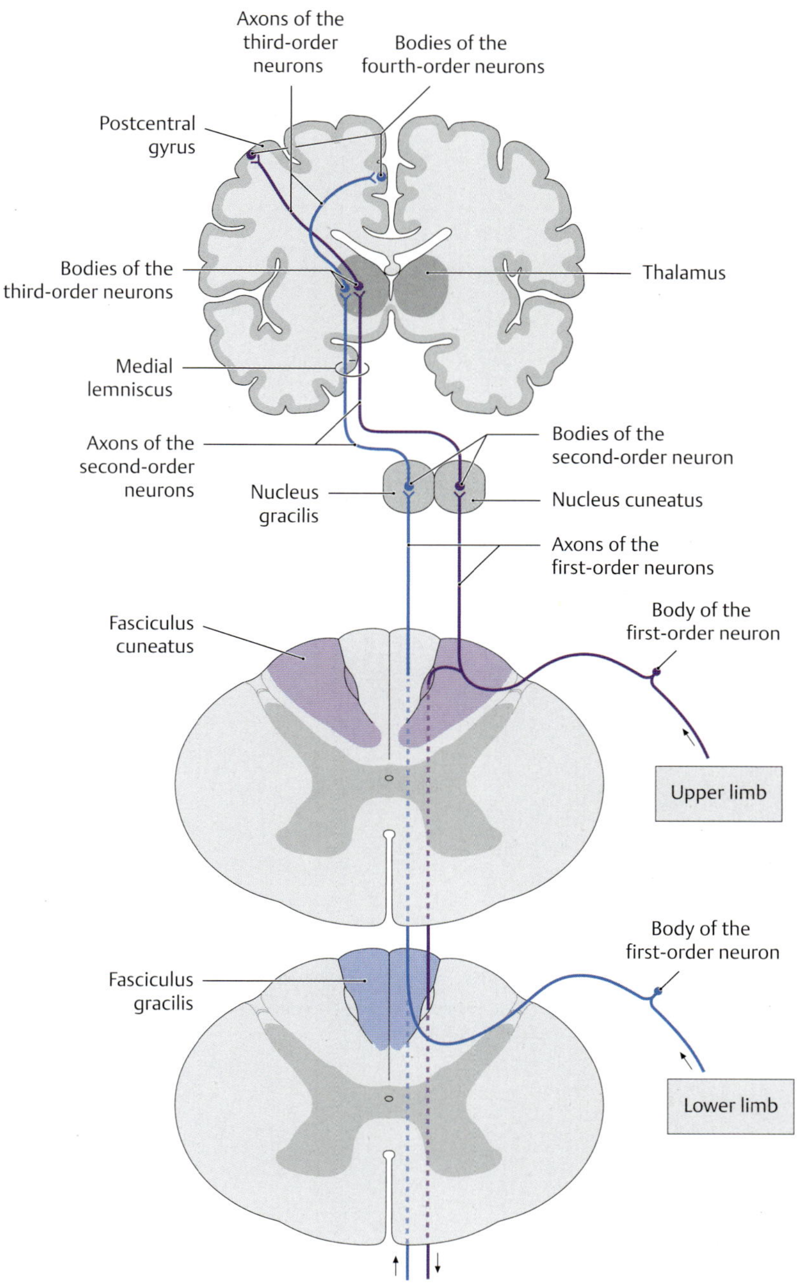

C Fasciculi gracilis and cuneatus and their central connections

- Just like in the case of the spinothalamic tract (see p. 402 f), the axons of the third-order neurons of the dorsal columns—medial lemniscus pathway—terminate in the somatosensory cortex of the telencephalon, the postcentral gyrus. That means that impulses carried by those tracts are also perceived *consciously* (conscious proprioception via muscle and tendon receptors as well as perception of vibration via Vater-Pacini corpuscles, fine touch via cutaneous receptors and so on).
- Just like in the case of the spinothalamic tract, the cell bodies of the first-order neurons are located in the dorsal root ganglia.
- The axons of the first-order neurons ascend uncrossed in the posterior columns to the gracilis and cuneatus nuclei (that contain the cell bodies of the second-order neurons) located in the caudal part of the medulla oblongata.
- The axons of the second-order neurons cross the midline and form the medial lemniscus that ascends through the brainstem to the thalamus (where they synapse with the third-order neurons).

Note: A lesion to the gracilis and cuneatus fasciculi leads to reduced or total loss of fine touch and conscious proprioception. The disturbance caused by this lesion is always localized on the side of the body where the cell body of the first-order neuron (thus the peripheral neuron in the dorsal root ganglion) of the tract is located. This finding is explained by the above mentioned crossing of the axons of the second-order neuron that occurs in the medulla oblongata (while the second-order neurons of other sensory pathways are located in the spinal cord!). For example, symptoms on the left side of the body are associated with lesions to the first-order neuron or the body of the second-order neuron on the left side or lesions to the medial lemniscus, the third-order neuron or the postcentral gyrus on the right side.

11.7 Ascending Tracts of the Spinal Cord: Spinocerebellar Tracts

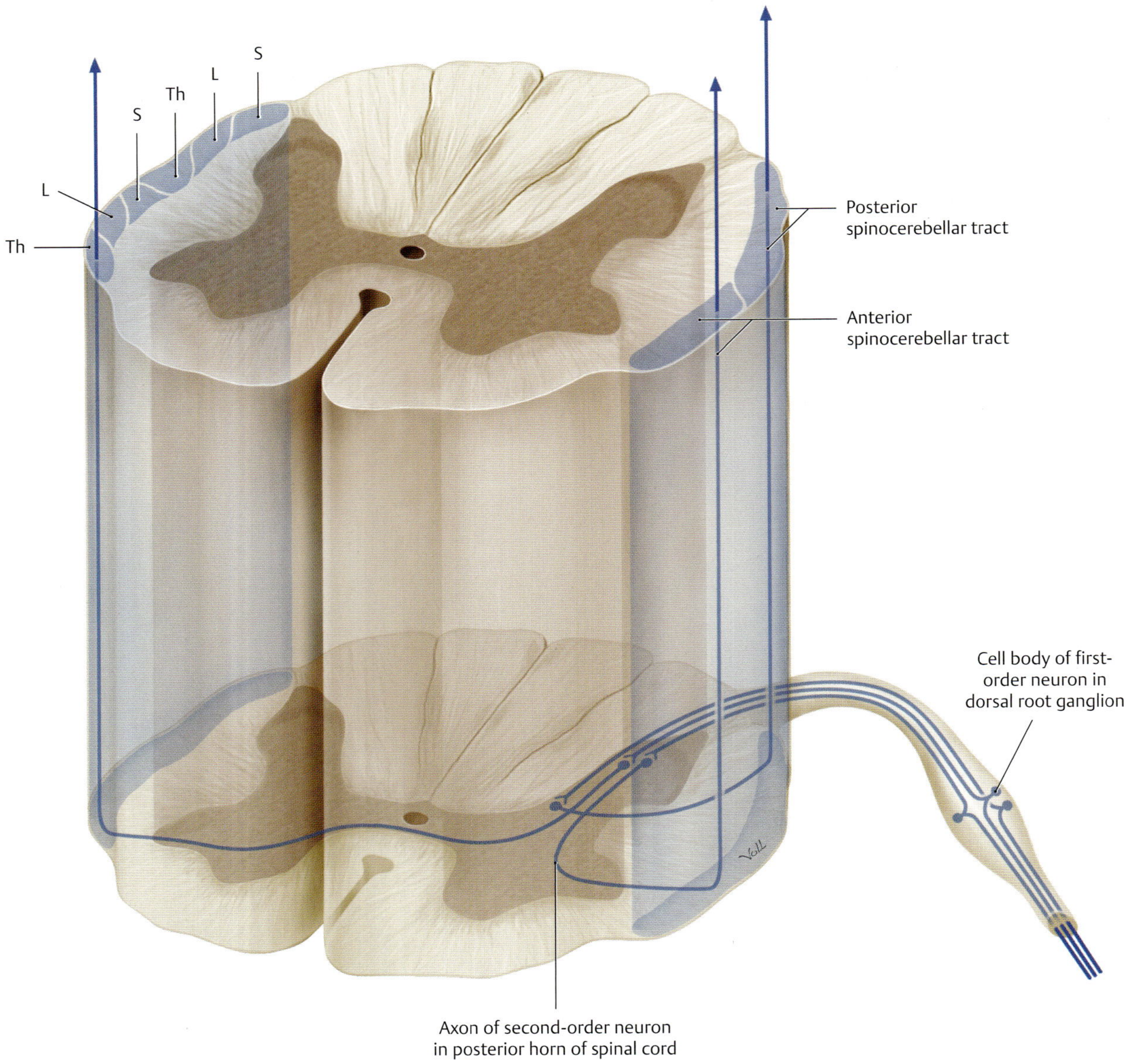

A Anterior and posterior spinocerebellar tracts
The spinocerebellar tracts are located in the *lateral funiculus* of the spinal cord and unlike the previously mentioned ascending tracts of the spinal cord don't carry their information toward the cerebral cortex (via thalamus) but to the *cerebellum*. That means that the impulses they carry are *not consciously* perceived. Their afferent input is involved in the unconscious coordination of motor activities such as running or bike riding (unconscious proprioception). Both tracts have the same somatotopy from ventral to dorsal (represented clockwise on the figure):

- thoracic (Th)
- lumbar (L)
- sacral (S)

Fibers with similar function from the cervical region pass through the fasciculus cuneatus to the accessory cuneate nucleus and continue as cuneocerebellar fibers to the cerebellum. However, they do not pass through the posterior spinocerebellar tract, which contains no fibers from the cervical cord.

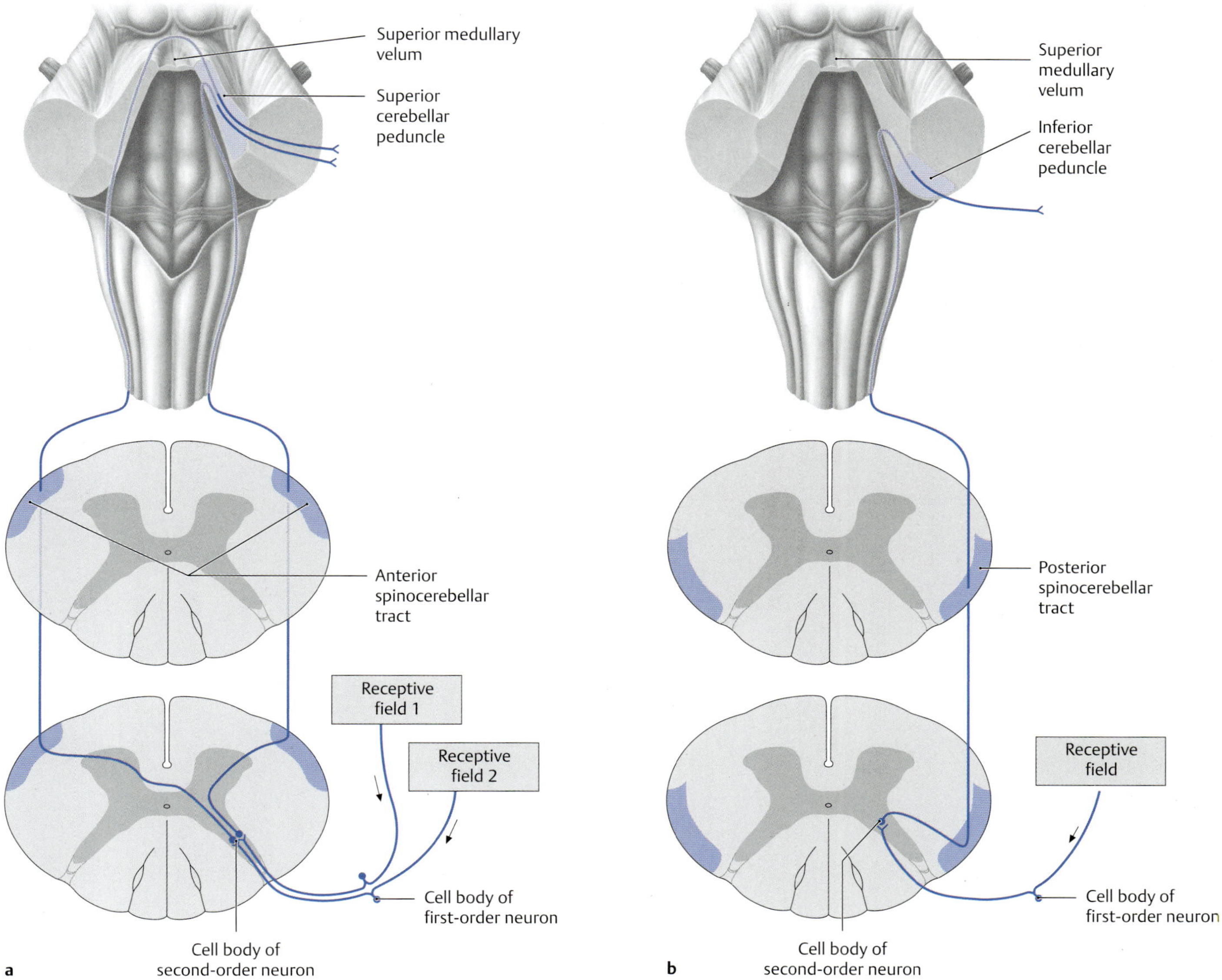

B Anterior and posterior spinocerebellar tracts and their central connections

a Anterior spinocerebellar tract; **b** Posterior spinocerebellar tract.

- Unlike the previously mentioned ascending tracts, both spinocerebellar tracts end in the cerebellum (no conscious processing of information!) mainly in the vermis, which due to the input from the spinal cord is functionally referred to as "*Spinocerebellum*." However, they reach the cerebellum via different cerebellar peduncles:
  - the anterior spinocerebellar tract via the *superior* cerebellar peduncle
  - the posterior spinocerebellar tract via the *inferior* cerebellar peduncle
- Like with all other ascending tracts, the cell bodies of the first-order neurons of both tracts are located in the dorsal root ganglia. Their axons are IA fibers, which are rapidly conducting, myelinated fibers. They convey the information from muscle spindles and tendon receptors to the second-order neurons, which for both tracts are located in the *posterior horn of the spinal cord* albeit at different places:
  - The second-order neuron of the *anterior* spinocerebellar tract is located in the middle of the posterior horn.
  - The second-order neuron of the *posterior* spinocerebellar tract is located in the Clarke's nucleus, which extends from C8 to L2.

The axons of the *posterior* spinocerebellar tract ascend *only* ipsilaterally to the cerebellum; the axons of the *anterior* spinocerebellar tract, however, only partly ascend ipsilaterally. A part of the fibers cross in the spinal cord and then run contralaterally to the brainstem. These contralateral fibers then cross in the superior medullary velum back to their original side and thus reach the same side of the cerebellum as the uncrossed fibers.

11.8 Descending Tracts of the Spinal Cord: Pyramidal (Corticospinal) Tracts

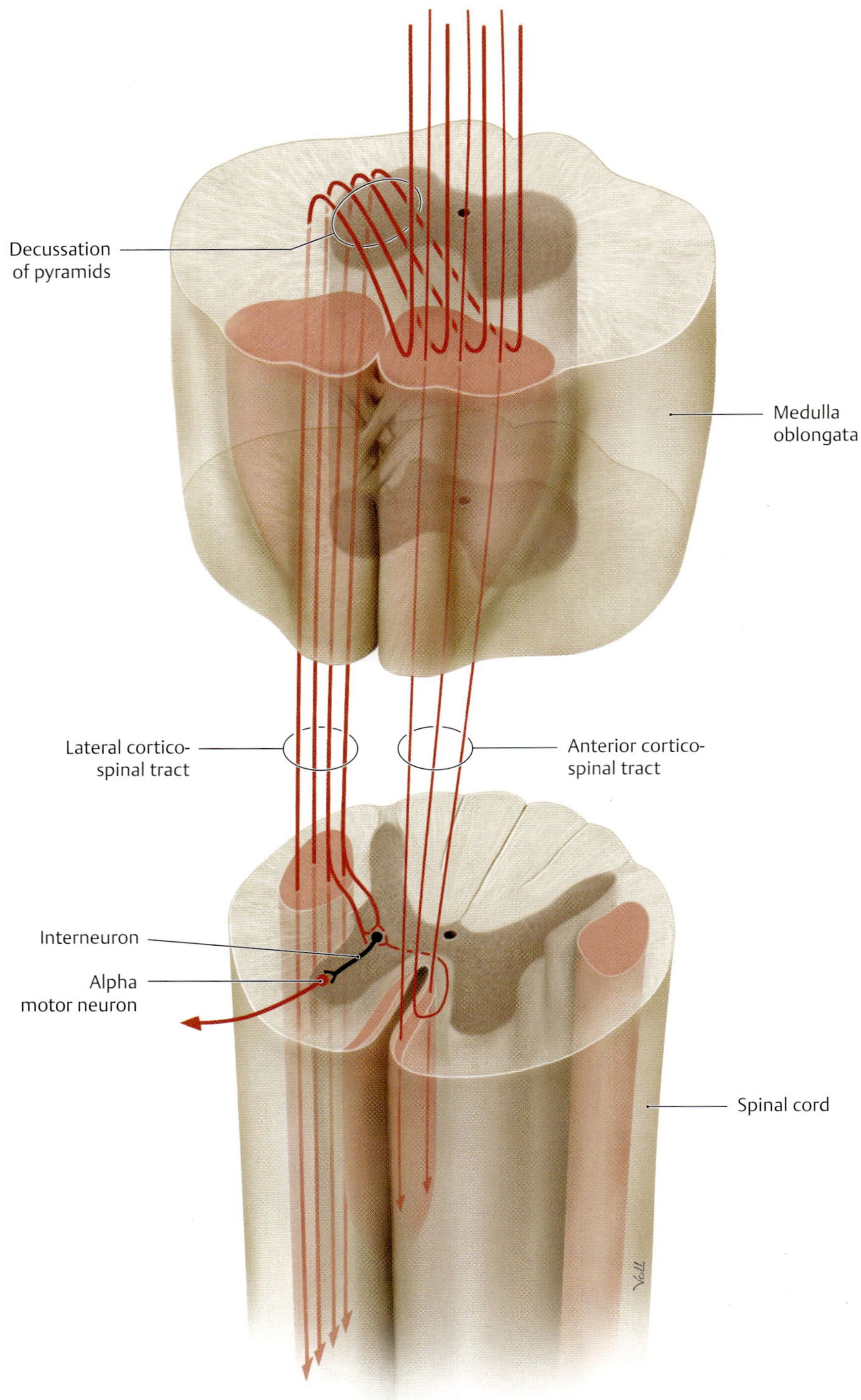

A Course of the anterior and lateral corticospinal tracts (pyramidal tract) in the lower medulla oblongata and spinal cord
The pyramidal tract, which begins in the motor cortex, is the most important pathway for voluntary motor function. Some of its axons, the *corticonuclear fibers*, terminate at the cranial nerve nuclei while others, the *corticospinal fibers*, terminate on the motor anterior horn cells of the spinal cord (see **B** for further details). A third group, the *corticoreticular fibers*, are distributed to nuclei of the reticular formation.

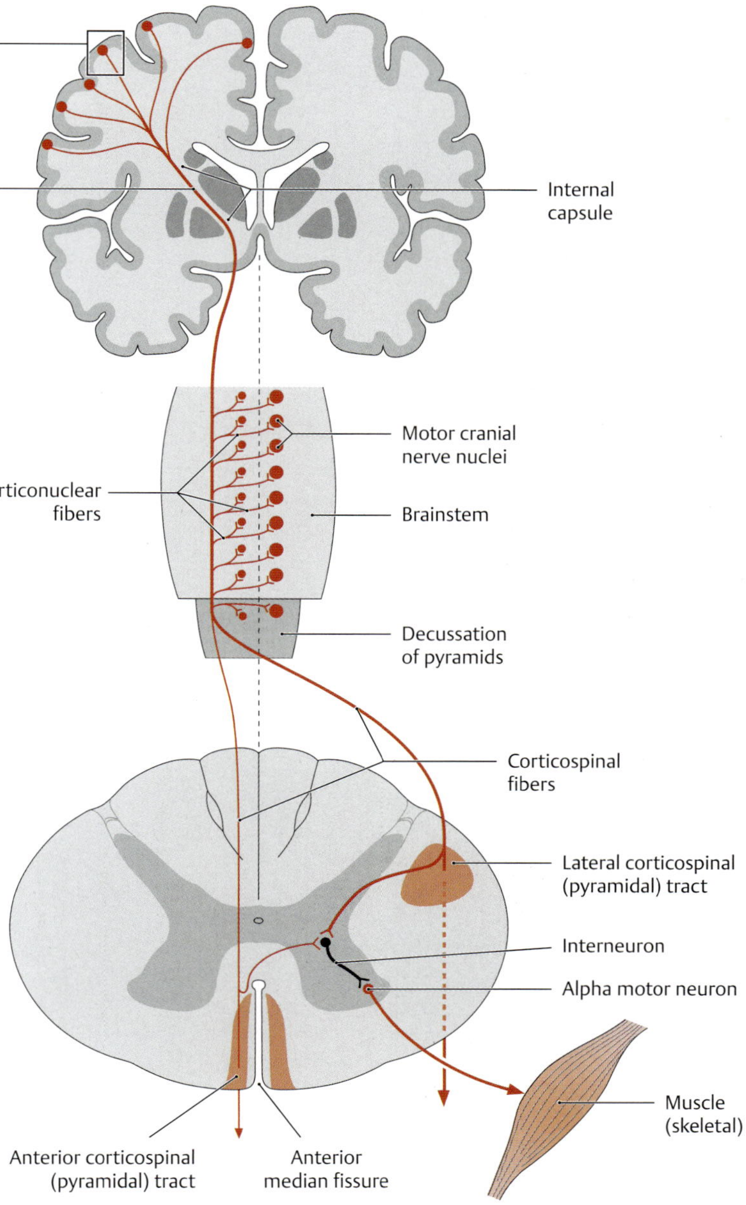

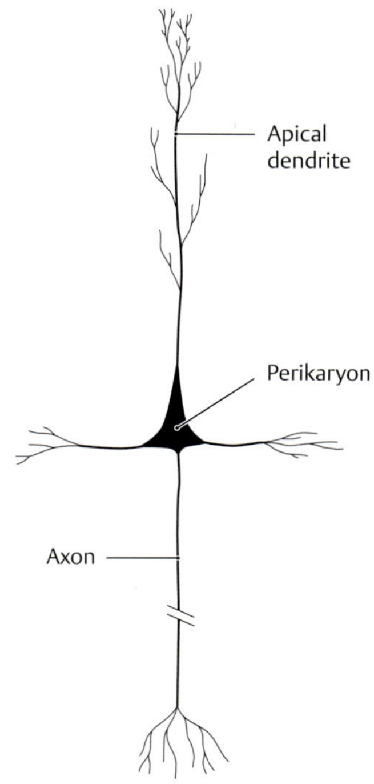

C Silver-impregnation (Golgi) method staining of pyramidal cell
This method produces a silhouette of the stained neurons. The axons of the pyramidal cells form the pyramidal tract. Approximately 40% are located in the motor cortex (Brodmann area 4, see p. 328).

B Course of the pyramidal tract

- The pyramidal tract originates in the motor cortex at the pyramidal cells (large afferent neurons with pyramid-shaped cell bodies, see **C**). The pyramidal tract has three components:
  - *Corticonuclear fibers* for the cranial nerve nuclei
  - *Corticospinal fibers* for the spinal cord
  - *Corticoreticular fibers* to the reticular formation
- All three components pass through the internal capsule from the telencephalon, continuing into the brainstem and spinal cord.
- In the brainstem, the *corticonuclear* fibers are distributed to the motor nuclei of the cranial nerves.
- The *corticospinal* fibers descend to the decussation of the pyramids in the lower medulla oblongata, where approximately 80% of them cross to the opposite side. The fibers continue into the spinal cord, where they form the lateral corticospinal tract, which has a somatotopic organization: the fibers for the **sacral cord** are the most lateral, while the fibers for the cervical cord are the most medial.
- The remaining 20% of *corticospinal* fibers continue to descend without crossing, forming the anterior *corticospinal tract*, which borders the anterior median fissure in a transverse section of the spinal cord. The anterior corticospinal tract is particularly well developed in the cervical cord, but is not present in the lower thoracic, lumbar, or sacral cords.
- Most fibers of the *anterior corticospinal tract* cross at the segmental level to terminate on the same motor neurons as the *lateral corticospinal tract*. The axons of the pyramid cells terminate via intercalated cells on alpha and gamma motor neurons, Renshaw cells, and inhibitory interneurons (not shown).

Lesions of the pyramidal tract are discussed on p. 461. Other motor tracts are closely applied to the pyramidal tract in the region of the internal capsule and will be described in the next unit. While the pyramidal tract controls *conscious* movement (voluntary motor activity), *supplementary motor tracts* are essential for involuntary muscle processes (e.g., standing, walking, running; see p. 460).

11.9 Descending Tracts of the Spinal Cord: Extrapyramidal and Autonomic Tracts

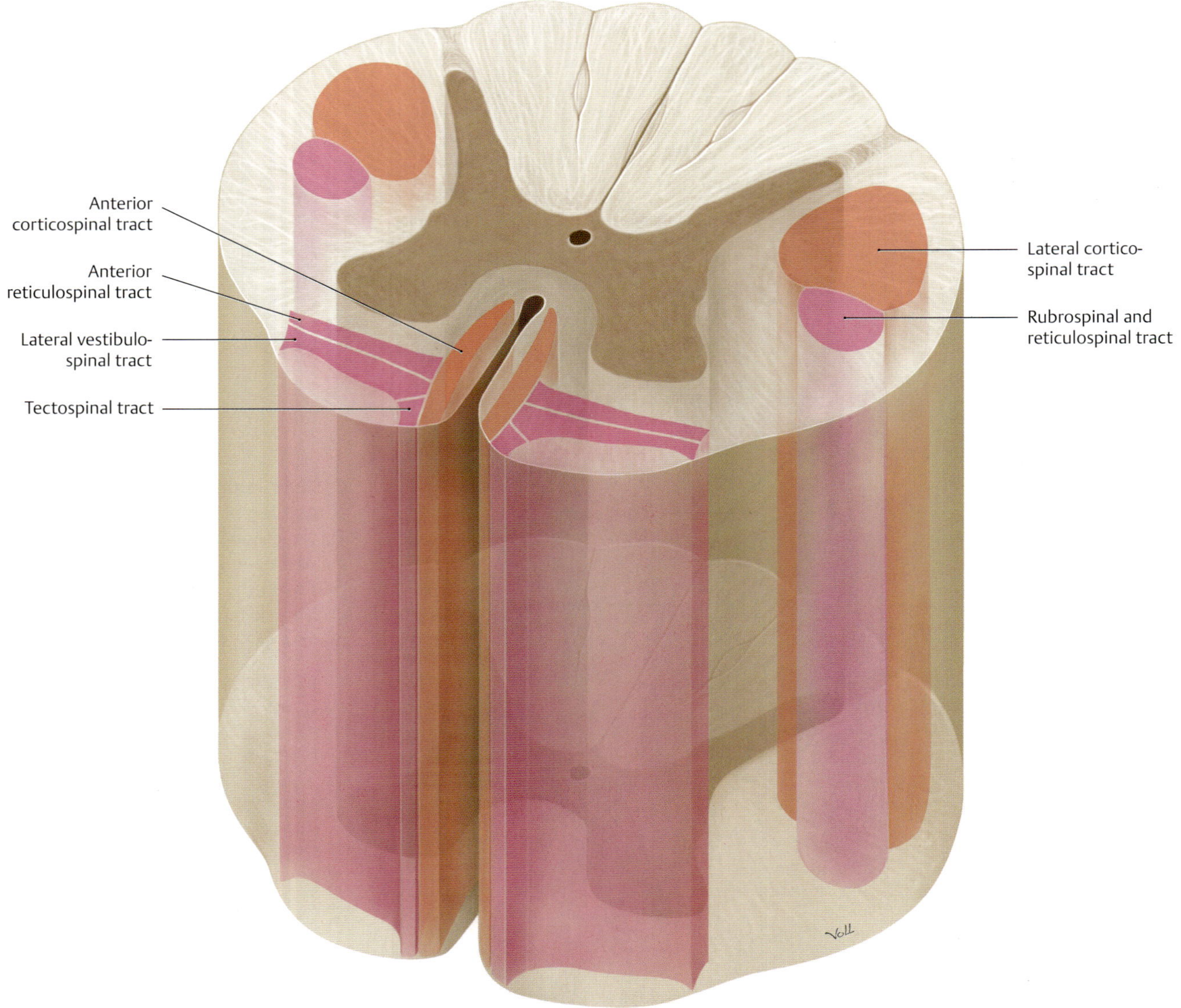

A Tracts of the extrapyramidal motor system in the spinal cord
Unlike the pyramidal tract, which controls conscious, voluntary motor activities (e.g., raising a cup to the mouth), the *extra*pyramidal motor system (cerebellum, basal nuclei, and motor nuclei of the brainstem) is necessary for *automatic* and *learned* motor processes (e.g., walking, running, cycling). The division into a pyramidal and extrapyramidal system has proven useful in clinical practice. For central circuitry see **B**. As the pyramidal tract and extrapyramidal tracts are closely integrated with one another and course adjacent to each other, injuries generally involve both simultaneously (see p. 394). Isolated lesions of the one system or the other at the spinal cord level are virtually unknown. A recent classification that combines the classic pyramidal and extrapyramidal tracts differentiates lateral and medial topographic and functional systems. The lateral system includes two tracts, the lateral corticospinal tract (lateral pyramidal tract) and the rubrospinal tract. The lateral system projects to the distal musculature of the upper extremity and is responsible for the fine motor function of the hand and arm (in humans the rubrospinal tract probably extends only as far as the superior spinal cord). The medial system consists of three tracts, the anterior reticulospinal tract, the lateral vestibulospinal tract, and the tectospinal tract. This system is responsible for motor function in the torso and for postural motor function.

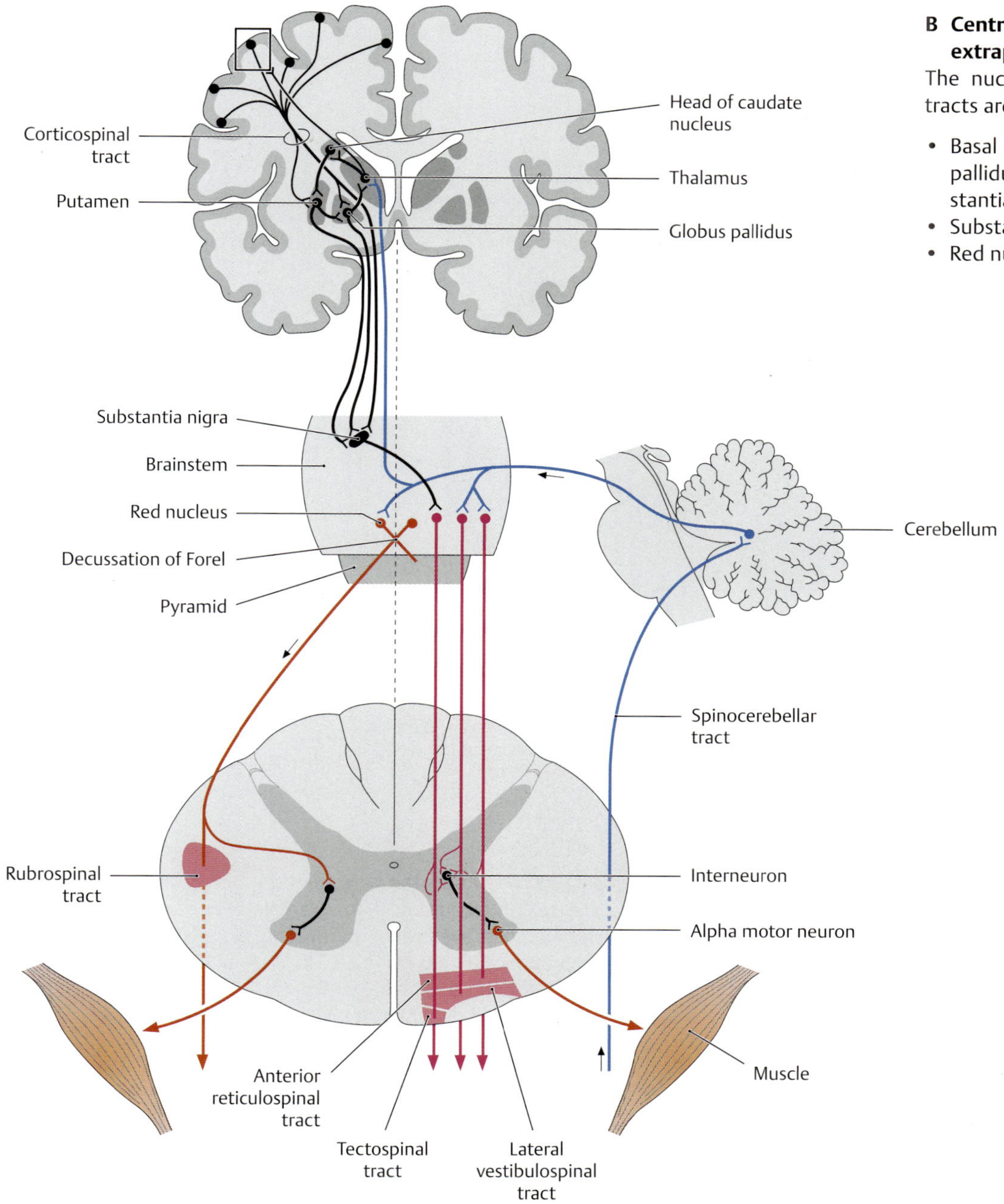

B Central origin and course of the extrapyramidal tracts

The nuclei of origin of the extrapyramidal tracts are as follows:

- Basal nuclei (corpus striatum and globus pallidus, which act in relation with the substantia nigra)
- Substantia nigra
- Red nucleus

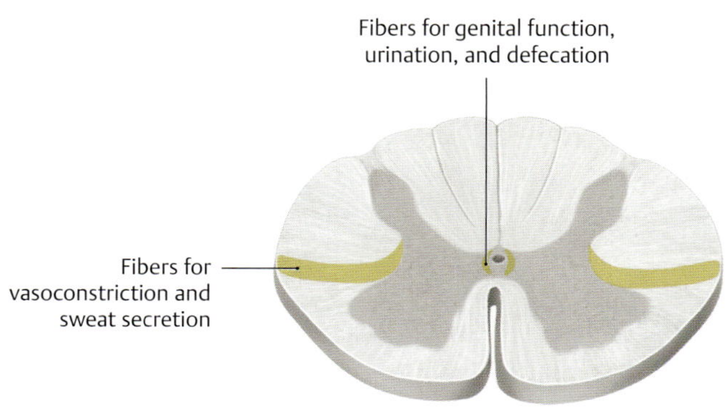

C Autonomic pathways of the spinal cord

Autonomic pathways have a somewhat diffuse arrangement in the spinal cord and rarely form closed tract systems. There are two exceptions:

1. The descending central sympathetic tract for vasoconstriction and sweat secretion borders the pyramidal tract anteriorly and shows the same somatotopic organization as the pyramidal tract.
2. The parependymal tract runs on both sides of the central canal and contains both ascending and descending fibers. Passing from the spinal cord to the hypothalamus, this tract is concerned with urination, defecation, and genital functions.

11.10 Tracts of the Spinal Cord, Overview

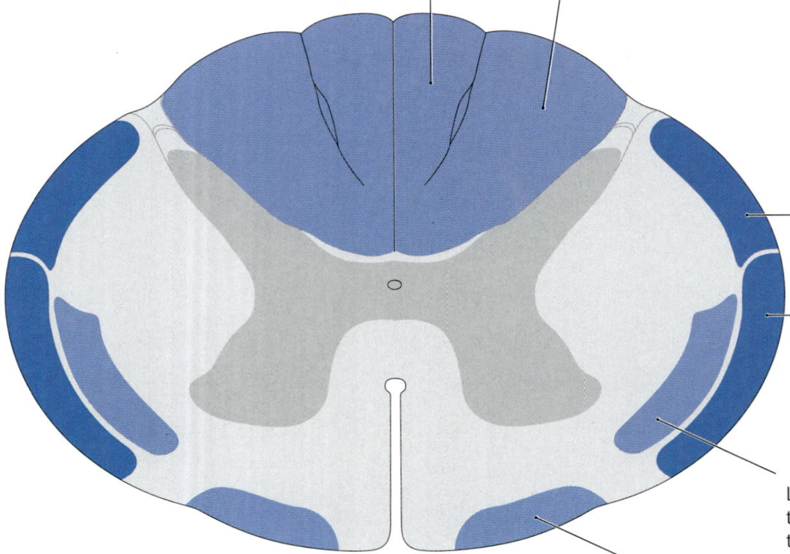

A Ascending tracts in the spinal cord
Transverse section through the spinal cord. Ascending tracts are afferent (= sensory) pathways that carry information from the trunk and limbs to the brain. The most important ascending tracts and their functions are listed below.

Spinothalamic tracts
- Anterior spinothalamic tract (coarse touch sensation)
- Lateral spinothalamic tract (pain and temperature sensation)

Tracts of the posterior funiculus (dorsal column)
- Fasciculus gracilis (fine touch sensation, conscious proprioception of the *lower* limb)
- Fasciculus cuneatus (fine touch sensation, conscious proprioception of the *upper* limb).

Spinocerebellar tracts
- Anterior spinocerebellar tract (unconscious proprioception to the cerebellum)
- Posterior spinocerebellar tract (unconscious proprioception to the cerebellum)

Proprioception involves the perception of limb position in space ("position sense"). It lets us know, for example, that our arm is in front of or behind our chest even when our eyes are closed. The information involved in proprioception is complex. Thus, our position sense tells us where our joints are in relation to one another while our motion sense tells us the speed and direction of joint movements. We also have a "force sense" by which we can perceive the muscular force that is associated with joint movements. Moreover, proprioception takes place on both a conscious (I know that my hand is making a fist in my pants pocket without seeing it) and an unconscious level, enabling us to ride a bicycle and climb stairs without thinking about it. The table on p. 445 gives a comprehensive review of all the ascending tracts.

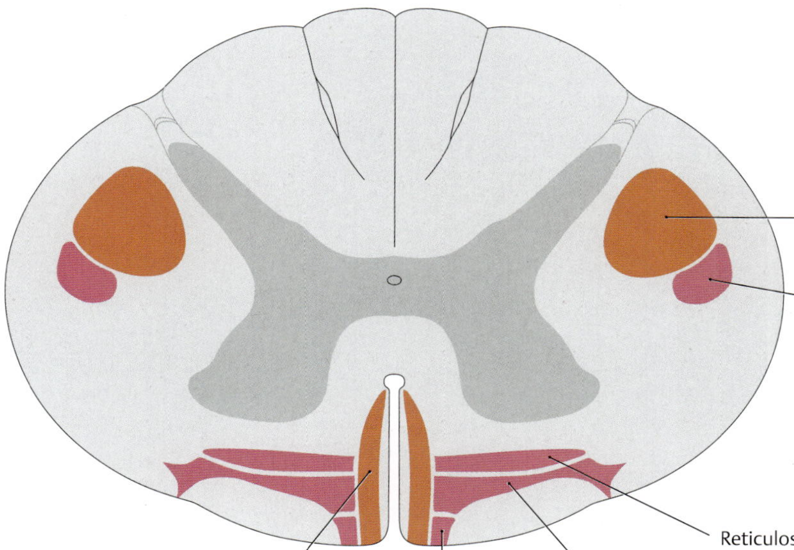

B Descending tracts in the spinal cord
Transverse section through the spinal cord. The descending tracts of the spinal cord are concerned with motor function. They convey information from higher motor centers to the motor neurons in the spinal cord. According to a relatively recent classification (not yet fully accepted in clinical medicine), the descending tracts of the spinal cord can be divided into two motor systems:

- **Lateral motor system** (concerned with fine, precise motor skills in the hands):
- – Pyramidal tract (anterior and lateral corticospinal tract)
- – Rubrospinal tract

- **Medial motor system** (innervates medially situated motor neurons controlling trunk movement and stance):
- – Reticulospinal tract
- – Tectospinal tract
- – Vestibulospinal tract

Except for the pyramidal tract, which may be represented as a monosynaptic pathway in a simplified scheme, it is difficult to offer a simple and direct classification of the motor system because sequences of movements are programmed and coordinated in multiple feedback mechanisms called "motor loops" (see p. 459). There is no point, then, in listing the various tracts in a simplified table. While the tracts can be distinguished rather clearly from one another at the level of the spinal cord, their fibers are so intermixed at the higher cortical levels that isolated motor disturbances (unlike sensory disturbances) essentially do not occur at the level of the spinal cord.

11.11 Blood Vessels of the Spinal Cord: Arteries

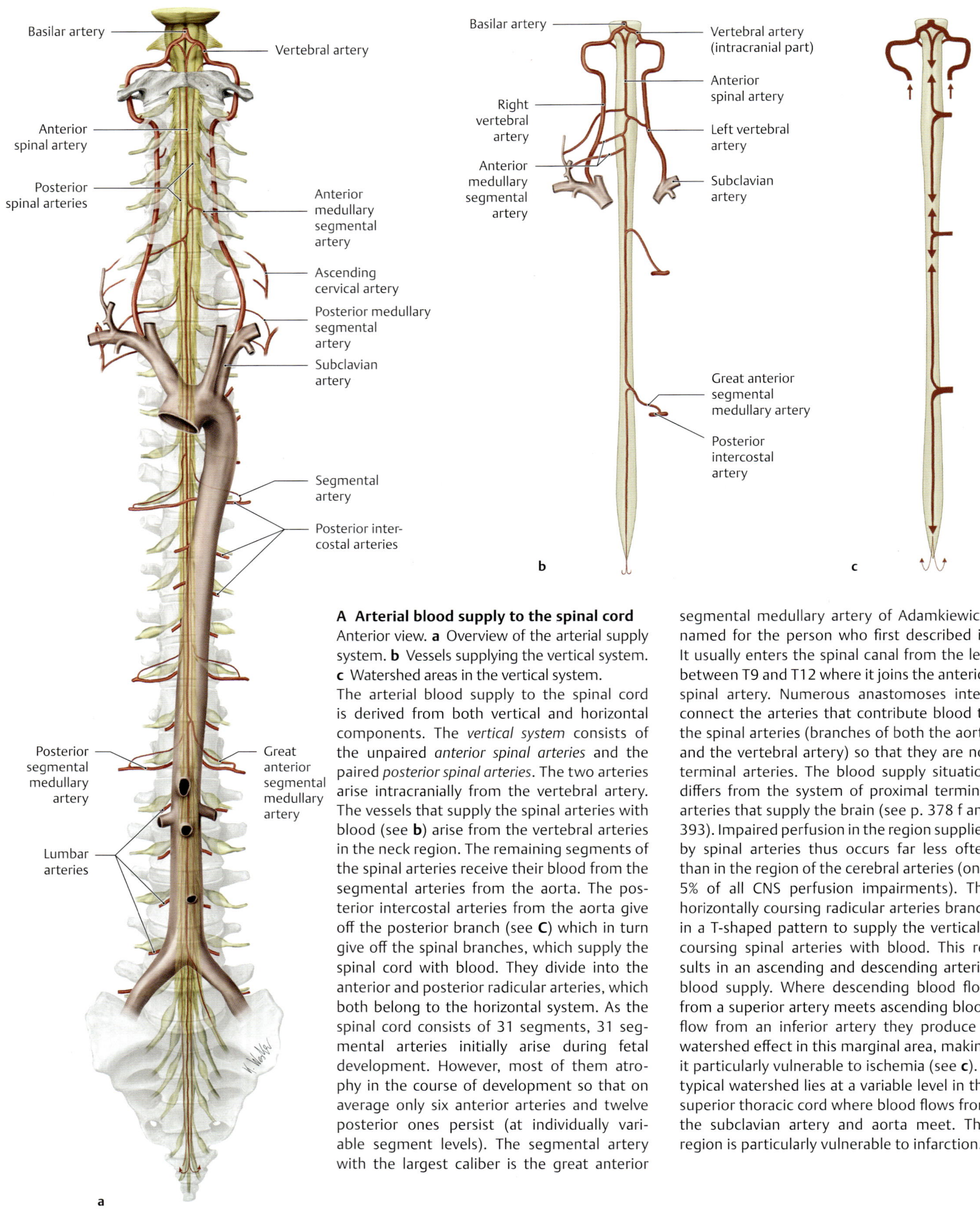

A Arterial blood supply to the spinal cord

Anterior view. **a** Overview of the arterial supply system. **b** Vessels supplying the vertical system. **c** Watershed areas in the vertical system.

The arterial blood supply to the spinal cord is derived from both vertical and horizontal components. The *vertical system* consists of the unpaired *anterior spinal arteries* and the paired *posterior spinal arteries*. The two arteries arise intracranially from the vertebral artery. The vessels that supply the spinal arteries with blood (see **b**) arise from the vertebral arteries in the neck region. The remaining segments of the spinal arteries receive their blood from the segmental arteries from the aorta. The posterior intercostal arteries from the aorta give off the posterior branch (see **C**) which in turn give off the spinal branches, which supply the spinal cord with blood. They divide into the anterior and posterior radicular arteries, which both belong to the horizontal system. As the spinal cord consists of 31 segments, 31 segmental arteries initially arise during fetal development. However, most of them atrophy in the course of development so that on average only six anterior arteries and twelve posterior ones persist (at individually variable segment levels). The segmental artery with the largest caliber is the great anterior segmental medullary artery of Adamkiewicz, named for the person who first described it. It usually enters the spinal canal from the left between T9 and T12 where it joins the anterior spinal artery. Numerous anastomoses interconnect the arteries that contribute blood to the spinal arteries (branches of both the aorta and the vertebral artery) so that they are not terminal arteries. The blood supply situation differs from the system of proximal terminal arteries that supply the brain (see p. 378 f and 393). Impaired perfusion in the region supplied by spinal arteries thus occurs far less often than in the region of the cerebral arteries (only 5% of all CNS perfusion impairments). The horizontally coursing radicular arteries branch in a T-shaped pattern to supply the vertically coursing spinal arteries with blood. This results in an ascending and descending arterial blood supply. Where descending blood flow from a superior artery meets ascending blood flow from an inferior artery they produce a watershed effect in this marginal area, making it particularly vulnerable to ischemia (see **c**). A typical watershed lies at a variable level in the superior thoracic cord where blood flows from the subclavian artery and aorta meet. This region is particularly vulnerable to infarction.

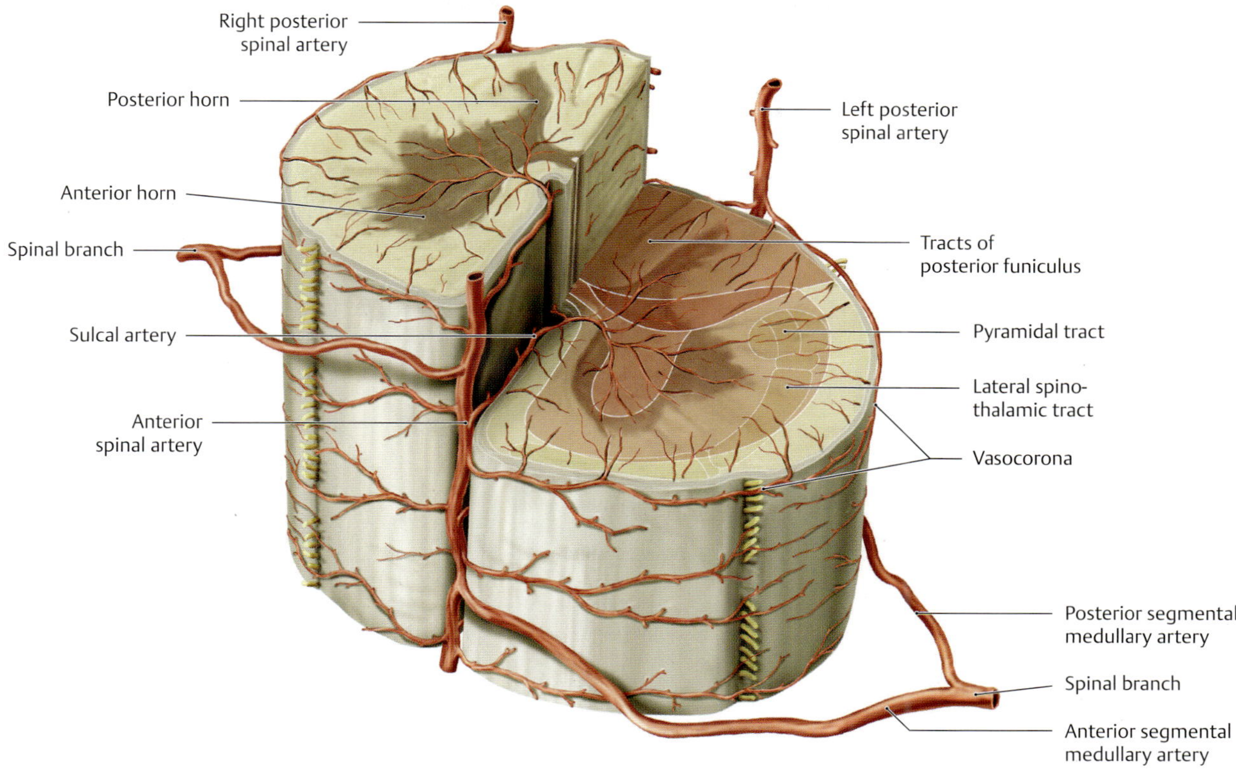

B Blood supply to the spinal cord segments

In each spinal cord segment, the *anterior spinal artery* gives off several (5–9) **sulcal arteries** which course posteriorly in the anterior median fissure. Typically, each sulcal artery enters one half of the spinal cord, supplying the anterior horn, base of the posterior horn, and the anterior and lateral funiculi (approximately two-thirds of the total area) in that half; the sulcal arteries tend to alternate direction (left or right) to supply both halves of the spinal cord segment. The paired *posterior spinal arteries* provide the blood supply to the posterior one-third of the cord, including the posterior horn and funiculus. All three spinal arteries contribute numerous delicate anastomosing **vasocorona** on the pial surface of the spinal cord which in turn send branches into the periphery of the cord. The sulcal arteries are the only end-arteries within the spinal cord, and their occlusion may produce clinical symptoms. Occlusion of the anterior spinal artery at segmental levels may damage the anterior horn and ventral roots resulting in flaccid paralysis of the muscles supplied by these segments. If the pyramidal tract in the lateral funiculus is involved, spastic paralysis will develop below the lesion level. An occlusion of the posterior spinal arteries in one or more segments will affect the posterior horn and funiculus leading to disturbances of proprioception, vibration, and pressure sensation.

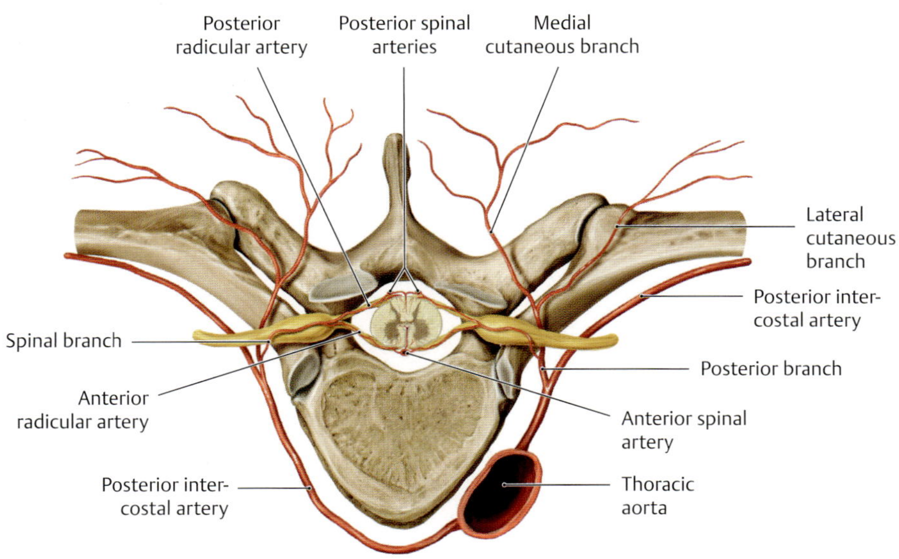

C Blood vessels supplying the spinal cord

Thoracic vertebra viewed from above. The spinal branches arise from the posterior branches of segmental arteries and divide into an anterior and a posterior radicular artery. The radicular arteries supply the dorsal and ventral roots, and peripheral portions of the dorsal and ventral horns; they also communicate with the vasocorona. These arteries have a better developed connection with the anterior spinal artery at some levels and with the posterior spinal artery at other levels.

11.12 Blood Vessels of the Spinal Cord: Veins

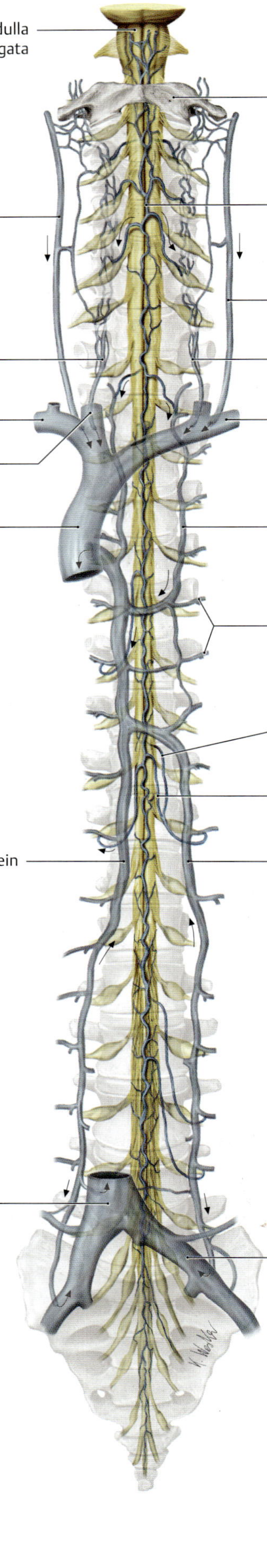

A Venous drainage of the spinal cord
Anterior view. Analogous to the arterial supply, the venous drainage of the spinal cord consists of a *horizontal system* (venous rings, see **B**) and a vertical system that drains the venous rings. The vertical system is illustrated here. While the arterial blood supply is based on three vessels, the interior of the spinal cord drains through venous plexuses into only two unpaired vessels: an anterior and a posterior spinal vein (see **B**). The *anterior* spinal vein communicates superiorly with veins of the brainstem. Its lower portion enters the filum terminale (a glial filament extending from the conus medullaris to the sacral end of the dural sac, where it is attached). The larger *posterior* spinal vein communicates with the **radicular veins** at the cervical level and ends at the conus medullaris. The radicular veins connect these veins, which lie within the pia mater, with the internal vertebral venous plexus (see **C**). Blood from the cord drains into the **vertebral veins**, which open into the superior vena cava. Blood from the thoracic cord drains into the **intercostal veins**, which drain into the superior vena cava via the azygos and hemiazygos system. Radicular veins are present at only certain segments, as shown. Their distribution varies among individuals.

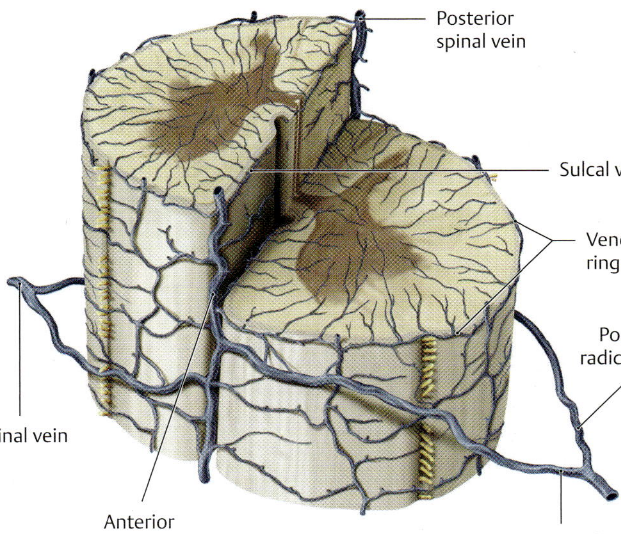

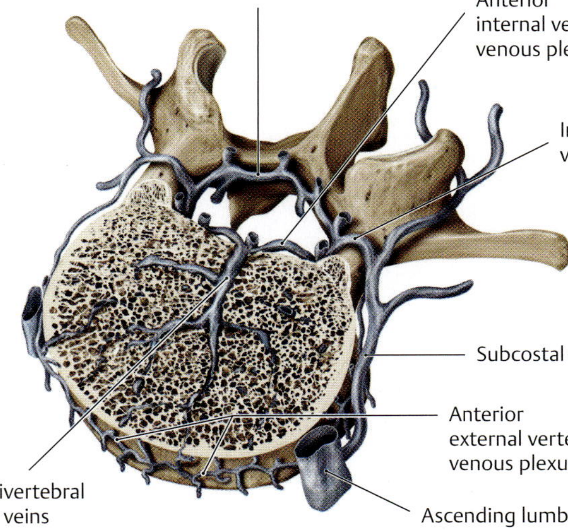

B Venous drainage of a spinal cord segment

Anterior view from upper left. A spinal cord segment is drained by the anterior and posterior spinal veins. These vessels are located within the pia mater and are interconnected by an anastomotic venous ring. Both veins channel blood through the radicular veins to the internal vertebral venous plexus (see **C**). Unlike the radicular veins, the veins *inside* the spinal cord have no valves. As a result, venous stasis may cause a hazardous rise of pressure in the spinal cord. A typical cause of increased intramedullary venous pressure is an arteriovenous fistula, which is an abnormal communication between an artery and vein in the spinal cord. Because the pressure in the arteries is higher than in the veins, arterial blood tends to enter the veins of the spinal cord through the fistulous connection. The fistula will remain asymptomatic as long as the intramedullary veins maintain an adequate drainage capacity. But if the flow across the fistula outstrips their drainage capacity, the functions of the spinal cord will be impaired by the increased pressure. This is manifested clinically by disturbances of gait, spastic paralysis, and sensory disturbances. Untreated, the decompensated fistula will eventually cause a complete functional transection of the spinal cord. The treatment of choice is surgical correction of the fistula.

C Vertebral venous plexus

Transverse section viewed obliquely from upper left. The veins of the spinal cord and its coverings are connected to the internal vertebral venous plexus via the radicular and spinal veins. Located in the fatty tissue of the epidural space, this plexus occupies the inner circumference of the vertebral canal. The internal plexus is connected to the external vertebral venous plexus by the *inter*vertebral and *basi*vertebral veins. Anastomoses exist between the tributary regions of the anterior and posterior spinal veins. Oblique anastomoses are located in the interior of the spinal cord and may extend over several segments (not shown). These connections are particularly important in maintaining a constant intramedullary venous pressure.

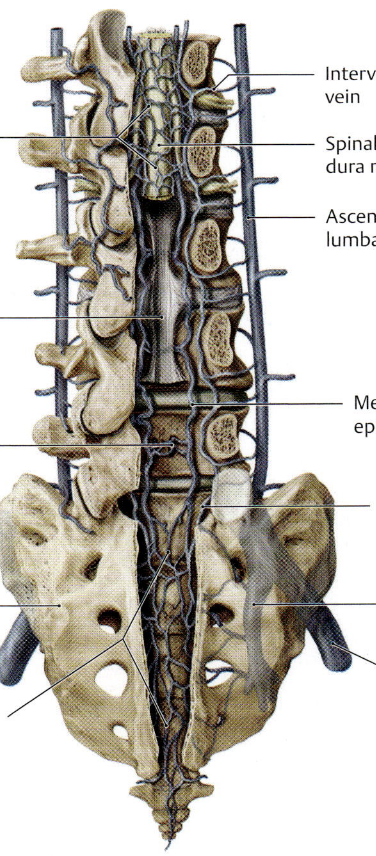

D Epidural veins in the sacral and lumbar vertebral canals

Posterior view (vertebral canal windowed). The internal veins of the spinal cord are valveless up to the point at which they emerge from the spinal dura mater. The internal vertebral venous plexus is connected by other valveless veins (not shown here) to the venous plexus of the prostate. It is relatively easy for prostatic carcinoma cells to pass along the veins of the prostatic venous plexus to the sacral venous plexus and destroy the surrounding tissue. For this reason, prostatic carcinoma frequently metastasizes to this region and destroys the surrounding bone, resulting in severe pain.

11.13 Spinal Cord, Topography

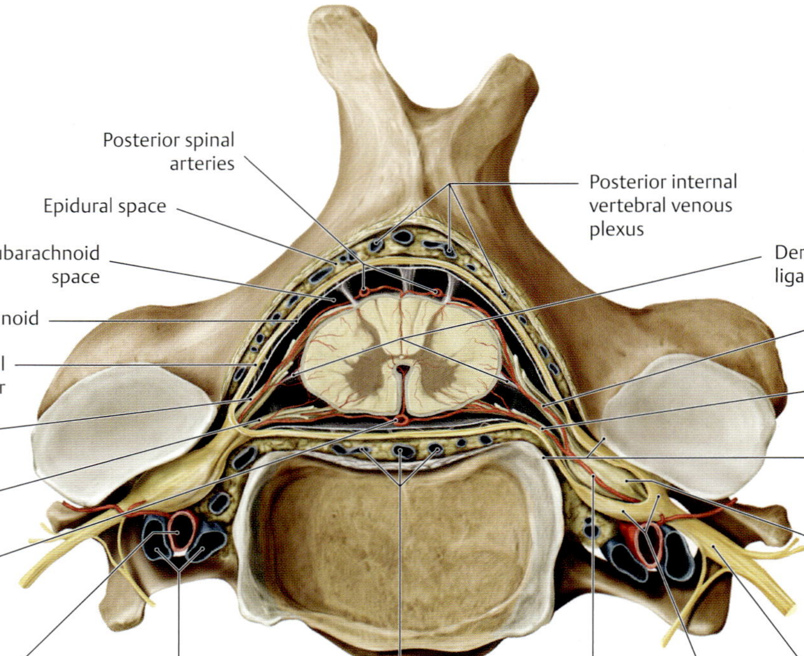

A Spinal cord and spinal nerve in the vertebral canal at the level of the C 4 vertebra

Transverse section viewed from above. The spinal cord occupies the center of the vertebral foramen and is anchored within the subarachnoid space to the spinal dura mater by the denticulate ligament. The root sleeve, an outpouching of the dura mater in the intravertebral foramen, contains the spinal ganglion and the dorsal and ventral roots of the spinal nerve. The spinal dura mater is bounded externally by the epidural space, which contains venous plexuses, fat, and connective tissue. The epidural space extends upward as far as the foramen magnum, where the dura becomes fused to the cranial periosteum (see p. 311).

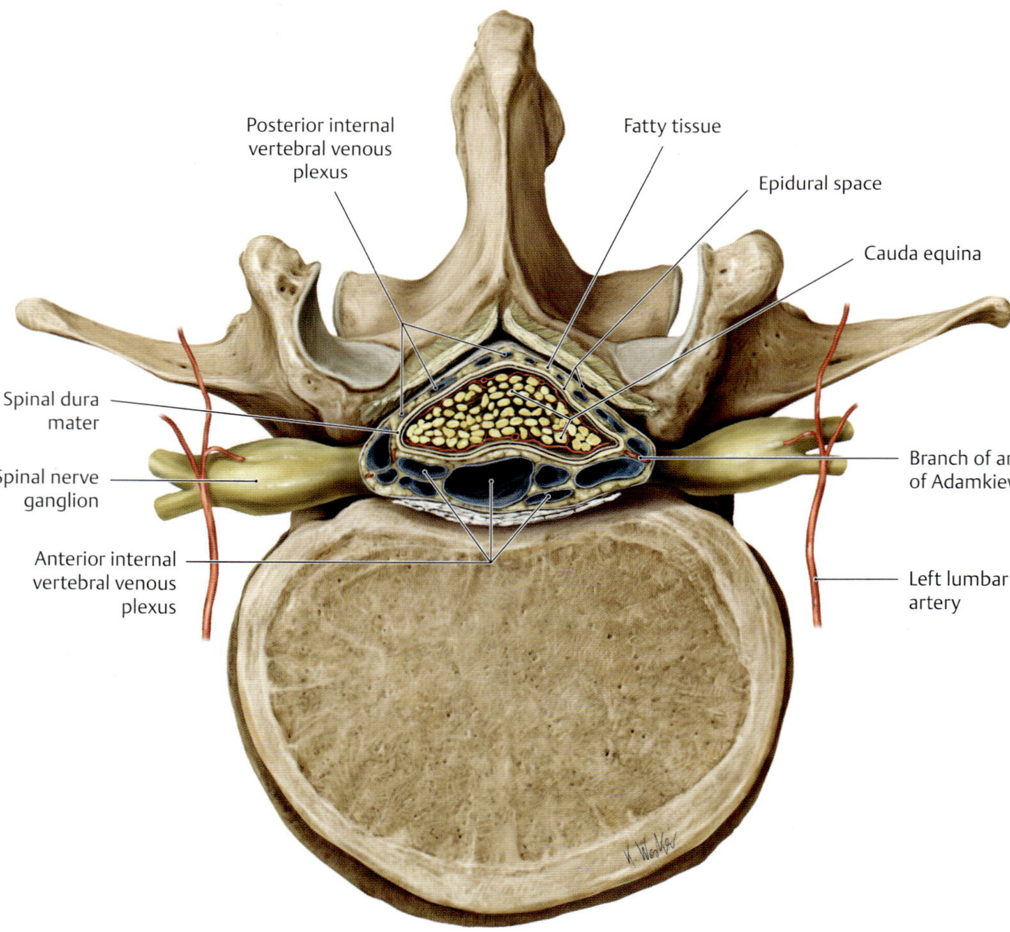

B Cauda equina at the level of the L 2 vertebra

Transverse section viewed from below. The spinal cord usually ends at the level of the first lumbar vertebra (L 1). The space below the low-er end of the spinal cord is occupied by the cauda equina and filum terminale in the dural sac (lumbar cistern, see p. 311), which ends at the level of the S 2 vertebra (see **C** and **D**). The epidural space expands at that level and contains extensive venous plexuses and fatty tissue.

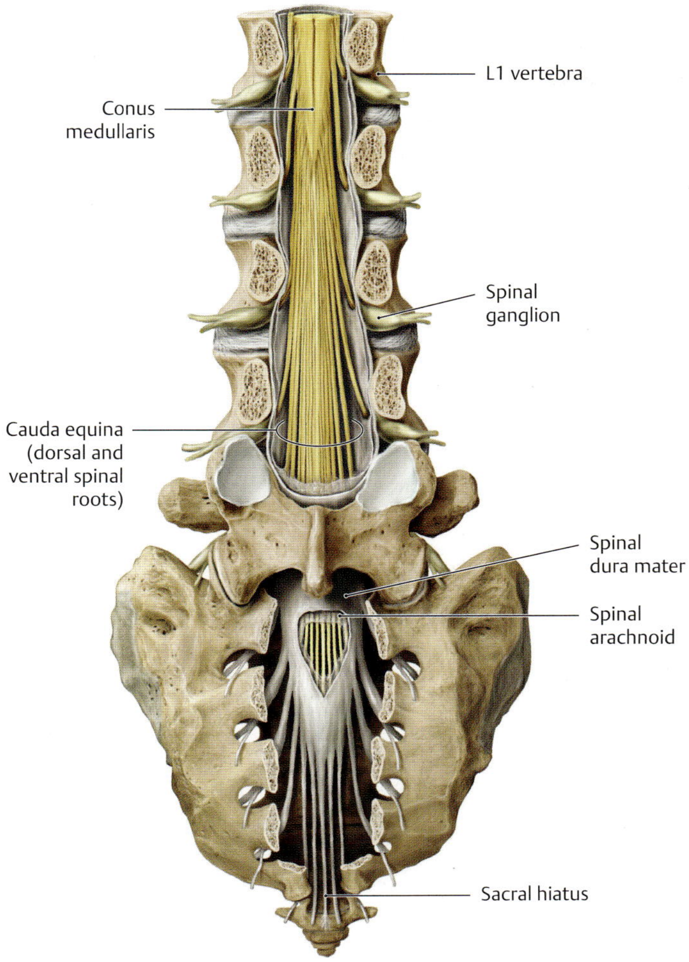

C Cauda equina in the vertebral canal
Posterior view. The laminae and the dorsal surface of the sacrum have been partially removed. The spinal cord in the adult terminates at approximately the level of the first lumbar vertebra (L1). The dorsal and ventral spinal nerve roots extending from the lower end of the spinal cord (conus medullaris) are known collectively as the cauda equina. During lumbar puncture at this level, a needle introduced into the subarachnoid space (lumbar cistern) normally slips past the spinal nerve roots without injuring them.

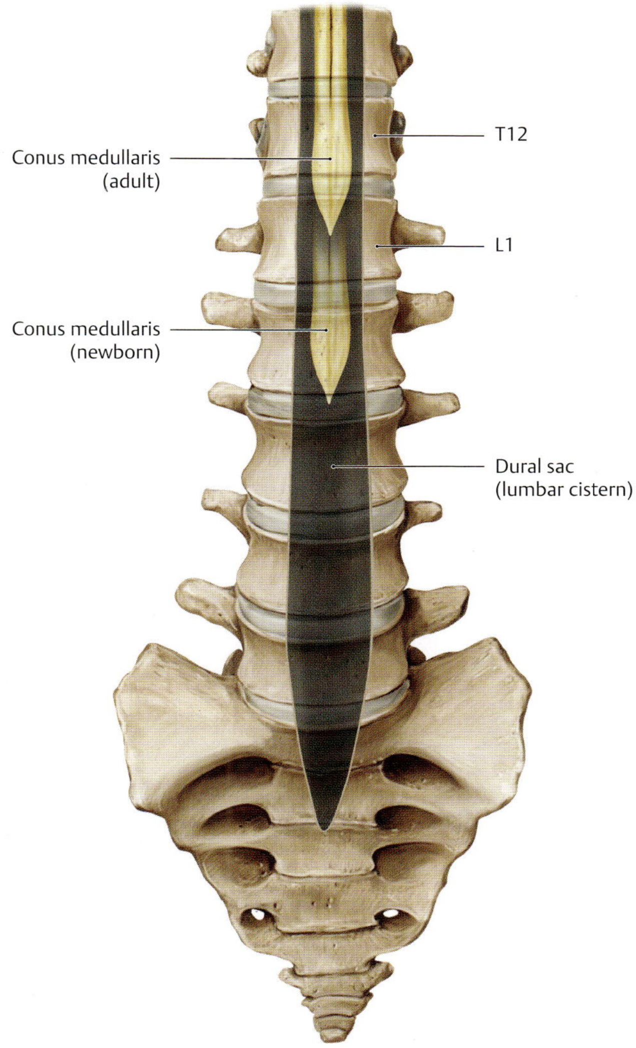

D The spinal cord, dural sac, and vertebral column at different ages
Anterior view. As an individual grows, the longitudinal growth of the spinal cord increasingly lags behind that of the vertebral column. At birth the distal end of the spinal cord, the conus medullaris, is at the level of the L3 vertebral body (where lumbar puncture is contraindicated). The spinal cord of a tall adult ends at the T12/L1 level, while that of a short adult extends to the L2/L3 level. The dural sac always extends into the upper sacrum. It is important to consider these anatomical relationships during lumbar puncture. It is best to introduce the needle at the L3/L4 interspace.

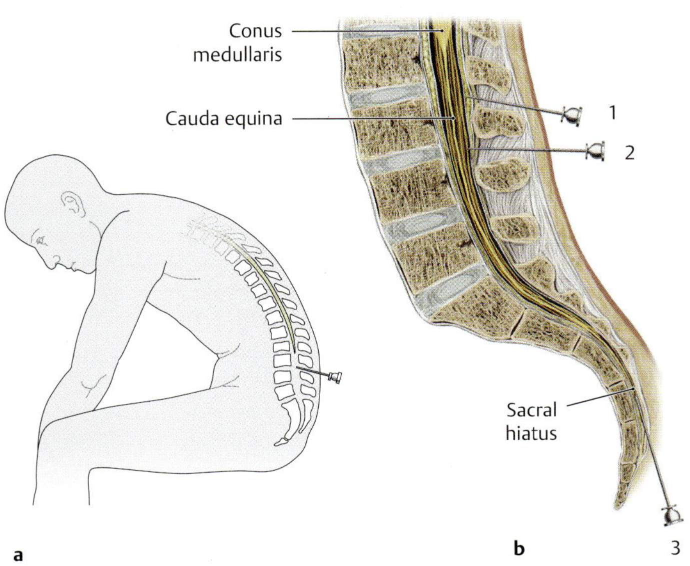

E Lumbar puncture, epidural anesthesia, and lumbar anesthesia
In preparation for a **lumbar puncture**, the patient bends far forward to separate the spinous processes of the lumbar spine. The spinal needle is usually introduced between the spinous processes of the L 3 and L 4 vertebrae. It is advanced through the skin and into the dural sac (lumbar cistern) to obtain a cerebrospinal fluid sample. This procedure has numerous applications, including the diagnosis of meningitis. For **epidural anesthesia**, a catheter is placed in the epidural space without penetrating the dural sac (1). **Lumbar anesthesia** is induced by injecting a local anesthetic solution into the dural sac (2). Another option is to pass the needle into the epidural space through the sacral hiatus (3).

12.1 Coronal Sections: I and II (Frontal)

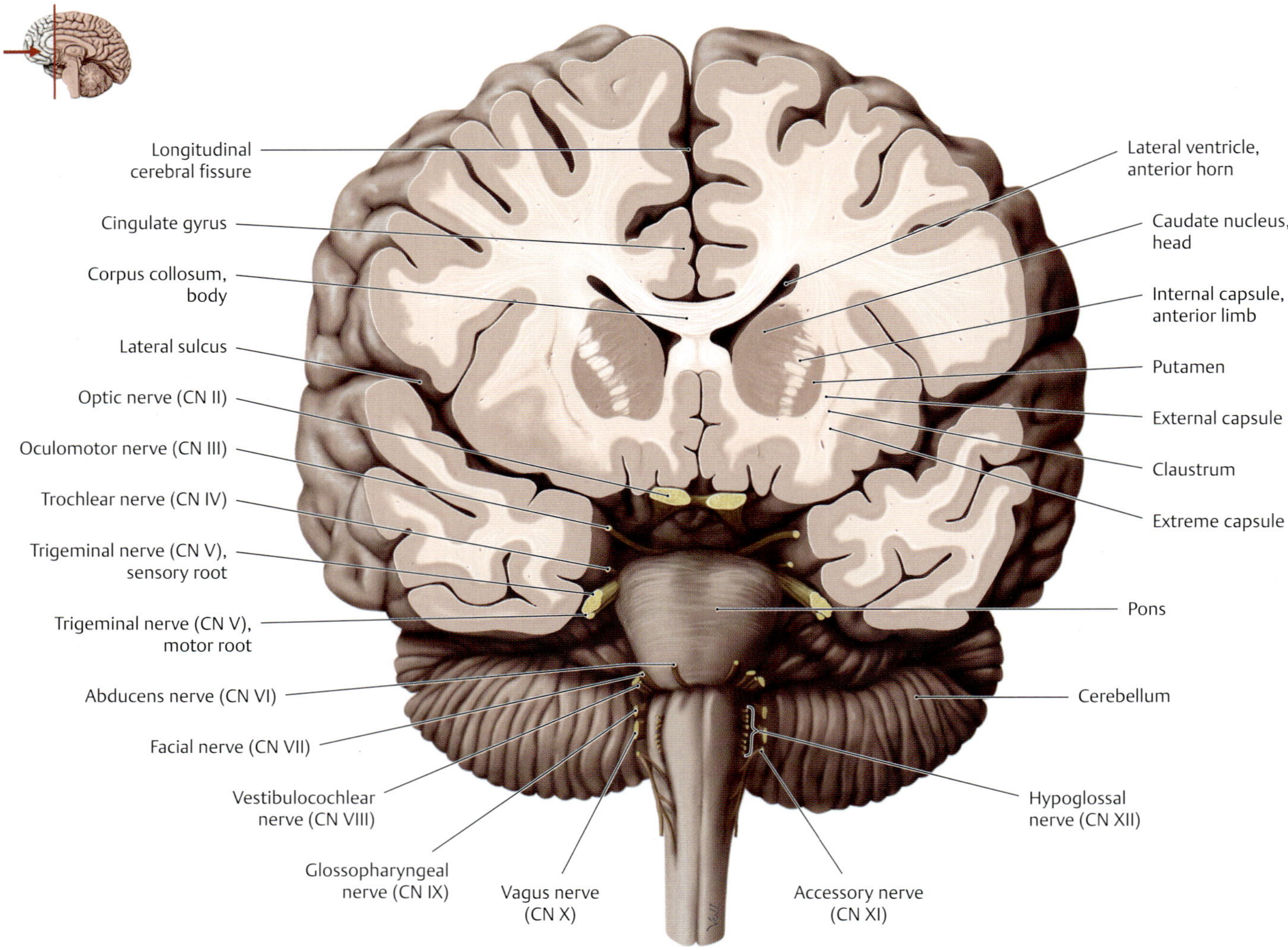

General remarks on sectional brain anatomy
The series of sections (coronal, transverse, and sagittal) in this chapter is intended to help the reader gain an appreciation of the three-dimensional anatomy of the brain. This is necessary for the correct interpretation of modern sectional imaging modalities (CT and MRI for the investigation of suspected stroke, brain tumors, meningitis, and trauma). In offering this synoptic perspective, we assume that the reader has read the previous chapters and has gained at least a general appreciation of the functional and descriptive anatomy of the brain. The legends and especially the small accompanying schematic diagrams are intended to facilitate a three-dimensional understanding of the two-dimensional sections (the plane of the section in each figure is indicated by a red line in the small, inset image).
The planes of section have been selected to display the structures of *greatest clinical importance* more clearly than can be done in actual tissue sections, which are not always optimally fixed and preserved. Because the sections were modeled on specimens taken from different individuals, some structures will not be found at the same location in every figure. The structures of the brain were assigned to specific ontogenetic regions in previous chapters, and these relationships are summarized in **B**, p. 443, at the end of this chapter.
Note the relationship of the sectional planes to the Forel axis in the anterior part of the brain and to the Meynert axis in the brainstem region (see **B**, p. 270).

A Coronal section I
The body (trunk) of the *corpus callosum*, which interconnects the two cerebral hemispheres, is prominently displayed in this coronal section. Superior to the corpus callosum is the *cingulate gyrus*, which also appears in subsequent sections. Inferior to the corpus callosum is the *caudate nucleus*, which appears particularly large because this section passes through the widest portion of its head (see **C**). The nucleus appears different in later sections because it tapers occipitally to a narrow tail (see p. 422 f). The schematic lateral view (**C**) shows how the caudate nucleus is closely applied to the *lateral ventricle* and follows its concavity (shown in green). The caudate nucleus and the *putamen* together form the *corpus striatum*, whose "striation" is formed by the anterior limb of the internal capsule, a streak of white matter. The putamen still appears quite small at this level because the section passes only through its anterior tip. It becomes larger as the planes of section move further occipitally. The structures *anterior* to this plane consist of the cortex and white matter of the frontal lobe, both of which are easily identified. The temporal lobes, which still appear to be separate, detached structures, join the rest of the telencephalon in more occipital sectional planes (see p. 421).

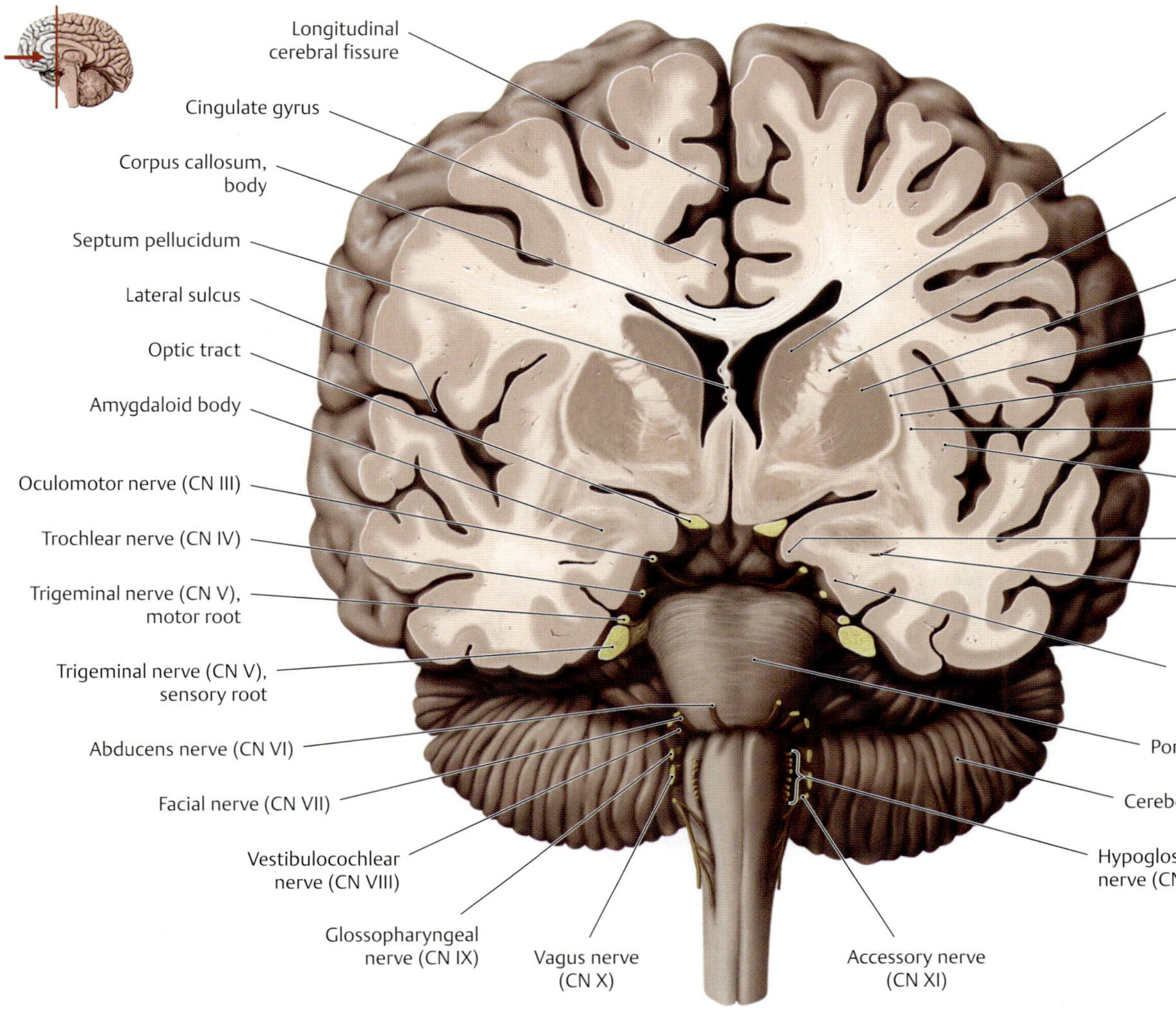

B Coronal section II
This section contains essentially the same structures as in **A**. The plane no longer passes through the *head* of the caudate nucleus, instead passing through its slender body. The *inferior horn* (temporal horn) of the lateral ventricle appears as a slitlike structure and also provides a useful landmark: ventral to the inferior horn is a portion of the *parahippocampal gyrus*. Superior and medial to the inferior horn is the *amygdala*.

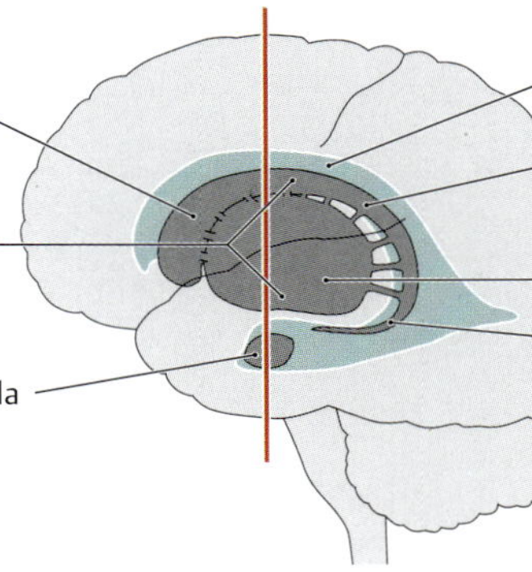

C Relationship between the caudate nucleus and lateral ventricle
Left lateral view.

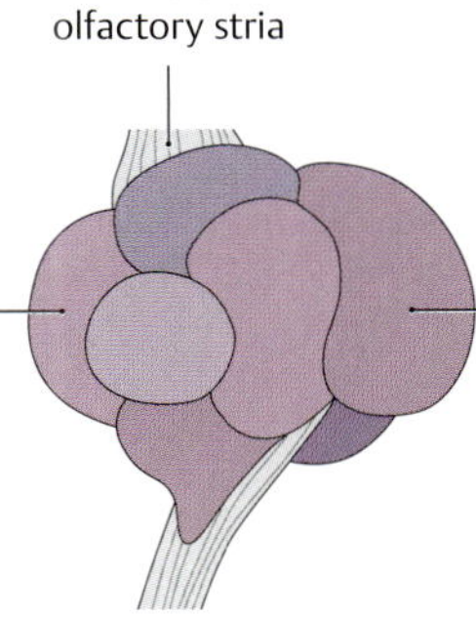

D Amygdala
Right lateral view.

12.2 Coronal Sections: III and IV

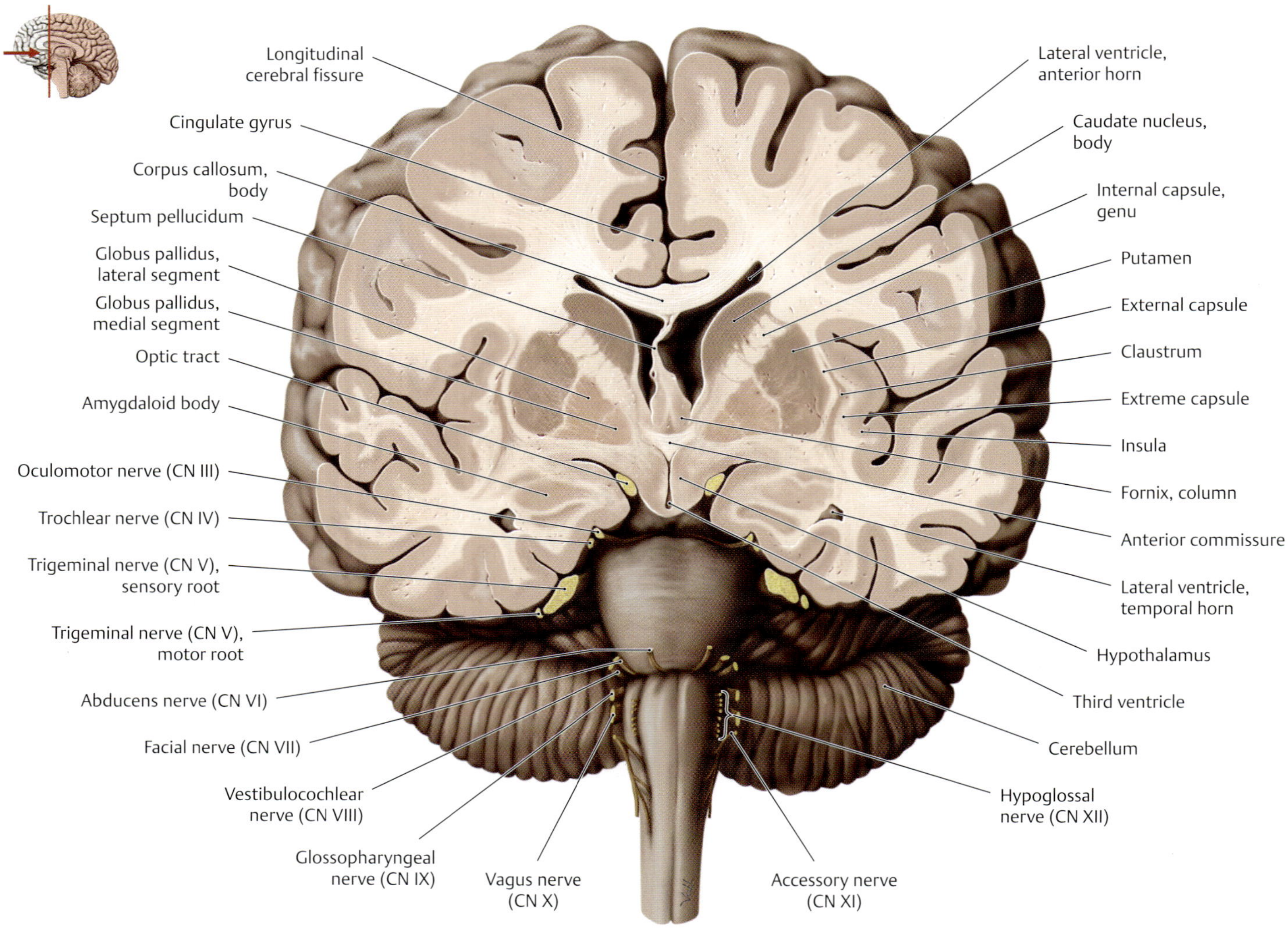

A Coronal section III
The inferior (temporal) horn of the lateral ventricle appears somewhat larger in the plane of this section. In the ventricular system, we can now see the floor of the *third ventricle* (see **B**) and the surrounding hypothalamus. The thalamus cannot yet be seen given that it lies slightly above and behind the hypothalamus. The *anterior commissure* appears in this plane as does the *globus pallidus*, which consists of a medial and a lateral segment. The large descending pathway, the corticospinal tract, passes through the *internal capsule*, which has a somatotopic organization. The genu of the internal capsule transmits axons of the corticonuclear tract. The course of these axons is shown schematically in **C** (the fornix appears in **D**).

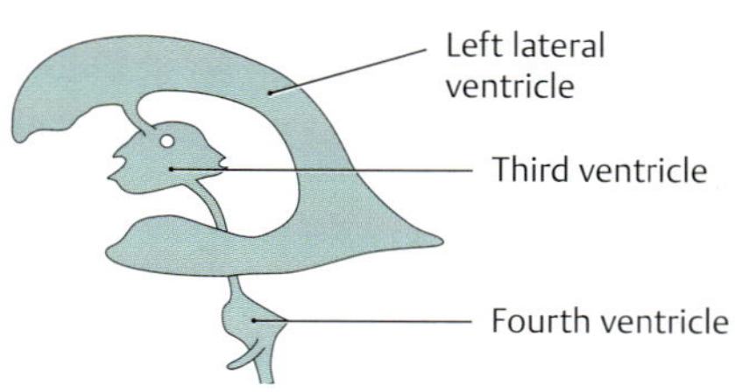

B Ventricular system
Left lateral view.

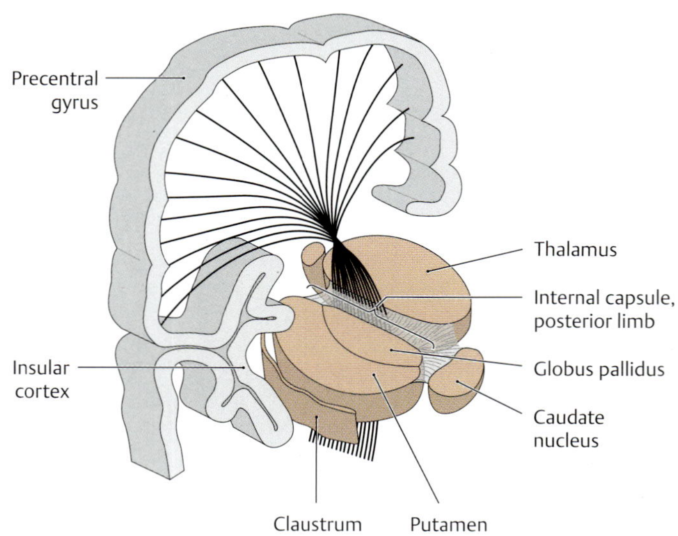

C Course of the pyramidal tract in the internal capsule
Left anterior view.

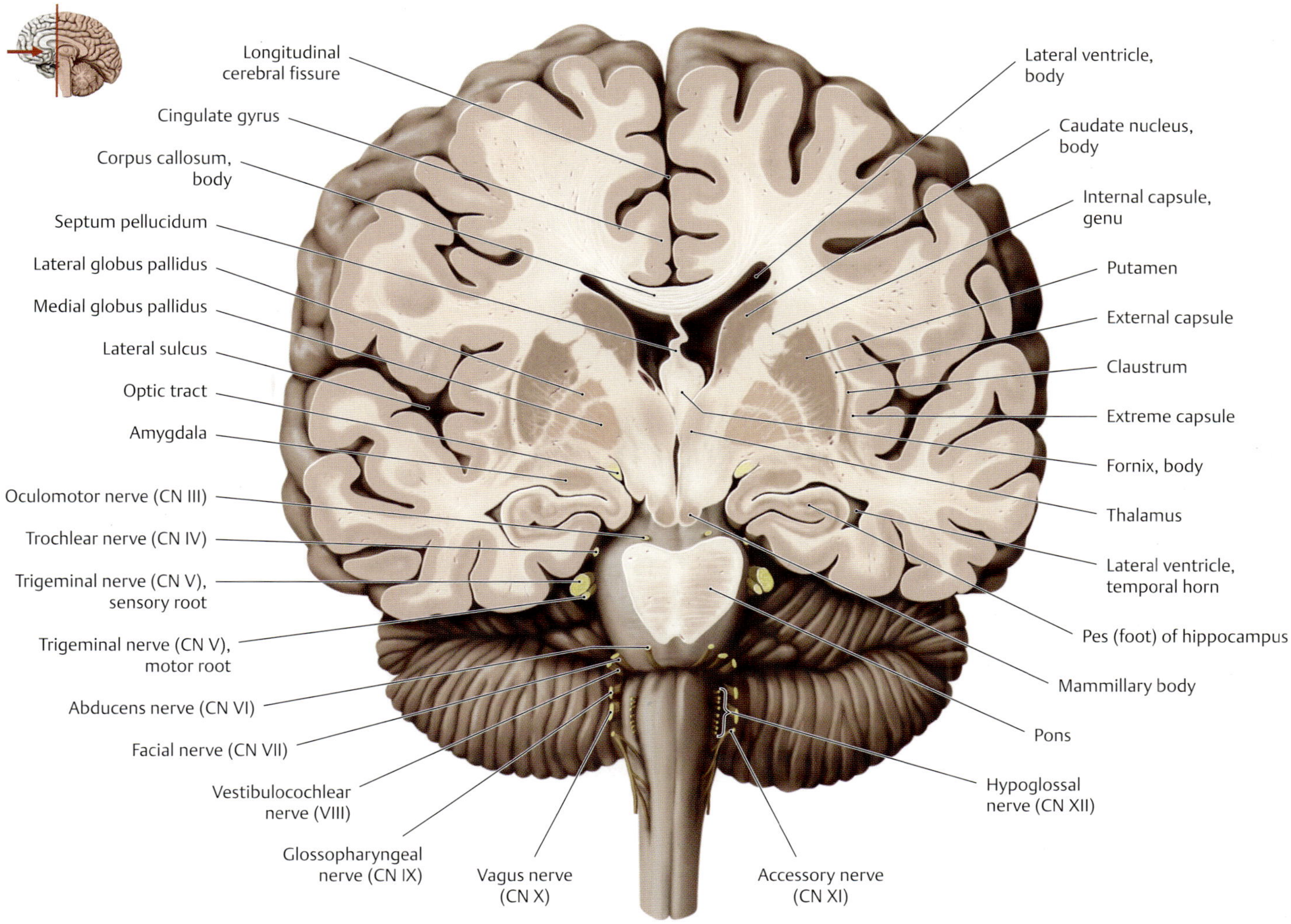

D Coronal section IV

The division of the globus pallidus into medial and lateral segments can now be seen clearly. This section displays the full width of both the inferior horn of the lateral ventricle and the *claustrum* (believed to be important in the regulation of sexual behavior). While the plane in **A** passed through the anterior commissure, this more occipital plane slices the *mammillary bodies* (see **E**). Pathological changes in the mammillary bodies can be found during autopsy of chronic alcoholics. The mammillary bodies are flanked on each side by the *foot of the hippocampus*.

An important part of the limbic system, the mammillary bodies are connected to the hippocampus by the *fornix* (see **F**). Due to the anatomical curvature of the fornix, its *columns* are visible in more frontal sections (see **A**), while its *crura* appear as widely separated structures in more occipital sections (see **C**, p. 427). The *septum pellucidum* stretches between the fornix and corpus callosum, forming the medial boundary of the lateral ventricles (see **A** and **D**).

The first structure of the brainstem, the *pons*, can also be identified in this section.

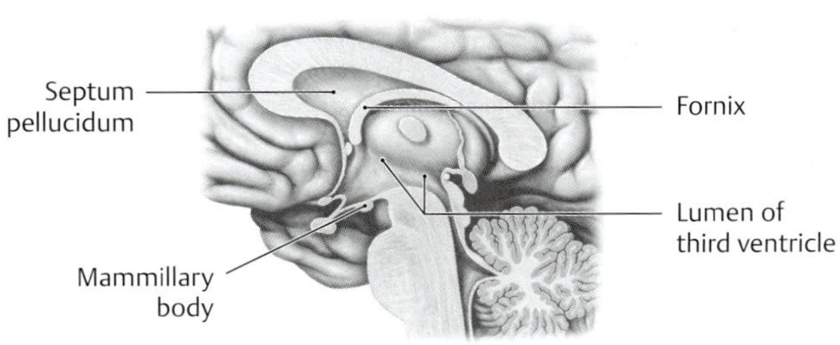

E Midsagittal section through the diencephalon and brainstem
Lateral view.

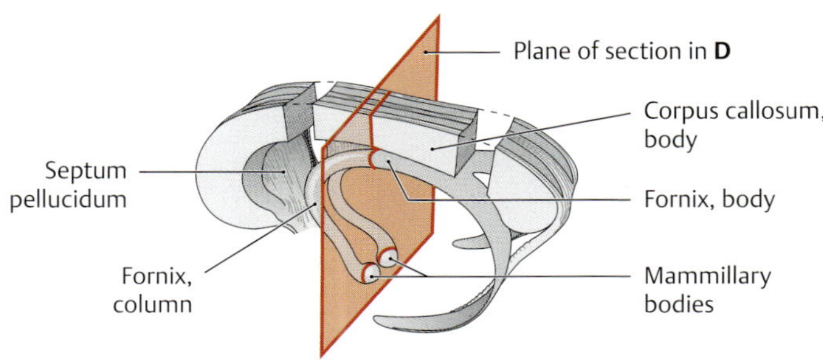

F Mammillary bodies and fornix

12.3 Coronal Sections: V and VI

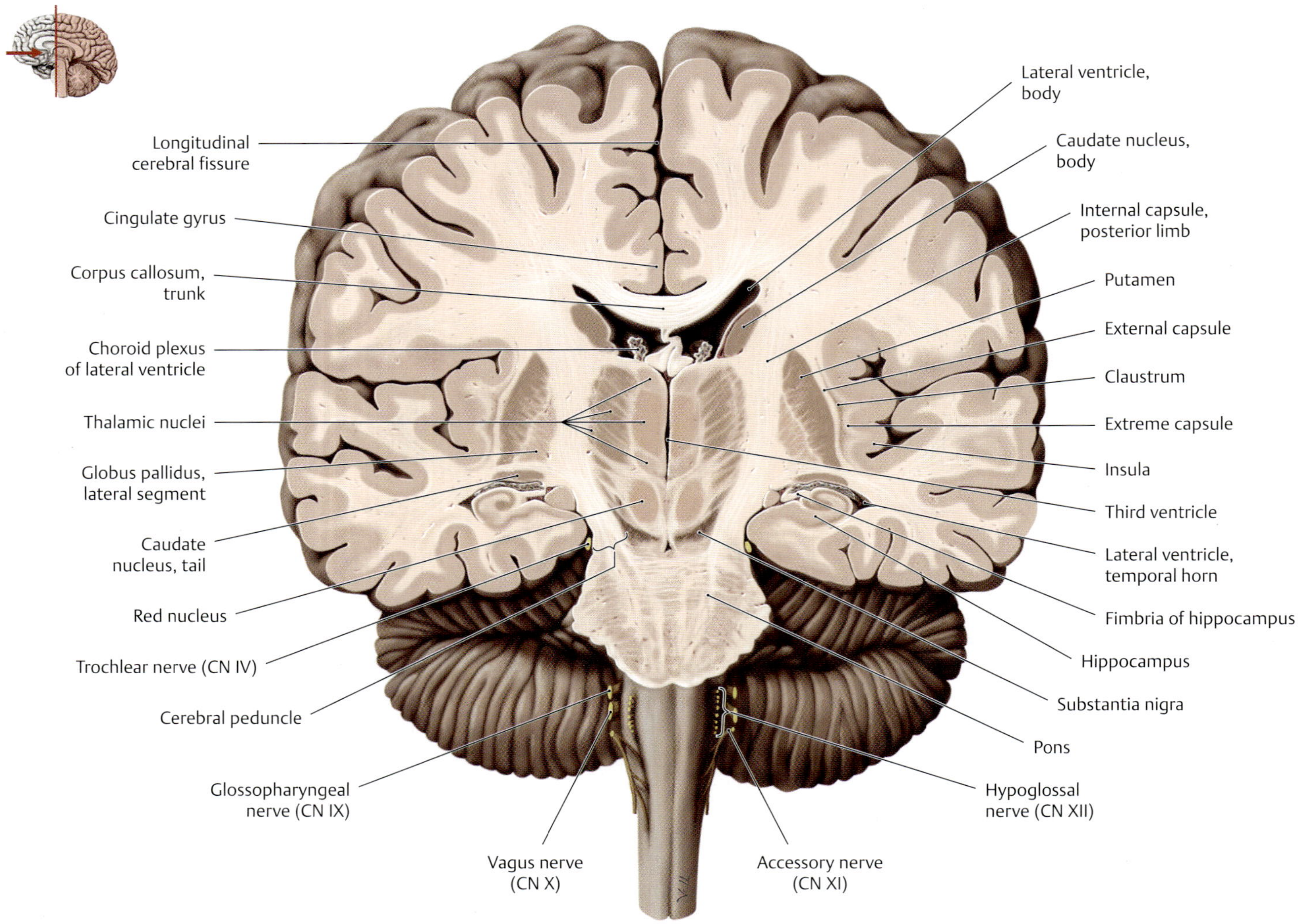

A Coronal section V

The appearance of the central nuclear region has changed markedly. The *caudate nucleus* is cut twice by the plane of this section. Its body borders the body of the lateral ventricle, and a small portion of its tail borders the inferior horn of the ventricle (see **C** and **E**). Because the head and body of the caudate nucleus rim the lateral aspect of the anterior (frontal) horn and the body of the lateral ventricle, the caudate nucleus has a curved shape similar to that of the lateral ventricle (see **C**). Thus, the tail of the caudate nucleus is ventral and lateral in relation to its head and body. Panel **E** shows that a coronal section through the tail of the caudate nucleus cuts the occipital portions of the *putamen*. A section in a slightly more occipital plane may not contain any part of the basal nuclei at all (see **B**). The central part of the lateral horn has become much narrower due to the presence of the *thalamus*, showing here several thalamic nuclei. This is the first plane that displays the *choroid plexus*, which can be seen within the lateral ventricles. The choroid plexus extends from the interventricular foramen (not visible here) into the inferior horn. Because the foramen lies anterior to the thalamus, the plexus can be seen only in coronal sections that also pass through thalamic structures. Ventral to the thalamus are the *red nucleus* and *substantia nigra*; these are important midbrain structures that bulge into the diencephalon and extend almost to the level of the globus pallidus (not visible here; see **B**). The *hippocampus* indents the floor of the temporal horn, and its fimbria can be seen. This section also shows how the fibers of the corticospinal tract pass through the *posterior limb* of the internal capsule and continue into the cerebral peduncles and pons.

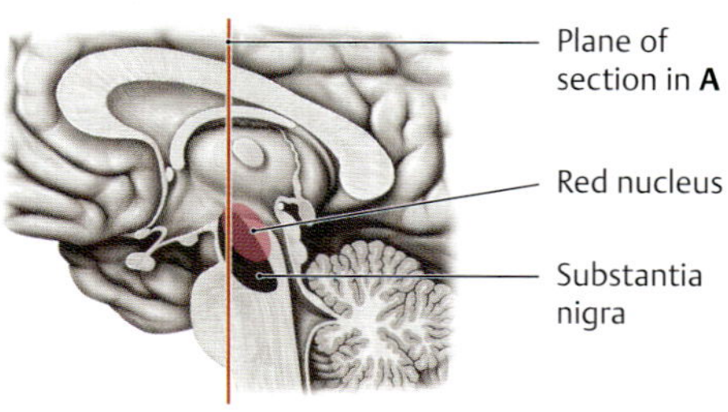

B Red nucleus and substantia nigra
Midsagittal section.

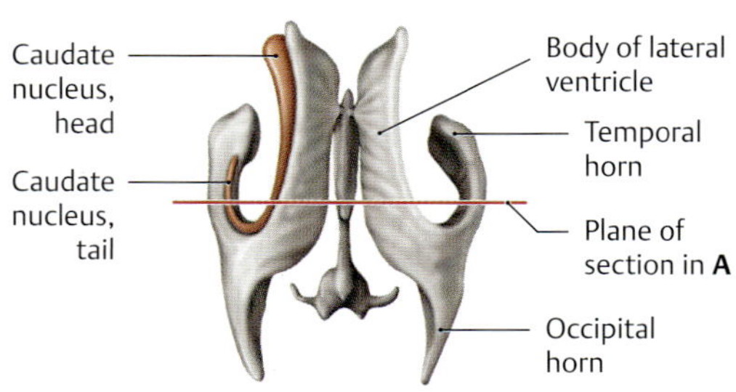

C Ventricular system
Superior view.

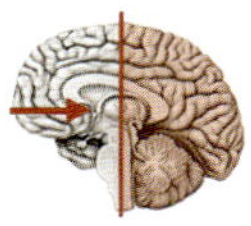

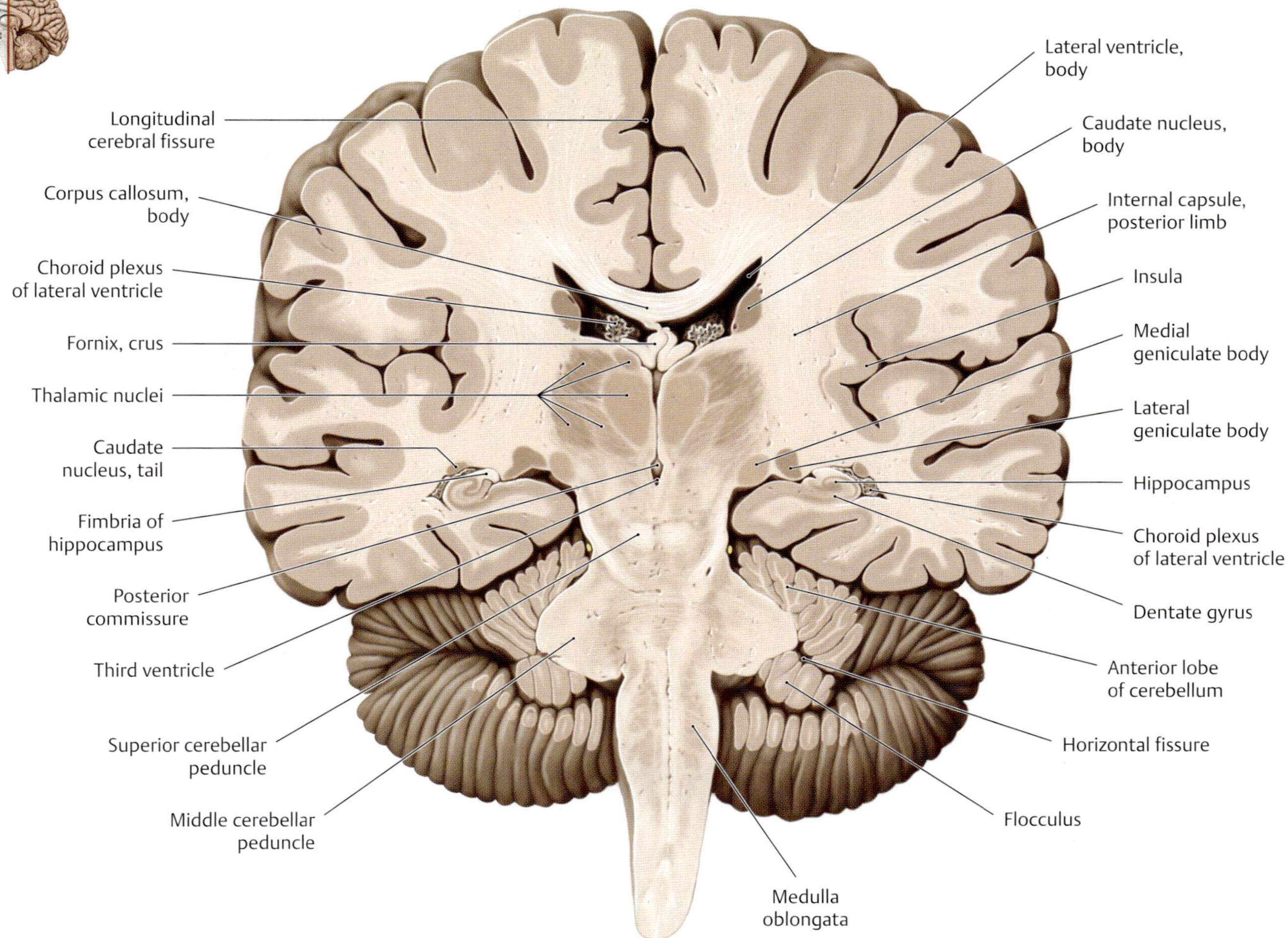

D Coronal section VI

The caudal thalamic nuclei are well displayed in this section, bordering the lateral ventricles from below and the third ventricle from the sides. The putamen lies at a more rostral level and is no longer visible in this plane (see the transverse section on p. 336). This section passes through the *posterior limb* of the internal capsule (see also **C**, p. 422) and the anterior part of the *posterior commissure* (see **A**, p. 426 and **D** p. 427).

The *medial* and *lateral geniculate bodies*, which are components of the auditory and visual pathways respectively, appear as two darker nuclei that flank the thalamus on the right and left sides at the same level as the commissure (see **F**). The crura of the fornix can be seen between the thalamus and corpus callosum. This is the first section that passes through parts of the *cerebellum*. Here the *middle cerebellar peduncle* passes laterally toward the cerebellar hemispheres.

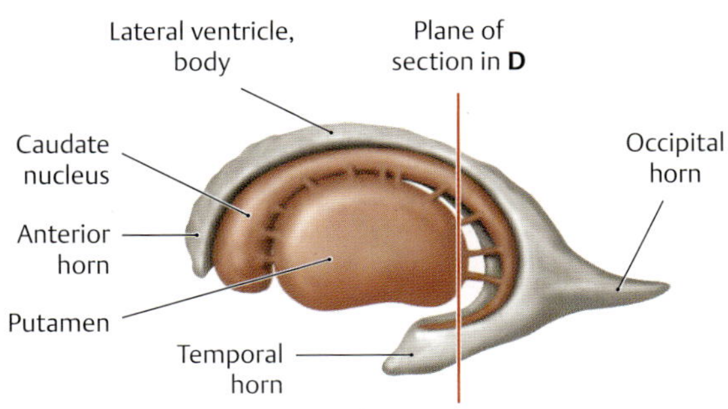

E Topographical relationship between the caudate nucleus and ventricular system

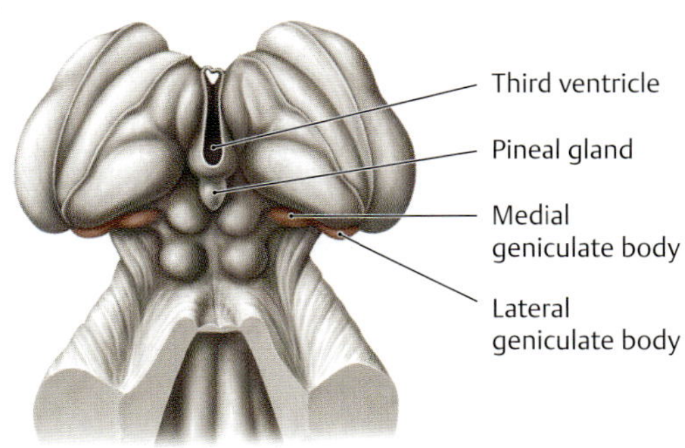

F The diencephalon (with geniculate bodies) and brainstem
Posterior view.

12.4 Coronal Sections: VII and VIII

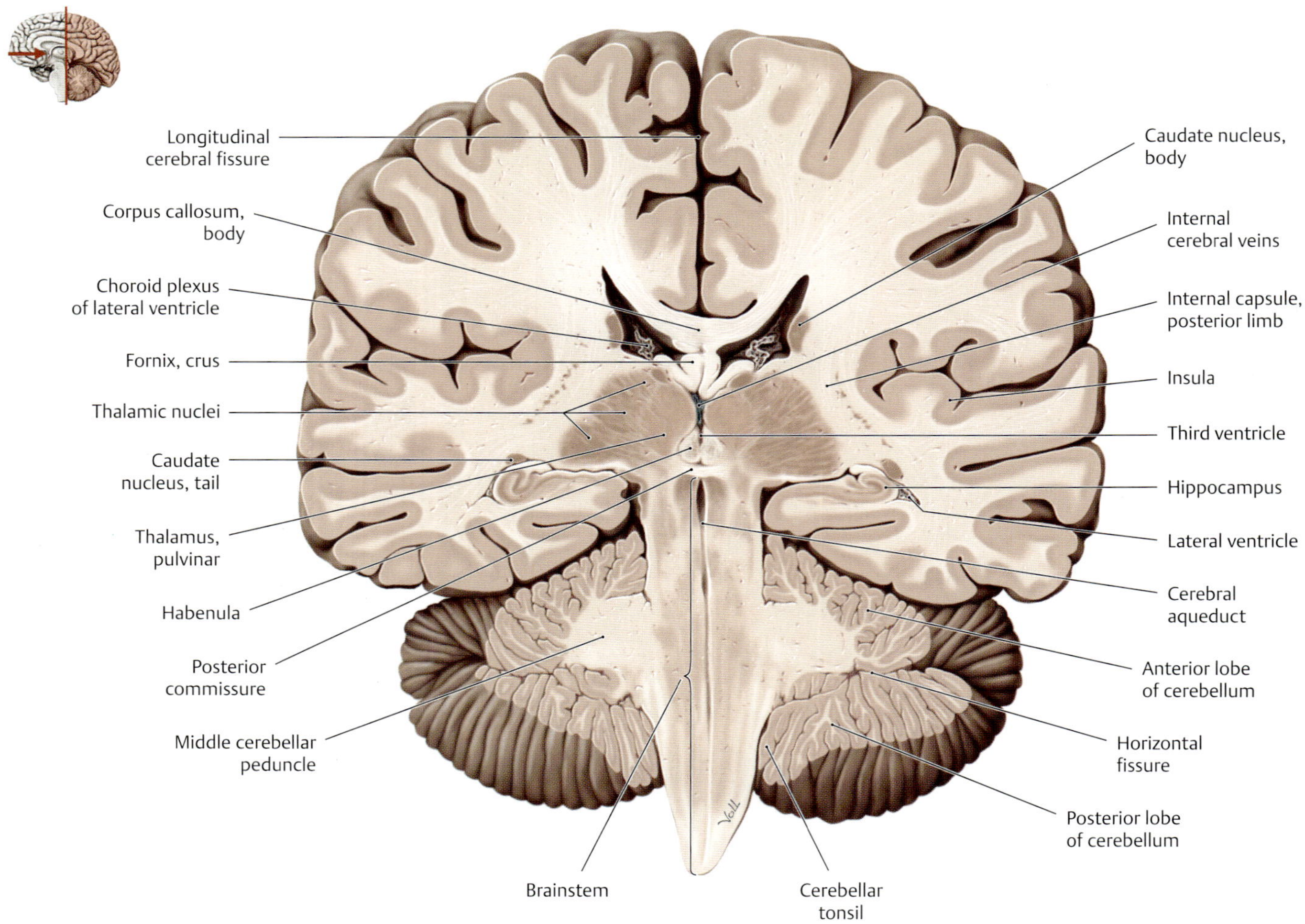

A Coronal section VII

Among the diencephalic and telencephalic nuclei, we can still identify the thalamus and occipital portions of the caudate nucleus, which become progressively smaller in the following sections until they finally disappear (see **C** and p. 428). The occipital part of the *hippocampus* can be seen below the medial wall of the lateral ventricle. This section cuts the brainstem along the *cerebral aqueduct* (see **C**). The cerebellum is connected to the brainstem by three white-matter stalks: the *superior cerebellar peduncle* (mainly efferent), *middle cerebellar peduncle* (afferent), and *inferior cerebellar peduncle* (afferent and efferent). Because the *middle* cerebellar peduncle extends further anteriorly than the other two peduncles (note its relationship to the brainstem axis), it is the first peduncle to appear in this frontal-to-occipital series of sections (see also **A**, p. 424, and **D**, p. 425). The *superior* cerebellar peduncle begins on the posterior side of the pons and thus appears in a later section (see **B**). There are no natural anatomical boundaries between the middle and inferior cerebellar peduncles, and therefore the latter is not separately labeled in the sections. The superficial veins were removed from the brain when this section was prepared, and only the internal cerebral veins appear in this and the following section.

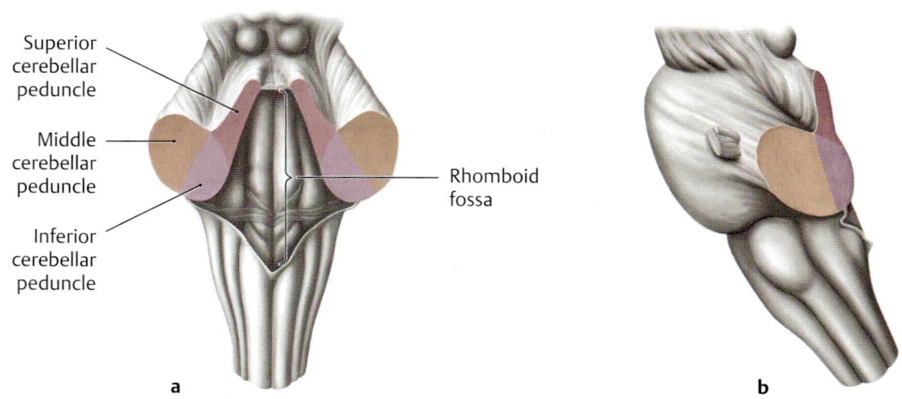

B Cerebellar peduncles on the brainstem
(**a**) Posterior view; (**b**) Lateral view.

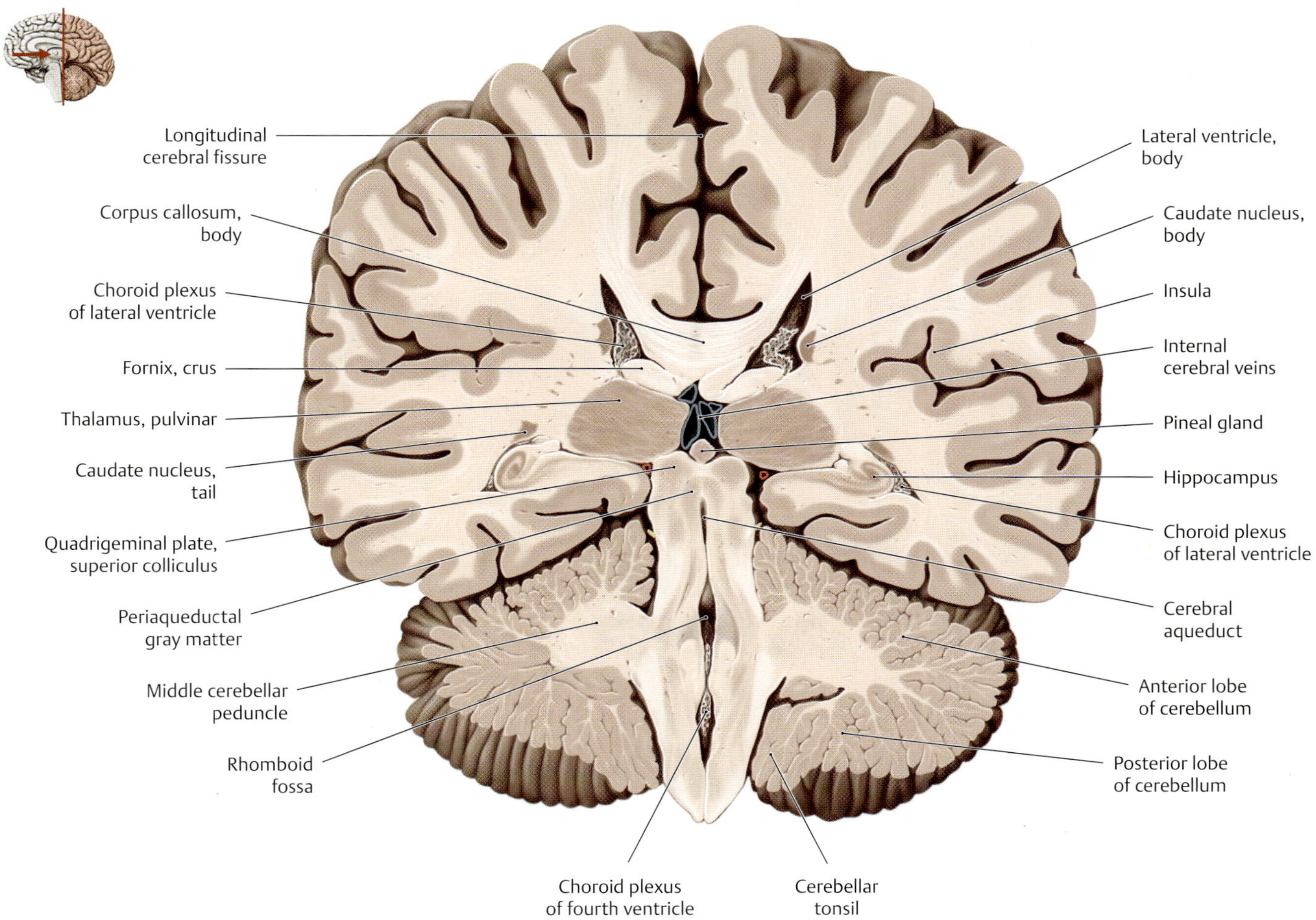

C Coronal section VIII

The thalamic nuclei appear smaller than in previous sections, and more of the cerebellar cortex is seen. This plane passes through part of the cerebral aqueduct. The *rhomboid fossa*, which forms the floor of the fourth ventricle, is clearly visible in the dorsal part of the brainstem (see **D** and **Ba**). The quadrigeminal plate (lamina tecti) is also visible. Its smaller *superior* colliculi are particularly well displayed in this section, while the *inferior* colliculi are more prominent in the next section (see **A**, p. 428).

The pineal gland is only partially visible because of its somewhat more occipital location (see **D**); a full cross-section can be seen in **A**, p. 428. The present section shows the division of the paired fornix tract into its two *crura*. The hippocampus here borders on the inferior horn of the lateral ventricle on each side, bulging into its floor from the medial side (see also **A** and **E**). The hippocampus is an important component of the limbic system and is one of the first structures to undergo detectable morphological changes in Alzheimer's disease.

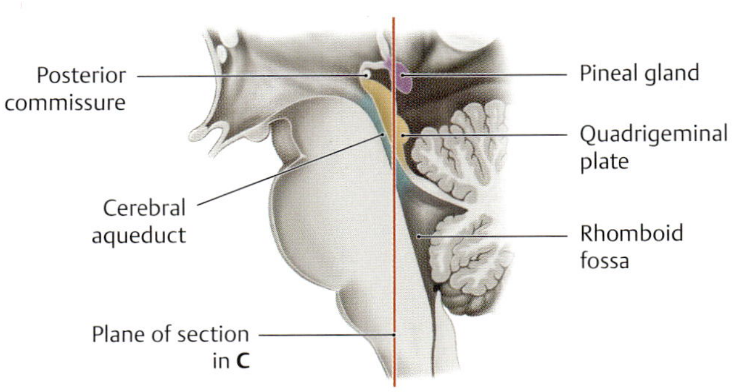

D Midsagittal section through the rhombencephalon, mesencephalon, and diencephalon

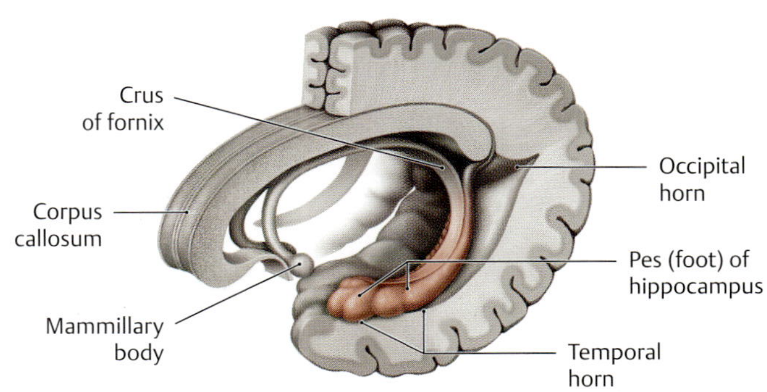

E Hippocampal formation

Left anterior and lateral oblique view.

12.5 Coronal Sections: IX and X

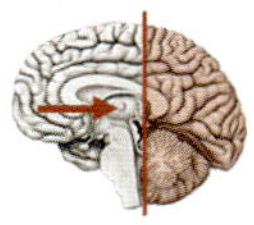

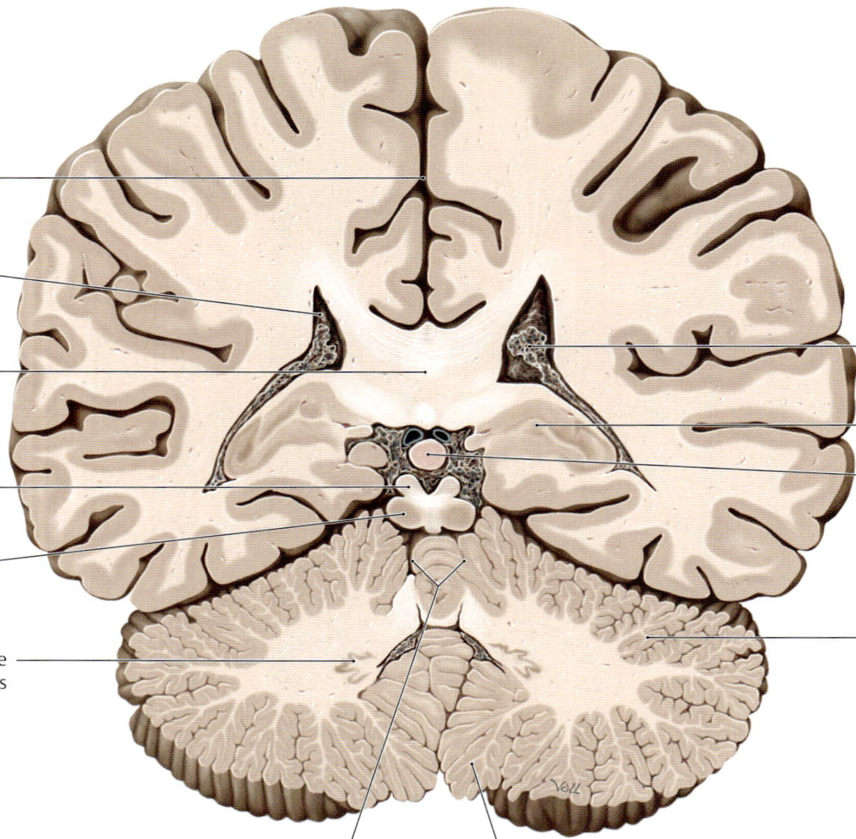

A Coronal section IX

The pineal gland, a control center for circadian rhythms, is here displayed in full cross-section (contrast with the previous section (see **C**, p. 427); see also **D**, p. 427). Below it lies the quadrigeminal plate, the dorsal part of the midbrain (note its relationship to the brainstem axis). The larger *inferior* colliculi of the quadrigeminal plate are more prominent here than in the previous section (the inclination of the brainstem gives them a more posterior location). The *inferior* colliculi are part of the auditory pathway, while the *superior* colliculi (more clearly seen in the previous section) are part of the visual pathway. At the level of the cerebellum, the *vermis* can be identified as an unpaired midline structure. The only cerebellar nucleus visible at this level is the *dentate nucleus*, which is surrounded by the cerebellar white matter. The other deep cerebral nuclei are not visible in the plane of this section.

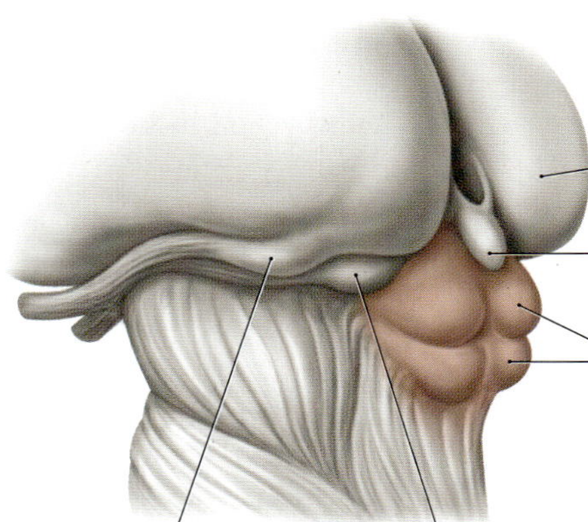

B Quadrigeminal plate (tectum)
Left posterior oblique view.

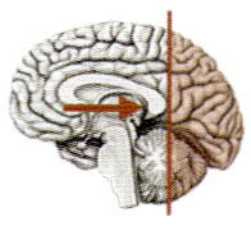

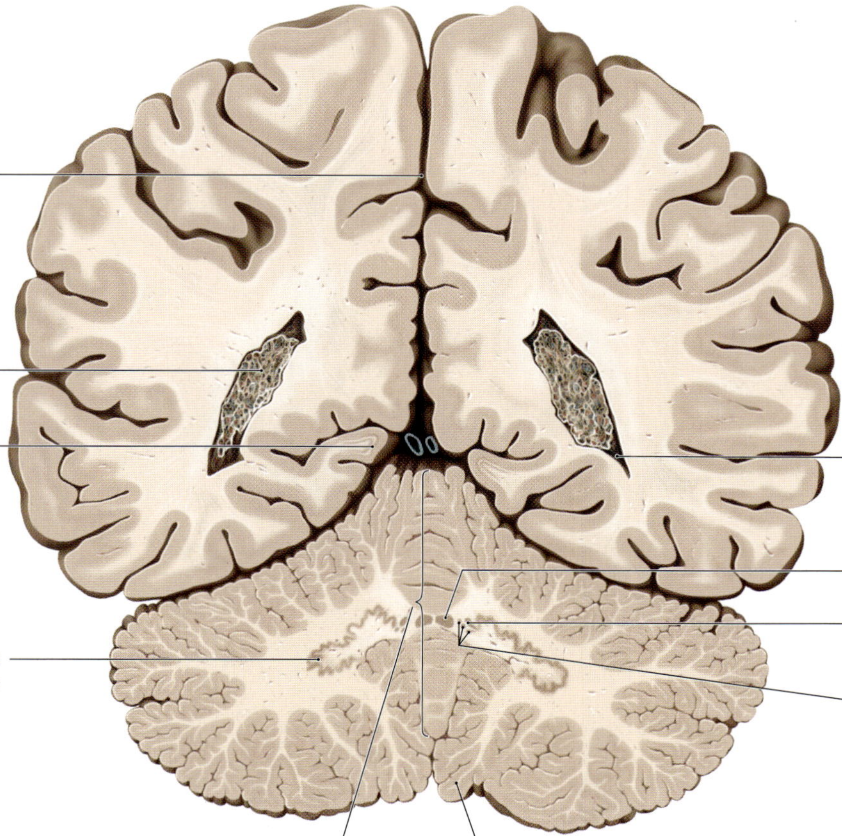

C Coronal section X
This plane presents the four *cerebellar nuclei*:

- Dentate nucleus (lateral cerebellar nucleus)
- Emboliform nucleus (anterior interpositus nucleus)
- Globose nucleus (posterior interpositus nucleus)
- Fastigial nucleus (medial cerebellar nucleus)

The longitudinally cut cerebellar vermis presents a larger area here than in the previous section. The fourth ventricle is no longer visible in the plane of this section.

12.6 Coronal Sections: XI and XII (Occipital)

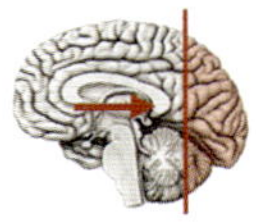

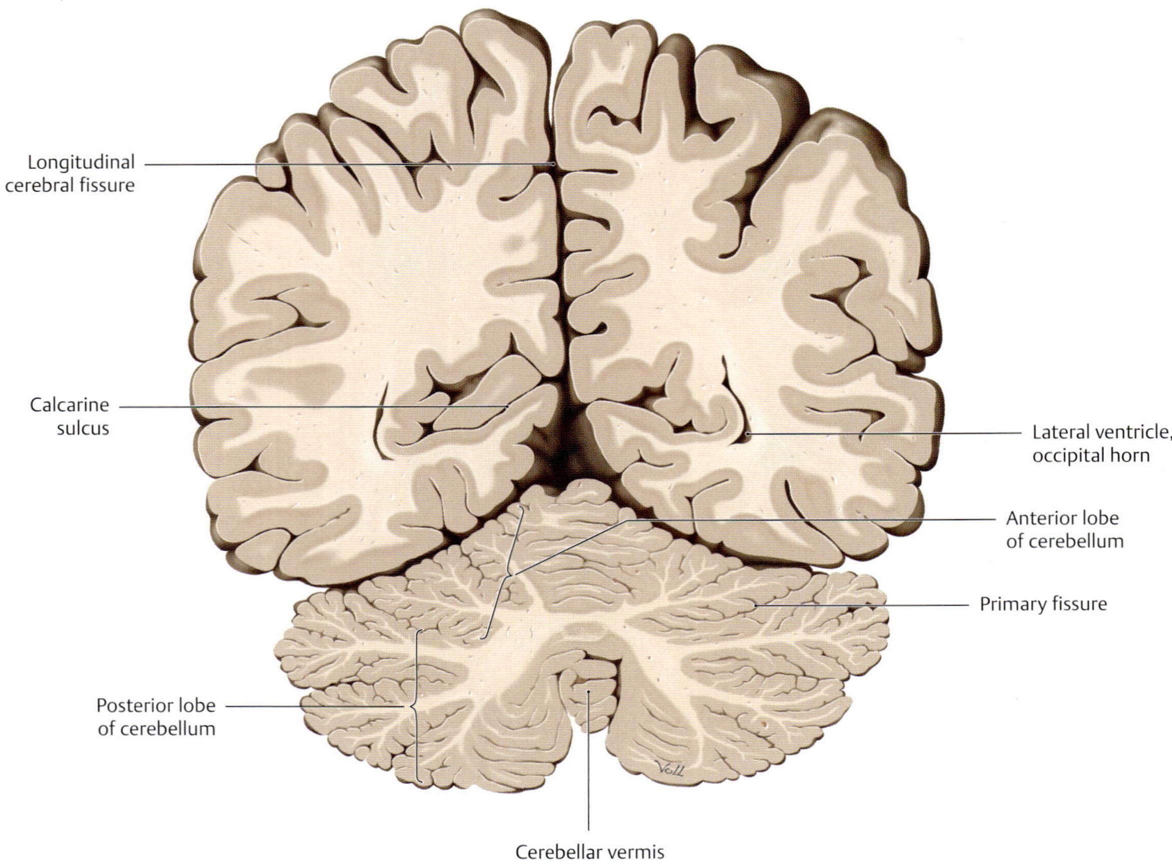

A Coronal section XI

The plane of this section clearly shows the posterior (occipital) horns of the lateral ventricles; these appear only as narrow slits in the next section (see **D**). The section also illustrates once again how the posterior horn is an extension of the inferior (temporal) horn (see **B**). Between the cerebellum and the occipital lobe of the cerebrum lies the *tentorium cerebelli* (see **C**). The tentorium contains the straight sinus, which passes to the confluence of the sinuses. It is one of the dural venous sinuses that drain blood from the brain, beginning at the confluence of the great cerebral vein and the inferior sagittal sinus (removed during preparation of the falx cerebri). Because the dura is removed from the brain in the preparation of most tissue sections, the sinuses enclosed by the dura mater also tend to be removed.

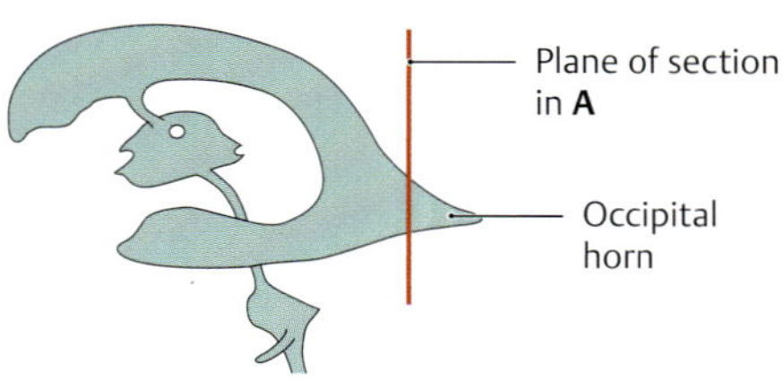

B Ventricular system viewed from the left side

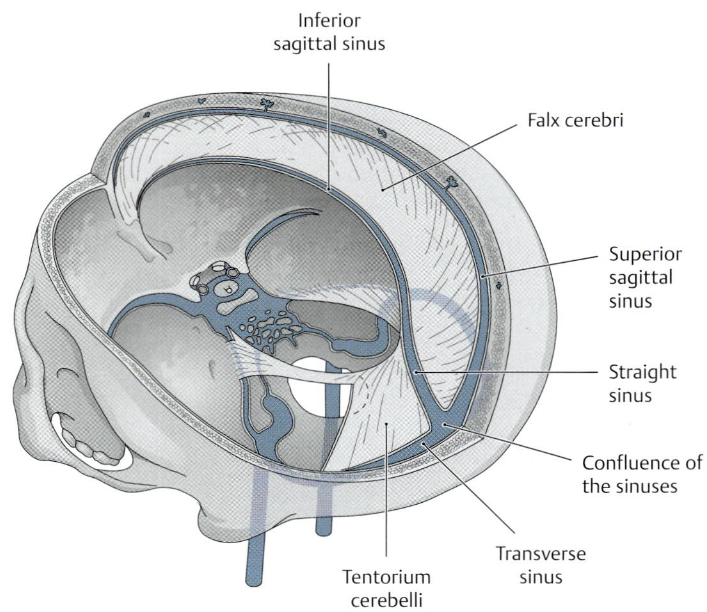

C The dural sinuses viewed from upper left

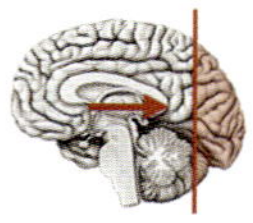

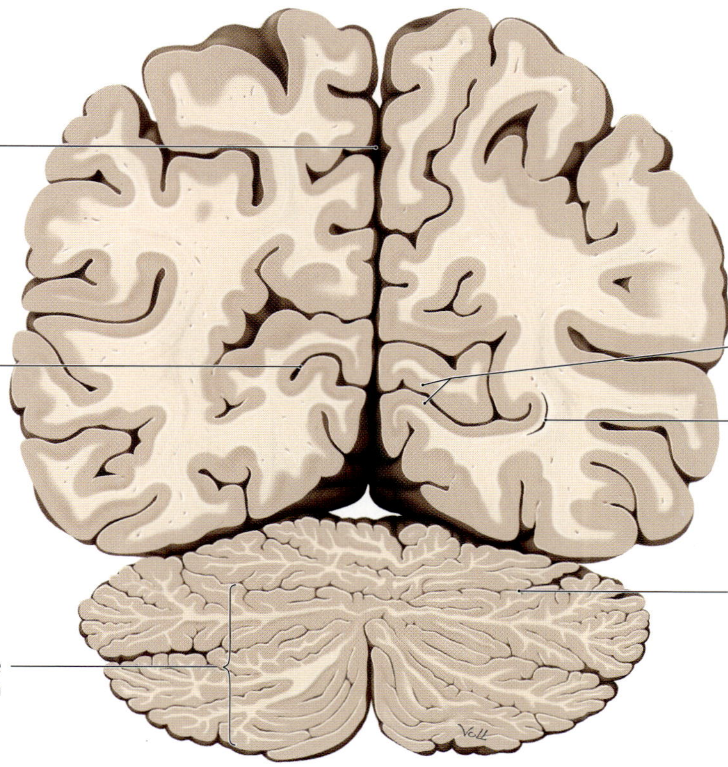

D Coronal section XII
In the plane of this section, the posterior (occipital) horn of the lateral ventricle has dwindled to a narrow slit. The relatively long *calcarine sulcus* is visible in the occipital lobe of the cerebrum, and also appears in several of the proceeding sections. It is surrounded by the *striate area* (primary visual cortex, also called area 17 in the Brodmann brain map), the size of which is best appreciated on the medial surface of the brain (see **E**). More occipital sections are not presented in this chapter, as they would show nothing but cortex and subcortical white matter.

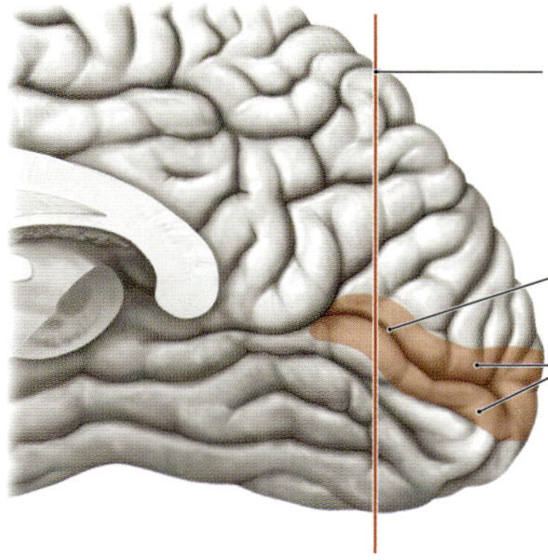

E Right striate area (visual cortex)
Medial surface of the right hemisphere, viewed from the left side.

12.7 Transverse Sections: I and II (Cranial)

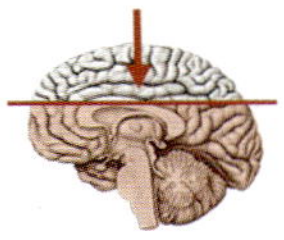

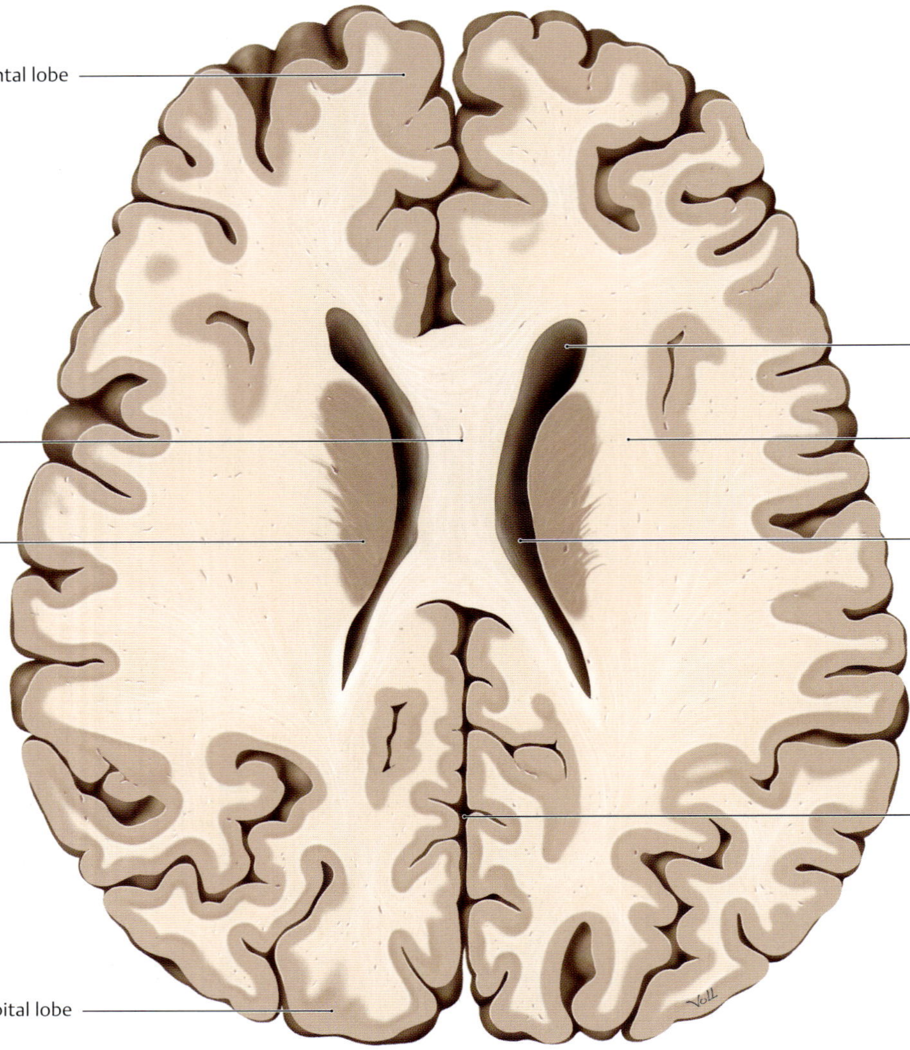

General remarks on transverse (axial, horizontal) brain sections
The sections in this series are viewed from above and behind the head (position of axes see p. 270); that is, the observer is looking at the surface of the slice as it would typically appear in a brain autopsy or during a neurosurgical operation. Thus, the left side of the brain appears on the left side of the drawing. This contrasts with the image orientation in CT and MRI, where brain slices are always viewed from below; that is, the left side of the brain appears on the right side of the image.

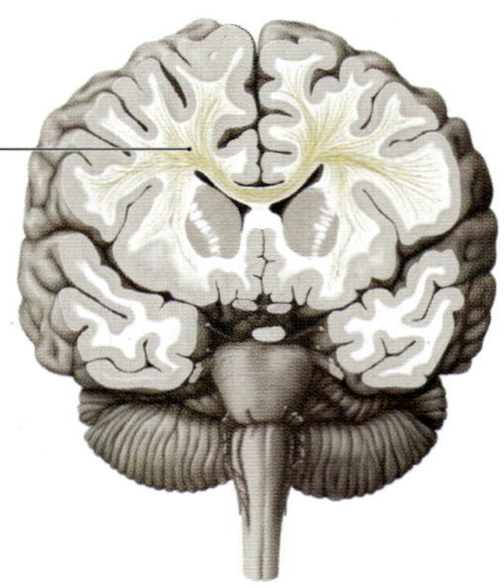

B Coronal section through the brain

A Transverse section I
This highest of the transverse brain sections passes through frontal, parietal, and occipital structures of the telencephalon. Each of the two *lateral ventricles* is bordered laterally by the body of the caudate nucleus, and medially by the *body of the corpus callosum*. The corpus callosum transmits fiber tracts which interconnect areas in both hemispheres that serve the same function (*commissural tracts*). When viewed in cross section, the corpus callosum appears to be interrupted by the ventricles and caudate nucleus, when, in fact, it arches over these structures, forming the roof of the lateral ventricles. The course of the tracts that pass through the corpus callosum can be appreciated by looking at a coronal section (see **B**).

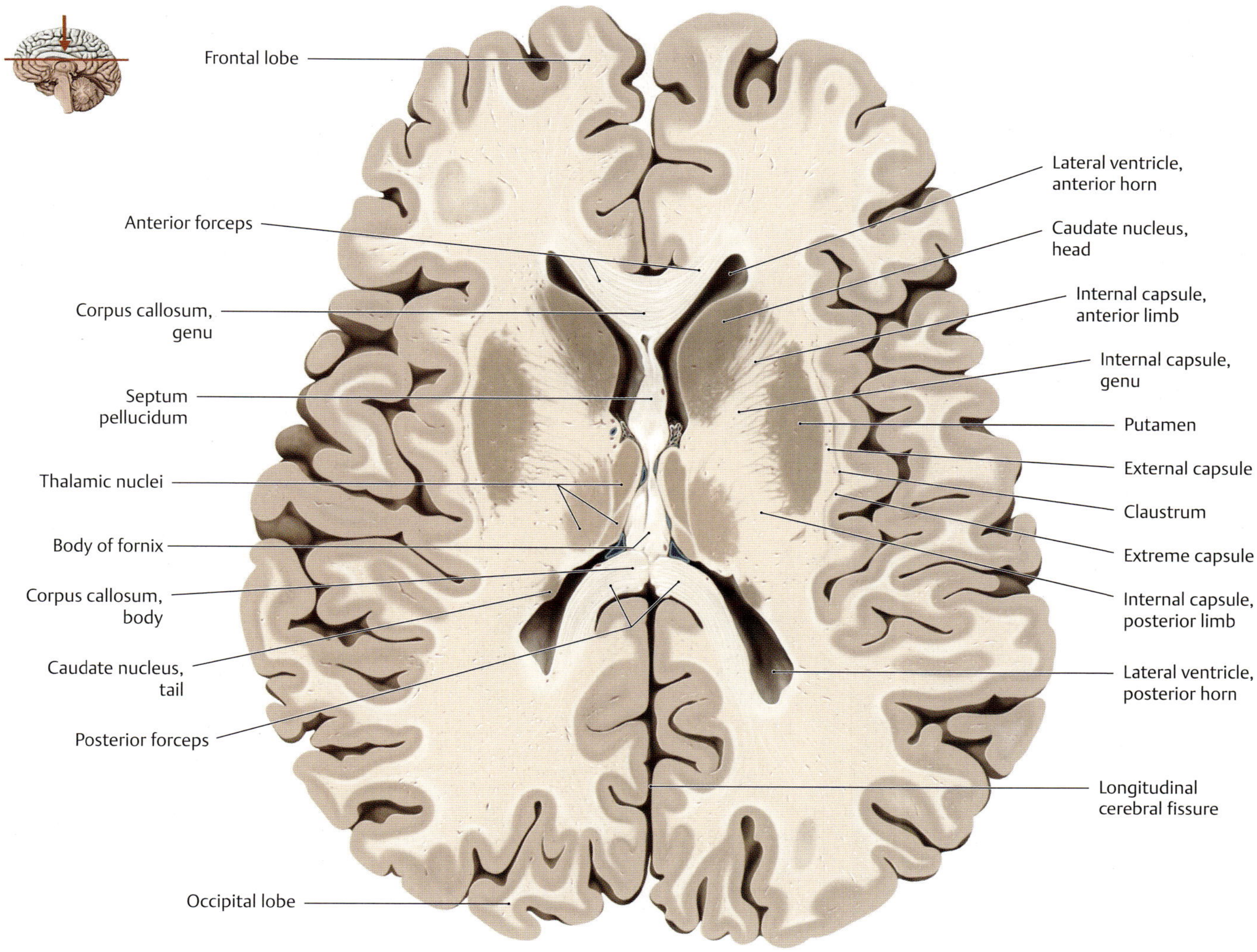

C Transverse section II

In this section, unlike the previous one, each *lateral ventricle* appears divided in two. Because this section is at a lower level, it cuts the anterior and posterior horns of the lateral ventricle separately, missing the body of the ventricle (see **D**). It also cuts a broad swath of the *internal capsule* with its genu and anterior and posterior limbs. The optic radiation, which runs in the white matter of the occipital lobe, is not labeled here because it has no grossly visible anatomical boundaries. The *corpus callosum* also appears divided into two parts: the genu anteriorly and the body more posteriorly. This apparent division results from a second curvature of the corpus callosum at its genu ("knee"), where it is anteriorly convex. The diagram in **E** demonstrates why this section passes successively through the genu of the corpus callosum, the septum pellucidum, the body of the fornix, and finally the body of the corpus callosum. The septum pellucidum forms the anteromedial wall of both lateral ventricles. The septum itself contains small nuclei. Sections of the thalamic nuclei (ventral lateral, lateral dorsal, and anterior nuclei) are also visible along with the putamen and caudate nucleus. The head and tail of the caudate nucleus appear separately in the section (see also p. 336). The putamen, caudate nucleus, and intervening fibers of the internal capsule are collectively called the corpus striatum.

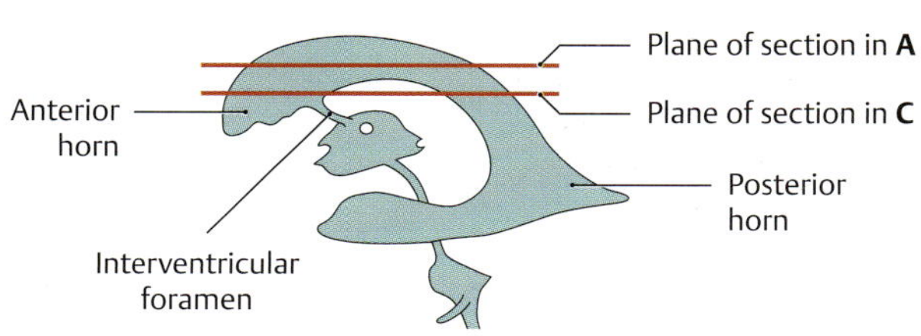

D Lateral view of the ventricular system

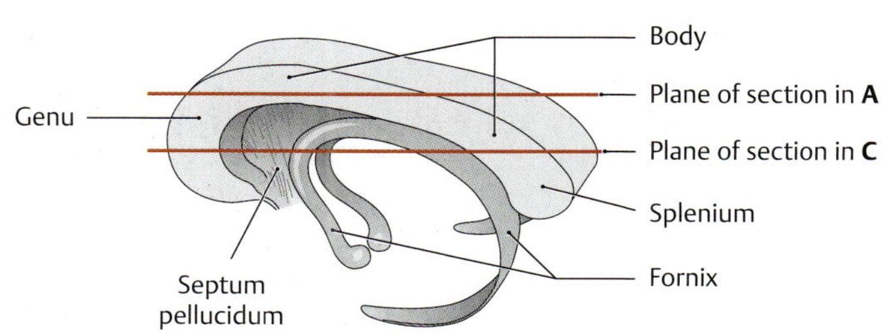

E Corpus callosum and fornix

12.8 Transverse Sections: III and IV

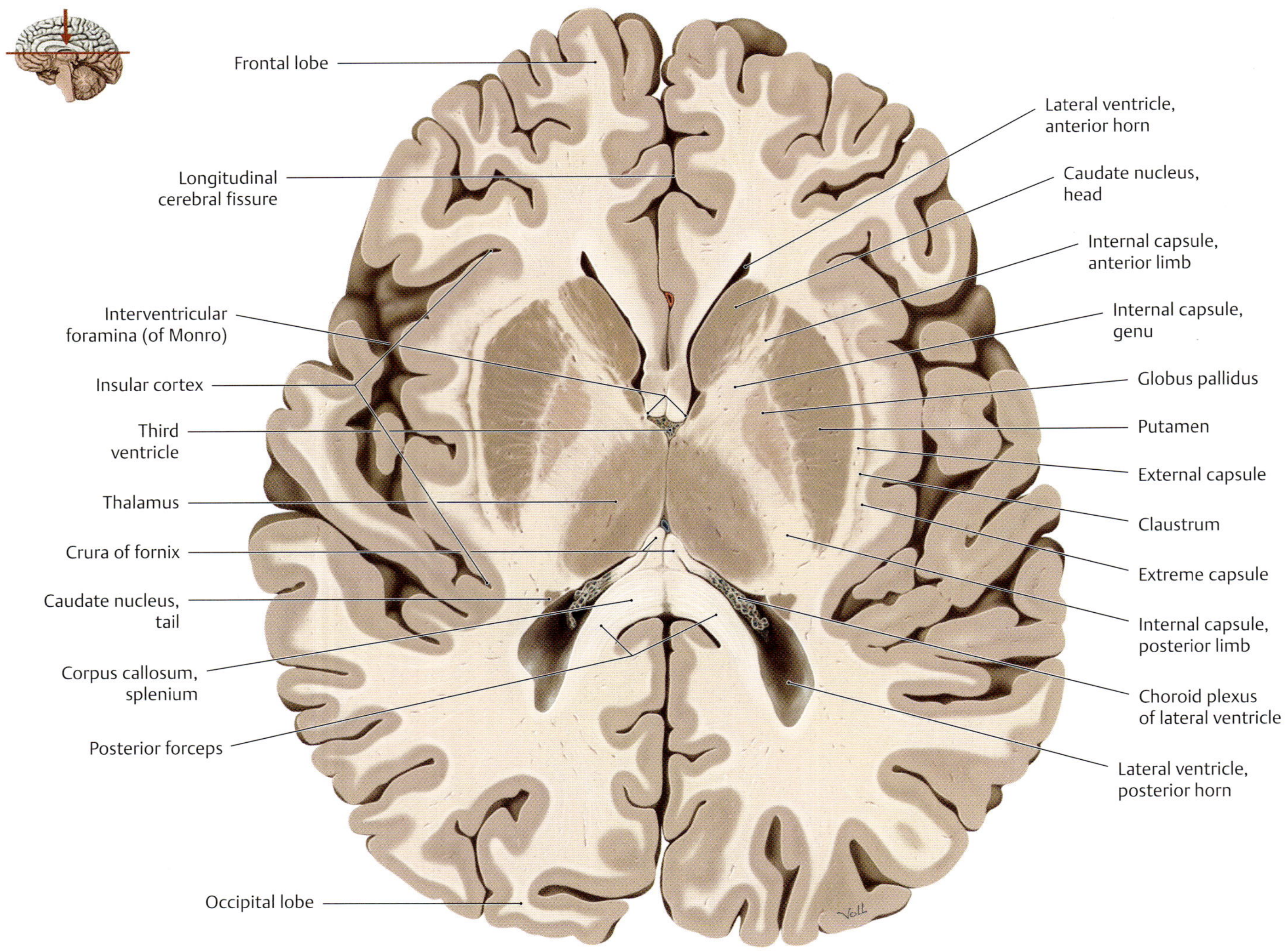

A Transverse section III

The lateral ventricles communicate with the third ventricle through the *interventricular foramina* (of Monro). They are located directly anterior to the thalamus (see **D**, p. 433). The nuclei of the telencephalon make up the deep gray matter of the cerebrum. The spatial relationship between the caudate nucleus and thalamus is illustrated in **B**. The caudate nucleus is larger frontally, and the thalamus larger occipitally. While the caudate nucleus and putamen of the motor system belong to the telencephalon, the thalamus of the sensory system belongs to the diencephalon. This transverse section passes through the caudate nucleus twice due to the anatomical curvature of the nucleus. This is the first transverse section that displays the globus pallidus, part of the motor system. The insular cortex is seen with the *claustrum* medial to it. The *crura* of the *fornix* are seen as posterior to the thalamus (see also **E**, p. 433). They unite at a slightly higher level to form the *body of the fornix*, which lies just below the corpus callosum and was visible in the previous section (see **C**, p. 433). The course of the internal capsule is visible in both this section and the last.

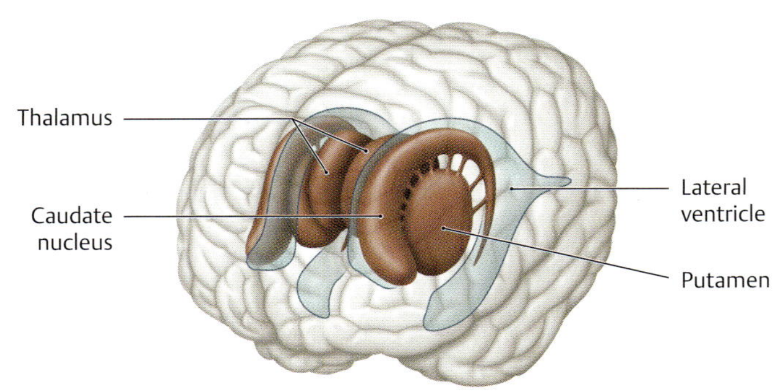

B Spatial relationships of the caudate nucleus, putamen, thalamus, and lateral ventricles

Left anterior oblique view.

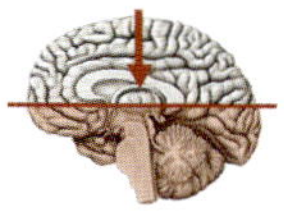

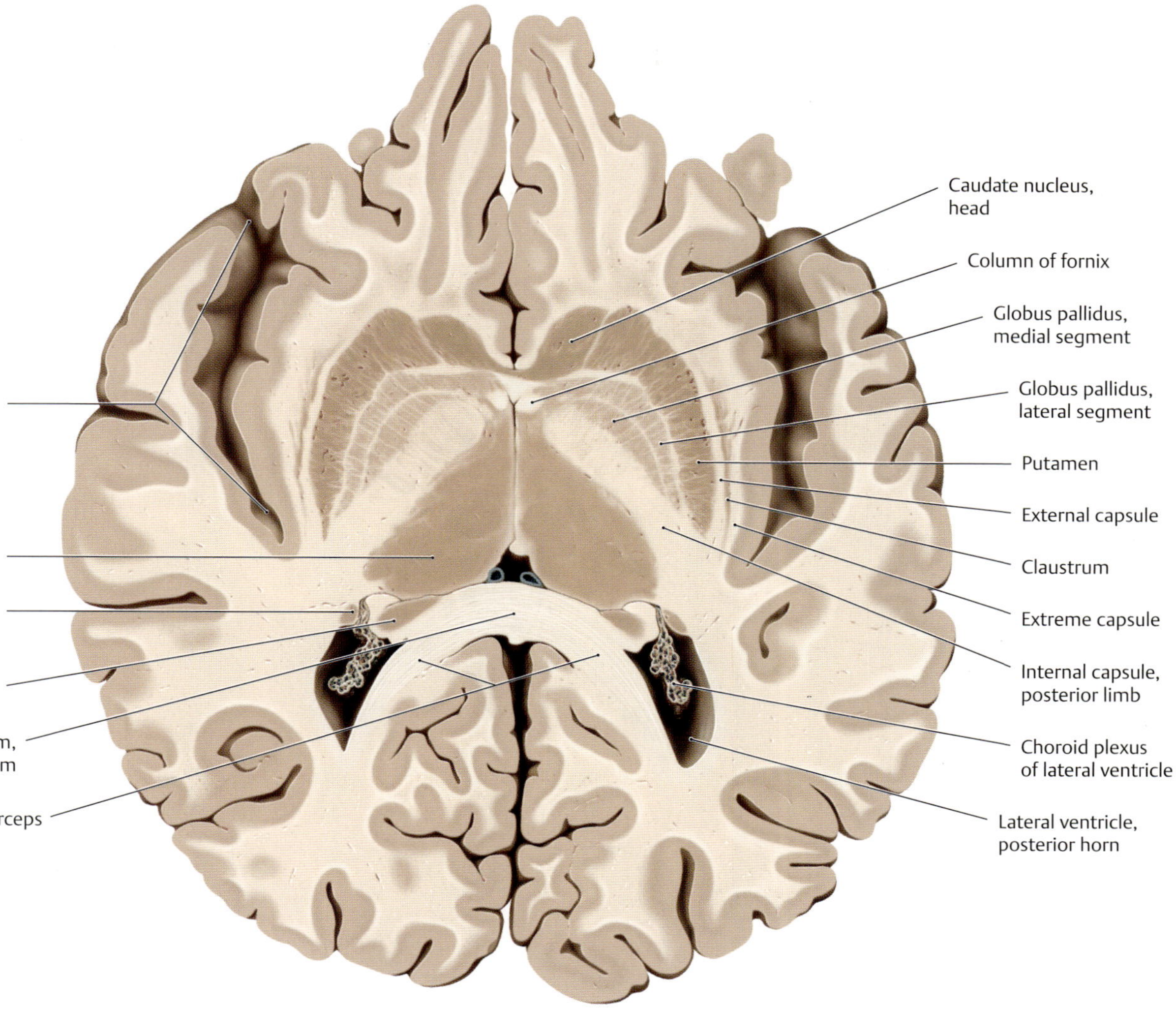

C Transverse section IV

The nuclei shown in the previous section here appear as a roughly circular mass at the center of the brain, surrounded by the gray matter of the cerebral cortex, also called the *pallium* ("cloak") for obvious reasons. The choroid plexus is here visible in both lateral ventricles. This section cuts the occipital part of the corpus callosum, the *splenium*, as well as the basal portion of the *insular cortex* (see **E**, p. 433). The insula is a cortical region that lies below the surface and is covered by the opercula. The insular cistern should be used as a reference point, for example, when comparing this section to **A** and **D**.

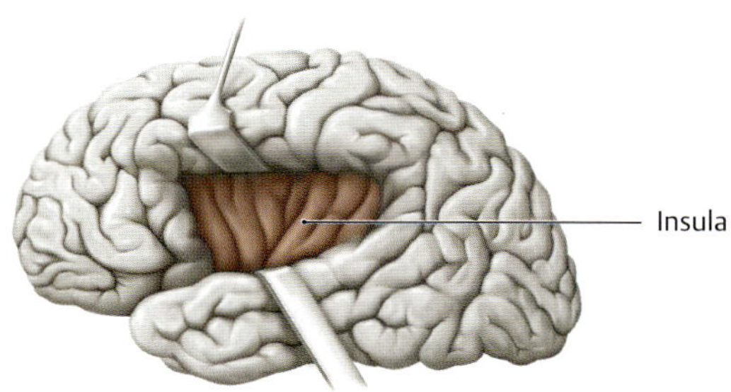

D Left insular region
Lateral view.

12.9 Transverse Sections: V and VI (Caudal)

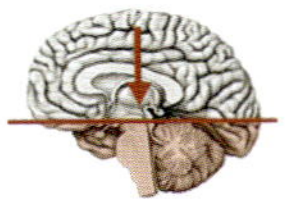

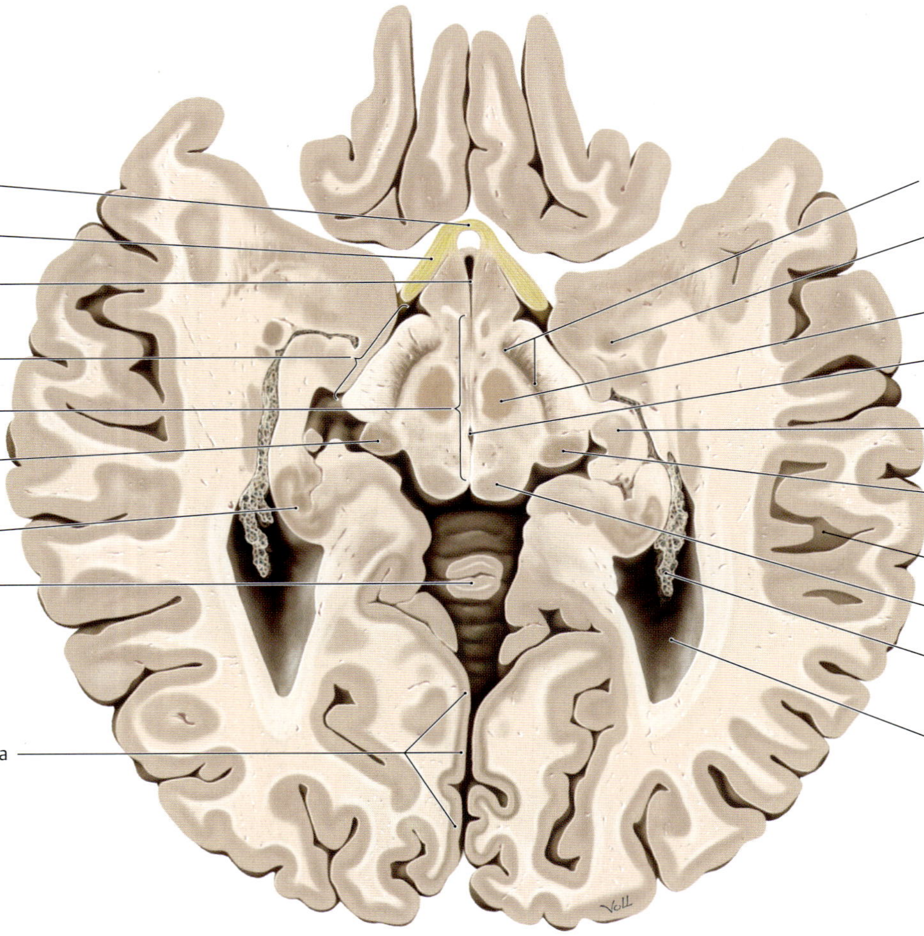

A Transverse section V

Structures visible in this section include the cerebral aqueduct, the basal part of the third ventricle (see also **B**, p. 422), and the *optic recess*. While the third ventricle is slitlike at this level, the section cuts a very large area of the ventricular system where it opens into the two posterior horns. This is the first transverse section that displays the midbrain (*mesencephalon*), passing through its oral portion. The cerebral peduncles (*crura cerebri*), the *substantia nigra*, and the *superior colliculi* of the quadrigeminal plate can also be seen. Visible structures of the *diencephalon* in this plane include the *medial* and *lateral geniculate bodies* (appearing only on the right side, see **B**) and the *optic tract*, which is an extension of the diencephalon.

Note: Closely adjacent structures in the brain may belong to different ontogenetic regions. For example, the medial and lateral geniculate bodies are part of the diencephalon, while the superior and inferior colliculi (the latter is not visible), which make up the quadrigeminal plate, are part of the mesencephalon. It should be recalled, however, that the lateral geniculate body and superior colliculus are part of the visual pathway while the medial geniculate body and inferior colliculus are part of the auditory pathway.

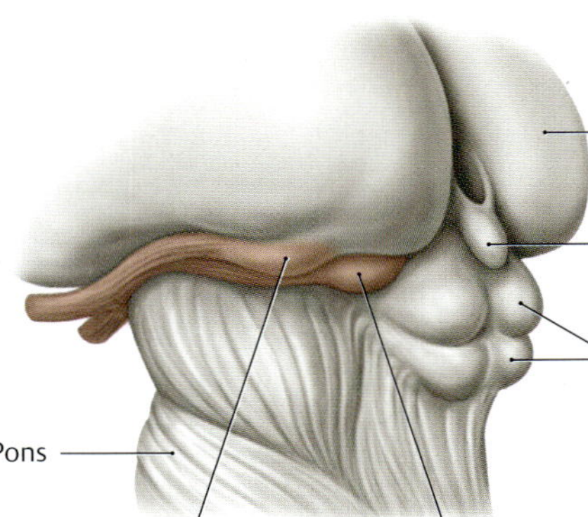

B Pons, midbrain, and adjacent diencephalon
Left posterior oblique view.

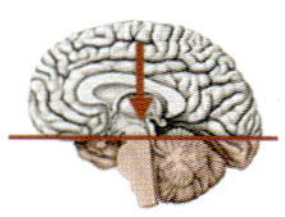

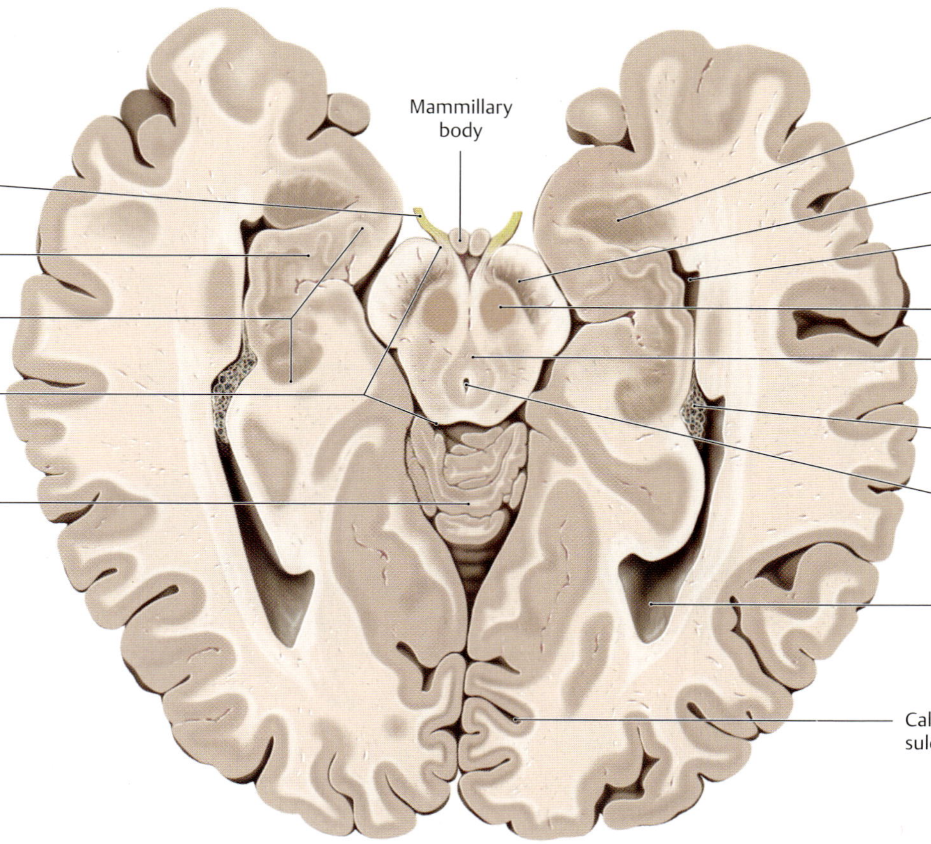

C Transverse section VI

The structures that occupy the largest area at this level are the telencephalon, the medial portions of the mesencephalon, and the cerebellum. The nuclei located on the anteromedian aspect of each temporal lobe of the telencephalon are the *amygdalae*. The lower part of the section cuts the *calcarine sulcus* with the surrounding visual cortex. This section also passes through the choroid plexus of the lateral ventricles, whose *posterior* and *inferior horns* are displayed. Important structures of the *mesencephalon* are the substantia nigra and red nucleus, both of which are part of the motor system. The mammillary bodies are part of the *diencephalon* and are connected by the fornix (not visible in this section) to the hippocampus, which is part of the *telencephalon*. The mammillary bodies lie in the same horizontal plane as the hippocampus and the same coronal plane as its pes (foot). These relationships result from the curved shape of the fornix (see **D**). More transverse sections at lower levels would supply little additional information on the cerebrum; therefore our series of transverse sections ends here. The brainstem structures lying below the mesencephalon are displayed in a separate group of sections (see p. 362 ff).

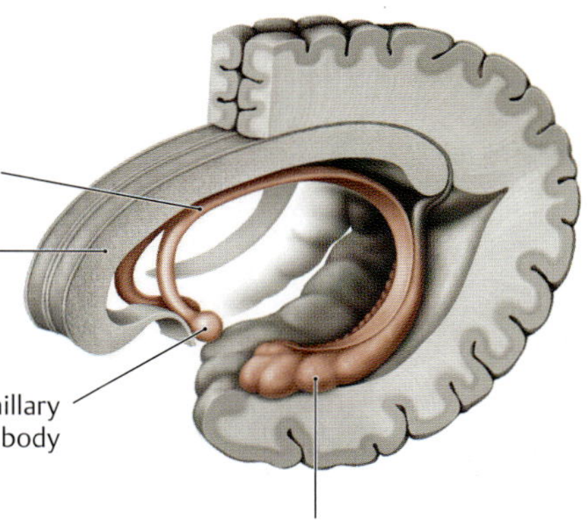

D Fornix

Left anterior oblique view.

12.10 Sagittal Sections: I–III (Lateral)

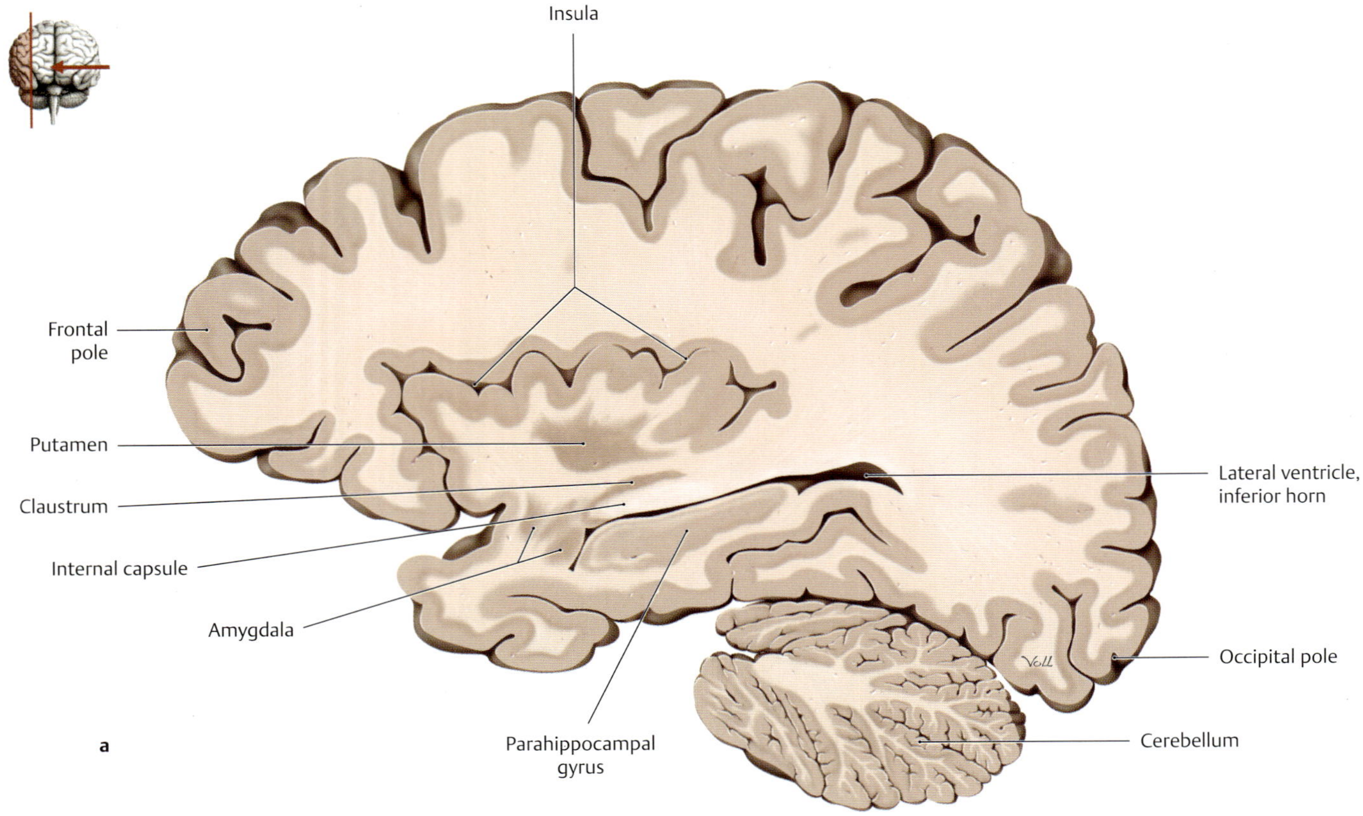

A Sagittal sections I–III

Left lateral view. The plane of section (**a**) passes through the *inferior* (*temporal*) *horn* of the lateral ventricle; the more medially situated *posterior* (*occipital*) *horn* is seen in **b** and **c** (see **C**, p. 424 for relative position of both horns). The *amygdala*, which is directly anterior to the inferior horn, lies in the same sagittal plane as the parahippocampal gyrus (**a–c**; see also **C**, p. 437). The internal capsule can also be seen in sections **a–c**; the long ascending and descending tracts pass through this structure. The most lateral section (**a**) offers the only view of the *insular cortex*, a part of the cerebral cortex that has sunk below the surface of the hemisphere (compare with the coronal sections on p. 421 and the following pages). The *putamen*, the most laterally situated among the basal nuclei of the telencephalon (see also **A**, p. 424) is also found in **a**, but appears larger in the more medial sections (**b**, **c**). A portion of the *claustrum* can be seen ventral to the putamen (**a**), although most of the claustrum is lateral to the putamen (see **A**, p. 424) and outside the plane of the section. Section **b** just cuts the tail of the *caudate nucleus*, which is situated more laterally than its head and body (see also **C**, p. 424 and **E**, p. 425). The most medial section in this series (**c**) cuts the *calcarine sulcus* (see p. 440) and the *lateral geniculate body* which lies at the edge of the thalamus. The lateral segment of the globus pallidus can also be seen (**c**): the segments of the *globus pallidus* are actually medial to the putamen (see **D**, p. 423), but can be visualized here due to their concentric arrangement.

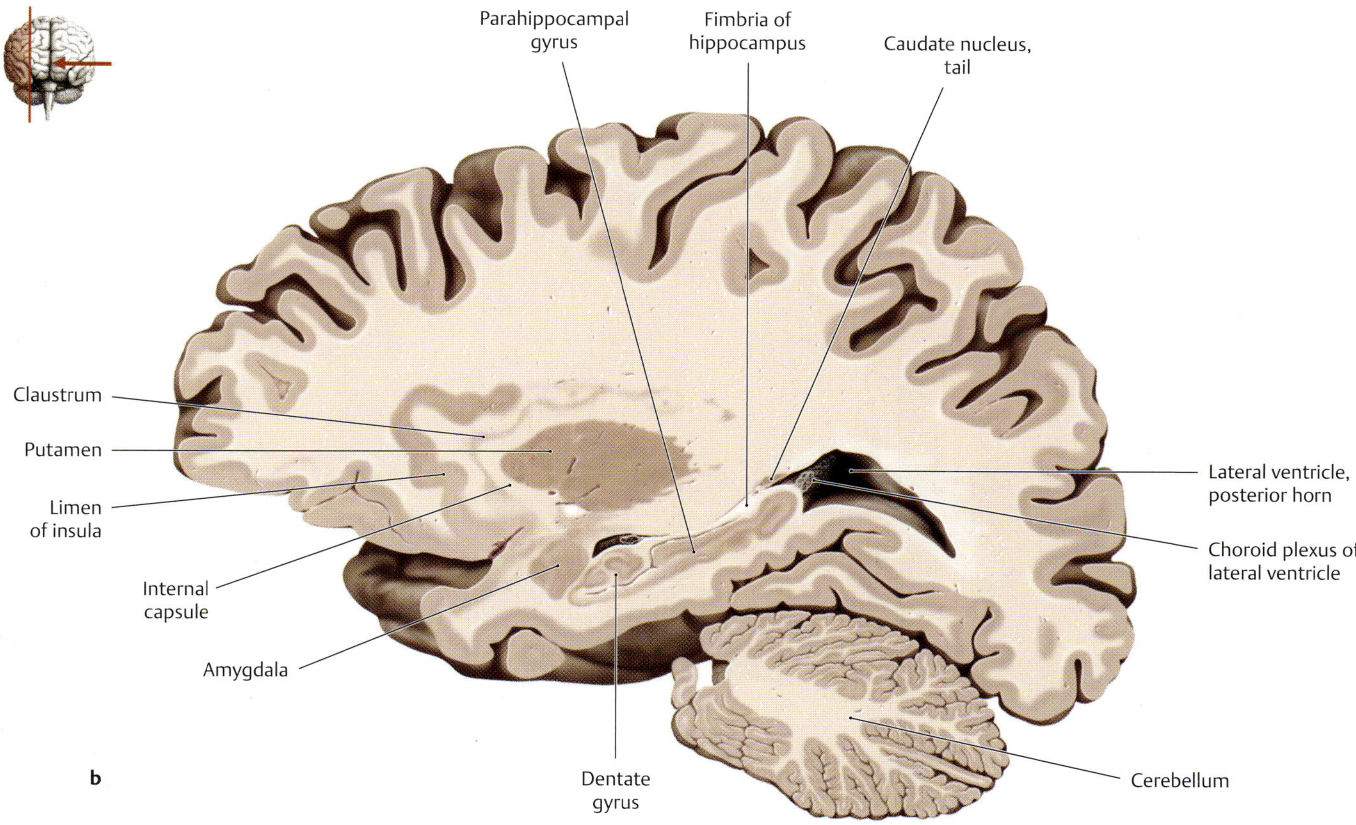
Parahippocampal gyrus
Fimbria of hippocampus
Caudate nucleus, tail
Claustrum
Putamen
Limen of insula
Internal capsule
Amygdala
Lateral ventricle, posterior horn
Choroid plexus of lateral ventricle
Dentate gyrus
Cerebellum

b

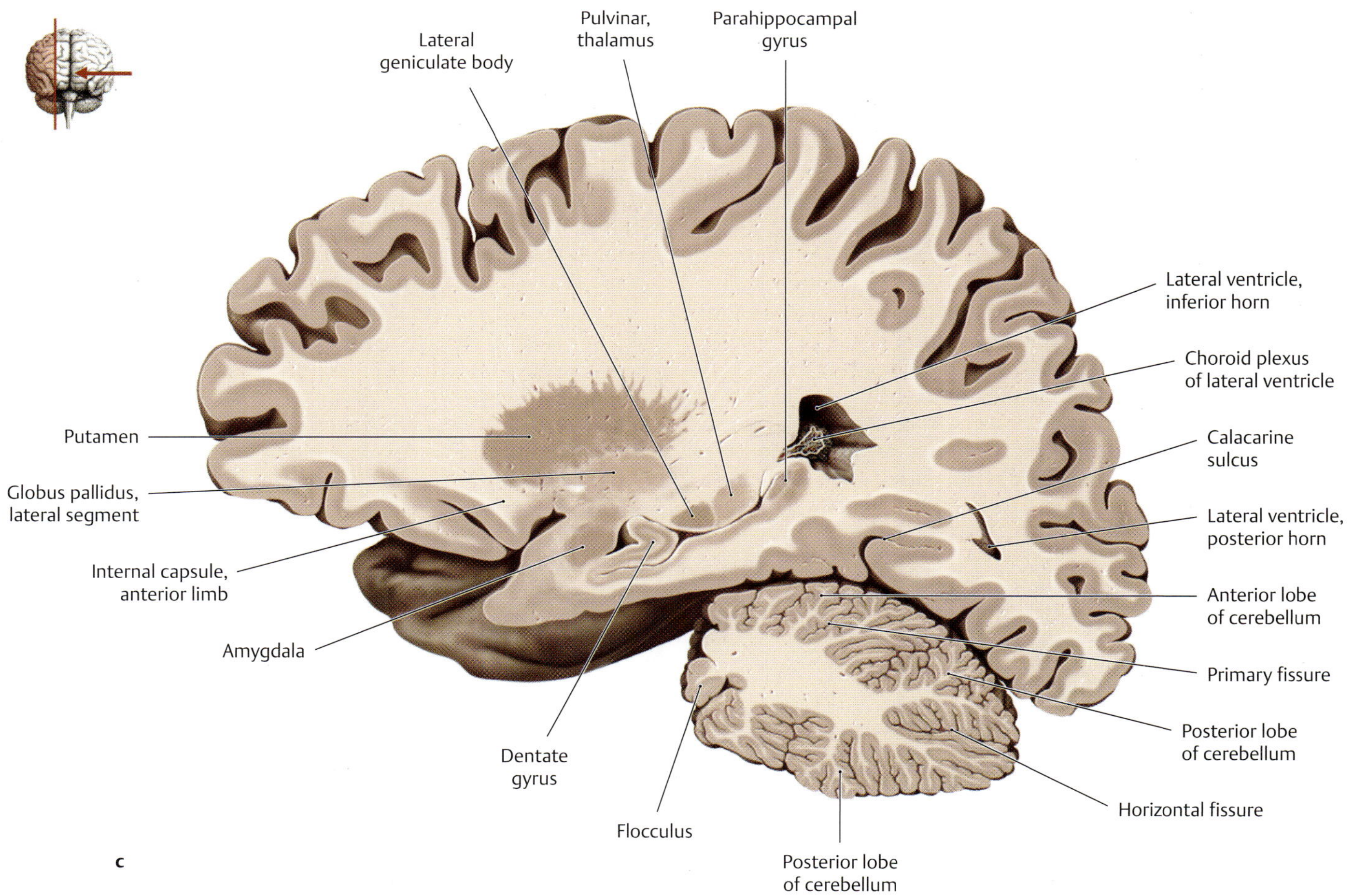
Lateral geniculate body
Pulvinar, thalamus
Parahippocampal gyrus
Putamen
Globus pallidus, lateral segment
Internal capsule, anterior limb
Amygdala
Lateral ventricle, inferior horn
Choroid plexus of lateral ventricle
Calacarine sulcus
Lateral ventricle, posterior horn
Anterior lobe of cerebellum
Primary fissure
Posterior lobe of cerebellum
Horizontal fissure
Dentate gyrus
Flocculus
Posterior lobe of cerebellum

c

12.11 Sagittal Sections: IV–VI

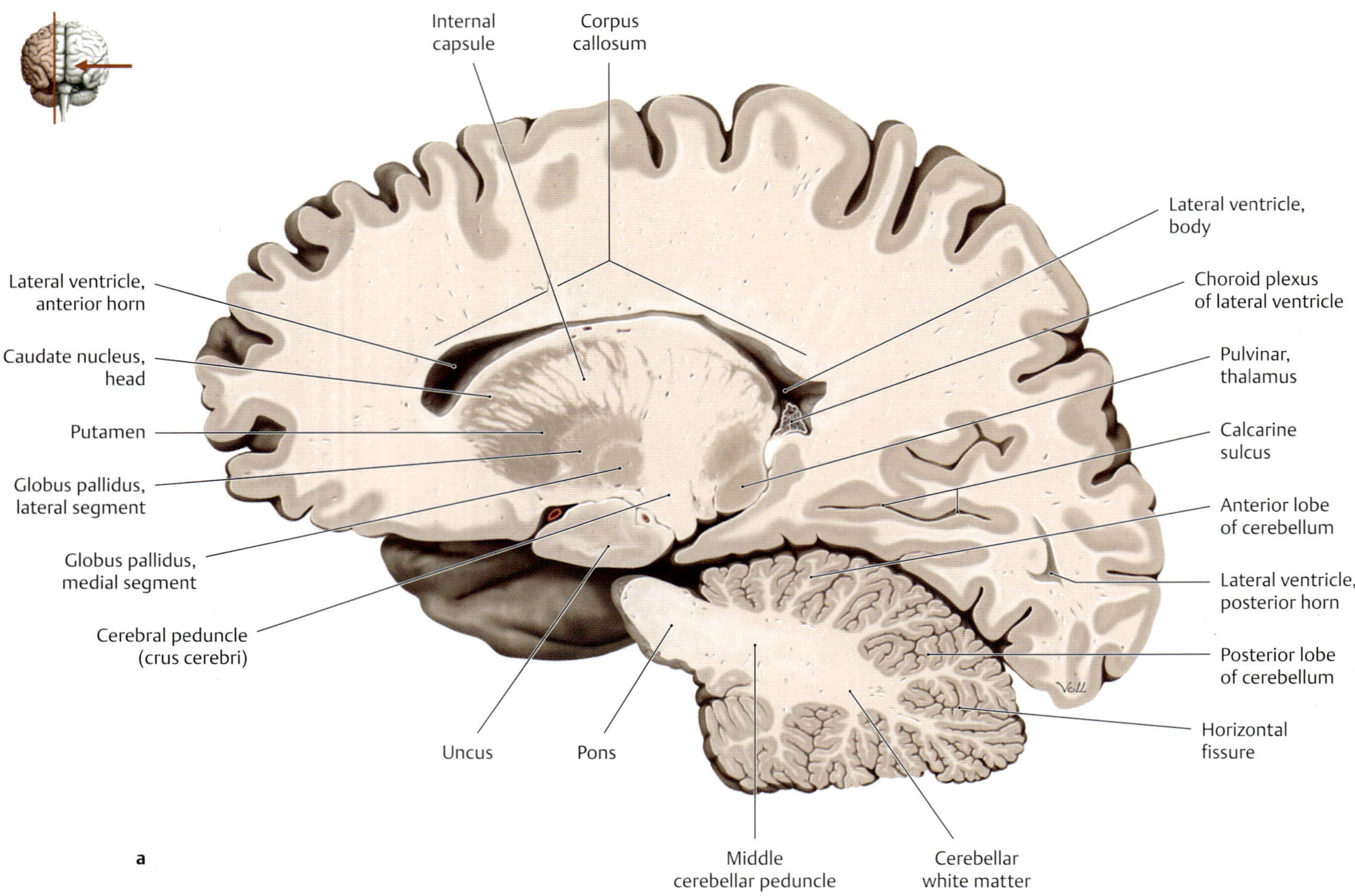

A Sagittal sections IV–VI

Left lateral view. The dominant ventricular structures in all three of these sections are the anterior horn and body of the *lateral ventricle* (the junction with the laterally situated posterior horn appears only in **a**). The *corpus callosum*, which connects functionally related areas of the two cerebral hemispheres (commissural tracts), can be identified in the cerebral white matter although it is not sharply delineated (**a–c**). As the sections move closer to the midline, the putamen grows smaller while the caudate nucleus becomes increasingly prominent (**a–c**). These two bodies are known collectively as the *corpus striatum*, and their characteristic striations are seen particularly well in **a** (the white matter that separates the gray-matter streaks of the corpus striatum is the *internal capsule*). The previous sagittal sections showed only the lateral segment of the *globus pallidus* (see p. 439), but its medial segment is displayed in both **a** and **b**. As the globus pallidus disappears and the putamen becomes less prominent, the nuclei of the medially situated thalamus become visible below the lateral ventricle (**c**; the subthalamic nuclei include the anterior, posterior, and lateral ventral nuclei of the diencephalon). The location of the thalamus explains why it is sometimes referred to as the *dorsal thalamus*. Section **c** also shows the *substantia nigra* in the mesencephalon (below the diencephalon), the inferior olivary nucleus in the underlying medulla oblongata, and the *dentate nucleus* of the cerebellum. The ascending and descending tracts previously visible only in the internal capsule can now be seen in the pons, part of the brainstem (**c**, corticospinal tract). The only visible portion of the fourth ventricle, barely sectioned in **c**, is its lateral recess.

The sectioned nucleus accumbens in **c** is an important part of the brain's reward system, which for example controls addictive behavior and can be affected in case of severe depression.

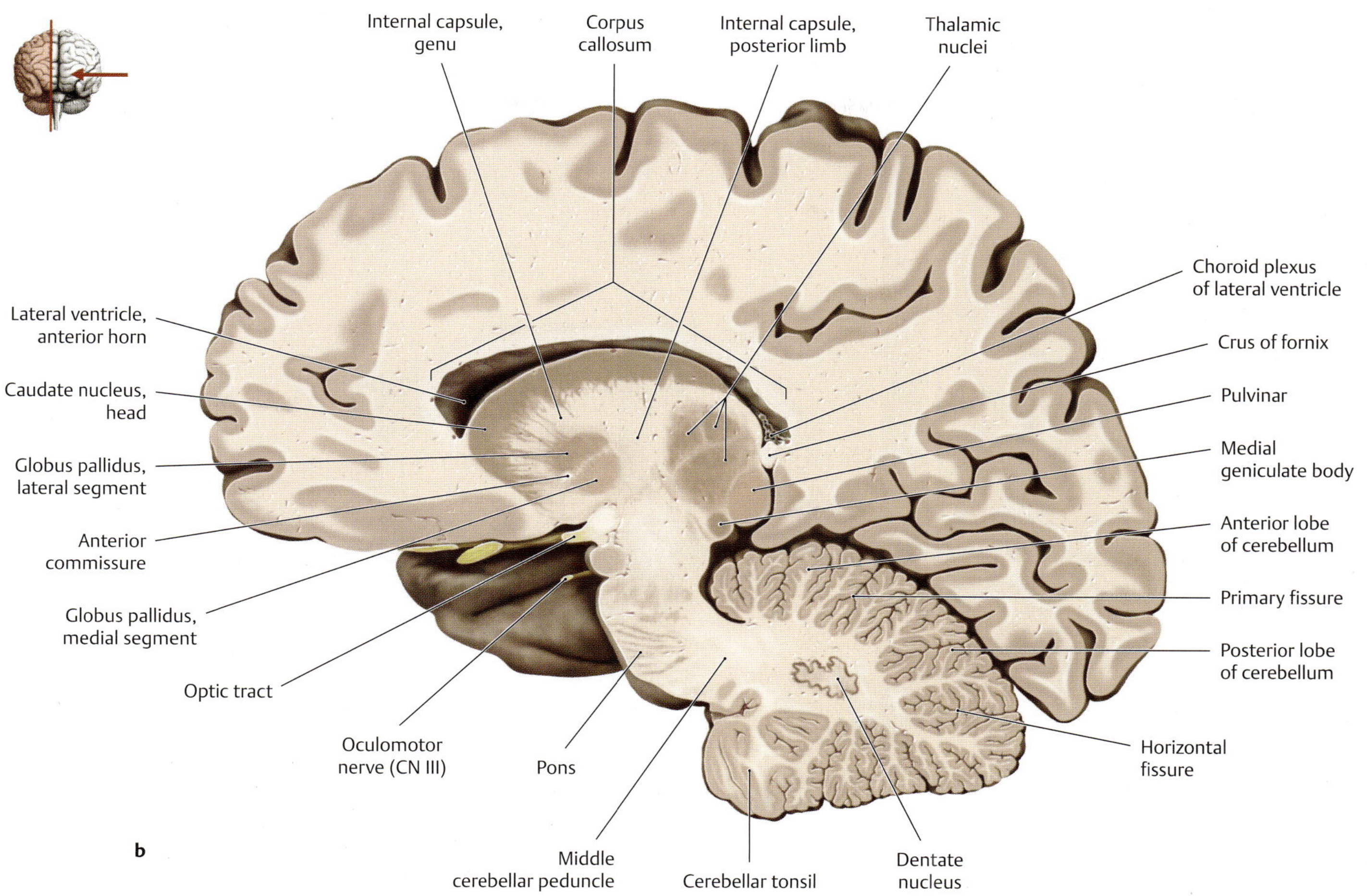
Internal capsule, genu
Corpus callosum
Internal capsule, posterior limb
Thalamic nuclei
Lateral ventricle, anterior horn
Caudate nucleus, head
Globus pallidus, lateral segment
Anterior commissure
Globus pallidus, medial segment
Optic tract
Oculomotor nerve (CN III)
Pons
Middle cerebellar peduncle
Cerebellar tonsil
Dentate nucleus
Choroid plexus of lateral ventricle
Crus of fornix
Pulvinar
Medial geniculate body
Anterior lobe of cerebellum
Primary fissure
Posterior lobe of cerebellum
Horizontal fissure

b

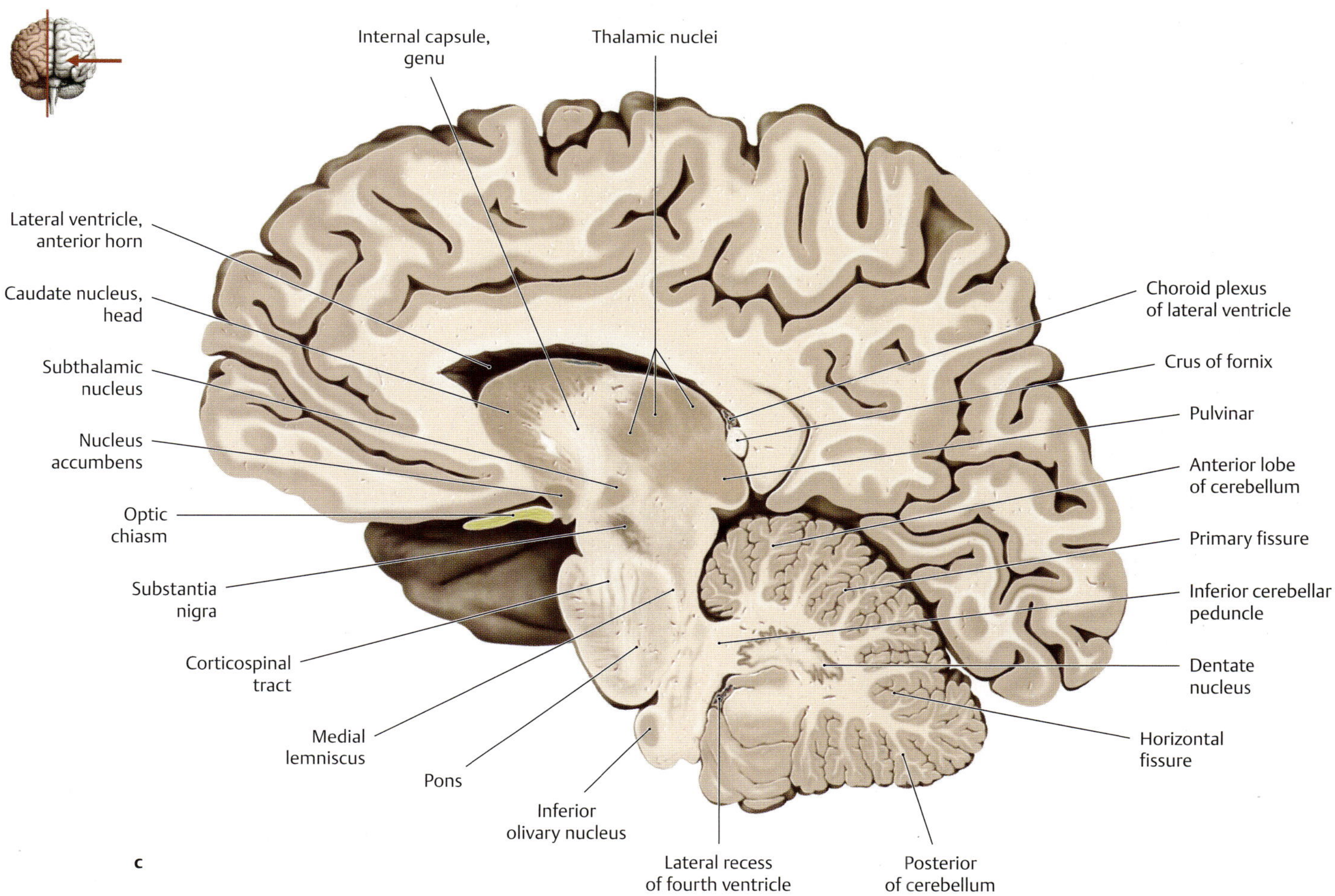
Internal capsule, genu
Thalamic nuclei
Lateral ventricle, anterior horn
Caudate nucleus, head
Subthalamic nucleus
Nucleus accumbens
Optic chiasm
Substantia nigra
Corticospinal tract
Medial lemniscus
Pons
Inferior olivary nucleus
Lateral recess of fourth ventricle
Posterior of cerebellum
Choroid plexus of lateral ventricle
Crus of fornix
Pulvinar
Anterior lobe of cerebellum
Primary fissure
Inferior cerebellar peduncle
Dentate nucleus
Horizontal fissure

c

12.12 Sagittal Sections: VII and VIII (Medial)

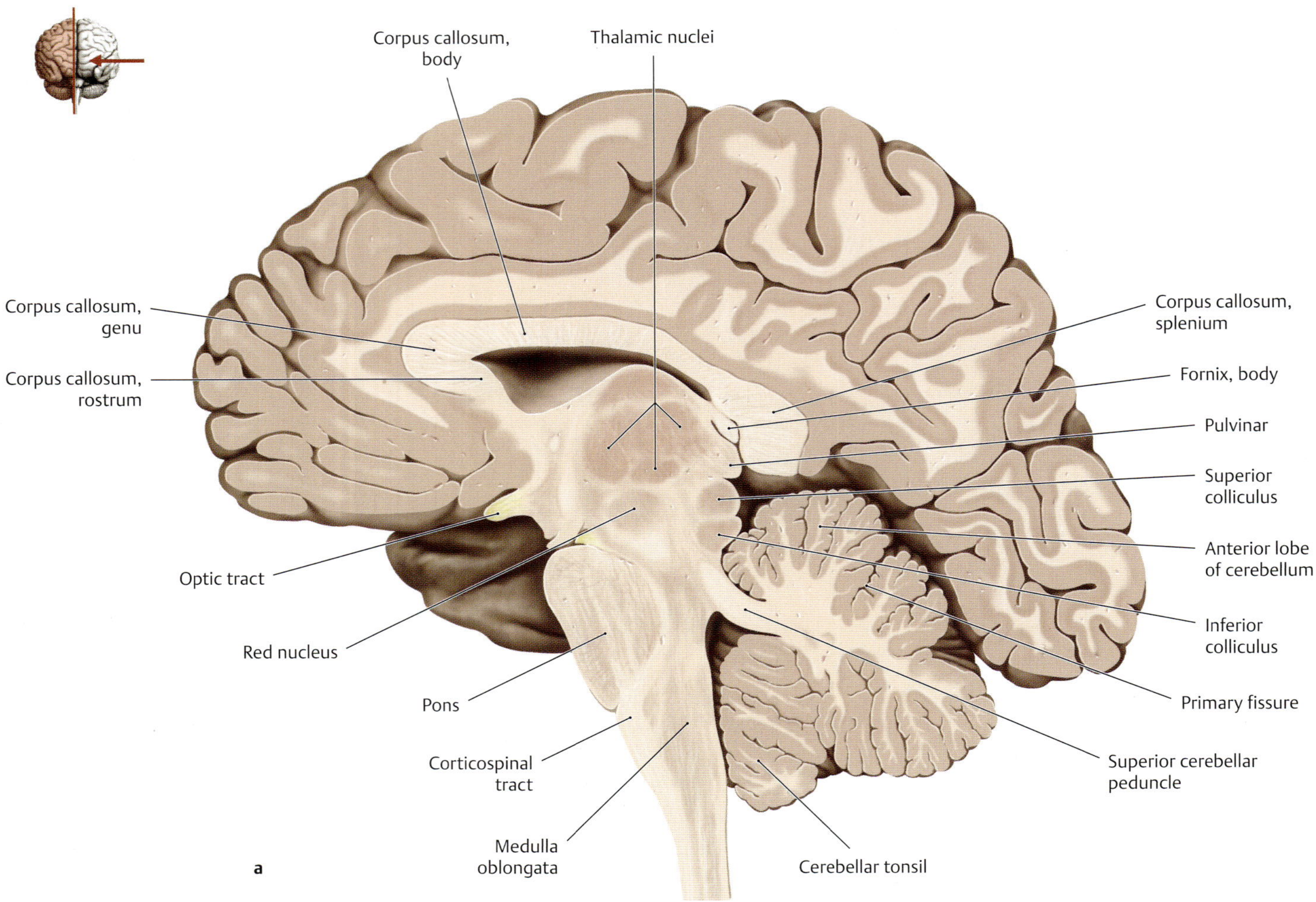

A Sagittal sections VII und VIII

Left lateral view. This section (**a**) is so close to the midline that it passes through the principal paramedian structures: the substantia nigra, the red nucleus, and one each of the paired superior and inferior colliculi. The pyramidal tract (corticospinal tract) runs in front of the inferior olive in the medulla oblongata. A complete sagittal section of the corpus callosum is displayed, and most of the fornix tract is displayed in longitudinal section (**b**). The cerebellum has reached its maximum extent and forms the roof of the fourth ventricle (**b**). A portion of the *septum pellucidum*, which stretches between the fornix and corpus callosum, is also displayed.

When the brain is removed, the pituitary gland, which appears in **b**, remains in the sella turcica; that is, it is always torn from the brain at its stalk when the brain is removed.

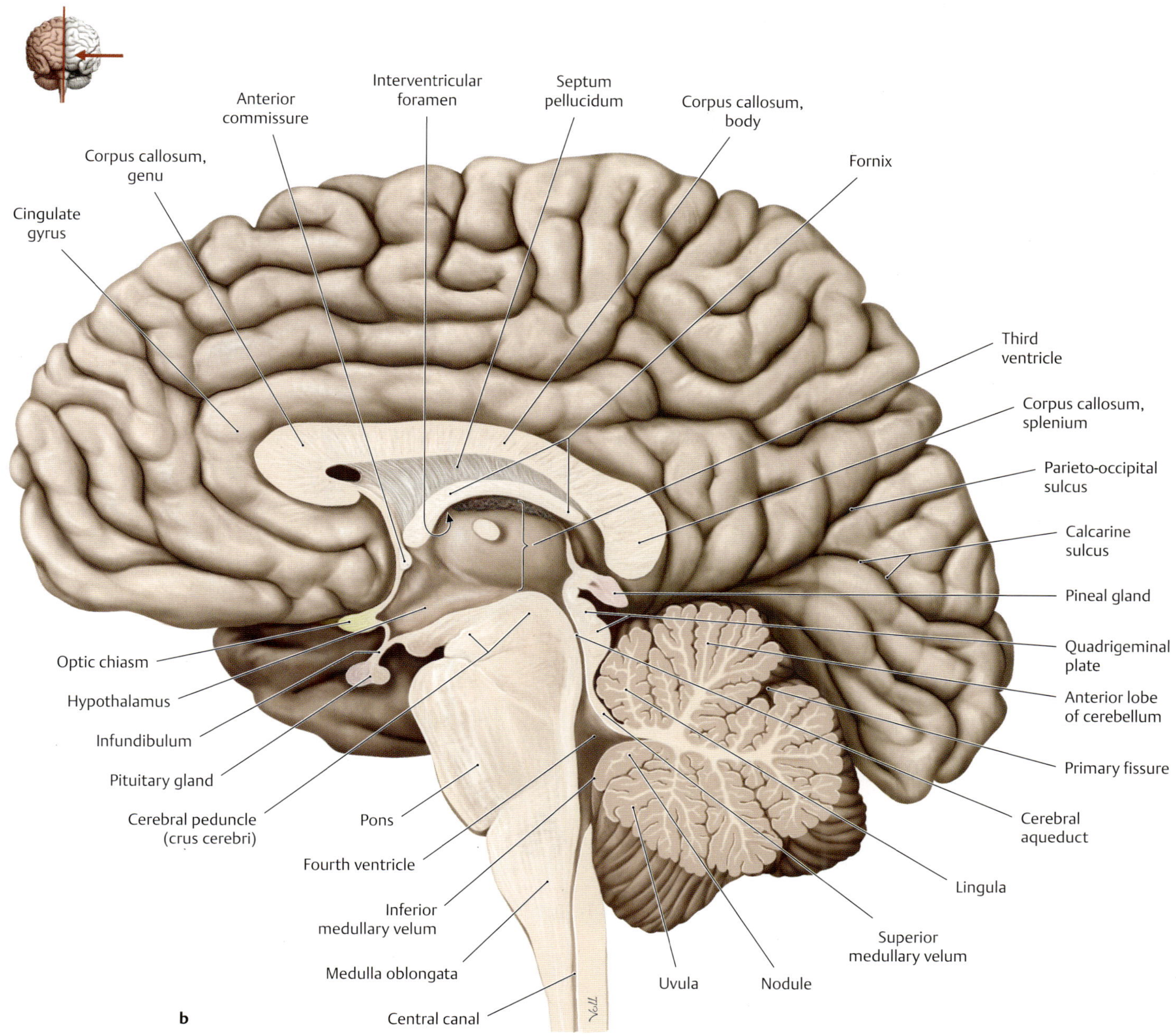

b

B Principal structures in the serial sections

The major structures seen in the serial sections are here assigned to their corresponding brain regions. Within each region, the structures are listed from most rostral to most caudal.

Telencephalon (endbrain)
- External capsule
- Extreme capsule
- Internal capsule
- Claustrum
- Anterior commissure
- Amygdala
- Corpus callosum
- Fornix
- Globus pallidus
- Cingulate gyrus
- Hippocampus
- Caudate nucleus
- Putamen
- Septum pellucidum

Diencephalon (interbrain)
- Lateral geniculate body
- Medial geniculate body
- Pineal gland
- Pulvinar of thalamus
- Thalamus
- Optic tract
- Mammillary body
- Hypothalamus
- Subthalamic nucleus

Mesencephalon (midbrain)
- Cerebral aqueduct
- Quadrigeminal plate (lamina tecti)
- Superior colliculus
- Inferior colliculus
- Red nucleus
- Substantia nigra
- Cerebral peduncle (crus cerebri)

13.1 Somatosensory System: Synopsis of the Pathways

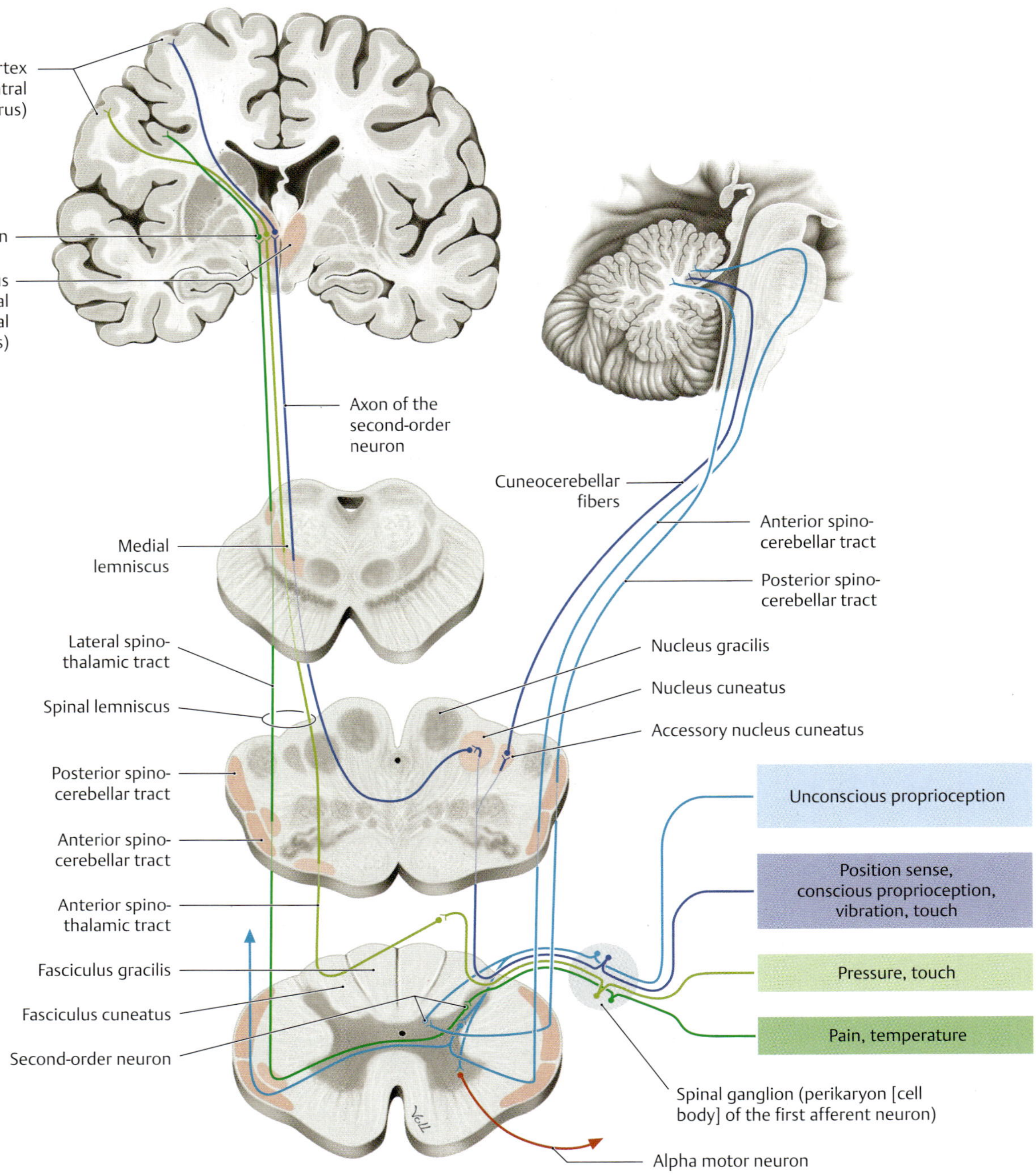

A Simplified diagram of the somatosensory pathways of the spinal cord

Stimuli generate impulses in various receptors in the periphery of the body which are transmitted to the cerebrum and cerebellum along the sensory (afferent) pathways or tracts shown here (see **B** for details). **Proprioception** is concerned with the perception of the position of the limbs in space (position sense). The types of *information* involved in proprioception (depth sense) are complex: position sense (the position of the limbs in relation to one another) is distinguished from motion sense (speed and direction of joint movements) and force sense (the muscular force associated with joint movements). We also distinguish between conscious and unconscious proprioception.

- Information on *conscious proprioception* travels in the posterior funiculus of the spinal cord (fasciculus gracilis and fasciculus cuneatus) and is relayed through their nuclei (nucleus gracilis and nucleus cuneatus) to the *thalamus*. From there it is conveyed to the *sensory cortex* (postcentral gyrus), where the information rises to consciousness ("I know that my left hand is making a fist, even though my eyes are closed").
- *Unconscious proprioception,* which enables us to ride a bicycle and climb stairs without thinking about it, is conveyed by the spinocerebellar tracts to the *cerebellum,* where it remains at the unconscious level.

Sensory information from the head is mediated by the trigeminal nerve and is not depicted here (see p. 448).

B Synopsis of somatosensory pathways

The impulses generated by various stimuli in different receptors are transmitted via peripheral nerves to the spinal cord. The cell body of the first afferent neuron which is connected with the receptors for all pathways is located in the dorsal root ganglion. The axons from the ganglion pass along various tracts in the spinal cord to the second neuron. The axon of the second neuron either passes directly to the cerebellum or reaches the thalamus where it synapses with the third order neurons that project to the cerebral cortex.

Name of pathway	Sensory quality	Receptor	Course in the spinal cord	Central course (rostral to the spinal cord)
Spinothalamic tracts				
Anterior spinothalamic tract	• Crude touch	• Hair follicles • Various skin receptors	The cell body of the second neuron is located in the posterior horn and may be up to 15 segments above or 2 segments below the entry of the first neuron. Its axons cross in the white commissure (see p. 402)	The axons of the second neuron (spinal lemniscus) terminate in the ventral posterolateral nucleus of the thalamus (see **D**, p. 347). There they synapse onto the third neuron, whose axons project to the postcentral gyrus
Lateral spinothalamic tract	• Pain and temperature	• Mostly free nerve endings	The cell body of the second neuron is in the substantia gelatinosa. Its axon crosses at the same level in the anterior commissure (see p. 402)	The axons of the second neuron (spinal lemniscus) terminate in the ventral posterolateral nucleus of the thalamus, where they synapse with the third neuron, whose axons project to the postcentral gyrus
Tracts of the posterior funiculus (dorsal column)				
Fasciculus gracilis	• Fine touch • Conscious proprioception of *lower* limb	• Vater-Pacini corpuscles • Muscle and tendon receptors	The axons of the first neuron pass to the nucleus gracilis in the caudal medulla oblongata (second neuron) (see p. 404 and **B**, p. 361)	The axons of the second neuron cross in the brainstem and traverse the medial lemniscus (see **B**, p. 361) to the ventral posterolateral nucleus of the thalamus. There they synapse with the third neuron, whose axons project to the postcentral gyrus
Fasciculus cuneatus	• Fine touch • Conscious proprioception of *upper* limb	• Vater-Pacini corpuscles • Muscle and tendon receptors	The axons of the first neuron pass to the nucleus cuneatus in the caudal medulla oblongata (second neuron) (see p. 404 and **B**, p. 361)	The axons of the second neuron cross in the brainstem and travel in the medial lemniscus (see **B**, p. 361) to the ventral posterolateral nucleus of the thalamus. There they synapse with the third neuron, whose axons project to the postcentral gyrus
Spinocerebellar tracts				
Anterior spinocerebellar tract (of Gowers)	• Unconscious crossed and uncrossed extero- and proprioception to the cerebellum	• Muscle spindles • Tendon receptors • Joint receptors • Skin receptors	The second neuron is located in the posterior horn of the spinal cord. The axons of the second neuron run directly to the cerebellum, both crossed and uncrossed, (see p. 406)	The axons of the second neuron pass through the superior cerebellar peduncle to the vermian part of the spinocerebellum (no third neuron) (see also p. 371)
Posterior spinocerebellar tract (of Flechsig)	• Unconscious uncrossed extero- and proprioception to the cerebellum	• Muscle spindles • Tendon receptors • Joint receptors • Skin receptors	The second neuron is located in the Clarke column (Stilling nucleus) in the gray matter at the base of the posterior horn. The axons of the second neuron run directly to the cerebellum without crossing (see p. 406)	The axons of the second neuron pass through the inferior cerebellar peduncle to the vermian part of the spinocerebellum (no third neuron) (see also p. 371)

13.2 Somatosensory System: Stimulus Processing

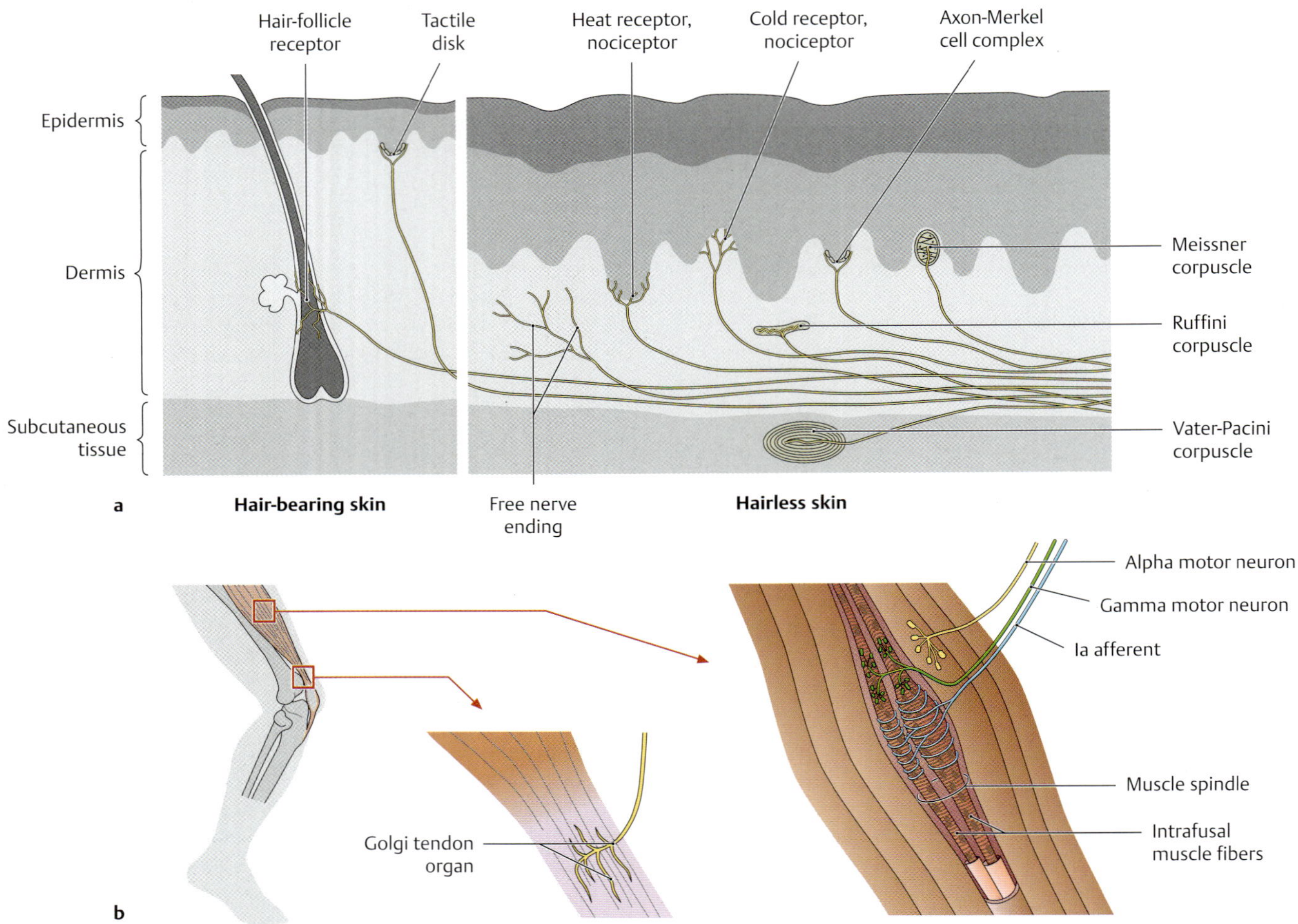

A Receptors of the somatosensory system

a Skin receptors: Various types of stimuli generate impulses in different receptors in the periphery of the body (illustrated here in sections through hair-bearing and hairless skin). These impulses are transmitted through peripheral nerves to the spinal cord, from which they are relayed and carried by specific tracts to the thalamus and then the somatosensory cortex (see p. 445). Sensory modalities cannot always be uniquely assigned to specific receptors. The figure does not indicate the prevalence of the different receptor types. Nociceptors (pain receptors), like heat and cold receptors, consist of free nerve endings. Nociceptors make up approximately 50% of all receptors.

b Joint receptors: Proprioception encompasses position sense, motion sense, and force sense. Proprioceptors include muscle spindles, tendon sensors, and joint sensors (not shown).

B Receptive field sizes of cortical modules in the upper limb of a primate

Sensory information is processed in cortical "modules" (see **C**, p. 327). This drawing shows the size of the receptive fields supplied by modules. In areas where high resolution of sensory information is not required (e.g., the forearm), one module supplies a large receptive field. In areas that require finer tactile sensation (e.g., the fingers), one module supplies a much smaller receptive field. The size of these fields determines the overall proportions of the sensory homunculus (see **C**). Because one skin area may be innervated by several neurons, many of the receptive fields overlap. Information is transmitted from the receptive field to the cortex by a chain of neurons and their axons. These neurons and axons are located at specific sites in the CNS (topographical principle).

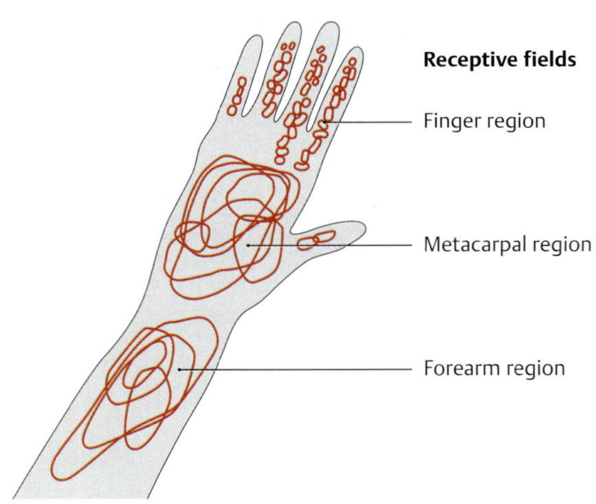

C Somatotopic organization of the somatosensory cortex: the sensory homunculus

Right anterosuperior view of the right postcentral gyrus. The axons of sensory neurons that are connected in the thalamus pass through the internal capsule (especially in the posterior limb) and are projected over a wide area onto the primary somatosensory cortex in the postcentral gyrus. There the information reaches the conscious level. The postcentral gyrus has a somatotopical organization; i.e., each body region is represented in a particular cortical area. Because the body regions vary in their sensitivity (meaning their required “circuit density” varies), they are represented in areas of varying size on the somatosensory cortex. This creates what may be called a sensory homunculus whose body proportions are accordingly distorted.

Note: The postcentral gyrus always projects the contralateral half of the body so that the right gyrus projects the left half and vice versa. The cortical area of the head is separated from the rest of the body. In contrast to the “headless” torso, the representation of the head is upright. The jaw, teeth, tongue, and pharynx have their own cortical areas beneath the head area. The lower limb and genitals are here represented on the medial surface of the brain on the posterior paracentral gyrus beneath the margin of the mantle (cf. Coolen R. L. et al. 2020). Other depictions of the sensory homunculus represent the genitals at the level of the torso (Michels L. et al. 2010). Descending motor pathways from the motor cortex also course within the internal capsule. The close proximity of the motor and sensory pathways explains why damage to the internal capsule (such as can occur in a stroke) often simultaneously produces sensory and motor deficits, always on the side opposite the lesion (cf. motor homunculus, **B**, p. 457).

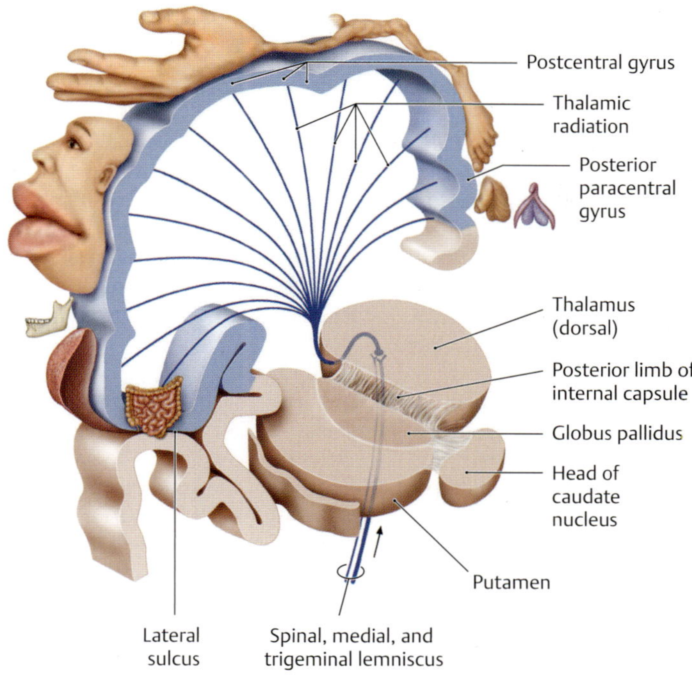

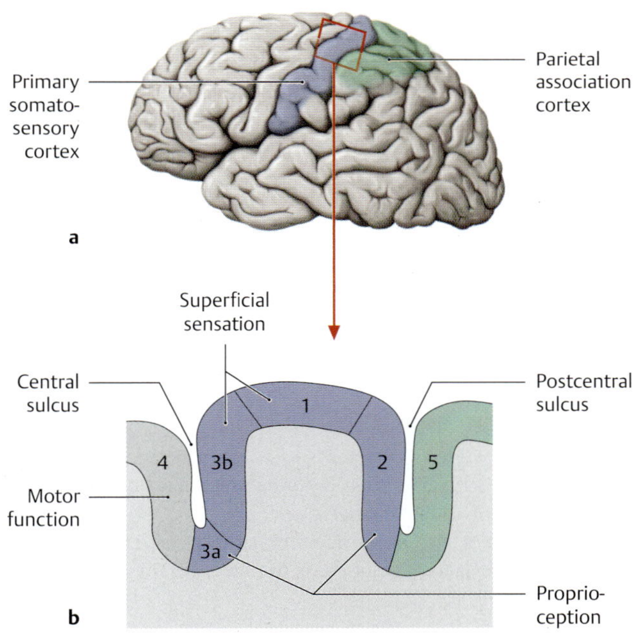

D Primary somatosensory cortex and parietal association cortex

a Left lateral view. The Brodmann areas are numbered in the sectional view (**b**). The contralateral half of the body is represented in the primary somatosensory cortex (except the perioral region, which is represented bilaterally). This area of the cortex is concerned with somatosensory perception. The parietal association cortex receives information from both sides of the body. Thus, the processing of stimuli becomes increasingly complex in these cortical areas.

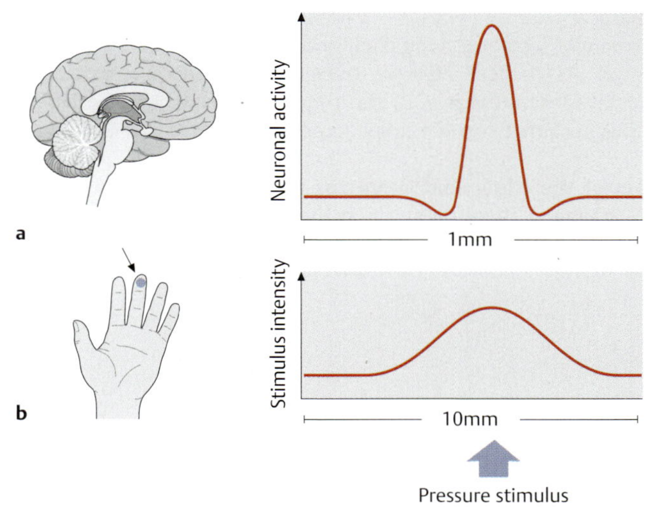

E Activity of cortical cell columns in the primary somatosensory cortex

a Amplitude of the neuronal response in the primary somatosensory cortex in response to a peripheral pressure stimulus. The intensity of the stimulus is shown in **b**. The diagrams illustrate the principle of sensory information processing in the cortex. When approximately 100 intensity detectors in the fingertip are stimulated by pressure, approximately 10,000 neurons in the corresponding cell column in the primary somatosensory cortex (see columnar organization of the cortex, **C**, p. 327) respond to the stimulus. Because the intensity of the peripheral pressure stimulus is maximal at the center and fades toward the edges, it is processed in the cortex accordingly. Cortical processing amplifies the contrast between the greater and lesser stimulus intensities, resulting in a sharper peak (**a**). While the stimulated area on the fingertip measures approximately 100 mm^2, the information is processed in only a 1 mm^2 area of the primary somatosensory cortex.

13.3 Somatosensory System: Lesions

A Sites of occurrence of lesions in the somatosensory pathways (after Bähr and Frotscher)

The central portions of the somatosensory pathways may be damaged at various sites from the spinal root to the somatosensory cortex as a result of trauma, tumor mass effect, hemorrhage, or infarction. The signs and symptoms are helpful in determining the location of the lesion. This unit deals strictly with lesions in conscious pathways. The innervation of the trunk and limbs is mediated by the spinal nerves. The innervation of the head is mediated by the trigeminal nerve, which has its own nuclei (see below).

Cortical or subcortical lesion (1, 2): A lesion at this level is manifested by paresthesia (tingling) and numbness in the corresponding regions of the trunk and limbs on the *opposite side* of the body. The symptoms may be most pronounced distally because of the large receptive fields on the fingers and the relatively small receptive fields on the trunk (see p. 447). The motor and somatosensory cortex are closely interlinked because fibers in the sensory tracts from the thalamus also terminate in the motor cortex, and because the cortical areas are adjacent (pre- and postcentral gyrus).

Lesions caudal to the thalamus (3): All sensation is abolished in the *contralateral* half of the body (thalamus = "gateway to consciousness"). A partial lesion that spares the pain and temperature pathways **(4)** is characterized by hypesthesia (decreased tactile sensation) on the *contralateral* face and body. Pain and temperature sensation are unaffected. As cortical afferents travel crossed and uncrossed to the principal sensory nucleus of the trigeminal nerve, it is possible that epicritic sensitivity could remain intact in a unilateral lesion.

Lesion of the trigeminal lemniscus and lateral spinothalamic tract (5): Damage to these pathways in the brainstem causes a loss of pain and temperature sensation in the *contralateral* half of the face and body. Other sensory modalities are unaffected.

Lesion of the medial lemniscus and anterior spinothalamic tract (6): All sensory modalities on the *opposite* side of the body are abolished except for pain and temperature. The medial lemniscus transmits the axons of the second neurons of the anterior spinothalamic tract and both tracts of the posterior funiculus. The axons of the second neuron of the anterior spinothalamic tract connect to the medial lemniscus in the medulla oblongata.

Lesion of the trigeminal nucleus, spinal tract of the trigeminal nerve, and lateral spinothalamic tract (7): Pain and temperature sensation is abolished on the *ipsilateral* side of the face (uncrossed axons of the first neuron from the trigeminal ganglion) and on the *contralateral* side of the body (axons of the crossed second neuron in the lateral spinothalamic tract).

Lesion of the posterior funiculi (8): This lesion causes an *ipsilateral* loss of position sense, vibration sense, and two-point discrimination. Because coordinated motor function relies on sensory input that operates in a feedback loop, the lack of sensory input leads to ipsilateral sensory ataxia.

Posterior horn lesion (9): A circumscribed lesion involving one or a few segments causes an *ipsilateral* loss of pain and temperature sensation in the affected segment(s), because pain and temperature sensation are relayed to the second neuron within the posterior horn. Other sensory modalities including crude touch are transmitted in the posterior funiculus and relayed to the dorsal column nuclei; hence they are unaffected. The effects of a posterior horn lesion are called a "dissociated sensory deficit."

Dorsal root lesion (10): This lesion causes *ipsilateral,* radicular sensory disturbances that may range from pain in the corresponding dermatome to a complete loss of sensation. Concomitant involvement of the ventral root leads to segmental weakness. This clinical situation may be caused by a herniated intervertebral disk (see p. 463).

B Terminology of the lemnisci

Lemniscus (= ribbon) is a purely morphologic term for a sensory pathway in the brainstem. There are historical reasons for this term. Structurally, it does not represent a "new" pathway, rather the continuation of an existing pathway under another name. Four lemnisci are distinguished:

- *Medial lemniscus:* Epicritic somatic sensation of the torso and extremities; it is the continuation of the fasciculus gracilis and fasciculus cuneatus.
- *Spinal lemniscus:* Protopathic somatic sensation of the torso and extremities; it is the continuation of the anterior spinothalamic tract and lateral spinothalamic tract.
- *Trigeminal lemniscus:* Epicritic and protopathic sensation of the area innervated by the trigeminal nerve.
- *Lemniscus lateralis:* Part of the auditory pathway ("specific somatosensitivity"). The lateral lemniscus is not shown in the figure on p. 449.

The four lemnisci are described in greater detail on p. 539.

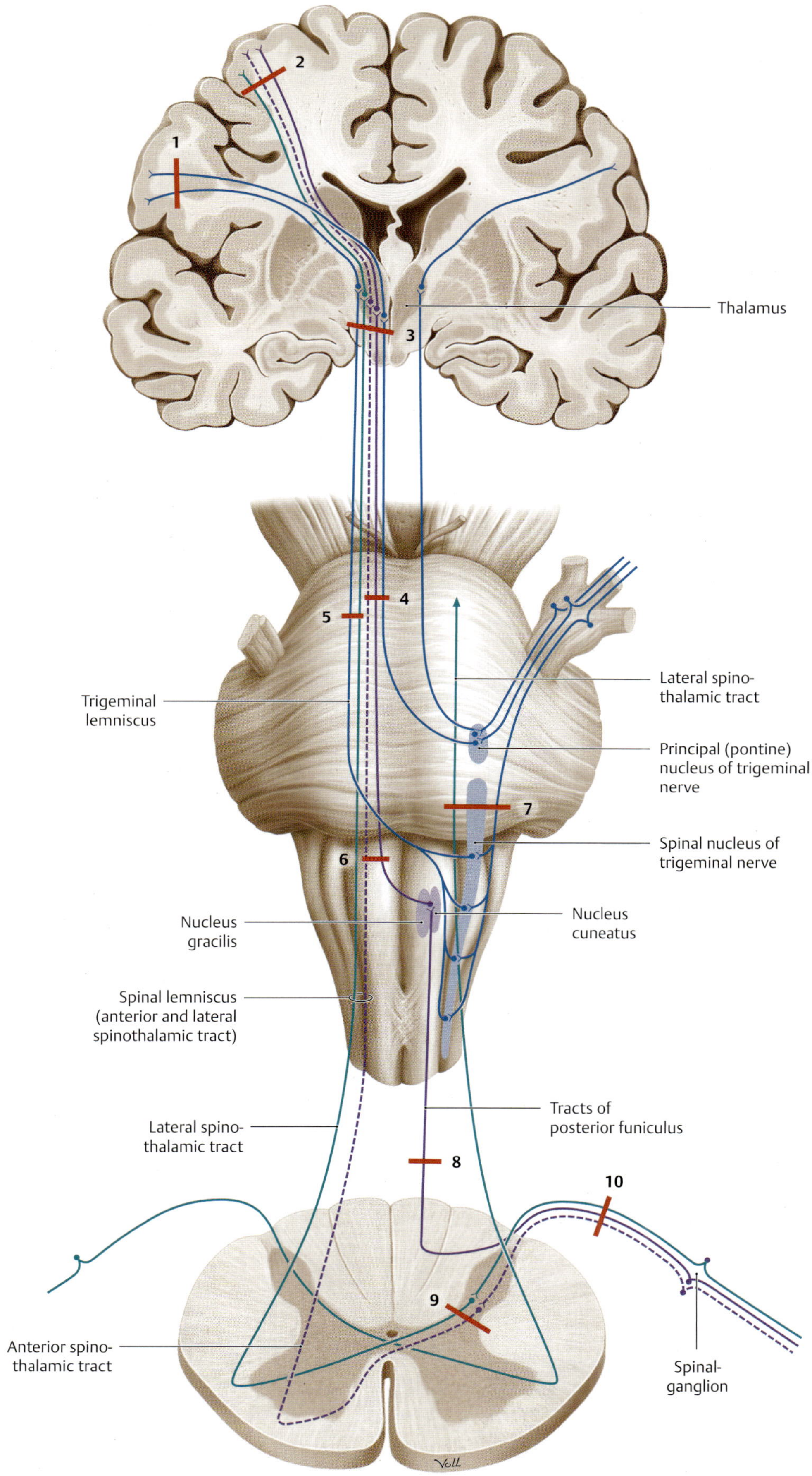
2
1
Thalamus
3
5
4
Lateral spino-
thalamic tract
Trigeminal
lemniscus
Principal (pontine)
nucleus of trigeminal
nerve
7
Spinal nucleus of
trigeminal nerve
6
Nucleus
gracilis
Nucleus
cuneatus
Spinal lemniscus
(anterior and lateral
spinothalamic tract)
Tracts of
posterior funiculus
Lateral spino-
thalamic tract
8
10
9
Anterior spino-
thalamic tract
Spinal-
ganglion

13.4 Somatosensory System: Pain Conduction

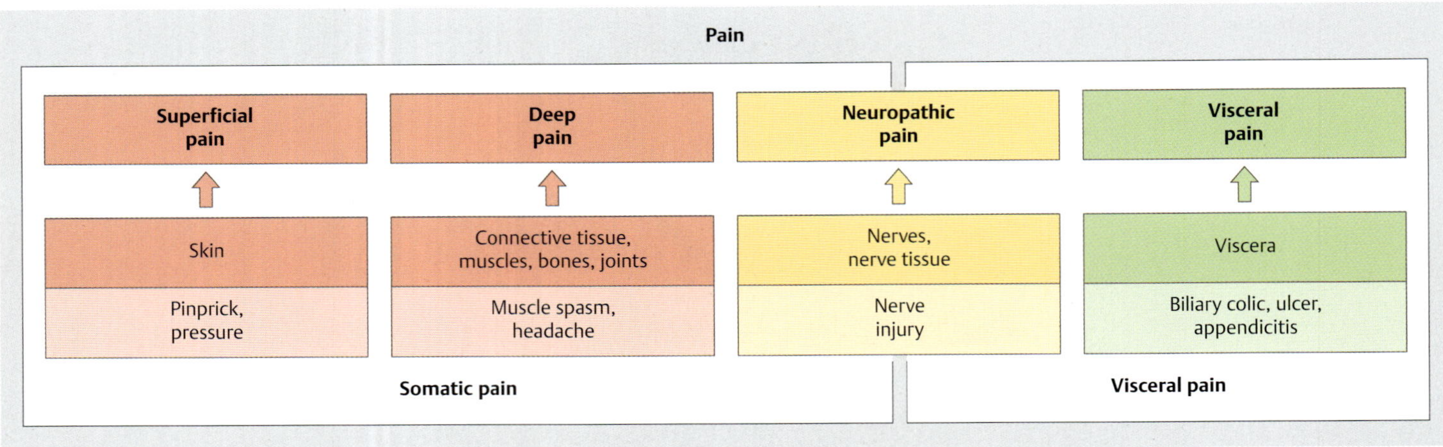

A Synopsis of pain modalities
The International Association for the Study of Pain defines pain as "an unpleasant sensory and emotional experience associated with actual or potential tissue damage, or described in terms of such damage." Pain is classified by its site of origin as *somatic* or *visceral*. Somatic pain generally originates in the trunk, limbs, or head, while visceral pain originates in the internal organs. *Neuropathic* pain is caused by damage to the nerves themselves. It may involve nerves of the somatic and/or autonomic nervous system. The somatic pain fibers described below travel with the spinal or cranial nerves, while the visceral pain fibers travel with the autonomic nerves (see p. 302).

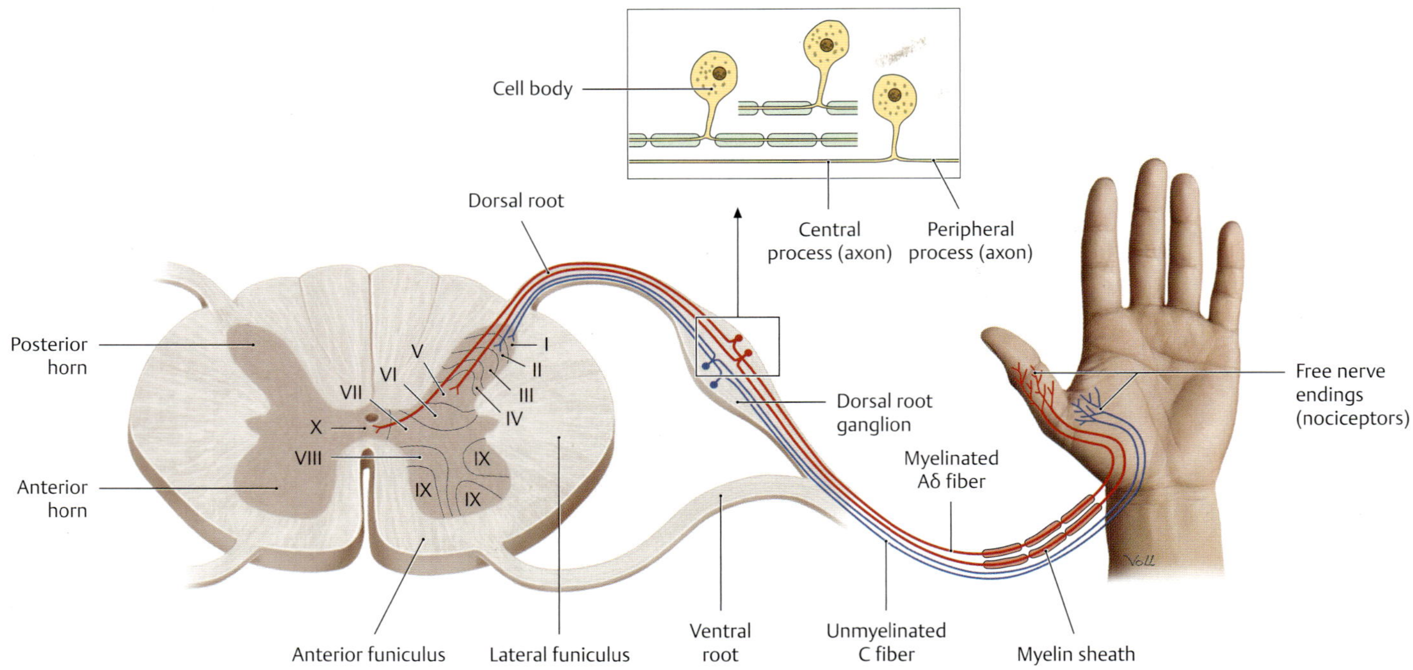

B Peripheral somatic pain conduction (after Lorke)
Somatic pain impulses from the trunk and limbs are conducted by myelinated Aδ fibers (temperature, pain, position) and unmyelinated C fibers (temperature, pain). The cell bodies of these afferent nerve fibers are located in the dorsal root ganglion (pseudounipolar neurons). Their axons terminate in the posterior horn of the spinal cord, chiefly in the Rexed laminae I, II, and IV–VI. The nociceptors, afferent fibers ascend after synapsing in the posterior horn (see **C**).
Note: Most somatosensory pain fibers are myelinated, while the viscerosensory fibers are unmyelinated.

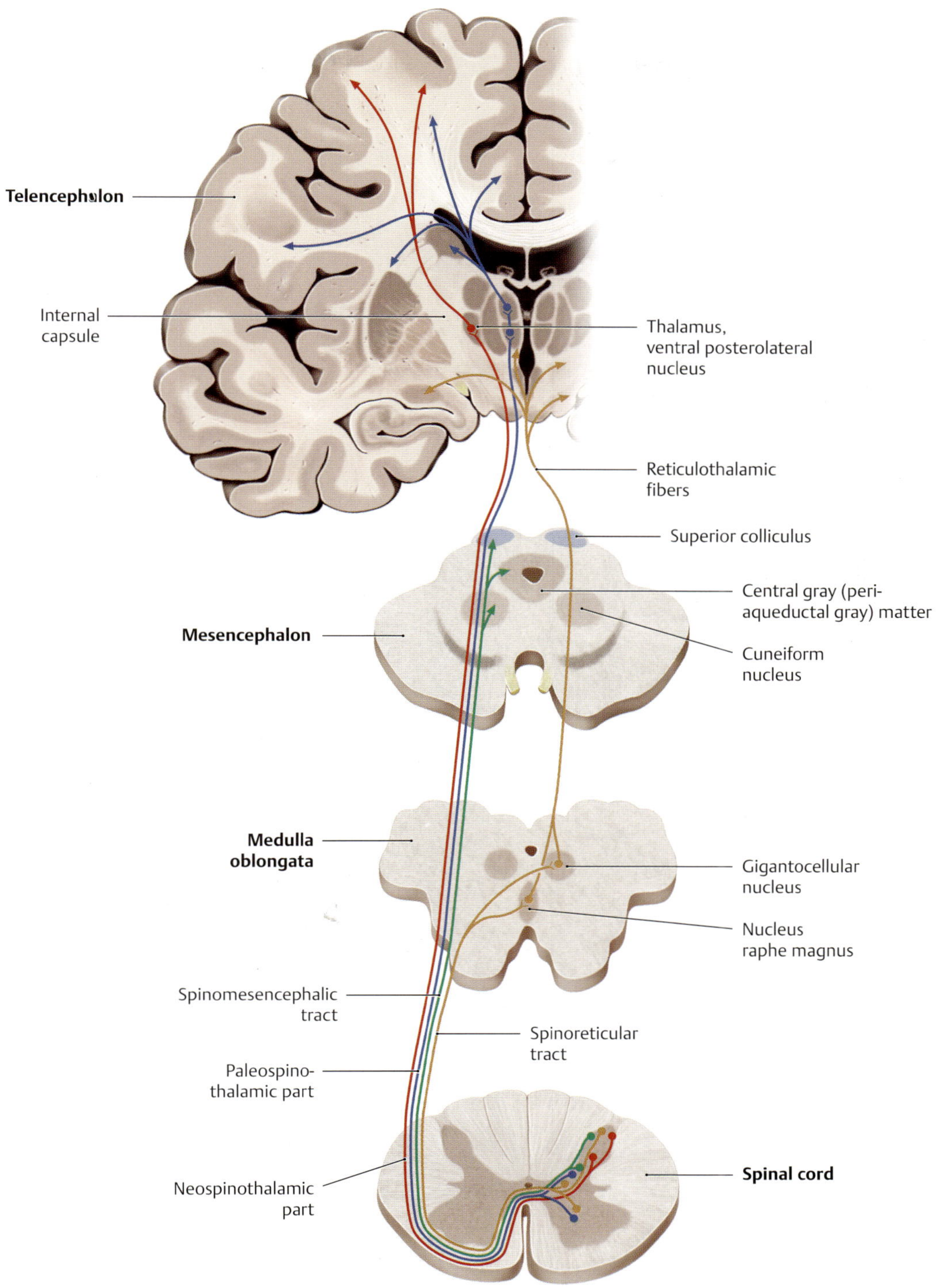

C Ascending pain pathways from the trunk and limbs

The axons of the primary afferent neurons for pain sensation in the trunk and limbs terminate on the neurons (shown above) located in the posterior horn of the spinal cord. The lateral spinothalamic tract is subdivided into a neo- and paleospinothalamic part. The second neuron of the *neospinothalamic part* of the pain pathway (red) terminates in the ventral posterolateral nucleus of the thalamus. The third neuron projects from there to the primary somatosensory cortex (postcentral gyrus) of the brain. The second neuron of the *paleospinothalamic tract* (blue) terminates in the intralaminar and medial nuclei of the thalamus, whose third neuron then projects to a variety of brain regions. This pain pathway is mainly responsible for the emotional component associated with pain. In addition to these pain pathways that end on the cerebral cortex, there are also pain pathways that end in *subcortical* regions—the spinomesencephalic tract and spinoreticular tract. The second neuron of the *spinomesencephalic tract* (green) terminates mainly in the central gray (periaqueductal gray) matter. Other axons terminate in the cuneiform nucleus or anterior pretectal nucleus. The second neuron of the *spinoreticular tract* (orange) ends in the reticular formation, represented here by the nucleus raphes magnus and the gigantocellular nucleus. Reticulothalamic fibers transmit the pain impulses onward to the medial thalamus, hypothalamus, and limbic system.

13.5 Somatosensory System: Pain Pathways in the Head and the Central Analgesic System

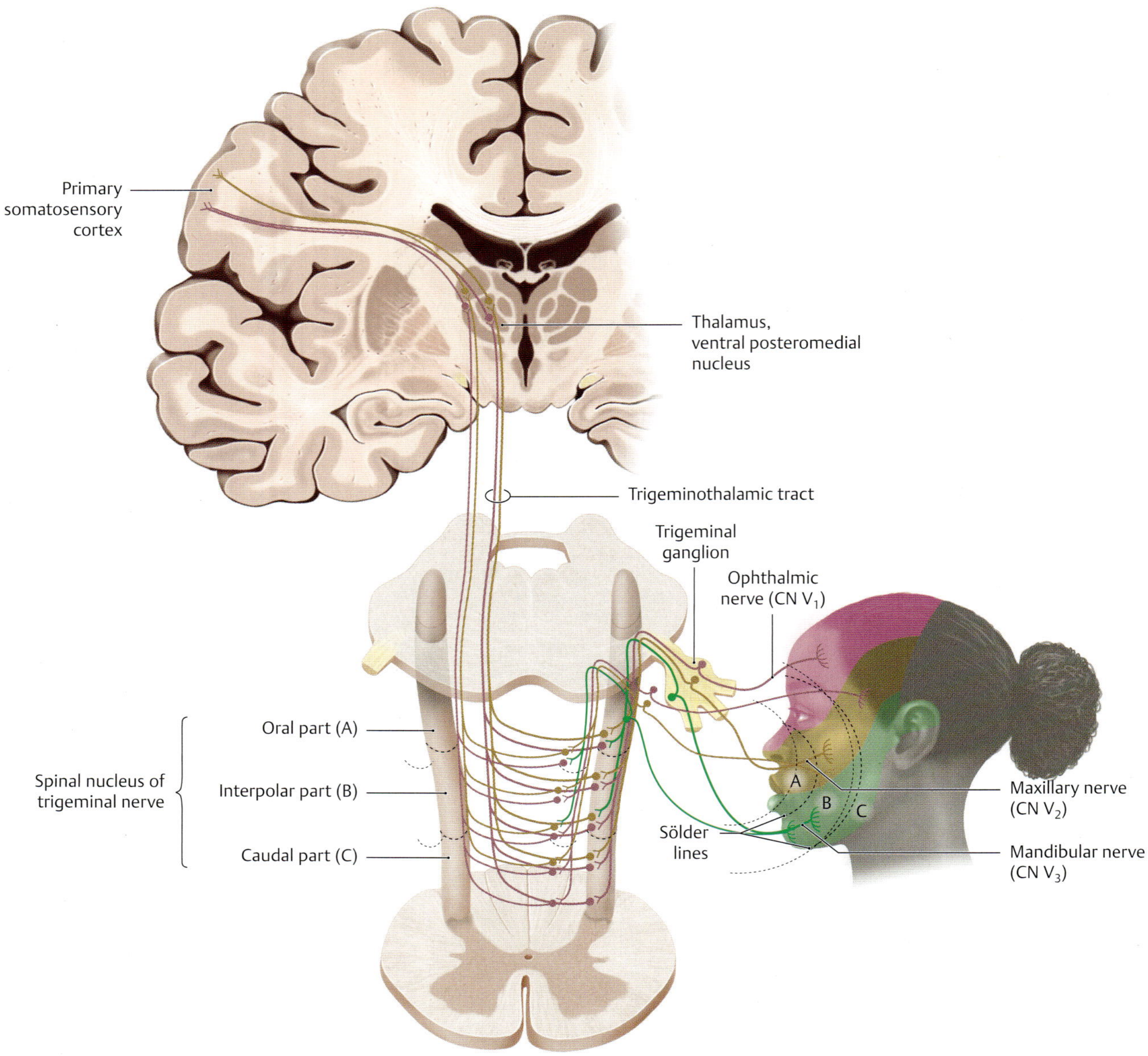

A Pain pathways in the head (after Lorke)
The pain fibers in the head accompany the principal divisions of the trigeminal nerve (CN V$_1$–V$_3$). The cell bodies of these primary afferent neurons of the pain pathway are located in the trigeminal ganglion. Their axons terminate in the spinal nucleus of the trigeminal nerve.
Note the somatotopic organization of this nuclear region: The perioral region (**a**) is cranial and the occipital region (**c**) is caudal. Because of this arrangement, central lesions lead to deficits that are distributed along the Sölder lines (see **D**, p.121).

The axons of the second-order neurons cross the midline and travel in the trigeminothalamic tract to the ventral posteromedial nucleus and to the intralaminar thalamic nuclei on the opposite side, where they terminate. The third-order (thalamic) neuron of the pain pathway ends in the primary somatosensory cortex. Only the pain fibers of the trigeminal nerve are pictured in the diagram. In the trigeminal nerve itself, the other sensory fibers run parallel to the pain fibers but terminate in various trigeminal nuclei (see p. 120).

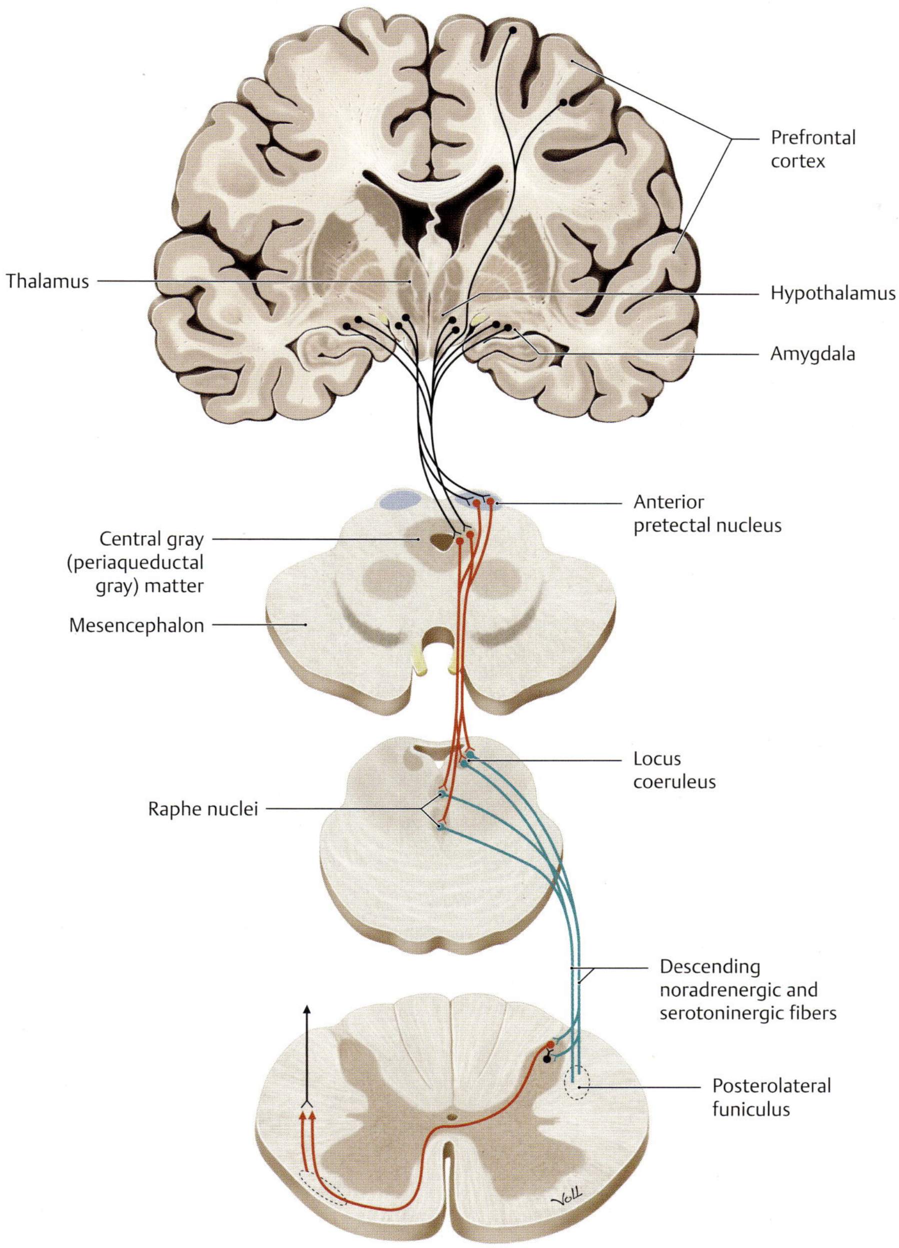

B Pathways of the central descending analgesic system (after Lorke)

Besides the ascending pathways that carry pain sensation to the primary somatosensory cortex, there are also descending pathways that have the ability to suppress pain impulses. The central relay station for the descending analgesic (pain-relieving) system is the central gray (periaqueductal gray) matter of the mesencephalon. It is activated by afferent input from the hypothalamus, the prefrontal cortex, and the amygdaloid bodies (part of the limbic system, not shown). It also receives afferent input from the spinal cord (see p. 450). The axons from the excitatory glutamatergic neurons (red) of the central gray matter terminate on serotoninergic neurons in the raphe nuclei and on noradrenergic neurons in the locus ceruleus (both shown in blue). The axons from both types of neuron descend in the posterolateral funiculus. They terminate directly or indirectly (via inhibitory neurons) on the analgesic projection neurons (second afferent neuron of the pain pathway), thereby inhibiting the further conduction of pain impulses.

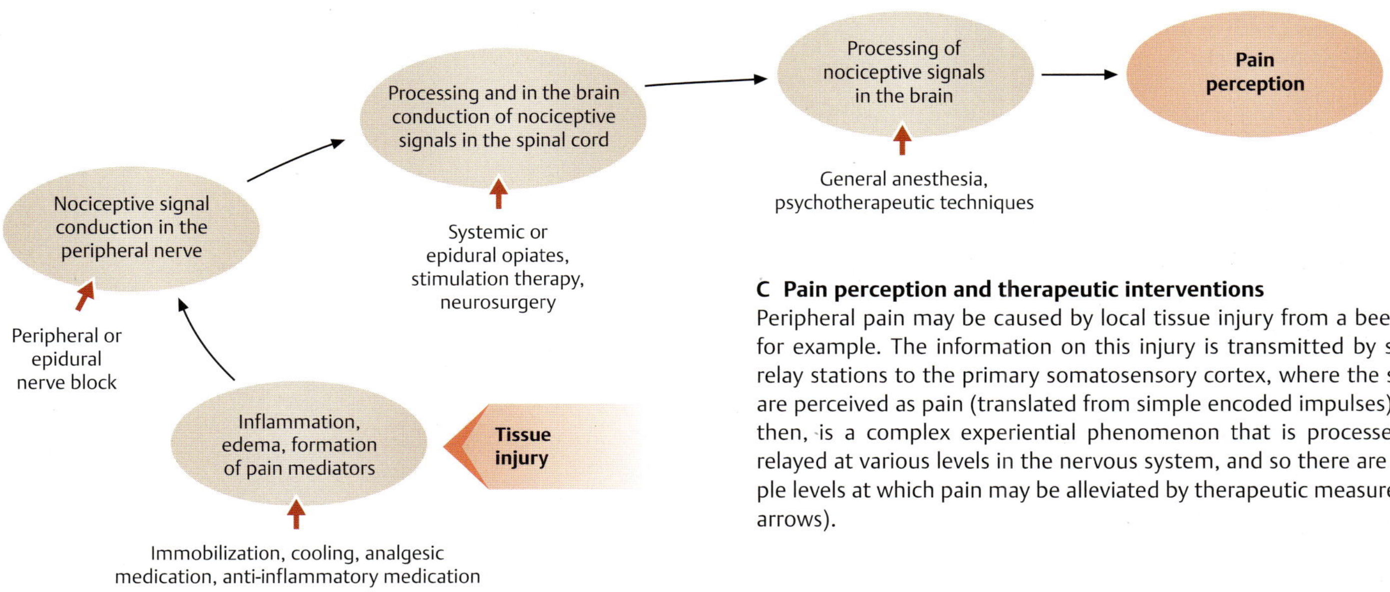

C Pain perception and therapeutic interventions

Peripheral pain may be caused by local tissue injury from a bee sting, for example. The information on this injury is transmitted by several relay stations to the primary somatosensory cortex, where the signals are perceived as pain (translated from simple encoded impulses). Pain, then, is a complex experiential phenomenon that is processed and relayed at various levels in the nervous system, and so there are multiple levels at which pain may be alleviated by therapeutic measures (red arrows).

13.6 Motor System, Overview

A Simplified representation of the anatomical structures involved in a voluntary movement (pyramidal motor system)
(after Klinke and Silbernagl)

The first step in performing a voluntary movement is to plan the movement in the association cerebral cortex (e.g., goal: "I want to pick up my coffee cup"). The cerebellar hemispheres and basal nuclei work in parallel to program the movement and inform the premotor cortex of the result of this planning. The premotor cortex passes the information to the primary motor cortex (M1), which relays the information through the *pyramidal tract* to the alpha motor neuron (*pyramidal motor system*). The alpha motor neuron then transmits the information to the skeletal muscle, which transforms the program into a specific voluntary movement. Sensorimotor functions provide important feedback during this process (How far has the movement progressed? How strong is my grip on the cup handle?—different from gripping an eggshell, for example). Although some of the later figures portray the primary motor cortex as the starting point for a voluntary movement, this diagram shows that many motor centers are involved in the execution of a voluntary movement (including the *extrapyramidal motor system,* see **C** and **D**; cerebellum). For practical reasons, however, the discussion commonly begins at the primary motor cortex (M1).

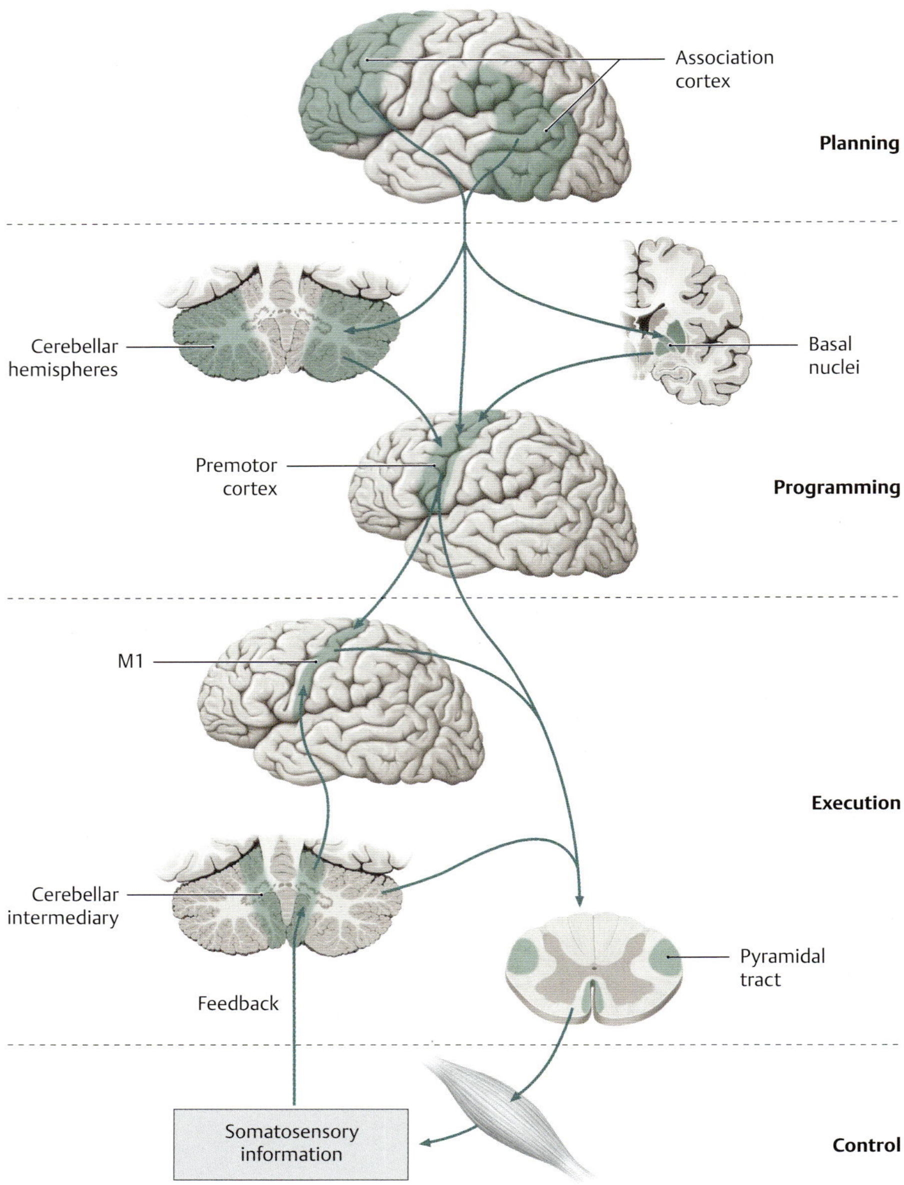

B Cortical areas with motor function: initiating a movement

Lateral view of the left hemisphere. The initiation of a voluntary movement (reaching for a coffee cup) results from the interaction of various cortical areas. The *primary motor cortex* (M1, Brodmann area 4) is located in the precentral gyrus (execution of a movement). The rostrally adjacent area 6 consists of the lateral premotor cortex and medial supplementary motor cortex (initiation of a movement). Association fibers (see p. 334) establish close functional connections with sensory areas 1, 2, and 3 (postcentral gyrus with primary somatosensory cortex, S1) and with areas 5 and 7 (posterior parietal cortex), which have an associative motor function. These areas provide the cortical representation of space, which is important in precision grasping movements and eye movements.

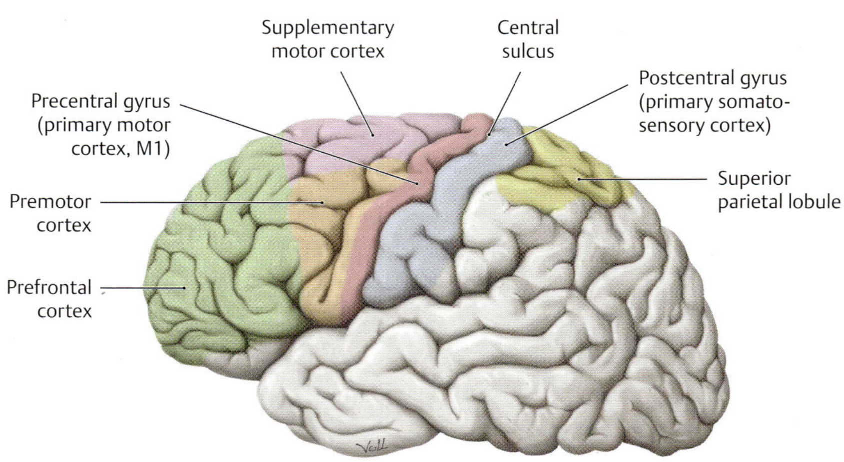

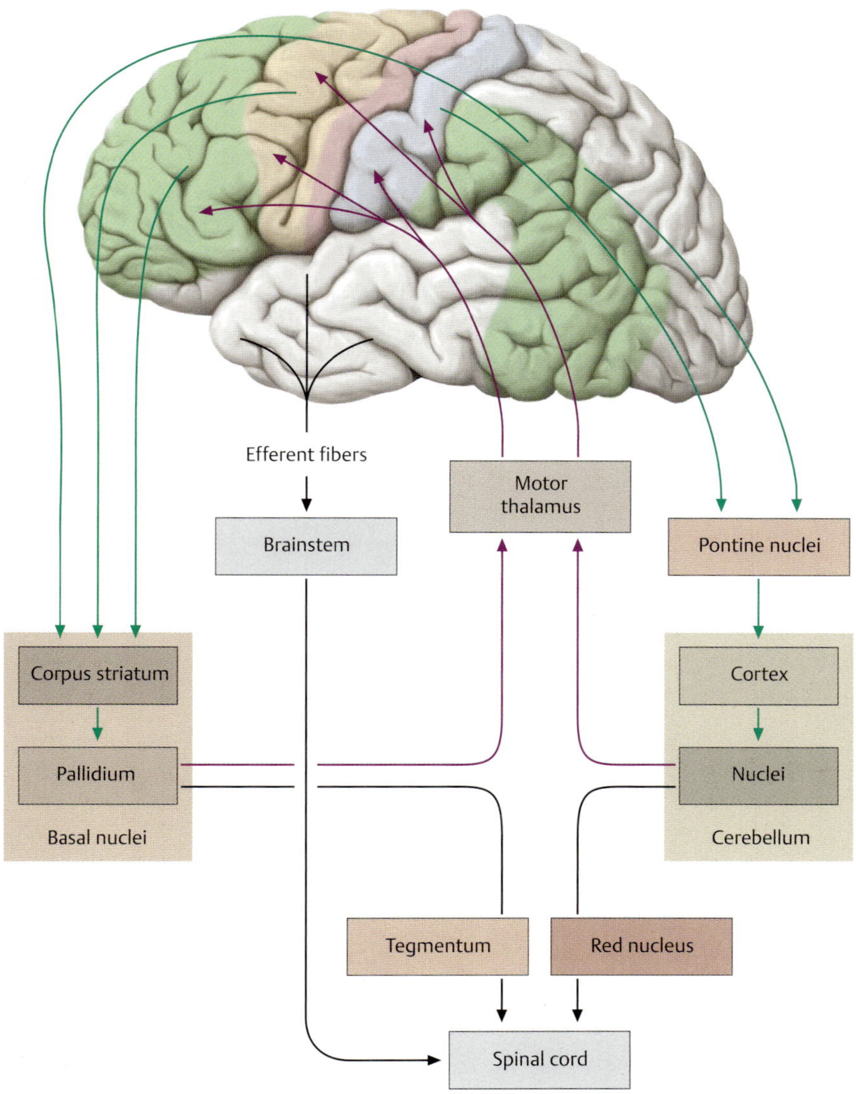

C Connections of the cortex with the basal nuclei and cerebellum: programming of complex movements

The pyramidal motor system (the primary motor cortex and the pyramidal tract arising from it) is assisted by the basal nuclei and cerebellum in the planning and programming of complex movements. While afferent fibers of the motor nuclei (green) project directly to the basal nuclei (left) without synapsing, the cerebellum is indirectly controlled via pontine nuclei (right; see **C**, p. 361). The motor thalamus provides a feedback loop for both structures (see p. 459). The efferent fibers of the basal nuclei and cerebellum are distributed to lower structures including the spinal cord. The importance of the basal nuclei and cerebellum in voluntary movements can be appreciated by noting the effects of lesions in these structures. While diseases of the basal nuclei impair the initiation and execution of movements (e.g., in Parkinson's disease), cerebellar lesions are characterized by uncoordinated movements (e.g., the reeling movements of inebriation, caused by a temporary toxic insult to the cerebellum).

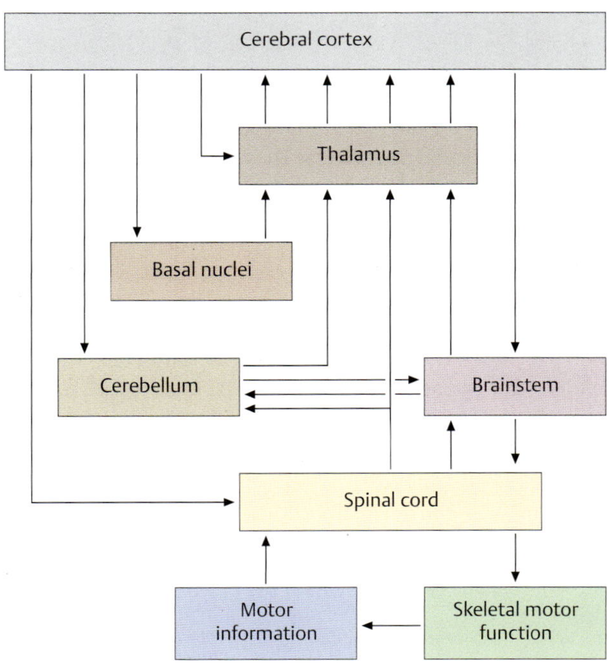

D Simplified block diagram of the sensorimotor system in the control of movement

Voluntary movements require constant feedback from the periphery (muscle spindles, tendon organs) in order to remain within the desired limits. Because the motor and sensory systems are so closely interrelated functionally, they are often described jointly as the sensorimotor system. The spinal cord, brainstem, cerebellum, and cerebral cortex are the three control levels of the sensorimotor system. All information from periphery, cerebellum, and the basal nuclei passes through the thalamus on its way to the cerebral cortex. The clinical importance of the sensory system in movement is illustrated by the sensory ataxia that may occur when sensory function is lost (see **D**, p. 471). The oculomotor component of the sensorimotor system is not shown.

13.7 Motor System: Pyramidal (Corticospinal) Tract

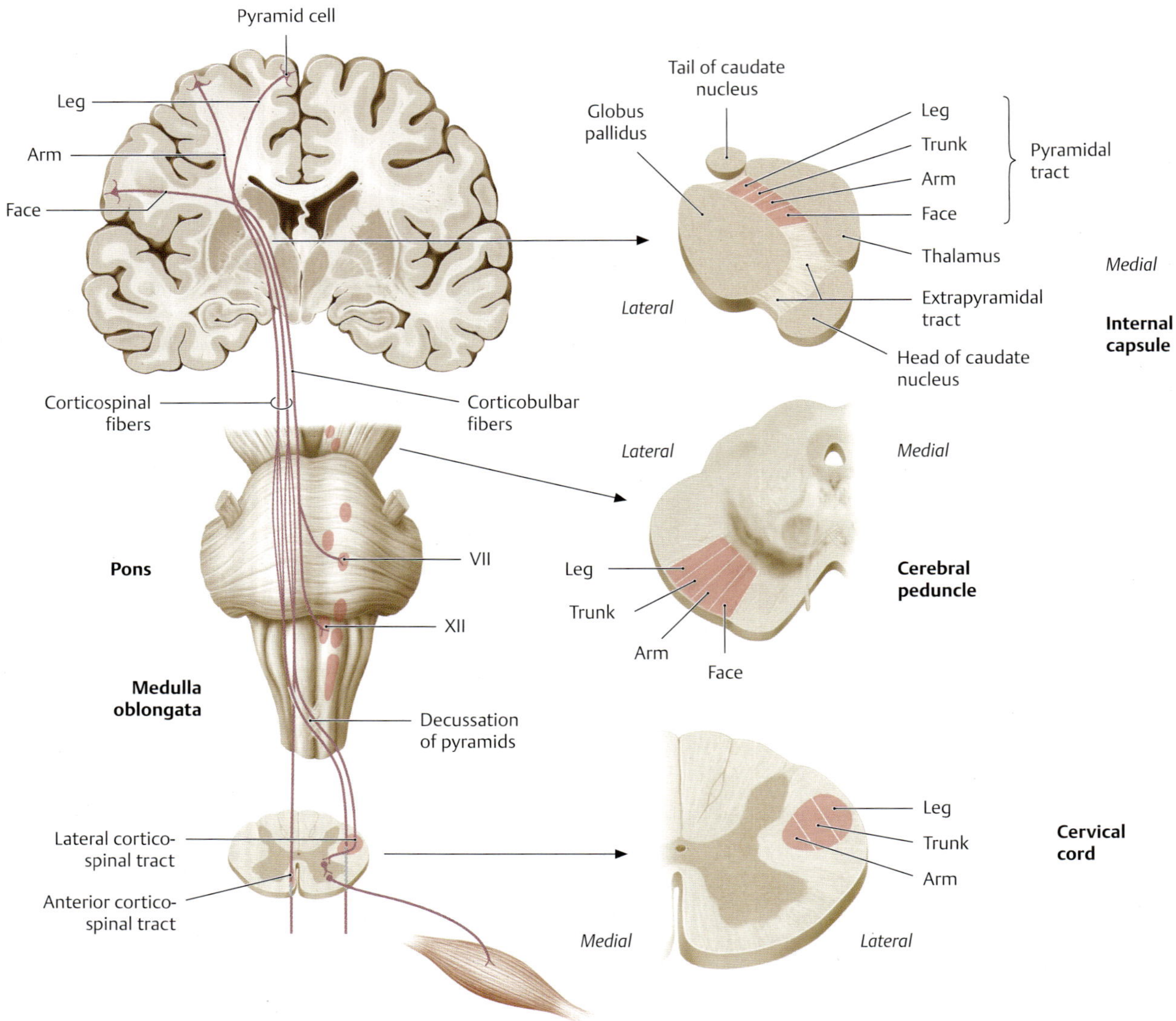

A Course of the pyramidal (corticospinal) tract
The pyramidal tract consists of three fiber systems: corticospinal fibers, corticonuclear fibers, and corticoreticular fibers (the latter are not shown here; they pass to the gigantocellular nucleus of the reticular formation in the brainstem and will not be further discussed). These groups of fibers constitute the descending motor pathways from the primary motor cortex. The corticospinal fibers pass to the motor neurons in the anterior horn of the spinal cord, while the corticonuclear fibers pass to the motor nuclei of cranial nerves.
Corticospinal fibers: Only a small percentage of the axons of the corticospinal fibers originate from the large pyramidal neurons in lamina V of the precentral gyrus (the laminar structure of the motor cortex is shown in **D**). Most of the axons arise from small pyramidal cells and other neurons in laminae V and VI. Other axons originate from adjacent brain regions. All of them descend through the internal capsule. Eighty percent of the fibers *cross the midline* at the level of the medulla oblongata (decussation of the pyramids) and descend in the spinal cord as the *lateral corticospinal (pyramidal) tract.* The *uncrossed* fibers descend in the cord as the *anterior corticospinal (pyramidal) tract* and cross later at the segmental level. Most of the axons terminate on intercalated cells whose synapses end on motor neurons.

Note: The basic pattern of somatotopic organization described earlier at the spinal cord level is found at all levels of the pyramidal tract. This facilitates localization of the lesion in the pyramidal tract.
Corticonuclear fibers: The motor nuclei and motor segments of the cranial nerves receive their axons from pyramidal cells in the facial region of the premotor cortex. These corticonuclear fibers terminate in the contralateral motor nuclei of cranial nerves III–VII and IX–XII in the brainstem (the fibers to other brainstem nuclei are shown in **C**). Besides this contralateral supply, axons also pass to several cranial nerve nuclei on the same (ipsilateral) side, resulting in a bilateral innervation pattern (not shown here). This dual supply is clinically important in lesions of the facial nerve, for example (upper versus lower face) (see **D**, p. 125).
Notes on the "pyramidal tract": Some authors interpret this term as applying strictly to the portion of the tract below the decussation of the pyramids, while other authors apply the term to the entire tract. Most publications, including this atlas, use "pyramidal tract" as a collective term for all of the fiber tracts described here. Some authors derive the term not from the decussation of the pyramids but from the giant pyramidal cells (Betz cells) in the cerebral cortex (see **C** and p. 409).

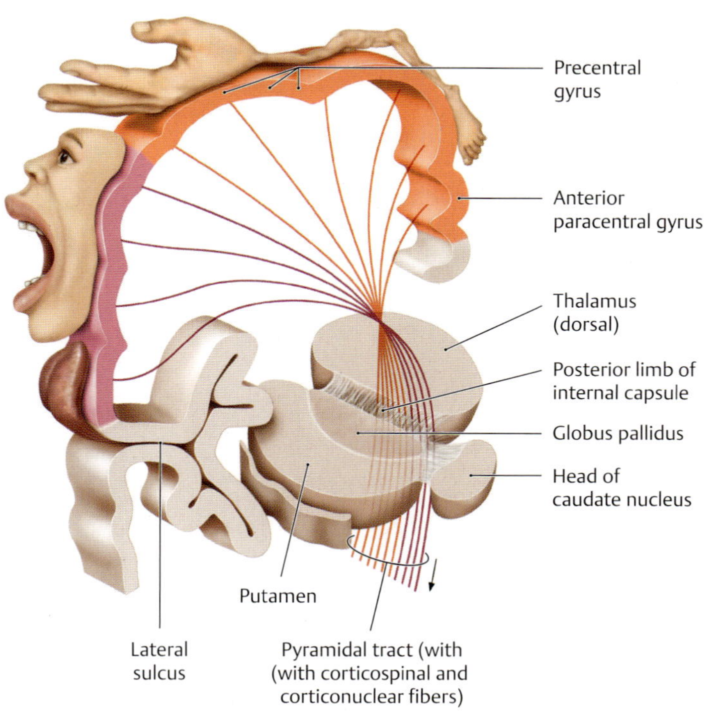

B Somatotopic organization of the somatomotor cortex: the motor homunculus

Anterosuperior view of the right precentral gyrus. Axons of neurons of the primary somato*motor* cortex in the precentral gyrus extend as the pyramidal tract to the motor neurons in the brainstem and spinal cord. The axons pass through the internal capsule (primarily the posterior crus) and course as cortico*nuclear* fibers to the cranial nerves (*nuclei*) or as the anterior or lateral corticospinal tract to the *spinal cord*. The precentral gyrus exhibits *somatotopic organization*. Specific cortical areas control the motor function of specific parts of the body. The result is a "motor representation" of the body, a *motor homunculus*. Body parts with complex motor function such as the hands or head (facial expression) require a large number of cortical neurons and are represented in large regions on the cortex regardless of their actual physical size. The precentral gyrus always controls the motor function of the contralateral half of the body. The cortical area of the skull is separated from the rest of the body. In contrast to the "headless" torso, the skull is upright. The leg is represented on the medial surface of the brain beneath the margin of the mantle. A few motor functions *only on the skull* are also represented bilaterally (see **D**, p. 125). Compare this with the illustration of the sensory homunculus on p. 447.

Note: The continuation of the precentral gyrus on the medial surface of the brain is known as the anterior paracentral gyrus.

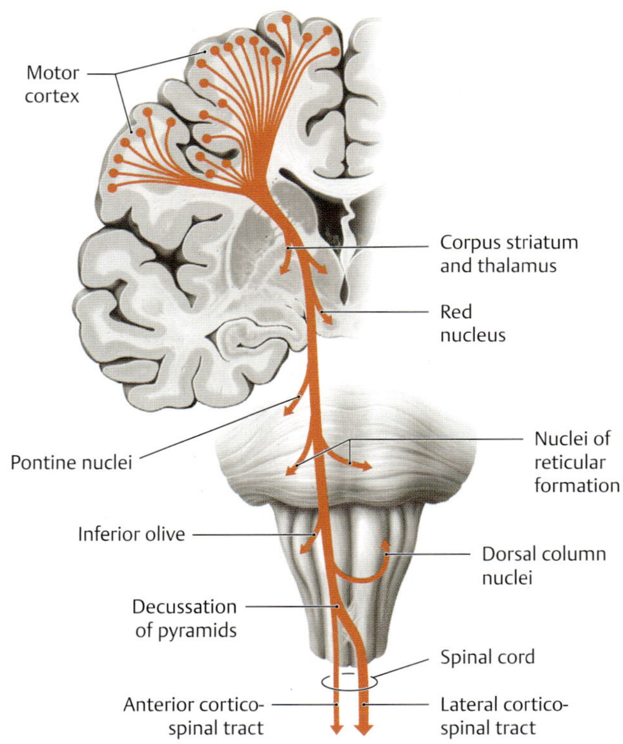

C Variety of cortical efferent fibers

Anterior view. Besides the corticospinal and corticonuclear fibers described above, a variety of axons descends from the cortex to various subcortical regions and into the spinal cord. The following subcortical regions also receive cortical efferent fibers: the corpus striatum, thalamus, red nucleus, pontine nuclei, reticular formation, inferior olive, dorsal column nuclei (these nuclear regions are described on p. 460), and spinal cord. The supraspinal efferent fibers listed above consist partially of axon collaterals from pyramidal tract neurons and partially of separate axons.

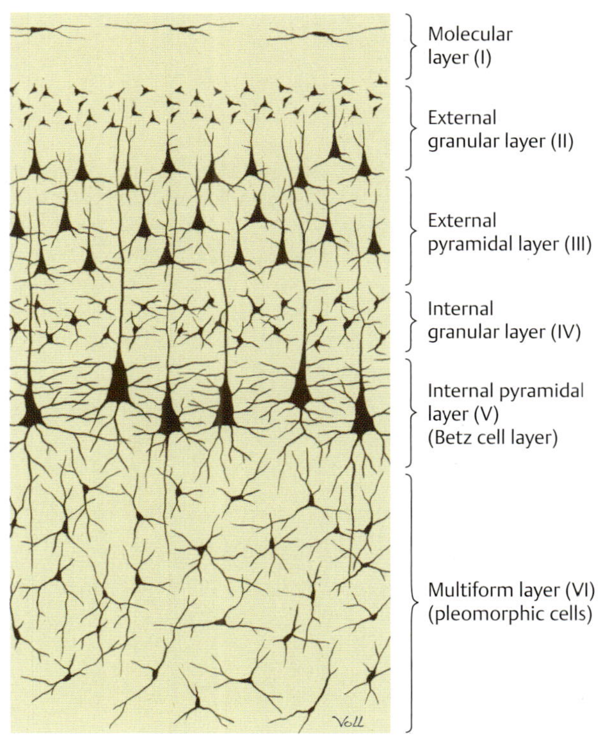

D Laminar structure of the motor cortex (= area 4 in the precentral gyrus)

The axons from giant pyramidal cells (Betz cells) in lamina V account for only a small percentage (< 4%) of the axons that make up the corticospinal tract. Small pyramidal cells and other neurons from laminae V and VI contribute the rest. In all, however, only about 40% of the axons of the pyramidal tract originate in area 4. The remaining 60% come from neurons in the supplementary motor fields and other cortical areas (see p. 454).

13.8 Motor System: Motor Nuclei

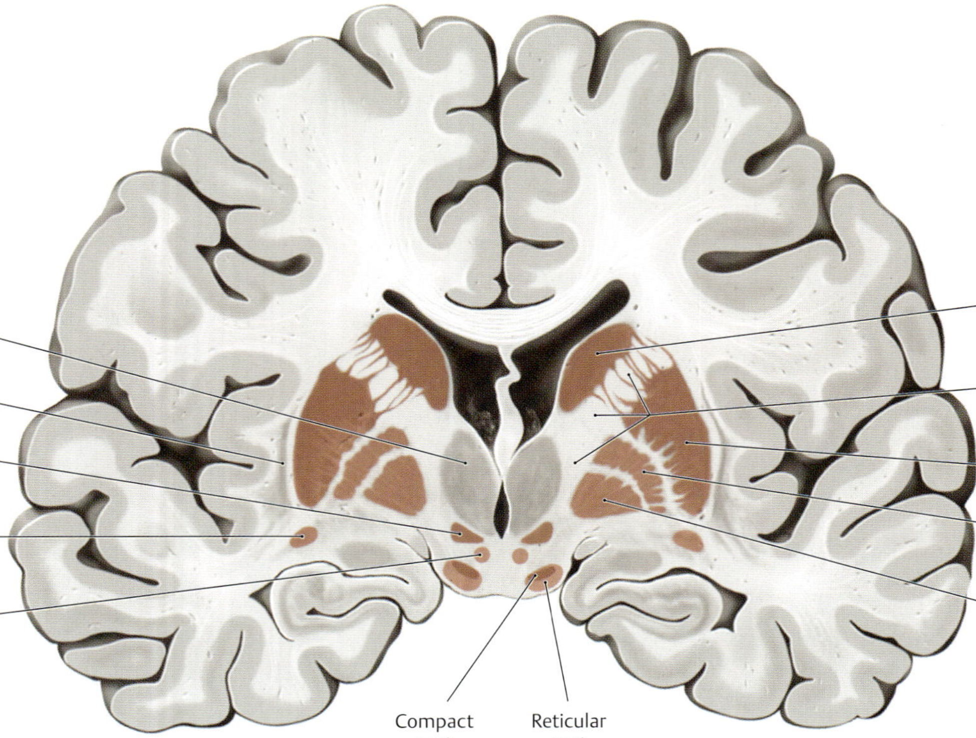

A Motor nuclei
Coronal section. The basal nuclei (ganglia) are subcortical nuclei of the telencephalon that have a role in the planning and execution of movements. They are the central relay station of the *extrapyramidal motor system* and make up almost all the central gray matter of the cerebrum. The only other central gray-matter structure is the thalamus, which is primarily sensory ("gateway to consciousness") and is involved only secondarily, through feedback mechanisms, in motor sequences. The three largest motor nuclei are as follows:

- Caudate nucleus
- Putamen
- Globus pallidus (developmentally, part of the diencephalon)

These three nuclei are sometimes known by varying collective designations:

- The *lentiform nucleus* is formed by the putamen, globus pallidus, and intervening fiber tracts.
- The *corpus striatum consists* of the putamen, caudate nucleus, and intervening streaks of gray matter. In addition to these three nuclei, there are other nuclei that are considered functional components of the motor system (also shown here).

In a strictly anatomical sense, only the telencephalic structures listed above are constituents of the basal nuclei (ganglia). Some textbooks include the *subthalamic nucleus* of the diencephalon (see p. 352) and the *substantia nigra* of the mesencephalon (see p. 357) among the basal nuclei because of their close functional relationship to nuclei. Functional disturbances of the basal nuclei are characterized by movement disorders (e.g., Parkinson's disease).
The nucleus accumbens is part of the reward circuit. For instance, when stimulated, it translates desires into action.

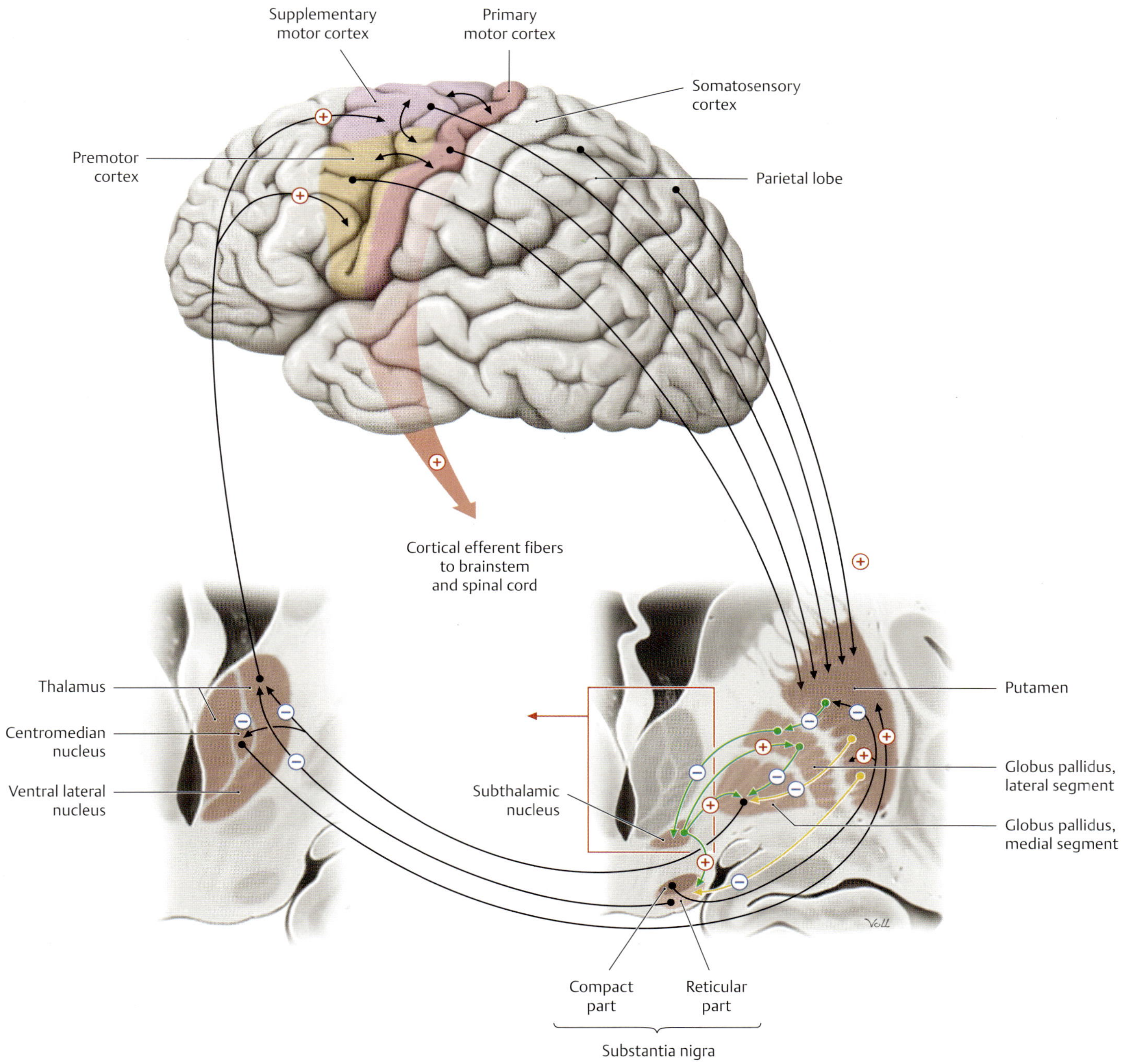

B Flow of information between motor cortical areas and basal nuclei: motor loop

The basal nuclei are concerned with the controlled, purposeful execution of fine voluntary movements (e.g., picking up an egg without breaking it). They integrate information from the cortex and subcortical regions, which they process in parallel and then return to motor cortical areas via the thalamus (feedback). Neurons from the premotor, primary motor, supplementary motor, and somatosensory cortex and from the parietal lobe send their axons to the putamen (see p. 337). Initially, there is a direct (yellow) and indirect (green) pathway for relaying the information out of the putamen. Both pathways ultimately lead to the motor cortex by way of the thalamus. In the *direct pathway* (yellow), the neurons of the putamen project to the medial globus pallidus and to the reticular part of the substantia nigra. Both nuclei then return feedback signals to the motor thalamus, which projects back to motor areas of the cortex. The *indirect* pathway (green) leads from the putamen through the lateral globus pallidus and subthalamic nucleus to the medial globus pallidus, which then projects to the thalamus. An alternate indirect route leads from the subthalamic nucleus to the reticular part of the substantia nigra, which in turn projects to the thalamus. When inhibitory dopaminergic neurons in the compact part of the substantia nigra cease to function, the indirect pathway is suppressed and the direct pathway is no longer facilitated. Both effects lead to the increased inhibition of thalamocortical neurons, resulting in decreased movements (*hypokinetic disorder,* e.g., in Parkinson's disease). Conversely, reduced activation of the internal part of the globus pallidus and the reticular part of the substantia nigra leads to increased activation of the thalamocortical neurons, resulting in abnormal spontaneous movements (*hyperkinetic disorder,* e.g., Huntington's disease). The diagram at lower left shows a close-up view of the boxed area (thalamus).

13.9 Motor System: Extrapyramidal Motor System and Lesions

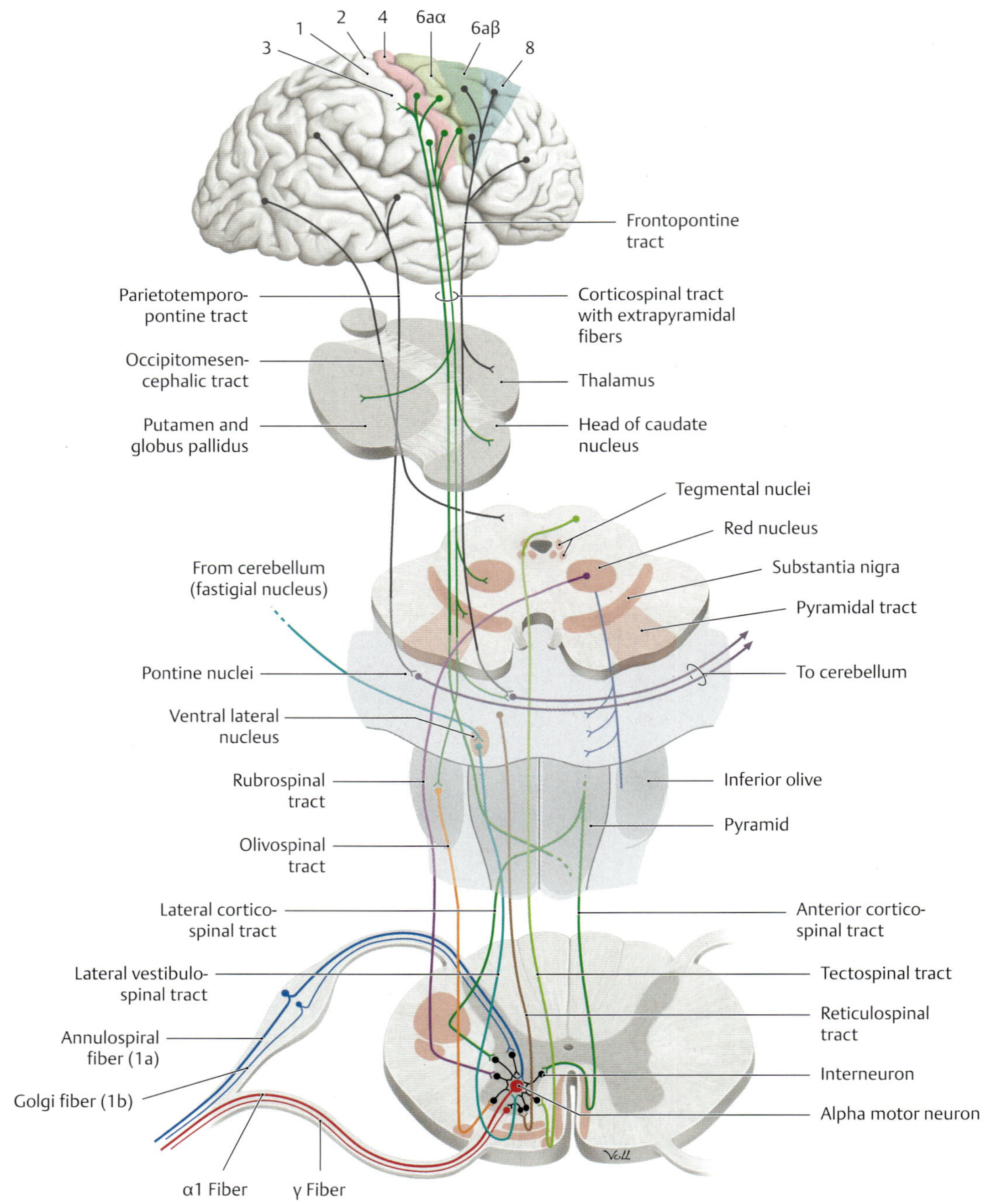

A Descending tracts of the extrapyramidal motor system

The neurons of origin of the descending tracts of the extrapyramidal motor system* arise from a heterogeneous group of nuclei that includes the basal nuclei (putamen, globus pallidus, and caudate nucleus), the red nucleus, the substantia nigra, and even motor cortical areas (e.g., area 6). The following descending tracts are part of the extrapyramidal motor system:

- Rubrospinal tract
- Olivospinal tract
- Vestibulospinal tract
- Reticulospinal tract
- Tectospinal tract

These long descending tracts terminate on interneurons which then form synapses onto alpha and gamma motor neurons, which they control. Besides these long descending motor tracts, the motor neurons additionally receive sensory input (blue). All impulses in these pathways are integrated by the alpha motor neuron and modulate its activity, thereby affecting muscular contractions. The functional integrity of the alpha motor neuron is tested clinically by reflex testing.

* The term "extrapyramidal motor system" has been criticized because its functional and anatomical components are so closely linked to the pyramidal motor system that the distinction seems arbitrary in an anatomical sense—particularly since the system does not include cerebellar tracts that are also involved in the control of motor function.

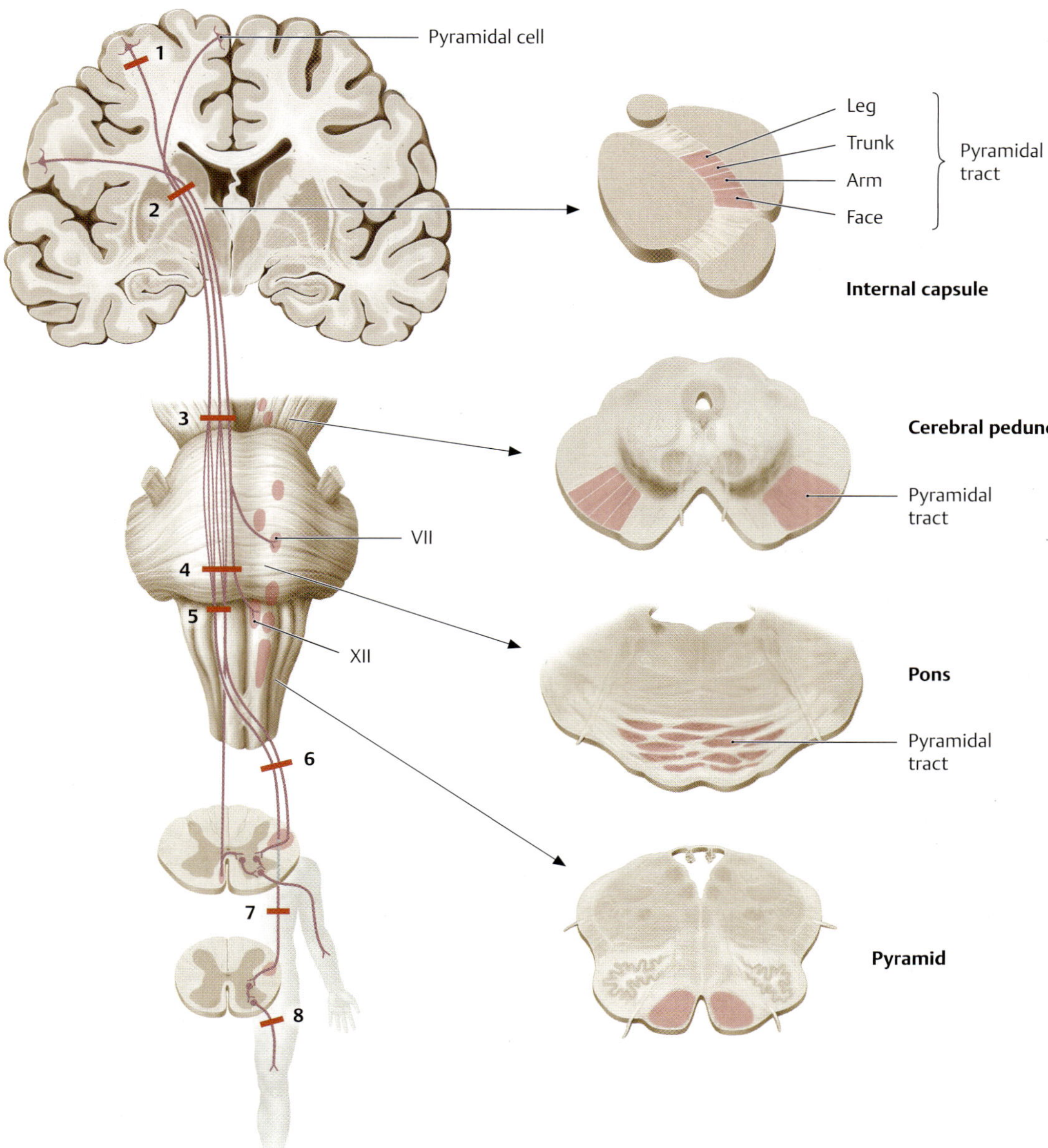

B Lesions of the central motor pathways and their effects

Lesion near the cortex (1): paralysis of the muscles innervated by the damaged cortical area. Because the face and hand are represented by particularly large areas in the motor cortex (see **B**, p. 457), paralysis often affects primarily the arm and face ("brachiofacial" paralysis). The paralysis invariably affects the side opposite the lesion (due to decussation of the pyramids) and is flaccid and partial (*paresis*) rather than complete because the extrapyramidal fibers are not damaged. If the extrapyramidal fibers were also damaged, the result would be contralateral *complete spastic paralysis* (see below).

Lesion at the level of the internal capsule (2): This leads to chronic, contralateral, spastic hemi*plegia* (complete paralysis) because the lesion affects both the pyramidal tract and the extrapyramidal motor path-ways,* which mix with pyramidal tract fibers in front of the internal capsule. Stroke is a frequent cause of lesions at this level.

Lesion at the level of the cerebral peduncle (crus cerebri) (3): contralateral spastic hemi*paresis.*

Lesion at the level of the pons (4): contralateral hemiparesis or bilateral paresis, depending on the size of the lesion. Because the fibers of the pyramidal tract occupy a larger cross-sectional area in the pons than in the internal capsule, not all of the fibers are damaged in many cases. For example, the fibers for the facial nerve and hypoglossal nerve are usually unaffected because of their dorsal location. Damage to the abducens nucleus may cause ipsilateral damage to the trigeminal nucleus (not shown).

Lesion at the level of the pyramid (5): Flaccid contralateral paresis occurs because the fibers of the extrapyramidal motor pathways (e.g., the rubrospinal and tectospinal tract) are more dorsal than the pyramidal tract fibers and are therefore unaffected by an isolated lesion of the pyramid.

Lesion at the level of the spinal cord (6, 7): A lesion at the level of the cervical cord (6) leads to ipsilateral spastic hemiplegia because the fibers of the pyramidal and extrapyramidal system are closely interwoven at this level and have already crossed to the opposite side. A lesion at the level of the thoracic cord (7) leads to spastic paralysis of the ipsilateral leg.

Lesion at the level of the peripheral nerve (8): This lesion damages the axon of the alpha motor neuron, resulting in flaccid paralysis.

* Thus, spastic paralysis is actually a sign of extrapyramidal motor damage. This fact was unknown when pyramidal tract lesions were first described, however, and it was assumed that a *pyramidal tract lesion* led to spastic paralysis. Because this fact has few practical implications, spasticity is still described in some textbooks as the classic sign of a pyramidal tract lesion. In most cases it would be better simply to regard spastic paralysis as a form of central paralysis.

13.10 Radicular Lesions: Sensory Deficits

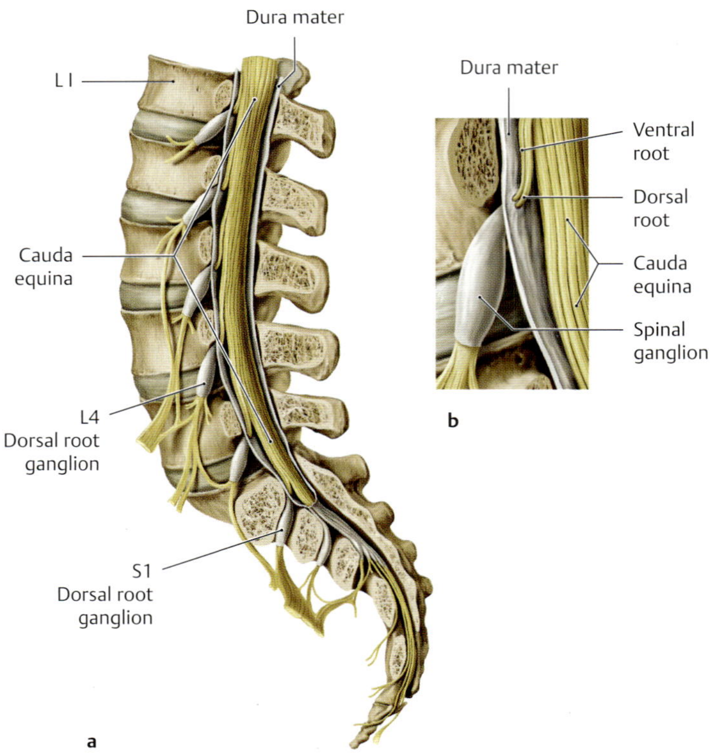

A Caudal end of the spinal cord and cauda equina in the vertebral canal
Midsagittal section viewed from the left side. The spinal cord ends approximately at the L 1 level, and the neural tissue in the vertebral canal below that level consists only of ventral and dorsal roots (see also p. 397). The ventral motor root and dorsal sensory root unite in the intervertebral foramen to form the spinal nerve. The roots enter and emerge from the spinal dural sac through two separate openings (**b**). This is the anatomical basis for the fact that sensory deficits (pain, loss of sensation) and motor deficits (muscular weakness ranging to paralysis) may develop separately in patients with nerve root compression (see **E**).

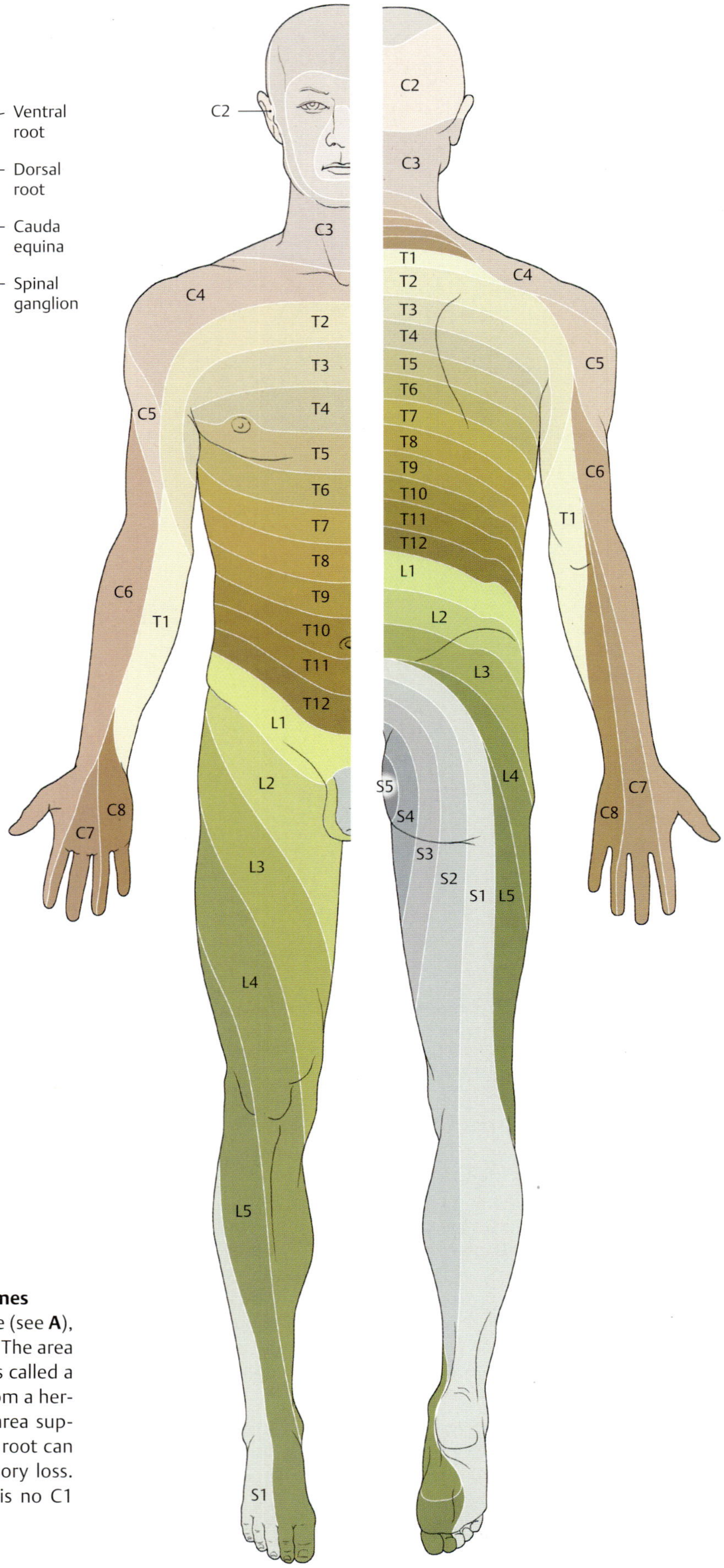

B Projection of radicular innervation to the skin: dermatomes
After the dorsal and ventral roots unite to form the spinal nerve (see **A**), their nerve fibers are distributed to their respective territories. The area of skin that is innervated by the fibers of a single dorsal root is called a *dermatome*. If the dorsal root is damaged (e.g., by pressure from a herniated intervertebral disk), sensation may be altered in the area supplied by the root. As a result, the level of the damaged nerve root can be identified by noting the dermatome affected by the sensory loss. Because the C1 segment contains only motor fibers, there is no C1 dermatome.

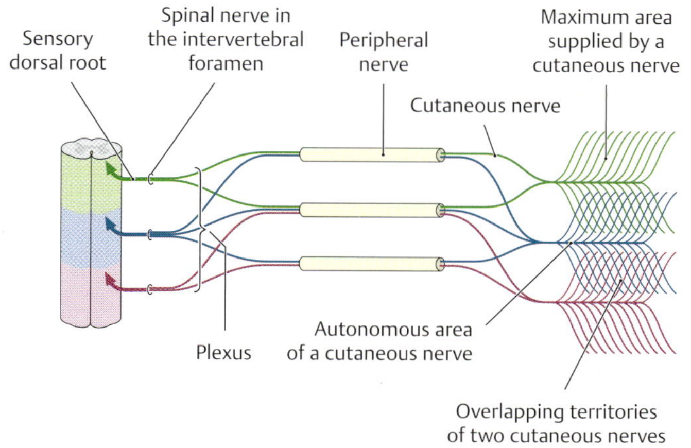

C Location of a radicular lesion

BA radicular lesion is located on the ventral motor root or dorsal sensory root between its site of emergence from the spinal cord and the union of both roots to form a peripheral nerve. Accordingly, a lesion of the ventral root leads to motor deficits (see p. 464) while a dorsal root lesion leads to sensory disturbances in the corresponding dermatome. The dermatomes on the limbs are shifted because of migratory processes during embryonic development, but the dermatomes on the trunk retain their segmental pattern of innervation (see **B** and **D**). Due to the overlap between adjacent dermatomes, the sensory loss that results from damage to a dermatome may be smaller than the size of the dermatome as it appears in the diagram. The brain does not "know" the location of the lesion; it processes information as if the lesion were located in the area supplied by the nerve (i.e., in the dermatome).

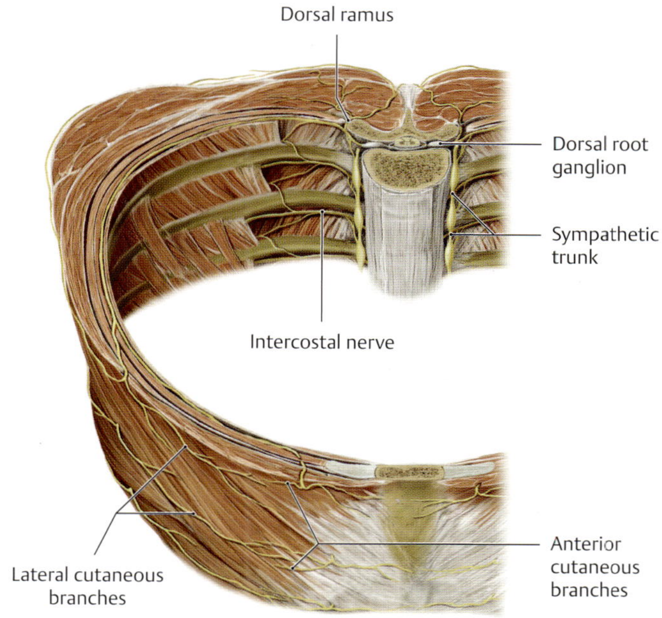

D Radicular innervation of the trunks

The segmental arrangement of the musculature is preserved in the trunk, and so the trunk retains a segmental (radicular) innervation pattern. Because the nerves in the trunk do not form plexuses, the radicular innervation pattern continues into the peripheral territory of a cutaneous nerve (T 2–T 12; see **B**). It can be seen that afferent fibers from the sympathetic trunk reach the peripheral nerves distal to the roots. This explains why radicular lesions are usually not associated with autonomic deficits in the affected dermatomes.

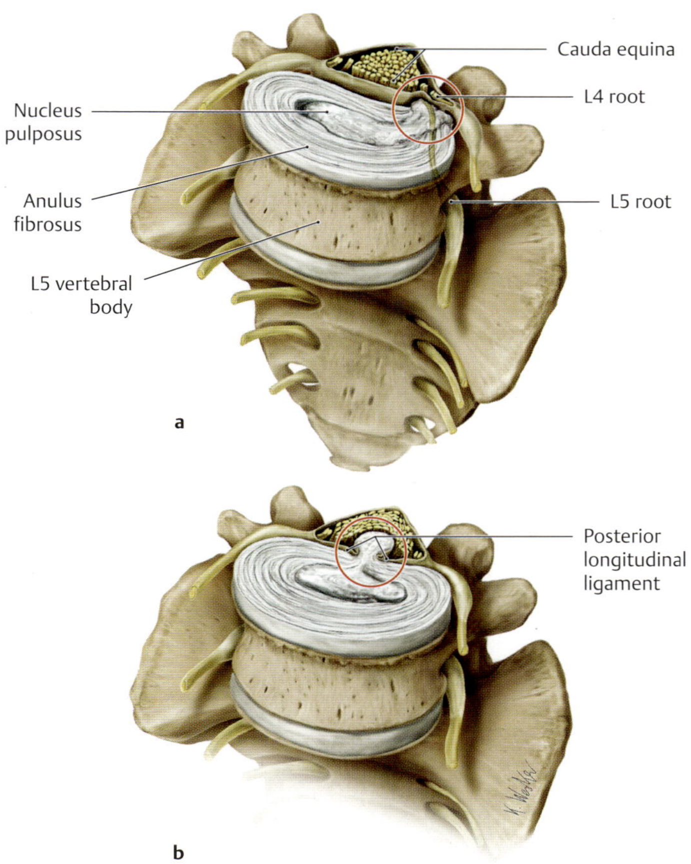

E Pressure on spinal nerve roots from a herniated lumbar disk of L 4/5

A herniated intervertebral disk may exert pressure on the spinal nerve root or cauda equina. The disk consists of a central gelatinous core (nucleus pulposus) and a peripheral ring of fibrocartilage (anulus fibrosus). When the anulus fibrosus is damaged, material from the gelatinous core may be extruded through the ring defect and impinge upon the root at its entry into the intervertebral foramen. This is a frequent cause of radicular symptoms, which have two grades of severity:

- Irritation of the nerve root in the region of the intervertebral foramen. This leads to pain in the low back (lumbago), potentially accompanied by pain radiating into the lower limb in the dermatome of the affected root (sciatica).
- A large disk herniation may compress the dorsal and/or ventral spinal nerve root, causing severe pain in addition to sensory deficits and (if the ventral root is affected) motor deficits.

a Posterolateral disk herniation at the L 4/5 level. This damages the L 5 root passing behind the herniated disk but not the descending L 4 root, which has already entered the intervertebral foramen at that level. As a result, the sensory deficits are manifested in the L 5 dermatome (see **B**). Only a far lateral disk herniation will damage the root that exits at the same level as the affected disk.

b Posteromedial disk herniation at the L 4/5 level. The material herniates through the posterior longitudinal ligament and impinges on the cauda equina. *Cauda equina syndrome* may develop if a lesion in this region compresses multiple roots. The locations of the deficits associated with specific root lesions are described on p. 464.

13.11 Radicular Lesions: Motor Deficits

A Indicator muscles of radicular lesions—limb muscles and diaphragm

While a lesion of the sensory dorsal roots leads to sensory disturbances in specific dermatomes (see p. 462 and **C**, p. 463), a lesion of the *motor ventral roots* will cause weakness to develop in specific muscles. Just as the affected dermatome indicates the site of the sensory root lesion, the affected muscle indicates the level of the damaged spinal cord segment or its root. The muscles that are predominantly supplied by a particular spinal cord segment are called its *indicator muscles* (analogous to the dermatomes for the dorsal roots). Because indicator muscles are supplied predominantly but, as a rule, not exclusively by a single segment, a lesion in one segment or spinal nerve root usually causes weakness (paresis) of the affected muscle rather than complete paralysis (plegia). Slight weakness may also be noted in muscles that receive some innervation from the affected segment but are not principally supplied by it. The indicator muscles in the upper and lower limbs are listed in the tables below. Whereas sensory (dorsal) root lesions may occur in isolation, motor (ventral) root lesions usually occur in association with dorsal root lesions, and therefore the dermatomes are also listed in the tables.

Note: Because the nerves of the trunk are derived directly from the spinal nerve roots without any intervening plexuses, the pattern of segmental innervation in the trunk is identical to the pattern of peripheral innervation.

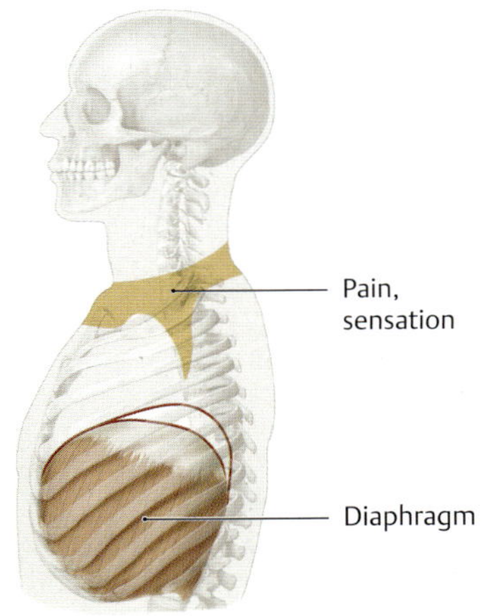

C4

Location of pain or sensory disturbance	Shoulder
Indicator muscle	Diaphragm
Reflexes abolished by a segmental lesion	None

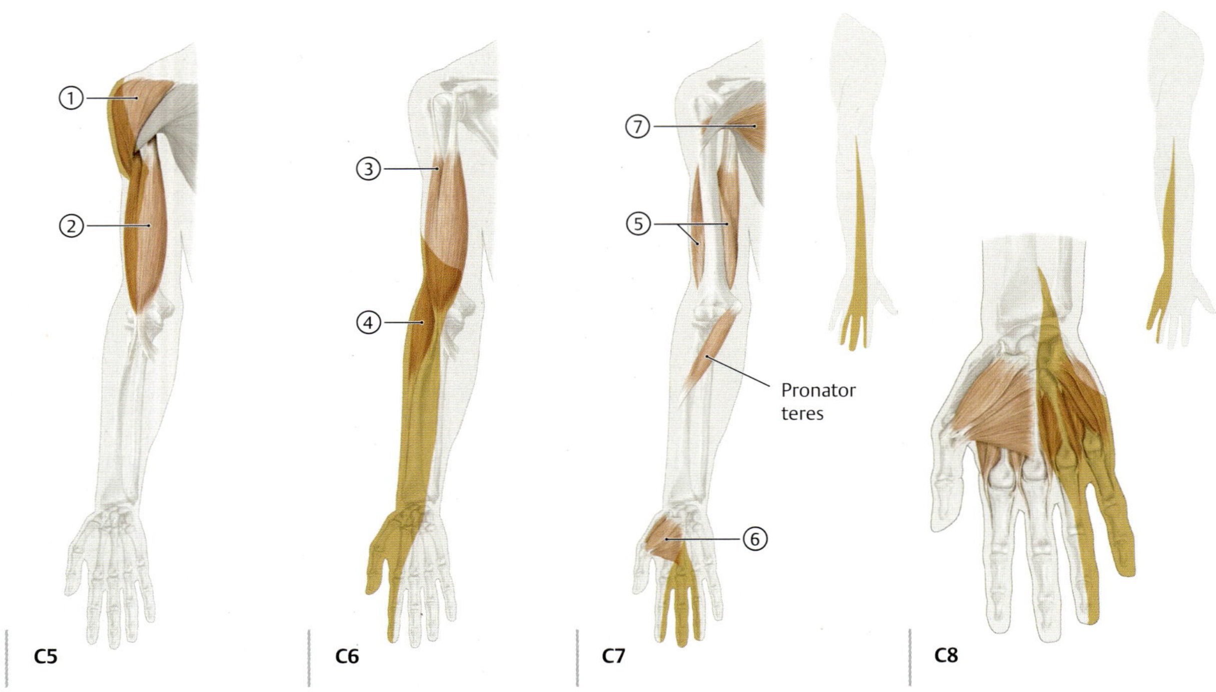

	C5	C6	C7	C8
Location of pain or sensory disturbance	Lateral and posterior side of shoulder, anterolateral side of proximal forearm	Dorsoradial upper arm, radial forearm → thumb	Posterior side of upper arm, extensor side of forearm → second/third (fourth) finger	Ulnar side of hand extending to small finger and ring finger
Indicator muscle (and other affected muscles)	① Deltoid ② (Biceps brachii)	③ Biceps brachii ④ (Brachioradialis)	⑤ Triceps brachii, hand and digital flexors and extensors ⑥ Thenar muscles ⑦ Pectoralis major (atrophy of sternocostal part)	Hypothenar, ulnar digital flexors (Triceps brachii, pectoralis major—abdominal part)
Reflexes affected by a segmental lesion	Biceps reflex (Brachioradialis reflex)	Biceps reflex (Brachioradialis reflex)	Triceps reflex (Trömner reflex)	Triceps reflex (Trömner reflex)

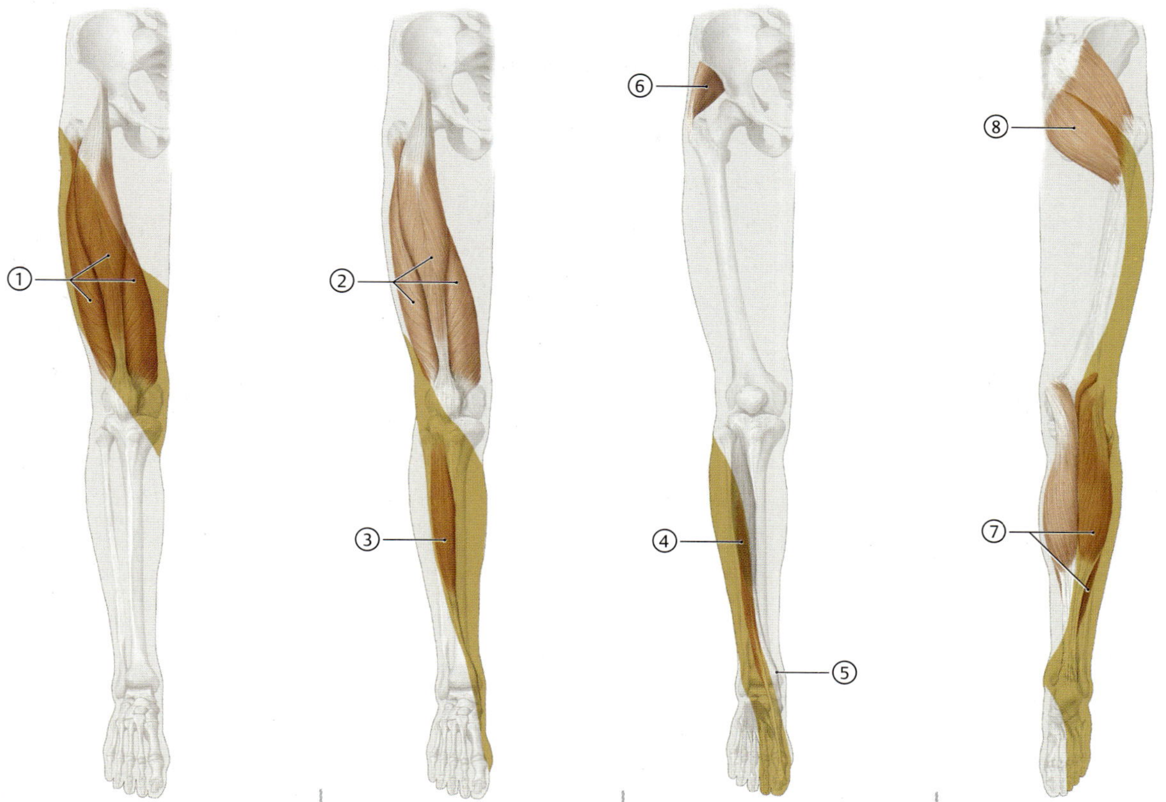

	L3	L4	L5	S1
Location of pain or sensory disturbance	Anterior side of thigh, passing obliquely downward from the approximate level of the trochanter to the medial side of the knee	Posterolateral thigh, extensor side of knee to anteromedial side of lower leg	Posterior side of thigh, lateral side of knee, antero-lateral lower leg, dorsum of foot to big toe	Lateral surface of thigh and calf, heel to lateral edge of foot
Indicator muscle (and other affected muscles)	① Quadriceps femoris (Adductors)	② Quadriceps femoris, especially the vastus medialis ③ (Tibialis anterior, adductors)	④ Extensor hallucis longus ⑤ Tibialis anterior ⑥ Gluteus medius	⑦ Triceps surae, peronei, thigh flexors ⑧ Gluteus maximus
Reflexes affected by a segmental lesion	Quadriceps reflex (= patellar tendon reflex = knee-jerk reflex)	Quadriceps reflex (Adductor reflex)	Tibialis posterior reflex	Triceps surae reflex (= Achilles tendon reflex = ankle-jerk reflex)

B Principal indicator muscles of the spinal cord segments
The table lists the typical indicator muscles for each cord segment.

Cord segment	Indicator muscle
C4	Diaphragm
C5	Deltoid
C6	Biceps brachii
C7	Triceps brachii
C8	Hypothenar muscles, flexor digitorum profundus on ulnar side
L3	Quadriceps femoris
L4	Quadriceps femoris, vastus medialis
L5	Extensor hallucis longus, tibialis anterior
S1	Triceps surae, peronei, gluteus maximus

C Clinical manifestations of nerve root irritation

- Pain in the affected dermatome
- Sensory losses in the affected dermatome
- Increased pain during coughing, sneezing, or straining
- Pain fibers more severely affected than other sensory fibers
- Motor deficits in the indicator muscles of the segment
- Reflexes associated with the affected segment are absent or diminished

13.12 Lesions of the Brachial Plexus

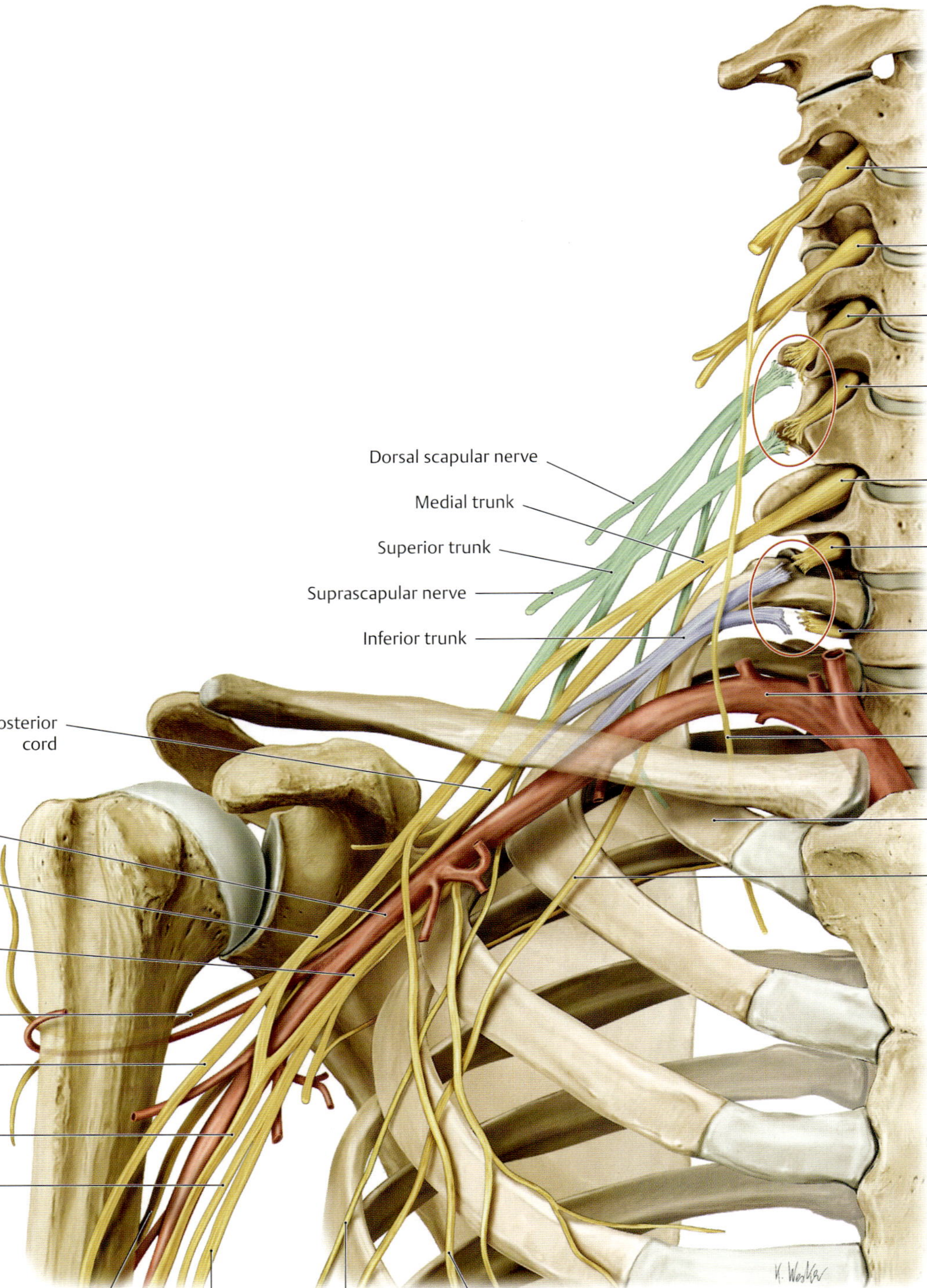

A Brachial plexus paralysis
Anterior view of the right side. Lesions are circled. By definition, two forms of brachial plexus paralysis are distinguished: *upper brachial plexus paralysis,* which is caused by a lesion of the C 5 and C 6 ventral rami (see **C**), and *lower brachial plexus paralysis,* which is caused by a lesion of the C 8 and T 1 ventral rami (see **D**). C 7 forms a "watershed" between the two forms of paralysis and is typically unaffected by either form. A complete lesion of the brachial plexus may also occur in severe trauma.

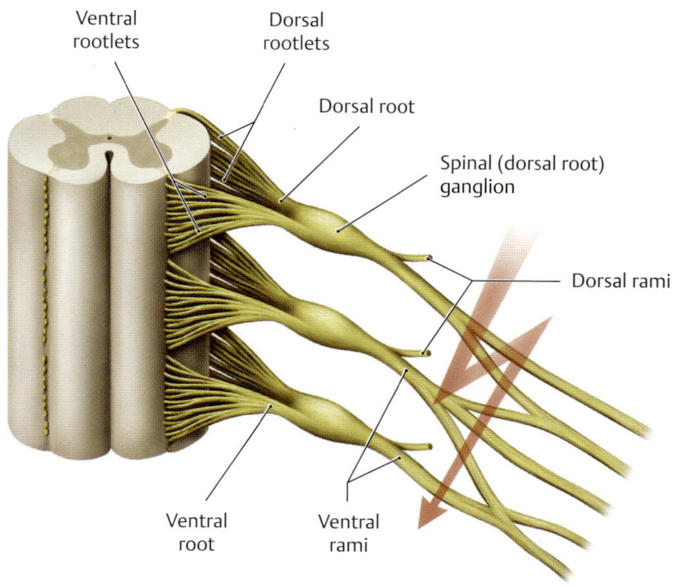

B Site of lesion in brachial plexus paralysis

A brachial plexus lesion affects the ventral rami of several spinal nerves, which transmit afferent signals to the plexus. Because the ventral rami carry both motor and sensory fibers, a brachial plexus lesion always causes a combination of motor and sensory deficits. The resulting paralysis (see **C**) is always of the flaccid type because of its peripheral nature (lesion of the second motor neuron).

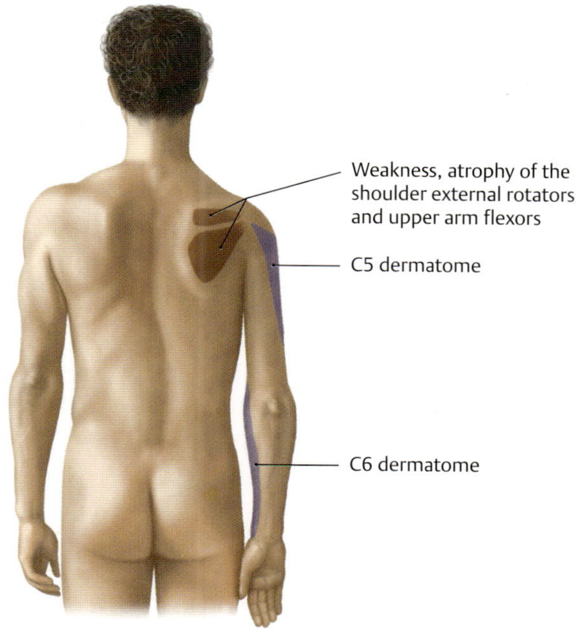

C Example: upper brachial plexus paralysis (Erb's palsy)

This condition results from a lesion of the ventral rami of the C 5 and C 6 spinal nerves, causing paralysis of the abductors and external rotators of the shoulder joint and of the upper arm flexors and supinator. The arm hangs limply at the side (loss of the upper arm flexors), and the palm faces backward (loss of the supinator with dominance of the pronators). There may also be partial paralysis of the extensor muscles of the elbow joint and hand. Typical cases present with sensory disturbances on the lateral surface of the upper arm and forearm, but these signs may be absent. A frequent cause of upper brachial plexus paralysis is obstetric trauma.

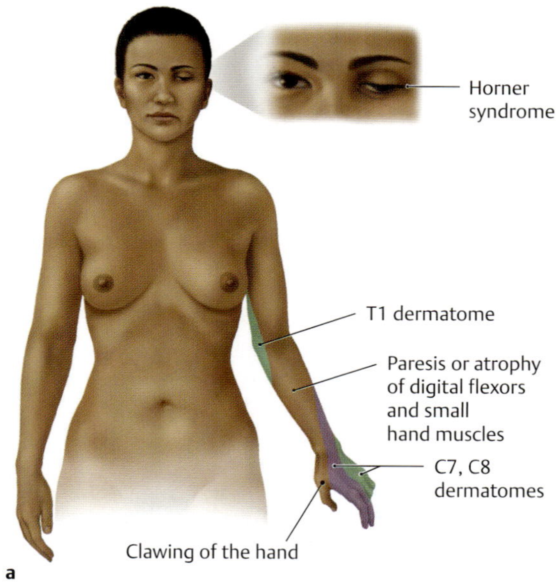

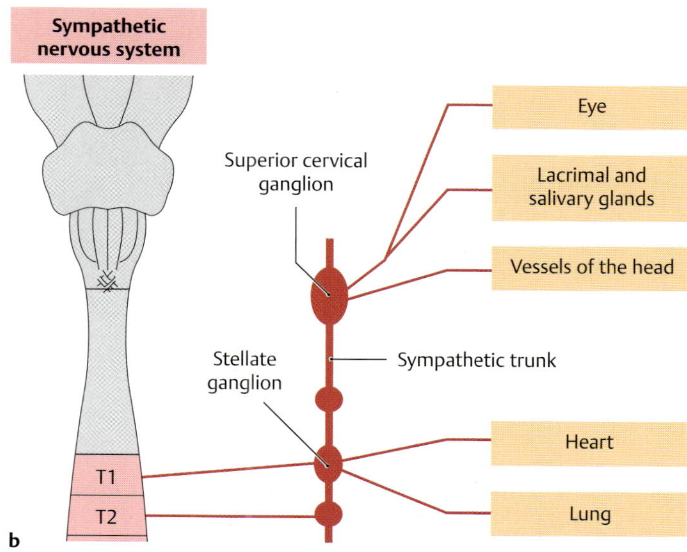

D Example: lower brachial plexus paralysis (Dejerine–Klumpke palsy)

This paralysis results from a lesion of the ventral rami of the C 8 and T 1 spinal nerves (see **A**). It affects the hand muscles, the digital flexors, and the flexor muscles in the wrist (claw hand with atrophy of hand muscles, **a**). Sensory disturbances affect the ulnar surfaces of the forearm and hand. Because the sympathetic fibers for the head leave the spinal cord at T 1 (**b**), the sympathetic innervation of the head is also lost. This is manifested by a *unilateral Horner syndrome,* characterized by miosis (contracted pupil due to paralysis of the dilator pupillae) and narrowing of the palpebral fissure (not ptosis) due to a loss of sympathetic innervation to the superior and inferior tarsal muscles. The narrowed palpebral fissure mimics enophthalmos (sinking of the eyeball into the orbit).

13.13 Lesions of the Lumbosacral Plexus

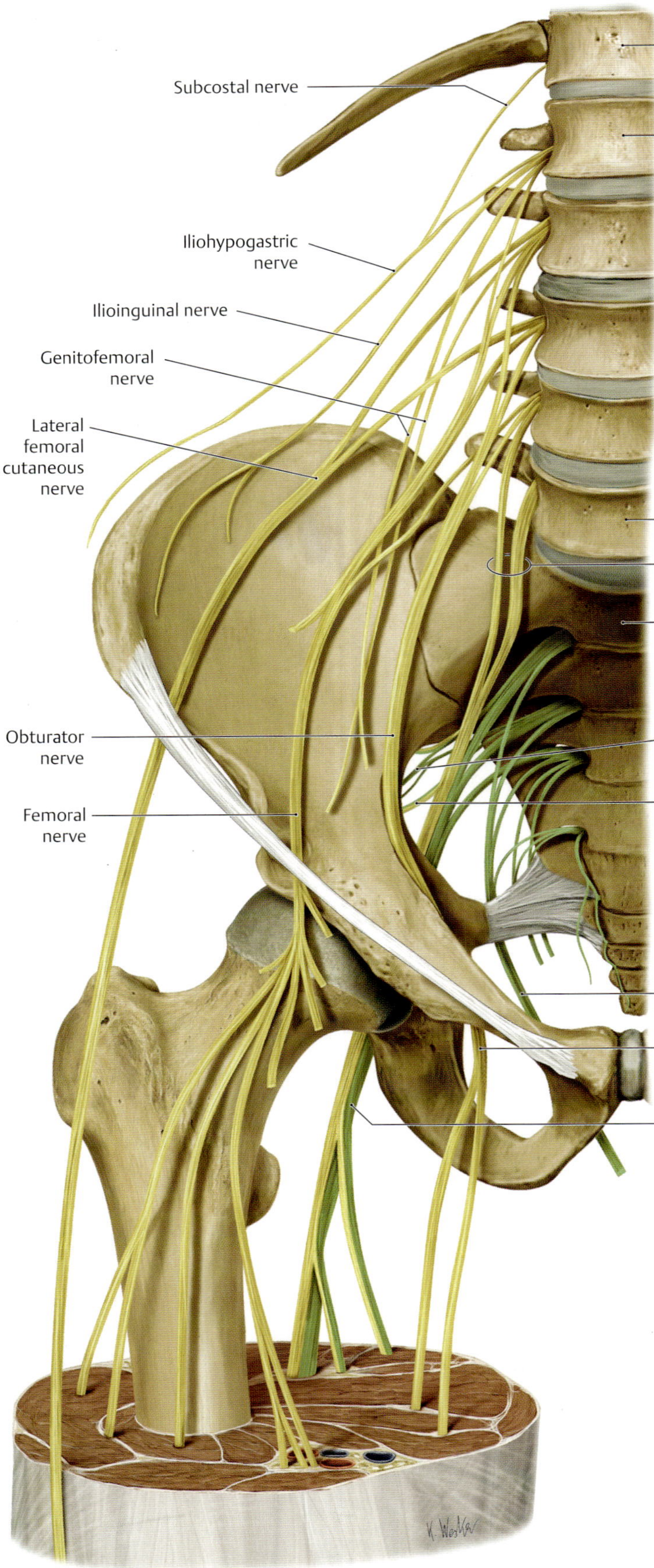

A Lumbosacral plexus
Anterior view. The lumbosacral plexus is divided into a lumbar plexus (T 12–L 4) and sacral plexus (L 5–S 4). The inferior fibers of L4 as well as all fibers of L 5 merge to form the lumbosacral trunk, which is the connection to the sacral plexus. The latter runs in dorsal direction.
Note: Most nerves of the lumbar component run in ventral direction whereas the nerves from the sacral component run in dorsal direction. Since the lumbosacral plexus lies very protected deep inside the pelvis, it is less frequently affected by lesions than the brachial plexus which runs closer to the surface. Lesions to the lumbosacral plexus occur in case of fractures of the pelvis ring, sacrum or hip and as a result of hip replacement.

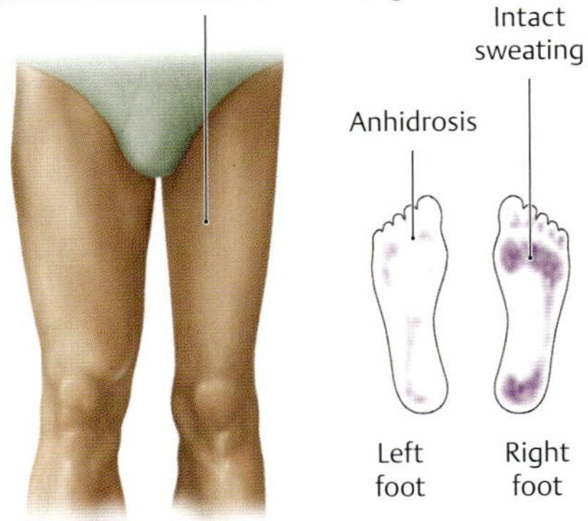

B Lesion of the left lumbar plexus (T 12–L 4)
The dominant feature of this condition is femoral nerve paralysis affecting the hip flexors, knee extensors, and the external rotators and adductors of the thigh (**a**). A sensory deficit is found on the anteromedial aspect of the thigh and calf. The lesion also disrupts the sympathetic fibers for the leg, which arise from the lumbar cord and pass through the lumbar plexus. The clinical manifestations (**b**) include increased warmth of the foot (loss of sympathetic vasoconstriction) and anhidrosis on the sole of the foot (sweating is absent because of loss of sympathetic innervation to the sweat glands). When sweating is intact, the ninhydrin test is positive (footprint on a sheet of paper stains purple with 1% ninhydrin solution).
Note: Manifestations in the limbs are recognized by comparison with the unaffected side.

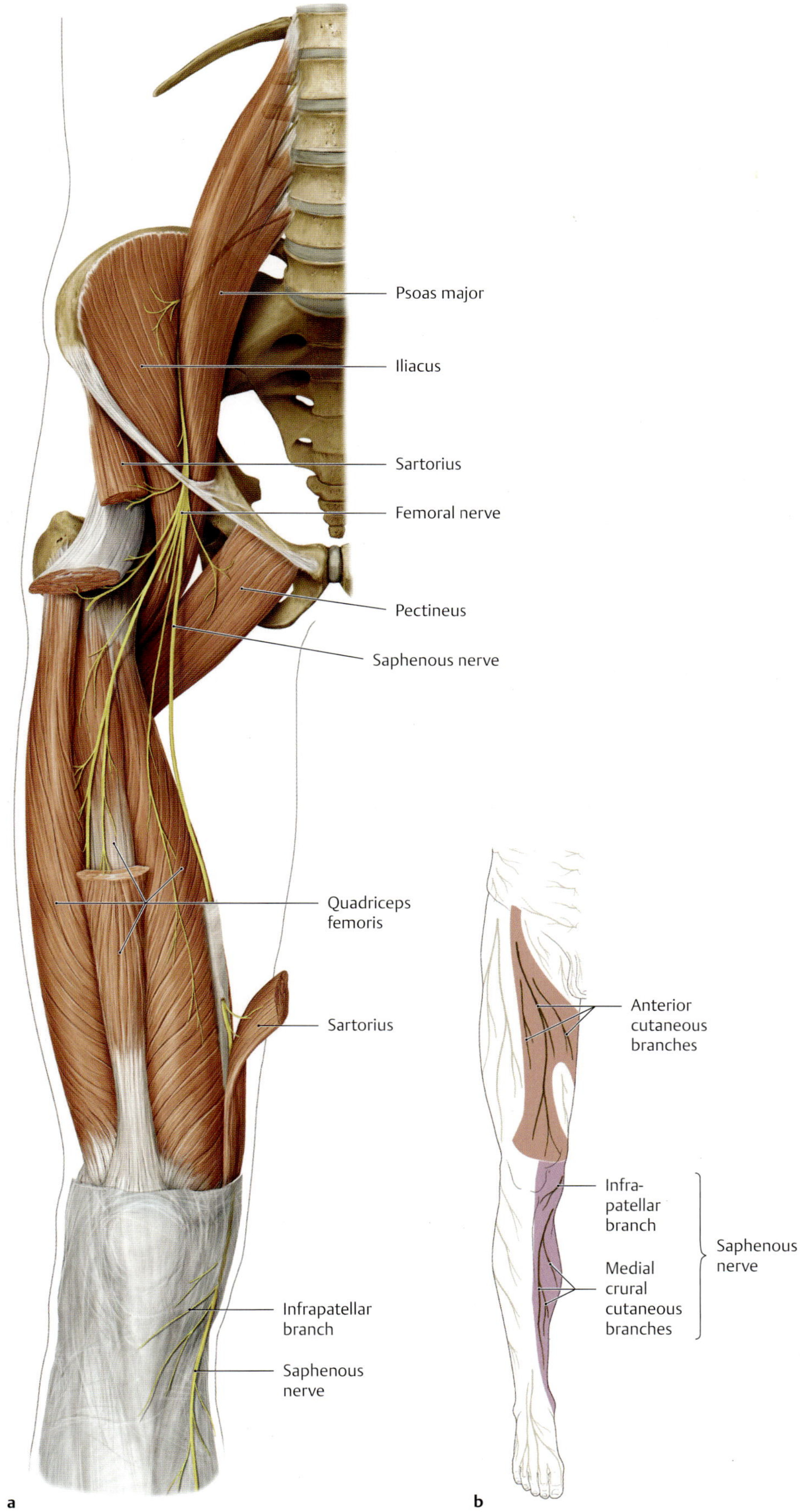

C Muscular and cutaneous distribution of the femoral nerve (L 1–L 4)
Anterior view.

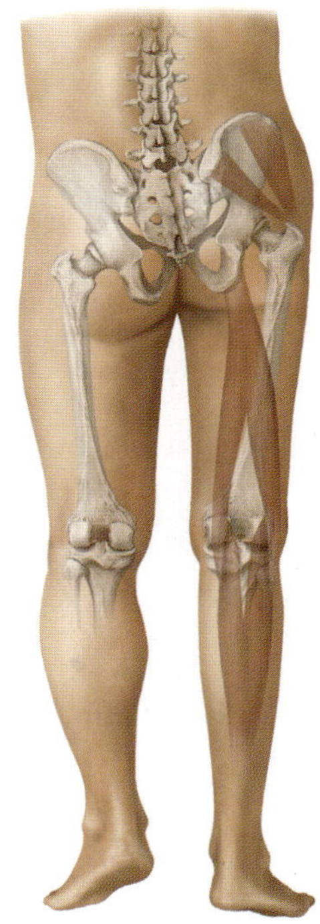

D Lesion of the right sacral plexus (L 5–S 4)
This lesion presents clinically with *paralysis of the sciatic nerve* and its two main branches, the tibial and common fibular nerves, which are jointly affected. The results are loss of plantar flexion (tibial nerve paralysis, inability to walk on the toes) and paralysis of the foot and toe extensors (common fibular nerve, steppage gait: the patient must raise the knee abnormally high while walking to avoid dragging the toes on the ground). Sensory disturbances are noted on the posterior surfaces of the thigh, lower leg, and foot. Because the *superior gluteal nerve* is involved, the gluteus medius and minimus are also paralyzed. These two muscles stabilize the pelvis of the stationary side during gait. When they are paralyzed, the pelvis tilts toward the swinging leg, producing a "waddling" gait (known also as a positive Trendelenburg sign). The superior gluteal nerve also innervates the tensor fasciae latae, which normally acts in the same manners as the two gluteal muscles. Specific categories of peripheral nerve lesions are described in the volume on *General Anatomy and Musculoskeletal System.*

13.14 Lesions of the Spinal Cord and Peripheral Nerves: Sensory Deficits

Overview of the next three units (after Bähr and Frotscher)
Two questions should be addressed in the diagnostic evaluation of spinal cord lesions:

1. What structure(s) within the *cross-section* of the spinal cord is (are) affected? This is determined systematically by proceeding from the periphery of the cord toward the center.
2. At what level of the spinal cord (in longitudinal section) is the lesion located?

In these units we will first correlate various deficit patterns (syndromes) with the structures in the cross-section of the spinal cord. We will then discuss the level of the lesion in the longitudinal or craniocaudal dimension. Since these syndromes present with deficits that result from damage to specific anatomical structures, they can be explained in anatomical terms. Based on the lesions and syndromes described here, the reader can test his or her ability to relate what has already been learned to the locations and effects of spinal cord lesions.

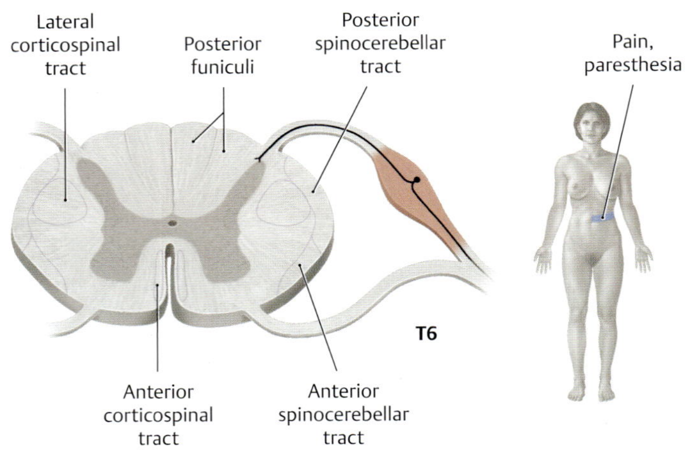

A Spinal ganglion syndrome illustrated for an isolated lesion of T 6
As part of the dorsal roots, the dorsal root (spinal) ganglia are concerned with the transmission of sensory information. (Recall that the ganglia contain the cell bodies of the first sensory neurons.) When only a single spinal ganglion is affected (e.g., by a viral infection such as herpes zoster), the resulting pain and paresthesia are limited to the sensory distribution (dermatome) of the ganglion. Because the dermatomes show considerable overlap, adjacent dermatomes can assume the function of the affected dermatome. As a result, the area that shows absolute sensory loss, called the “autonomous area” of the dermatome, may be quite small.

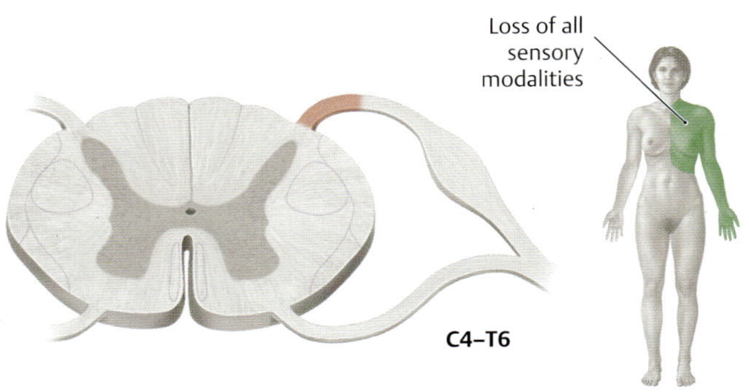

B Dorsal root syndrome illustrated for a lesion at the C 4–T 6 level
When a lesion (trauma, degenerative spinal changes, tumor) affects multiple successive dorsal roots as in this example, complete sensory loss occurs in the affected dermatomes. When this sensory loss affects the afferent limb of a reflex, that reflex will be absent or diminished. If the sensory dorsal roots are irritated but not disrupted, as in the case of a herniated intervertebral disk, severe pain may sometimes be perceived in the affected dermatome. Because pain fibers do not overlap as much as other sensory fibers, the examiner should have no difficulty in identifying the affected dermatome, and thus the corresponding spinal cord segment, from the location of the pain.

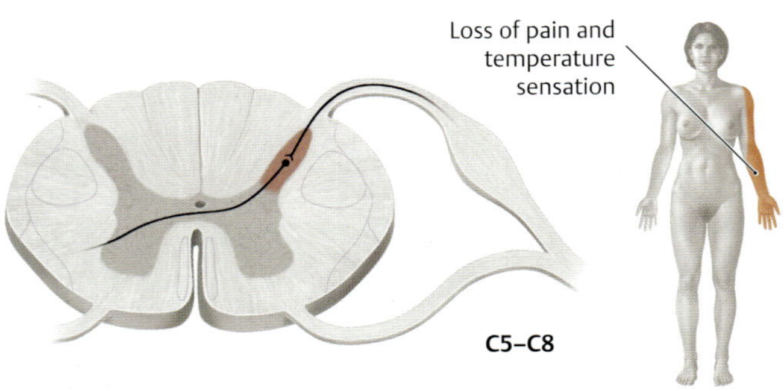

C Posterior horn syndrome illustrated for a lesion at the C 5–C 8 level
This lesion, like a dorsal root lesion of the spinal nerves, is characterized by a segmental pattern of sensory disturbance. But with a posterior *horn* lesion of the spinal cord, unlike a dorsal *root* lesion, the resulting sensory deficit is incomplete. Pain and temperature sensation are abolished in the dermatomes on the ipsilateral side because the first peripheral/afferent neuron of the lateral spinothalamic tract arrives to the posterior horn, which is within the damaged area. Position sense and vibration sense are unaffected because the fibers for these sensory modalities are both conveyed in the posterior funiculus. Bypassing the posterior horn, these fibers pass directly via the posterior funiculi and ascend to the nucleus gracilis or nucleus cuneatus where they synapse (see p. 404 f). A lesion of the anterior spinothalamic tract does not produce striking clinical signs. The deficit (loss of pain and temperature sensation with preservation of position and vibration sense) is called a *dissociated sensory loss.* Pain and temperature sensation are preserved below the lesion because the tracts in the white matter (lateral spinothalamic tract) are undamaged. This type of dissociated sensory loss occurs in syringomyelia, a congenital or acquired condition in which there is an expanded cavity in or near the central canal of the spinal cord. (According to the strictest terminology, expansion of the central canal itself = hydromyelia).

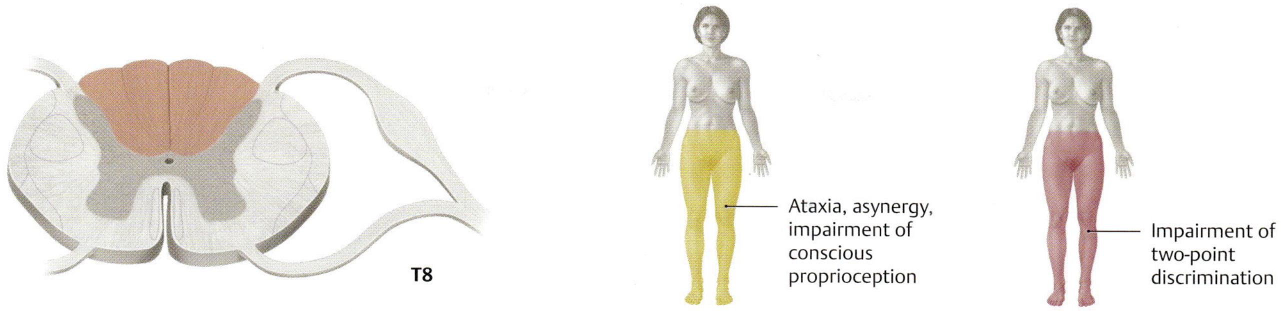

D Lesion of the posterior funiculi at the T 8 level

A lesion of the posterior funiculi (see also p. 404 f) is characterized by a loss of

- Position sense,
- Vibration sense, and
- Two-point discrimination.

These deficits occur distal to the lesion, hence they involve the legs and lower trunk when the lesion is at the T 8 level. When the legs are affected, as in the present example, the loss of position sense (mediated by proprioception, see p. 290) leads to an unsteady gait (ataxia). When the arm is affected (not shown here), the only clinical finding is sensory impairment. The lack of feedback to the motor system also prevents the precise interaction of different muscle groups during fine movements (asynergy). Ataxia results from the fact that information on body position is essential for carrying out movements. Vision can (partly) compensate for this loss of information when the eyes are open, and so the ataxia worsens when the eyes are closed (Romberg's sign). This *sensory ataxia* differs from *cerebellar ataxia* in that the latter cannot be compensated by visual control.

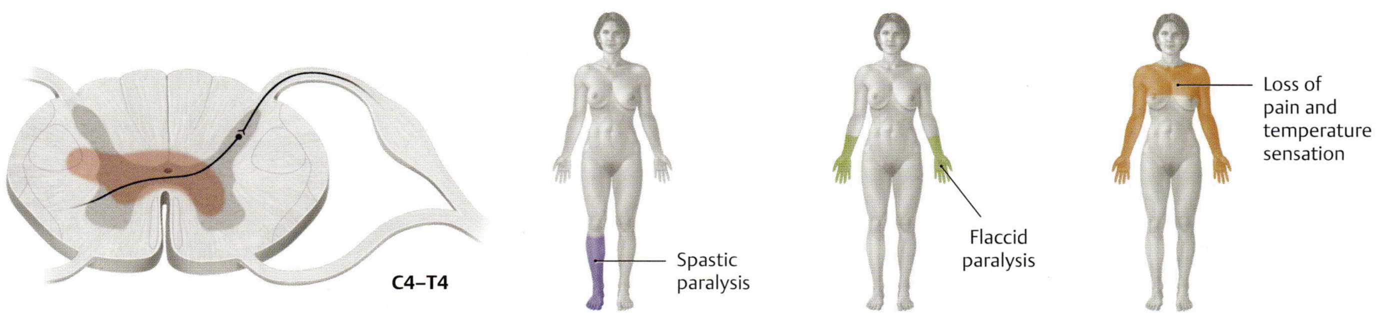

E Gray matter syndrome illustrated for a lesion at the C 4–T 4 level

This syndrome results from a pathological process (e.g., a tumor) in and around the central canal. All tracts that cross through the gray matter are damaged, i.e., the anterior and lateral spinothalamic tracts. The result is a dissociated sensory loss (loss of pain and temperature sensation with preservation of position, vibration, and touch), in this case involving the arms and upper chest (compare with **C**). A relatively large lesion may additionally affect the anterior horns, which contain the alpha motor neuron, causing a flaccid paralysis in the distal portions of the upper limb. An even larger lesion may concomitantly affect the pyramidal tract, causing spastic paralysis of the distal muscles (here in the legs). This syndrome may result from syringomyelia (see **C**) or tumors located near the central canal.

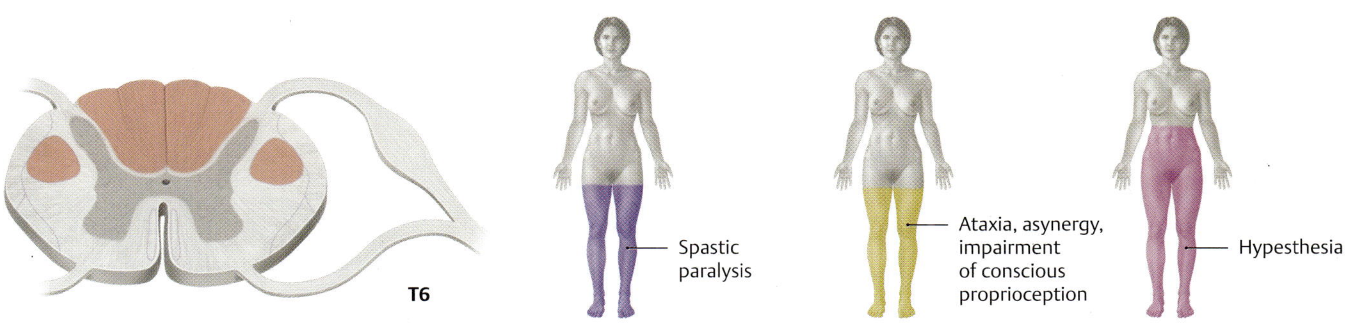

F Combined disease of the posterior funiculi and pyramidal tract illustrated for a lesion at the T 6 level

A *lesion of the posterior funiculi* leads to loss of position and vibration sense. A concomitant *pyramidal tract lesion* additionally leads to spastic paralysis of the legs and abdominal muscles below the affected dermatome (i.e., below T 6 in the example). This predominantly cervicothoracic lesion typically occurs in funicular myelosis (vitamin B12 deficiency), in which the posterior funiculi are affected initially, followed by the pyramidal tract. This disease is characterized by degeneration of the myelin sheaths.

13.15 Lesions of the Spinal Cord and Peripheral Nerves: Motor Deficits

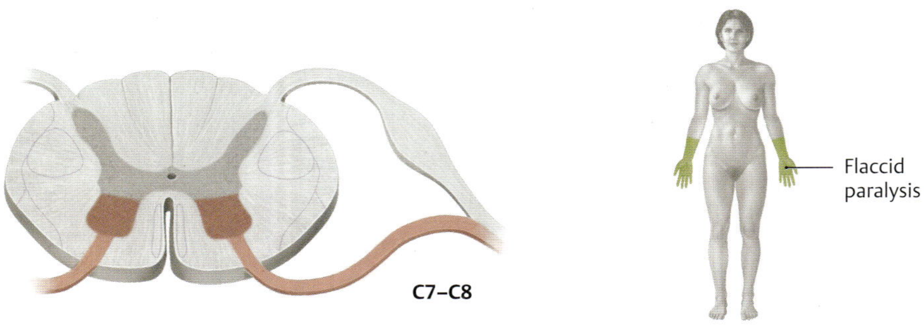

A Anterior horn syndrome illustrated for a lesion at the C 7–C 8 level

Damage to the motor anterior horn cells leads to ipsilateral paralysis, in this case involving the hands and forearm muscles because the lesion is at C 7–C 8 and these segments innervate the muscles in this region. The paralysis is flaccid because the alpha motor neuron that supplies the muscles (lower motor neuron) has ceased to function. Because larger muscles are supplied by motor neurons from more than one segment (see **A**, p. 398), damage to a single segment may lead only to muscular weakness (paresis) rather than complete paralysis of the affected muscle group. When the lateral horns are additionally involved, decreased sweating and vasomotor function will also be noted because the lateral horns contain the cell bodies of the sympathetic neurons that subserve these functions. This type of lesion may occur in poliomyelitis or in spinal muscular atrophy, for example. These relatively rare diseases are relentlessly progressive.

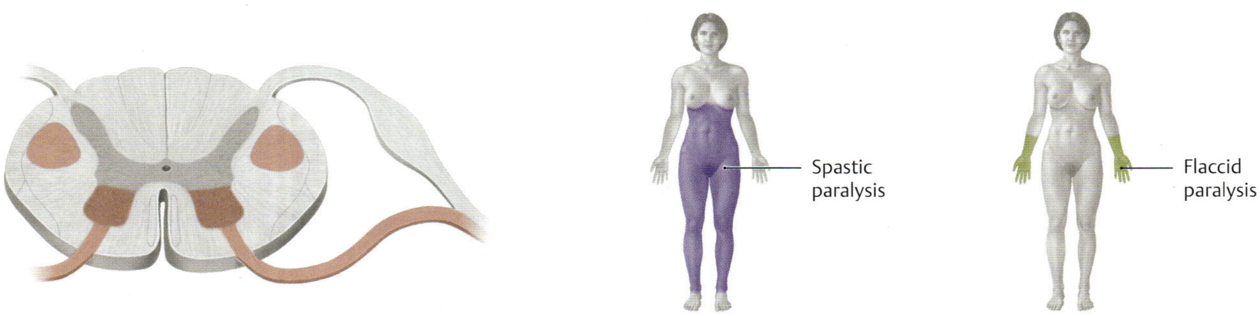

B Combined lesions of the anterior horn and lateral corticospinal tract

These lesions produce a combination of flaccid and spastic paralysis. Damage to the motor anterior horns or lower motor neuron causes flaccid paralysis, while a lesion of the lateral corticospinal tract or upper motor neuron causes spastic paralysis. The degree of injury to both types of neuron may be highly variable. In the example shown, an anterior horn lesion at the C 7–C 8 level has caused flaccid paralysis of the forearm and hand. By contrast, a lesion of the lateral corticospinal tract at the T 5 level would cause spastic paralysis of the abdominal and leg muscles.

Note: When the second motor neuron in the anterior horn is already damaged (flaccid paralysis), an additional lesion of the lateral corticospinal tract at the level of the same segment will not produce any noticeable effects.

This lesion pattern occurs in amyotrophic lateral sclerosis, in which the first cortical motor neuron (pyramidal tract lesion) and second spinal motor neuron (anterior horn lesion) both undergo progressive degeneration (etiology unclear). The end stage is marked by additional involvement of the motor cranial nerve nuclei, with swallowing and speaking difficulties (bulbar paralysis).

C Corticospinal tract syndrome

Progressive spastic spinal paralysis (Erb-Charcot disease) is characterized by a progressive degeneration of the cortical neurons in the motor cortex with increasing failure of the corticospinal pathways (axonal degeneration of the first motor neuron). The course of the disease is marked by a progressive spastic paralysis of the limbs that begins in the lower limbs and eventually reaches the upper limbs.

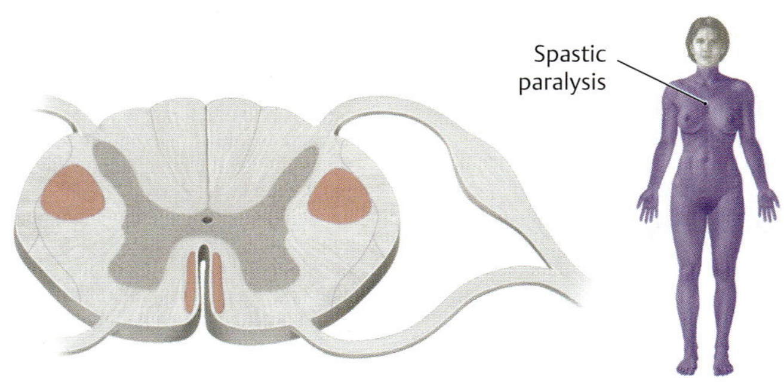

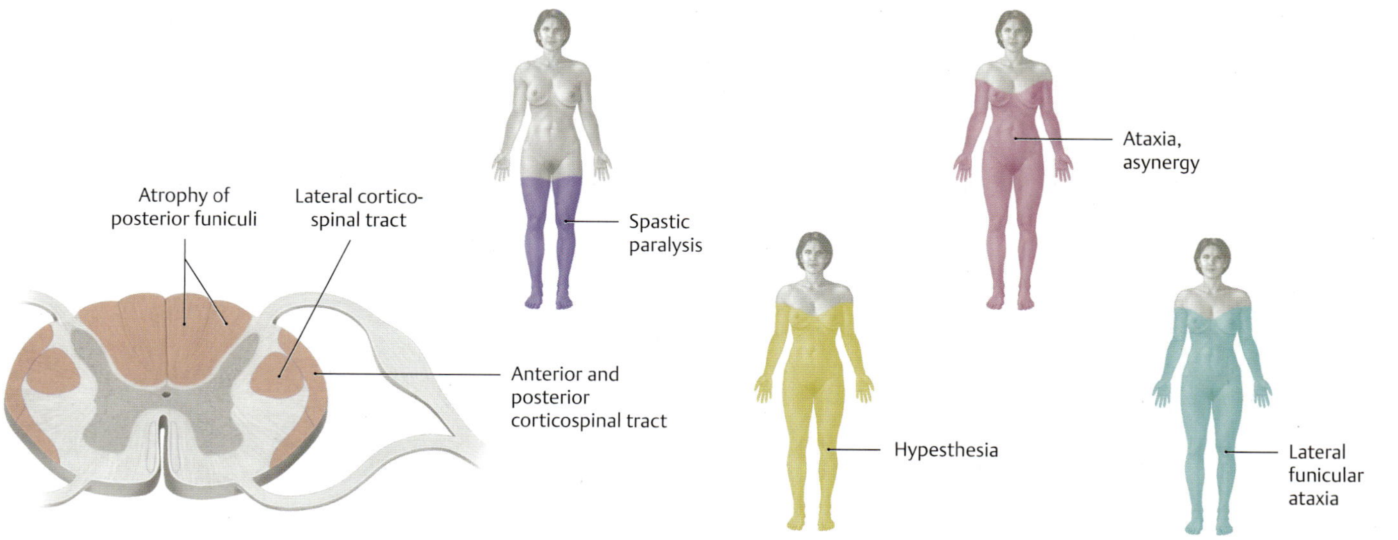

D Combined lesions of the posterior funiculus, spinocerebellar tracts, and pyramidal tract

This syndrome begins with destruction of the neurons in the dorsal root (spinal) ganglia, which transmit information on conscious position sense (loss: ataxia, asynergy), vibration sense, and two-point discrimination. This neuronal destruction leads to atrophy of the posterior funiculi. There is little or no impairment of pain and temperature sensation, which are still transmitted to higher centers in the unaffected lateral spinothalamic tract. The loss of conscious proprioception alone is sufficient to cause sensory ataxia (lack of feedback to the motor system, see **D**, p. 471). But the lesions additionally affect the spinocerebellar tracts (unconscious proprioception), injury to which suffices to cause ataxia, and so this dual injury causes a particularly severe loss of conscious and unconscious proprioception. This is the main clinical feature of the disease. Spastic paralysis also develops as a result of pyramidal tract dysfunction. The prototype of this disease is hereditary Friedreich ataxia, which has several variants. The gene has been localized on chromosome 19.

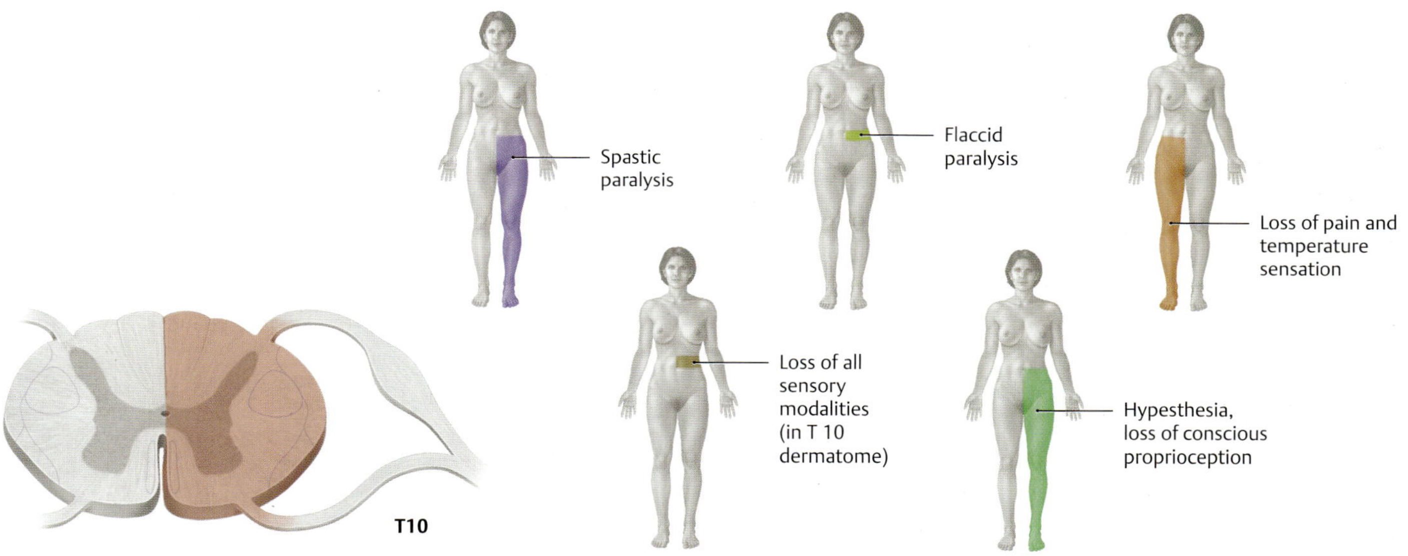

E Spinal hemisection syndrome (Brown–Séquard syndrome) illustrated for a lesion at the T 10 level on the left side

Hemisection of the spinal cord, though uncommon (e.g., in stab injuries), is an excellent model for testing our understanding of the function and course of the nerve tracts in the spinal cord. Spastic paralysis due to interruption of the lateral corticospinal tract (see footnote on p. 461) occurs on the side of the lesion (and below the level of the lesion). The interruption of the posterior funiculi (pathways for conscious proprioception) causes a loss of position and vibration sense and two-point discrimination on the side of the lesion. After spinal shock has subsided, spastic paralysis develops below the level of the lesion (here affecting the left lower limb). Of course, this paralysis does not produce an ataxia like that described following interruption of the posterior funiculi. Destruction of the alpha motor neurons in the locally damaged segment (in this case T 10) leads to ipsilateral flaccid paralysis associated with this segment. Because the axons of the lateral spinothalamic tract have already crossed to the unaffected side below the lesion, pain and temperature sensation is preserved on the *ipsilateral* side below the lesion. These two types of sensation are lost on the *contralateral* side, however, because the crossed axons on the opposite side have been interrupted at the level of the lesion. If spinal root irritation occurs at the level of the lesion, radicular pain may occur because of the descending course of the sensory (and motor) roots in the segment above the lesion (see **E**, p. 463).

13.16 Lesions of the Spinal Cord, Assessment

A Deficits caused by complete cord lesions at various levels

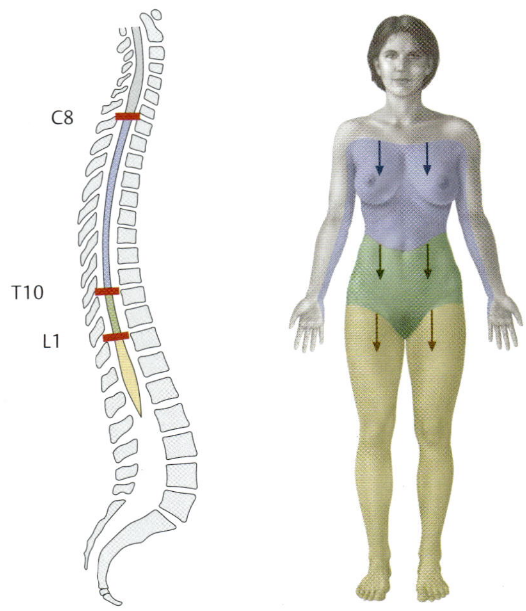

Having explored the manifestations of lesions at different sites in the cross-section of the spinal cord, we will now consider the effects of lesions at various levels of the cord. An example is the paralysis caused by a *complete spinal cord lesion,* which occurs acutely after a severe injury and is considerably more common than the incomplete lesions described earlier (see **E**, p. 473). A complete cord lesion following acute trauma is initially manifested by *spinal shock,* the pathophysiology of which is not yet fully understood. This condition is marked by complete flaccid paralysis below the site of the lesion, with a loss of all sensory modalities from the level of the lesion downward. Loss of bladder and rectal function and impotence are also present. Because the lesion also interrupts the sympathetic fibers, sweating and thermoregulation are impaired. The gray matter of the spinal cord recovers over a period ranging from a few days to eight weeks. The spinal reflexes return, and the flaccid paralysis changes to a spastic paralysis. There is a recovery of bladder and rectal function, but only at a reflex level since voluntary control has been permanently lost. Impotence is permanent. **Lesions of the cervical cord** above C 3 are swiftly fatal because they disrupt the efferent supply of the phrenic nerve (main root at C 4), which innervates the diaphragm and maintains abdominal respiration, while innervation to the intercostal muscles is also lost, causing a failure of thoracic respiration. A complete lesion of the lower cervical cord causes paralysis of all four limbs (quadriplegia), and respiration is precarious because of paralysis of the intercostal muscles. **Lesions of the upper thoracic cord** (T 2 downward) spare the arms but respiration is compromised because of paralysis of the intercostal muscles. A lesion of the **lower thoracic cord** (the exact site is unimportant) has little or no effect on the abdominal muscles, and respiration is not impaired. If the sympathetic splanchnic nerves are also damaged, there may be compromise of visceral motor function ranging to paralytic ileus (see p. 304). With **lesions of the lumbar cord**, a distinction is drawn between epiconus syndrome (L 4–S 2) and conus (conus medullaris) syndrome (S 3 downward). *Epiconus syndrome* is characterized by a flaccid paralysis of the legs (only the roots are affected, causing peripheral paralysis), and reflex but not conscious emptying of the bladder and rectum is preserved. Sexual potency is lost. In *conus syndrome,* the legs are not paralyzed and only the foregoing autonomic disturbances are present. The motor deficits described here are also associated with sensory deficits (see **B**).

B Deficits associated with complete spinal cord lesions at various levels (after Rohkamm)

Level of lesion	Motor deficits	Sensory deficits	Autonomic deficits
C 1–C 3 (high cervical cord lesion)	• Quadriplegia • Paralysis of nuchal muscles • Spasticity • Respiratory paralysis (immediate death if not artificially ventilated)	• Sensory loss from occiput or mandibular border downward • Pain in occipital region, back of neck, and shoulder region	• Reflex visceral functions (bladder, bowel) with no voluntary control • Horner syndrome
C 4–C 5	• Quadriplegia • Diaphragmatic respiration only	• Sensory loss from clavicle or shoulder downward	• See above
C 6–C 8 (lower cervical cord lesion)	• Quadriplegia • Diaphragmatic respiration • Spasticity	• Sensory loss from upper chest wall and back downward, and on the arms (sparing the shoulders)	• See above
T 1–T 5	• Paraplegia • Decreased respiratory volume	• Sensory loss from inside of forearm, upper chest wall and back	• Reflex function of bladder and rectum • Erection without voluntary control
T 5–T 10	• Paraplegia, spasticity	• Sensory loss from affected level in chest wall and back	• See above
T 11–L 3	• Paraplegia	• Sensory loss from groin region or front of thigh, depending on site of lesion	• See above
L 4–S 2 (epiconus, spinal nerve roots paralyzed)	• Distal paraplegia	• Sensory loss from front of thigh, dorsum of foot, sole of foot, or back of thigh, depending on site of lesion	• Flaccid paralysis of bladder and rectum • Impotence
S 3–S 5 (conus)	• No deficit	• Sensory loss in perianal region and inside of thigh	• See above

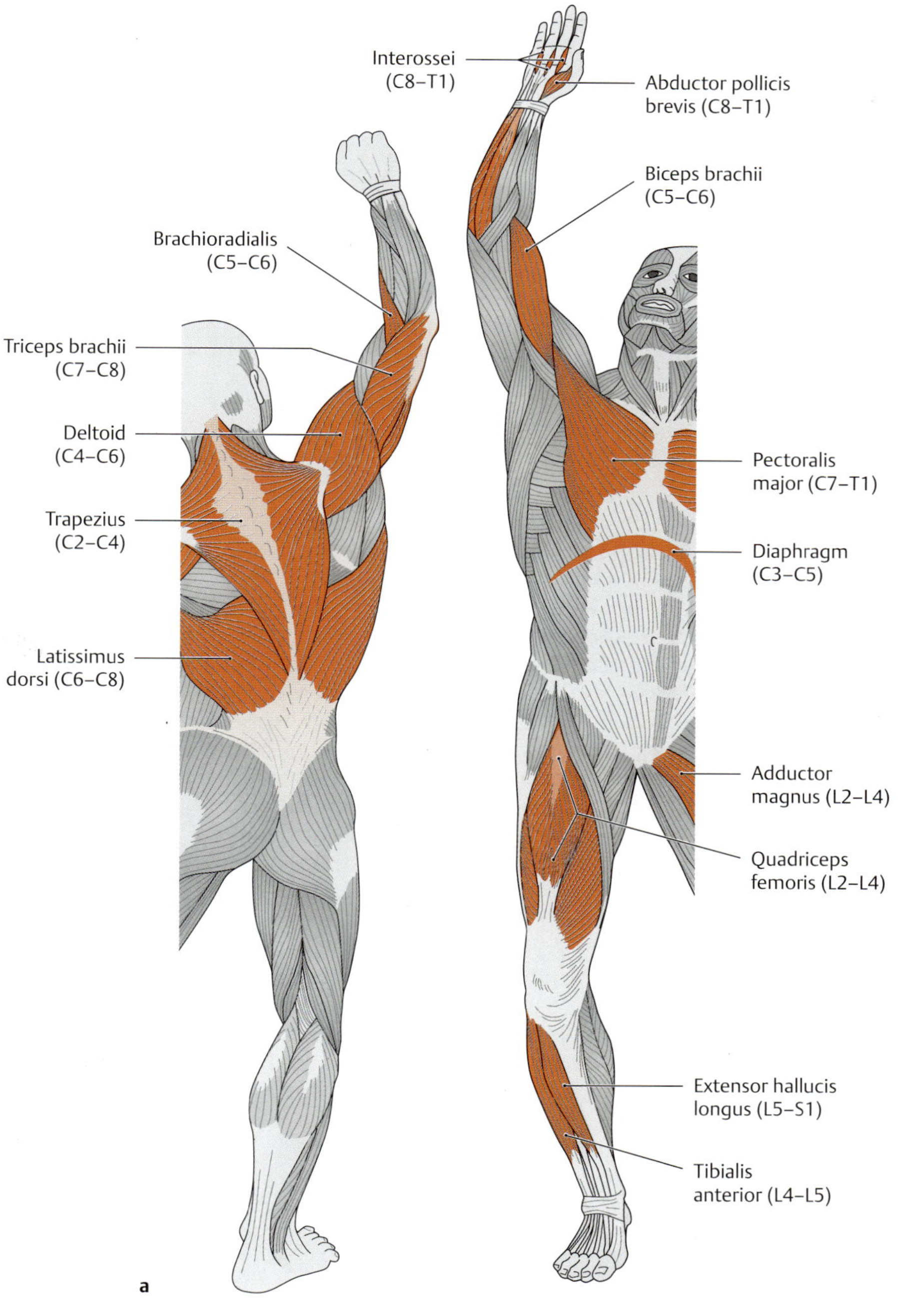

a

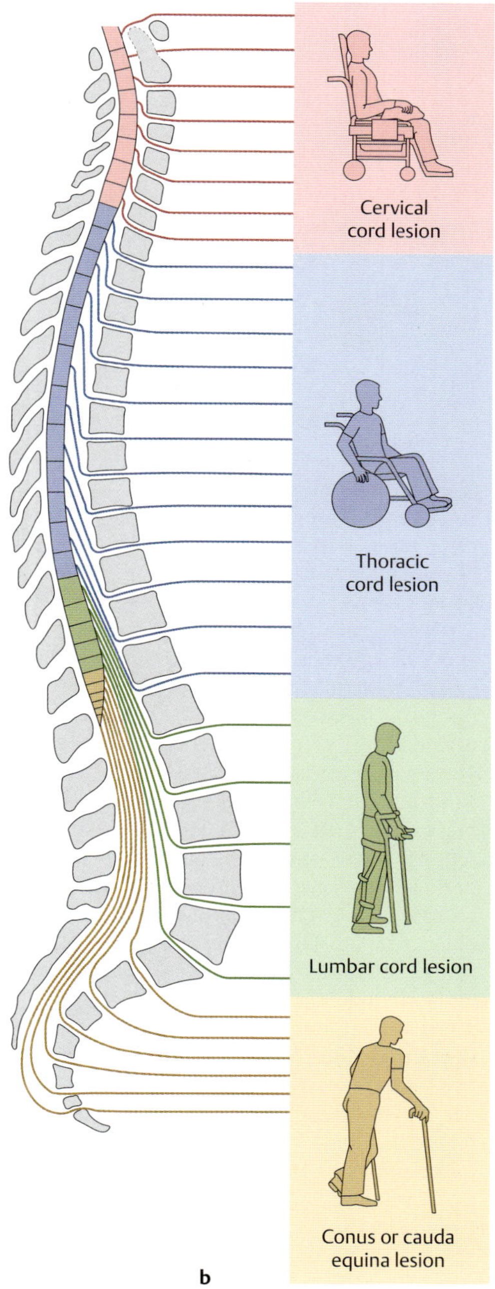

b

C Determining the level of spinal cord lesions

a Muscles and the spinal cord segments that innervate them. Most muscles are multisegmental, that is they receive innervation from several spinal cord segments. Thus, for example, a lesion at the C 7 level will not necessarily cause complete paralysis of the latissimus dorsi, because that muscle is also innervated by C 6. This is not the case with the "indicator muscles," which are supplied almost exclusively by a single segment (see B, p. 465). A lesion at the L 3 level, for example, will cause almost complete paralysis of the quadriceps femoris because that muscle is innervated almost entirely by L 3.

b The degree of disability varies, depending on the level of the complete cord lesion.

13.17 Visual System: Overview and Geniculate Part

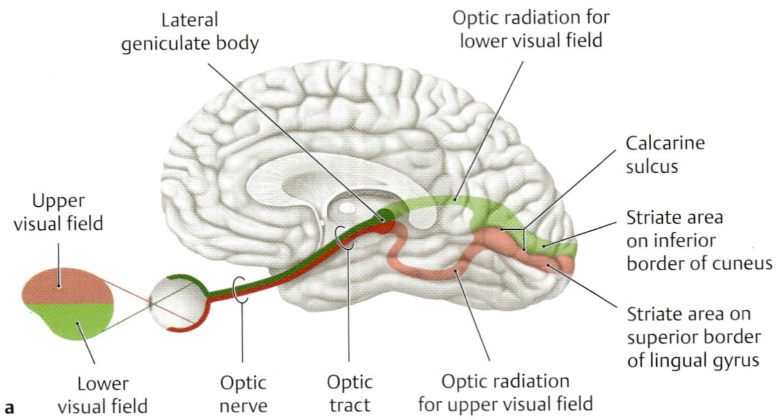

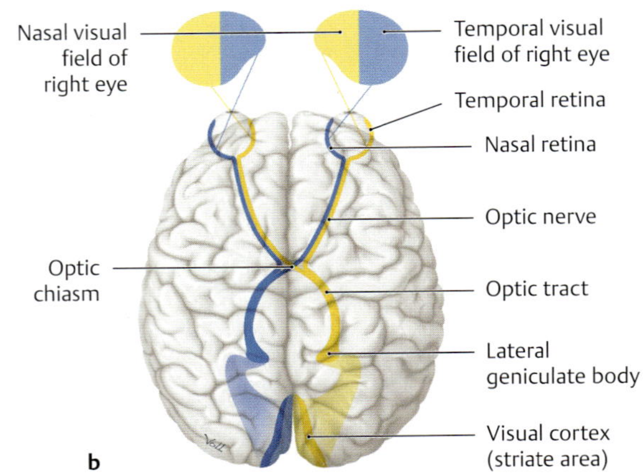

A Overview of the visual pathway

Left lateral view of the right cerebral hemisphere (**a**) and superior view through a transparent cerebrum (**b**).

The visual pathway begins in the retina (initial neuronal processing of visual stimuli, see **B**). The retina lies behind the pupil. This small aperture in the eye has the effect of projecting light rays incident from above onto the lower retina and light rays incident from below onto the upper retina (**a**). The same applies to light rays incident on the left and right (**b**). Thus, the image on the retina is upside down and reversed left to right, producing a **camera obscura or pinhole image effect**.

The retina and visual field are divided into four quadrants, which are connected in a very specific manner to the four quadrants of the primary visual cortex (see **C**). The axons of the third neuronal layer in the retina form the optic nerve (second cranial nerve) of each eye. The two optic nerves leave the respective orbit through the optic canal. Posterior to it they come together in the optic chiasm at the base of the diencephalon. Here the axons of the *nasal* retina cross to the contralateral side (see **b**). The fibers of the *temporal* retina continue on the ipsilateral side. This has the following effect on vision: Because the nasal halves of the retina look outward (temporal visual field, see **b**), the respective "outer half" of the visual world is conducted to the respective contralateral half of the brain whereas the "inner half" of the visual world (nasal visual field) remains in the ipsilateral half of the brain. This means that for the left half of the brain (see blue markings in **b**), it looks to the right with the *temporal* retina of the left eye (nerve fibers do *not cross*) and also looks to the right with the nasal retina of the right eye (fibers cross).

Note: Therefore, one half of the brain (in contrast to one eye, which sees the left *and* right world) only perceives the contralateral world. The upper and lower "worlds" are perceived as follows: Regardless of whether the fibers cross or not, information from the *upper* half of the retina (but from the lower visual field) ends in the *upper* visual cortex (above the calcarine sulcus at the lower border of the cuneus), whereas information from the *lower* half of the retina ends in the *lower* visual cortex (beneath the calcarine sulcus on the upper border of the lingual gyrus, see **a**). The upper portions of the visual cortex thus look down and vice versa. The pathway posterior to the optic chiasm, is no longer referred to as the "optic nerve" but is called the **"optic tract."** The vast majority of the optic nerve fibers (90%) course further in this tract to a nucleus in the thalamus, the **lateral geniculate** body (the *genicular portion* of the visual pathway), where they are again connected (fourth neuron). The neurons in the lateral geniculate body project the conscious visual perception onto the primary visual cortex on the occipital pole of the brain. The remaining 10% of the axons of the third neuron do not end in the lateral geniculate body (*non-genicular portion* of the visual pathway, see **B**, p. 479) and do not produce a conscious visual perception. The path from the neurons in the lateral geniculate body to the visual cortex (fifth neuron) is referred to as the **optic radiation**. It extends in a band over the lower and posterior horn of the lateral ventricle.

Note: Like the retina, the optic nerve, optic chiasm, and optic tract all belong to the CNS, specifically to the diencephalon. They are invested in meninges. The optic nerve is thus not a true nerve but a diencephalic pathway that has migrated anteriorly out of the brain.

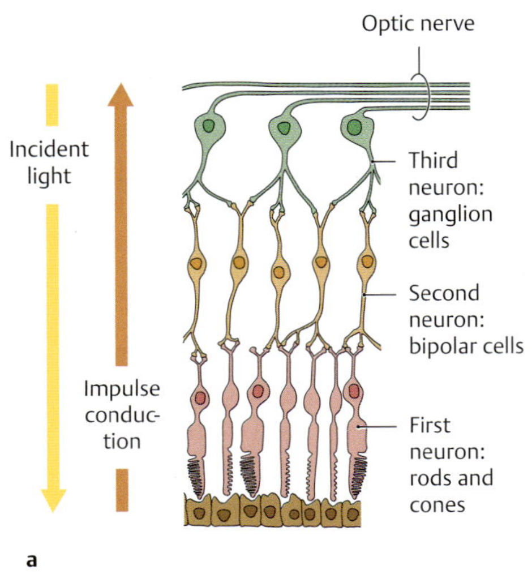

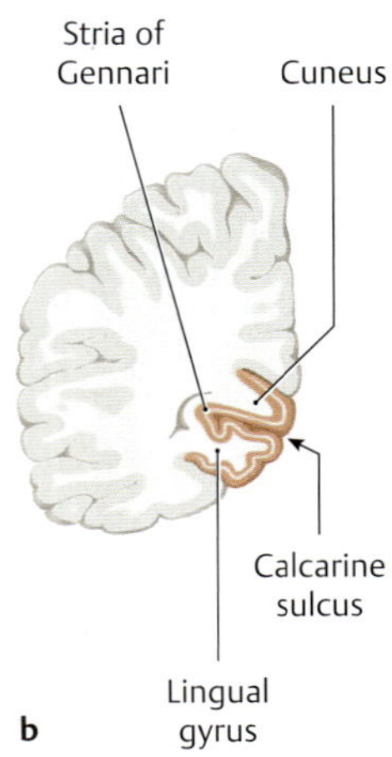

B Structure of the retina and visual cortex

a Circuitry of the retina; **b** coronal section through the occipital lobe.

Three layers of neurons connected in series form the retina. The first neuron is also a photoreceptor for black and white perception (rods) or color perception (cones). It is connected via bipolar cells (second neuron) with the third neuron, the ganglion cells. Its axons form the optic nerve.

Note: The photosensitive photoreceptors lie on the side of the retina facing away from the light (inversion of the retina).

A strong convergence of signal processing occurs during this connection; 125 million photoreceptor cells interact with 4 million ganglion cells. The entire primary visual cortex (striate area, area 17 after Brodmann) is subdivided into four quadrants; the longitudinal fissure divides the visual cortex into left and right halves (see **Ab**). The calcarine sulcus (see **Aa**) in turn divides each half into an upper portion (at the cuneus) and a lower portion (at the lingual gyrus). Within the visual cortex the fibers of the optic radiation are bundled together to form a macroscopically visible layer of white matter, the stria of Gennari.

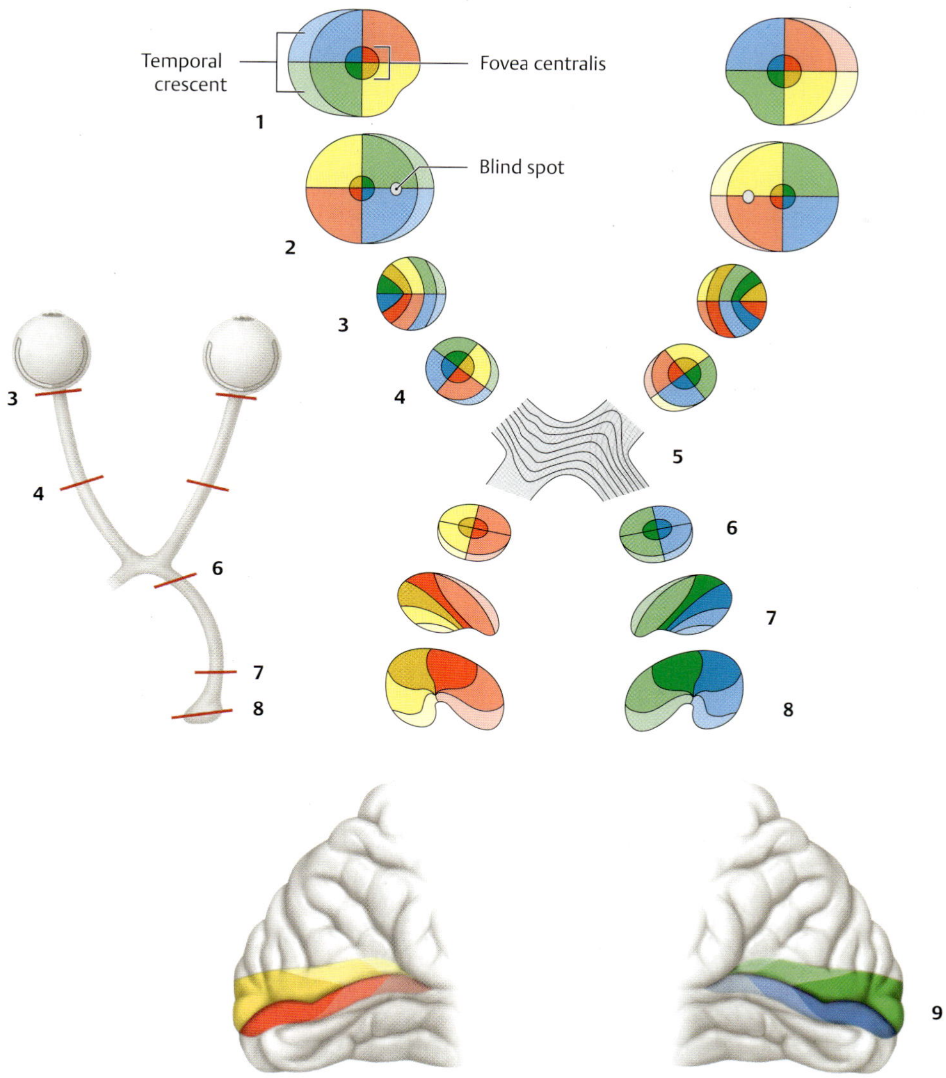

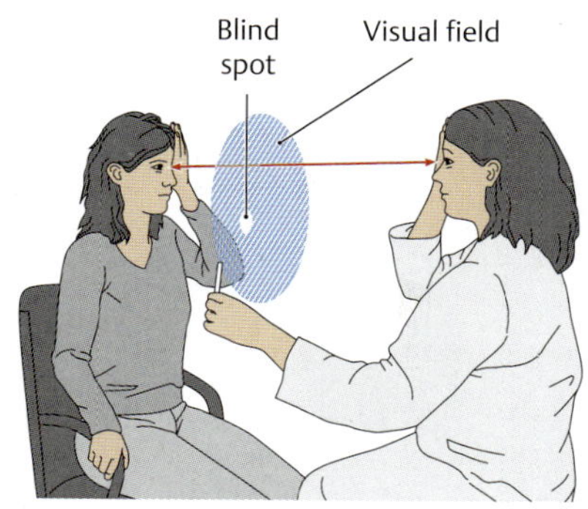

D Roughly determining the visual field with the confrontation test

Determining the visual field is an essential step in diagnosing impairments of the visual pathway (see **A**, p. 478). The confrontation test is a *rough* test for detecting visual field defects. The examiner (with an intact visual field) and the patient sit face-to-face. The physician and patient each fix their gaze on the other's open eye, creating identical visual axes. The examiner then moves his or her index finger or a stick from the outer edge of the visual field toward the center. The patient signals as soon as he or she can see the finger or stick. The *precise* extent of the respective visual field can be determined by perimetry, in which points of light replace the examiner's finger.

C Topographic organization of the geniculate part of the visual pathway

The fovea centralis, the point of maximum visual acuity on the retina, has a high receptor density. Accordingly, a great many axons pass centrally from its receptors, and so the fovea centralis is represented by an exceptionally large area in the visual cortex. Other, more peripheral portions of the retina contain fewer receptors and therefore fewer axons, resulting in a smaller representational area in the visual cortex. The figure is intended to illustrate this as well as showing the course of the nerve fibers from the various parts of the retina to the visual cortex.

1 **Representation of the visual field as measured by a perimeter:** The zones, which each correspond to a specific **field of view** (= left), are each marked on the left with decreasing color intensity
- The smallest and darkest zone is at the center of the fovea centralis; it corresponds to the central visual field.
- The largest zone is the macular visual field, which also contains the "blind spot" (= optic disk, see **2**).
- The "temporal crescent" represents the temporal, monocular part of the visual field.
- Note that the lower nasal quadrant of each visual field is indented by the nose (small medial depression).

2 **Retina:** Because the pupil acts as a pinhole aperture (see **Aa**), the image on the retina is inverted and reversed temporal to nasal.

3, 4 In the initial part of the **optic nerve**, the fibers that represent the macular visual field first occupy a lateral position (**3**) and then move increasingly toward the center of the nerve (**4**).

5 In traversing the **optic chiasm**, the nasal fibers of the optic nerve cross the midline to the opposite side.

6 At the **start of the optic tract**, the fibers from the corresponding halves of the retinae unite—the right halves of the retinae in the right tract, the left halves in the left tract. The impulses from the right visual field finally terminate in the left striate area. Initially the macular fibers continue to occupy a central position in the optic tract.

7 At the **end of the optic tract**, just before it enters the lateral geniculate body, the fibers are collected to form a wedge.

8 In the **lateral geniculate body**, the wedge shape is preserved, the macular fibers occupying almost half the wedge. These fibers synapse with the fourth neurons, which project to the posterior end of the occipital pole (visual cortex).

9 This figure shows that the central part of the visual field is represented by the largest area in the **visual cortex** compared with other portions of the field. This is due to the large number of axons that run to the optic nerve from the fovea centralis. This large proportion of axons is continued into the visual cortex, establishing a point-to-point (retinotopic) correlation between the fovea centralis and the visual cortex. The other parts of the visual field also show a point-to-point correlation but have fewer axons. The other visual fields also have point-to-point connections but send out significantly fewer axons. The central *lower* half of the visual field is represented by a large area on the occipital pole *above* the calcarine sulcus, while the central *upper* half of the visual field is represented *below* the sulcus. The region of central vision also occupies the largest area within the lateral geniculate body (see **8**).

13.18 Visual System: Lesions and Nongeniculate Part

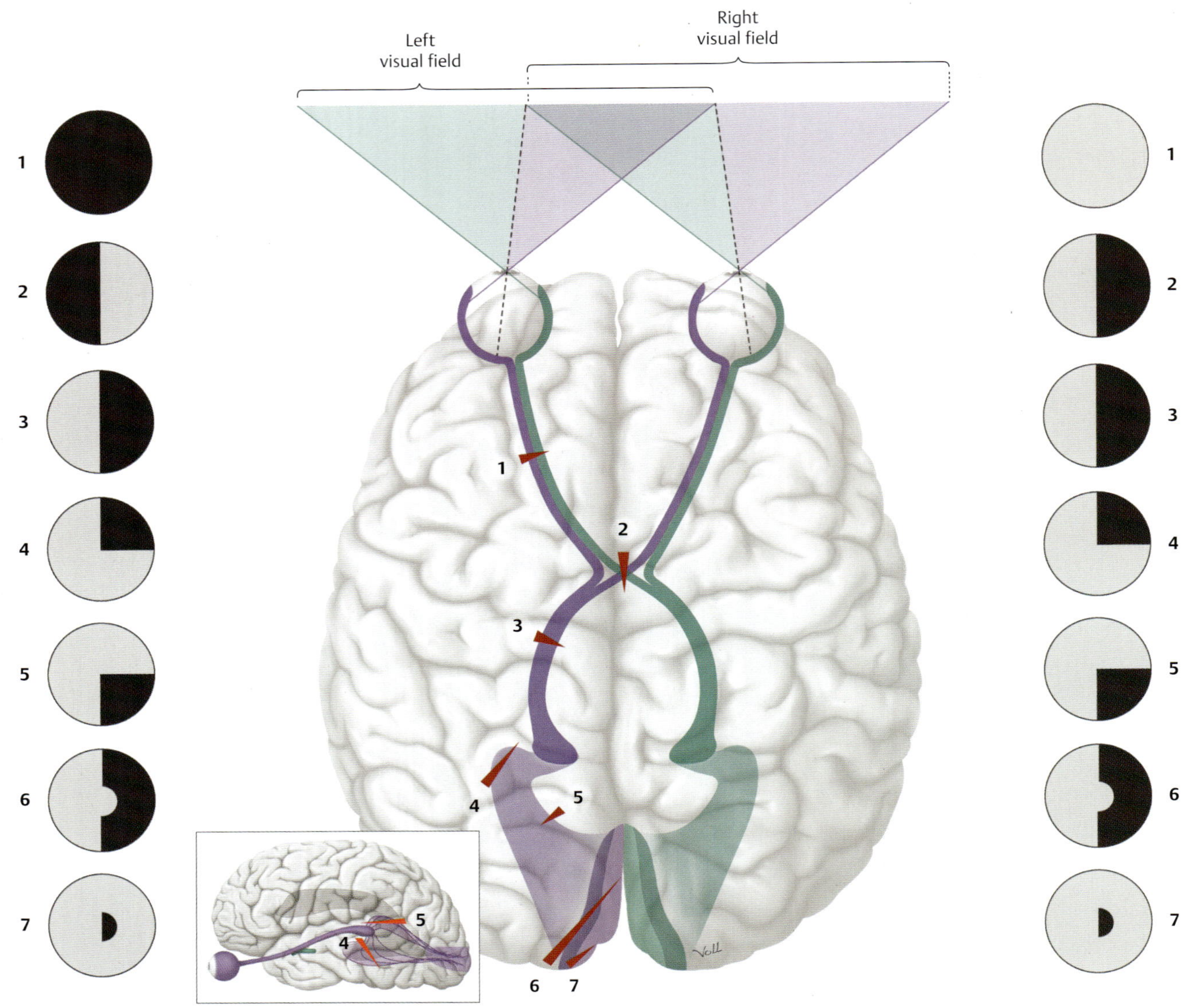

A Visual field defects (scotomata) and their location along the visual pathway

Visual field defects and lesion sites are illustrated here for the left visual pathway. Lesions of the visual pathway may result from a large number of neurological diseases. The patient perceives the lesion as a visual disturbance. Because the nature of the visual field defect often points to the location of the lesion, it is clinically important to know the patterns of defects that may be encountered. Division of the visual field into four quadrants is helpful in determining the location of a lesion. The quadrants are designated as upper and lower temporal, and upper and lower nasal (see also p. 477).

1 A unilateral optic nerve lesion produces blindness (amaurosis) in the affected eye only.
2 A lesion of the optic chiasm causes bitemporal hemianopia (as in a horse wearing blinders) because it interrupts the fibers from the nasal portions of the retina (the only ones that cross in the optic chiasm), which represent the temporal visual fields
3 A unilateral lesion of the optic tract causes contralateral homonymous hemianopia because it interrupts fibers from the temporal portions of the retina on the ipsilateral side and the nasal portions on the opposite side. Thus the right or left half of the visual field is affected in each eye.

Note: All homonymous visual field defects are caused by a retrochiasmal lesion.

4 A unilateral lesion of the optic radiation in the anterior temporal lobe (Meyer's loop) leads to contralateral upper quadrantanopia (a "pie-in-the sky" deficit). This occurs because the affected fibers wind around the inferior horn of the lateral ventricle in the temporal lobe and are separated from the fibers that come from the lower half of the visual field (see p. 476).
5 A unilateral lesion in the medial part of the optic radiation in the parietal lobe leads to contralateral lower quadrantanopia. This occurs because the fibers course superior to those for the upper quadrant in Meyer's loop (see p. 476).
6 A lesion of the occipital lobe leads to homonymous hemianopia. Because the optic radiation fans out widely before entering the visual cortex, lesions of the occipital lobe have been described that spare foveal vision. These lesions are most commonly due to intracerebral hemorrhage. The visual field defects may vary considerably because of the variable size of the hemorrhage.
7 A lesion confined to the cortical areas of the occipital pole, which represent the macula, is characterized by a homonymous hemianopic central scotoma.

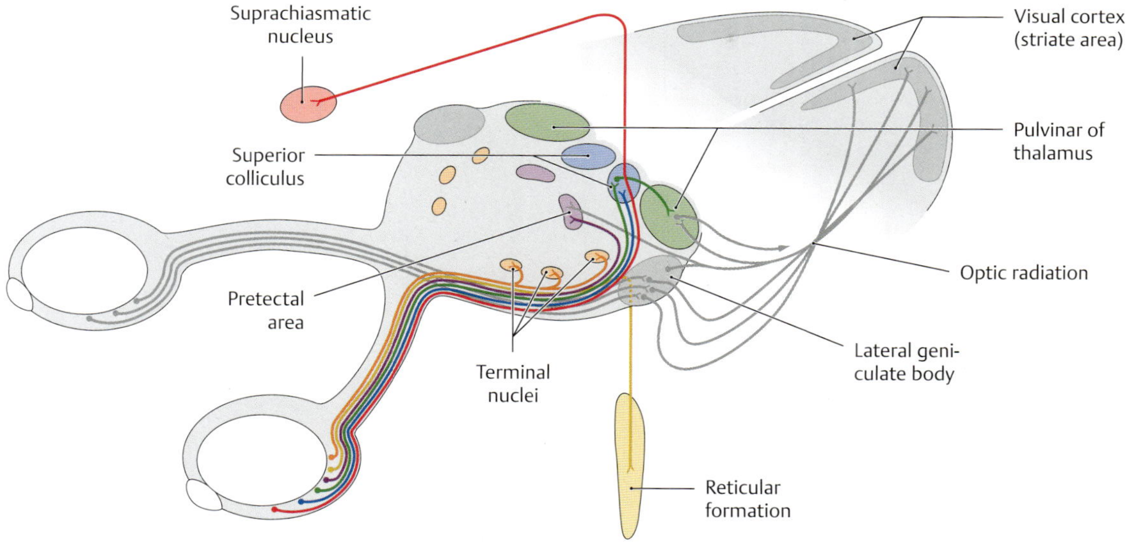

B Nongeniculate part of the visual pathway

Approximately 10% of the axons of the optic nerve do not terminate on neurons in the lateral geniculate body for projection to the visual cortex. They continue along the medial root of the optic tract, forming the *nongeniculate part* of the visual pathway. The information from these fibers is not processed at a conscious level but plays an important role in the unconscious regulation of various vision-related processes and in visually mediated reflexes (e.g., the afferent limb of the pupillary light reflex). Axons from the nongeniculate part of the visual pathway terminate in the following regions:

- Axons to the superior colliculus: transmit kinetic information that is necessary for tracking moving objects by unconscious eye and head movements (retinotectal system).
- Axons to the pretectal area: afferents for pupillary responses and accommodation reflexes (retinopretectal system). Subdivision into specific nuclei has not yet been accomplished in humans, and so the term "area" is used.
- Axons to the suprachiasmatic nucleus of the hypothalamus: influence circadian rhythms.
- Axons to the thalamic nuclei (optic tract) in the tegmentum of the mesencephalon and to the vestibular nuclei: afferent fibers for optokinetic nystagmus (jerky, physiological eye movements during the tracking of fast-moving objects). This has also been called the "accessory visual system."
- Axons to the pulvinar of the thalamus: visual association cortex for oculomotor function (neurons are relayed in the superior colliculus).
- Axons to the parvocellular nucleus of the reticular formation: arousal function.

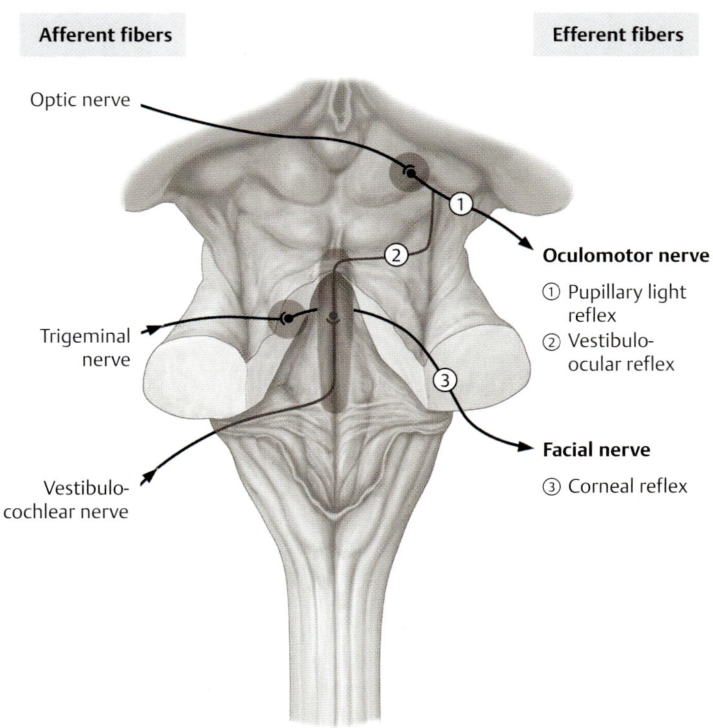

C Brainstem reflexes: clinical importance of the nongeniculate part of the visual pathway

Brainstem reflexes are important in the examination of comatose patients. Loss of all brainstem reflexes is considered evidence of brain death. Three of these reflexes are described below:

Pupillary light reflex: The pupillary light reflex relies on the nongeniculate parts of the visual pathway (see p. 481). The afferent fibers for this reflex come from the optic nerve, which is an extension of the diencephalon (since the diencephalon is not part of the brainstem, "brainstem reflex" is a somewhat unfortunate term). The efferents for the pupillary reflex come from the accessory nucleus of the oculomotor nerve (CN III), which is located in the brainstem. Loss of the pupillary reflex may signify a lesion of the diencephalon or mesencephalon (midbrain).

Vestibulo-ocular reflex: Irrigating the ear canal with cold water in a normal individual evokes nystagmus that beats toward the opposite side (afferent fibers are conveyed in the vestibulocochlear nerve: CN VIII, efferent fibers in the abducens and oculomotor nerves: CN VI and III). When the vestibuloocular reflex is absent or altered in a comatose patient, it is considered a poor sign because this reflex is the most reliable clinical test of brainstem function.

Corneal reflex: This reflex is not mediated by the visual pathway. The afferent fibers for the reflex (elicited by stimulation of the cornea, as by touching it with a sterile cotton wisp) travel in the trigeminal nerve and the efferent fibers (contraction of the orbicularis oculi in response to corneal irritation) in the facial nerve. The relay center for the corneal reflex is located in the pontine region of the brainstem.

13.19 Visual System: Reflexes

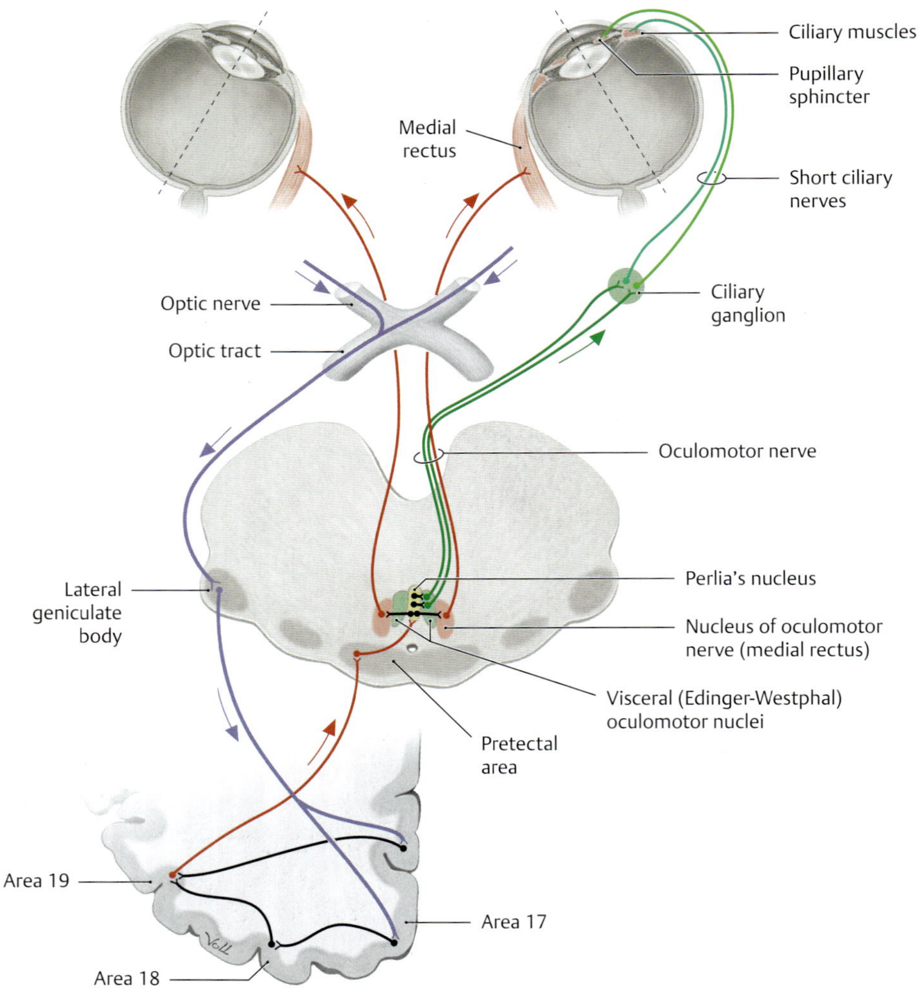

A Pathways for convergence and accommodation

When the head moves closer to an object, the visual axes of the eyes must move closer together (convergence) and *simultaneously* the lenses must adjust their focal length (accommodation). Both processes are necessary for a sharp, three-dimensional visual impression. Three subprocesses can be identified in convergence and accommodation:

1. In **convergence**, the two medial rectus muscles move the ocular axis inward to keep the image of the approaching object on the fovea centralis.
2. In **accommodation**, the curvature of the lens is increased to keep the image of the object sharply focused on the retina. The lens is flattened by contraction of the lenticular fibers, which are attached to the ciliary muscle. When the ciliary muscle contracts during accommodation, it relaxes the tension on the lenticular fibers, and the intrinsic pressure of the lens causes it to assume a more rounded shape.
3. The pupil is constricted by the sphincter pupillae to increase visual acuity.

Convergence and accommodation may be conscious (fixing the gaze on a near object) or unconscious (fixing the gaze on an approaching automobile). Most of the axons of the third neuron in the visual pathway course in the optic nerve to the lateral geniculate body. There they are relayed to the fourth neuron, whose axons project to the primary visual cortex (area 17). Axons from the secondary visual area (19) finally reach the pretectal area by way of synaptic relays and interneurons. Another relay occurs at that level, and the axons from these neurons terminate in Perlia's nucleus, which is located between the two Edinger-Westphal nuclei (visceral oculomotor nuclei). Two functionally distinct groups of neurons are located in Perlia's nucleus:

- For accommodation, one group of neurons relays impulses to the *somatomotor* oculomotor nucleus, whose axons pass directly to the medial rectus muscle.
- The other group relays the neurons responsible for accommodation and pupillary constriction to the *visceromotor* (parasympathetic) accessory nuclei of the oculomotor nerve (parasympathetic innervation is illustrated here for one side only).

After synapsing in this nuclear region, the preganglionic parasympathetic axons pass to the ciliary ganglion, where they synapse with the postganglionic parasympathetic neurons. Again, two groups of neurons are distinguished: one passes to the ciliary muscle (accommodation) and the other to the pupillary sphincter (pupillary constriction). The pupillary sphincter light response is abolished in tertiary syphilis, while accommodation (ciliary muscle) and convergence are preserved. This phenomenon, called an Argyll Robertson pupil, suggests that the connections to the ciliary and pupillary sphincter muscles are mediated by different tracts, although the anatomy of these tracts is not yet fully understood.

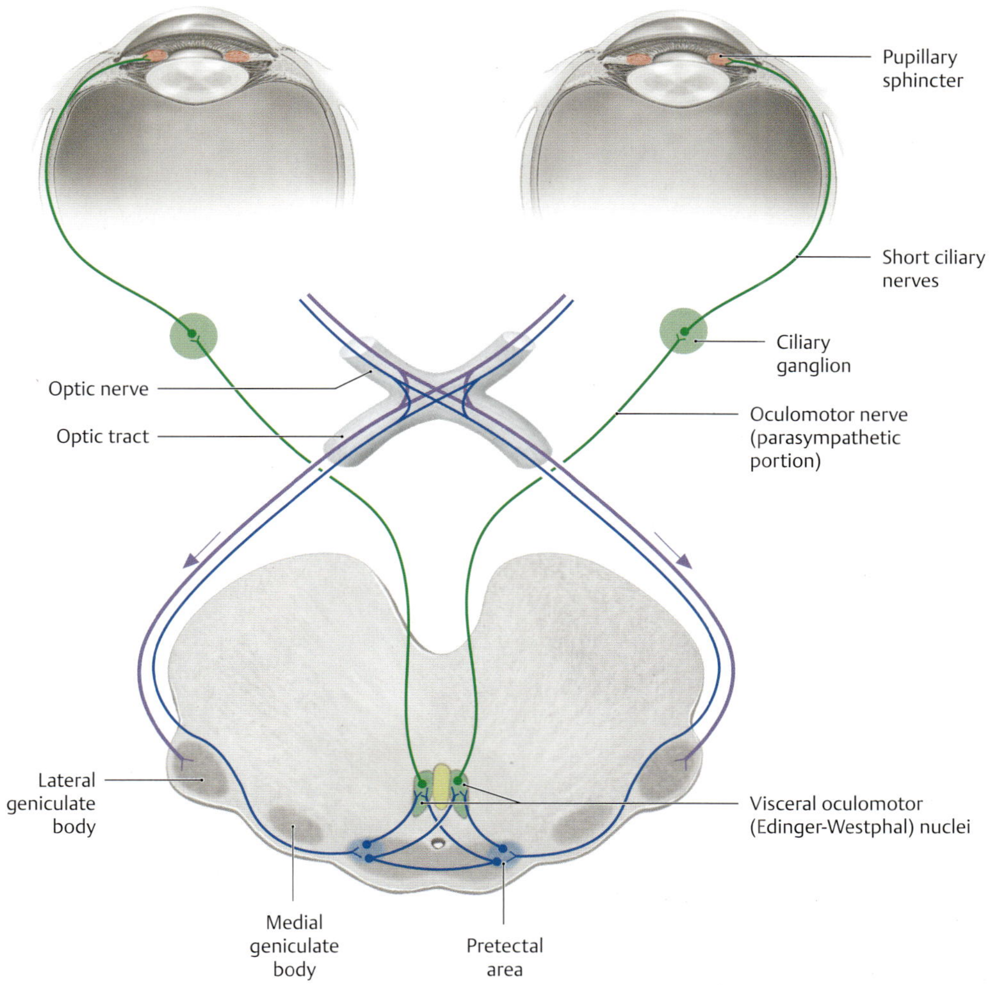

B Regulation of pupillary size—the light reflex

The pupillary light reflex enables the eye to adapt to varying levels of brightness. When a large amount of light enters the eye, like the beam of a flashlight, the pupil constricts (to protect the photoreceptors in the retina); when the light fades, the pupil dilates. As the term "reflex" implies, this adaptation takes place without conscious input (*nongeniculate* part of the visual pathway).

Afferent limb of the light reflex: The first three neurons (first neurons: rods and cones; second neurons: bipolar cells; third neurons: ganglion cells) in the *afferent* limb of the light reflex are located in the retina. The axons from the ganglion cells form the optic nerve. The axons responsible for the light reflex (blue) pass to the pretectal area (nongeniculate part of the visual pathway) in the medial root of the optic tract. The other axons pass to the lateral geniculate body (purple). After synapsing in the pretectal nucleus, the axons from the fourth neurons pass to the parasympathetic nuclei (accessory nuclei of the oculomotor nerve: Edinger-Westphal nuclei) of the oculomotor nerve. Because *both* sides are innervated, a *consensual light response* will occur (see below).

Efferent limb of the light reflex: The neurons located in the Edinger-Westphal nucleus (preganglionic parasympathetic neurons) distribute their axons to the ciliary ganglion. There they are relayed to postganglionic parasympathetic neurons that send their axons to the pupillary sphincter.

The *direct* pupillary light response is distinguished from the consensual (indirect) response:

The **direct light response** is tested by covering both eyes of the conscious, cooperative patient and then uncovering one eye. After a short latency period, the pupil of the light-exposed eye will contract.

To test the **indirect light response**, the examiner places his hand on the bridge of the patient's nose, shading one eye from the beam of a flashlight while shining it into the other eye. The object is to test whether shining the light into one eye will cause the pupil of the shaded eye to contract as well (*consensual light response*).

Loss of the light response due to certain lesions: With a unilateral optic nerve lesion, shining a light into the affected side will induce no direct light response on the affected side. The consensual light response on the opposite side will also be lost because of impairment of the afferent limb of the light response on the affected side. Illumination of the unaffected side will, of course, elicit pupillary contraction on that side (direct light response). A consensual light response is also present because the afferent signals for this reflex are mediated by the unaffected side while the efferent signals are not mediated by the optic nerve. With a lesion of the parasympathetic oculomotor nucleus or ciliary ganglion, the efferent limb of the reflex is lost. In either case the patient has no direct or indirect pupillary light response on the affected side. A lesion of the optic radiation or visual cortex (*geniculate* part of the visual pathway) does not abolish this reflex given that it will affect only the geniculate part of the visual pathway.

13.20 Visual System: Coordination of Eye Movement

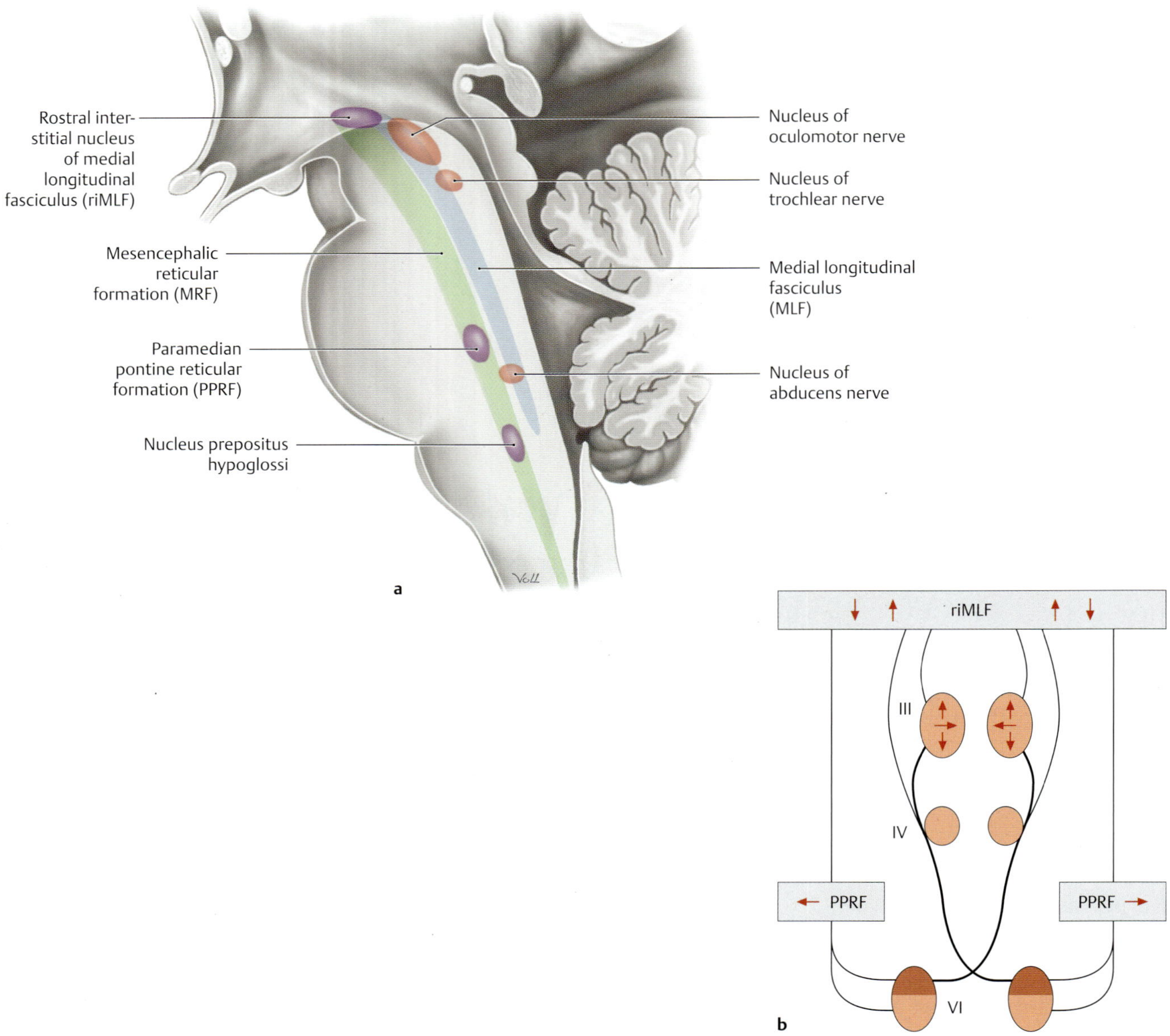

A Oculomotor nuclei and their higher connections in the brainstem

a Midsagittal section viewed from the left side. **b** Circuit diagram showing the supranuclear organization of eye movements.

When we shift our gaze to a new object, we swiftly move the axis of vision of our eyes toward the intended target. These rapid, precise, "ballistic" eye movements are called *saccades*. They are preprogrammed and, once initiated, cannot be altered until the end of the saccadic movement. The nuclei of all the nerves that supply the eye muscles (nuclei of cranial nerves III, IV, and VI, shaded red) are involved in carrying out these movements. They are interconnected for this purpose by the *medial longitudinal fasciculus* (shaded blue; see **B** for its location). Because these complex movements essentially involve all of the extraocular muscles and the nerves supplying them, the activity of the nuclei must be coordinated at a higher or *supranuclear level*. This means, for example, that when we gaze to the right with the *right* eye, the right lateral rectus muscle (CN VI, abducens nucleus activated) must contract while the right medial rectus muscle (CN III, oculomotor nucleus inhibited) must relax. For the *left* eye, the left lateral rectus (CN VI) must relax while the left medial rectus (CN III) must contract. Movements of this kind that involve both eyes are called *conjugate eye movements*. These movements are coordinated by several centers (premotor nuclei, shaded purple). Horizontal gaze movements are programmed in the nuclear region of the paramedian pontine reticular formation (PPRF), while vertical gaze movements are programmed in the rostral interstitial nucleus of the medial longitudinal fasciculus (riMLF). Both gaze centers establish bilateral connections with the nuclei of cranial nerves III, IV, and VI. The tonic signals for maintaining the new eye position originate from the nucleus prepositus hypoglossi (see **a**).

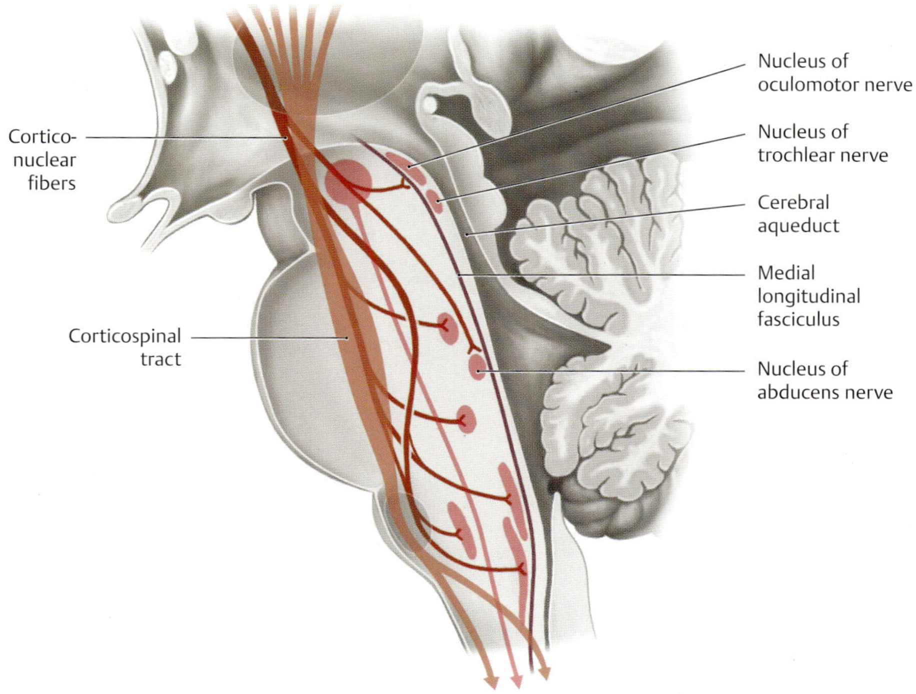

B Course of the medial longitudinal fasciculus in the brainstem

Midsagittal section viewed from the left side. The medial longitudinal fasciculus runs anterior to the cerebral aqueduct on both sides and continues from the mesencephalon to the cervical spinal cord. It transmits fibers for the coordination of conjugate eye movements. A lesion of the MLF results in internuclear ophthalmoplegia (see **C**).

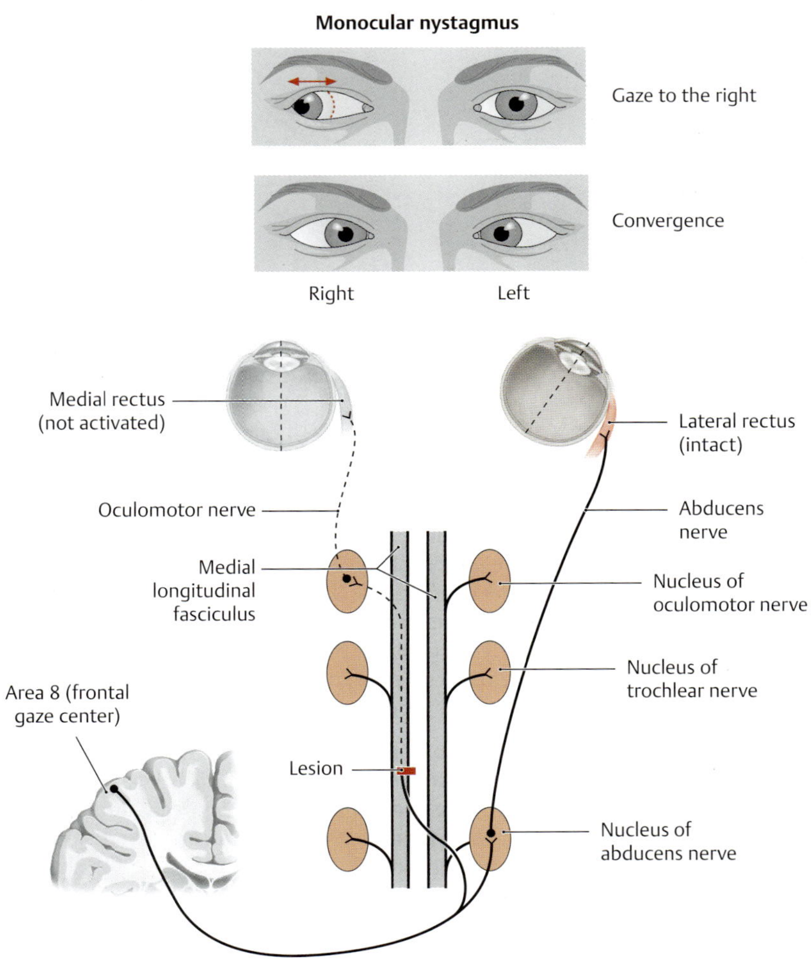

C Lesion of the medial longitudinal fasciculus and internuclear ophthalmoplegia

The medial longitudinal fasciculus interconnects the oculomotor nuclei and also connects them with the opposite side (**b**). When this "information highway" is interrupted, internuclear ophthalmoplegia develops. This type of lesion most commonly occurs between the abducens nucleus and the oculomotor nucleus. It may be unilateral or bilateral. Typical causes are multiple sclerosis and diminished blood flow. The lesion is manifested by the loss of conjugate eye movements (**a**). With a lesion of the left medial longitudinal fasciculus, as shown here, the left medial rectus muscle is no longer activated during gaze to the right. The eye cannot be moved *inward* on the side of the lesion (loss of the medial rectus), and the opposite eye goes into an abducting nystagmus (lateral rectus is intact and innervated by the abducent nerve). Reflex movements such as convergence are not impaired because there is no peripheral or nuclear lesion and this reaction is not mediated by the medial longitudinal fasciculus.

13.21 Auditory Pathway

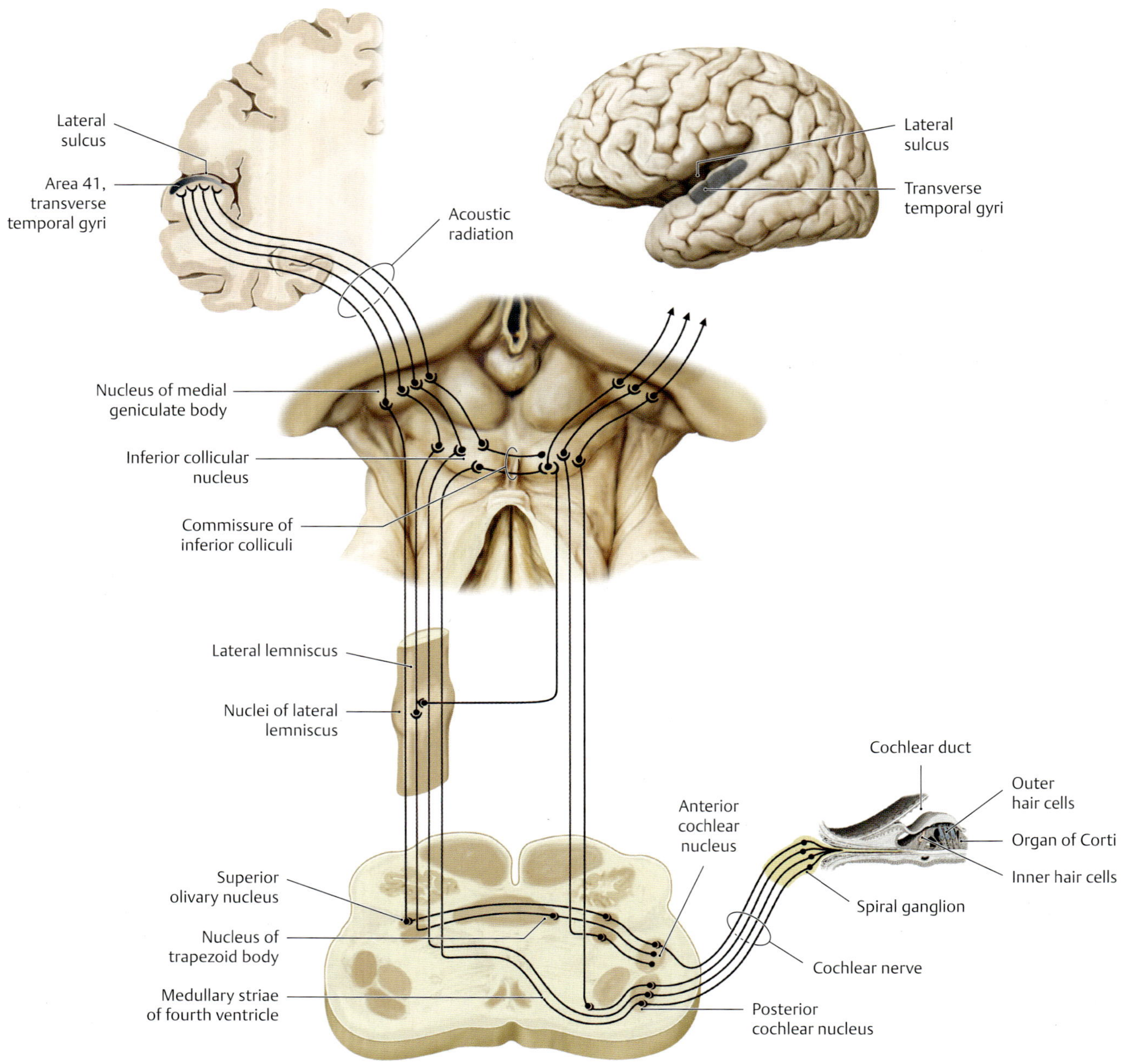

A Afferent auditory pathway of the left ear

The receptors of the auditory pathway are the inner hair cells of the organ of Corti. Because they lack neural processes, they are called *secondary sensory cells.* They are located in the cochlear duct of the basilar membrane and are studded with stereocilia, which are exposed to shearing forces from the tectorial membrane in response to a traveling wave. This causes bowing of the stereocilia (see p. 153). These bowing movements act as a stimulus to evoke cascades of neural signals. Dendritic processes of the bipolar neurons in the spiral ganglion pick up the stimulus. The bipolar neurons then transmit impulses via their axons, which are collected to form the cochlear nerve, to the anterior and posterior cochlear nuclei. In these nuclei the signals are relayed to the second neuron of the auditory pathway. Information from the cochlear nuclei is then transmitted via 4–6 nuclei to the primary auditory cortex, where the auditory information is consciously perceived (analogous to the visual cortex). The primary auditory cortex is located—somewhat hidden in the lateral sulcus—in the transverse temporal gyri (Heschl gyri, Brodmann area 41). The auditory pathway thus contains the following key stations:

- Inner hair cells in the organ of Corti
- Spiral ganglion
- Anterior and posterior cochlear nuclei
- Nucleus of the trapezoid body and superior olivary nucleus
- Nucleus of the lateral lemniscus
- Inferior collicular nucleus
- Nucleus of medial geniculate body
- Primary auditory cortex in the temporal lobe (transverse temporal gyri: Heschl gyri or Brodmann area 41)

The individual parts of the cochlea are correlated with specific areas in the auditory cortex and its relay stations. This is known as the *tonotopic organization of the auditory pathway.* This organizational principle is similar to that in the visual pathway. Binaural processing of the auditory information: stereo hearing) first occurs at the level of the superior olivary nucleus. At all further stages of the auditory pathway there are also interconnections between the right and left sides of the auditory pathway (for clarity, these are not shown here). A cochlea that has ceased to function can sometimes be replaced with a cochlear implant.

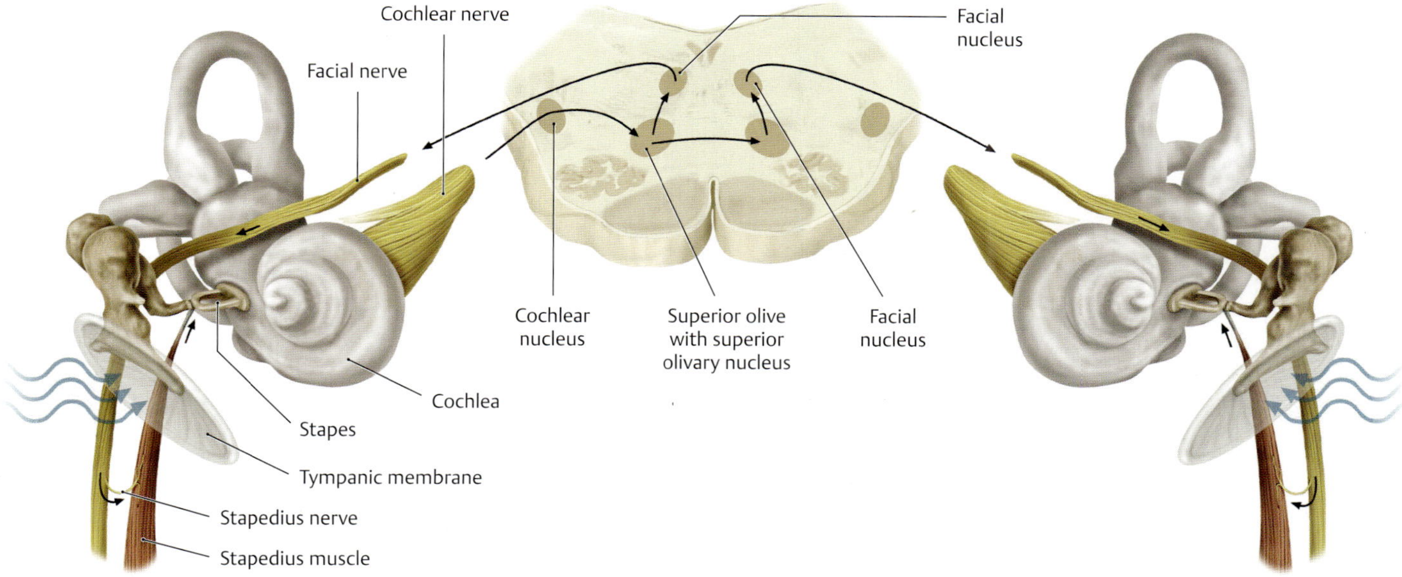

B The stapedius reflex
When the volume of an acoustic signal reaches a certain threshold, the stapedius reflex triggers a contraction of the stapedius muscle. This reflex can be utilized to test hearing without the patient's cooperation ("objective" auditory testing). The test is done by introducing a sonic probe into the ear canal and presenting a test noise to the tympanic membrane. When the noise volume reaches a certain threshold, it evokes the stapedius reflex and the tympanic membrane stiffens. The change in the resistance of the tympanic membrane is then measured and recorded. The *afferent* limb of this reflex is in the cochlear nerve. Information is conveyed to the facial nucleus on each side by way of the superior olivary nucleus. The *efferent* limb of this reflex is formed by special visceromotor fibers of the facial nerve.

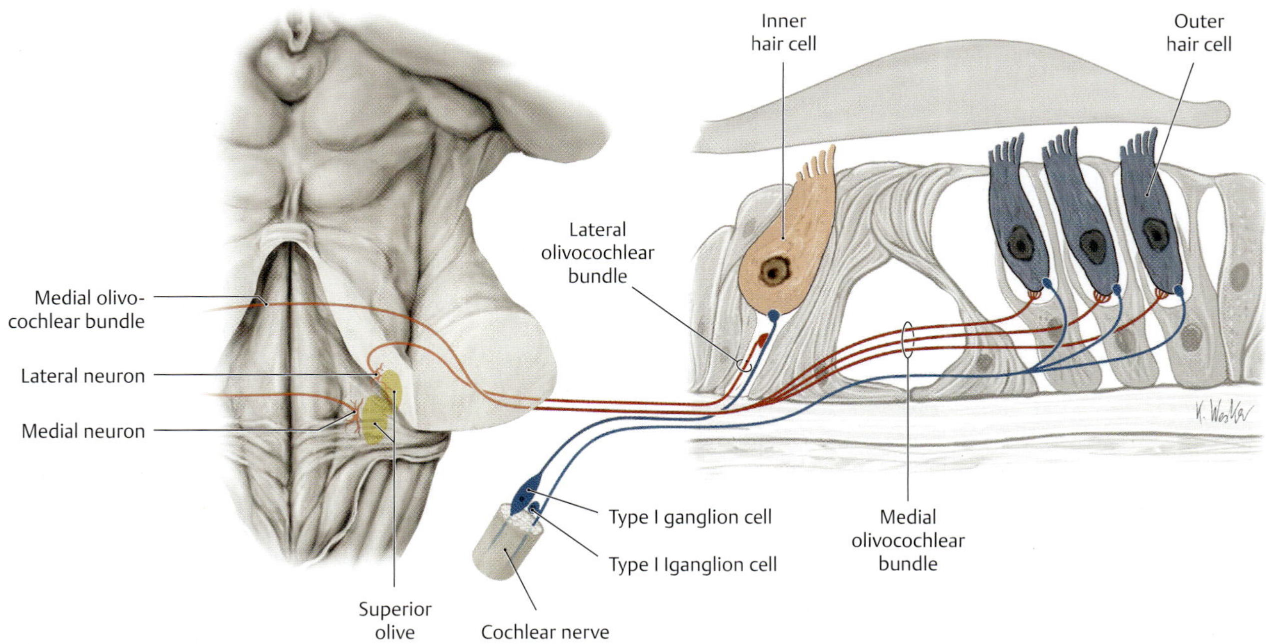

C Efferent fibers from the olive to the Corti organ
Besides the afferent fibers from the organ of Corti (see **A**, shown here in blue), which form the vestibulocochlear nerve, there are also efferent fibers (red) that pass to the organ of Corti in the inner ear and are concerned with the active preprocessing of sound ("cochlear amplifier") and acoustic protection. The efferent fibers arise from neurons that are located in either the lateral or medial part of the superior olive and project from there to the cochlea (lateral or medial olivocochlear bundle). The fibers of the lateral neurons pass *uncrossed* to the dendrites of the *inner* hair cells, while the fibers of the medial neurons cross to the opposite side and terminate at the base of the *outer* hair cells, whose activity they influence. When stimulated, the outer hair cells can actively amplify the traveling wave. This increases the sensitivity of the inner hair cells (the actual receptor cells). The activity of the efferents from the olive can be recorded as otoacoustic emissions (OAE). This test can be used to screen for hearing abnormalities in newborns.

13.22 Vestibular System

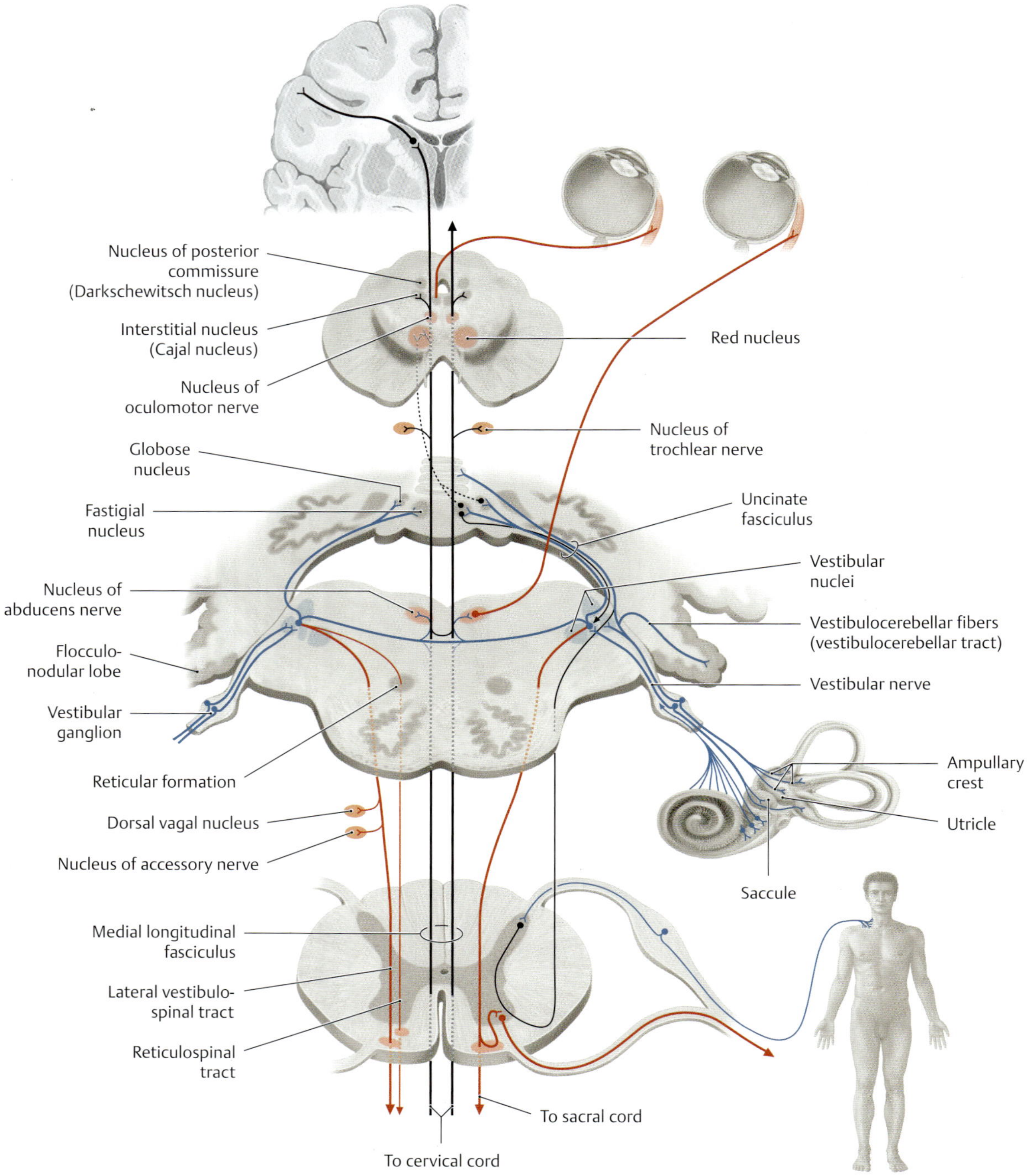

A Central connections of the vestibular nerve

Three systems are involved in the regulation of human balance:

- Vestibular system
- Proprioceptive system
- Visual system

The latter two systems have already been described. The peripheral receptors of the *vestibular system* are located in the membranous labyrinth (see petrous bone, pp. 142, 154), which consists of the utricle and saccule and the ampullae of the three semicircular canals. The maculae of the utricle and saccule respond to linear acceleration, while the semicircular canal organs in the ampullary crests respond to angular (rotational) acceleration. Like the hair cells of the inner ear, the receptors of the vestibular system are *secondary* sensory cells. The basal portions of the secondary sensory cells are surrounded by dendritic processes of bipolar neurons with their bodies located in the vestibular ganglion. The axons from these neurons form the vestibular nerve and terminate in the four vestibular nuclei (see **C**). Besides input from the vestibular apparatus, these nuclei also receive sensory input (see **B**). The vestibular nuclei show a topographical organization (see **C**) and distribute their efferent fibers to three targets:

- Motor neurons in the spinal cord via the lateral vestibulospinal tract. These motor neurons help to maintain upright stance, mainly by increasing the tone of extensor muscles
- Flocculonodular lobe of the cerebellum (direct sensory input to the cerebellum) via vestibulocerebellar fibers
- Ipsilateral and contralateral oculomotor nuclei via the ascending part of the medial longitudinal fasciculus

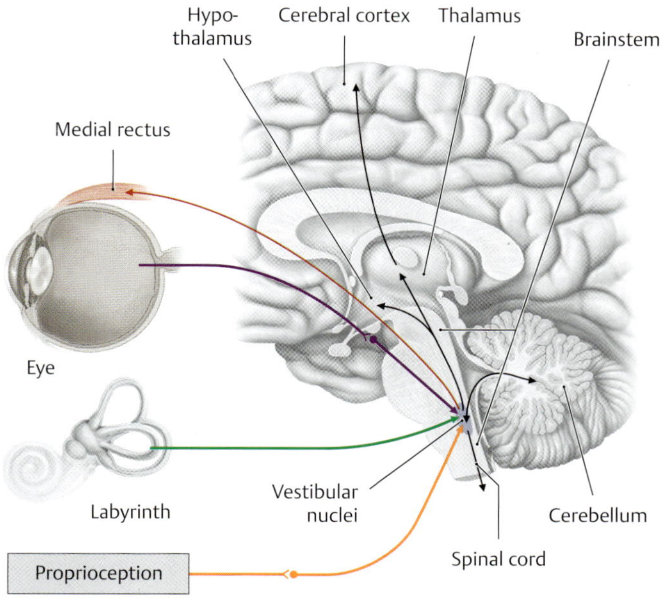

B Central role of the vestibular nuclei in the maintenance of balance

The afferent fibers that pass to the vestibular nuclei and the efferent fibers that emerge from them demonstrate the central role of these nuclei in maintaining balance. The vestibular nuclei receive afferent input from the vestibular system, proprioceptive system (position sense, muscles, and joints), and visual system. They then distribute efferent fibers to nuclei that control the motor systems important for balance. These nuclei are located in the

- Spinal cord (motor support),
- Cerebellum (fine control of motor function), and
- Brainstem (oculomotor nuclei for oculomotor function).

Efferents from the vestibular nuclei are also distributed to the following regions:

- Thalamus and cortex (spatial sense)
- Hypothalamus (autonomic regulation: vomiting in response to vertigo)

Note: Acute failure of the vestibular system is manifested by rotary vertigo.

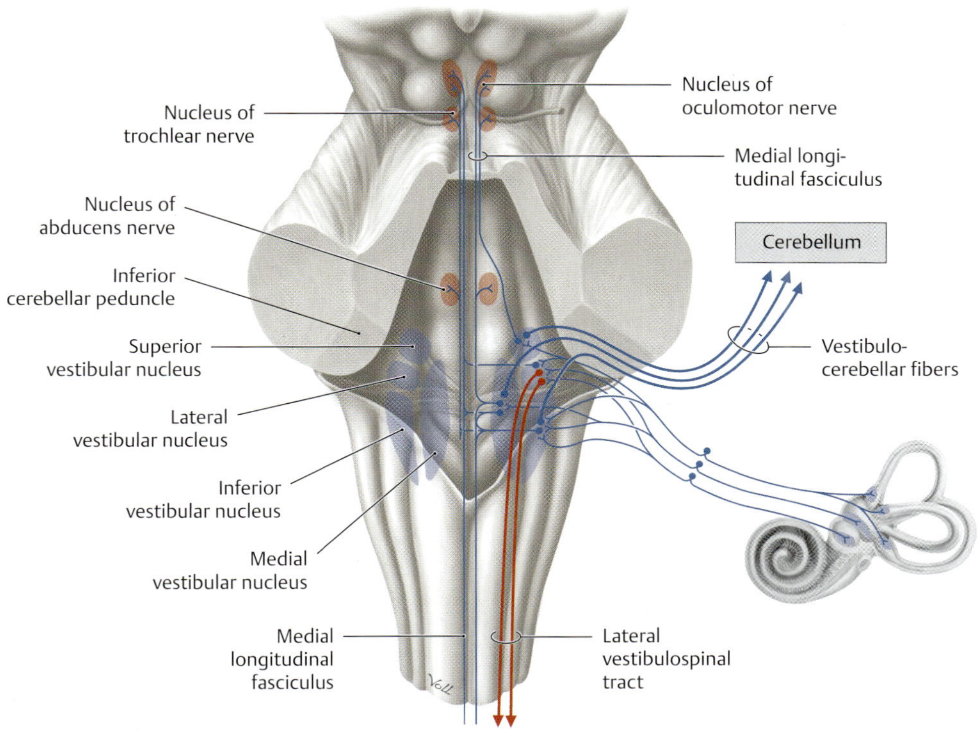

C Vestibular nuclei: topographic organization and central connections

Four nuclei are distinguished:

- Superior vestibular nucleus (of Bechterew)
- Lateral vestibular nucleus (of Deiters)
- Medial vestibular nucleus (of Schwalbe)
- Inferior vestibular nucleus (of Roller)

The vestibular system has a topographic organization:

- The afferent fibers of the saccular macula terminate in the inferior vestibular nucleus and lateral vestibular nucleus.
- The afferent fibers of the utricular macula terminate in the medial part of the inferior vestibular nucleus, the lateral part of the medial vestibular nucleus, and the lateral vestibular nucleus.
- The afferent fibers from the ampullary crests of the semicircular canals terminate in the superior vestibular nucleus, the upper part of the inferior vestibular nucleus, and the lateral vestibular nucleus.

The efferent fibers from the lateral vestibular nucleus pass to the lateral vestibulospinal tract. This tract extends to the sacral part of the spinal cord, its axons terminating on motor neurons. Functionally it is concerned with keeping the body upright, chiefly by increasing the tone of the extensor muscles. The vestibulocerebellar fibers from the other three nuclei act through the cerebellum to modulate muscular tone. All four vestibular nuclei distribute ipsilateral and contralateral axons via the medial longitudinal fasciculus to the three motor nuclei of the nerves to the extraocular muscles (i.e., the nuclei of the abducens, trochlear, and oculomotor nerves).

13.23 Gustatory System (Taste)

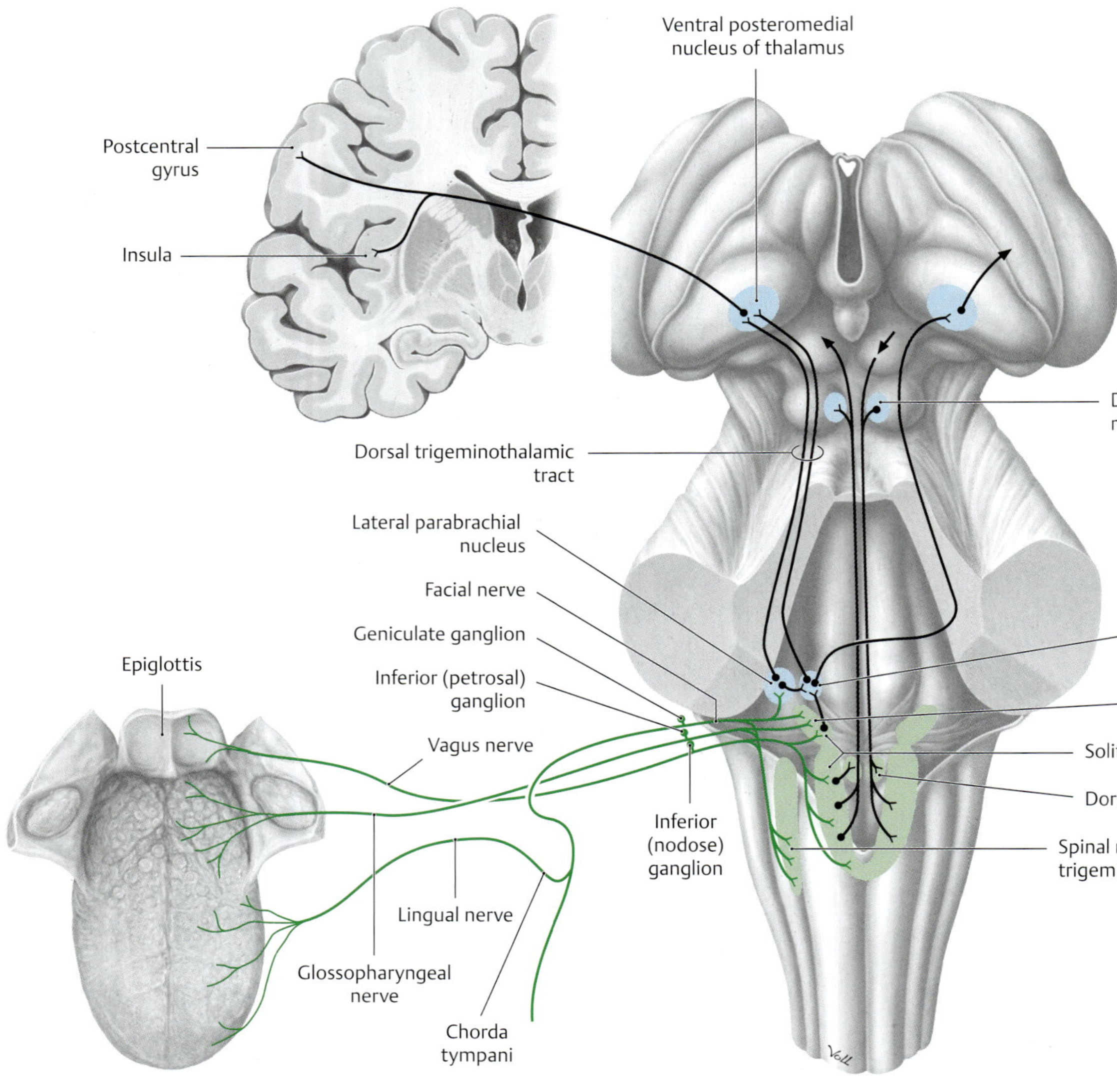

A Gustatory pathway
The receptors for the sense of taste are the taste buds of the tongue (see **B**). Unlike other receptor cells, the receptor cells of the taste buds are specialized epithelial cells (secondary sensory cells given that they do not have an axon). When these epithelial cells are chemically stimulated, the base of the cells releases glutamate, which stimulates the peripheral processes of afferent cranial nerves. These different cranial nerves serve different areas of the tongue. It is rare, therefore, for a complete loss of taste (ageusia) to occur.

- The *anterior two-thirds of the tongue* are supplied by the facial nerve (CN VII), the afferent fibers first passing in the lingual nerve (branch of the trigeminal nerve) and then in the chorda tympani to the geniculate ganglion of the facial nerve.
- The *posterior third of the tongue* and the *vallate papillae* are supplied by the glossopharyngeal nerve (CN IX).
- The *epiglottis* is supplied by the vagus nerve (CN X).

Peripheral processes from pseudounipolar ganglion cells (which correspond to pseudounipolar spinal ganglion cells) terminate on the taste buds. The central portions of these processes convey taste information to the gustatory part of the nucleus of the solitary tract. Thus, they function as the first afferent neuron of the gustatory pathway. Their cell bodies are located in the geniculate ganglion for the facial nerve, in the inferior (petrosal) ganglion for the glossopharyngeal nerve, and in the inferior (nodose) ganglion for the vagus nerve. After the first neurons synapse with the second neurons in the gustatory part of the nucleus of tractus solitarius (and some in the lateral parabrachial nucleus), some of the axons of the second neurons run ipsilaterally and contralaterally with the trigeminothalamic tract to the ventral posteromedial (VPM) nucleus of the thalamus, where they terminate on the third neurons. These neurons then project to the postcentral gyrus and the insular cortex. However, some of the axons of the second neurons travel to an additional intermediate station in the brainstem, the medial parabrachial nucleus, which in turn projects (as third neurons) to the thalamus, which further projects (as fourth neurons) to the insular cortex and postcentral gyrus. Collaterals from the first and second neurons of the gustatory afferent pathway are distributed to the superior and inferior salivatory nuclei. Afferent impulses in these fibers induce the secretion of saliva during eating ("salivary reflex"). The parasympathetic preganglionic fibers exit the brainstem via cranial nerves VII and IX (see the descriptions of these cranial nerves for details). Besides this purely gustatory pathway, spicy foods may also stimulate trigeminal fibers (not shown), which contribute to the sensation of taste. Finally, olfaction (the sense of smell), too, is a major component of the sense of taste as it is subjectively perceived: patients who cannot smell (anosmosia) report that their food tastes abnormally bland.

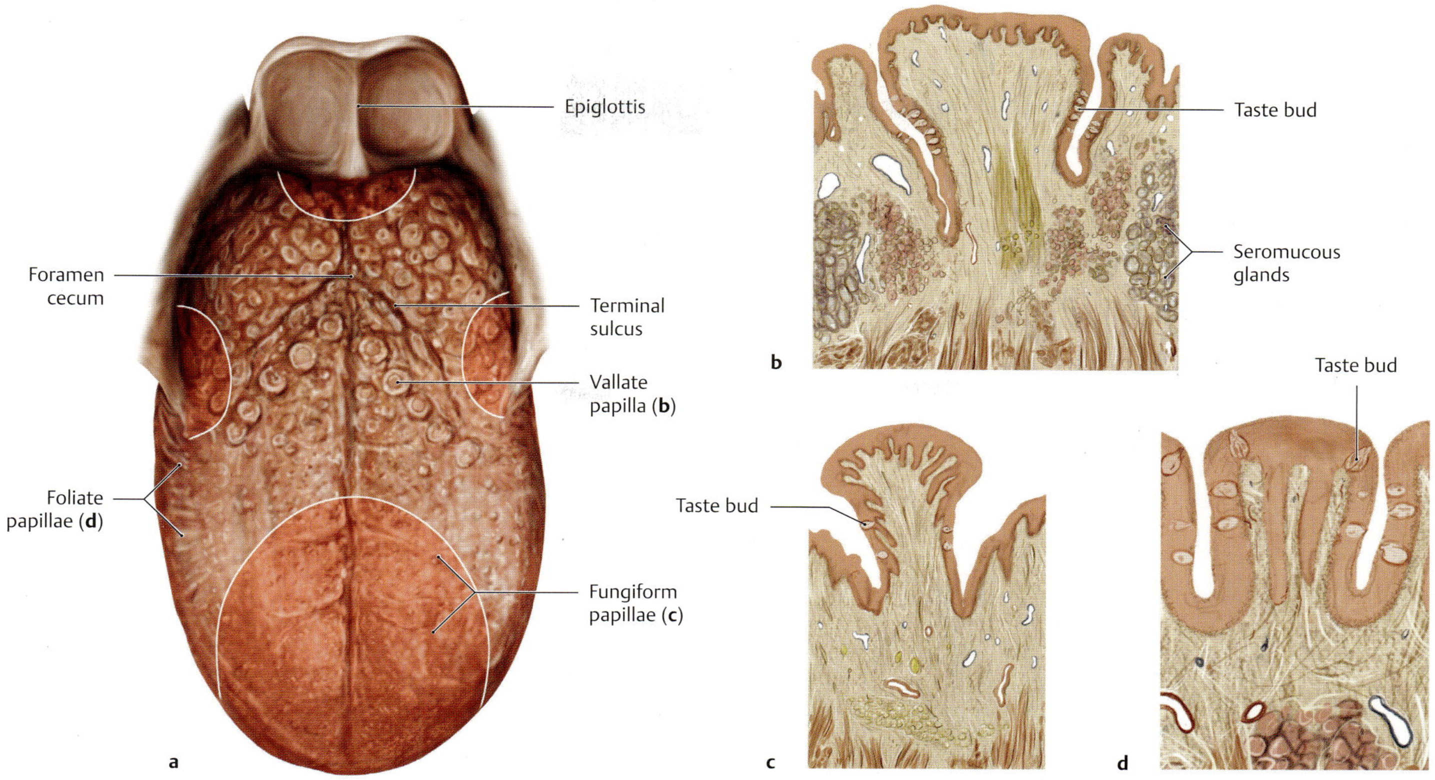

B Organization of the taste receptors in the tongue
The human tongue contains approximately 4600 taste buds in which the secondary sensory cells for taste perception are collected. They are concentrated in the white bordered areas. The taste buds (see **C**) are embedded in the epithelium of the lingual mucosa and are located on the surface expansions of the lingual mucosa—the vallate papillae (principal site, **b**), the fungiform papillae (**c**), and the foliate papillae (**d**). Additionally, isolated taste buds are located in the mucous membranes of the soft palate and pharynx. The surrounding serous glands of the tongue (Ebner glands), which are most closely associated with the vallate papillae, constantly wash the taste buds clean to allow for new tasting. Humans can perceive five basic tastes: sweet, sour, salty, bitter, and a fifth "savory" taste, called umami, which is activated by glutamate (a taste enhancer).

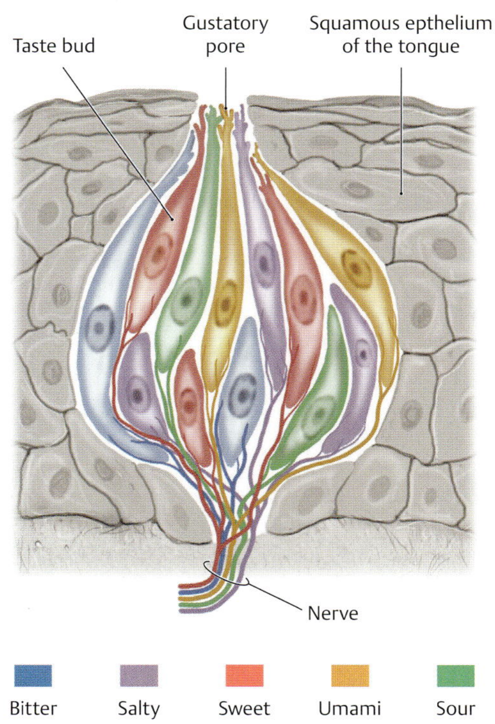

C Microscopic structure of a taste bud
Nerves induce the formation of taste buds in the oral mucosa. Processes of neurons of the three above mentioned cranial nerves, which grow into the oral mucosa from the basal side, induce the epithelium to differentiate into the depicted taste cells (modified epithelial cells). Their microvilli extend to the gustatory pore. Specialized taste receptor proteins in the cell membrane of the micorvilli are responsible for taste perception (for details, see physiology textbooks). After low-molecular-weight flavored substances bind to the receptor proteins, a signal transduction is induced, which causes the release of glutamate. This in turn excites the peripheral processes of the pseudounipolar neurons with the bodies in the ganglia of the mentioned three cranial nerves. Based on their features, each receptor cell is specialized in one of the five tastes (see color coding); the entire range of the perception of taste qualities is coded within each individual taste bud. This explains why the old notion that particular areas of the tongue are sensitive to specific taste qualities is incorrect.

13.24 Olfactory System (Smell)

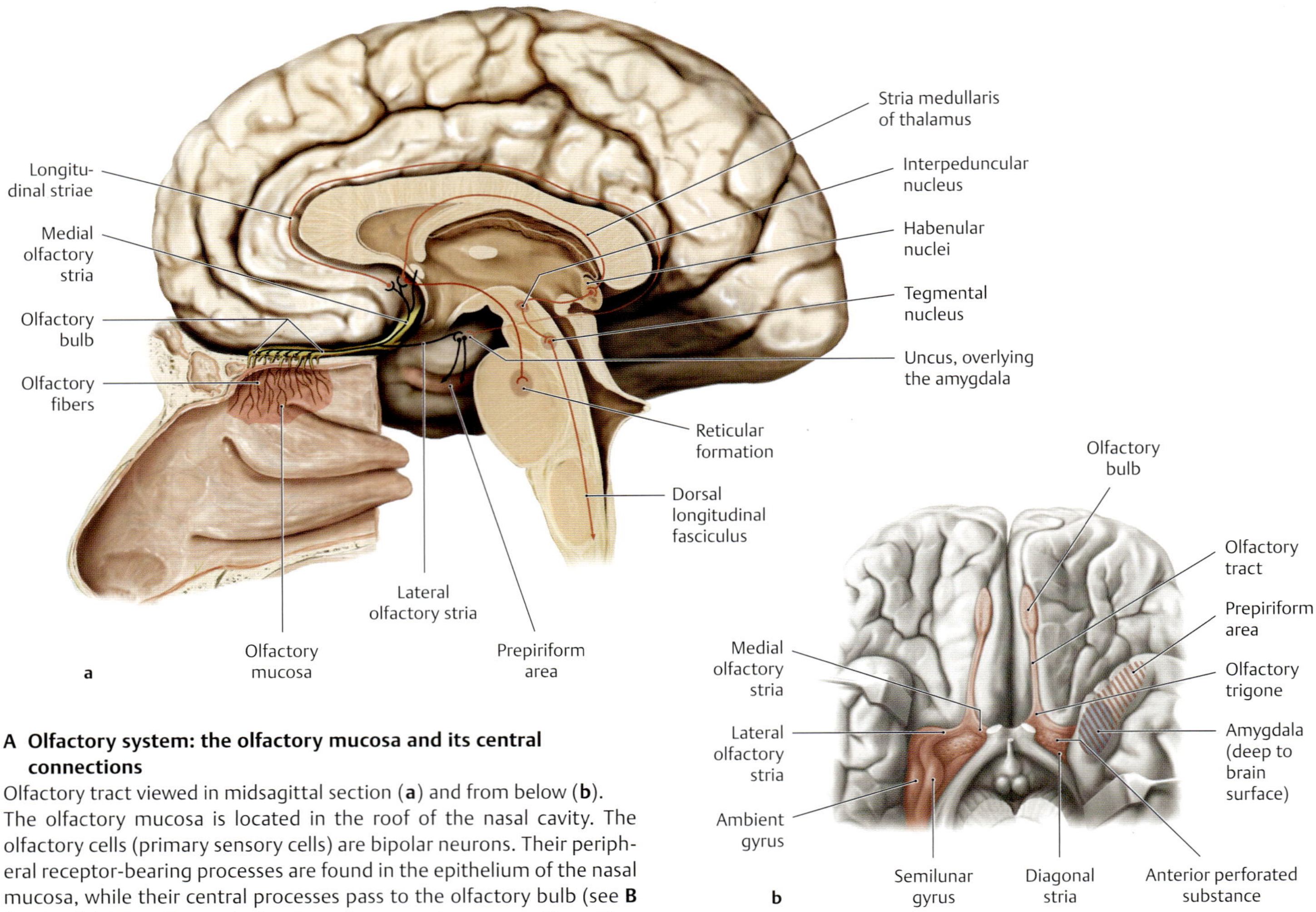

A Olfactory system: the olfactory mucosa and its central connections

Olfactory tract viewed in midsagittal section (**a**) and from below (**b**).
The olfactory mucosa is located in the roof of the nasal cavity. The olfactory cells (primary sensory cells) are bipolar neurons. Their peripheral receptor-bearing processes are found in the epithelium of the nasal mucosa, while their central processes pass to the olfactory bulb (see **B** for details). The *olfactory bulb,* where the second neurons of the olfactory pathway (mitral and tufted cells) are located, is considered an extension of the telencephalon. The axons of these second neurons pass centrally as the *olfactory tract.* In front of the anterior perforated substance, the olfactory tract widens to form the olfactory trigone and splits into the lateral and medial olfactory striae.

- Some of the axons of the olfactory tract run in the **lateral olfactory stria** to the olfactory centers: the amygdala, semilunar gyrus, and ambient gyrus. The prepiriform area (Brodmann area 28) is considered to be the primary olfactory cortex in the strict sense. It contains the third neurons of the olfactory pathway.
  Note: The prepiriform area is shaded in b, lying at the junction of the basal side of the frontal lobe and the medial side of the temporal lobe.
- Other axons of the olfactory tract run in the **medial olfactory stria** to nuclei in the septal (subcallosal) area, which is part of the limbic system (see p. 492), and to the olfactory tubercle, a small elevation in the anterior perforated substance.
- Yet other axons of the olfactory tract terminate in the **anterior olfactory nucleus**, where the fibers that cross to the opposite side branch off and are relayed. This nucleus is located in the olfactory trigone, which lies between the two olfactory striae and in front of the anterior perforated substance.

Note: None of these three tracts are routed through the thalamus. Thus, the olfactory system is the only sensory system that is not relayed in the thalamus before reaching the cortex. There is, however, an indirect route from the primary olfactory cortex to the neocortex passing through the thalamus and terminating in the basal forebrain. The olfactory signals are further analyzed in these basal portions of the forebrain (not shown).
The olfactory system is linked to other brain areas well beyond the primary olfactory cortex, with the result that olfactory stimuli can evoke complex emotional and behavioral responses. Noxious smells may induce nausea, while appetizing smells evoke watering of the mouth. Presumably these sensations are processed by the hypothalamus, thalamus, and limbic system (see p. 492) via connections established mainly by the medial forebrain bundle and the medullary striae of the thalamus. The medial forebrain bundle distributes axons to the following structures:

- Hypothalamic nuclei
- Reticular formation
- Salivatory nuclei
- Dorsal vagal nucleus

he axons that run in the medullary striae of the thalamus terminate in the habenular nuclei. This tract also continues to the brainstem, where it stimulates salivation in response to smell.

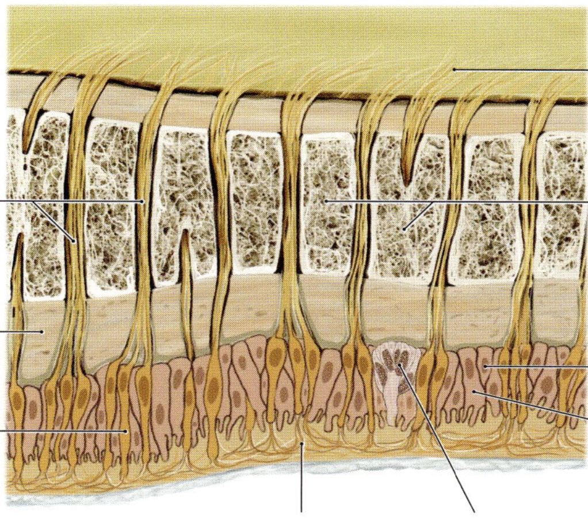

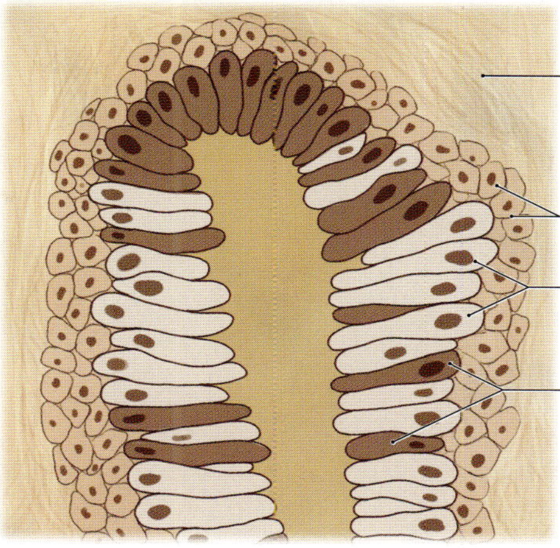

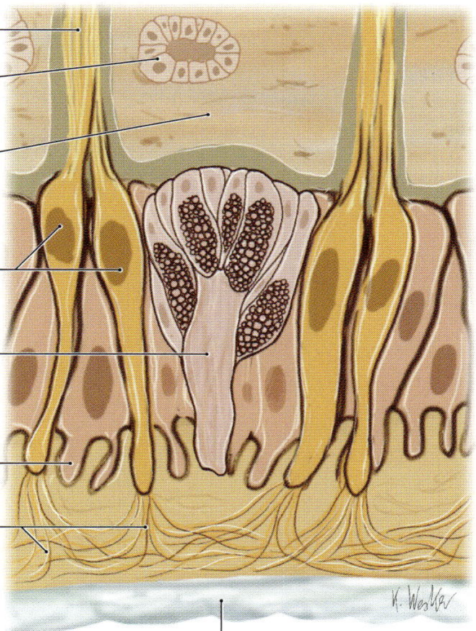

B Olfactory mucosa and vomeronasal organ (VNO)

The **olfactory mucosa** occupies an area of approximately 2 cm^2 on the roof of each nasal cavity, and 10^7 primary sensory cells are concentrated in each of these areas (**a, b**). At the molecular level, the olfactory receptor proteins are located in the cilia of the sensory cells (**b**). Each sensory cell has only one specialized receptor protein that mediates signal transduction when an odorant molecule binds to it. Although humans are microsmatic, having a sense of smell that is feeble compared with other mammals, the olfactory receptor proteins still make up 2% of the human genome. This underscores the importance of olfaction in humans. The primary olfactory sensory cells have a life span of approximately 60 days and regenerate from the basal cells (lifelong division of neurons). The bundled central processes (axons) from hundreds of olfactory cells form olfactory fibers (**a**) that pass through the cribriform plate of the ethmoid bone and terminate in the *olfactory bulb* (see **C**), which lies above the cribriform plate. The **vomeronasal organ** (**c**) is located on both sides of the anterior nasal septum. Its central connections in humans are unknown. It responds to steroids and evokes unconscious reactions in subjects (possibly influences the choice of a mate). Mate selection in many animal species is known to be mediated by olfactory impulses that are perceived in the vomeronasal organ.

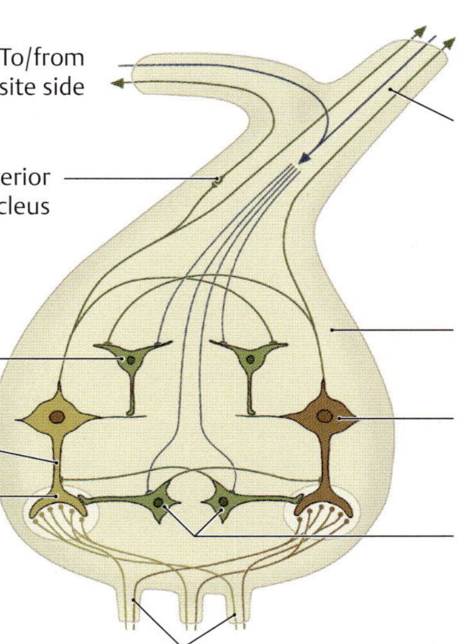

C Synaptic patterns in an olfactory bulb

Specialized neurons in the olfactory bulb, called mitral cells, form apical dendrites that receive synaptic contact from the axons of thousands of primary sensory cells. The dendrite plus the synapses make up the *olfactory glomeruli.* Axons from sensory cells with the same receptor protein form glomeruli with only one or a small number of mitral cells. The basal axons of the mitral cells form the olfactory tract. The axons that run in the olfactory tract project primarily to the olfactory cortex but are also distributed to other nuclei in the CNS. The axon collaterals of the mitral cells pass to granule cells: both granule cells and periglomerular cells inhibit the activity of the mitral cells, causing less sensory information to reach higher centers. These inhibitory processes are believed to heighten olfactory contrast, which aids in the more accurate perception of smells. The tufted cells, which also project to the primary olfactory cortex, are not shown.

13.25 Limbic System

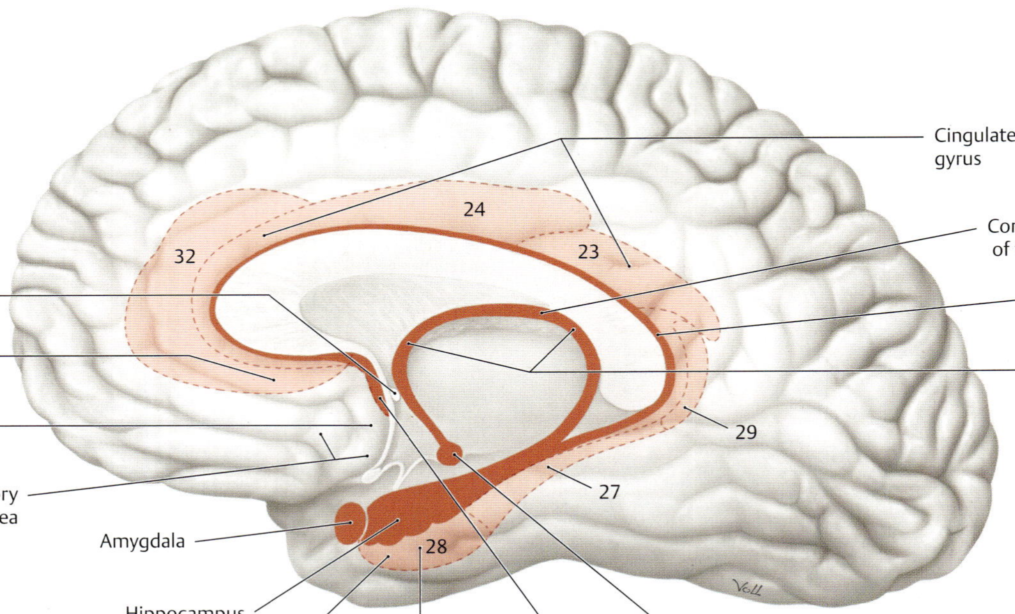

A Limbic system viewed through the partially transparent cortex
Medial view of the right hemisphere. The term "limbic system" (Latin limbus: "border" or "fringe") was first used by Broca in 1878, who collectively described the gyri surrounding the corpus callosum, diencephalon, and basal nuclei as the *grand lobe limbique.* The limbic system encompasses neocortical, archicortical, and paleocortical regions as well as subcortical nuclei. The extent of the limbic system is such that it can exchange and integrate information between the telencephalon (cerebral cortex), diencephalon, and mesencephalon. Viewed from the medial aspect of the cerebral hemispheres, the limbic system is seen to consist of an inner arc and an outer arc.

The **outer arc** is formed by
- Parahippocampal gyrus,
- Cingulate gyrus (also called the limbic gyrus),
- Subcallosal area.

Some classifications also include the paraolfactory area in the outer arc.
The **inner arc** is formed by
- Hippocampal formation,
- Fornix,
- Septal area (also known simply as the septum),
- Diagonal band of Broca (not visible in this view), and
- Paraterminal gyrus.

The limbic system also includes the amygdalae and mammillary bodies. The following nuclei are also considered part of the limbic system but are not shown: the anterior thalamic nucleus, habenular nucleus, dorsal tegmental nucleus, and interpeduncular nucleus.
The limbic system is concerned with the regulation of drive and affective behavior and plays a crucial role in memory and learning. The numbers in the diagram indicate the Brodmann areas.

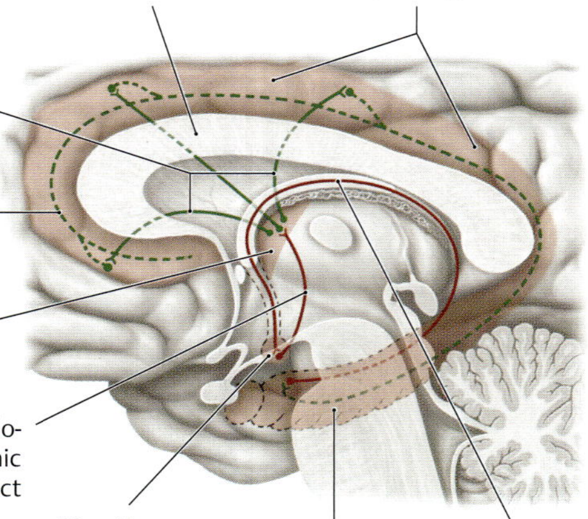

B Neuronal circuit (Papez circuit)
View of the medial surface of the right hemisphere. Several nuclei of the limbic system are interconnected by a *neuronal circuit* (see below) called the Papez circuit after the anatomist who first described it. MacLean later (1949) expanded the concept by introducing the term limbic system. The sequence below indicates the nuclei (normal print) and tracts (*italic print*) that are the successive stations of this neuronal circuit:

Hippocampus → *fornix* → mammillary body → *mammillothalamic tract* (Vicq d'Azyr bundle) → anterior thalamic nuclei→ *thalamocingular tract (radiation)* → cingulate gyrus → *cingulohippocampal fibers* → hippocampus.

This neuronal circuit interconnects ontogenically distinct parts of the limbic system. It establishes a connection between information stored in the unconscious and conscious behavior.

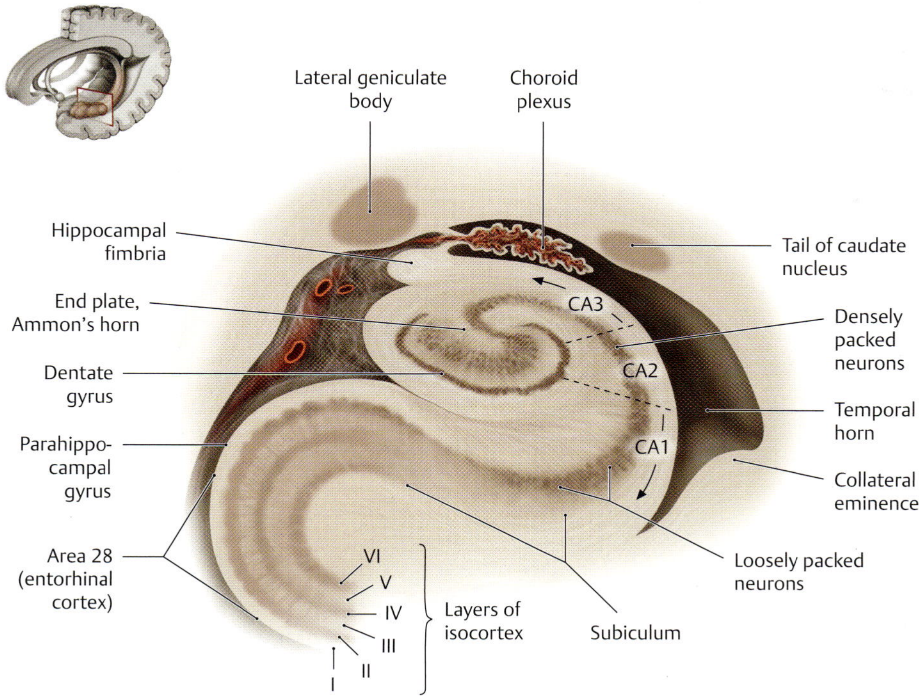

C Cytoarchitecture of the hippocampal formation (after Bähr and Frotscher)
View from anterior left.
Note: The hippocampal formation has a three-layered allocortex instead of a six-layered isocortex (lower left in diagram). It is a phylogenetically older structure than the isocortex. At the center of the allocortex is a band of neurons that forms the neuronal layer of the hippocampus (hippocampus proper [Ammon's horn]). The neurons in this layer are mainly pyramidal cells. Three regions, designated CA 1–CA 3, can be distinguished based on differences in the density of the pyramidal cells. *Region CA 1,* called also the "Sommer sector," is important in neuropathology because the death of neurons in this sector is the first morphologically detectable sign of cerebral hypoxia. Besides the hippocampus proper, we can also identify the cellular sheet of the dentate gyrus (dentate fascia), which consists mainly of granule cells.

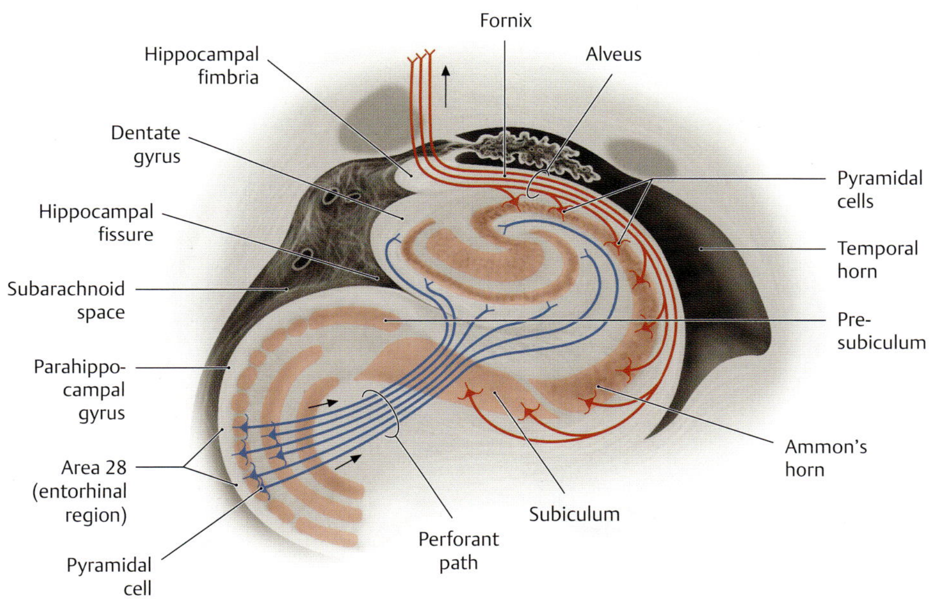

D Connections of the hippocampus
Left anterior view. The most important afferent pathway to the hippocampus is the *perforant path* (blue), which extends from the entorhinal region (triangular pyramidal cells of Brodmann area 28) to the hippocampus (where it ends in a synapse). The neurons that project from area 28 into the hippocampus receive afferent input from many brain regions. Thus, the entorhinal region is considered the gateway to the hippocampus. The pyramidal cells of Ammon's horn (triangles) send their axons into the fornix, and the axons transmitted via the fornix continue to the mammillary body (Papez neuronal circuit) or to the septal nuclei.

E Important definitions pertaining to the limbic system

Archicortex
Phylogenetically old structures of the cerebral cortex; does not have a six-layered architecture

Hippocampus (retrocommissural)
Ammon's horn (hippocampus proper), dentate gyrus (dentate fascia), subiculum (some authors consider it part of the hippocampal formation rather than the hippocampus itself)

Hippocampal formation
Hippocampus plus the entorhinal area of the parahippocampal gyrus

Limbic system
Important coordinating system for memory and emotions. Includes the following *telencephalic* structures: cingulate gyrus, parahippocampal gyrus, hippocampal formation, septal nuclei, and amygdala. Its *diencephalic* components include the anterior thalamic nucleus, mammillary bodies, nucleus accumbens, and habenular nucleus. Its *brainstem* components are the raphe nuclei. The medial forebrain bundle and the dorsal longitudinal fasciculus contribute to the fiber tracts of the limbic system.

Periarchicortex
A broad transitional zone around the hippocampus, consisting of the cingulate gyrus, the isthmus of the cingulate gyrus, and the parahippocampal gyrus

13.26 Brain: Functional Organization

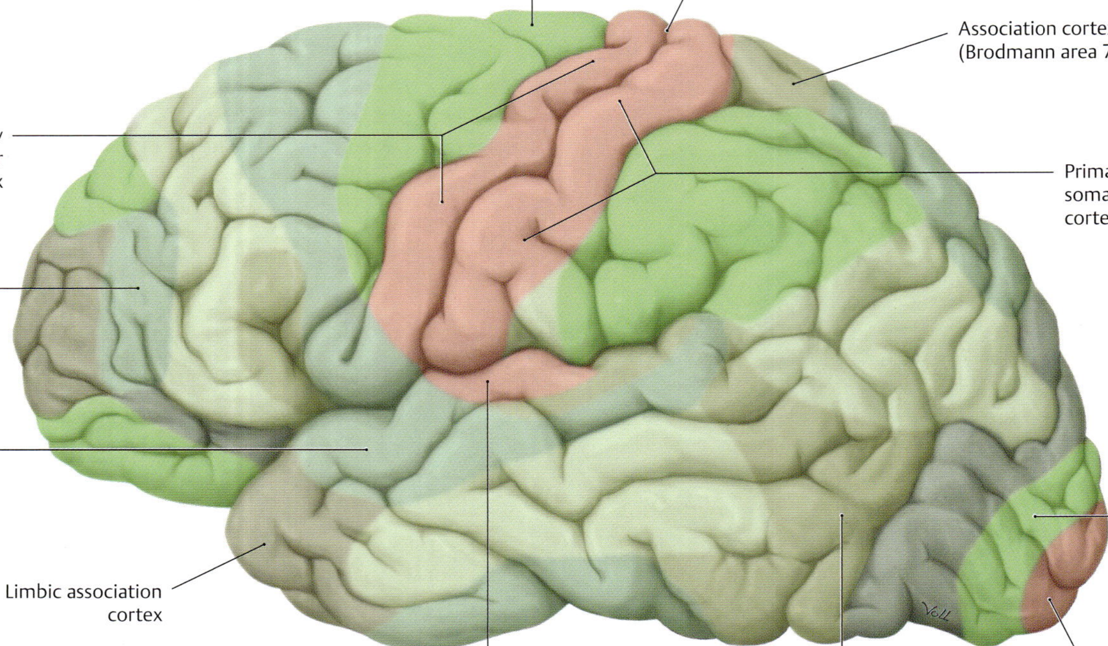

A Functional organization of the neocortex
Left lateral view. The primary sensory and motor areas are shown in red, and the areas of the association cortex are shown in different shades of green. Projection tracts begin or end, respectively, in the primary motor or sensory areas. More than 80% of the cortical surface area is association cortex, which is secondarily connected to the primary sensory or primary motor areas. The neuronal processing of differentiated behavior and intellectual performance takes place in the association cortex, which has increased greatly in size over the course of human evolution. The functional organization pattern shown here, such as the localization of the primary motor cortex in the precentral gyrus, can be demonstrated in living subjects with modern imaging techniques. The results of such studies are illustrated in the figures below. Interestingly, the correlations described in these studies correspond reasonably well with the cortical areas defined by Brodmann.

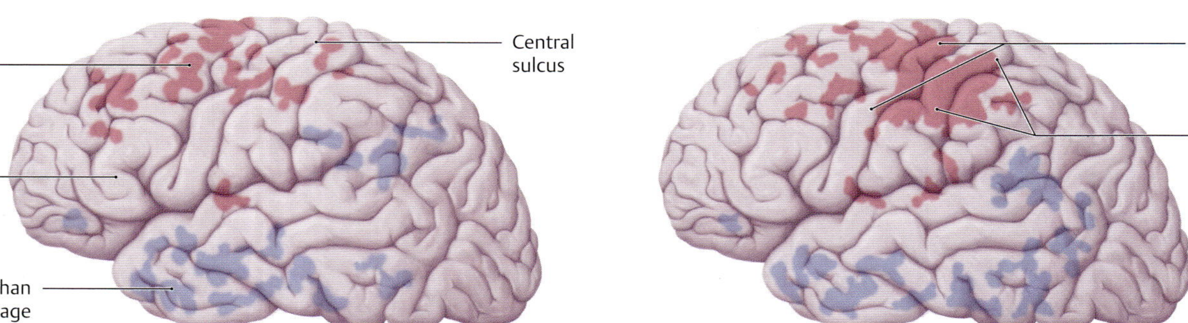

B Analysis of brain function based on studies of regional cerebral blood flow
Left lateral view of the brain. When neurons are activated they consume more glucose and oxygen, which must be delivered to them via the bloodstream. This may produce a detectable increase in regional blood flow. These brain maps illustrate the local patterns of cerebral blood flow at rest (**a**) and during movement of the right hand (**b**). When the right hand is moved, increased blood flow is recorded in the left precentral gyrus, which contains the motor representation of the right hand (see motor homunculus in **B** on p. 457). Simultaneous activation is noted in the sensory cortex of the postcentral region, showing that the sensory cortex is also active during motor function (feedback loop).

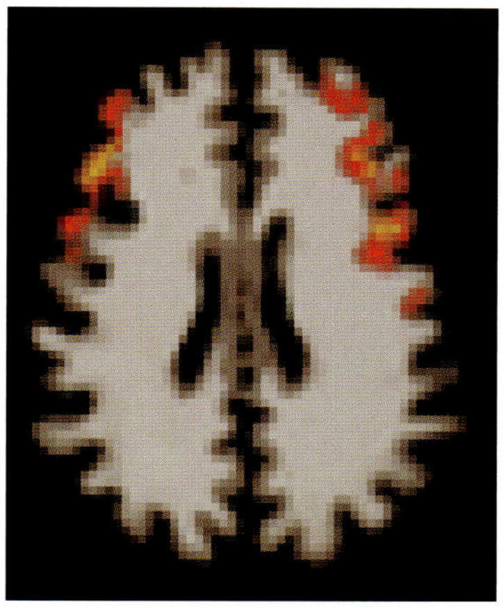

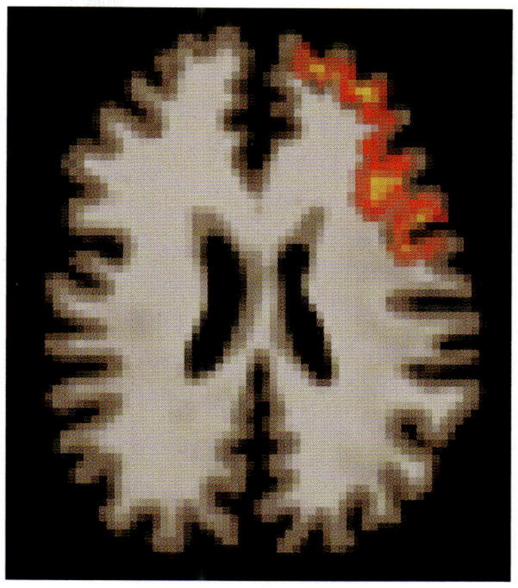

C Gender differences in neuronal processing
Patterns of brain activity can also be demonstrated by functional magnetic resonance imaging (fMRI). This provides a noninvasive method for investigating the metabolic activity of the brain. Because no human brain is identical to any other, a comparison of several brains will show slight variations in the distribution of specific functions. By superimposing the results of examinations in different brains, we can produce a generalized map that shows the approximate distribution of brain functions. Compare the summation map for female brains on the left with a map for male brains on the right. Both groups of subjects were given phonological tasks based on recognizing differences in the meaning of spoken sounds. While the female subjects activated both sides of their brain when solving the tasks, the male subjects activated only the left side (the sectional images are viewed from below).

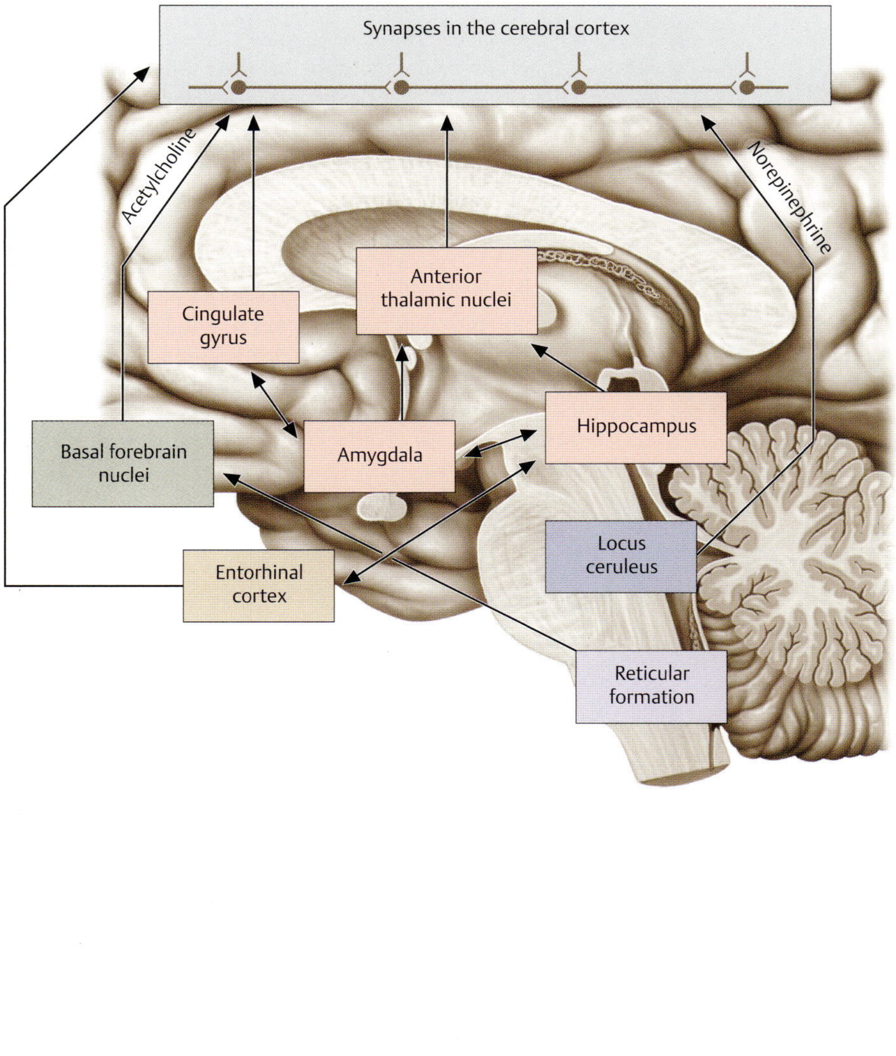

D Modulating subcortical centers
The cerebral cortex, the seat of our conscious thoughts and actions, is influenced by various subcortical centers. The parts of the limbic system that are crucial for learning and memory are indicated in light red.

13.27 Brain: Hemispheric Dominance

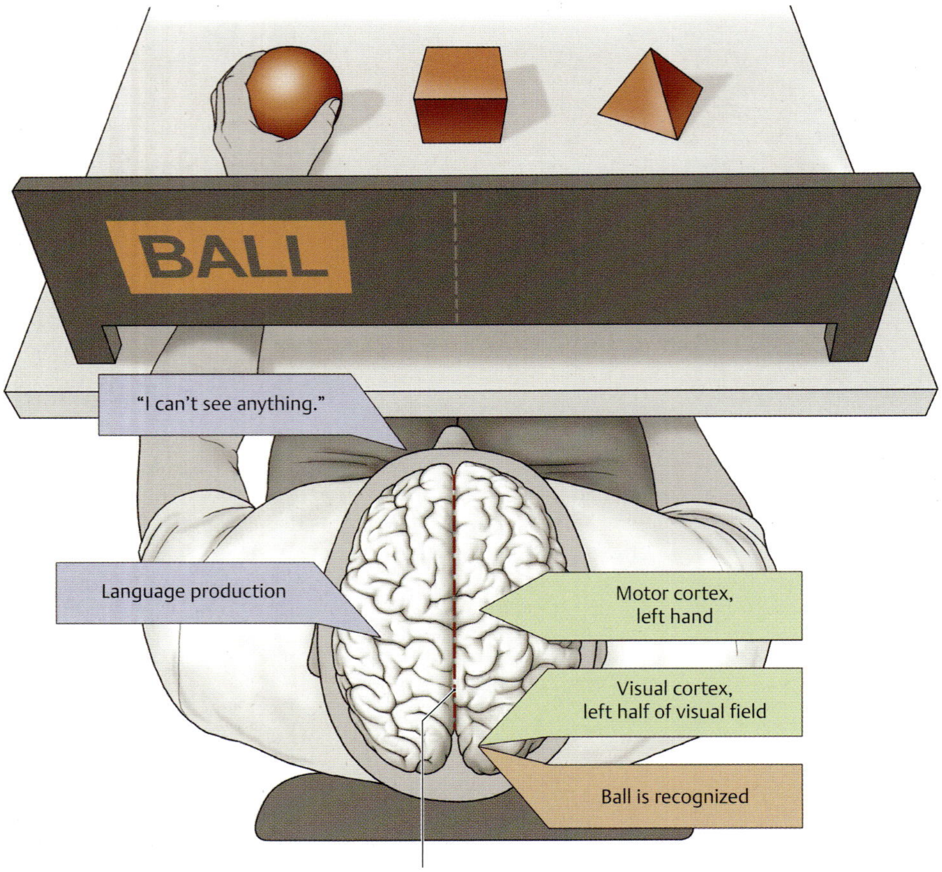

A Demonstration of hemispheric dominance for language in split-brain patients (after Klinke, Pape, and Silbernagl)

The corpus callosum is by far the most important commissural tract, interconnecting areas of like function in both hemispheres of the brain. Because lesions of the corpus callosum were once considered to have no clinical effects, surgical division of the corpus callosum was commonly performed at one time in epileptic patients to keep epileptic seizures from spreading across the brain. This operation interrupts the connections in the *upper telencephalon* while leaving intact the more deeply situated *diencephalon,* which contains the optic tract. Patients who have undergone this operation are called "split-brain patients." They have no obvious clinical abnormalities, but special neuropsychological tests reveal deficits, the study of which has improved our understanding of brain function. In one test the patient sits in front of a screen on which words are projected. Meanwhile, the patient can grasp objects behind the screen without being able to see them. When the word "Ball" is flashed briefly on the left side of the screen, the patient perceives it in the visual cortex on the right side (the optic tract has not been cut). Because language production resides in the *left* hemisphere in 97% of the population, the patient cannot verbalize the projected word out loud because communication between the hemispheres has been interrupted at the level of the telencephalon (seat of speech production). But the patient is still able to feel the ball manually and pick it out from other objects. The function of the corpus callosum is to enable both hemispheres (which can function independently to a degree) to communicate with each other when the need arises. Because of the phenomenon of hemispheric dominance, the corpus callosum in humans is more elaborately developed than in other animal species. The male and female brain differs in the assignment of functional roles to the cortical areas. In the male, only one hemisphere participates in the execution of linguistic tasks whereas females activate both hemispheres (see **C**, p. 495). This fact is believed to also have an impact on the structure of the corpus callosum. According to several studies, the number of axons in the isthmus of the corpus callosum is said to be larger in the female (approximately 25% larger isthmus area), who are supposed to show better speech comprehension ability than males. However, these findings are highly controversial.

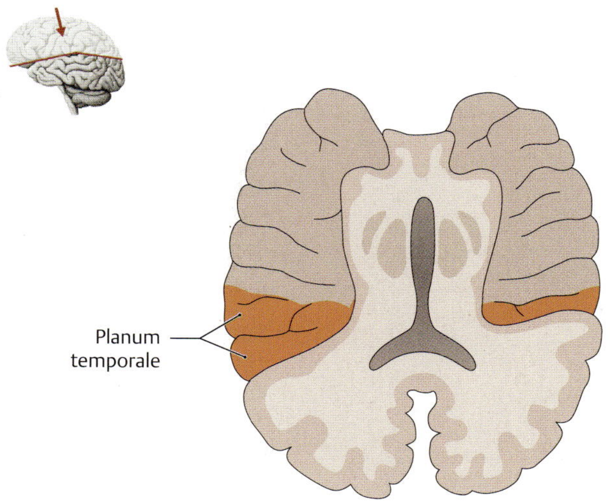

B Hemispheric asymmetry (after Klinke and Silbernagl)
Superior view of the temporal lobe of a brain that has been taken apart (i.e., the frontal lobes have been removed) along the lateral fissure. The *planum temporale,* located on the posterior and superior surface of the temporal lobe, has different contours on the two sides of the brain, being more pronounced on the left side than on the right in two-thirds of individuals. The functional significance of this asymmetry is uncertain. We cannot explain it simply by noting that Wernicke's speech area is located in that part of the temporal lobe, because while temporal asymmetry is present in only 67% of the population, the speech area is located on the left side in 97%.

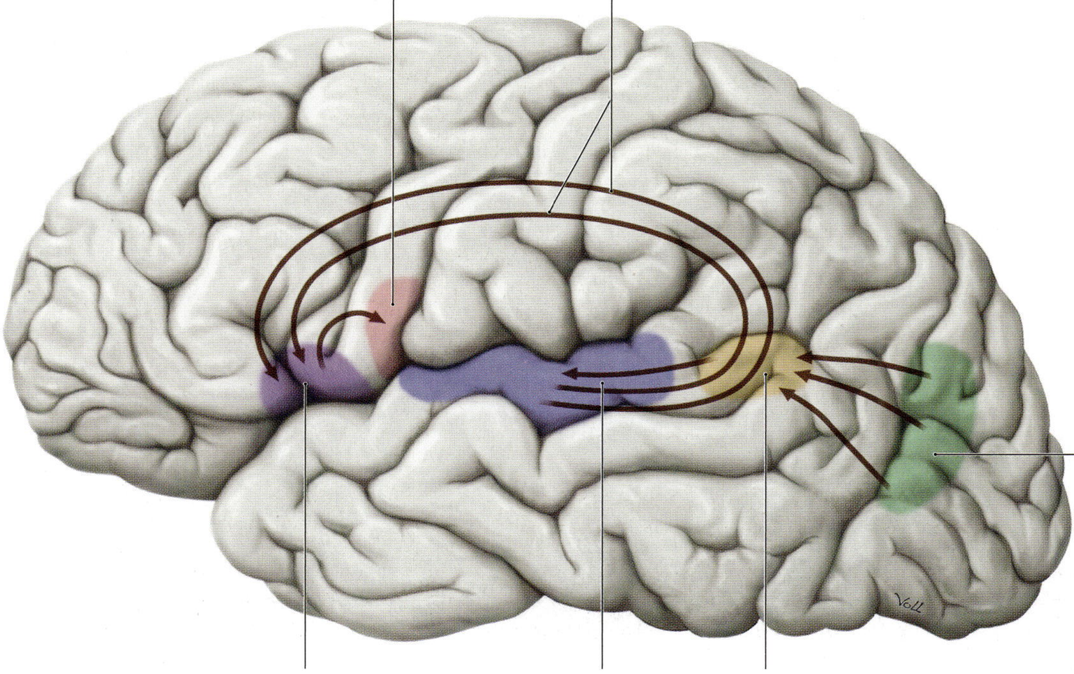

C Language areas in the normally dominant left hemisphere
Lateral view. The brain contains several language areas whose loss is associated with typical clinical symptoms. *Wernicke's area* (the posterior part of area 22) is necessary for language comprehension, while *Broca's area* (area 44) is concerned with language production. The two areas are interconnected by the superior longitudinal (arcuate) fasciculus. Broca's area activates the mouth and tongue region of the motor cortex for the articulation of speech. The angular gyrus coordinates the inputs from the visual, acoustic, and somatosensory cortices and relays them onward to Wernicke's area.

13.28 Brain: Clinical Findings

The figures in this unit illustrate the correlations that have been discovered between specific brain areas and clinical findings. Studies of this kind have enabled us to link particular patterns of behavior, some abnormal, and particular clinical symptoms to specific areas in the brain.

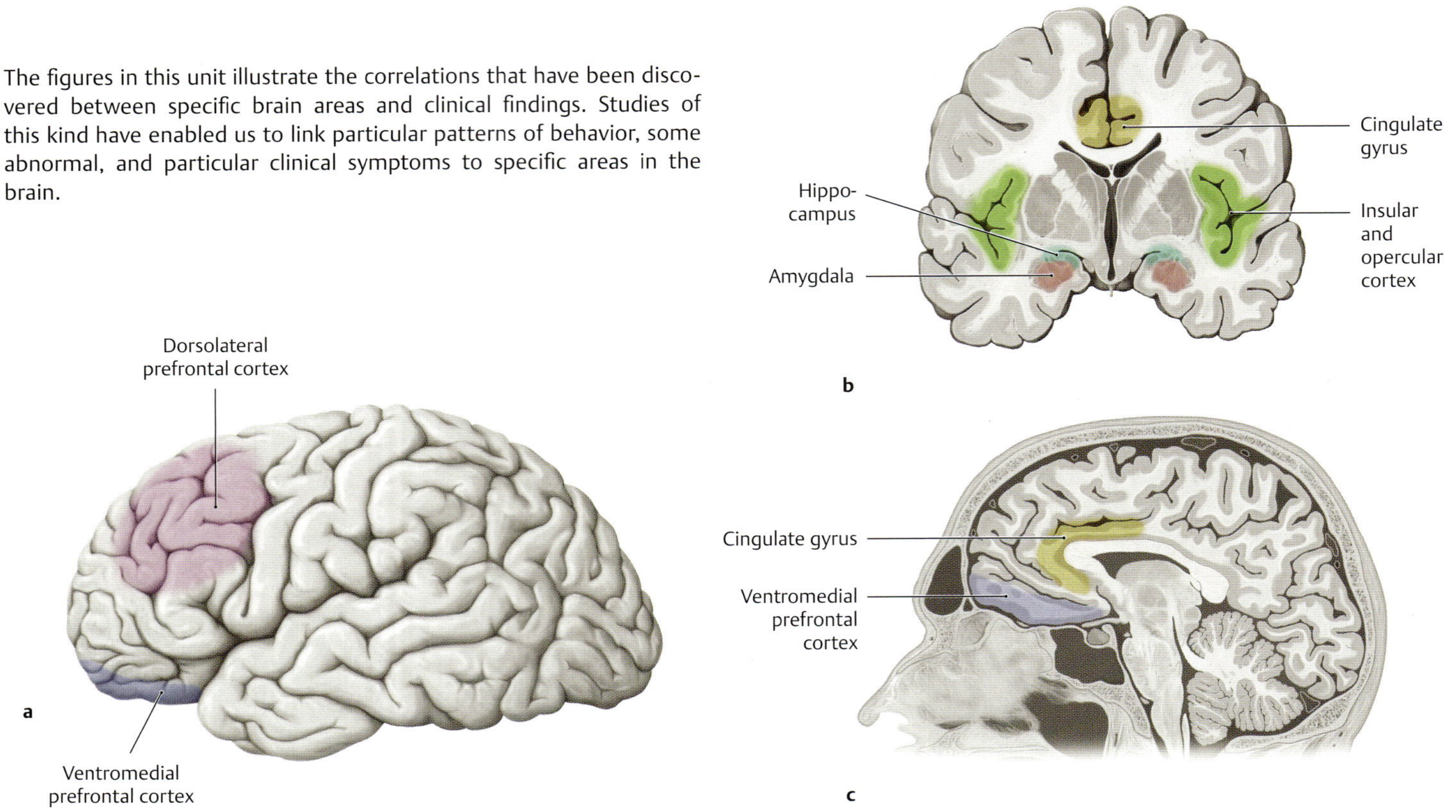

A Neuroanatomy of emotions

a Lateral view of the left hemisphere. **b** Anterior view of a coronal section through the amygdala. **c** Midsagittal section of the right hemisphere, medial aspect.

Emotion is linked to specific regions of the brain. The ventromedial prefrontal cortex is connected primarily to the amygdaloid bodies and is believed to modulate emotion, while the dorsolateral prefrontal cortex is connected primarily to the hippocampus. This is the area of the cortex in which memories are stored along with their emotional valence. Abnormalities of this network are believed to play a role in depression.

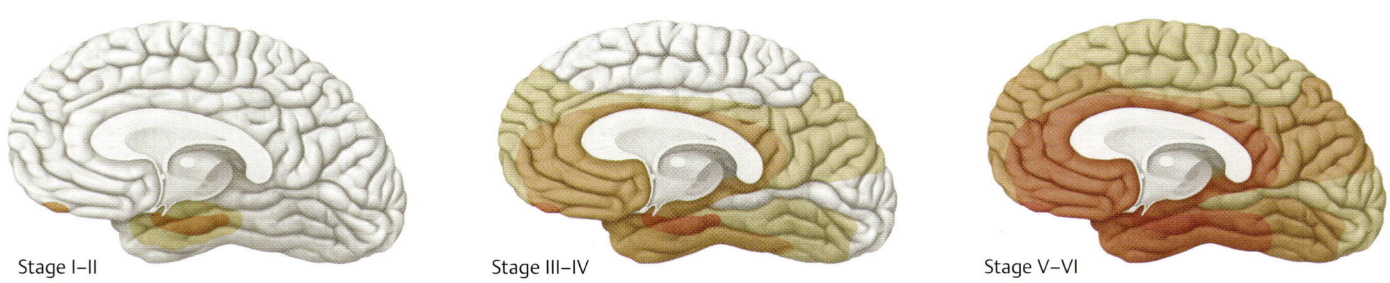

B Spread of Alzheimer's disease through the brain after Braak and Braak

Medial view of the right hemisphere. Alzheimer's disease is a relentlessly progressive disease of the cerebral cortex that causes memory loss and, eventually, profound dementia. The progression of the disease can be demonstrated with special staining methods and can be divided into stages using the classification of Braak and Braak:

- Stages I–II: the appearance of the nerve cells is altered in the periphery of the entorhinal cortex (= transentorhinal region), which is considered part of the allocortex (see p. 330). These stages are still asymptomatic.
- Stages III–IV: the lesions have spread to involve the limbic system (also part of the allocortex), and initial clinical symptoms appear. These stages may be detectable by imaging studies in some cases.
- Stages V–VI: the entire isocortex is involved, and the clinical manifestations are fully developed.

Thus, the allocortex is important in brain pathophysiology as the site of origin of Alzheimer's dementia, even though it makes up only 5% of the cerebral cortex.

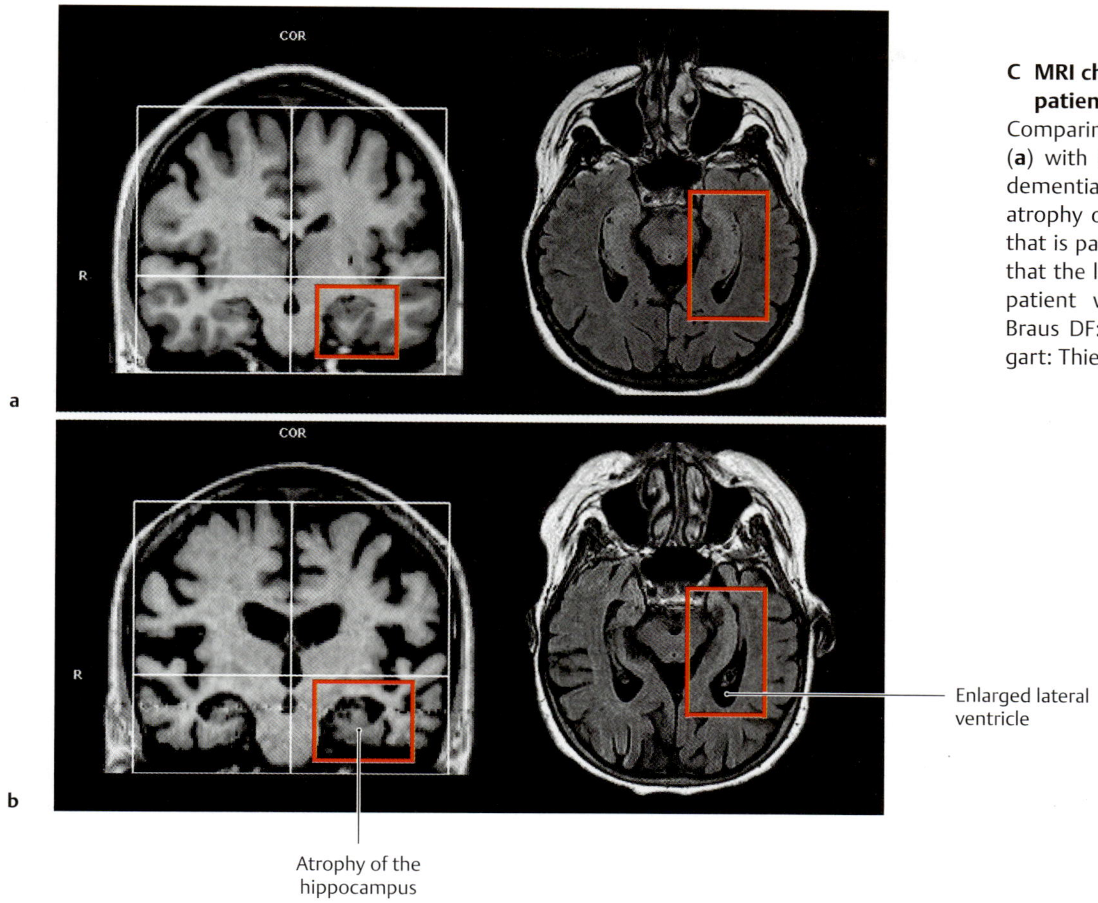

C MRI changes in the hippocampus in a patient with Alzheimer's dementia

Comparing the brain of a healthy subject (**a**) with that of a patient with Alzheimer's dementia (**b**), we notice that the latter shows atrophy of the hippocampus, a brain region that is part of the allocortex. We notice, too, that the lateral ventricles are enlarged in the patient with Alzheimer's dementia (from Braus DF: *Ein Blick ins Gehirn.* 3rd ed. Stuttgart: Thieme; 2014).

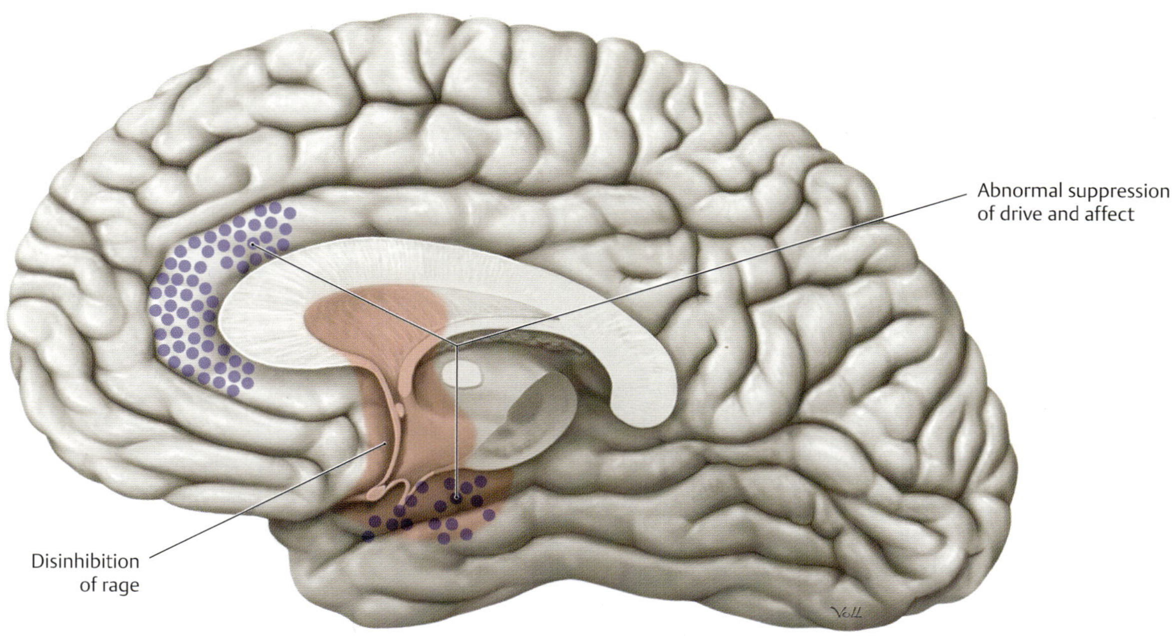

D Lesions of certain brain areas and associated behavioral changes

Medial view of the right hemisphere. Bilateral lesions of the medial temporal lobe and the frontal part of the cingulate gyrus (blue dots) lead to a suppression of drive and affect. This structural abnormality in the limbic system produces clinical changes that include apathy, a blank facial expression, monotone speech, and a dull, nonspontaneous mode of behavior. The condition may be caused by tumors, decreased blood flow, or trauma. On the other hand, tumors involving the septum pellucidum and hypothalamus (pink-shaded area) and certain forms of epilepsy may cause a disinhibition of anger, and the patient may respond to seemingly trivial events with attacks of "hypothalamic rage" accompanied by screaming and biting. This outburst is not directed against any particular person or object and persists for some time.

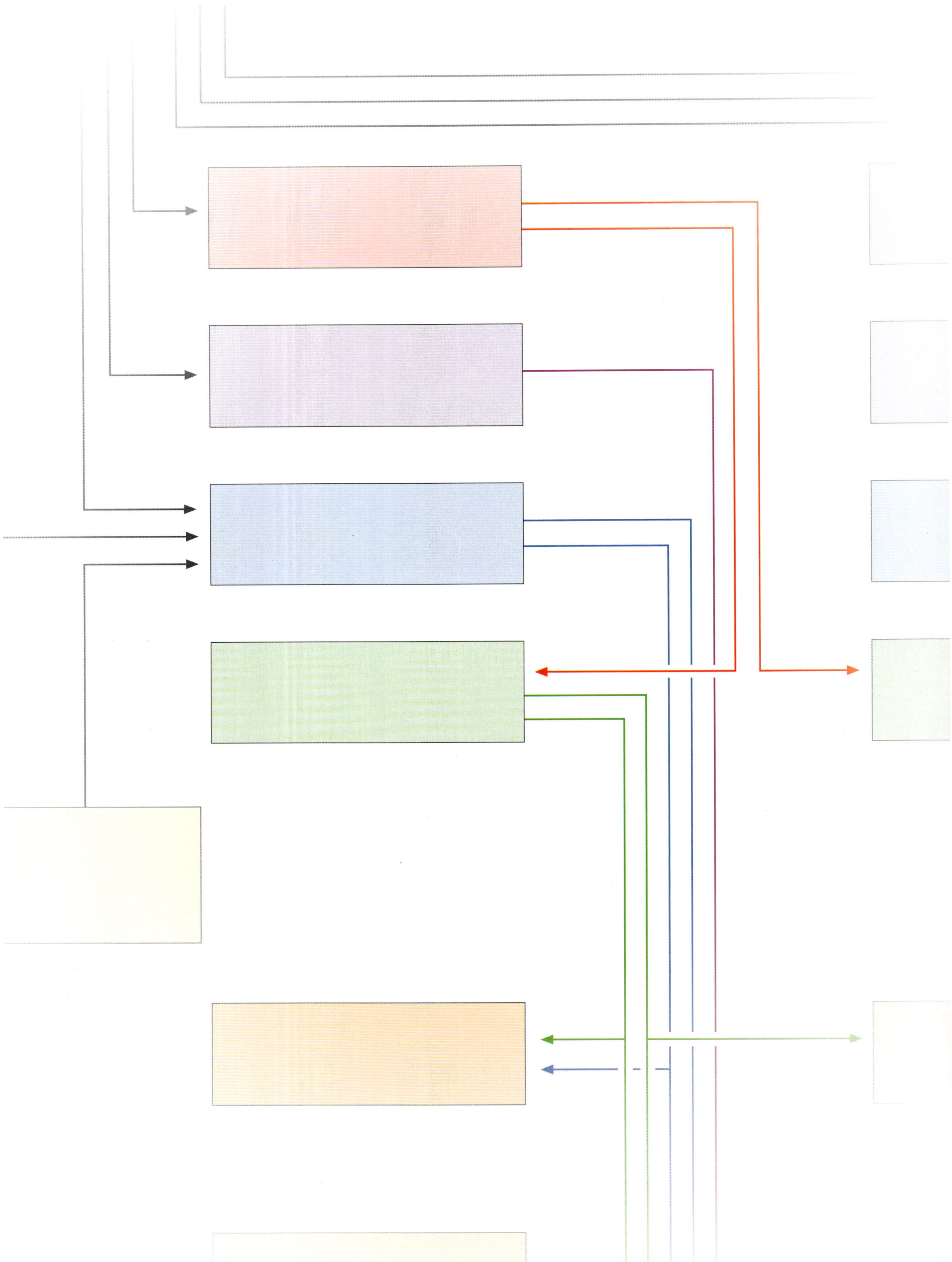

C Glossary and Synopsis

1.1 Gray Matter (Substantia grisea)

- **Definition of "gray matter":** collection of neuronal cell bodies (perikarya, somata)
- **Distribution:**
  - in the CNS as cortex and nuclei
  - in the PNS the equivalent of gray matter is known as ganglia (sensory or autonomic)

Gray matter in the CNS, morphological terms

Cortex
- *Definition:* layered arrangement of neuronal cell bodies at the outer surface of the CNS and thus visible from outside, in the majority of cases
- *Distribution:*
  - telencephalon (cerebral cortex)
  - cerebellum (cerebellar cortex)

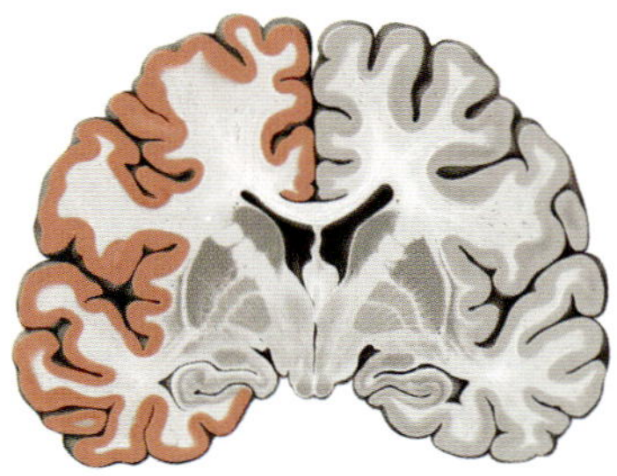

Cortex cerebri

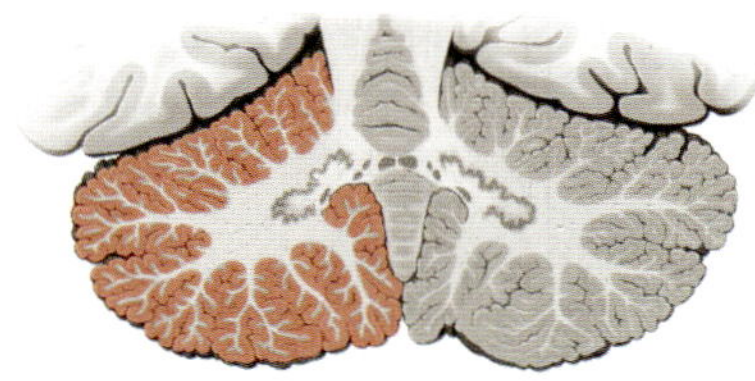

Cortex cerebelli

Nucleus:
- *Definition:* localized collection of neuronal cell bodies within the white matter (see p. 504f), thus visible only in sections
- *Distribution:* all parts of the CNS, in the spinal cord also in specific morphological arrangements:
  - as column: term used for three-dimensional representation of the clusters of neuron cell bodies arranged in nuclei or horn, respectively: term used for two-dimensional representation, thus a cross-section of the column. On a cross-section, all columns of gray matter give the typical butterfly shape of the spinal cord.
  - as reticular formation (reticulum = net): net-like arrangement of numerous, very small nuclei, which, based on their small size are morphologically hardly identifiable as nuclei; therefore the gray and white matter appear "mixed" in a net-like pattern. Reticular formation also exists in the brainstem.

Note: Per definition, nuclei exist only in the CNS, not in the PNS!

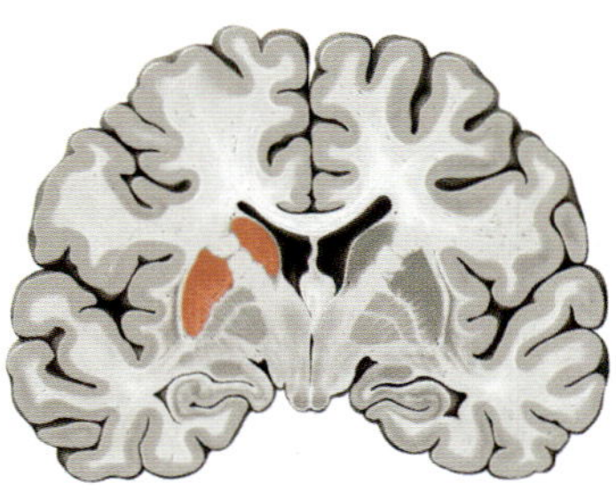

Nuclei in the telencephalon (example of basal nuclei)

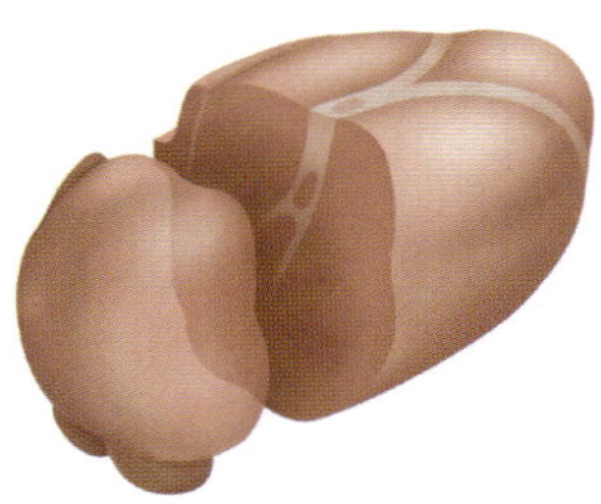

Nucleus in the diencephalon (here: thalamus as collection of nuclei = nuclear area)

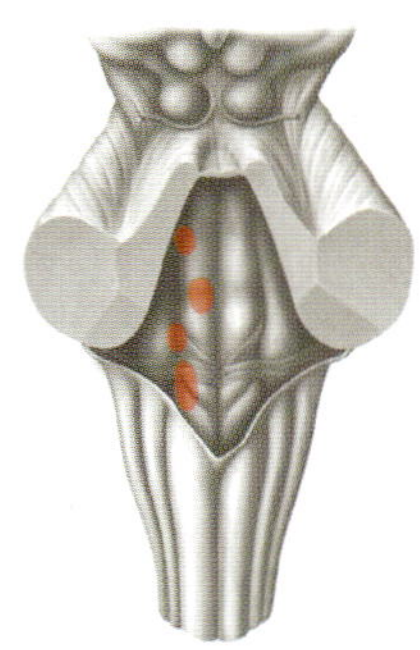

Nuclei in the brainstem (here: some of the cranial nerve nuclei)

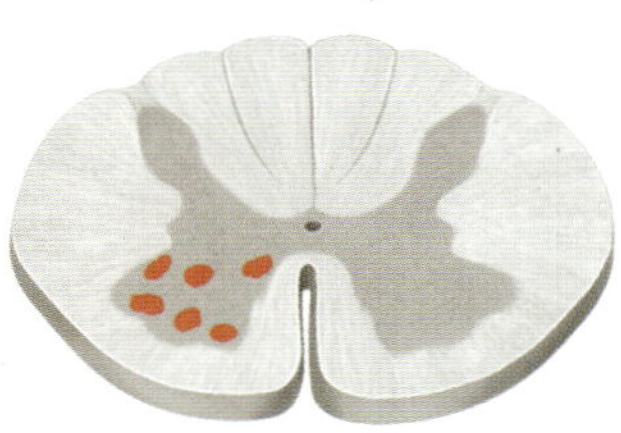

Nuclei in the spinal cord

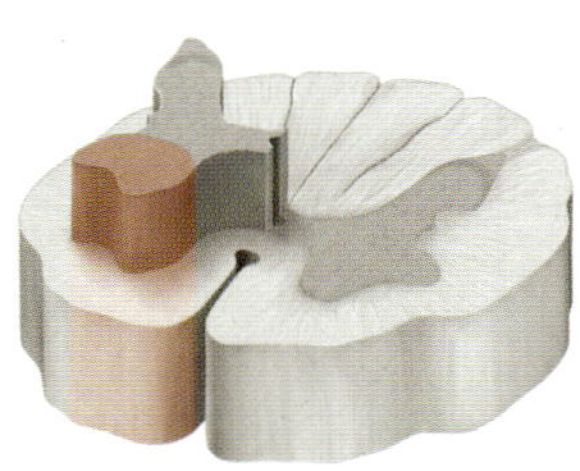

Arrangement of gray matter in columns in the spinal cord

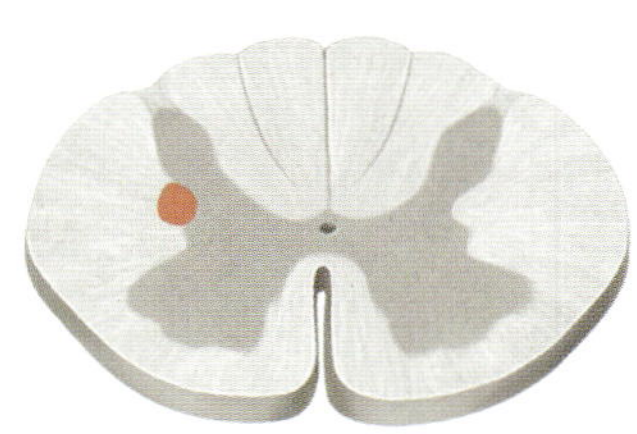

Arrangement resembling a "net" in the spinal cord

Lamina:

- *Definition:* layered arrangement of neurons; microscopically or barely macroscopically visible. In the cerebellum and at the hippocampus, the layers are also referred to as stratum/strata.
- *Distribution:* cortex and nuclei (not in all nuclei!) and spinal cord. The lamina in the spinal cord are classified cytomorphologically according to Rexed, even if they don't always feature a classical layer pattern.

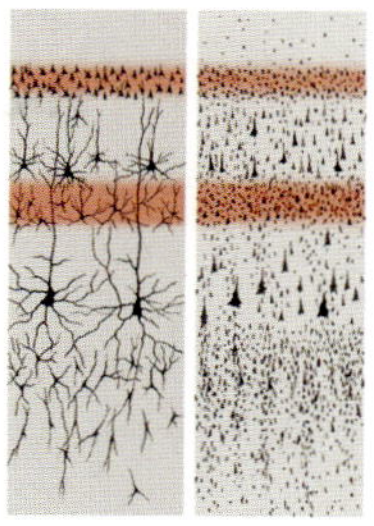

Cerebral cortex
(here: isocortex)

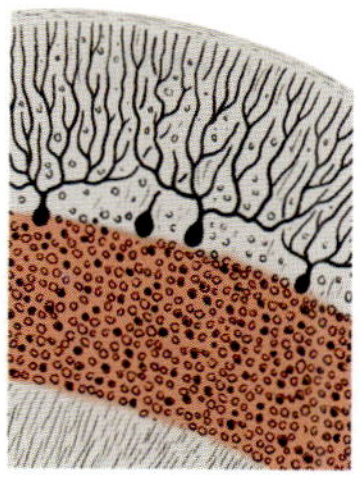

Cerebellar cortex

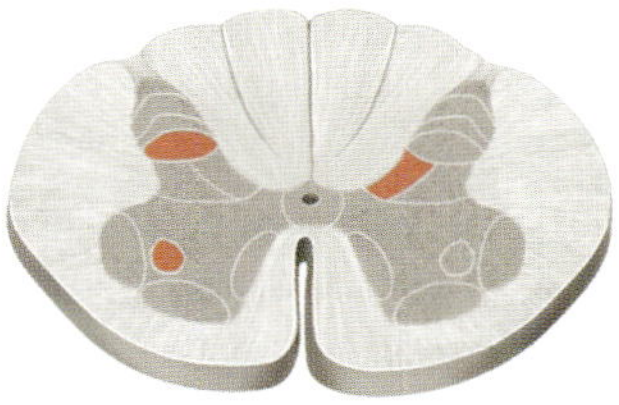

Spinal cord:
Laminae according to Rexed

Gray matter in the CNS, functional terms: nuclei of origin and terminali

- **Nucleus of origin [A]:**
  a tract originates from it (originating neuron)
- **Terminal nucleus [B]:**
  at which a fiber tract ends (terminating neuron)
- **Motor nucleus**
  is always the originating nucleus, from which a motor fiber emerges.
  Note: Not every nucleus of origin is a motor nucleus!
- **Sensory nucleus**
  is always a terminal nucleus, at which a sensory tract or afferent fibers from cranial or spinal nerves end.
  Note: Not every terminal nucleus is a sensory nucleus!

Gray matter in the CNS, terminology aspects

Note: For historical reasons, some nuclei are not called "nucleus" but have proper names. Notable examples:

- **Telencephalon**
  - Putamen
  - Globus pallidus
  - Claustrum
- **Diencephalon**
  - Thalamus
  - Zona incerta
- **Midbrain (mesencephalon)**
  - Substantia nigra
- **Brainstem**
  - Substantia grisea centralis

The equivalent of gray matter in the PNS, morphological terms

Ganglion: cluster of neuronal cell bodies in the PNS. Based on their function (see below), ganglia are divided into

- Sensory ganglion (somatic nervous system) and
- Autonomic ganglion (autonomic nervous system).

Note: Per definition, ganglia are found only in the PNS. Thus, the term "basal ganglia" is incorrect. Accurately, they are basal nuclei, which is also expressed in the Latin term "Nuclei basales."

Sensory ganglion:
Ganglion of the somatic nervous system, which would be

- Dorsal root ganglion, on the posterior root of the spinal nerve in the proximity of the spinal cord or as
- Sensory ganglion of a cranial nerve along the course of the sensory component of a cranial nerve.

Note: Synapses are found only in autonomic ganglia, not in sensory ones.

Autonomic ganglion:
Ganglion of the autonomic nervous system, which could be

- Sympathetic ganglion either paravertebral in the sympathetic trunk or prevertebral (only in abdomen and pelvis);
- Parasympathetic ganglion, which is close to the target organs; usually very small.

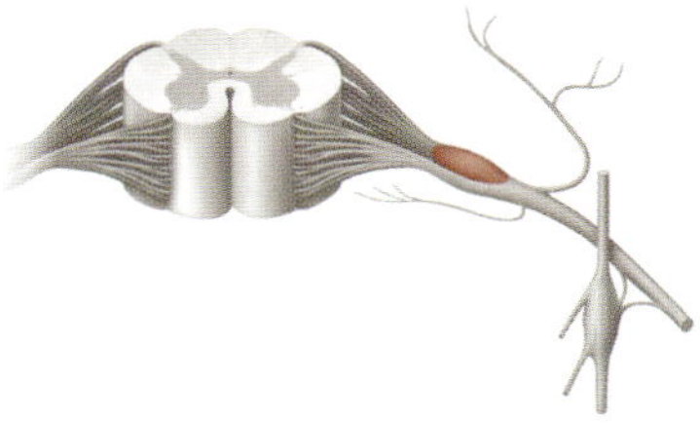

Dorsal root ganglion

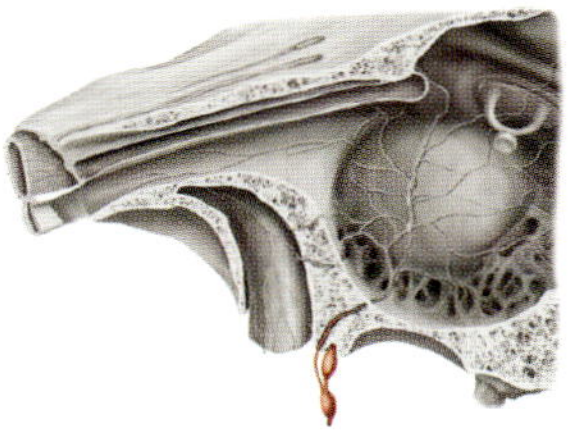

Sensory ganglia of the glossopharyngeal nerve

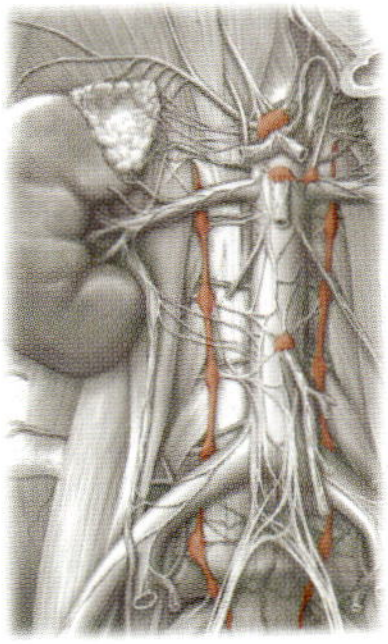

Sympathetic ganglia: sympathetic trunk and prevertebral ganglia

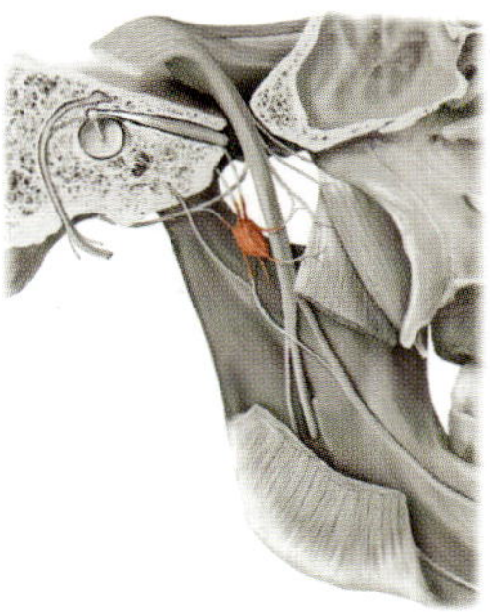

Parasympathetic ganglion: pterygopalatine ganglion

1.2 White matter (Substantia alba)

- **Definition of "white matter":**
  Accumulation of bundled and myelinated neuronal processes, which appear white in the unstained cross-section specimens, because the myelin sheaths mainly consist of lipids
- **Distribution:**
  - in the telencephalon and cerebellum as subcortical white matter (located underneath the cortex); it appears morphologically homogeneous, yet functionally it is divided into microscopically detectable tracts,
  - in the PNS, the equivalent of white matter consists of nerve fibers.

The distinction between the following terms is not always clearly defined and is not consistently used.

Morphological terms

Funiculus (cord) or column
- Cord-like strand, morphologically loose arrangement of white matter
- Example: Dorsal column in the spinal cord

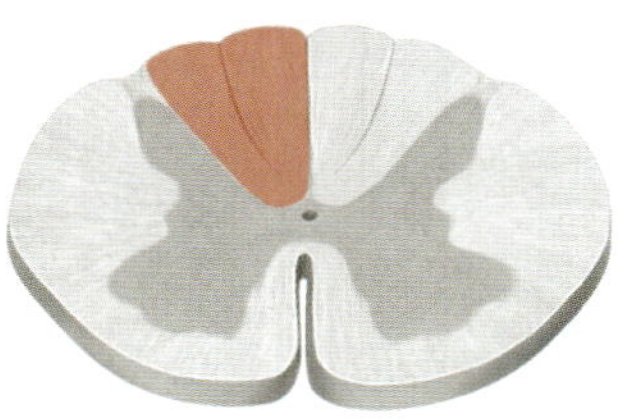

Tract:
- Group of nerve fibers with a common origin and destination
- Example: spinothalamic tract that runs from the spinal cord to the thalamus

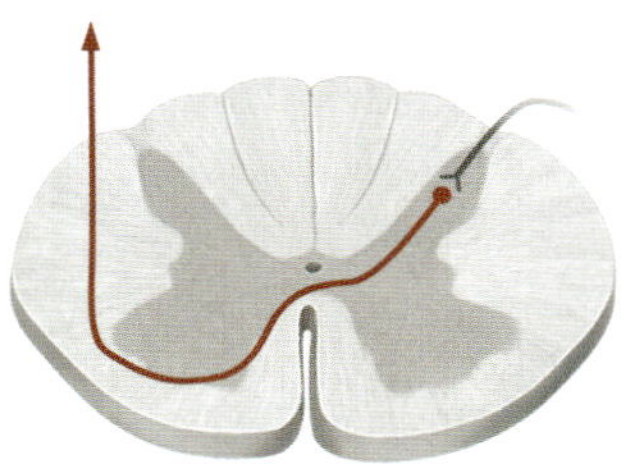

Fasciculus (bundle):
- Morphologically clearly defined accumulation of neuronal processes; contains at least one, p.r.n. multiple tracts
- Example: Fasciculus cuneatus

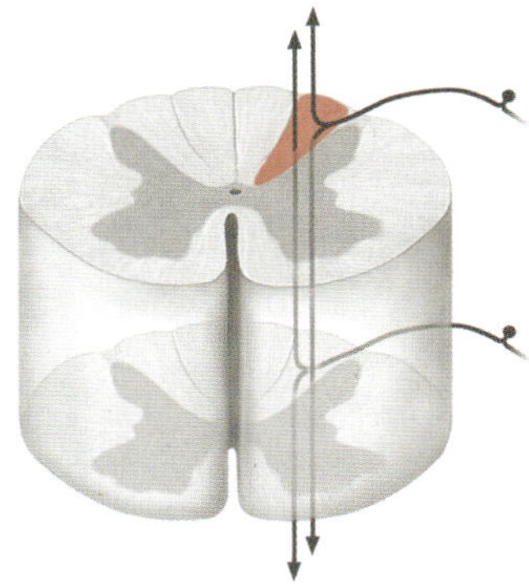

Stria (strand):
- Strandlike accumulation of bundles of white matter
- Example: Corpus striatum in the basal nuclei of the telencephalon: Due to their rapid growth, the bundles of white matter "break up" the clusters of neuronal cell bodies that form nuclei, creating a "zebra stripe" pattern.

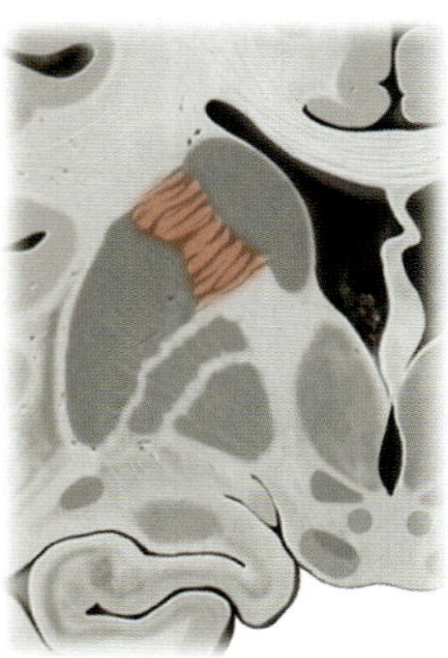

Lemniscus (ribbon):
Historically used term, specifically for four sensory tracts in the brainstem, which exhibit a ribbon-like course: medial, lateral, spinal and trigeminal lemniscus

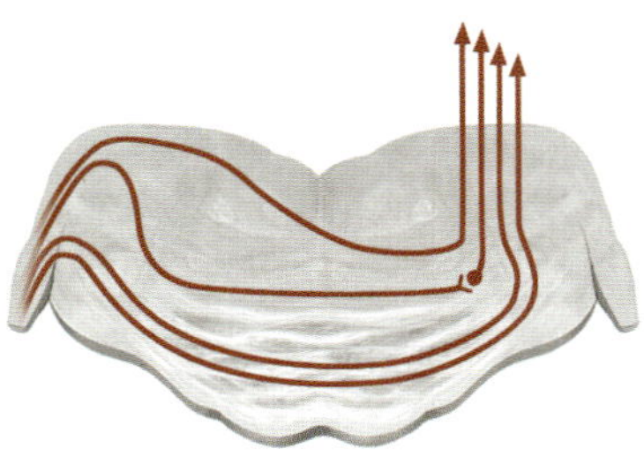

Course:
Everywhere in the CNS, particularly in the spinal cord and the brainstem, a distinction is made between the ascending (running from caudal to cranial) and descending (running from cranial to caudal) trajectory

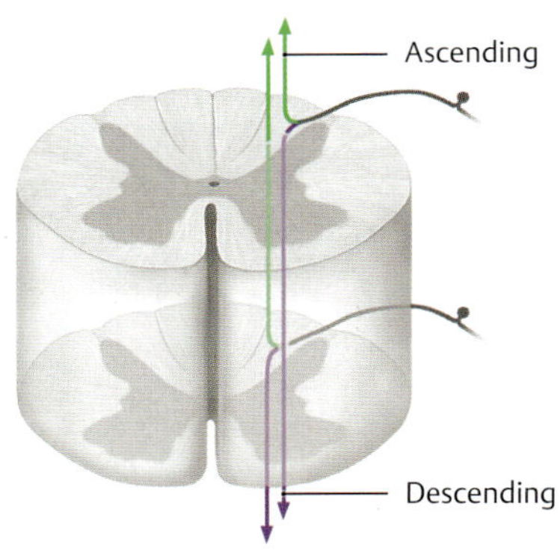

Terminological particularities regarding tracts

Note: For historical reasons, some tracts are not termed "tract" or "fasciculus," but have proper names. Notable examples:

- **In the telencephalon:** internal, external and extreme capsule; corpus callosum
- **Diencephalon and telencephalon:** fornix (vault)
- **Brainstem:** lemniscus (ribbon)

White matter in the CNS, functional terms

Projection fibers:
- All tracts within the CNS that connect areas of different levels of organization such as the cerebral cortex (Co) with subcortical centers (sc), but also tracts connecting the lower levels among themselves without *involvement of the cortex* (such as brainstem and spinal cord).
- *Corticofugal* projection tracts course away from the cortex (such as the pyramidal tract); *corticopetal* tracts course toward the cortex (such as the thalamocortical fibers).

Note: One projection fiber conveys information in only one direction.

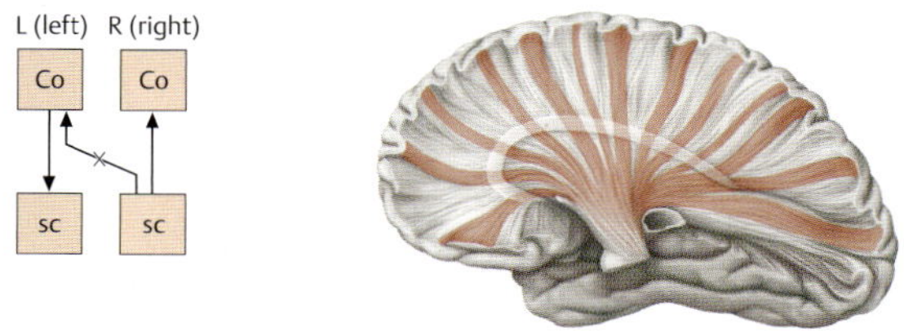

Target neuron ispi- or contralateral to the originating neurons

Association fibers:
- White matter bundles that connect different cortical parts of the same cerebral hemisphere (cf. p. 530)
- Example: superior longitudinal fasciculus

Note: An association fasciculus usually conveys information bidirectionally.

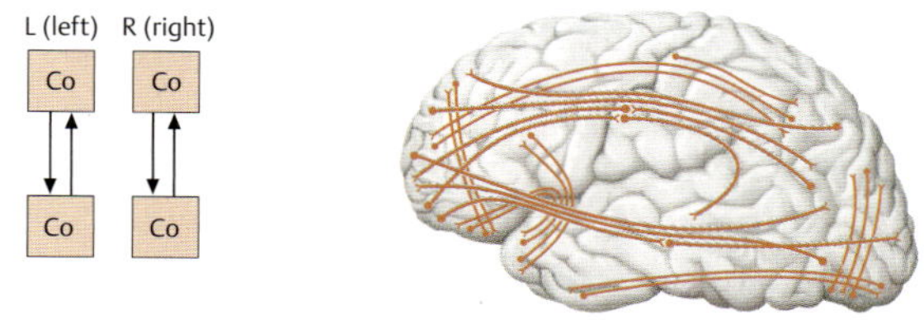

Target neuron *ipsi*lateral to the originating neuron

Commissure:
- Tracts that connect similar structures on the left and right side of the CNS
- Example: anterior commissure (cf. p. 540)
- **Commissural fibers:** the fibers that form of a commissure

Note: Commissures always convey information bidirectionally.

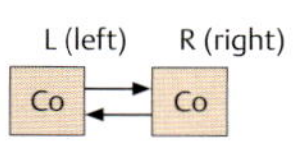

Target neuron *contra*lateral to the originating neuron

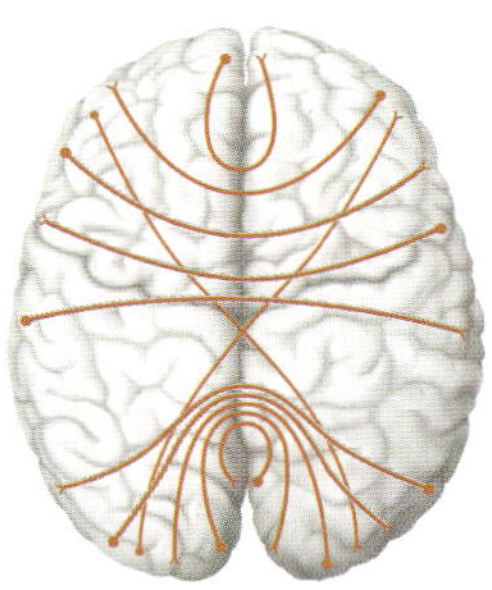

Decussation (crossing):
- Nerve fibers crossing the midline to the opposite side of the CNS
- Connecting different structures
- Example: pyramidal decussation (crossing of the pyramidal tract; cf. p. 547)

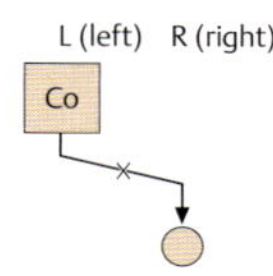

Target neuron *contra*lateral to the originating neuron

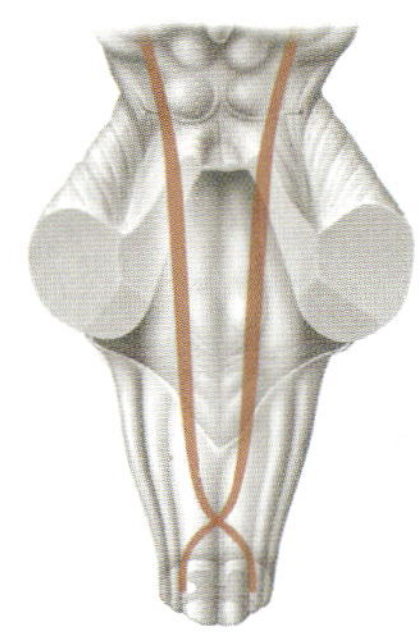

Nerve fibers in the PNS, functional terms

Afferent fibers (blue): nerve fibers bundled in one nerve, carrying impulses toward the CNS

Efferent fibers (red): nerve fibers bundled in one nerve, carrying impulses away from the CNS

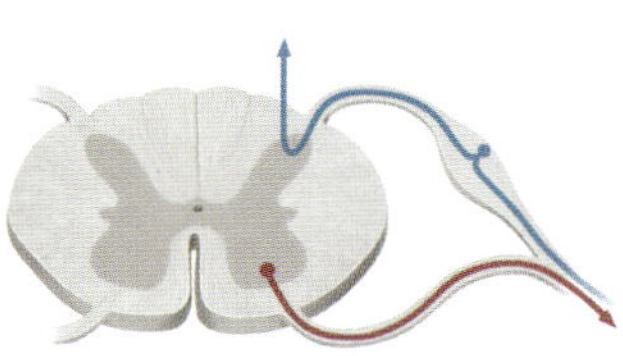

Somatic fibers: Fibers that innervate skeletal muscles and the skin

Autonomic fibers: Fibers that innervate the internal organs (not shown here)

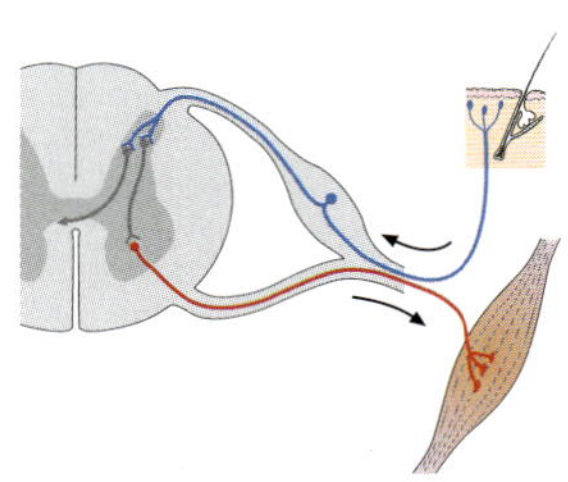

Autonomic plexus:
- Network of autonomic fibers
- Example: inferior hypogastric plexus

Visceral plexus:
- Specific part of an autonomic plexus, directly at the organ
- Example: rectal plexus

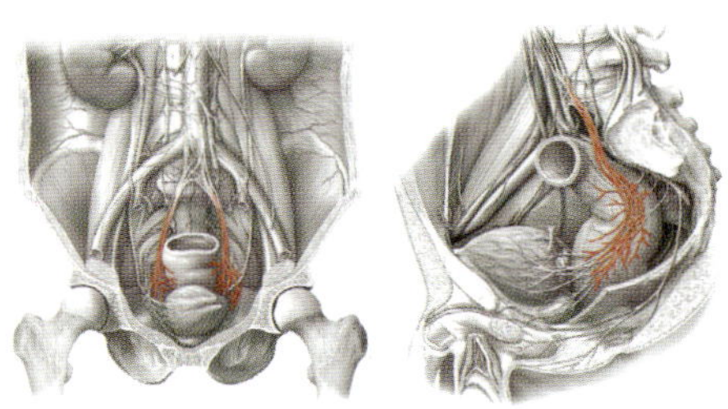

Preganglionic fibers (purple):
- Nerve fibers from the CNS to the autonomic ganglion
- In the sympathetic nervous system as white ramus communicans to the paravertebral ganglion (sympathetic chain) or as thoracic or lumbar splanchnic nerve to the prevertebral ganglion
- In the parasympathetic nervous system in the composition of certain cranial nerves or as pelvic splanchnic nerves

Postganglionic fibers (green):
- Nerve fibers from the autonomic ganglion to the target organ
- In the sympathetic nervous system as gray ramus communicans to the spinal nerve or as autonomic plexus to the target organ

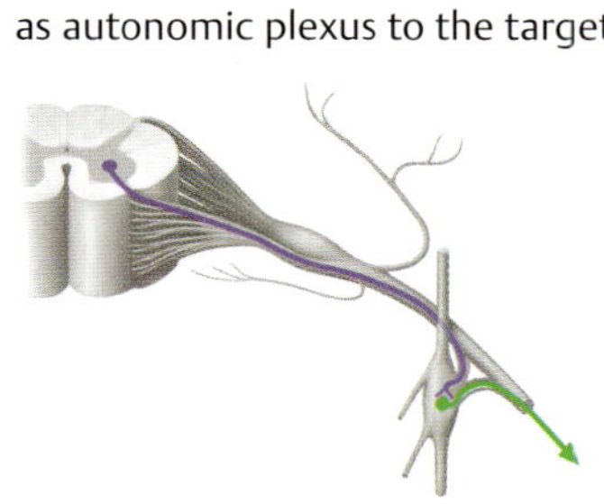

1.3 Sensory and Motor Functions: Overview of the Spinal Cord and Spinal Cord Tracts

A Sensory and motor functions in the CNS and PNS: general terminology

Sensory functions of the CNS and PNS	Motor functions of the CNS and PNS
Somatosensation: • General somatosensation: including the following: – *Exteroception* (external perception, or superficial sensation): transmission of impulses from the skin – *Proprioception* (self-perception, or deep sensation), transmission of impulses from muscle spindles and stretch receptors in tendons and articular capsules (via the sensory components of the cranial and spinal nerves) • Based on the type of sensation, exteroception is further divided into – *Epicritic sensation* (fine touch, vibration; two-point discrimination and pressure) and – *Protopathic sensation* (diffuse touch and pressure; temperature and pain). • Special somatosensation: Processing of impulses from the retina (vision) and inner ear (hearing; acceleration) via the optic nerve and vestibulocochlear nerve respectively	**Somatomotor:** The innervation of striated muscles of the trunk, limbs, neck, and extra-ocular muscles is provided by the somatomotor component of the corresponding spinal and cranial nerves.
Visceral sensation: • General visceral sensation: Transmission of impulses from the internal organs and blood vessels (e.g., wall tension, blood pressure, oxygen saturation); via afferent autonomic fibers, (especially sympathetic fibers), mainly via the splanchnic nerves, but also via the cranial nerves IX and X; • Special visceral sensation: Transmission of impulses from the taste buds (via the cranial nerves VII, IX and X) and the olfactory mucosa (via the olfactory nerves, bulbs and tracts). *Note:* The perikarya of the pseudounipolar neurons, which convey visceral sensation, are located in the sensory ganglia of spinal or cranial nerves (e.g., of vagal nerve).	**Visceromotor** (innervation of the "internal organs"): • General visceromotor Innervation of the smooth muscles of the organs (viscera) and the blood vessels as well as glands and the heart. It is conveyed through the vegetative nervous system via parasympathetic and sympathetic nerve fibers, which partly run with spinal or cranial nerves (in case of the latter only parasympathetic) and partly independently (e.g., as splanchnic nerves). • Special visceromotor Embryology concept. They supply the striate muscles innervated by the nerves of branchial arches: mastication (V_3); facial expression (VII); pharynx and larynx (IX and X) as well as craniofugal muscles (XI). (From a phylogenetic perspective, it refers to somatomotor innervation of muscles that were "visceral muscles" in fish).

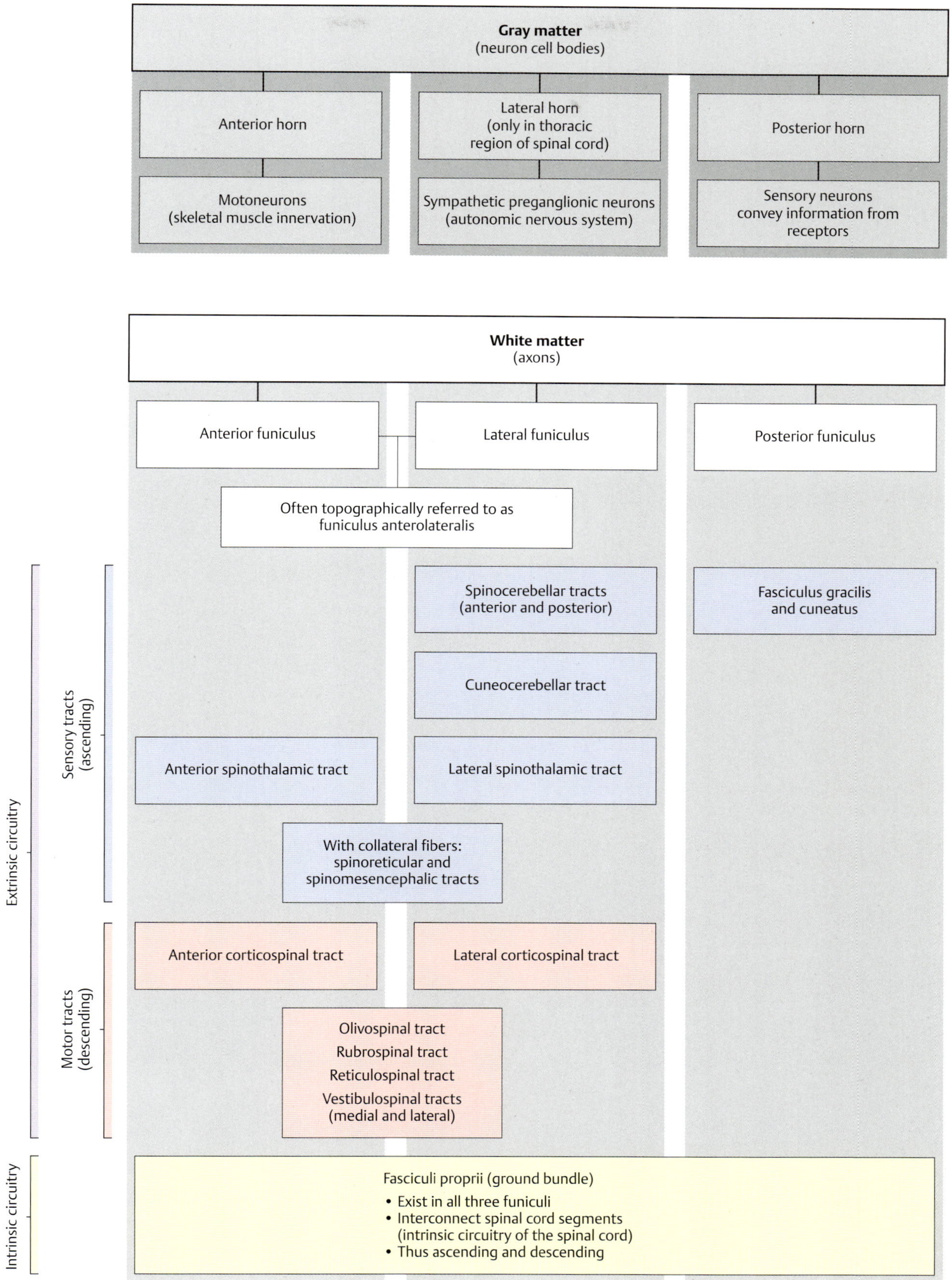

B Overview of spinal cord and spinal cord tracts
Note: In the brainstem, the spinothalamic tract is known as the spinal lemniscus, while the medial lemniscus contains the axons of neurons with their cell bodies located in the gracilis and cuneatus nuclei, see p. 508 f.

2.1 Sensory Tracts of the Spinal Cord

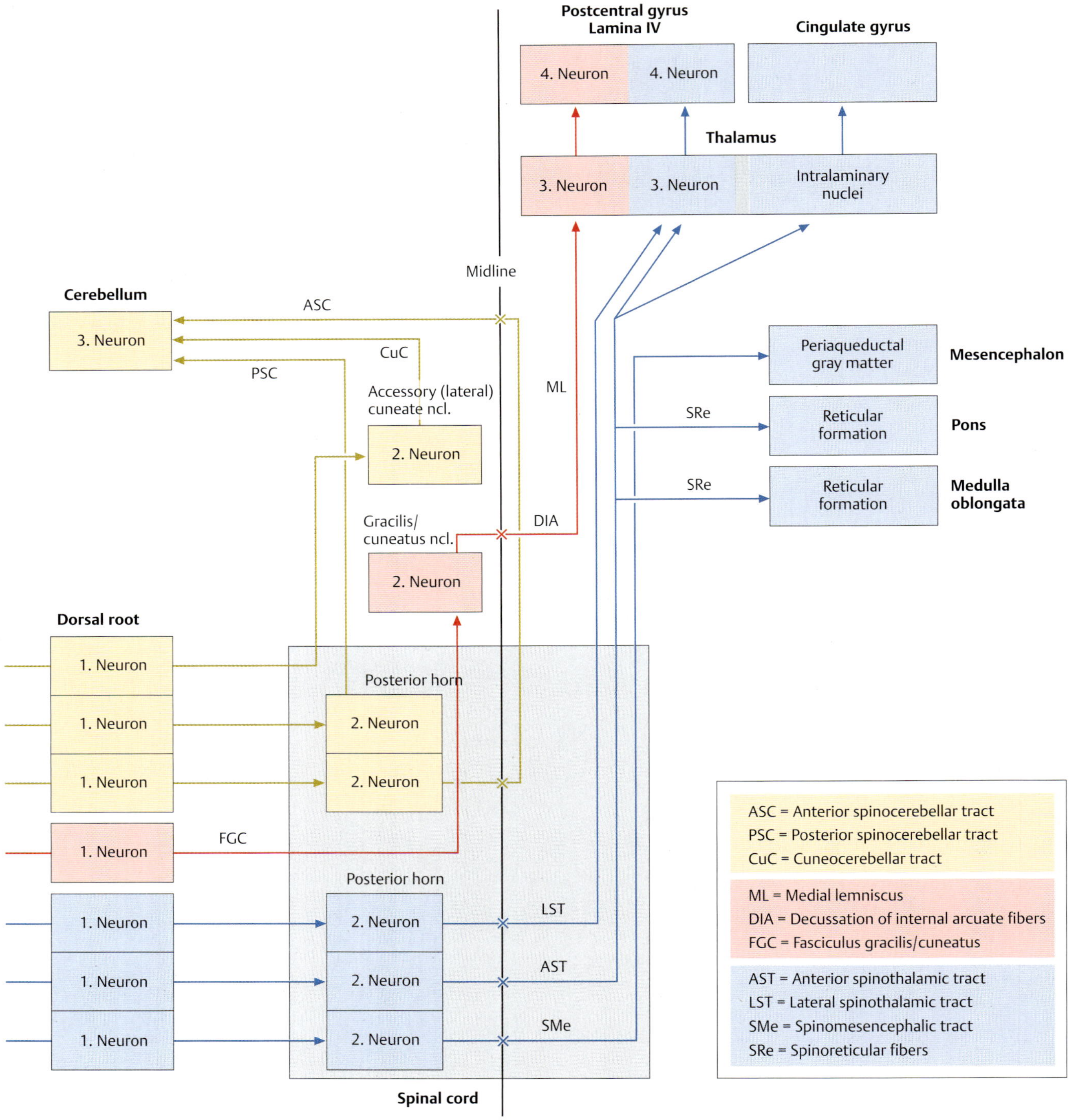

Definition and function

The sensory tracts in the spinal cord carry all somatosensory modalities related to the trunk, neck, and limbs to the cerebellum or to the telencephalon. Since they share very important features, they are presented together in this chapter. The clearest classification of the tracts is the one based on the type of information they transmit:

- The type of sensation that can be perceived consciously reaches the telencephalon via the thalamus (*spinocortical*) and is transmitted through a four-neuron chain.
- The type of sensation that is unconscious ascends to the cerebellum (*spinocerebellar*) without thalamic involvement and is transmitted through a three-neuron chain.

Note: Pathways to the telencephalon always cross; pathways to the cerebellum terminate on the same side with the point of origin. Even the anterior spinocerebellar tract eventually ends ipsilaterally, as it crosses the midline twice.

Qualities of somatosensation

- Exteroception (conscious external sensation through the skin):
  - epicritic sensation is carried in the *fasciculus gracilis* and *cuneatus* (dorsal column)
  - protopathic sensation is carried in the *anterior and lateral spinothalamic tracts*; important collaterals exist for this tract (see below).
- Proprioception (largely unconscious), the responsible tracts run to the cerebellum as
  - *anterior* and *posterior spinocerebellar tracts* (responsible for the lower part of the body and lower limb) and
  - *cuneocerebellar tract* (responsible for the upper part of the body and upper limb, see below).
- Information related to conscious proprioception is carried by the *fasciculi gracilis* and *cuneatus* (thus fasciculi gracilis/cuneatus carry extero- and proprioceptive information).

Neural wiring and topography of tracts

4 (spinocortical) or 3 (spinocerebellar) consecutive neurons. For all tracts, the first-order neuron is located in the dorsal root ganglion. For the tracts ascending to the telencephalon, the third-order and sometimes the fourth-order neuron have the same location.

First-order neuron
Pseudounipolar neuron in the dorsal root ganglion: Its peripheral process receives the information from a receptor (for pain transmission, the receptor is the ending of the neuronal process itself) and the axon (central process) carries it with via the dorsal root of the spinal nerve to the spinal cord.

Second-order neuron:

- *Fasciculus gracilis* and *cuneatus* consist of axons of the first-order neurons. They end in the ipsilateral nucleus gracilis and cuneatus respectively (in the medulla oblongata) where the bodies of the second-order neurons are located. After crossing the midline immediately rostral to the nuclei (at the lemniscal decussation), the axons of the second-order neurons form the medial lemniscus, thus reaching the third-order neuron in the contralateral thalamus.
- *Anterior* and *lateral spinothalamic tracts*: The second-order neurons' cell bodies are in the ispilateral posterior horn of the spinal cord. The axons of the second-order neurons cross the midline and ascend in the contralateral anterolateral funiculus to the thalamus. In the brainstem, the axons of the second-order neurons are refferred to as the spinal lemniscus. Axons of the second-order neurons can also ascend to the reticular formation (*spinoreticular fibers*) or to the mesencephalon (*spinomesencephalic fibers*) for the subcortical processing of painful stimuli (e.g., reacting to painful stimuli);
- *Anterior* and *posterior spinocerebellar tracts*: The cell bodies of the second-order neurons that form the posterior spinocerebellar tract are located at the base of the *ipsilateral posterior horn* in the dorsal nucleus of Clarke. These axons remain uncrossed and travel in the lateral funiculus of the spinal cord to the ipsilateral brainstem. The cell bodies of the second-order neurons that form the anterior spinocerebellar tract are located in the middle of the ipsilateral posterior horn. Their axons run in the lateral funiculus either crossed (at the anterior white commissure) or uncrossed and reach the brainstem. The axons of the *posterior* spinocerebellar tract travel via the inferior cerebellar peduncle to the ipsilateral cerebellum.

  Note: Collaterals of the posterior spinocerebellar tract reach to a brainstem nucleus ("Nucleus Z"; adjacent to nucleus gracilis), which further projects via the medial lemniscus to the thalamus (VPL nucleus), which in turn projects to the postcentral gyrus (ensuring conscious proprioception of the lower part of the body, not shown here). The axons of the anterior spinocerebellar tract reach the mesencephalon and then the cerebellum through the superior cerebellar peduncle. The fibers in this tract that crossed in the spinal cord, cross back to their original side.
- *Cuneocerebellar tract*: The second-order neurons are located in the accessory (lateral) cuneate nucleus, which is immediately next to the nucleus cuneatus of the medulla oblongata. The axons of the second-order neurons travel uncrossed through the ipsilateral inferior cerebellar peduncle to the cerebellum. Similar to posterior spinocerebellar tract, collaterals from the cuneocerebellar tract project to the thalamus, which in turn projects to the telencephalon (ensuring conscious proprioception for the upper body).

Third-order neuron:

- *Fasciculus gracilis/cuneatus* and *anterior/lateral spinothalamic tract:* The body of the third-order neuron is located in the ventral posterolateral nucleus (VPL) of the thalamus. Their axons travel to the cerebral cortex (to the fourth-order neurons) in the thalamic radiations in the posterior limb of the internal capsule.
- *Only for the spinothalamic tracts:* Bodies of third-order neurons are also located in the thalamic intralaminar nuclei, which project to the cingulate gyrus (limbic system; emotional meaning of pain).
- *Spinocerebellar* and *cuneocerebellar tracts:* Bodies of third-order neurons are located in the cerebellum, either in the cerebellar nuclei (mainly the emboliform and globose nuclei) or as granule cells in the cortex of the spinocerebellum (in the anterior lobe, vermis, paramedial zone) that synapse with mossy fibers.

Fourth-order neuron:

- *Fasciculus gracilis/cuneatus* and *spinothalamic tracts:* The body of fourth-order neurons are located in the internal granular layer (layer IV) of the postcentral gyrus. In case of the spinothalamic pathway, bodies of fourth-order neurons are also located in the cingulate gyrus.
- Tracts running to the cerebellum don't have a fourth-order neuron.

Somatotopic organization of tracts

Fibers corresponding to the sacral spinal segments are located medial or dorsal, while those corresponding to the cervical segments are positioned lateral or ventral.

Symptoms

- Dysfunction of fasciculus gracilis leads to impaired perception of touch, pressure, vibration, and position sense.
- Dysfunction of the spinothalamic tracts leads to impaired perception of pain and temperature.
- Dysfunction of spinocerebellar tracts leads to gross motor functional and gait impairment (sensory ataxia).

2.2 Motor Tracts of the Spinal Cord

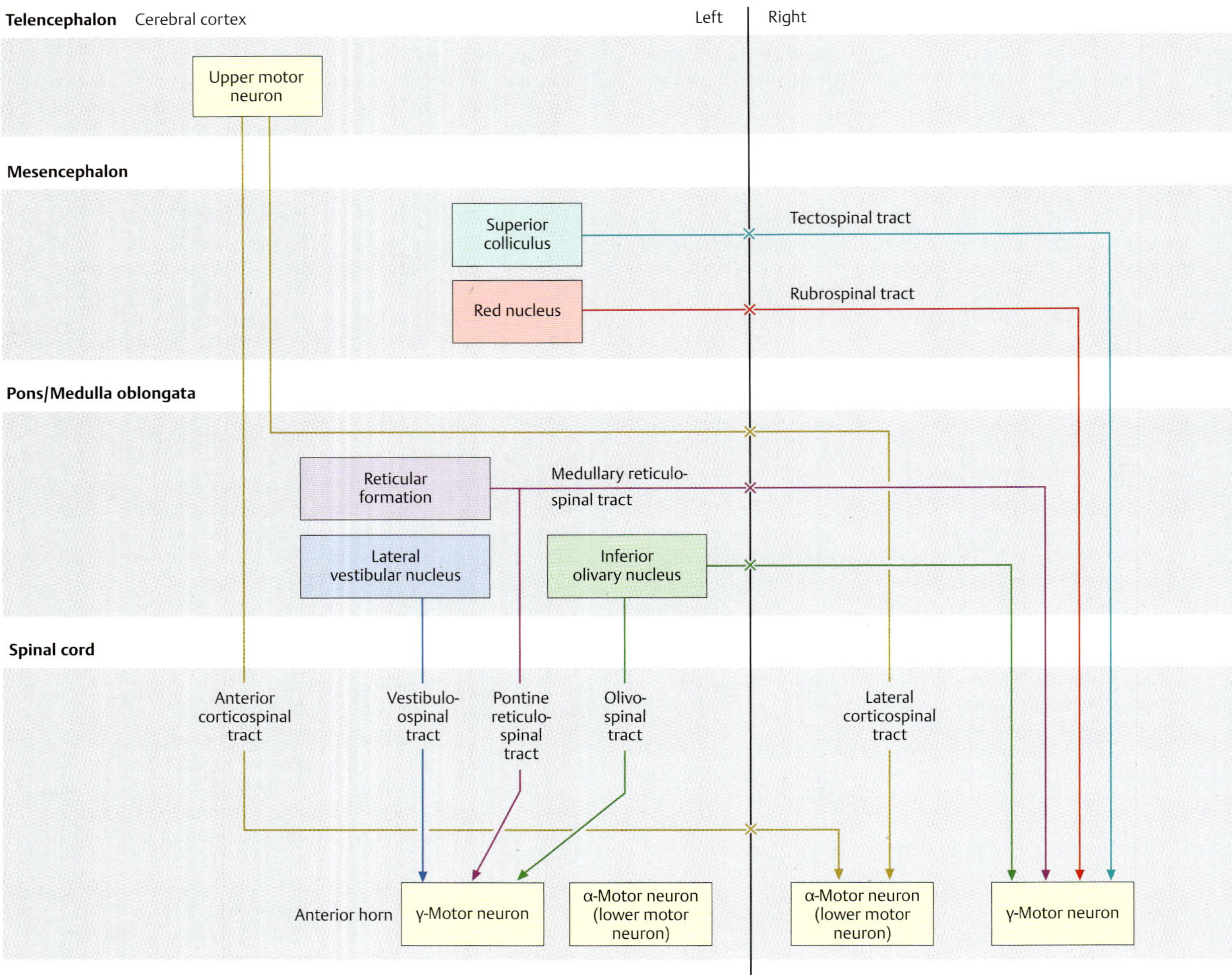

Definition and function

Motor tracts of the spinal cord can be divided into two groups:

- Pyramidal fibers (passing through the pyramid in the medulla oblongata)
- Extrapyramidal fibers (don't run in caudal direction in the pyramid, but in the tegmentum)

Pyramidal fibers originate in the cerebral cortex; extrapyramidal tracts originate in nuclei of the brainstem. A rough classification based on their functions, which is still used in the clinic, is analogous to the tracts, as one refers to pyramidal and extrapyramidal motor functions. However, physiologically, both systems work closely together.

Pyramidal fibers in the spinal cord (Anterior and lateral corticospinal tracts)

Definition and function:

- Major motor tract (voluntary motor function, conscious movement control of neck, trunk and limbs)
- The part of the *pyramidal tract*, which extends from the primary motor cortex to the spinal cord. Only when it reaches the spinal cord, is it called *corticospinal tract*; before entering the spinal cord, the fibers of this descending tract are usually referred to as *corticospinal fibers*. Like the other fibers of the pyramidal tract (fibers in the cortico*bulbar* tract to the cranial nerve nuclei and cortico*reticular* fibers to the reticular formation), they include axons of the large pyramidal cells.

Pathway characteristics:
Somatomotor; descending; efferent.
Note: Per definition, the corticonuclear and corticoreticular fibers should not be referred to as part of the pyramidal tract, since they end above the pyramid which means they don't pass through it. On functional grounds, they are considered in the same category as the corticospinal fibers and based on their neurons of origin, they are usually considered part of the "pyramidal fibers."

Neural wiring and topography of the tract (corticospinal fibers): total of two neurons:

Upper motor neuron:
Large pyramidal cells in the internal pyramidal layer (layer V) of the precentral gyrus (primary motor cortex); 40% of which are located in the Brodmann area 4; the remaining 60% are located in neighboring brain regions.

Course of the axons of the upper motor neurons: On their descending way from the telencephalon, to the decussation of the pyramids the *corticospinal fibers* travel through the

- Primary motor cortex → posterior limb of the internal capsule, → cerebral peduncles of the midbrain → base of the pons (basal pons) → medullary pyramid
- At the pyramidal decussation (thus above the spinal cord), 80% of fibers cross to the opposite side. From there
  - The uncrossed 20% run *ipsilaterally* in the spinal cord as the *anterior* corticospinal tract; they cross in the anterior white commissure only at the level of the spinal segment where those fibers end. This component of the tract ends at about the middle of the thoracic region.
  - The crossed fibers run *contralaterally* in the spinal cord as the *lateral* corticospinal tract (all spinal cord segments contain a portion of this tract).

Lower motor neuron:
α- or γ-motor neurons in the anterior horn of the spinal cord, largely in the laminae A-C after Rexed, on which the axons of the corticospinal tract terminate. The axon terminals form excitatory synapses. Axons of the lower motor neuron end on target organs, in this case striate muscles. The neurotransmitter is acetylcholine.
Note: The corticospinal tract ends on the lower motor neuron. The axons of the lower motor neurons form the somatomotor fibers in the composition of the spinal nerve.

Extrapyramidal fibers in the spinal cord

Definition and function:
Major motor pathways (mainly for fine movement control).

Pathway characteristics:
Somatomotor; descending; efferent.
The extrapyramidal pathways originate as upper motor neurons in brainstem nuclei and the premotor cortex, end mostly on γ-motor neurons in the spinal cord (as lower motor neurons), and are usually collectively called "extrapyramidal motor" pathways. They are responsible for fine-tuning motor function and subcortical preparation of a cortically initiated movement. Topographically, they run in the anterior or lateral funiculi.

Major extrapyramidal pathways are as follows:
- Lateral/Medial vestibulospinal tracts: originate in the vestibular nuclei.
- Olivospinal tract: originates in the inferior olivary nucleus.
- Ponto- and medullary reticulospinal tracts: originate in the reticular formation nuclei of the pons and medulla oblongata respectively
- Rubrospinal tract: originates in the red nucleus.
- Tectospinal tract: originates in superior colliculus nucleus of the tectum. This tract is detectable only in the cervical spinal cord.

Extrapyramidal pathways largely cross (either completely or partially). Only the lateral vestibulospinal tract has not been verified to cross.

Somatotopic organization of the anterior and lateral corticospinal tracts
(not known for extrapyramidal pathways in humans)

- In the posterior limb of the internal capsule: cervical fibers rostral; sacral fibers occipital
- In the cerebral peduncles (midbrain): cervical fibers medial; sacral fibers lateral
- In the spinal cord: cervical fibers medial; sacral fibers lateral

Symptoms

Dysfunction of the corticospinal tract leads to impaired voluntary movement of the neck, trunk, and limbs. Depending on the extent of the damage, it can result in paresis (loss of crude voluntary movement) or plegia (complete paralysis) of muscles or muscle groups. Since damage of the corticospinal fibers or tract as a result of the mechanism of injury (e.g., impairment of blood flow in the brainstem; spinal cord transection) usually also affects the *extrapyramidal pathways* which exert an inhibitory influence on spinal cord excitation, the paralysis (dysfunction of the tractus corticospinalis) is accompanied by spasticity (increased muscle tone, increased reflexes).
Note: Damage to the upper motor neuron of the pyramidal tract leads to spastic paralysis. Damage to the lower motor neuron leads to flaccid paralysis (same as in the loss of motor fibers in a peripheral nerve).

2.3 Sensory Trigeminal Pathway

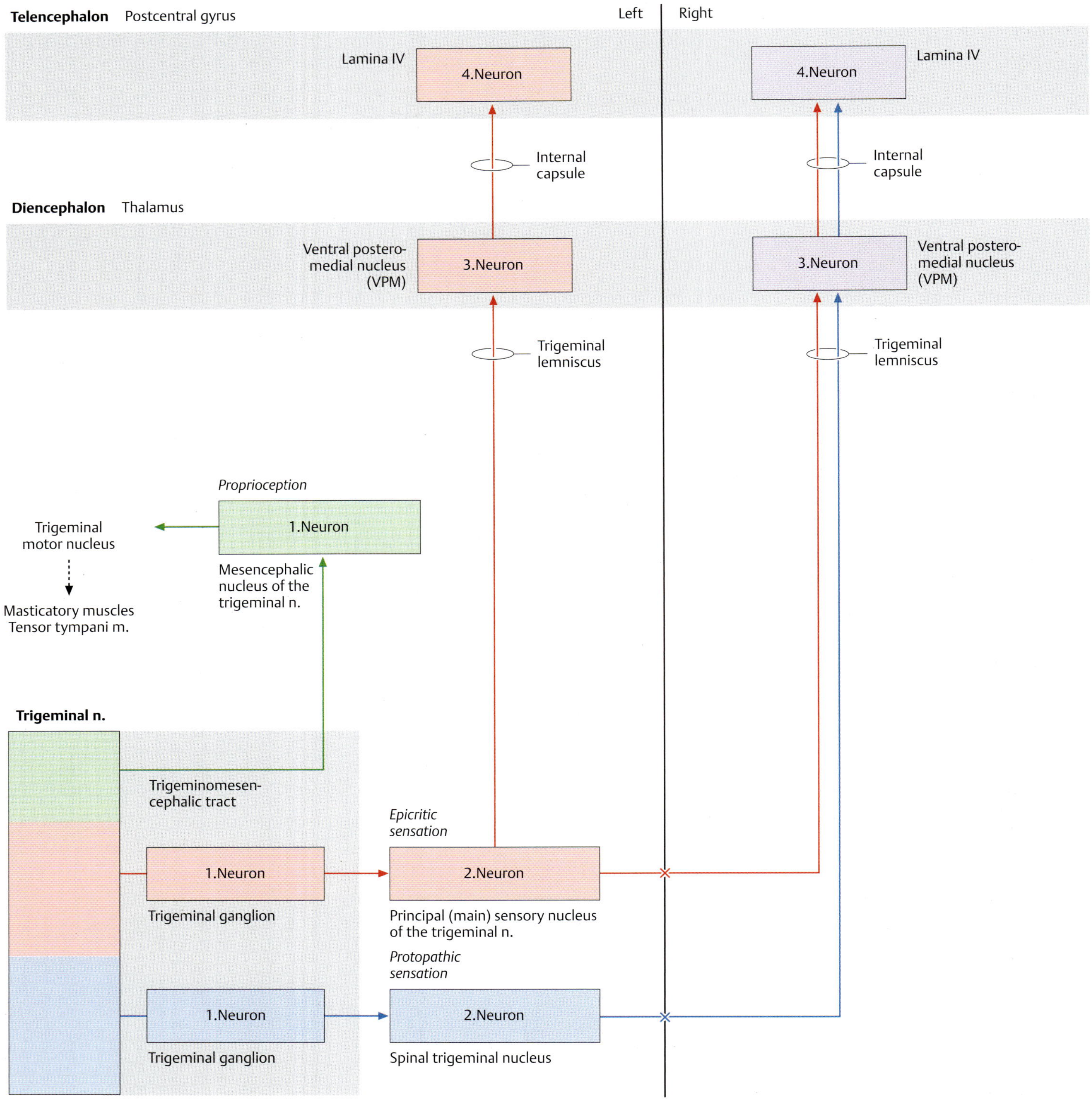

Definition and function

Major pathway of superficial sensation and (partially conscious) deep sensation.

- Superficial sensation (exteroception): information received from specific receptors on the skin surface and mucous membranes is carried to the telencephalon for conscious perception of
  - light touch, two-point discrimination and vibration (*epicritic* perception) as well as
  - crude touch and pressure, pain and temperature (*protopathic* perception). In addition to the skin surface and mucosae, pain receptors are also found in the meninges.
- Deep sensation (proprioception); information from receptors of muscles, tendons, and articular capsules located within the skull is carried to the telencephalon for conscious perception (and also unconscious perception) of increased muscle tension (*proprioceptive* perception).

Pathway characteristics

Somatosensory, ascending; afferent.
Note: All information concerning superficial and deep sensation from the head is transmitted via one single sensory trigeminal pathway. For the trunk and limbs, however, the respective information is conducted via two pathways: anterolateral system (protopathy, thus pain and temperature) and posterior column (epicritic, conscious proprioception).

Neural wiring and topography of the tract

A total of 4 serially connected neurons:

- **First-order neuron:** Pseudounipolar cell in the trigeminal ganglion located in the middle cranial fossa. It receives the stimulus via its peripheral process and carries it to the brainstem via the central process (that enters the pons) to the ipsilateral second-order neuron in the trigeminal nuclei.
  Note: The first-order neuron for the quality of "proprioception" is not located in the trigeminal ganglion but in mesencephalic nucleus of the trigeminal nerve. The mesencephalic nucleus is per definition a trigeminal ganglion which is positioned in the CNS and consists of pseudounipolar cells.
- **Second-order neuron:** For the epicritic sensation principal or main nucleus of the trigeminal nerve (located in the pons); for the protopathic sensation in the spinal nucleus of the trigeminal nerve (located in the medulla oblongata and extending into the spinal cord). The axons of the second-order neurons ascend as part of the trigeminothalamic tract to the thalamus. These fibers are called the trigeminal lemniscus and join the medial lemniscus.
  Note: The axons of the second-order neuron of the principal nucleus travel both uncrossed and crossed to the thalamus; those of the spinal nucleus travel crossed. The stimuli about epicritic sensation through the trigeminal nerve reaches both contra- and ipsilateral postcentral gyri.
- **Third-order neuron:** In the ventral posteromedial (VPM) nucleus of the ipsi and contralateral thalamus. From there, the axons of the third-order neurons travel in the thalamic radiations in the posterior limb of the internal capsule to the fourth-order neuron.
- **Fourth-order neuron:** In the telencephalon in the internal granular layer (layer IV) of the postcentral gyrus.

Note: The trigeminal nerve also has a motor nucleus that provides its motor component for the muscles of mastication and the tensor tympani muscle in the middle ear. However, the cortical control of this motor nucleus is an exception which is why it is not discussed here but as part of the "control of the motor nuclei of cranial nerves," see p. 520 f.

Somatotopic organization of the pathway

The fibers of the fourth-order neuron end in the postcentral gyrus in the area which begins superior to the central sulcus and extends toward the parietal cortex to the middle of the postcentral gyrus.

Symptoms

A dysfunction of the sensory trigeminal pathway (e.g., as a result of vascular disorders, cranial fractures or tumors) leads to impaired conscious perception of crude and light pressure, crude and light touch, pain, temperature and proprioception.
Note: Due to the (partial) crossing of the tract in the brainstem

- A lesion of the tract from the trigeminal nerve all the way to the second-order neuron leads to ipsilateral loss of sensation;
- A lesion of the tract from the thalamus to the postcentral gyrus leads to
  - contralateral disorder for the entirely contralateral projection of protopathic sensation
  - ipsi- and contralateral dysfunction in terms of epicritic sensation but usually not a complete loss due to the representation on the postcentral gyrus on both sides

2.4 Auditory Pathway

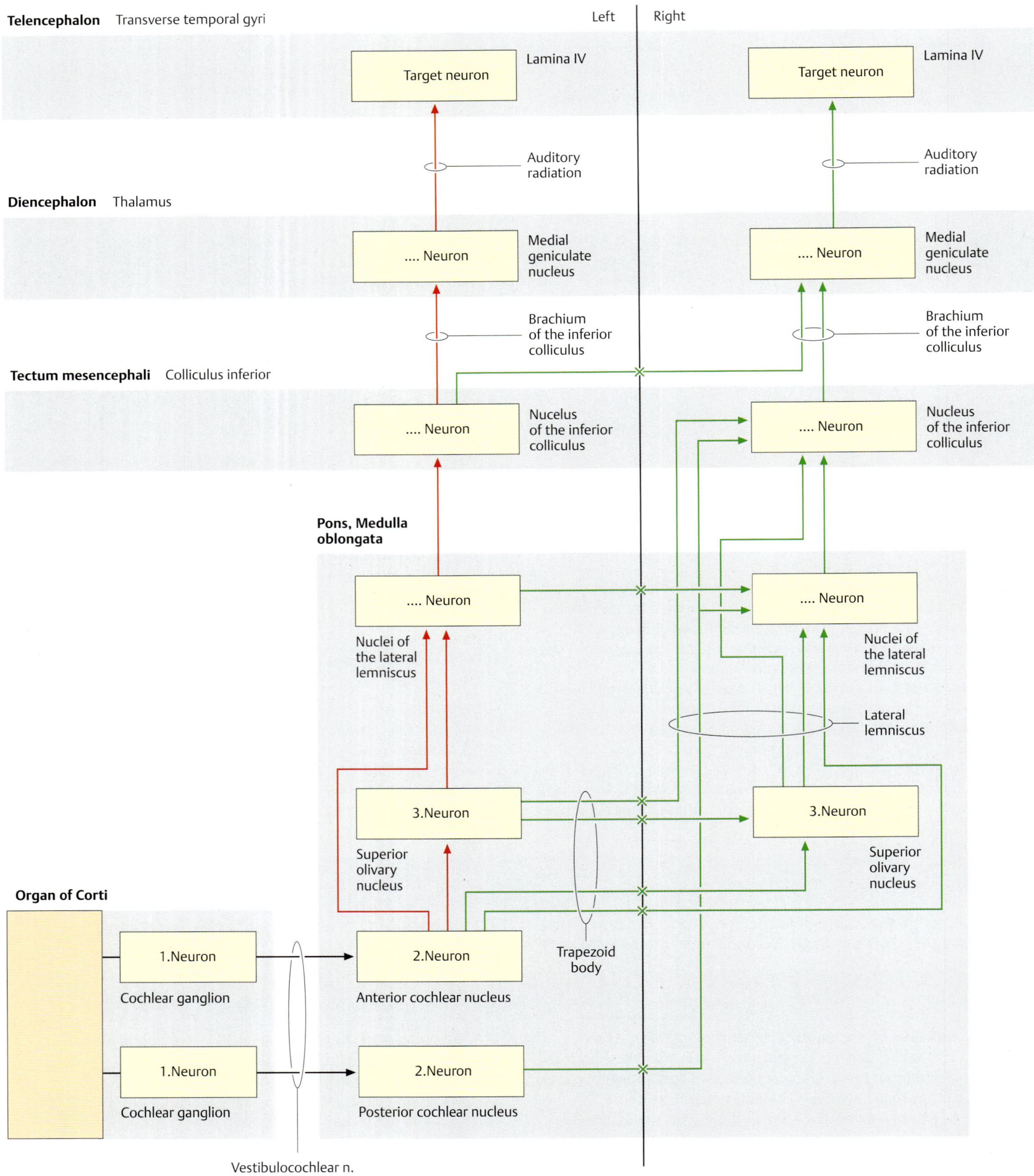

Definition and function

Pathway for the perception of acoustic stimuli including information about the amplitude, frequency and spatial location of a sound.

Characteristics of pathway

(special) somatosensory (sensory); afferent.
Note: The information is processed by a sensory organ (organ of Corti) in the cochlea (in the temporal bone), which contains specialized sensory cells (hair cells). The mechanic stimulation of these cells result in impulses that are transmitted via the cochlear part of the vestibulocochlear nerve (VIII).

Neural wiring and topography of the pathway

A total of at least six serially connected neurons:

- **First-order neuron:** Bipolar neuron in the cochlear ganglion (spiral ganglion). It receives the information from the receptor cells (inner hair cell in the organ of Corti). The axon travels via the eights cranial nerve and enters the brainstem at the cerebellopontine angle.
- **Second-order neuron:** Is located in the ipsilateral anterior/posterior cochlear nuclei of the brainstem, in the floor of the fourth ventricle close to the lateral recess. Axons of the second-order neurons travel crossed and uncrossed to the third-order neuron. All ascending fibers that leave the cochlear nuclei are collectively called lateral lemniscus.
- **Third-order neuron:** Superior olivary nucleus (axons of the second-order neuron predominantly originate in the anterior cochlear nucleus). From the superior olivary nucleus and the anterior cochlear nucleus, fibers travel to the opposite side. When crossing over, they can (but not necessarily have to) terminate in a small nuclear group (not shown) called trapezoid body nuclei. All of these small nuclei together with the crossing fibers are collectively called the trapezoid body.

Note: One characteristic of the auditory pathway is that the successive stations of this neuronal circuit are not always followed by all parts of the tract. Groups of axons can bypass individual neural relay stations shown here. Only first (in the cochlear ganglion), second (in the cochlear nuclei), and last (cortical neuron; see target neuron) are constant stations of this neuronal circuit. Thus, a strict neuron enumeration after the third-order neuron of this particular pathway is no longer useful.

- **Additional stations of the neuronal circuit:**
  - Nuclei of the lateral lemniscus (receive input from both cochlear nuclei)
  - Nucleus of the inferior colliculus (in the inferior colliculus of the mesencephalon); from here, axons travel to the thalamus via the brachium of the inferior colliculus.
  - Medial geniculate nucleus (in the medial geniculate body of the thalamus). From here, axons travel as acoustic radiation to the primary auditory cortex.
- **Target neuron:** Primary auditory cortex, internal granular layer (layer IV) in the transverse temporal gyri (Heschl's gyri), Brodmann area 41

Note: The pattern of crossing of axons of the the second-order neuron and the following neurons of the pathway leads to the primary auditory cortex receiving information from both cochlear organs, which substantially contributes to the auditory spatial perception.

Somatotopic (= in this case tonotopic) organization of pathway

The tonotopic organization of the auditory cortex adapts to the structure of Heschl's gyri. In the primary auditory cortex, high frequencies are rather located near the occipital bone, and low frequencies more anteriorly.

Symptoms

Unilateral damage to the auditory pathway proximal to the cochlear nuclei leads to impaired auditory spatial perception. Bilateral damage leads to deafness. Unilateral damage distal to the cochlear nuclei results in unilateral deafness (on the affected side).

2.5 Gustatory Pathway

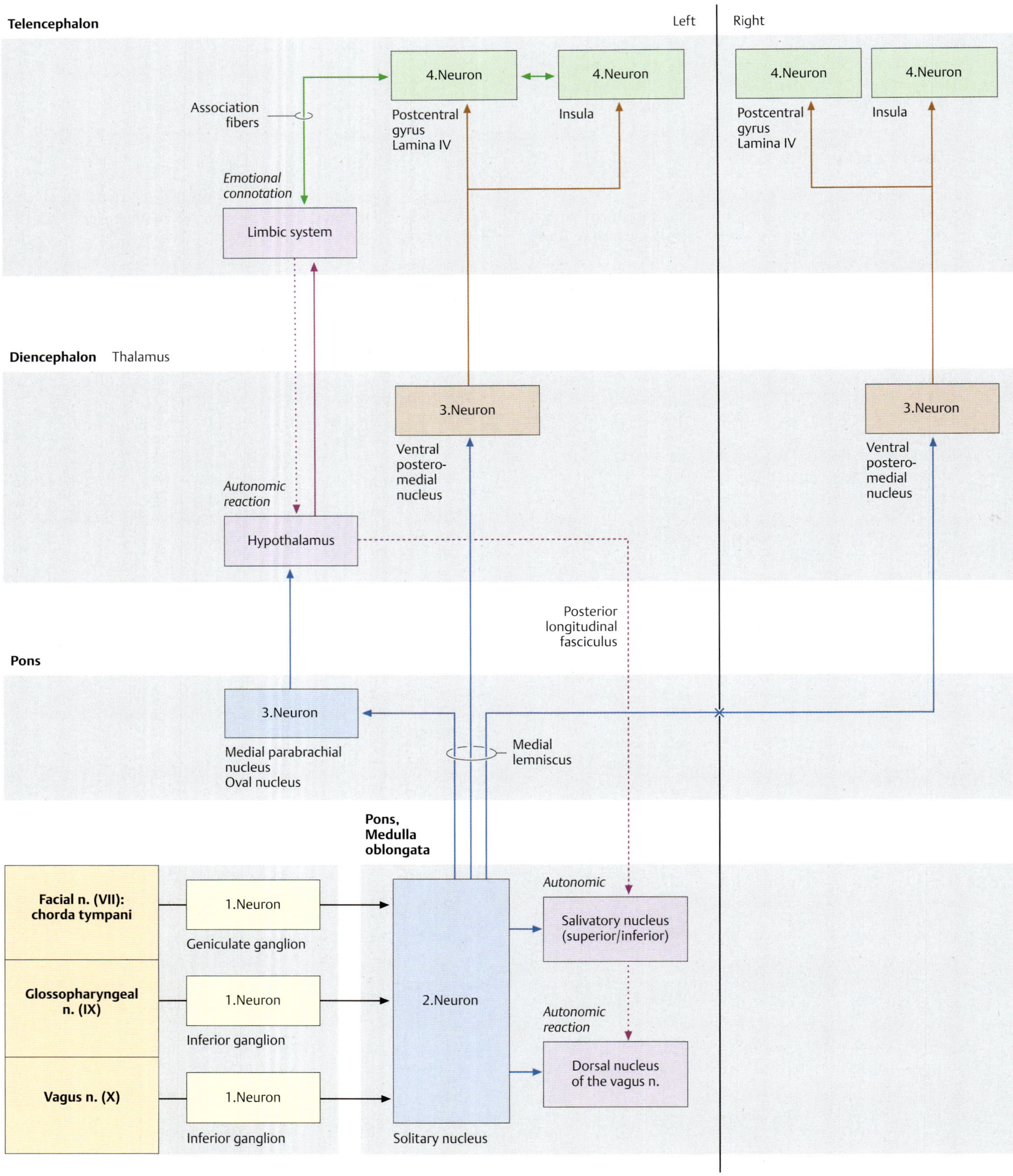

Definition and function

Pathway for the conscious taste sensation from the tongue (sensation of sweet, sour, salty, bitter, umami)

Characteristics of pathway

(special) viscerosensory (sensory); afferent.
Note: Taste information is conveyed via three cranial nerves: facial n. (VII), glossopharyngeal n. (IX) and vagus n. (X). They all pick up signals from taste receptors on the tongue surface and carry them first to a common, centrally located nucleus, the *solitary nucleus* (nucleus of the solitary tract). This pathway ends in two different cortical locations: insula and postcentral gyrus.

Neural wiring and topography of the pathway

- **First-order neuron:** Pseudounipolar neuron with the cell body *in the ganglion of the corresponding cranial nerve*. Its peripheral process receives the information from a taste receptor. The central process of the pseudounipolar neuron with the body in the cranial nerve ganglion ascends ipsilaterally to the brainstem where it synapses with the second-order neuron in the solitary nucleus.
  Note: The afferent fibers of the facial n. initially run with the lingual n., then with the chorda tympani n. before joining the facial n. in the facial canal of the temporal bone and traveling as part of the facial nerve to the brainstem.
- **Second-order neuron:** In the medulla oblongata ipsilateral in the solitary nucleus (pars gustatoria). The axons of the second-order neurons ascend uncrossed to the pons (where they terminate on third-order neurons) or bypass the pontine nuclei and directly join the ipsilateral medial lemniscus (and apparently to a lesser degree the contralateral one) on the way to the thalamus (where the third-order neurons are located in this case).
- **Third-order neuron:**
  - in the *pons*: in a pontine nuclear group close to the lateral recess of the fourth ventricle: parabrachial nucleus and oval nucleus. From there, the pathway ascends uncrossed to the hypothalamus and further to parts of the limbic system.
  - in the *thalamus*: located in the ventral posteromedial nucleus. From there, fibers of the thalamic radiation ascend in the posterior limb of the internal capsule.
- **Fourth-order neuron** in the postcentral gyrus (internal granular layer [IV]) or the insular cortex**.**

Note: Thus, the gustatory pathway ends on two cortical regions, where apparently different type of information is processed. Collaterals of the parabrachial nucleus and oval nucleus reach the hypothalamus (autonomic reaction) and areas of the limbic system (gustatory sensation and their emotional connotations). From the second-order neuron, the collaterals ascend to the salivary nuclei (reflex of salivation). Via the posterior longitudinal fasciculus (PLF), the hypothalamus can control autonomic reactions by influencing the autonomic nuclei of the brainstem.

Somatotopic organization of pathway

Not known.

Clinical correlations

A dysfunction of the gustatory pathway leads to a loss of taste sensation (ageusia). It is extremely rare, since a bilateral peripheral lesion of the cranial nerves VII, IX, and X is highly unlikely and a central lesion, in the brainstem for instance, would affect so many other structures that the clinical presentation would be dominated by more severe manifestations.

2.6 Olfactory Pathway

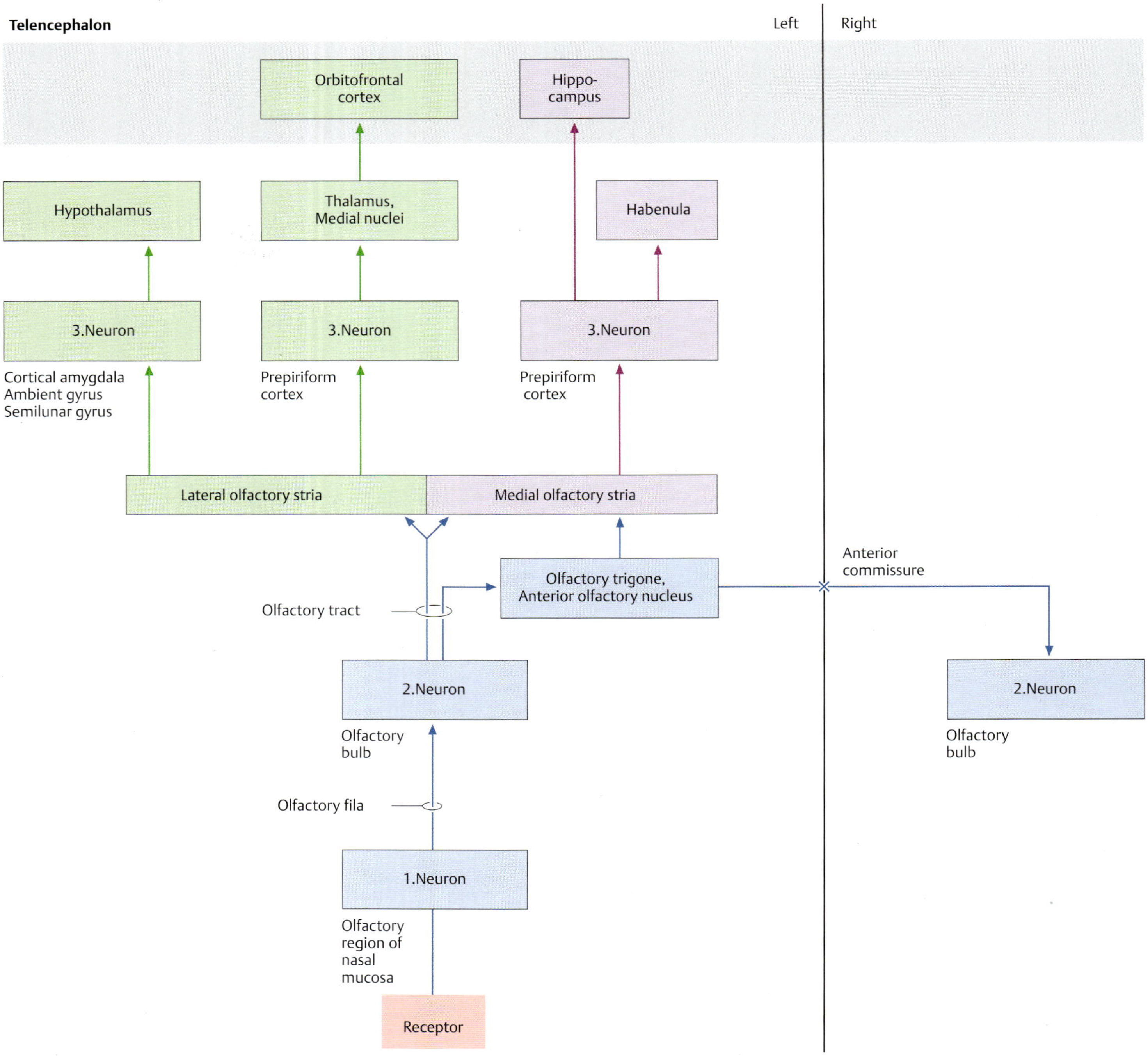

Definition and function

Pathway of conscious sensation of the olfactory system for the perception of olfactory stimuli.

Characteristics of pathway

(special) viscerosensory (sensory); afferent.
Note: Part of the olfactory pathway is represented by the first cranial nerve (olfactory n.). The olfactory n., however, is not a true cranial nerve but, per definition, an extension segment of the telencephalic cortex (in this case paleocortex), that is the CNS:

- Therefore, it is surrounded by meninges,
- it is bathed in cerebrospinal fluid,
- the axons of the neurons contained in them are surrounded by central glia (oligodendrocytes).

The olfactory nerve on the other hand does not represent a coherent structure but consists of the sum of the numerous individual olfactory filaments. The olfactory filaments are the axons of the primary sensory cells (receptor cells) of the olfactory epithelium. The olfactory nerve is by definition a component of the peripheral nervous system.

Neural wiring and topography of the pathway

A total of 3 serially connected neurons:

- **First-order neuron:** lies as receptor cell (primary sensory cell) in the roof of the nasal cavities. The peripheral process has at its end a receptor located in the nasal mucosa. The central process (part of olfactory fila or filaments) passes through the cribriform plate of the ethmoid bone to reach the second-order neuron.
- **Second-order neuron:** in the olfactory bulb, located on the ethmoid bone, in the anterior cranial fossa. There are two types of second-order neurons: mitral cells and tufted cells. The axons of the second-order neurons travel via the olfactory tract that divides into a medial and a lateral olfactory stria.
- **Third-order neuron:** projects to successive neurons, and is found in three locations:
  - for the lateral olfactory stria: in the *prepiriform area* (Brodmann area 28); it conveys information via the thalamus (medial nuclei) to the orbitofrontal cortex or neurons in the *cortex surrounding the amygdala* (semilunar and ambient gyri); further to the hypothalamus;
  - for the medial olfactory stria: nuclei in the subcallosal area (with septal nuclei) convey information to the habenula and hippocampus. Both connections remain ipsilateral;
  - for crossed fibers: anterior olfactory nucleus (in the olfactory trigone) conveys information to the olfactory bulb.

Note: The second-order neuron in the the lateral olfactory stria reaches cortical areas without thalamic participation. The olfactory pathway is thus, according to present knowledge, the only afferent pathway that can reach telencephalic neurons without passing through the thalamus. The extensive projection of the stria olfactoria to neurons of the limbic system (mainly the cortex surrounding the amygdala) explains the strong emotional connotations of olfactory impressions. The projection to the hypothalamus is responsible for autonomic reactions (e.g., nausea, p.r.n. vomiting) related to unpleasant olfactory sensations.

Somatotopic organization of pathway

Not known.

Clinical correlations

Olfactory pathway dysfunction leads to anosmia. It can result from damages to both olfactory bulbi or both olfactory tracts in the case of basal skull fracture.

2.7 Control of Motor Nuclei of Cranial Nerves

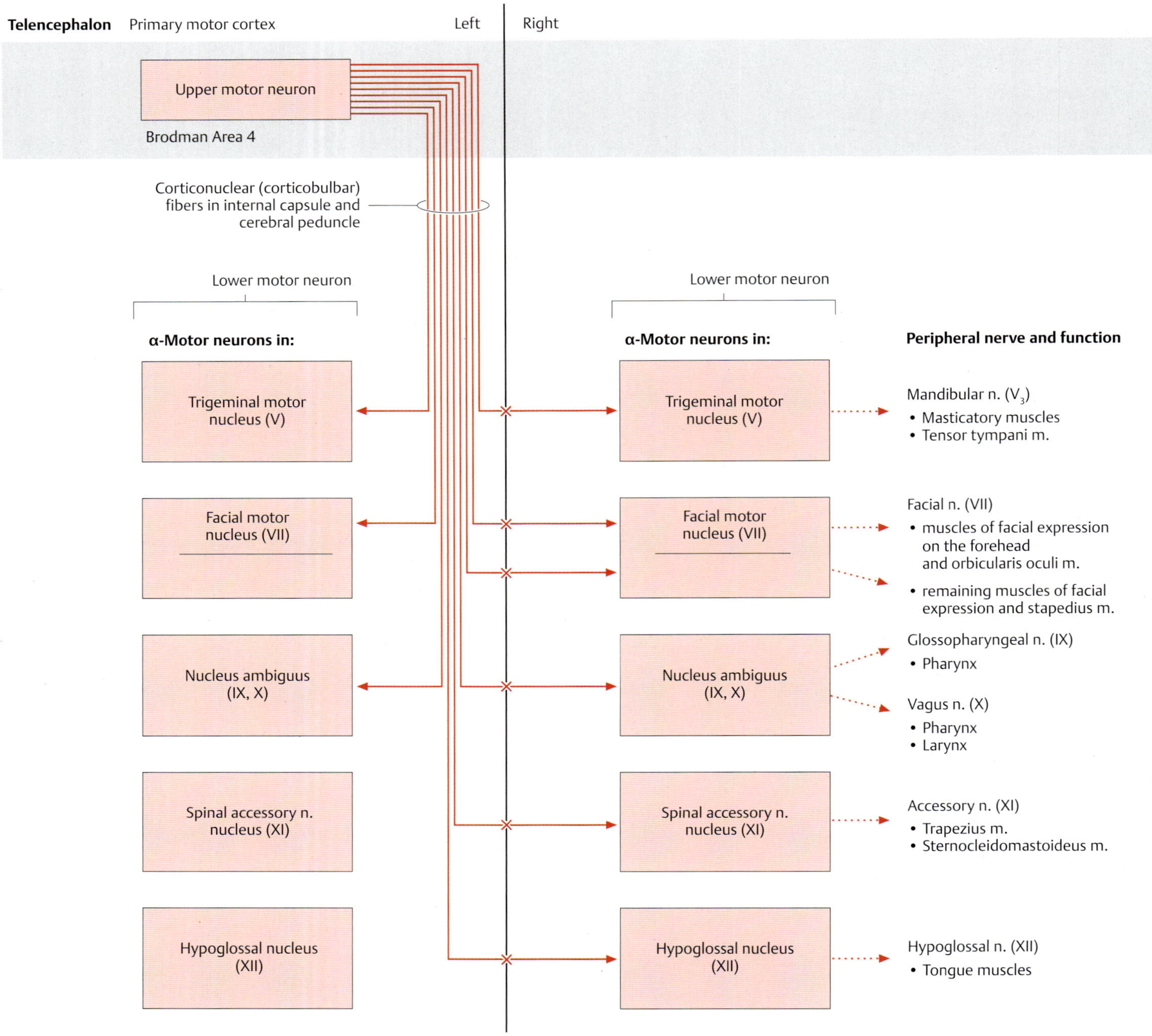

Organization of the motor nuclei of cranial nerves

Based on their function, they are divided into two groups:

- Nuclei for the motor function of eye muscles (III, IV, and VI) and
- Nuclei for the other motor functions controlled by cranial nerves (Vmotor; VII, IX, X, XI, and XII).

Usually, the cortical control is mediated via a common pathway, the corticonuclear or corticobulbar tract (fibers). This pathway, however, differentiates into two parts: one for the eye muscles, one for the other motor functions. Control of eye movement is mediated through one section of the tract via multiple centers in the brainstem before the eye muscle nuclei are reached, via the medial longitudinal fasciculus (see "control of motor functions of eye muscles," p. 522 f). Only the control of the other cranial nerve motor nuclei is explained here, those that are reached *directly* by the second part of the corticonuclear tract. This is analogous to the corticospinal fibers that project to motor neurons in the spinal cord.

Definition and function of the corticonuclear fibers for the control of the motor nuclei of cranial nerves

- Major pathway for voluntary motor function: conscious movement control of masticatory muscles, muscles of facial expression, tongue, other muscles attached to the skull, as well as subconscious motor control of pharyngeal and laryngeal muscles
- The part of the *pyramidal tract* between the primary motor cortex and the motor nuclei in the brainstem. Similar to the other fibers of the pyramidal tract (i.e., cortico*spinal* fibers to the spinal cord and cortico*reticular* fibers to the reticular formation), these fibers are axons of the large pyramidal neurons.

Characteristics of pathway

Somatomotor; descending; efferent

Neural wiring and topography of the pathway

Total of two serially connected neurons:

- **Upper motor neuron:** large pyramidal cells in the internal pyramidal layer (layer V) of the precentral gyrus (primary motor cortex); they are located in the Brodmann area 4. Most other neurons originate in neighboring cortical regions. On their descending way from the telencephalon to the brainstem, the axons of the upper motor neurons pass through the following structures:

  Primary motor cortex → genu of the internal capsule → cerebral peduncle (mesencephalon) → pontine tegmentum

  Decussation of the upper motor neuron axons: partial crossing (largely in the pons), thus resulting in crossed and uncrossed projections from the motor cortex to the lower motor neurons

  Axons of the upper motor neurons terminate only *contralaterally* on
  - Portion of the facial motor nucleus that controls the facial expression of the lower face,
  - Accessory nerve nucleus,
  - Hypoglossal nucleus.

  Axons of the upper motor neurons terminate both *contra-* and *ipsilaterally* on the
  - Motor nucleus of the trigeminal nerve,
  - Motor nucleus of the facial nerve that controls the superior part of the face (muscles of the forehead and orbicularis oculi m.),
  - Nucleus ambiguus (innervation of pharynx and larynx).

- **Lower motor neurons:** α-motor neurons in the
  - Motor nucleus of the trigeminal n. (masticatory muscles and tensor tympani m.),
  - Motor nucleus of the facial n. (muscles of facial expression),
  - Nucleus ambiguous that projects via the glossopharyngeal and vagus nerves (pharynx and larynx),
  - Nucleus of the accessorii n. (trapezius and sternocleidomastoid muscles), and
  - Hypoglossal nucleus (most muscles of the tongue).

  The axons of the corticonuclear fibers end as excitatory synapses on these nuclei. The axons of the lower motor neurons terminate in the target organ, in this case the muscles; therefore they represent the motor component of the respective cranial nerve. The neurotransmitter is acetylcholin.
  Note: The corticonuclear fibers end on the lower motor neurons. The axons of the lower motor neurons forms the motor component of the respective cranial nerve.

Somatotopic organization of the pathway

- Internal capsule: in the genu, rostral to the corticospinal fibers that run in the posterior limb
- Mesencephalon: in the cerebral peduncles; medial to the corticospinal fibers.

Clinical correlations

Dysfunction of the corticonuclear fibers leads to impaired voluntary movement related to chewing (trigeminal n.), facial expression (facial n.), turning the head and shrugging the shoulder (accessory n.) and movements of the tongue (hypoglossal n.).
Note: Dysfunction of the upper motor neurons leads to a *central* type of palsy and dysfunction of the lower motor neurons to a *peripheral* palsy (similar to a lesion to the motor fibers in the cranial nerve).
Since only one part of the facial nucleus is innervated ipsi- and contralaterally, a distinction can be made between a nuclear or infranuclear lesion palsy (lower motor neuron or peripheral nerve is affected) vs. a supranuclear lesion palsy (upper motor neuron is affected):

- In case of a palsy due to a peripheral nerve lesion, all fibers are affected (including those that control forehead muscles and the orbicularis oculi m.).
- In case of a supranuclear palsy, the forehead muscles and part of the orbicularis oculi m. are not paralyzed because the lower motor neurons controlling these muscles are influenced by fibers arriving from the ipsilateral motor cortex as well.

2.8 Ocular Motor Control

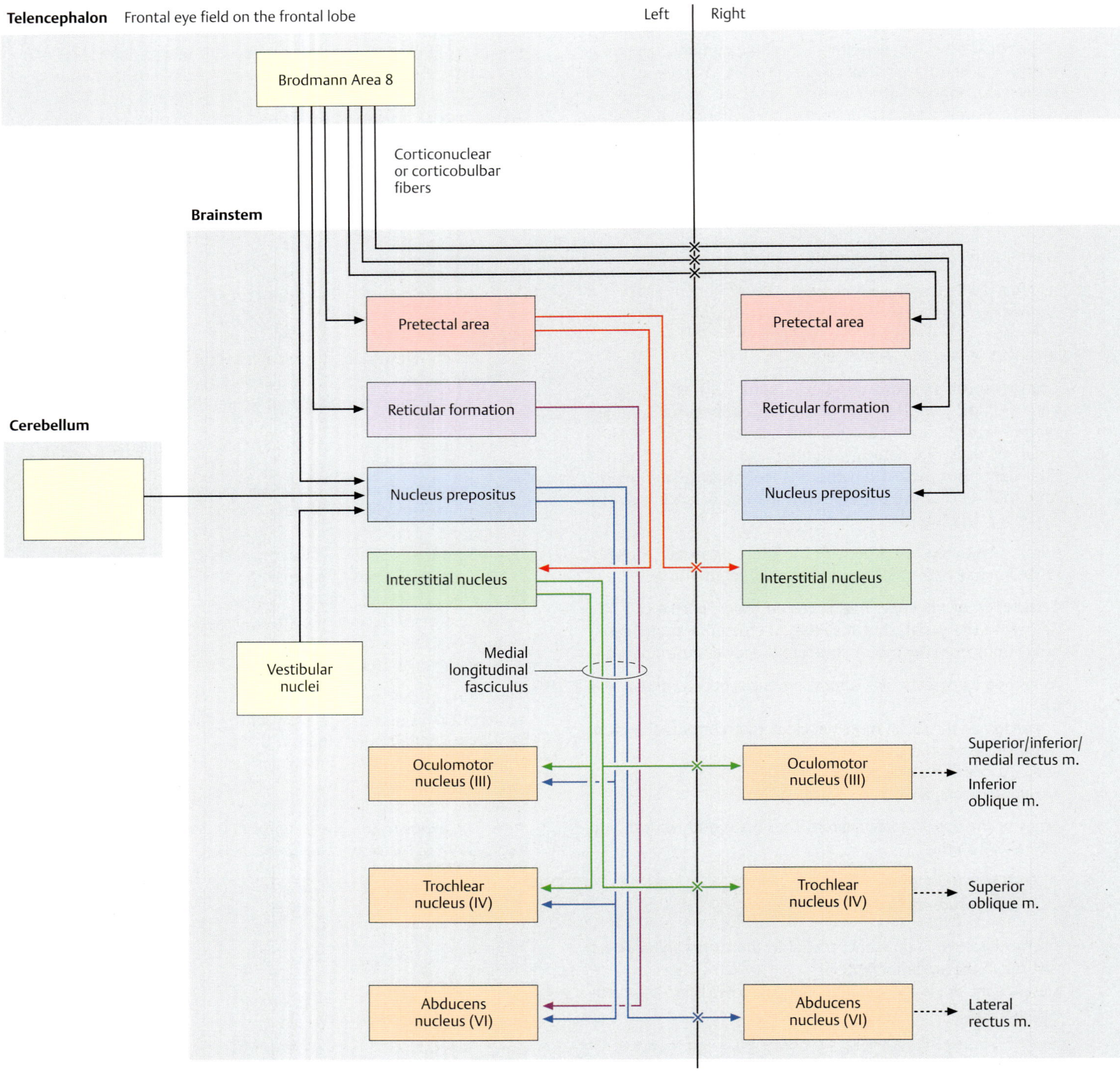

Definition and function

The control of eye movements is extremely complex. In order to guarantee an unambiguous visual impression, images fall on corresponding areas of the retina. This requires that both eyes move in a coordinated way. If that doesn't happen and light rays don't fall on the corresponding retinal points, double vision results. The ocular motor control is mainly a reflexive response mediated by subcortical centers (see "projections of the retina," p. 526 f). Voluntary eye movements are possible. However, they are not initiated by the precentral gyrus (somatomotor function) but are controlled by a specialized command center in the frontal lobe (as opposed to the precentral gyrus), called the frontal eye field (part of Brodmann area 8). Unlike the precentral gyrus, the frontal eye field doesn't send its efferents directly to α-motor neurons in nuclei of the cranial nerves but they reach control centers in the brainstem (midbrain and pons), which further project to the motor nuclei responsible for eye movements.

Characteristics of pathway

Somatomotor; descending; efferent.

Neural wiring and topography of pathway

The originating neurons are located in the frontal eye field (in this case, neurons are usually not numbered, thus the term "originating neuron"). Their axons travel along with axons of neurons of the precentral gyrus in the internal capsule as corticonuclear fibers. The neurons from area 8 project ipsi- and contralaterally to neurons in the pretectal area (at the diencephalic-mesencephalic junction) and to the reticular formation and nucleus prepositus. Neurons from the pretectal area project bilaterally to the interstitial nucleus. The prepositus and interstitial nuclei further project to the motor nuclei of cranial nerves III, IV, and VI as listed below.

- Nucleus prepositus projects ipsilaterally to all nuclei and contralaterally to the nucleus of cranial nerve VI.
- The interstitial nucleus projects ipsi- and contralaterally to the nuclei of cranial nerves III and IV,
- Neurons of the reticular formation in the brainstem project ipsilaterally to the nucleus of cranial nerve VI.

The connections between the cerebellum and the vestibular nuclei, especially the nucleus prepositus, coordinate the movements that maintain balance with the help of eye movements (e.g., vestibular nystagmus—involuntary eye movement during head turning, for example, when driving a car).

In the brainstem, the medial longitudinal fasciculus contains fibers responsible for interconnecting the nuclei responsible for eye muscles with the command centers and with the vestibular system (see also "brainstem pathways," p. 524 f).

Clinical correlations

- Only dysfunction of a single motor nucleus that controls eye muscles leads to dysfunction of a single muscle or muscle group in one eye.
- Dysfunction of command centers (e.g., in case of vascular lesions in the brainstem or lesions in the area surrounding the frontal eye field) are always associated with complex eye movement dysfunctions affecting both eyes.

2.9 Brainstem Pathways

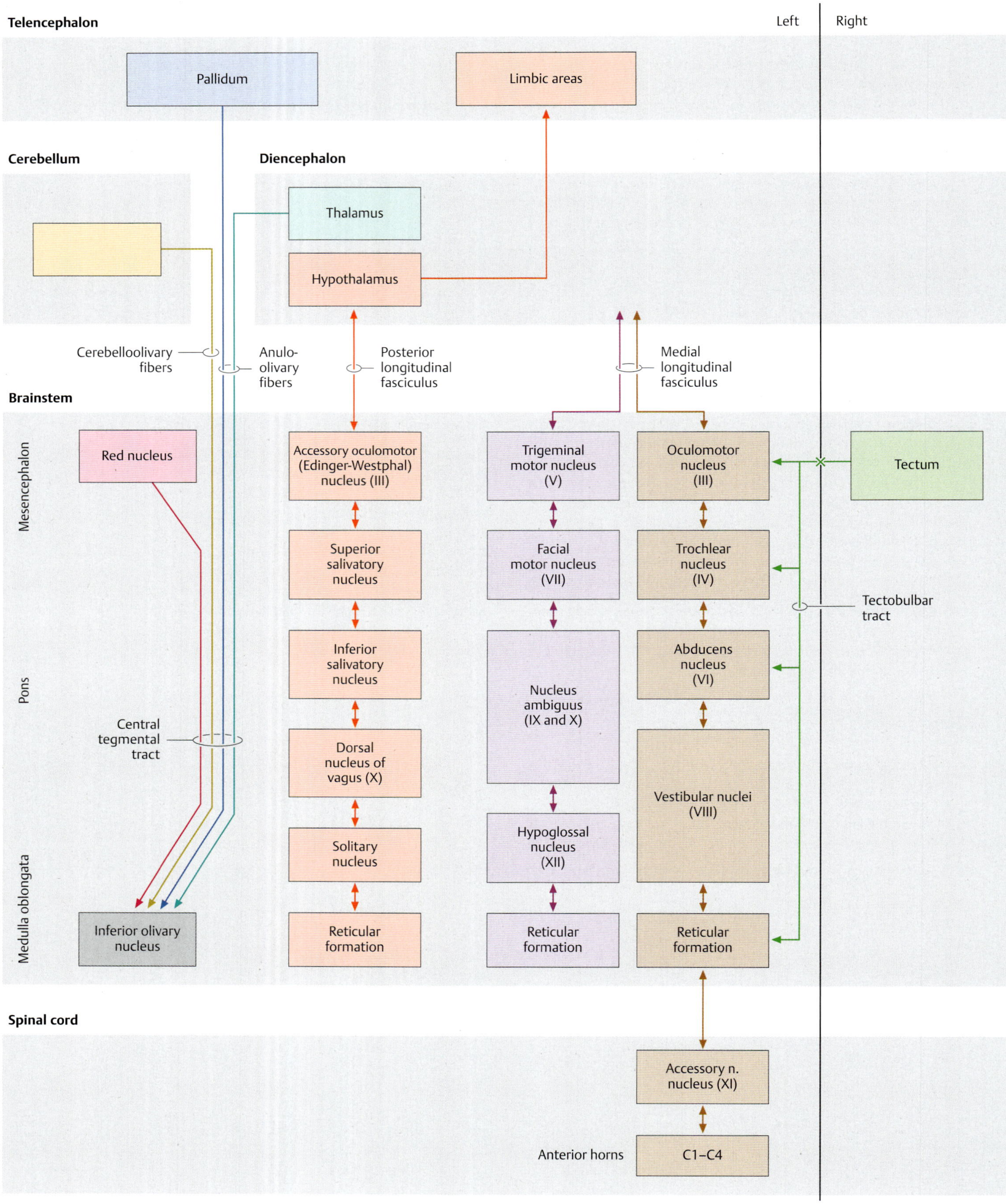

Essentially, brainstem pathways can be divided into two groups:

- Longitudinal pathways that exclusively or mainly pass through the brainstem
- Pathways that interconnect nuclei of the brainstem

The four major brainstem interconnections are explained below.

Longitudinal pathways (not shown here)

Either descending, thus mainly somatomotor or visceromotor, or ascending, thus mainly sensory:

- Descending pathways
  - **Pyramidal tract** (with its different parts, see p. 510 f)
  - **Corticopontine tract** as part of the corticopontocerebellar pathway (see p. 510 f);
- Ascending pathways: the four lemnisci:
  - **Medial lemniscus** (continuation of the pathway includes the posterior column, see p. 508)
  - **Spinal lemniscus** (continuation of the sensory anterolateral system, see p. 508)
  - **Trigeminal lemniscus** (continuation of trigeminal pathway) (see p. 512 f)
  - **Lateral lemniscus** (part of the auditory pathway) (see p. 514 f)

Interconnecting pathways

- **Central tegmental tract:** Descending pathway, most important pathway of the extrapyramidal system in the brainstem. Formed by several pathways: fibers originate from the telencephalon (pallidum), diencephalon (thalamus), cerebellum and—from the brainstem itself—the red nucleus. These individual pathways combine to form the central tegmental tract that ends in the inferior olivary nucleus. The inferior olivary nucleus is therefore a central relay nucleus of the extrapyramidal motor system.
- **Posterior longitudinal fasciculus:** This pathway contains both ascending and descending fibers and interconnects various parts of the autonomic nervous system. The hypothalamus as the main autonomic control center interconnects with parasympathetic nuclei and the gustatory nucleus. At the same time, there are collaterals reaching the motor nuclei of cranial nerves involved in chewing, swallowing, sucking, and gagging. The *reflex* motor activities related to these functions are carried on via the motor nuclei of cranial nerves V, VII, nucleus ambiguus (for the cranial nerves IX and X) and XII. The pathway crosses at multiple levels (not shown here).
- **Medial longitudinal fasciculus:** This functionally mixed pathway—which also contains both ascending and descending fibers—interconnects motor nuclei of the systems that control the movements of the eyes (III, IV, VI) and head (XI, anterior horn C1–C4) with vestibular nuclei (balance) for smooth pursuit eye movements but also motor nuclei of cranial nerves involved in the voluntary motor control of chewing, swallowing, sucking). The motor nuclei of cranial nerves are thus interconnected via both fasciculi. The pathway crosses at multiple levels (not shown here).
- **Tectobulbar tract:** Crossed pathway that originates in the nucleus of the superior colliculus (in the tectum) and projects to the motor nuclei responsible for eye movements and the reticular formation for *reflex* oculomotor activity.

2.10 Retinal Projections

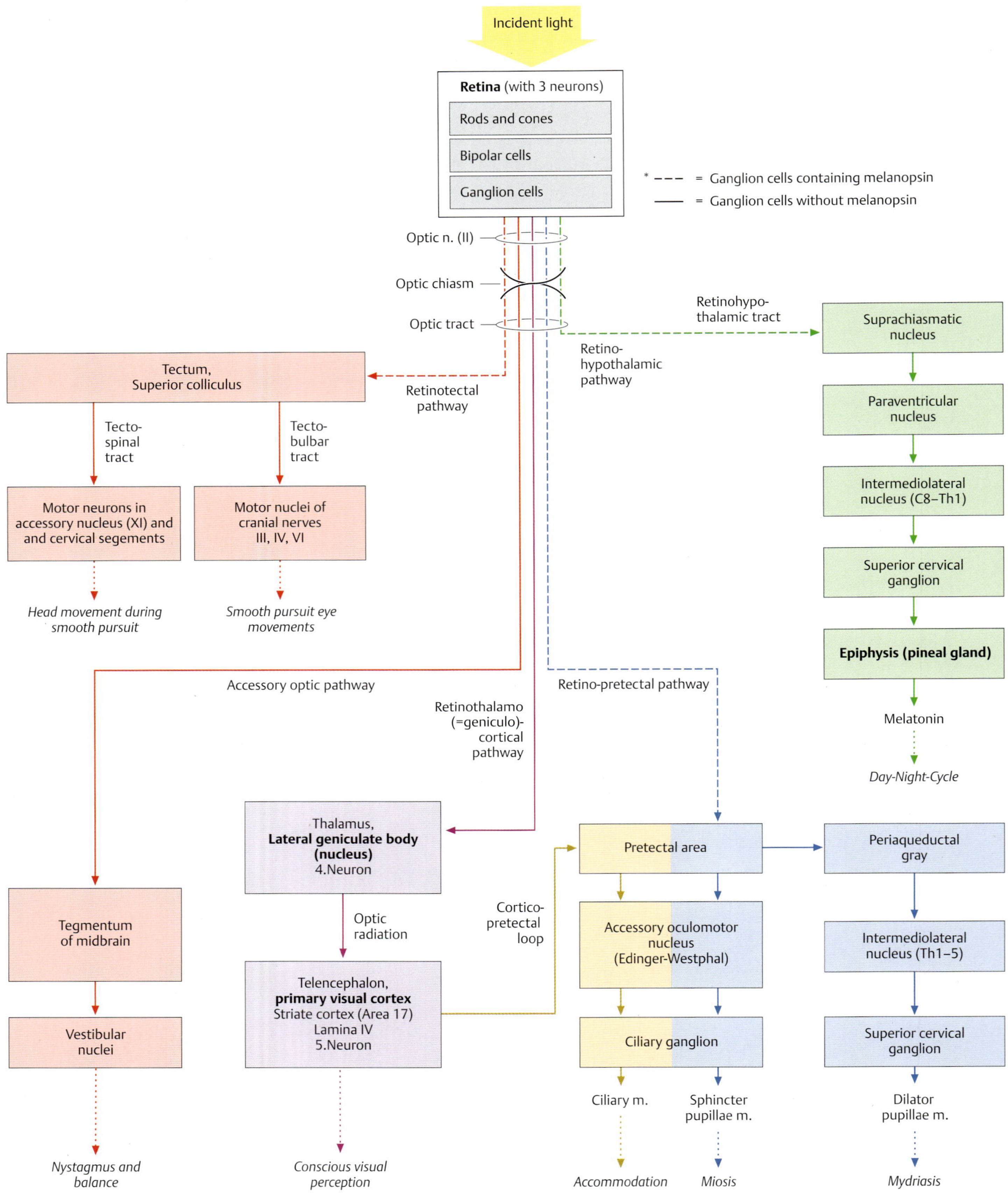

The visual system is responsible for processing visual stimuli. This includes not only the conscious perception of visual impressions but encompasses five different functions with the retina (a diencephalic derivative) as the common starting point.

Visual pathway

Mediates conscious perception and processing of visual impression (color, shape, size, position, movement, etc. of an object).

- Morphologically, largest part of the visual system.
- Passes through the *thalamus* (fourth-order neuron in the lateral *geniculate* body; first-order to third-order neurons in the retina) and from the thalamus to the primary visual *cortex*, where it ends above and below the calcarine sulcus in the striate cortex of cuneus and lingual gyrus.
- From the primary visual cortex, association pathways run to the secondary and tertiary visual cortical areas for further processing of complex visual information (not shown here).

Retinopretectal pathway

- Through control of the visceral motor innervation mediates the pupillary light reflex for which smooth muscles are responsible.
- Extends to the *pretectal area*, a nuclear region rostral to the superior colliculi of the mesencephalon, which topographically is part of the diencephalon (epithalamus).
- The pretectal area projects to the parasympathetic Edinger-Westphal nucleus in the mesencephalon and via the periventricular gray matter of the brainstem (periaqueductal gray) to sympathetic neurons in the spinal cord (C8–Th1). The Edinger-Westphal nucleus mediates pupil constriction (miosis) and lens accommodation and the sympathetic neurons are responsible for contraction of pupillary dilator muscle (mydriasis).
- The pretectal area, plays, therefore, a key functional role in two neuronal circuits: one *without* the participation of the thalamus and visual cortex (retinopretectal pathway) and one *involving* the participation of the visual cortex (corticopretectal loop). In the first case, the information is related to the *amount of light* that enters the eye, which causes the pupil to dilate or constrict. Since the cerebral visual cortex is not involved, this response can also be triggered in an *unconscious* patient. In the second case, information about *image sharpness* is transmitted which causes the lens to adjust to shift focus between near and far objects (and thus leads to focusing of the image). This requires a perception of the actual sharpness by the visual cortex, which means that only *fully conscious* people can respond adequately.

Retinotectal system

- Responsible for reflex tracking eye movements and accommodation.
- Passes through the superior colliculi of the mesencephalic *tectum* and the tectospinal and tectobulbar tracts to motor neurons that innervate various striate muscles, involved in head or eye movements. This way, the head and eyes automatically "follow" the moving object so that the image always falls on the site of the sharpest vision in both eyes.

Accessory optic system

Transmits visual information via the mesencephalon to the vestibular system (to analyze head motion). This way, balance and eye movements are coordinated (e.g., reflex head turning to compensate for eye movement). The accessory optic system thus supports (accessory) the retinotectal system.

Retino-hypothalamic system

Influences the circadian rhythm (e.g., day/night cycle) by measuring the daily light levels. Information relayed to the hypothalamus passes through several relay stations to reach the epiphysis (melatonin production and release).

Note: Axons from the nasal retina cross in the optic chiasm (approx. 48% of all fibers). Thus, for all above mentioned systems, axons from both eyes enter the respective relay stations, meaning bilateral processing of information. For a general overview, the diagram indicates only the junction of the optic chiasm, between the optic n. and optic tract. The crossed fibers are not displayed.

2.11 Autonomic and Sensory Ganglia of the Head

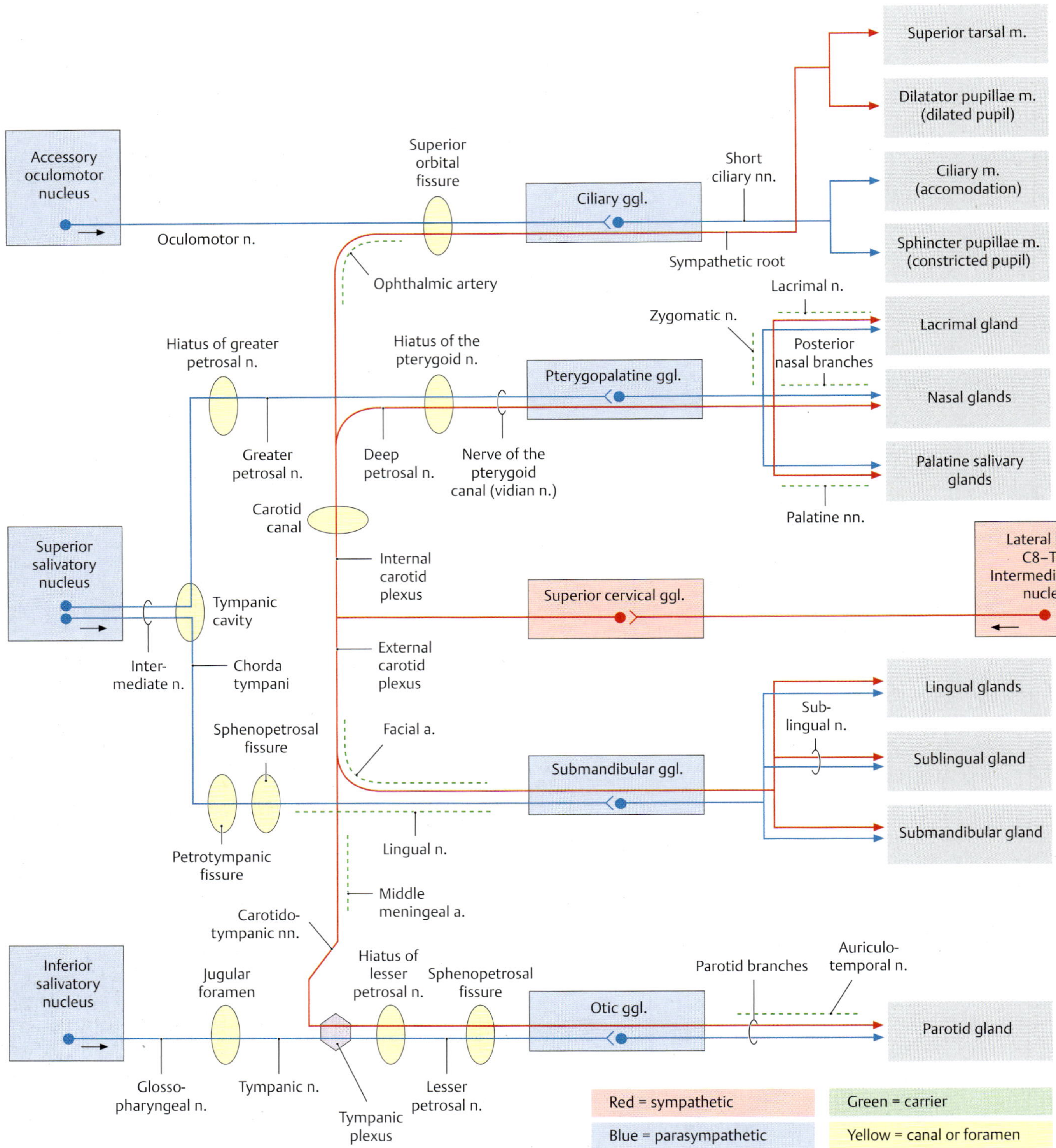

A Autonomic ganglia of the head

Autonomic and sensory ganglia of the head can be easily confused. This is why both types are depicted here along with the direction in which the respective ganglia relay impulses (see directional arrows). All autonomic ganglia of the head are parasympathetic. Inside the ganglia, fibers of parasympathetic preganglionic neurons arriving from the brainstem terminate at the perikaryon of the postganglionic neurons, which project their axons to the target organs. On their way to the target, the very thin and thus mechanically very sensitive fibers utilize other structures as a sort of "taxi" by traveling along them. Such structures include blood vessels or other nerves running to the same region as the autonomic fibers although they serve different functions. This is exactly what is initially confusing. This is why the autonomic fibers are represented here in blue (parasympathetic) or red (sympathetic) and the "main fibers," which have nothing to do with the autonomic fibers, are represented in green. All structures mentioned here pass through specific openings in the skull (canals and foraminae) which are represented in yellow.

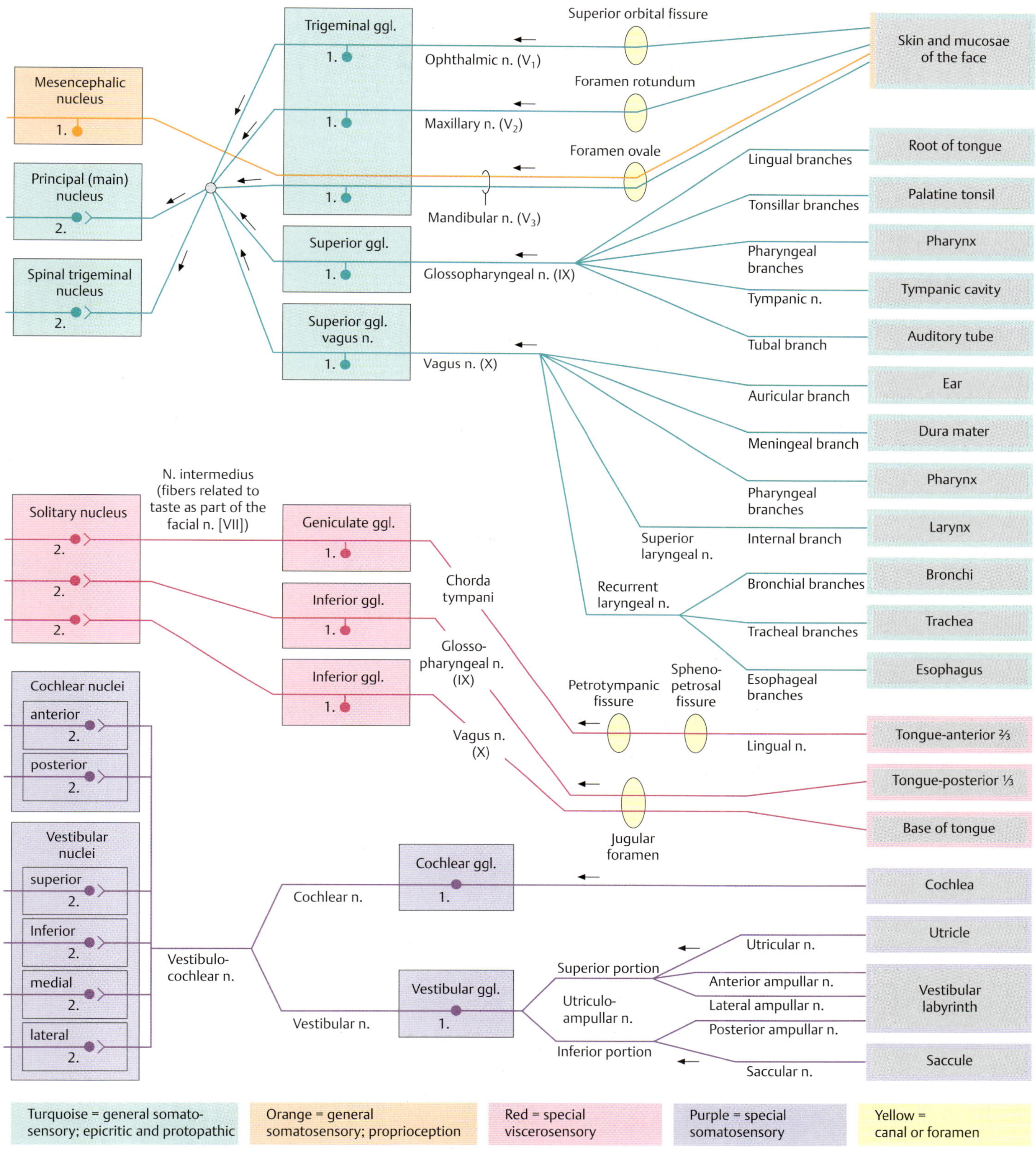

B Sensory ganglia of the head

Unlike the autonomic ganglia, the sensory ganglia contain no synapses. The sensory ganglia contain the bodies of the pseudounipolar or bipolar (in case of the vestibulocochlear n.) neurons (primary afferent neurons). Their peripheral processes bring impulses from a receptor, their central process synapse in the CNS. As an example, the glossopharyngeal n. carries taste information from the posterior third of the tongue, the fibers pass through the inferior ganglion and end in the solitary nucleus in the CNS. This specific information is *viscerosensory* (here represented in red). The glossopharyngeal n. also carries information from the pharynx, in this case general *somatosensory* information. Its fibers pass through the superior ganglion and end in the spinal nucleus of the trigeminal n., which conveys protopathic information from several cranial nerves (thus not only the trigeminal n. for which it is named). Temperature and pain sensation of the pharynx (e.g., very hot beverage) can thus be detected by the glossopharyngeal n. The vagus n. also conducts (via the superior ganglion of the vagus n.) protopathic information (mainly pain) from the larynx to the spinal nucleus of the trigeminal n. (e.g., pain caused by laryngitis).

2.12 Motor System Connectivity

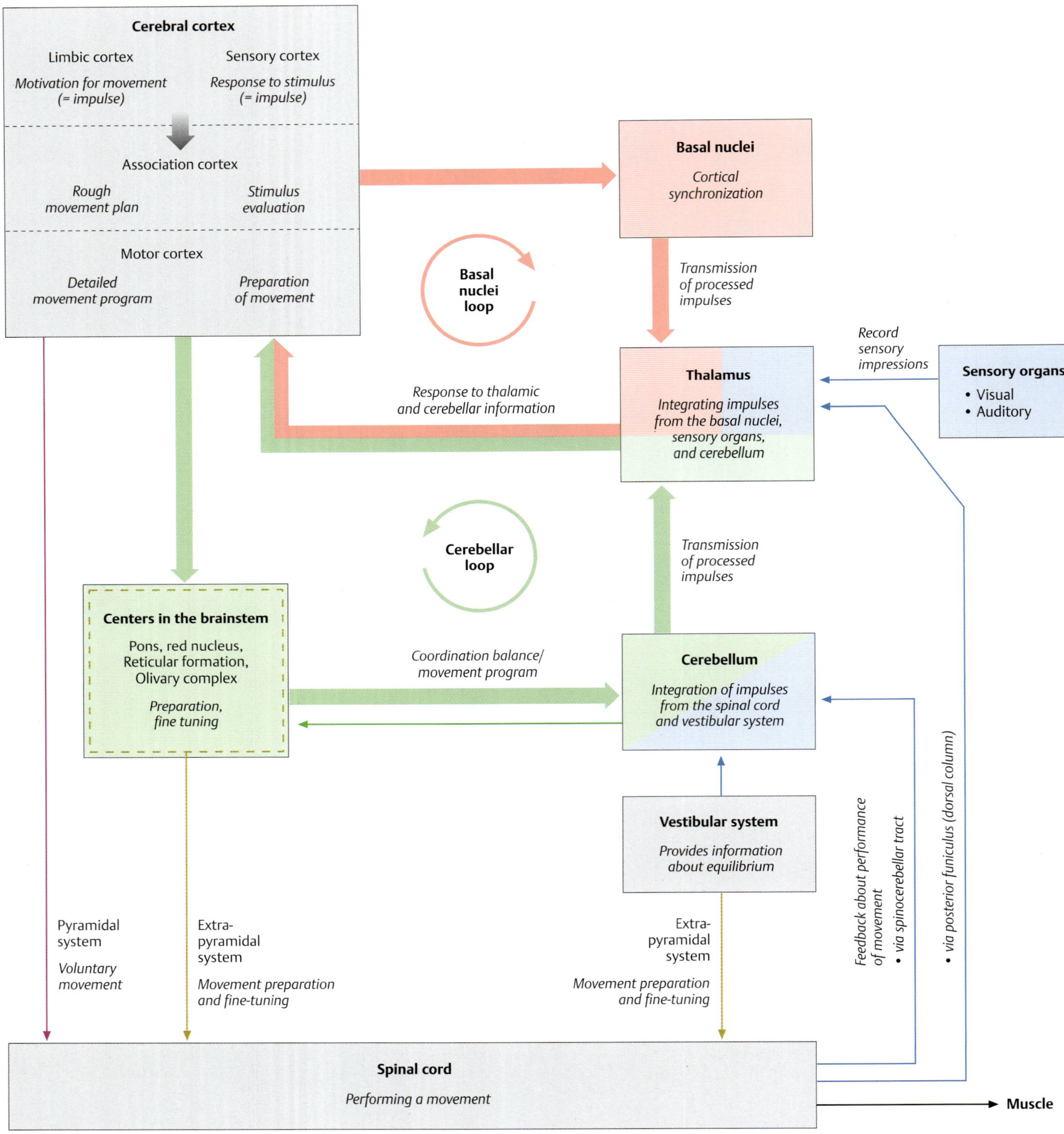

An overview of the functions of neurons, pathways and their interaction is depicted on the left, while the individual pathways, their structures, and nuclei are shown on the right.
Note: The cerebral cortex is the starting and ending point for two loops, the basal nuclei loop and the cerebellar loop. The thalamus participates in both loops ("motor thalamus"). It picks up signals from the basal nuclei and the cerebellum and relays the integrated impulse pattern to the motor cortex. At the same time, the thalamus receives input from the sensory organs ("sensory thalamus"). If these signals are relevant for movement, the thalamus feeds them into the impulse pattern as above. Thus, the thalamus is the major integration center for both loops as well as for sensory input.

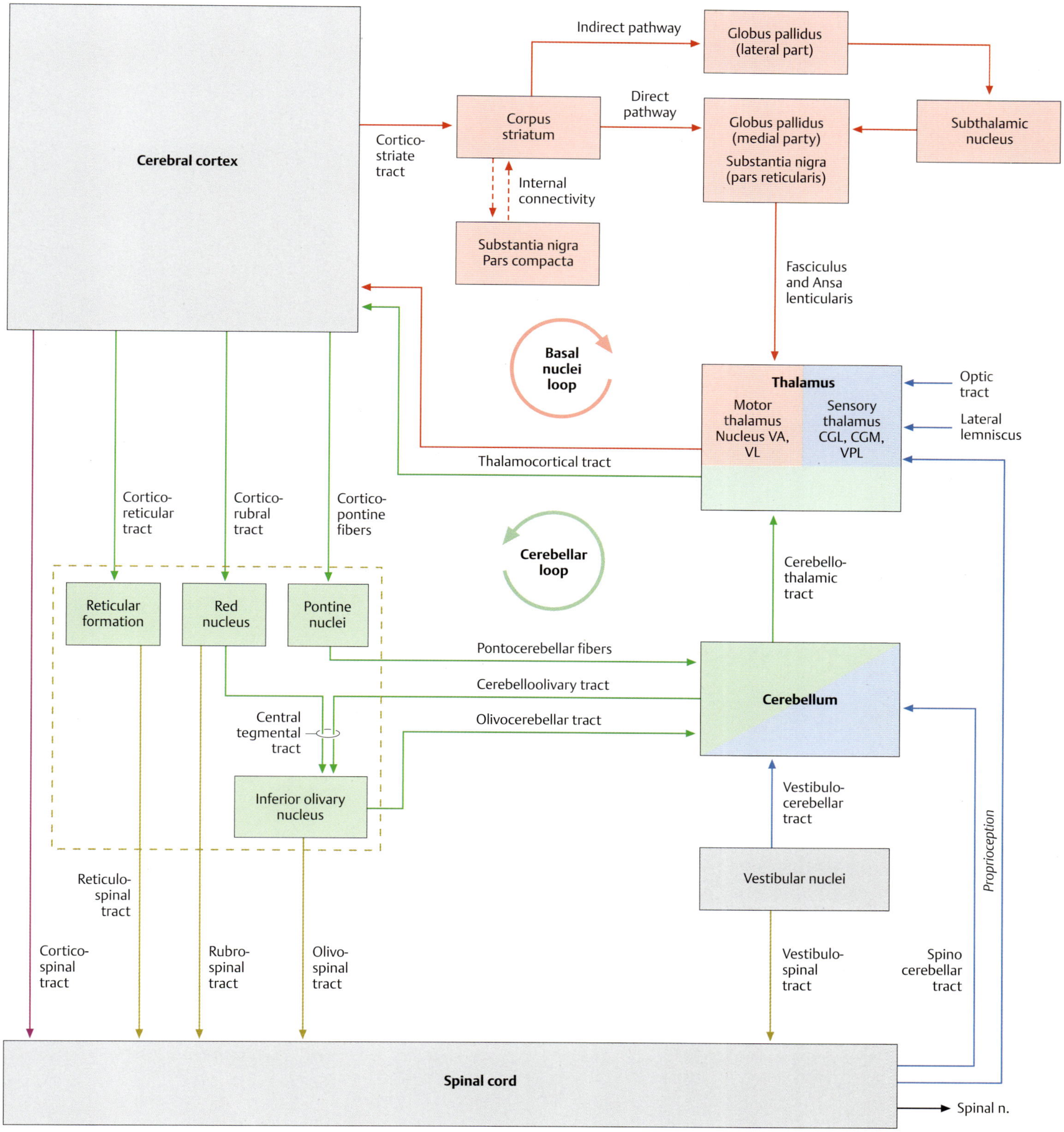

The thalamic impulses eventually generate a "complete" detailed movement program. It is relayed to brainstem centers (red nucleus, reticular formation, inferior olivary nucleus) for fine tuning. The inferior olivary nucleus represents a particularly significant connection of the cerebellar loop toward the spinal cord. The movement is ultimately initiated by impulses from the motor cortex (mostly precentral gyrus), which reach the spinal cord via the pyramidal tract (here corticospinal tract) (for voluntary movement).

The spinal cord itself executes the movement and sends the impulse via the spinal nerves to the corresponding muscles. Information about the execution of movement is sent via spinocerebellar tracts from the spinal cord to the cerebellum, which uses this information for constantly making postural adjustments in order to maintain balance. The cerebellum does not have direct efferent connections to the spinal cord but can indirectly influence the spinal cord via the inferior olivary nucleus.

2.13 Cerebellar Connectivity

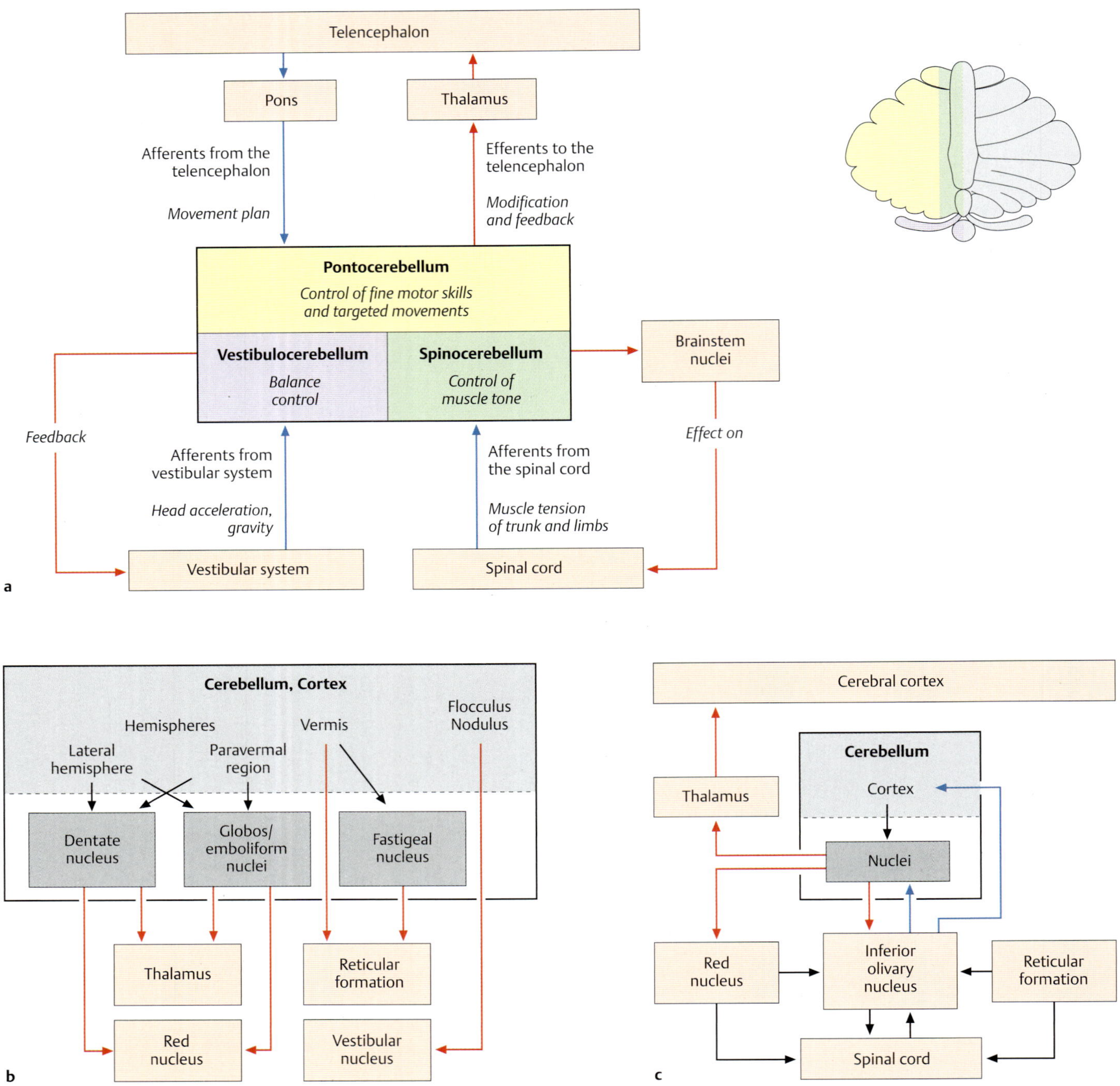

The functional organization of the cerebellum into ponto-, spino- and vestibulocerebellum (**a**) takes into account the **major afferents to the cerebellum:**

- From the telencephalon (via pons) for fine motor skills as part of planning of movements
- From the spinal cord for the regulation of muscle tone
- From the vestibular system for the control of head position and acceleration

Cerebellar efferent loops exist directly with the vestibular system and indirectly via the thalamus to the telencephalon and via nuclei of the brainstem to the spinal cord.

The **major cerebellar efferents** (**b**) usually don't originate from the cerebellar cortex but the cerebellar nuclei, which are largely assigned one particular cortical area. These nuclei project to the thalamus or to nuclei in the brainstem. The inferior olivary nucleus of the brainstem plays a significant role (**c**): It projects both to the cerebellum and to the spinal cord and receives afferents from both regions. Additionally, the inferior olive receives afferents from other brainstem nuclei (red nucleus and reticular formation). The olive thus integrates cerebellar and spinal impulses. The purpose of this complex wiring is to allow the cerebellum—indirectly via the brainstem nuclei—to influence the spinal cord's motor activity in order to maintain balance and to control fine and precise motor skills.

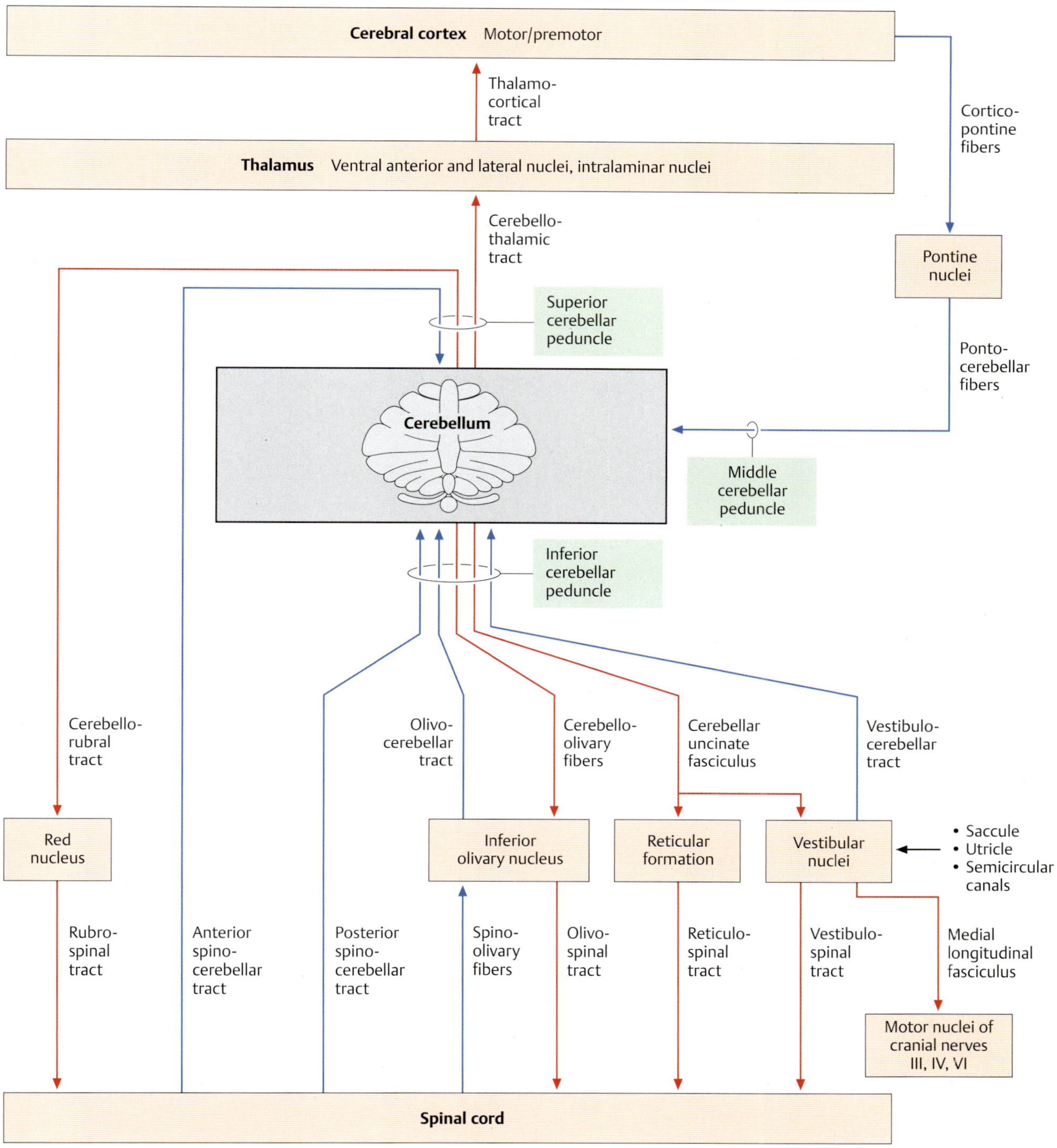

Cerebellar pathways
All pathways running to and from the cerebellum pass through one of the cerebellar peduncles. The middle cerebellar peduncle contains only afferents. All **afferents** end in the cortex with collaterals ending in cerebellar nuclei (not shown here). Histologically, the olivocerebellar tract is the only one that provides climbing fibers (they directly end on the Purkinje cells in the cerebellar cortex). All other afferents end as mossy fibers on the granule cells in the cerebellar cortex. The cerebellar **efferents** largely originate from the nuclei (see left side, **b**) and run either to the thalamus (feedback loop to the telencephalon (see left side, **a**) or to brainstem nuclei, which in turn project to the spinal cord via extrapyramidal tracts and thus control motor functions (cf. "pyramidal tract" and "brainstem pathways"). The projection from the vestibular nuclei to the nuclei that control eye movements help with compensatory eye movements during head movement.
Note: A direct projection of the cerebellum to the spinal cord has not been so far proven in humans.

2.14 Functional Cortical Areas

A Functional cortical areas

Functional lobes	Specialization	Localization	Symptoms in case of damage
Frontal lobe	Personality	① Orbital gyri	Abulia; impaired decision-making ability and absence of goal-oriented behavior; Witzelsucht (compulsive wisecracking) ("frontal lobe syndrome")
	Somatomotor function (primary motor cortex)	② Precentral gyrus	Contralateral paralysis; damage dependent on the localization of lesion on the cortex ("motor homunculus")
	Motor center for speech (Broca)	③ Inferior frontal gyrus (pars opercularis; pars triangularis) lateralization (dominant hemisphere mostly left)	Motor aphasia/Broca aphasia: inability to formulate more or less complex sentences
	Olfactory cortex	④ Anterior perforated substance, ambiens gyrus, semilunar gyrus	Anosmia
Parietal lobe	Somotosensation (primary somatosensory cortex)	⑤ Postcentral gyrus	Loss of tactile and temperature sensation and/or pain localization
	Abstract (non-pictorial) thinking, reading	⑥ Angular gyrus and supramarginal gyri Lateralization (dominant hemisphere)	Abstract thinking, reading, inability to perform mathematical calculations
Occipital lobe	Visual cortex (primary visual cortex)	⑦ Above and below the calcarine sulcus, cuneus and lingual gyrus	Loss of half of the visual field (homonymous hemianopsia) on the opposite side or defect in one quadrant of the contralateral visual field (quadrantanopsia)
Temporal lobe	Auditory cortex (primary auditory cortex)	⑧ Transverse temporal gyri (Heschl)	Only in case of bilateral damage: impaired auditory perception
	Sensory speech center (Wernicke)	⑨ Superior temporal gyrus	Sensory aphasia/Wernicke aphasia: inability to comprehend sentences
Limbic lobe	Learning, memory, emotional reponse	⑩ Hippocampal formation	Only in case of bilateral damage Impaired explicit memory
Insula	Gustatory cortex	⑪ Insular gyri	P.r.n. ageusia

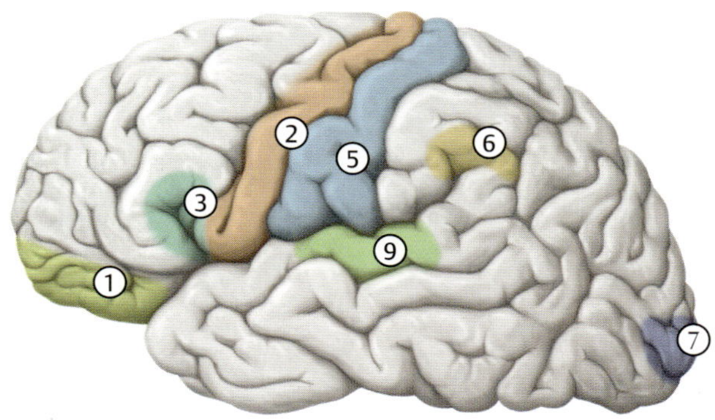

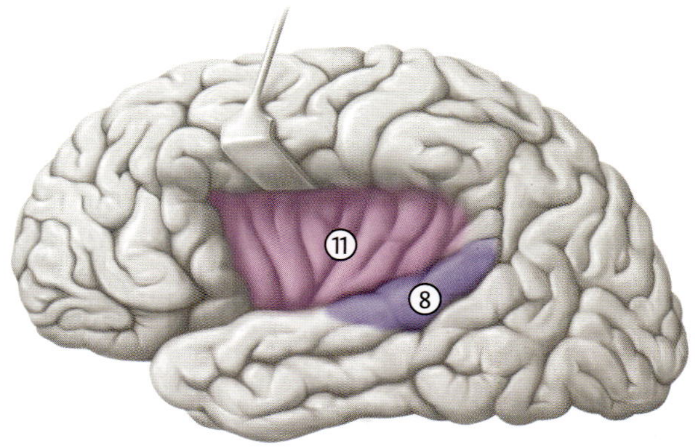

B Left hemisphere
a Lateral view; **b** lateral view, lateral sulcus widely open by retractors.

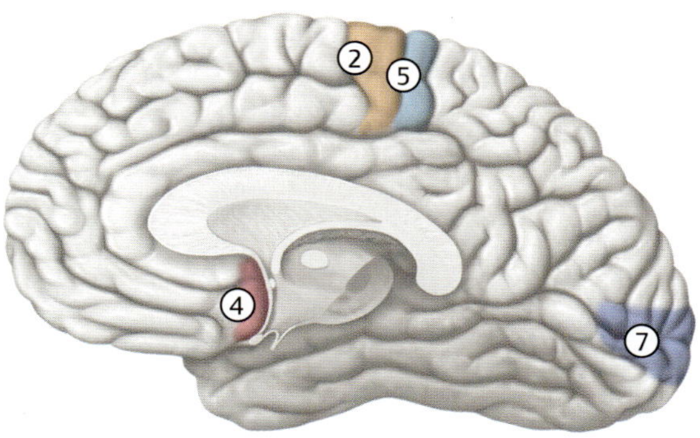

C Right hemisphere
Medial view.

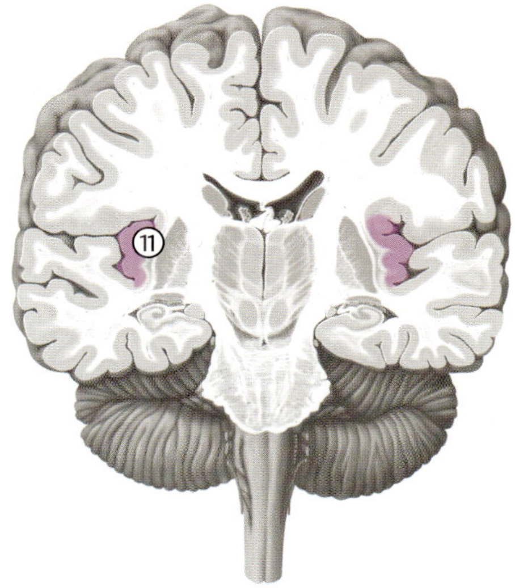

D Frontal section of the telencephalon
Anterior view.

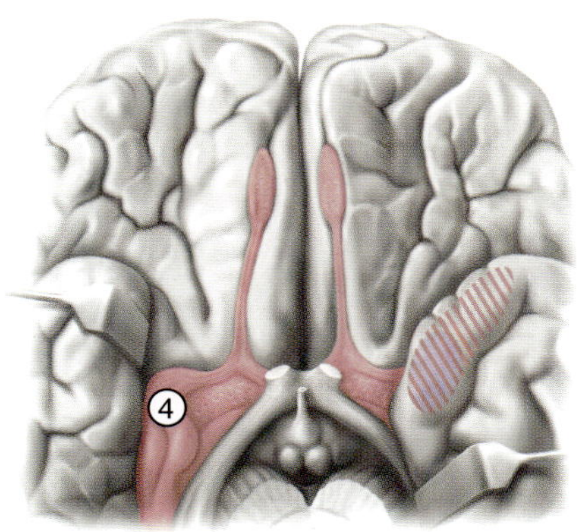

E Rostral part of the cerebral hemispheres
Basal view.

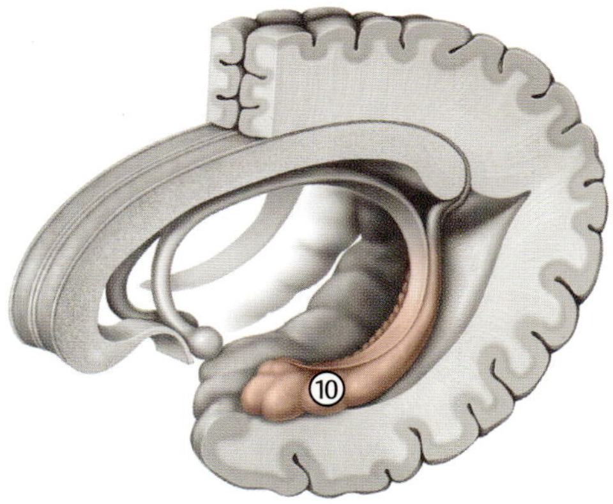

F Left hippocampal formation
Left anterior-superior view.

2.15 Association and Projection Pathways

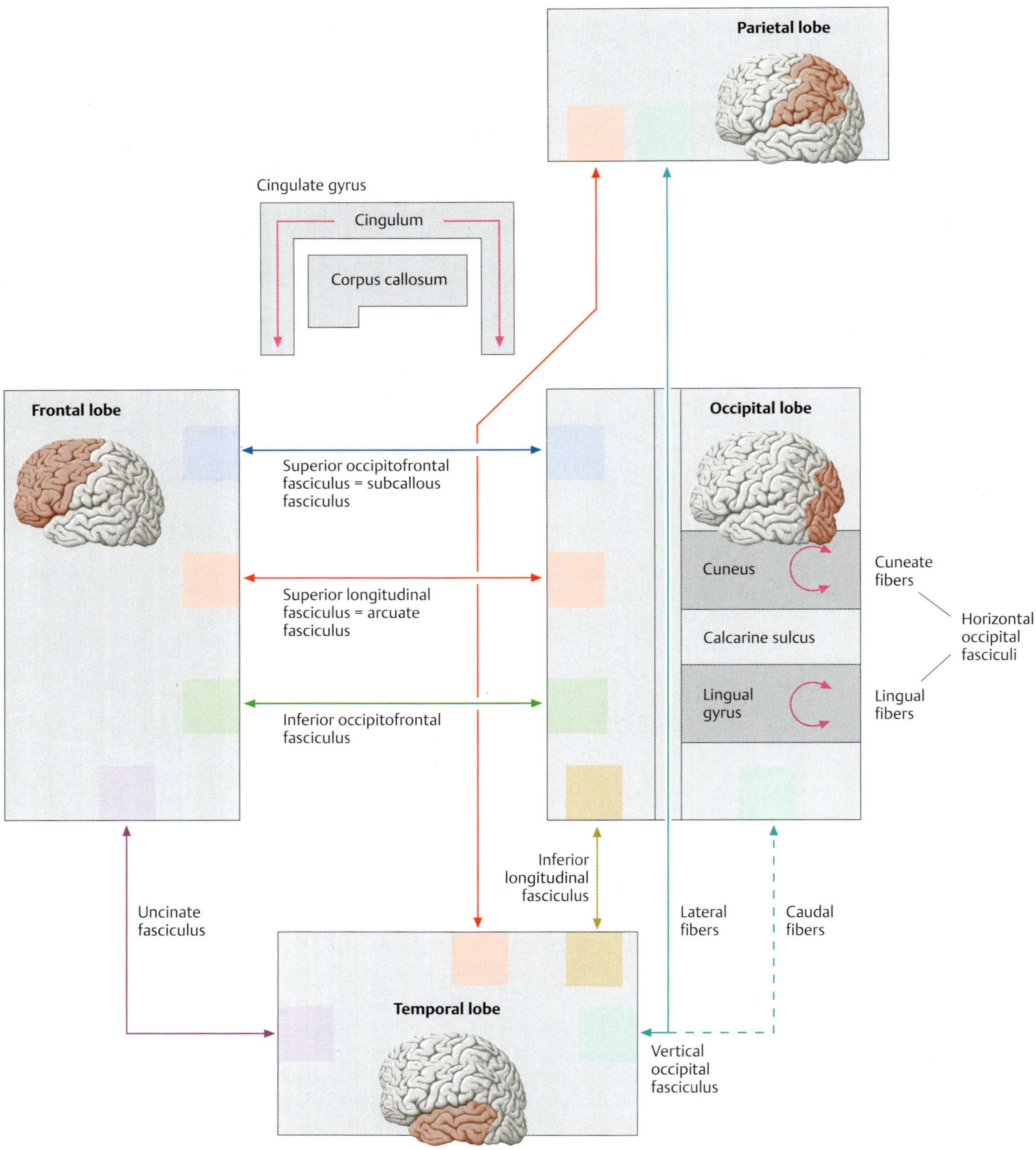

A Association pathways (association fibers in the telencephalon)
Association pathways connect different cortical regions, in order to, for instance, combine visual and acoustic information. Although such functional connections exist in all parts of the CNS, the term "association pathway" only refers to tracts of the telencephalon. There, association pathways connect different cortical areas of the same hemisphere (they never cross). There are three distinct type of association fibers:

- Arcuate fibers (not shown here) connect adjacent gyri.
- *Short* association fibers connect areas within one lobe (represented here are only the horizontal occipital fibers that connect lateral and medial parts of the occipital lobe).
- *Long* association fibers connect cortical areas of different lobes. These tracts are always individually named.

Note: The fibers of the vertical occipital fasciculi connect lateral temporal and parietal lobes and cross the occipital lobe.

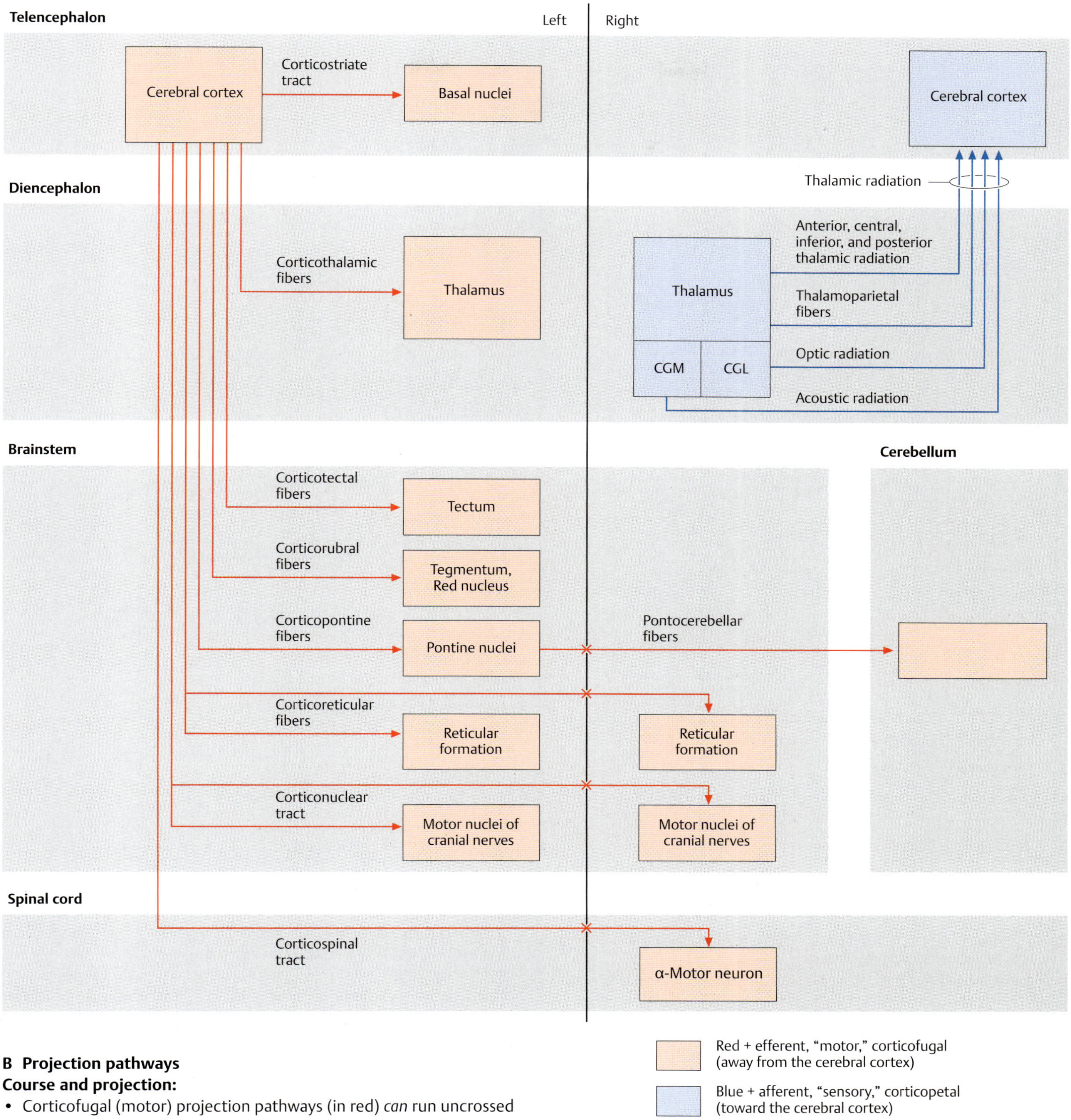

B Projection pathways

Course and projection:

- Corticofugal (motor) projection pathways (in red) *can* run uncrossed yet mostly cross. Motor impulses from the cerebral cortex thus travel to *contralateral* subcortical centers and influence motor activity of the contralateral side of the body.
- Corticopetal (sensory) projection pathways (in blue) *never cross*. Thus, they reach the cortex cerebri only from the ipsilateral thalamus. Yet, the thalamus itself, is reached by pathways of subordinate centers, most of which are located *contralaterally*. Subsequently, sensory impulses to the cerebral cortex originate mainly from the contralateral side of the body.

Exceptions to this basic principle:

- Motor function: cortical projections to individual motor nuclei of cranial nerves (see p. 520 f and 522 f)
- Somatosensation: innervation of the head via the trigeminal n. (see p. 512)
- Special senses: olfactory pathway, gustatory pathway, auditory pathway, visual pathway (see respective wiring diagram)

The following **major pathways** are distinguished:

- In the telencephalon: to the basal nuclei, particularly to the corpus striatum (corticofugal: corticostriate tract), not shown here, see "motor system connections," p. 530 f
- In the diencephalon: to and from the thalamus (corticofugal: corticothalamic fibers; corticopetal: thalamic radiations)
- To the brainstem: (e.g., corticopontine, corticonuclear, corticorubral, corticoreticular),
- In the spinal cord: corticospinal tract

2.16 Superior and Inferior Olive as well as the Four Lemnisci

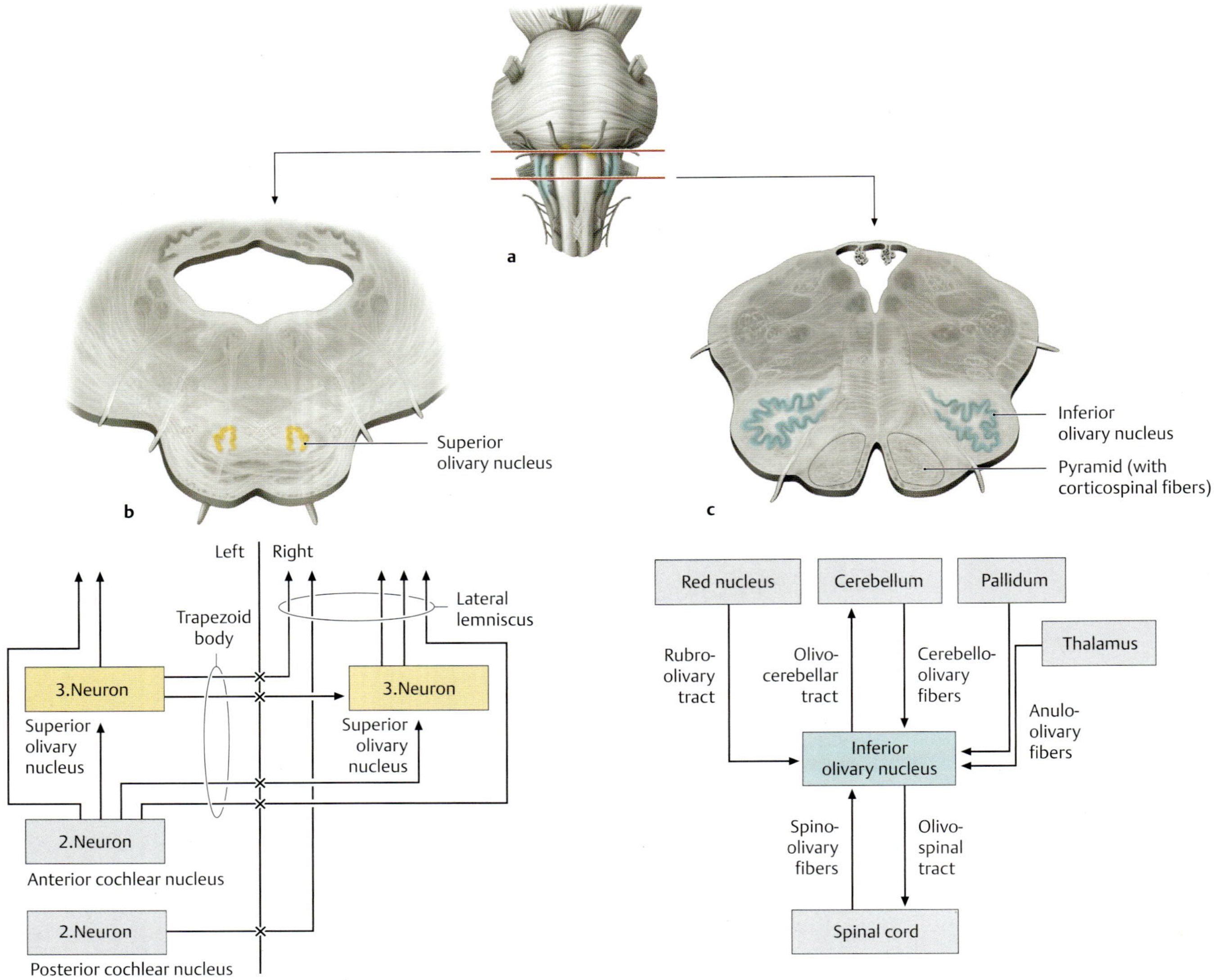

A Definition of the terms “olive,” “inferior,” and “superior olive” and connections of both olives

a Brainstem, ventral view; **b** Cross-section of the medulla oblongata near the pons—superior view; **c** Cross-section of medulla oblongata—inferior view.

- **Olive:** The olive is a distinct olive-shaped protrusion, located on the ventral aspect of the medulla oblongata. It lies lateral to the pyramid. The term “olive” is thus a descriptive macroscopic term.
- **Superior olive (Superior olivary nucleus):** The superior olive is significantly smaller than the inferior olive; it alone would not be identifiable as a protrusion. It is located inside the medulla oblongata, mediodorsal and largely cranial to the inferior olive and is thus clearly visible on cross-sections directly caudal to the pons (**b**). The superior olive continues into the most inferior parts of the pons. Due to the partial overlap of the inferior and superior olive, both nuclear complexes are sometimes visible on same cross-sections. Similar terms are used for the superior and inferior olive, which are adjacent topographically. Functionally, however they are not connected and have to be strictly separated.
- **Connections of the superior olive:** The superior olive is a major nucleus with role in the localization of sound and connections involved in the stapedius m. reflex (a protective reflex for the sense of hearing, see p. 485). It receives afferents from the anterior cochlear nucleus (both ipsi- and contralateral); both superior olives are connected and project via the lateral lemniscus to ipsi- and contralateral hierarchically upper nuclei of the auditory pathway. For more details see p. 484 f and 514.
- **Inferior olive** (*inferior olivary complex; inferior olivary nuclei*) (**c**): The inferior olive is located in the medulla oblongata. It consists of several nuclei; this is why it is also often referred to as “inferior olivary complex.” Due to its size, the inferior olivary complex gives the protrusion called the “olive” on the ventral aspect of the brainstem. Not all nuclei of the complex are visible to the naked eye.

Connections of the inferior olive: The inferior olive is involved in the coordination of motor activities and thus extensively connected to other neural regions concerned with motor functions:

- Olivocerebellar and cerebello-olivary tracts: connections with the cerebellum
- Olivospinal tract: pathway to the the anterior horn of the spinal cord
- Spino-olivary fibers: pathway originating in the spinal cord
- Anulo-olivary fibers: pathway from the basal nuclei and diencephalon (for more details see p. 514 and 537–539)

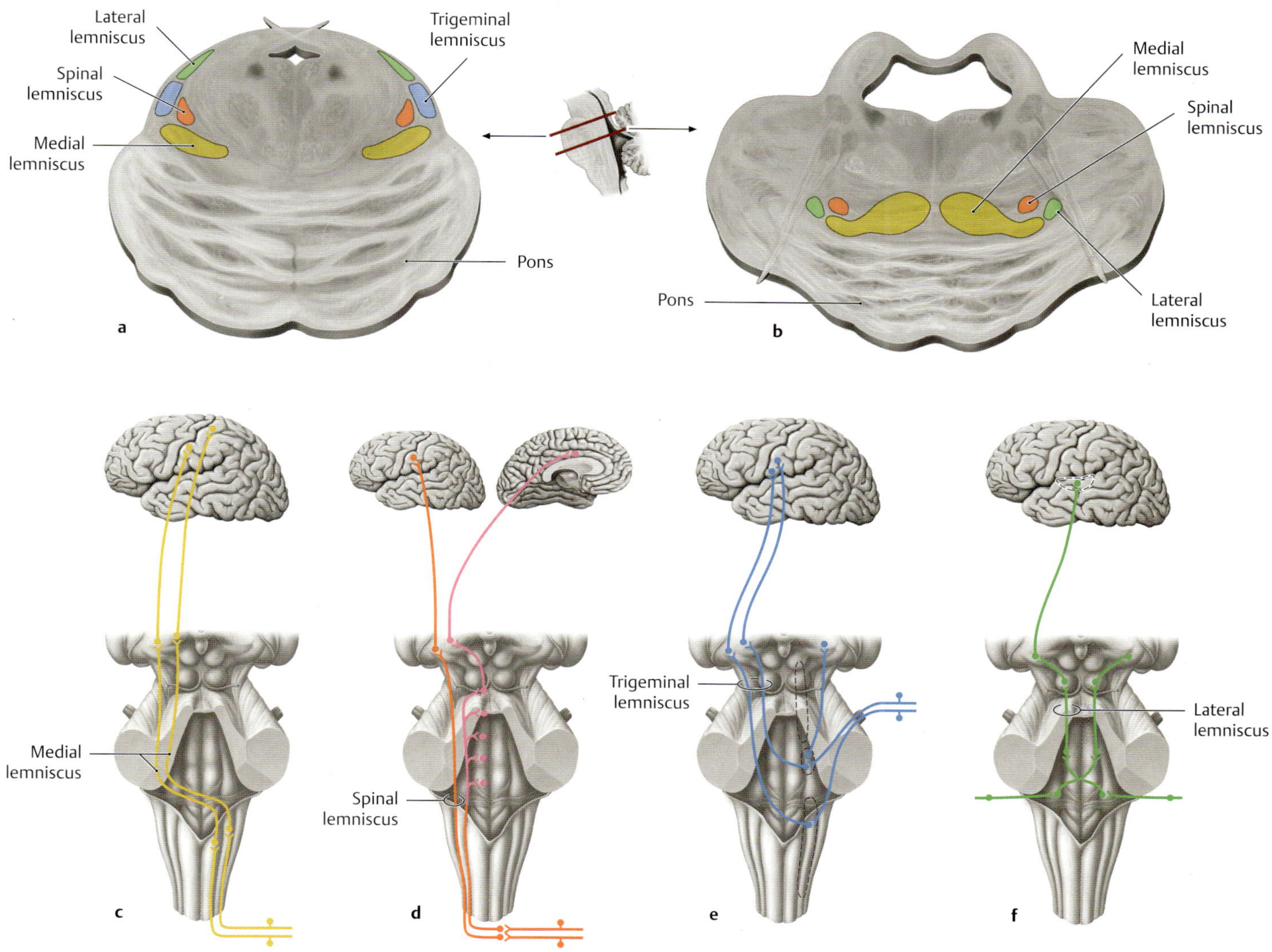

B The four lemnisci in the brainstem

a and **b** cross-section of the pons—superior and medial view respectively; **c–f** schematic representation of the four lemnisci.

The term lemniscus (ribbon) refers to the ribbon-like course of a total of four specific afferent (ascending) pathways in the brainstem. A lemniscus is not a "new" pathway but rather the name of a portion of a pathway. The specific **names of the individual lemnisci** are based on

- their location relative to each other in the brainstem (medial and lateral lemniscus),
- their origin in the spinal cord (spinal lemniscus), or
- their origin in a cranial nerve nucleus (trigeminal lemniscus).

The terms are historically related; they are not based on any classification. **a** and **b** display on two cross-section samples the respective location of the four lemnisci. A lemniscus contains axons of the second-order neuron which is located in the CNS. It starts with the course of the second axon in the brainstem and ends at the entry into the thalamic nucleus (diencephalon). Some fibers in all lemnisci are uncrossed. **Details follow:**

- *Medial lemniscus* (**c**): Continuation of the fasciculus gracilis or cuneatus. Second-order neurons (with the bodies in nucleus gracilis or cuneatus) are already in the brainstem. The entire lemniscus is formed by fibers that crossed in the decussation of the medial lemnisci and ends in the contralateral ventral posterolateral nucleus of the thalamus. It conveys epicritic sensation from the trunk, limbs, and back of the head.
- *Spinal lemniscus (***d***)* Continuation of the anterior and lateral spinothalamic tracts. The bodies of the second-order neurons are located in the posterior horn of the spinal cord and all of them decussate while still in the spinal cord; therefore the spinal lemniscus itself does not cross. It ends in the ventral posterolateral nucleus of the thalamus. The spinal lemniscus runs very close to the medial lemniscus in some parts of the brainstem; therefore an "individual" course is rarely described. It relays the protopathic sensation from trunk, limbs, and back of the head.
  Note: Unlike the other three terms, "spinal lemniscus" is not frequently used; occasionally it is used as a synonym for the *lateral* spinothalamic tract.
- *Trigeminal lemniscus* (trigeminothalamic tract; **e**): originates in the trigeminal nuclei. The second-order neurons (with the bodies in the principal nucleus or spinal nucleus) *cross only partially* and end in the contra- and ipsilateral ventral posteromedial nuclei of the thalamus. It conveys the epicritic and protopathic sensation from the head (not including the back of the head). Distinctive feature: it divides into an *anterior* trigeminothalamic tract (uncrossed fibers) and *posterior* (crossed fibers). Due to a particular role of the mesencephalic nucleus, which is discussed in a different chapter, this illustration depicts only a part of the trigeminal pathways.
- *Lateral lemniscus* (**f**): Auditory pathway. Second-order neurons (with the bodies in the anterior cochlear nucleus) in the brainstem; some cross and some remain ipsilateral; therefore they end in the contra- and ipsilateral *medial geniculate nucleus* (medial geniculate body) of the thalamus. It conveys information from the organs of hearing. *Distinctive feature*: the lemniscus contains "its own nuclei" (nuclei of the lateral lemniscus), which serve as relay stations for the auditory pathway. It terminates in the nucleus of the inferior colliculus of the mesencephalon.

2.17 Left to Right Connections in the CNS: Commissures and Decussations

A Commissures

Note: Commissures connect specific areas on the left side of the CNS with the analogous areas on the right side of the CNS and vice versa. For instance, they connect specific areas of the left and right visual cortex. Per definition, commissural projections are contralateral. The term commissure is generally used for the entire pathway. The site at which this pathway crossed the midline does not have a name. For further details see the term "decussation."

Name of pathway	Location/course	Structures connected by the pathway
Telencephalic commissures		
Corpus callosum • Frontal forceps (frontal lobe) • Occipital forceps (parietal and occipital lobes)	Roof and anterior wall of the lateral ventricles	Cerebral hemispheres with the exception of the temporal lobes; the temporal lobes are connected via the posterior part of the anterior commissure
Anterior commissure with an anterior and a posterior part	Adjacent to the lamina terminalis (anterior wall of the third ventricle)	• Anterior part: Olfactory nuclei • Posteror part: Medial and inferior temporal gyri
Commissura fornicis (Hippocampal commis-sure)	Border between telencephalon/ diencephalon, crus of fornix	Left and right hippocampus via the fimbria of the fornix
Diencephalic commissure (Diencephalon)		
Habenular commissure	Epithalamus, parietal to the pineal recess	Connection between left and right habenular nuclei
Commissures of the brainstem (truncus cerebri: medulla oblongata, pons, mesencephalon)		
Supraoptic commissure: ventral and dorsal	Parts of it pass through the diencephalon superior to the optic chiasm	Connection between the left and right pons and midbrain: the commissure thus passes through the diencephalon yet connects parts of the brainstem.
Posterior commissure	Connects midbrain nuclei	Connection between the light reflex tracts
Commissure of the superior colliculus	Midbrain, tectum	Superior colliculi
Commissure of the inferior colliculus	Midbrain, tectum	Inferior colliculi
Pontine cochlear commissure	Tegmentum of pons (trapezoid body)	Anterior cochlear nucleus
Cerebellar commissure		
Commissura cerebelli	Cerebellum; medulla; close to fastigial nucleus	Cerebellar hemispheres
Pathways of the spinal cord (medulla spinalis)		
Anterior/posterior white commissure	In each case between the anterior and posterior horns	Connection between symmetrical halves of the spinal cord; part of the fasciculi proprii (propriospinal fibers) The anterior white commissure contains axons of second-order neurons that cross the midline and carry information related to pain and temperature from one side of the body to the contralateral thalamus
Anterior/posterior gray commissure	Anterior and posterior to the central canal	Layer of gray matter; Not a real *functional* commissure.

B Decussation

Note: The term "decussations" refers to the crossover of tracts, not to analogous sites on the opposite side but to topographically different regions. For instance, the pyramidal tract runs from one cerebral hemisphere to contralateral half of the spinal cord. For theses tracts (which are called tracts, fasciculi, funiculi, or fibre), the site at which the tract crosses over—meaning it crosses the midline—lies in the median plane of the CNS, somewhere along the course of the the tract. This is in contrast to the commissures, for which the crossover point is located in the middle between left and right analogous structures. As a result, the crossover point of each crossing is individually named (cf. the term "commissure").

Name of decussation	Location	Name of the crossed pathway(s)	Structures connected by the pathway(s)
Anterior (ventral) tegmental decussation	Midbrain; tegmentum at the level of the superior colliculi	Fibers of the rubrospinal tracts	Connects the red nucleus in the midbrain with γ-motor neurons in the anterior horn of the spinal cord
Posterior (dorsal) tegmental decussation	Midbrain; tegmentum at the level of the superior colliculi	Fibers of the tectospinal and tectobulbar tracts	Connects the red nucleus in the midbrain with γ-motor neurons in the anterior horn of the spinal cord
Decussation of the superior cerebellar peduncles	Midbrain; tegmentum at the level of the inferior colliculi	Superior cerebellar peduncles (for more details see the information in right column)	• Anterior spinocerebellar tract: connects spinal cord with cerebellar cortex and cerebellar nuclei • Dentothalamic fasciculus: from the dentate nucleus of the cerebellum to the contralateral thalamus • Cerebellorubral fasciculus: from the cerebellar nuclei to the red nucleus in the midbrain
Decussation of trochlear nerve fibers	Midbrain; Tectum, in the white matter	Crossing of the axons of the trochlear nn.; This is the only crossing of a peripheral nerve.	The trochlear n. crosses at this level in order to innervate the opposite superior oblique m.
Decussation of the medial lemniscus (sensory decussation)	Medulla oblongata, at the level of the olive	Crossing of the axons originating in the gracile/cuneate nuclei (part of internal arcuate fibers)	Connect the gracile and cuneate nuclei with the ventral posterolateral nucleus of the thalamus
Pyramidal decussation	Medulla oblongata; ventral aspect, level of pyramids	About 80% of the pyramidal tract cross here	Connect the precentral gyrus and other areas of the cerebral cortex with α motor neurons in the anterior horn of the spinal cord

Note: With the exception of the trochlear n. (the only crossing of a peripheral n.), all the above mentioned decussations refer to crossings of pathways in the central nervous system.

2.18 Diencephalic Nuclei and Thalamic Nuclear Regions

A Diencephalic nuclei

Part of diencephalon	Nuclear region	Function
Epithalamus	• Habenular nuclei (in the habenula) • Pineal gland (epiphysis)	• Relay station for vegetative processing of olfactory impulses • Circadian rhythm and melatonin production
Thalamus	• Anterior nuclei • Medial nuclei • Intralaminar and midline nuclei • Reticular nuclei • Ventral posterolateral nucleus • Ventral posteromedial nucleus • Ventral anterior nucleus • Pulvinar • Medial geniculate nucleus • Lateral geniculate nucleus	• Limbic system • Emotional stability • Cerebellar connection • Interthalamic connection • Epicritic, protopathic, and proprioceptive information from trunk and limbs • Epicritic, protopathic, and proprioceptive information from the face • Cerebellar information • Functional relation to the association cortex • Relay station on the auditory pathway • Relay station on the visual pathway
Hypothalamus	• Infundibular nucleus • Mammillary body (with medial and lateral mammillary nuclei) • Paraventricular nucleus • Supraoptic nucleus • Suprachiasmatic nucleus	• Releasing and inhibiting hormones that act on the pituitary gland • Limbic system • Oxytocin • Antidiuretic hormone • Circadian rhythm
Subthalamus	• Subthalamic nucleus • Zona incerta	• (extrapyramidal) motor control

B Thalamic nuclear regions

Nuclear region	Afferent from	Efferent to	Function
Anterior nucleus	Medial and lateral mammillary nuclei of the mammillary body via the mammillothalamic tract	• Cingulate gyrus • Parahippocampal gyrus	• Limbic system • Part of the Papez circuit
Medial nuclei	• Amygdala • Olfactory cortex	Frontal cortical areas	Affective function
Median nuclei	• Telencephalon: cingulate gyrus • Diencephalon: hypothalamus • Brainstem: reticular formation	Cingulate gyrus; hippocampus; amygdala	Wakefulness; alertness
Ventral nuclei			
• Anterior/lateral ventral nucleus	• Globus pallidus; substantia nigra; cerebellar nuclei	• Motor cortical areas	• Motor functions
• Ventral posterolateral nucleus	• Medial lemniscus; spinothalamic tract	• Postcentral gyrus	• Sensation from limbs and trunk
• Ventral posteromedial nucleus	• Trigeminal lemniscus	• Postcentral gyrus	• Sensation from head/face
Dorsal nuclei			
• Pulvinar	• Pretectal area; superior colliculus	• Association cortex	• Control of eye movement
• Intralaminary nuclei	• Large parts of the cortex, brainstem; spinal cord	• Cortex; basal nuclei	• Motor system; alertness (ARAS)
• Reticular nucleus	• Cortex and other thalamic nuclei	• Thalamic nuclei	• Interthalamic connection (largely inhibition)

2.19 Nuclei of Cranial Nerves and Autonomic Nuclei

A Nuclei of the cranial nerves

Name of nucleus	Location	Course including nerve	Target organs
Somatic motor nuclei (general somatic efferent); the axons of these nerves end directly on target organs			
Oculomotor nucleus motor n.	Midbrain, at the level of the superior colliculus	Oculomotor n. (III)	Inferior oblique m., medial rectus m., superior and inferior recti mm., levator palpebrae superioris
Trochlear nucleus	Midbrain, at the level of the inferior colliculus	Trochlear n. (IV)	Superior oblique m.
Abducens nucleus	Midpons floor of the fourth ventricle	Abducens n. (VI)	Lateral rectus m.
Accessory n. nucleus	Cervical spinal cord (extending to C6 segment)	Accessory n. (spinal root) (XI)	Trapezius and sternocleidomastoid mm.
Hypoglossal nucleus	Medulla oblongata, floor of the fourth ventricle	Hypoglossal n. (XII)	Muscles of the tongue
Visceral motor nuclei (special visceral efferent or branchiomotor) (embryological term; control of skeletal muscles derived from pharyngeal or branchial arches); the axons in these nerves end directly on target organs			
Motor nucleus of the trigeminal n.	Midpons	Mandibular n. (V_3)	Muscles of mastication, tensor tympani m., tensor veli palatini m.; digastric m. (anterior belly); mylohyoid m.
Facial nucleus	Caudal pons	Facial n. (VII)	Muscles of facial expression, stapedius m.
Nucleus ambiguus	Medulla oblongata	• Glossopharyngeal n. (IX) • Vagus n. (X) • Accessory n., cranial root (XI)	• Pharyngeal muscles • Pharyngeal and laryngeal muscles • Laryngeal muscles, fibers ran back in the vagus nerve
Visceral efferent nuclei (general visceral motor) (control of smooth muscles of the internal organs, glands, and eyes) Accessory oculomotor nucleus; superior and inferior salivary nuclei; dorsal motor nucleus of the vagus, see **B**.			
Somatic sensory nuclei (general somatic afferent); with the exception of the mesencephalic nucleus of the trigeminal n., all these nuclei contain bodies of second-order neurons of afferent pathways, while the bodies of first neurons of the pathways are located in the respective sensory ganglia of cranial nerves.			
Principal (pontine, main) nucleus of trigeminal n.	Pons, rostral part	All three branches of the trigeminal n. First-order neuron in the trigeminal ggl.	Skin and mucosae: Epicritic sensation
Spinal trigeminal nucleus	Cervical spinal cord, extending to segment C6	All three branches of the trigeminal n.; First-order neuron in the trigeminal ggl.	Skin and mucosae: Protopathic sensation
Mesencephalic nucleus	Midbrain, tegmentum	Mandibular n. First-order neuron in the mesencephalic nucleus	Muscles of mastication, mandibular joint: proprioception
Medial, lateral, superior, and inferior vestibular nuclei	From pons to medulla oblongata	Vestibulocochlear n., vestibular part (VIII); first-order neuron in the vestibular ggl.	Cristae ampullares in the semicircular canals; Macula in the utricular and saccule; Balance
Anterior/posterior cochlear nuclei	Pontomedullary junction at the lateral recess of the fourth ventricle	Vestibulocochlear n., cochlear part (VIII); first-order neuron in the cochlear ggl.	Organ of Corti in the cochlea hearing
Visceral sensory nuclei (general and special visceral afferent); these nuclei contain second-order neurons of an afferent pathway, while the first-order neurons are located in the sensory ganglion of a cranial nerve			
Solitary nucleus (solitary tract nucleus) • Superior part • Inferior part	Medulla oblongata	• Special visceral afferent: N. VII; IX and X; first-order neuron in the geniculate ganglion and the inferior ganglia of IX and X respectively • General visceral afferent: N. IX and X; first-order neuron in the superior ggl. of IX and X	• Tongue papillae; taste • Lungs and carotid bifurcation; glomus caroticum; pulmonary stretch receptors

B Autonomic nuclei

Nuclear region	Preganglionic neuron (central), location and course of axons	Postganglionic neuron (peripheral), location of the ganglion and course of axons	Territory of distribution
Parasympathetic nuclei			
Accessory oculomotor nucleus (Edinger-Westphal nucleus)	Midbrain, tegmentum; travels with N. III	Orbit, ciliary ggl., then travels via the short ciliary nn.	Pupillary sphincter m.; ciliary m.
Superior salivary (salivatory) nucleus	Pons, tegmentum; travels initially with the intermediate n. (part of VII), then with chorda tympani	Submandibular ganglion; Rr. glandulares to the glands	Sublingual and submandibular glands
	Or as greater petrosal n.	Pterygopalatine ggl.; orbital branches; nasal branches; palatine nn.	Lacrimal gland; glands of the nose and palate
Inferior salivary (salivatory) nucleus	Pons, tegmentum; travels initially with N. IX then as tympanic n. And lesser petrosal n.	Otic ggl.; travels with the auriculotemporal n.	Parotid gland
Dorsal motor nucleus of the vagus	Pons/medulla oblongata; travel with N. X	Ganglia close to the target organs, from there as plexus	Organs from the neck to the abdomen, large intestine proximal to the left colic flexure
Sacral parasympathetic nuclei	Spinal cord, intermediolateral region, S2–4; splanchnic nn. pelvic	Ganglia close to the organs in the inferior hypogastric plexus	Urogenital system, large intestine distal to the left colic flexure
Sympathetic nuclei			
Intermediolateral and intermediomedial nuclei	Spinal cord, lateral horn, C8–L2		
	As white ramus communicans to the ganglia of the sympathetic trunk in the C8–L2 segments	All ganglia of the sympathetic trunk: *Gray* ramus communicans	Trunk and limbs: blood vessels, sweat glands
		T1–4 ganglia of the sympathetic trunk as cardiac plexus or cardiac nerves	Thoracic organs
	From the ganglia of the sympathetic trunk (without synapsing here) T5–12: Nn. splanchnici major and minor; L1–4: Nn. splanchnici lumbales	Prevertebral ganglia: Celiac ggl.; superior mesenteric ggl.; inferior mesenteric ggl. (plexus with various names)	Abdominal organs to the flexura coli sinistra
	S1–4: sacral splanchnic nn.	Inferior hypogastric plexus	Abdominal organs distal to the left colic flexure and urogenital system

2.20 Neurovascular Structures of the Nose

A Arteries and nerves of the nose
The arterial supply to the nose and the sensory innervation of the nasal mucosa follow common principles:
There are **two areas of supply** in the nasal cavity:

- the medial *nasal septum* (see **a** and **c**, left view) and
- the lateral *nasal wall* (see **b** and **d**, right view of the left lateral nasal wall).

Neurovascular structures enter the respective areas of supply via **two approaches:**

- *superiorly* (from the orbit) and
- *posteriorly* (from the pterygopalatine fossa through the sphenopalatine foramen).

Note: In the interest of clarity this depiction of the openings through which the neurovascular structures pass is neither drawn to scale nor is it topographically precise.

Arterial supply: The arteries of the nasal cavity arise from two flow tracts: the internal carotid artery (green) and the external carotid artery (orange).

- The *internal carotid artery* enters the cranial cavity through the carotid canal and gives off the ophthalmic artery. This artery passes through the optic canal into the orbit and there gives off the anterior and posterior ethmoidal arteries, which enter the nasal cavity through the anterior and posterior ethmoidal foramina. There they split into branches for the septum and lateral nasal wall. The ophthalmic artery thus supplies the nose *superiorly*.
- The *external carotid artery* gives off the maxillary artery whose branch—the sphenopalatine artery—enters the nasal cavity through the sphenopalatine foramen and also gives off branches for the septum and lateral nasal wall. The sphenopalatine artery supplies the nose *posteriorly*. This systematic separation of areas of supply is indicated by the dashed line.

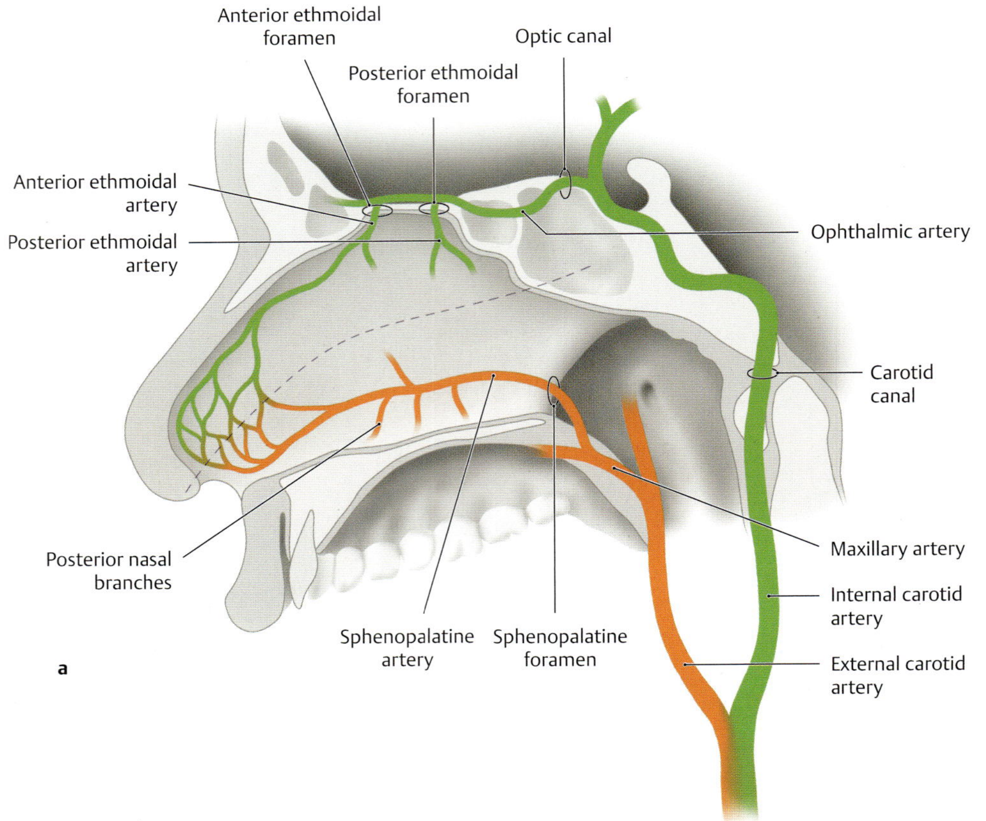

a

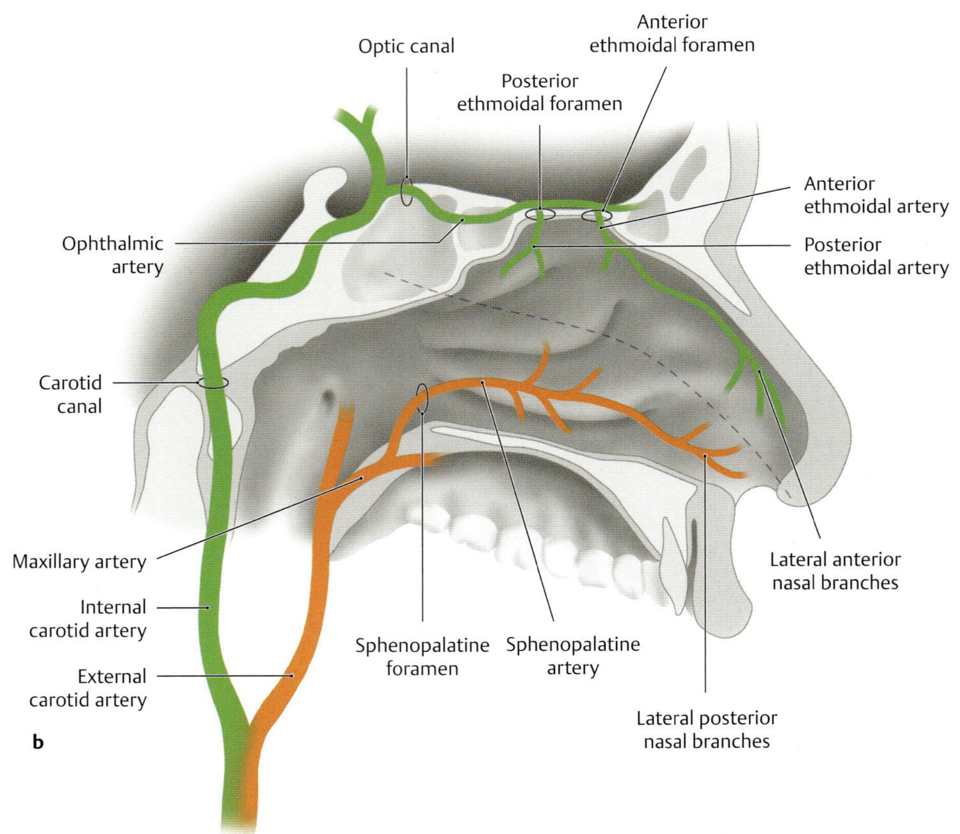

b

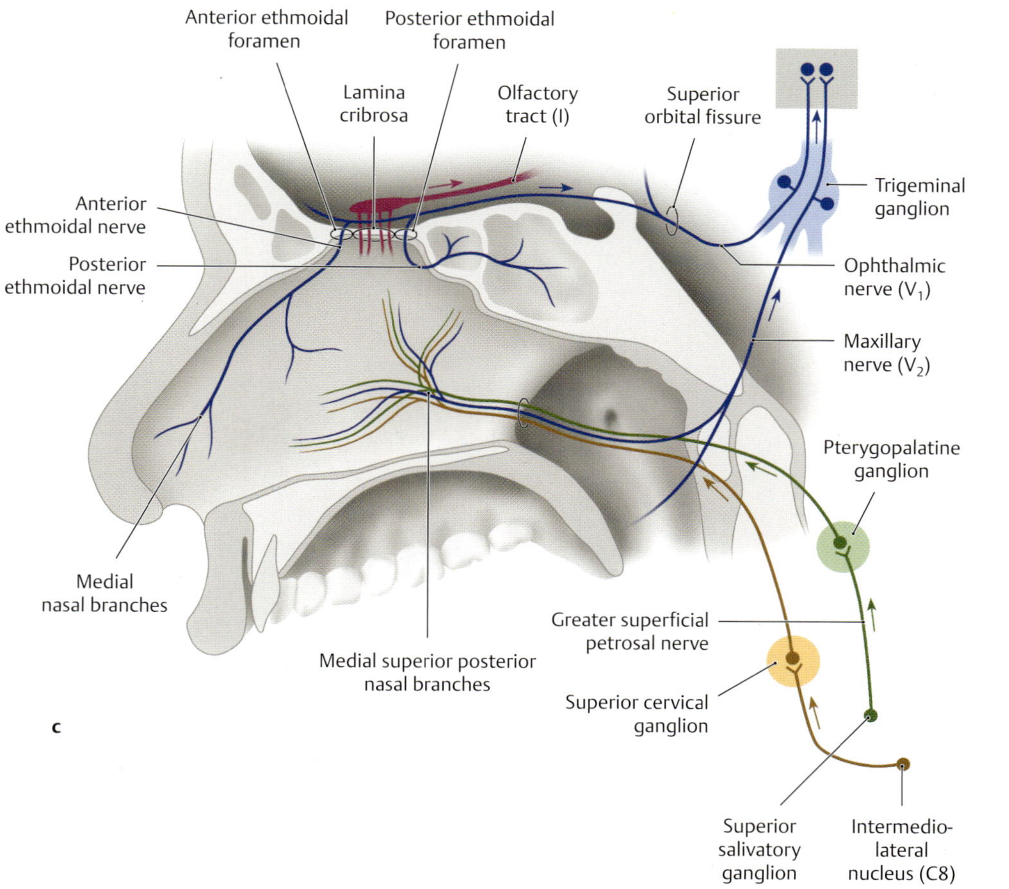

c

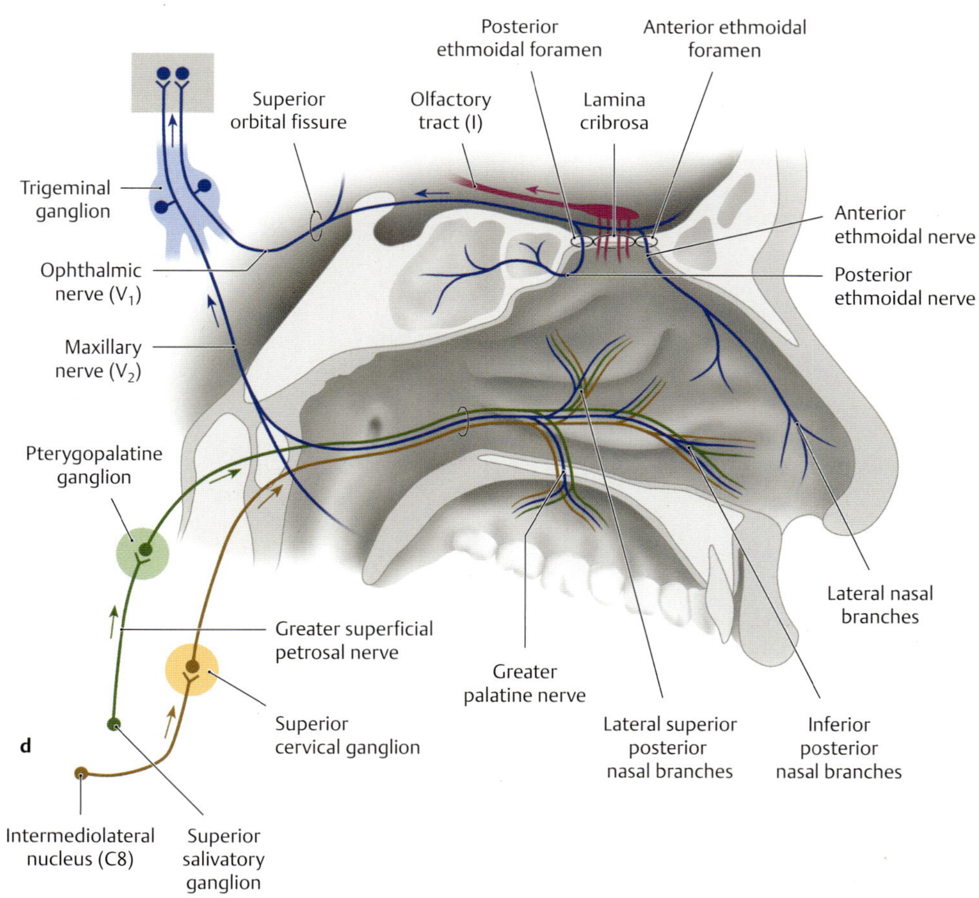

d

Sensory innervation:

- The anterior and posterior ethmoidal nerves pass through the anterior and posterior ethmoidal foramina to the ophthalmic nerve (V_1), which passes through the superior orbital fissure to the trigeminal ganglion. The ophthalmic nerve supplies the septal and lateral regions of the nose from *above*.
- Fine posterior nasal branches (medial and lateral superior branches) supply the septum and lateral nasal wall posteriorly, exit the nose through the sphenopalatine foramen, and extend to the maxillary nerve (V_2). The maxillary nerve supplies the nose *posteriorly*.

Note: The innervation for *smell* is provided *only superiorly* by the olfactory nerve (I), which passes through the ethmoid bone in the lamina cribrosa and reaches the olfactory region in the superior nasal cavity. The *autonomic innervation* of the nose is *only posterior*, whereby parasympathetic fibers from the pterygopalatine ganglion (green) and the superior cervical ganglion (brown) enter the nasal cavity posteriorly and separate in the lateral and septal wall to innervate the nasal glands.

Overview:

- Superior arterial supply and sensory innervation of the septum and lateral nasal wall: ophthalmic artery and nerve.
- Posterior arterial supply and sensory innervation of the septum and lateral nasal wall: sphenopalatine artery and maxillary nerve.

2.21 Vessels of the Orbit

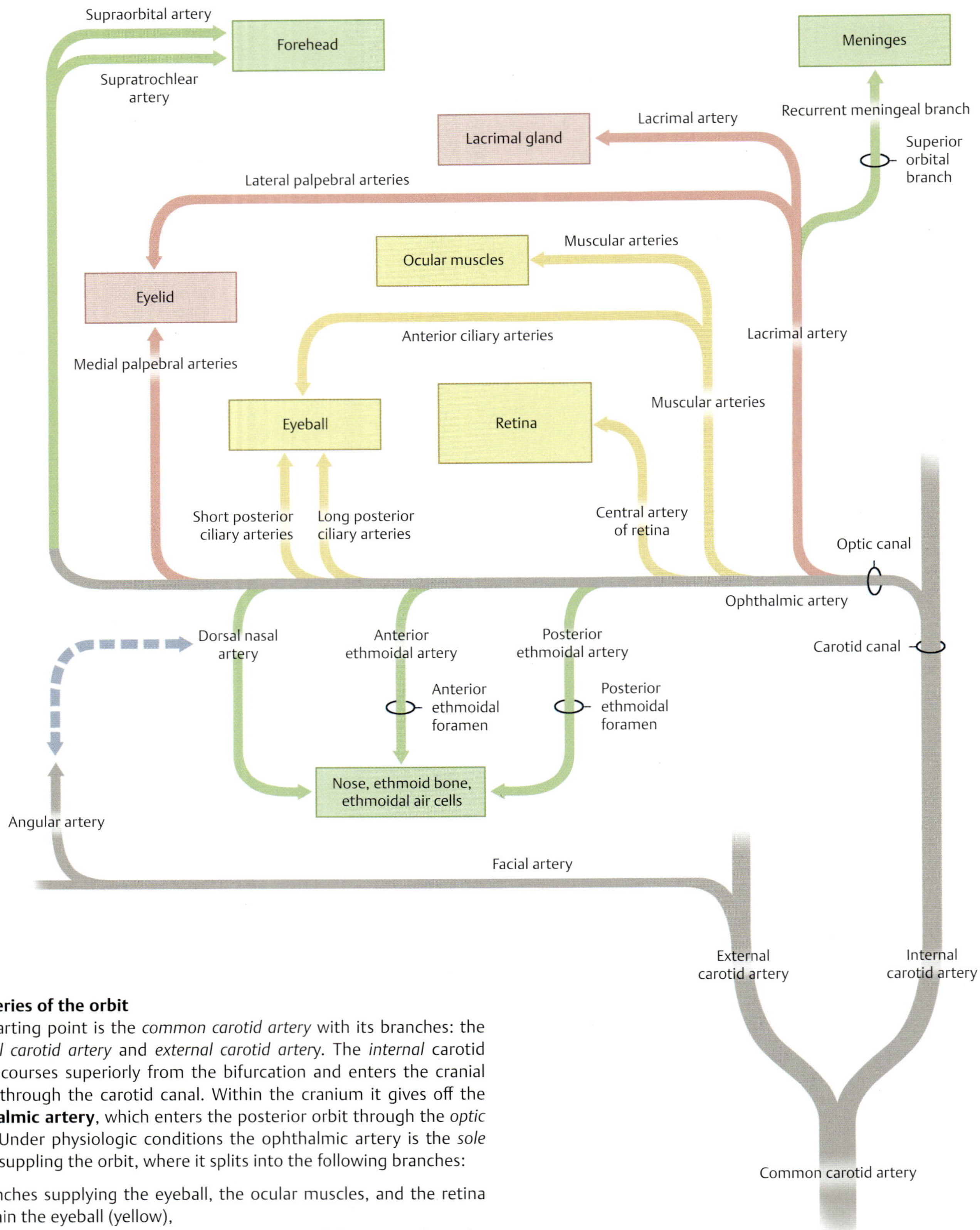

A Arteries of the orbit

The starting point is the *common carotid artery* with its branches: the *internal carotid artery* and *external carotid artery*. The *internal* carotid artery courses superiorly from the bifurcation and enters the cranial cavity through the carotid canal. Within the cranium it gives off the **ophthalmic artery**, which enters the posterior orbit through the *optic canal*. Under physiologic conditions the ophthalmic artery is the *sole* artery suppling the orbit, where it splits into the following branches:

- Branches supplying the eyeball, the ocular muscles, and the retina within the eyeball (yellow),
- Branches supplying the ancillary structures of the eye such as the eyelids and lacrimal gland (red),
- Branches supplying the region adjacent to the orbit: forehead, nose and paranasal sinuses, and meninges (green).

The *external* carotid artery only contributes to supplying the orbit under pathologic conditions when arterial supply via the ophthalmic artery is compromised. In such cases the *anastomosis* (see blue dashed line) between the *angular artery* (courses to the angle of the eye) and the *dorsal nasal* artery (branch of the ophthalmic artery) partially compensates the loss of arterial supply. The angular artery enters the frontal orbit.

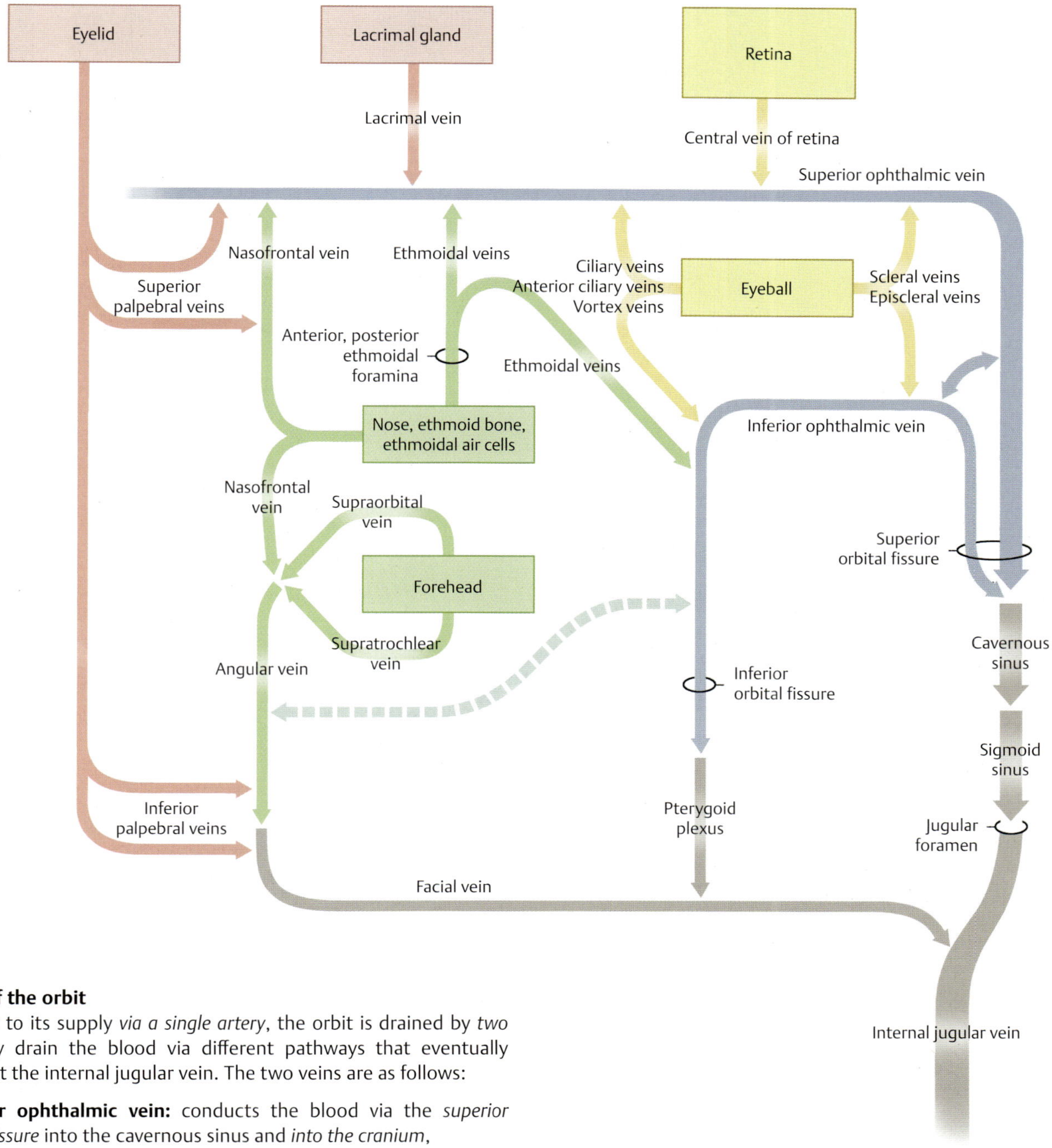

B Veins of the orbit

In contrast to its supply *via a single artery*, the orbit is drained by *two veins*. They drain the blood via different pathways that eventually converge at the internal jugular vein. The two veins are as follows:

- **Superior ophthalmic vein:** conducts the blood via the *superior orbital fissure* into the cavernous sinus and *into the cranium*,
- **Inferior ophthalmic vein:** similarly to the superior ophthalmic vein, it conducts the blood via the *inferior orbital fissure out of the cranium* and into the pterygoid plexus inferior to the base of the skull.

Venous drainage occurs via a network of vessels in contrast to the arterial supply, which resembles a one-way street. However, here too there are three major drainage areas with a corresponding system of branch veins:

- branches draining blood from the eyeball and the retina within the eyeball (yellow),
- branches draining blood from the region adjacent to the orbit: forehead, nose, and paranasal sinuses (green), and
- branches draining blood from the ancillary structures of the eye such as the eyelids and lacrimal glands (red).

The two ophthalmic veins are physiologically interconnected by an extensive anastomosis (see continuous blue line). There is also an anastomosis between the angular vein and the inferior ophthalmic vein as well as a connection between the angular vein and the superior ophthalmic vein via the nasofrontal vein. Both of these anastomotic systems are clinically significant. The low-pressure flow of blood through the valveless veins of the cranium can easily reverse direction. This means that there is a risk that, in infections in the nasal and facial region, blood from the area drained by the angular vein (especially skin in the nasal region) can flow in retrograde fashion to the ophthalmic vein, thus spreading germs into the orbit and further into the sinus system.

2.22 Nerves of the Orbit

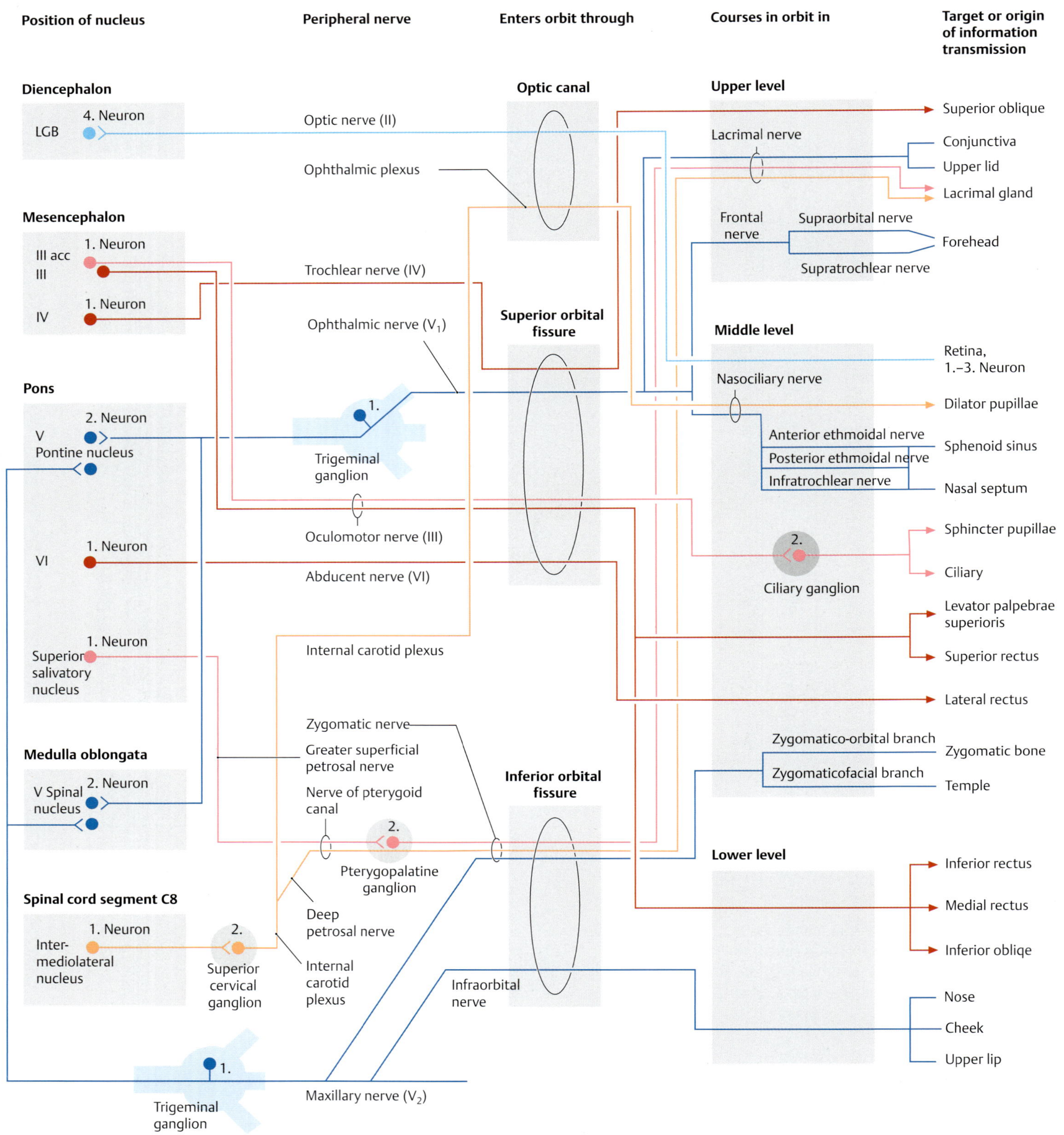

A Nerves of the orbit

The courses of nerves within the orbit are very complex. Achieving a comprehensive understanding of them requires an appreciation of their distinctive systematic, functional, and topographic features. This text is intended to help you orient yourself using the illustration much in the manner of a road map. This scheme divides the road map into five "information columns."

Topographical aspects

The orbit as a space (information column 4, "Courses in orbit in"): The orbit can be divided into *three levels*. Each level is schematically represented by a gray box. You will find important information for the topographical demarcation of the levels on p. 174. All neurovascular structures of the orbit, and therefore many nerves, course in one of the three levels. The *middle* level is by far the largest. It contains the eyeball as its salient landmark (see **A**, p. 174).

Access to the orbit (information column 3, "Enters orbit through"): The orbit is accessed posteriorly—from the left in the illustration—through *three openings, the optic canal and the superior and inferior orbital fissures* (see the ellipses in the gray boxes).

Note: The orbit and the cranial cavity communicate only through the optic canal and the *superior* orbital fissure. These two openings lie *superior* to the level of the skull base and give the orbit an *intracranial connection to the internal skull base*.

In contrast, the *inferior* orbital fissure lies *inferior* to the level of the skull base; it gives the orbit *extracranial access to the external skull base*. All neurovascular structures that enter or leave the orbit posteriorly must therefore pass through one of these three openings. To understand the course of the neurovascular structure, it is important to recognize that structures entering the orbit through the inferior orbital fissure can continue into the upper level; it is entirely possible to change levels. The orbital openings are shown in greater detail in Fig. **B**, p. 36.

Functional aspects

The relay stations (information column 1, "Position of nucleus"): The nerves of the orbit transmit motor and sensory information. This information is processed in the CNS in the diencephalon, the three segments of the brainstem (*mesencephalon, pons,* and *medulla oblongata*), and the spinal cord. In these segments of the CNS there are two **types of nuclei:**

- motor nuclei which send information, nuclei of origin, and
- sensory nuclei which receive information, terminal nuclei.

The **nuclei of origin** transmit information to the muscles and glands and are either *somato*motor nuclei (dark red, for the motor nuclei of cranial nerves **III**, **IV**, and **VI**) or *visceral* motor nuclei. Visceral motor nuclei belong to the parasympathetic system (pale red for **III acc**, accessory nucleus of the oculomotor nerve and superior salivatory nucleus) or to the sympathetic system (orange for the intermediolateral nucleus in spinal segment C8). The flow of information is conducted from left to right.

The **terminal nuclei** receive information in the visual system (*lateral geniculate body [LGB]*) from the retina or surface sensations from the skin, mucosa, or surface of the eye via two of the three branches of the trigeminal nerve (*pontine nucleus and spinal trigeminal nucleus* for epicritic and protopathic sensation). Sensory nuclei are shown in blue. The flow of information is conducted from right to left.

The effector organ (information column 5, "Target or origin of information transmission"): The source of the sensory information and target of the motor information are the "effector organs," which are shown on the far right.

Systematic aspects

Designation of the neurovascular structures (information column 2, "Peripheral nerve"): The information is transmitted via nerves named according to topographical, functional, or phenomenological criteria. They are shown in column 2. Sensory nerves include sensory ganglia along the course of the nerve (blue). Where information is conducted from right to left, these ganglia contain the first-order neuron of a neuron chain without synaptic connections. Autonomic ganglia are embedded for transmission of visceral motor information (gray circles). Where information is conducted from left to right, these ganglia contain the second-order neuron of a neuron chain (with synaptic relay).

You would like to

- learn the motor area of a somatomotor or visceral motor nucleus? Begin with information column 1 and follow the nerve to the right all the way to column 5. Note the gray ganglia in applicable cases;
- learn the nucleus for a sensory source area? Begin with information column 5 and follow the course of the nerve to the left all the way to column 1. Note the blue ganglia in applicable cases. The nerve may possibly split into branches within the orbit.
- Columns 2–4, which you will pass through as you follow the course of the nerve, inform you about the levels, openings, and names of the nerves.

2.23 Larynx

Arteries

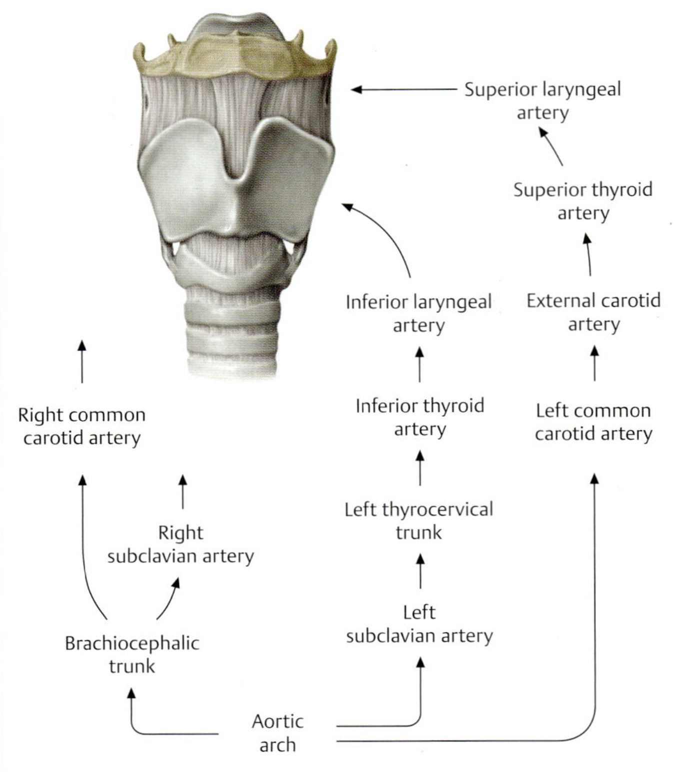

Veins

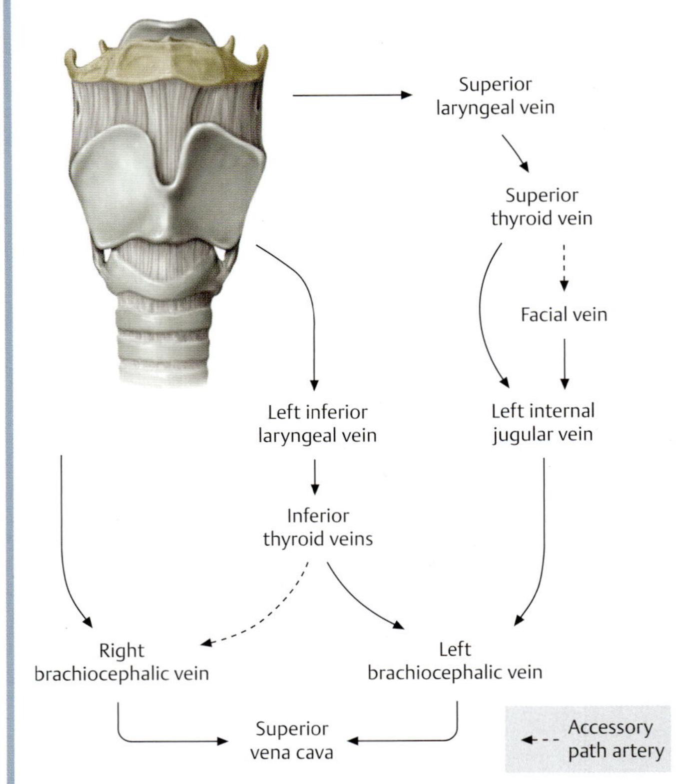

Lymph nodes

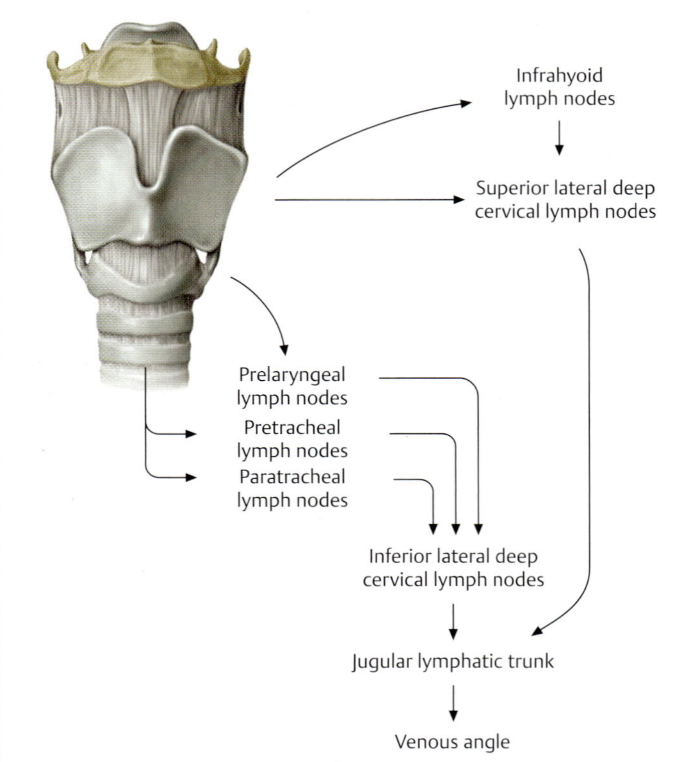

Innervation

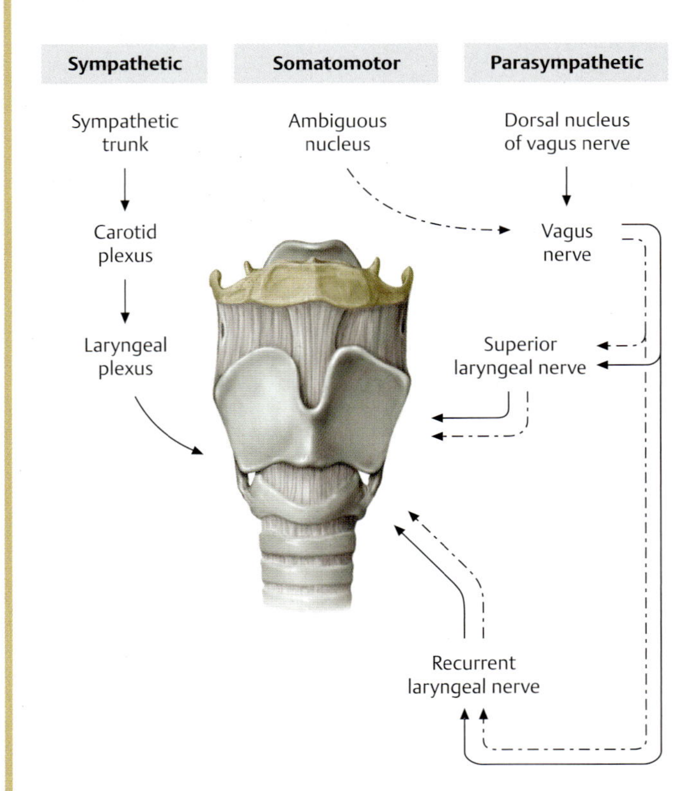

2.24 Thyroid Gland

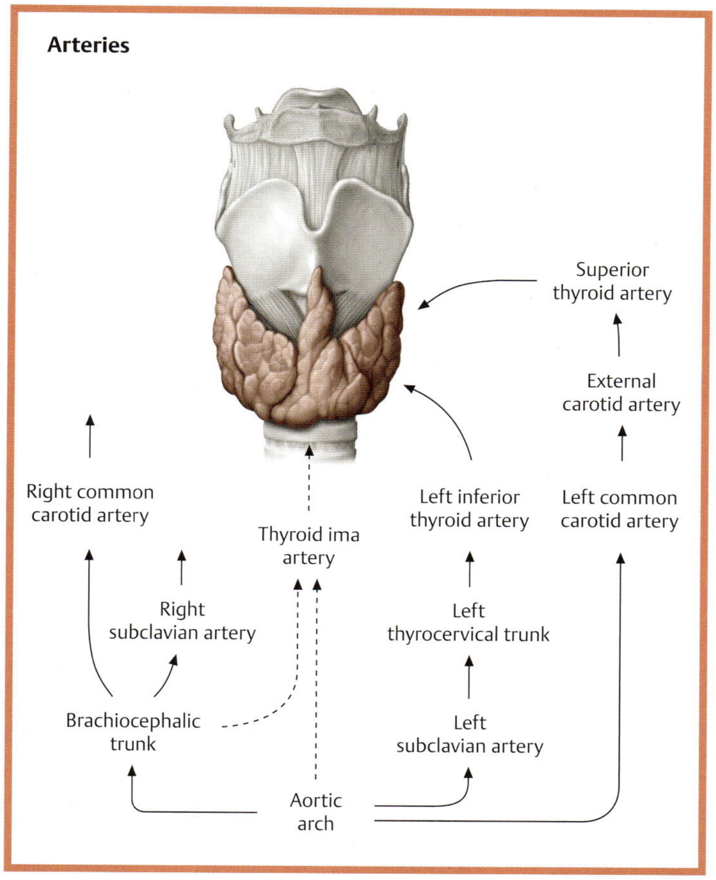

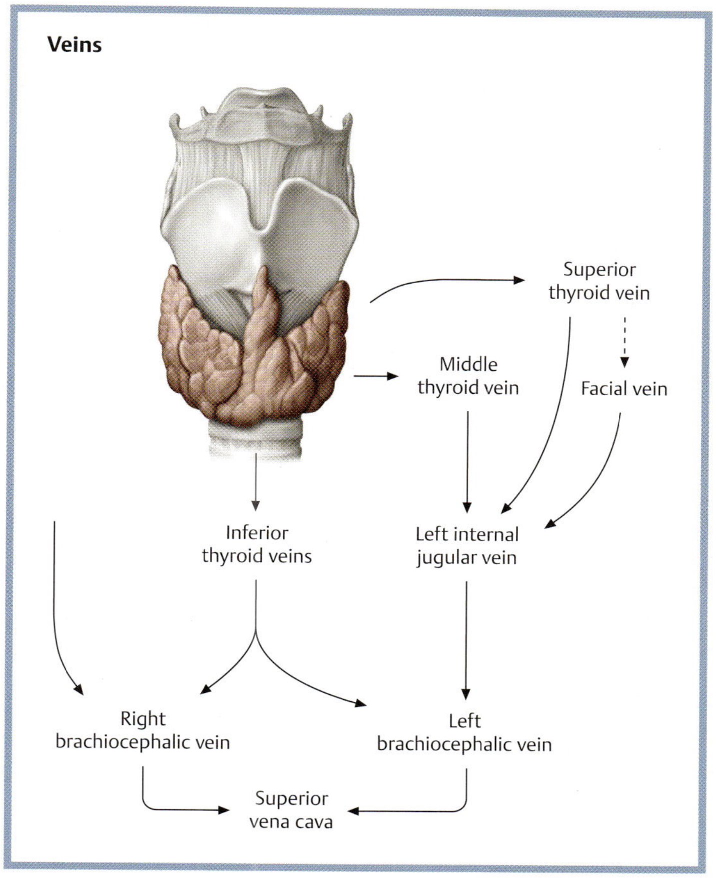

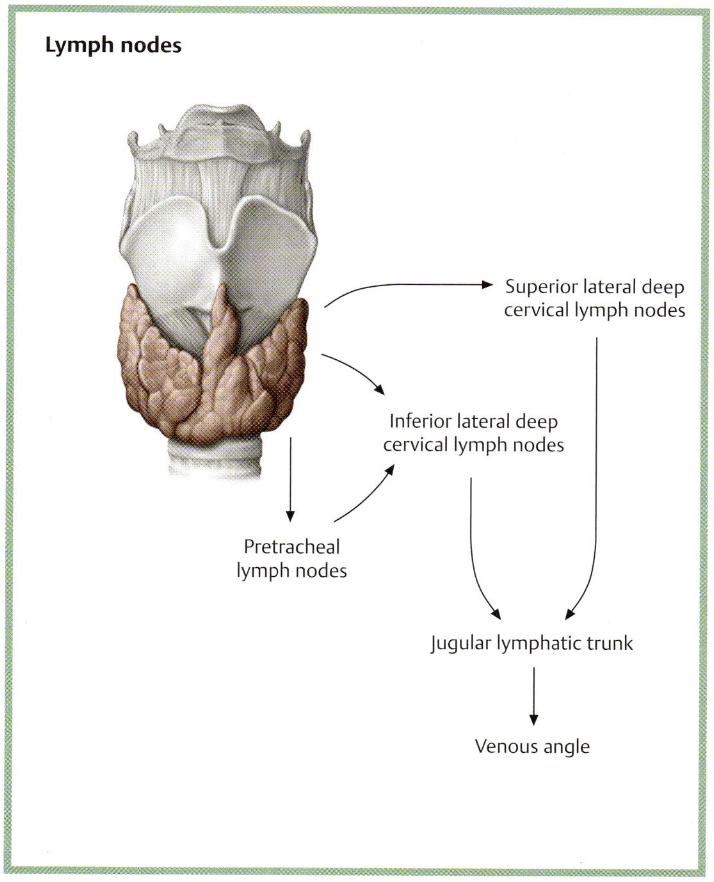

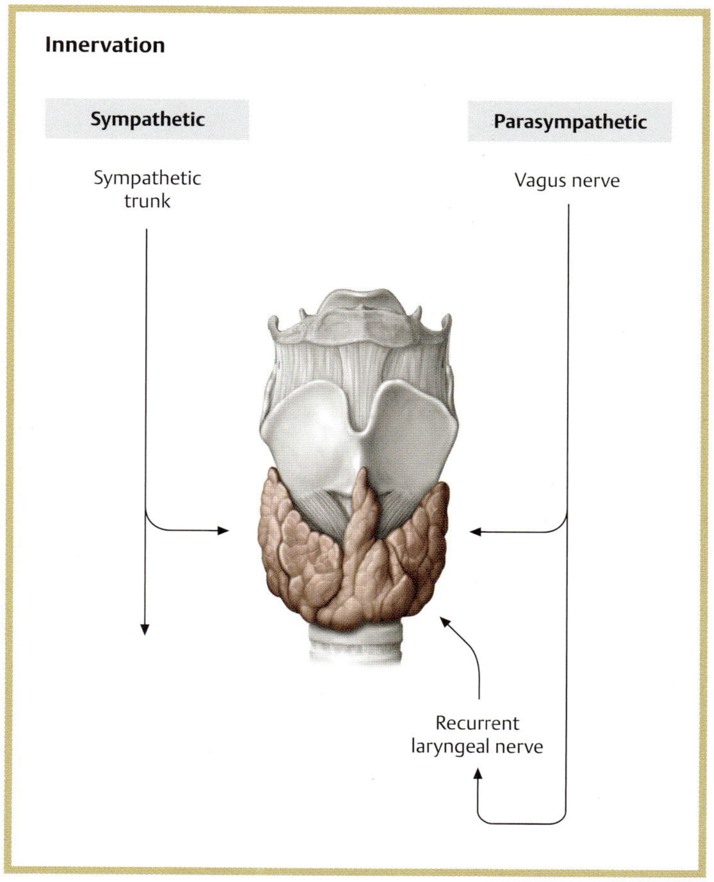

2.25 Pharynx*

Arteries

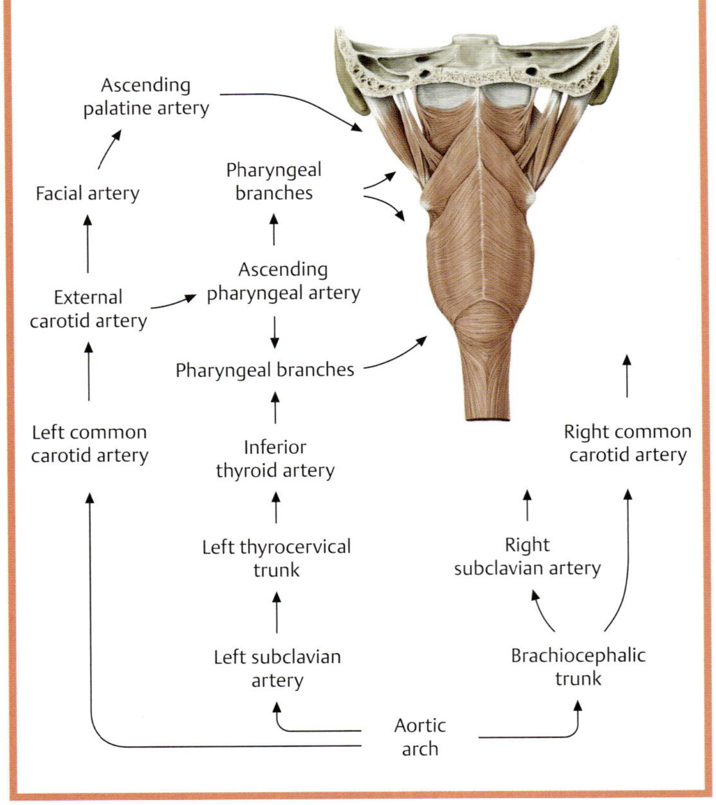

Veins

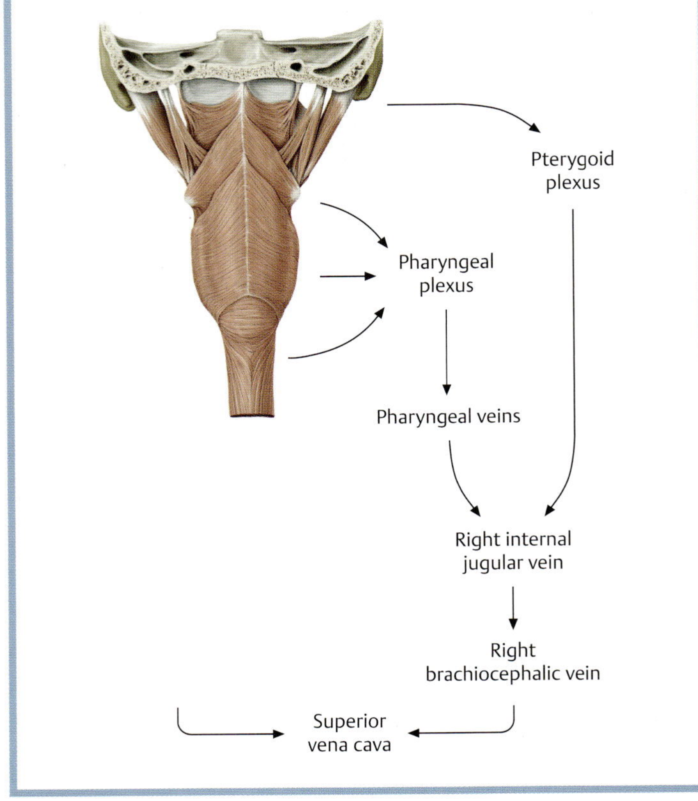

Lymph nodes

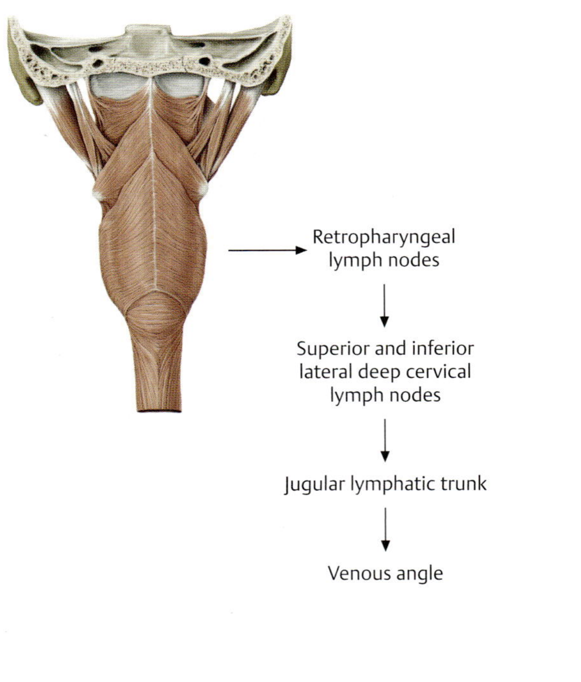

Innervation

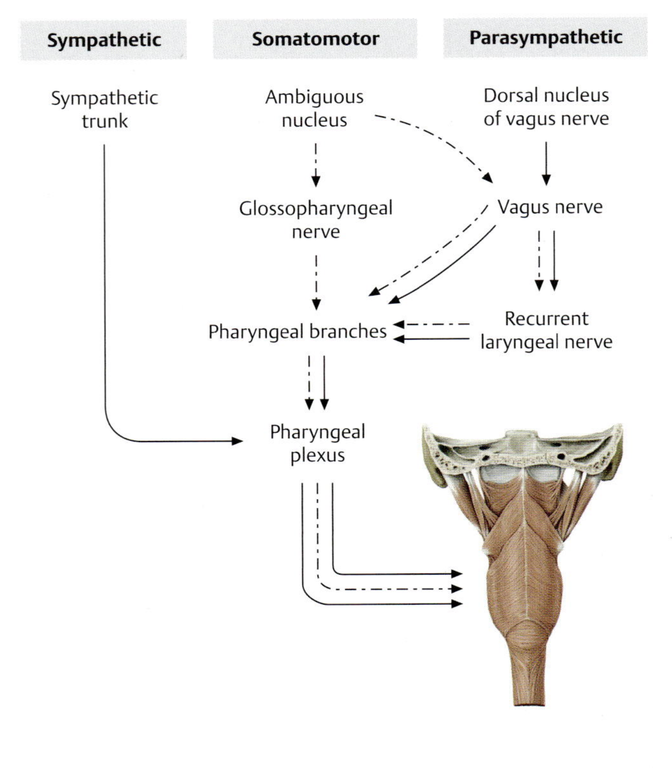

* Posterior view

Appendix

References

Abboud B. Anatomie topographique et vascularisation artérielle de parathyroides. Presse Med 1996; 25: 1156–61
Anschütz F. Die körperliche Untersuchung. 3rd ed. Heidelberg: Springer; 1978

Barr ML, Kiernan JA. The Human Nervous System. 5th ed. Philadelphia: JB Lippincott; 1988
Bähr M, Frotscher M. Neurologisch-topische Diagnostik. 10th ed. Stuttgart: Thieme; 2014
Bear MF, Connors BW, Paradiso MA. Neuroscience. Exploring the Brain. 2nd ed. Baltimore: Williams u. Wilkins; 2000
Becker W, Naumann HH, Pfaltz CR. Hals-Nasen-Ohren-Heilkunde. 2nd ed. Stuttgart: Thieme; 1983
Becker W, Naumann HH, Pfaltz CR. Ear, Nose and Throat Diseases. 2nd ed. Stuttgart: Thieme; 1994
Berghaus A, Rettinger G, Böhme G. Hals-Nasen-Ohren-Heilkunde. Duale Reihe. Stuttgart: Thieme; 1996
Blum HE, Müller-Wieland D (Hrsg.). Klinische Pathophysiologie. 10th ed. Stuttgart: Thieme; 2018
Bossy JG, Ferratier R. Studies of the spinal cord of Galago senegalensis, compared to that in man. J Comp Neurol 1968 Mar; 132(3): 485–98. PubMed PMID: 5657526
Braak H, Braak E. Neuroanatomie. In: Beyreuther K, Einhäupl KM, Förstl H, Kurz A, Hrsg. Demenzen. Stuttgart: Thieme; 2002: 118–129
Braus DF. EinBlick ins Gehirn. 3rd ed. Stuttgart: Thieme; 2014

Calabria G, Rolando M. Strutture e funzioni del film lacrimale. Genua: Proceedings of the 6th Symposium of the Italian Ophthalmological Society (S.O.I.); 1984: 9–35
Camper P. De Hominis Varietate (1792). Deutsche Fassung von S. Th. Sömmering (nach Kobes LWR. Quellenstudie zu Petrus Camper und der nach ihm benannten Schädelebene). Dtsch Zahnärztl Z; 1983: 38: 268–270
Carlsson GE, Haraldson T, Mohl ND. The dentition. In Mohl ND, Zarb GH, Carlsson GE, Rugh JD. A Textbook of Occlusion. Chicago: Quintessence Books; 1988
Chandrashekar J, Hoon MA, Ryba NJ, Zuker CS. The receptors and cells for mammalian taste. Nature 2006; 444: 288–294
Coolen RL et al. Curr Opin Urol 2020; 30: 480–485

Da Costa S, van der Zwaag W, Marques JP, Frackowiak RS, Clarke S, Saenz M. Human primary auditory cortex follows the shape of Heschl's gyrus. J Neurosci. 2011 Oct 5; 31(40): 14067-75. PubMed PMID: 21976491.
Dauber W. Bild-Lexikon der Anatomie. 10th ed. Stuttgart: Thieme; 2008

Faller A, Schünke M. Der Körper des Menschen. 17th ed. Stuttgart: Thieme; 2016
Frick H, Leonhardt H, Starck D. Allgemeine und spezielle Anatomie. Taschenlehrbuch der gesamten Anatomie. Bd. 1 and 2. 4th ed. Stuttgart: Thieme; 1992
Fritsch H, Kühnel W. Taschenatlas der Anatomie. Bd. 2. 11th ed. Stuttgart: Thieme; 2013
Füeßl HS, Middecke M. Anamnese und klinische Untersuchung. 6th ed. Stuttgart: Thieme; 2018

Gehlen W, Delank HW. Neurologie. 12th ed. Stuttgart: Thieme; 2010

Harvey R et al. The Olfactory Strip an Its Presvervation in Endoscopic Pituitary Surgery Maintains Smell and Sinonasal Function. In: Neurolog. Surg. B 2015; 76(06): 464–470
Hegglin J. Chirurgische Untersuchung. Stuttgart: Thieme; 1976
Hempelmann G, Krier C, Schulte am Esch J, Hrsg. Gesamtreihe ains. 4 Bände. Stuttgart: Thieme; 2001
Herrick JC. Brains of Rats and Men. Chicago: University of Chicago Press; 1926
Holodny et al. Diffusion tensor tractography of the motor white matter tracts in man – Current controversies and future directions. Ann NY Acad Sci 2005; 1064: 88–97

Ingvar DH. Functional landscapes of the dominant hemisphere. Brain Res 1976; 107: 181–197

Jänig W. Visceral afferent neurones: Neuroanatomy and functions, organ regulations and sensations. In: Vaitl D, Schandry R, eds. From the heart to the brain. Frankfurt am Main: Peter Lang; 1995: 5–34

Kahle W, Frotscher M. Taschenatlas der Anatomie. Bd. 3. 11th ed. Stuttgart: Thieme; 2013
Kell Ch A, von Kriegstein K, Rösler A, Kleinschmidt A, Laufs H. The Sensory Cortical Representation of the Human Penis: Revisiting Somatotopy in the Male Homunculus. J Neurosci Jun 2005; 25: 5984–5987
Kim et al. Corticospinal tract location in internal capsule of human brain: diffusion tensor tractography and functional MRI study. Neuroreport 2008; Vol 19, No 8
Kunze K. Lehrbuch der Neurologie. Stuttgart: Thieme; 1992
Kuwert T, Grünwald F, Haberkorn U, Krause T. Nuklearmedizin. 4th ed. Stuttgart: Thieme; 2008

Lang, G. Augenheilkunde. 5th ed. Stuttgart: Thieme; 2014
Lehmann KM, Hellwig E, Wenz H-J. Zahnärztliche Propädeutik. 13th ed. Köln: Deutscher Zahnärzte Verlag; 2015
Lippert H, Pabst R. Arterial Variations in Man. München: Bergman; 1985
Lorke D. Schmerzrelevante Neuroanatomie. In: Beck H, Martin E, Motsch J, Schulte am Esch J, Hrsg. ains. Bd. 4. Schmerztherapie. Stuttgart: Thieme; 2001: 13–28

Masuhr KF, Neumann M. Neurologie. Duale Reihe. 7th ed. Stuttgart: Thieme; 2013
Maurer J. Neurootologie. Stuttgart: Thieme; 1999
Meyer W. Die Zahn-Mund- und Kiefer-Heilkunde. Bd. 1. München: Urban & Schwarzenberg; 1958
Michels L et al. Neuroimage 2010; 49: 177–184
Mühlreiter F. Anatomie des menschlichen Gebisses. Leipzig: Felix; 1912
Müller-Vahl H, Mumenthaler M, Stöhr M. Läsionen peripherer Nerven und radikuläre Syndrome. 10th ed. Stuttgart: Thieme; 2014

Nieuwenhuys R, Voogd J, van Huijzen Chr. Das Zentralnervensystem des Menschen. 2nd ed. Berlin: Springer; 1991

Pape HC, Kurtz A, Silbernagl S. Physiologie. 8th ed. Stuttgart: Thieme; 2018
Platzer W. Atlas der topografischen Anatomie. Stuttgart: Thieme; 1982
Poeck K, Hartje W. Störungen von Antrieb und Affektivität. In: Hartje W, Poeck K, Hrsg. Klinische Neuropsychologie. 5th ed. Stuttgart: Thieme; 2002: 412–422
Poisel S, Golth D. Zur Variabilität der großen Arterien im Trigonum caroticum. Wiener medizinische Wochenschrift 1974; 124: 229–232

Probst R, Grevers G, Iro H. Hals-Nasen-Ohren-Heilkunde. 3rd ed. Stuttgart: Thieme; 2008
Rauber/Kopsch. Anatomie des Menschen. Bd. 1–4. Stuttgart: Thieme; Bd. 1, 2nd ed.; 1997, Bd. 2 and 3; 1987, Bd. 4; 1988
Robbins KT, Medina JE, Wolfe GT, Levine PA, Sessions RB, Pruet CW. Standardizing neck dissection terminology. Official report of the Academy's Committee for Head and Neck Surgery and Oncology. Arch Otolaryngol Head Neck Surg 1991 Jun; 117(6): 601-5. PubMed PMID: 2036180
Rohkamm R. Taschenatlas Neurologie. 4th ed. Stuttgart: Thieme; 2017
Romer AS, Parson TS. Vergleichende Anatomie der Wirbeltiere. 5th ed. Hamburg und Berlin: Paul Parey; 1983

Sachsenweger M. Augenheilkunde. 2nd ed. Stuttgart: Thieme; 2003
Sadler TW. Medizinische Embryologie. 12th ed. Stuttgart: Thieme; 2014
Scheibel ME, Scheibel AB. Activity cycles in neurons of the reticular formation. Recent Adv Biol Psychiatry. 1965; 8: 283–93
Schmidt F. Zur Innervation der Articulatio temporomandibularis. Gegenbaurs morphol Jb 1967; 110: 554–573
Schroeder HE. Orale Strukturbiologie. 3rd ed. Stuttgart: Thieme; 1987
Schumacher GH: Funktionelle Anatomie des orofazialen Systems. Heidelberg: Hüthig; 1985
Schumacher GH, Aumüller G. Topographische Anatomie des Menschen. 6. Aufl. Stuttgart: G. Fischer; 1994
Schumacher GH, Schmidt H. Anatomie und Biochemie der Zähne. Stuttgart: G. Fischer; 1976
Siegenthaler W. Klinische Pathophysiologie. 8th ed. Stuttgart: Thieme; 2000
Stammberger H, Hawke M. Essentials of functional endoscopic sinus surgery. 2nd ed. St. Louis: Mosby; 1993
Steiniger B, Schwarzbach H, Stachniss, V. Mikroskopische Anatomie der Zähne und des Parodonts. Stuttgart: Thieme; 2010
Strup JR, Türp JC, Witkowski S, Hürzeler MB, Kern M. Curriculum Prothetik (Band I). 2nd ed. Berlin Quintessenz 1999

Tillmann B. Farbatlas der Anatomie Zahnmedizin-Humanmedizin. Stuttgart: Thieme; 1997
Töndury G. Angewandte und topographische Anatomie. 5th ed. Stuttgart: Thieme; 1981

Vahlensieck M, Reiser M. MRT des Bewegungsapparates. 4th ed. Stuttgart: Thieme; 2014
Van Aken H, Wulf H (Hrsg.). Lokalanästhesie, Regionalanästhesie, Regionale Schmerztherapie. begr. von HCh Niesel. 3rd ed. Stuttgart: Thieme; 2010
von Lanz T, Wachsmuth W. Praktische Anatomie. Bd. 1/1B Kopf. Gehirn- und Augenschädel. Berlin: Springer; 2004
von Lanz T, Wachsmuth W. In: von Loeweneck u Feifel, Hrsg. Praktische Anatomie. Bd. 2, 6. Teil. Berlin: Springer; 1993
von Lanz T, Wachsmuth W. Praktische Anatomie. Bd. 1/2. Hals, Berlin: Springer; 1955
von Spee Graf F. Die Verschiebungsbahn des Unterkiefers am Schädel. Arch Anat Entwicklungsgesch. 1890; 285–294

Warshawsky H. The teeth. In Weiss L. Cell and Tissue Biology – a textbook of histology. 6. Aufl. München: Urban & Schwarzenberg; 1988
Wolpert L, Beddington R, Brockes J, Jessel T, Lawrence P, Meyerowitz E. Entwicklungsbiologie. Weinheim: Spektrum Verlag; 1999

Yim SH, Kim JH, Han Z-A, Jeon S, Cho JH, Kim GS, Choi S-A, Lee JH. Distribution of the corticobulbar tract in the internal capsule. Journal of the Neurological Sciences; Vol. 334; Issue 1-2; pp. 63–68: November 2013

Index

F

H

Q

R